Molecular Therapies of Cancer

Contents

Georg F. Weber

Molecular Therapies of Cancer

Springer

Georg F. Weber
University of Cincinnati College of Pharmacy
Cincinnati
Ohio
USA

ISBN 978-3-319-13277-8 ISBN 978-3-319-13278-5 (eBook)
DOI 10.1007/978-3-319-13278-5

Library of Congress Control Number: 2015930843

Springer Cham Heidelberg New York Dordrecht London

Printed on acid-free paper

Springer International Publishing AG Switzerland is part of Springer Science+Business Media (www.springer.com)

Foreword

Cancer pharmacotherapy has undergone dramatic changes. For centuries, trial and error attempts did not result in tangible success. From around 1945 through 1965, DNA damaging agents were generally used. However, their poisonous nature was dose limiting. The introduction of combination chemotherapy in 1965 led to improvements in reducing the serious adverse effects of this form of cancer chemotherapy. The approach to the drug treatment of cancer changed dramatically in the late 1990s, when molecularly targeted agents (predominantly small molecule kinase inhibitors and neutralizing antibodies) allowed the blockage of oncogene function, fairly selectively in cancer cells, as a first line of defense. This shift in treatment strategies rounded off 30 years of molecular cancer research that had been initiated with the discovery of the first endogenous oncogene, *src*, in 1976. The new therapeutic modalities demand a different approach to cancer diagnosis and classification than their predecessor treatments. The identification of a causative molecular defect, rather than the clinical presentation or histologic appearance, determines the most suitable drug therapy. Treatment in cycles of high dose chemotherapy followed by recovery phases has been the standard for classical chemotherapy. This is mandated by the need to reach near-toxic doses in order to eradicate most cancer cells, but the strain on the host cells makes breaks in the time lines unavoidable. For molecularly targeted drugs, treatment cycles are replaced by continuous ("metronomic") therapy. Often, these agents are taken without interruption until disease progression or unacceptable adverse effects occur. Despite the progress molecular biology has introduced into cancer management, the conventional combination chemotherapy will likely have a durable role as a second or third line of defense against advanced cancers. Likewise, the new generation molecularly targeted drugs are projected to have some continued benefit whenever medical research progresses to better treatment modalities in the future. While a lot has been written about anti-cancer drugs in various forums, a book that comprehensively and systematically reviews their molecular actions is much needed.

The molecular structures, targets, and mechanisms of action of anti-cancer drugs as well as their grouping into drug classes are the topic of this book. There has long been a separation between basic molecular research and clinical applications. One of our goals is to explain the clinical use of specific anti-cancer treatment regimens (exemplified in the text boxes) on the basis of the underlying molecular drug actions (discussed in the sections). While it is impossible to cover all classes of drugs that are in development, reference is made to some of the up and coming drugs and treatment approaches that may find clinical applications down the road. This inclusion should give the current edition a longevity it would not otherwise have. Drugs are referred to in the text with the most commonly used chemical name. Alternative names and code names are listed on first mention in separate parentheses. Trade names are given thereafter in angle brackets. Bullet points marked by hyphens are listings of facts, bullet points marked by filled circles list structurally or functionally related drugs. The inclusion of any compound in this book does not constitute a recommendation or endorsement. The administration of agents outside currently approved indications (off-label use) is considered experimental.

The history of cancer drug discovery and development is also the history of the people who participated in the process. It has highs and lows, bright and dark sides. The unique challenges of the subject have always attracted some of the most brilliant minds as well as some of the most self-absorbed egos. There are chapters in this history which are famous, others are infamous. To put the drug classes into the perspective of their origins, many of the descriptions in this book begin with a brief summary of the historical development that underlies the class of drugs to be discussed. Instead of reviewing the historical background in the first chapter, as I did in the predecessor book on molecular oncology [Georg F. Weber, Molecular Mechanisms of Cancer, Springer 2007], the stories are here woven into the main text. I tell them as they have been reported by public sources.

I am indebted to Drs. Jane Pruemer and Victor Warner for critically reading and providing feedback on the treatment sections and the chemical structures respectively. In comparison to the mentioned book on molecular oncology, which meticulously referenced the literature, the reference lists here are much less extensive. This is not a disregard for prior research accomplishments. Rather, it reflects the circumstance that drug information is widely available online without attribution of authorship, so that detailed citation is not a requirement. The inclusion of select references that cite key sources or are representative for further reading seems to be consistent with the aims and scope of a textbook. So, why a textbook that to a large extent repeats what the internet already provides? Research takes place on all levels of inquiry. A comprehensive review of existing knowledge accomplishes innovation through systematic classification and the derivation of new paradigms. The capsules printed in bold italics at the end of each chapter summarize key information on the drug classes discussed, some of which has not been explicit in the literature. May this book actively contribute to scholarship and education in the drug treatment of cancer.

Part VI Supportive Therapy

Introduction

The stigma that cancer equals death, originating in the experiences of Hippocrates, Galen, and Celsus, was attached to the disease for centuries. It led to the long respected dictum that doctors should not inform their patients of the diagnosis to avoid agony. Cancer continued to be regarded as largely incurable until the nineteenth century, when surgery was made more efficient through improved operating techniques and histological control. Also, anesthesia allowed surgery to flourish[1]. Classical cancer operations were devised by Bilroth (Germany), Handley (England), and Halsted (United States of America), who developed increasingly radical approaches to remove all of the tumor plus the regional lymph nodes. The complete excision of a cancer before its dissemination would be the only form of a cure for many decades. In light of this progress, the American Cancer Society was formed in 1913 to educate the public about the warning symptoms of cancer and to reduce their fatalistic fears. As a sign of continued progress, since the 1950s, the trend in surgery has been reversed toward progressively less invasive techniques.

Radiation therapy became the next feasible treatment available for cancer. In 1895, Wilhelm Conrad Röntgen, experimenting with electrical discharges in vacuum tubes (Crookes tubes), identified penetrating radiation that also produced fluorescence, and named it X-rays ("X" symbolizing the unknown). He published a total of 3 articles on X-rays between 1895 and 1897. By 1902, a case of radiation-induced cancer was reported, arising in an ulcerated area of the skin. Within a few years, a large number of such skin cancers had been observed, and the first report of leukemia in 5 radiation workers appeared in 1911. Nevertheless, the use of radiation to fight cancer was under study early on. The work by Maude Menton, Simon Flexner, and J.V. Jobling at the Rockefeller Institute lead to the publication of the monograph "Influence of Radium Bromide on a Carcinomatous Tumor of the White Rat" in 1910. This publication became one of the originating studies for radiation therapy. The invention of the linear accelerator in the first half of the twentieth century advanced radio-therapy from a palliative method to a cancer treatment with a curative intent. However, the lack of specificity and the inherent carcinogenicity of radiation exposure have rendered this modality a last resort for cancer treatment.

[1] In 1845, the traveling dentist Horace Wells demonstrated the use of nitrous oxide as an anesthetic at the Massachusetts General Hospital. Having chosen a particularly sturdy male volunteer, he provided insufficient anesthetic and the patient screamed in pain. After having been discredited, Wells turned into a traveling salesman for household items. Experimenting with gases, he later became addicted to chloroform. In a delirious state, he threw sulfuric acid at 2 prostitutes. He was jailed and committed suicide by slitting his femoral artery in 1848. In 1846 William Thomas Green Morton, a Boston dentist and business partner of Wells, found that diethyl ether was an alternative to nitrous oxide as an anesthetic. He successfully demonstrated his new technique for painless surgery at the Massachusetts General Hospital, in the surgical amphitheater now called the Ether Dome. Harvard professor Charles Thomas Jackson later claimed this use of ether was his idea given to Morton, and a lifelong dispute ensued. Independently of Wells and Morton, Crawford Long had noted that participants at ether frolics experienced bumps and bruises, but afterward had no recall of what had happened. In 1842, he administered ether to remove a cyst from a friend's neck, and further uses of ether ensued. The results of these trials were published in 1849 in The Southern Medical and Surgical Journal.

Surgery and radiation dominated the field of cancer therapy into the 1950s. Both surgery and radiation are, however, in most cases insufficient to control metastatic cancer.

In contrast to the above modalities, drug treatment can reach multiple sites within the body. Trial-and-error attempts at pharmacotherapy of cancer extend throughout the history of medicine, with many studies being intrinsically linked to naturally occurring substances. Chemical defense through cytotoxic or cytostatic mechanisms is widespread in the plant and animal kingdoms. However, potency rather than cell-type selectivity seems to be the main evolutionary driving force, and therefore only a small fraction of natural cytotoxic substances has found utility in medicine. Specifically, the usage of metals (preparations of silver, zinc, and mercury) and herbs as medication goes back to the ancient Indian system of ayurvedic medicine.

- In the tenth century, the Persian physician Rhazes introduced the use of chemicals such as vitriol, arsenic salts, and sal ammoniac for medical purposes. In 1865, Lissauer reported the use of potassium arsenite for two cases of leukemia. A textbook of medicine, written in 1894 by Osler, was the first publication to mention the administration of Fowler's solution (an arsenic containing medicinal) as a form of chemical treatment for lymphoma. Much later, metal agents found their revival with the discovery of platinum anti-cancer agents in 1965.
- Native cultures have used herbs to maintain health and treat illnesses. Some of the large number of herbs or extracts in traditional Chinese medicine may contain activity against cancers. The classic Chinese book on medicinal herbs was written during the Ming Dynasty (1152–1578) by Li Shi-Zhen. The aim is to restore the balance of Qi (the flow of energy in the body, which is essential for good health). Native Americans commonly applied poultices of roasted onions and bloodroot, which eroded the skin, to draw out cancers and other undesirable disease agents. Around the mid-nineteenth century, Native American herbs became popular in Europe. The Western herbal medicine focuses on a holistic approach. It uses remedies made from plants, which are believed to work due to the delicate chemical balance of the plant, or mixtures of plants, not one particular active ingredient. Today, herbal medicine is one of the most commonly used complementary and alternative therapies by people with cancer.

The term chemotherapy was first coined in the early 1900s by Paul Ehrlich, who defined it as using chemicals to treat disease (his focus was predominantly on syphilis, not cancer). He also documented the effectiveness of animal models to screen series of chemicals for their potential therapeutic activities. The systematic search for cancer chemotherapy began in the early twentieth century with attempts to narrow the plethora of natural and synthetic chemical compounds that might affect the disease by developing screening methods using transplantable tumors in small animals. A breakthrough in model development occurred in the early 1910s when George Clowes of the Roswell Park Memorial Institute in Buffalo, New York developed the first transplantable tumor systems in rodents. This advance allowed the standardization of model systems and the testing of large numbers of chemicals.

Conventional cancer chemotherapy has its main roots in the 1940s (see the historical summaries under alkylating agents and anti-metabolites below) (Fig. 1). The Cancer Chemotherapy National Service Center (CCNSC) was started in the U.S. in 1955. The Senate Appropriations Committee, at the urging by activist and philanthropist Mary Lasker, provided $ 5 million to the National Cancer Institute with a mandate for the establishment of the program. Ken Endicott became its first director. It was the mission of CCNSC to screen chemicals for cancer treatment on a large scale. The program faced the obstacle that, in the 1960s, medical oncology did not exist as a clinical specialty. At the time, the main issue of debate was whether cancer drugs caused more good than harm[2]. Progress was made however, and in

[2] At Yale, the first institution to have tested chemotherapy in humans in the modern era, the chemotherapist Paul Calabresi was forced to leave because he was involved in too much early testing of new anti-cancer drugs.

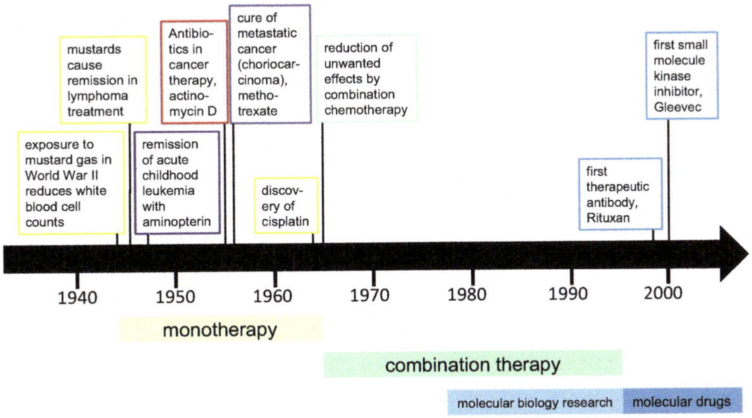

Fig. 1 Time line of cancer drug development. Three major phases cover monotherapy (~1946–1965, *yellow bar*), combination therapy (~1965–1997, *green bar*), and molecularly targeted therapy (since ~1997, *blue bar*). In the first phase, the discoveries of alkylating agents are boxed in *yellow*, the introduction of antibiotics is boxed in *wine red*, and milestones for anti-metabolites are boxed in *purple*. Attempts at cancer chemotherapy before ~1946 did not have any lasting impact

1966 the CCNSC was incorporated into the National Cancer Institute (NCI) structure as part of the chemotherapy program directed by Gordon Zubrod. Later named the Developmental Therapeutics Program, it was tightly linked to both the extramural clinical trials program and the NCI intramural program.

By 1970, combination chemotherapy had achieved lasting complete remissions in childhood leukemias and Hodgkin lymphoma. This provided the spark that was needed to gain widespread acceptance of cancer chemotherapy. Also in this time period, the adjuvant use of chemotherapy following surgery was pioneered to remove residual disease and reduce the risk of relapse. Early work on the combined treatment modality in breast cancer was done by Bernard Fisher in the U.S.A. and Gianni Bonadonna in Italy.

In 1971, the National Cancer Act, later referred to as "the war on cancer" (although this was never an official designation), was signed by then U.S. president Richard Nixon. It rang in decades of intensified research. In 1984, the U.S. National Cancer Institute started its investment in molecular biology.

In conjunction, chemotherapy, surgery, and radiation therapy constituted the 3 pillars of cancer therapy for the second half of the twentieth century. The beginning of the twenty first century has seen the introduction of molecularly targeted drugs, which have ushered in a new phase in chemotherapy as they target a specific defect and are administered continuously rather than in cycles. The approach to patient treatment has become more scientific with the introduction of clinical trials on a wide basis throughout the world. These clinical trials compare new treatments to standard treatments and contribute to a better understanding of benefits and risks.

Part I

General Principles

1 Principles of Molecular Cancer Treatment

The essential features of cancer cells are uncontrolled growth, extension of the cellular life span, invasiveness, and tumor specific or organ specific neoplasm-host interactions. The molecular mechanisms creating these phenotypic characteristics are potential anti-cancer drug targets.

Tumors consisting of fewer than 10^4 cells are likely small enough for elimination by host factors, including immune mechanisms. It takes about 10^9 cancer cells (mass approximately 1 g, diameter around 1 cm) for a tumor to be clinically detectable by palpation or radiography. The cells in such a tumor have undergone about 30 population doublings. Additional ten doublings are required for a 1 g tumor to reach 1 kg in mass (10^{12} cancer cells), which is frequently lethal. In its early stages, tumor growth is exponential because a large portion of the tumor cells is actively dividing (growth fraction). The doubling time (time required for the tumor to double in mass) is very short. As the tumor grows, the doubling time is slowed. The growth fraction is decreased due to the tumor outgrowing its blood and nutrient supplies.

The tumor burden impacts the response to chemotherapy. Because most anti-cancer agents have greater effect on rapidly dividing than on slowly dividing cells, tumors are most sensitive to the effects of chemotherapy when they are small and their growth fraction is high. The killing of tumor cells by drugs normally follows first order kinetics. The cell kill hypothesis (Skipper 1964) states that a certain percentage of cancer cells is killed with each course of chemotherapy. This means that there is always a fraction of tumor cells that are not eradicated, even after several treatment cycles. According to this hypothesis, the tumor burden never reaches zero (Fig. 1.1). The most achievable goal is the reduction of cells below about 10^4 to allow for the elimination by host factors. This hypothesis has influenced the clinical approach to dosing in favor of relatively aggressive uses of chemotherapy. The kinetics of tumor cell proliferation and death, combined with

- the almost inevitable presence of viable tumor cells at the end of therapy,
- the possibility of dormant tumor cells persisting without active proliferation,
- the tendency of cancer cells to acquire drug resistance through genetic instability,

has led to the reference to tumor regression as remission, not as a cure. Consistently, to assure near-complete cancer cell eradication, follow-up therapy is continued for years.

For many years, the complete resection of a tumor was the only prospect for a cure. Drug therapy (Table 1.1) could play a supportive role. When a growth could not be completely removed but the tumor burden could be reduced first by surgery, then chemotherapy was considered suitable to clear the remaining malignant cells, even if it would not have been potent enough to destroy the tumor in its entirety. This approach, first demonstrated as useful by Emil Frei, was termed adjuvant therapy. High doses of methotrexate prevented the recurrence of osteosarcoma following the surgical removal of the primary tumor. Bernard Fisher, chair of the National Surgical Adjuvant Breast and Bowel Project, and of Gianni Bonadonna, working in l'Istituto Nazionale Tumori di Milano, Italy, showed that adjuvant chemotherapy after complete surgical resection of breast tumors extended patient survival. Today, cancer chemotherapy may be indicated as a primary or secondary treatment. While the administration of cytotoxic drugs is the primary curative regimen for many blood cancers, most solid tumors are not curable with conventional chemotherapy alone. Chemotherapy in this setting is typically initiated for adjuvant, neoadjuvant, or palliative purposes.

- Adjuvant therapy is given to patients with potentially curable malignancies, who have no clinically detectable disease after surgery or radiation. Its effectiveness is reflected in reduced recurrence rates and prolonged patient survival.
- Neoadjuvant drug therapy is given preoperatively. Its goal is to facilitate surgery by reducing tumor burden and to destroy micro-metastases. Although chemotherapy can initially produce extensive remissions, most patients still harbor residual tumor cells. Therefore the ensuing surgery may be essential to protect from relapse.

G. F. Weber, *Molecular Therapies of Cancer*, DOI 10.1007/978-3-319-13278-5_1,

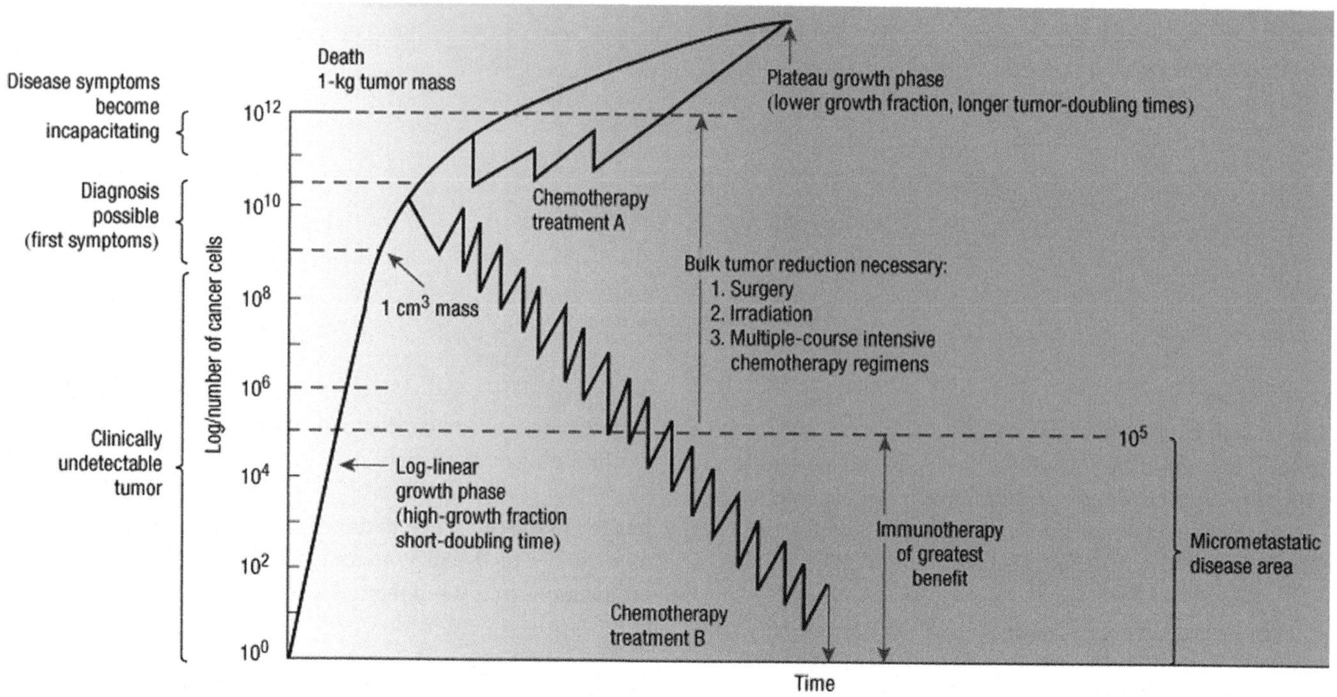

Fig. 1.1 Gompertzian growth curve. Shown is the growth kinetics in relationship to symptoms, diagnosis, and various treatment regimens. In the early stages, tumor growth is exponential, the doubling time of the tumor is constant. During this early phase, a large portion of the tumor cells is in the growth fraction of actively dividing cells. Because most anti-cancer agents have greater effect on rapidly dividing cells than on quiescent cells, tumors are most sensitive to the effects of chemotherapy when the tumor is small and the growth fraction is high. As the tumor grows, the doubling time is slowed and the growth fraction decreased. The sensitivity to chemotherapy tends to decline. (Buick 1994)

Table 1.1 Basic concepts of cancer chemotherapy

The traditional clinical use of cytotoxic chemotherapy is based on the concepts that
In the absence of mechanisms to revert tumor cells to normality, treatment requires the extensive eradication of tumor cells. Regimens that lead to tumor shrinkage may prolong survival
Cancer drugs typically exert their effects by first order kinetics. They kill a constant proportion of tumor cells rather than a constant number of cells. Therefore, the clinical results are improved if treatment is started early
Conventional cancer drugs suppress cell proliferation without having selectivity for the transformed cells, resulting in a narrow therapeutic index. Therefore, adverse effects mostly afflict tissues with a high fraction of dividing cells (intestines, hair, bone marrow)
The maximum tolerated dose (MTD) of conventional anti-cancer drugs has a higher probability of shrinking tumors (achieving remission) than any lower dose. The upper limit for dose escalation is the dose limiting toxicity (DLT) (Cristofanilli 2002)
Intermittent high doses are more effective at killing tumors, but require resting phases for the recovery of the patient
The high toxicity of conventional anti-cancer drugs makes it important to decrease the resulting adverse effects by administering combinations of drugs
Due to their genetic instability, tumors often develop drug resistance, resulting in relapse
Basic principles for molecularly targeted cancer therapy include
Cancers are caused by somatic mutations that result in altered biomolecules, which constitute drug targets that are unique for the tumor cells
Inhibition of the growth or survival pathways that are excessively active in cancer cells can control the disease. In the absence of mechanisms to revert tumor cells to normality, growth or survival pathway inhibitors need to be administered consistently
Due to their genetic instability, tumors often develop drug resistance, resulting in relapse

- When chemotherapy is only used to ameliorate the symptoms of the malignancy, it is palliative. Palliative treatment may retard tumor growth enough to reduce untoward symptoms caused by the tumor, but it does not achieve remission.

With increasing options for treating cancer patients, a treatment continuum defines a strategic approach that is tailored to the pathogenetic characteristics of each cancer.

Dose intensity is defined as the dose delivered to the patient over a specified period of time. The three main variables that determine delivered dose intensity are the dose per course, the interval between courses (dose density), and the total cumulative dose. The goal of dosing is the achievement of an effective drug concentration in the tumor without intolerable adverse effects to the patient. Dose intensity is particularly important in the setting of high dose chemotherapy with autologous hematopoietic stem cell support. Although lethal myelosuppression is avoided by administering hematopoietic stem cells, other severe toxicities emerge as the anti-neoplastic drug doses are increased.

The most suitable dose is determined, in part, by the tumor blood supply (access by drugs is facilitated by high vascularization) and the location of the tumor (drug delivery to "pharmacological sanctuaries", such as the brain or the pleural space is difficult). Due to diffusion gradients, the concentration of an injected anti-cancer drug decreases exponentially with the distance from the tumor blood vessels. This may cause a decrease to half its perivascular concentration at a distance of about 40–50 µm. With a mean distance from blood vessels to regions of hypoxia of 90–140 µm, many viable tumor cells are not exposed to active concentrations of drug following a single injection (Primeau 2005).

Two cardinal principles for anti-cancer drug treatment are safety and efficacy. The efficacy of anti-cancer chemotherapy is reflected in response rate (tumor shrinkage in response to drug treatment), time to progression or relapse, and survival.

An important element in the administration of molecularly targeted anti-cancer drugs is the application of biomarkers for patient selection (genostratification). Molecular disease classification in cancer has become consequential with the availability of molecularly targeted drugs. In situations, where clear treatment choices are available for distinct molecular pathologies, standardized tests can determine the presence of the critical genes or proteins. The co-development of diagnostics and therapeutics constitutes theranostics. For conventional anti-cancer drugs, which broadly inhibit cell proliferation rather than being specifically molecularly targeted, stratification is less feasible.

Biomarkers (molecular indicators of a disease state) are used to assess safety and efficacy. Polymorphisms in select genes can predict treatment response or treatment resistance to a wide spectrum of drugs. Such polymorphisms are undetectable in clinical assessment or in histological diagnosis. In some cases, the relevant genes for drug responses may be unrelated to the molecular defects that cause disease onset or influence disease manifestations. Molecular tests can determine the presence of such variants and support rational pharmacotherapy decisions, rather than empirical adjustments over time. Epithelial cells usually do not circulate in the blood stream. Their presence indicates a pathologic state, such as cancer, and may be a reflection of treatment success. Another aspect of the genetics of drug responses is the prediction of adverse drug effects due to genetic predisposition (toxicogenetics). It is important to exclude patients from specific treatments who are at high risk for encountering adverse effects. The prediction of such a risk, however, is often not possible without being based on reliable biomarkers. The concept of a "pharmacological audit trail", based on molecular markers, has been invoked to assess drug performance (Workman 2003).

References

Buick RN (1994) Cellular basis of chemotherapy. In: Von Hoff DD, Dorr RT (eds) Cancer chemotherapy handbook. Elsevier, New York, pp 3–14

Cristofanilli M, Charnsangavej C, Hortobagyi GN (2002) Angiogenesis modulation in cancer research: novel clinical approaches. Nat Rev Drug Discov 1:415–426

Primeau AJ, Rendon A, Hedley D, Lilge L, Tannock IF (2005) The distribution of the anticancer drug doxorubicin in relation to blood vessels in solid tumors. Clin Cancer Res 11:8782–8788

Skipper HE, Schabel FR Jr, Wilcox WS (1964) Experimental evaluation of potential anticancer agents. XII. On the criteria and kinetics associated with "curability" of experimental leukemia. Cancer Chemother Rep 35:1–111

Workman P (2003) How much gets there and what does it do? The need for better pharmacokinetic and pharmacodynamic endpoints in contemporary drug discovery and development. Curr Pharm Des 9:891–902

Part II

Molecular Basis of Anti-Cancer Drug Treatment

DNA Damaging Drugs

2

The classical anti-cancer agents comprise cytotoxic compounds. Mostly, these drugs act by exerting DNA damage. In essence, there are two major response phenotypes available to a cell upon DNA damage, such as a chemotherapeutic drug action,

- to arrest the cell cycle and repair the damage,
- to initiate a pathway to apoptosis (programmed cell death).

In either scenario, the uncontrolled growth of the tumor cells is curtailed. The major limitation of the cytotoxic anti-cancer drugs is the tumor non-specific action, and the suppression of all rapidly dividing cells[1].

> ***DNA damaging drugs interfere with transcription and reduplication.***
> ***Affected cells respond with cell cycle arrest or programmed cell death.***
> ***DNA damaging drugs are mutagenic, teratogenic, and carcinogenic.***
> ***Adverse effects are exerted on rapidly proliferating cells (skin—hair loss, gastrointestinal tract—nausea and vomiting, bone marrow—anemia causing fatigue/leukopenia causing infections/thrombocytopenia causing bleeding).***

2.1 Alkylating Agents

Alkylating agents[2] are electrophilic and bind covalently to electron-rich functional groups of various target molecules via first-order or second-order nucleophilic substitutions (nucleophiles are electron-rich molecules or ions, such as OH^-, H_2O, halogenides, alcohols, thiols and amines). The first order reactants include aromatic and aliphatic nitrogen and sulfur mustards. Second order reactants include ethylene imines and epoxides, alkylmethane sulfonates of the busulfan (Myleran) type, and α-halogenated acids, ketones, and their derivatives.

- For first-order reactions, the rate limiting step is the ionization of the alkylating agent to form a positively charged carbonium ion, which then rapidly reacts with water, or a negative center, or a nucleophilic center. Within DNA and RNA, the most reactive site is the *N*7 position of guanine (Fig. 2.1). In DNA, this is followed by *N*3 of adenine, *N*1 of adenine, *N*1 of cytosine, and *N*7 of adenine (Table 2.1). The rate limiting step of the reaction is the formation of positively charged cyclic immonium ions, whereas the rate of the reaction is essentially independent of the nature and concentration of the nucleophilic target being attacked.
- For second order nucleophilic substitutions, both reactants interact to form a transition complex. No carbonium ion is formed. The rate of the reaction depends on both concentrations, with bond strengths, electron affinity, and accessibility of both reagents being important (Knock 1967).

Alkylating agents exert cytotoxic effects by transferring alkyl groups to DNA, thereby damaging the DNA and interfering with DNA transcription and cell division. This class of drugs mainly works by three distinct mechanisms:

- The attachment of alkyl groups to DNA bases prevents DNA synthesis and RNA transcription, and it results in the DNA being fragmented by repair enzymes in a process to replace the altered bases.
- The two arms of mustard drugs can cross-link DNA strands. In this process, two bases are linked together. Bridges can be formed within a single molecule of DNA (intra-strand cross-links[3]) or a bridge may connect two DNA molecules (inter-strand cross-links). Cross-linking prevents DNA from being separated for reduplication or transcription. Although bifunctionality of alkylating

[1] Because the desired drug actions (damage to rapidly proliferating cancer cells) and the adverse effects (damage to rapidly proliferating healthy cells) are identical in targets and mechanisms, they are not separable.

[2] Alkyl designates a functional group (a "side chain") that consists solely of single-bonded carbon and hydrogen atoms. Alkylating anti-cancer agents attach alkyl groups to biomolecules.

[3] called limpet attachment of the drug molecule to the DNA.

G. F. Weber, *Molecular Therapies of Cancer*, DOI 10.1007/978-3-319-13278-5_2,

agents is not required for their mutagenic and carcinogenic properties, it is important for high anti-cancer activity.

- Alkylating agents can induce the mispairing of nucleotides, leading to mutations. Alkylated G bases may erroneously pair with Ts. If this altered pairing is not corrected by DNA repair it can result in permanent genetic change (Fig. 2.2).

Adverse Effects Due to the genetic damage exerted by the drug class, the treatment of cancer patients with alkylating agents is linked to an increased risk for secondary cancers. Alkylating agents can cause mutations not unlike those produced by radiation. These mutations occasionally lead to transformation. One form of cancer that may arise is a relatively rare type of acute non-lymphocytic leukemia (ANL). Highly treatment resistant cases appear as early as 2 years following initial therapy and peak around 5 years after exposure to alkylating agents. The risk of osteosarcomata may be elevated after the treatment of childhood cancers with alkylating agents.

Alkylating agents attach alkyl groups to DNA bases, leading to DNA fragmentation.
Alkylating agents cause intra- and inter-strand DNA cross-links.
Alkylating agents can induce mispairing of nucleotides, leading to mutations.
Alkylating agents exert cytotoxicity in all phases of the cell cycle.
Nitrogen mustards and chlorethylnitrosoureas have a preference for guanine-N7 alkylation.

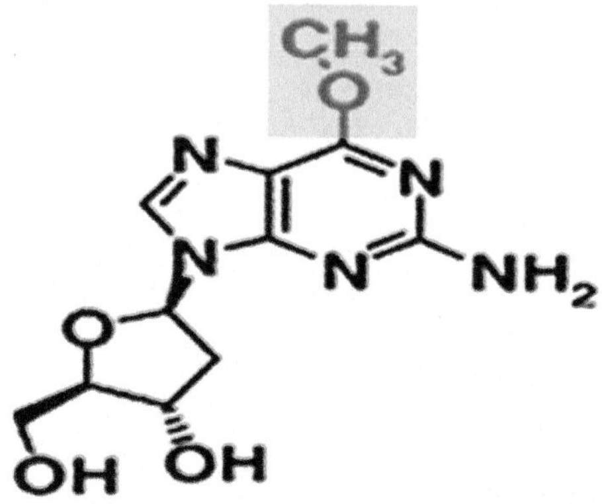

O⁶-mdGuo

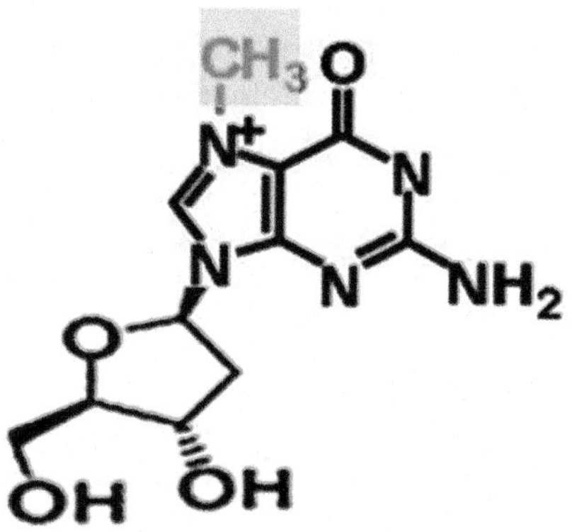

7-meGuo

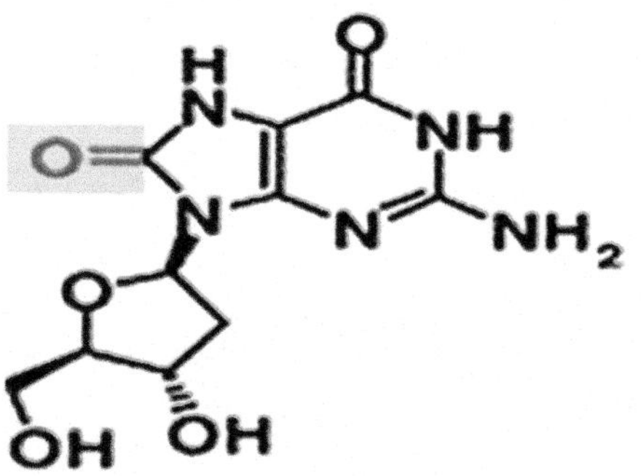

8-oxodGuo

Fig. 2.1 Common DNA adducts of guanosine. DNA damaging anticancer drugs may alter guanine residues to mutagenize and kill proliferating cells. O^6-methyl-2′-deoxyguanosine (*O^6-mdGuo*), N^7-methyl-guanosine (*7meGuo*), and 8-oxo-7,8-dihydro-2′-deoxyguanosine (*8-oxodGuo*) represent such DNA lesions. The modifications are highlighted in *pink*. (Adapted from Brink et al. 2006; Nay 2013)

2.1.1 Nitrogen Mustards

The beginning of the modern era of cancer chemotherapy is rooted directly in the discovery of nitrogen mustard. Mustard gas (sulfur mustard, H-gas) had been used as a chemical warfare agent during World War I, the first documented battlefield use being in Ypres, Belgium in 1917. The name assigned to the gas by the German military was Lost (referring to Lommel and Steinkopf, who in 1916 proposed the military use to the German Imperial General Staff). Exposure to mustard gas induces severe injuries to the eyes, skin, and respiratory tract. In 1917, Krumbhaar, a Captain in the U.S. Medical Corps, noted the development of profound leukopenia in individuals who survived a gas attack for several days (Krumbhaar 1919; Krumbhaar and Krumbhaar 1919). Following up on this observation, a group from the U.S. Office of Scientific Research and Development (OSRD) at Yale Medical School secretly studied the effects of nitrogen mustard on lymphomata. Milton Winternitz, who had worked on sulfur mustards in World War I, obtained the OSRD contract to study the chemistry of mustard compounds. He recruited the pharmacologists Louis S. Goodman and Alfred Gilman

Table 2.1 DNA target sites for alkylating anti-cancer agents

Base	Target	Drug	Class	Recognition sequence
Guanine	*N7*	Melphalan	Nitrogen mustard	
		Cyclophosphamide	Phosphoramide mustard	
		Temozolomide	Triazene	
		Cisplatin	Platinum drug	
		Fotemustine	Nitrosourea	3′ end of guanine tracts
Guanine	*N1*	Fotemustine	Nitrosourea	
Guanine	*N2*	Ecteinascidin-743	Minor groove binding antibiotic (G/C preference)	AGC, CGC, TGG
Guanine	*N3*	Duocarmycin A	Cyclopropylpyrroloindole antibiotic	5′-GCAATTGCG-CAATTGC-3′
Guanine	*O6*	Temozolomide	Triazene	
		Dacrbazine	Triazene	
		Laromustine	Hydrazine	
Guanine		Duocarmycin A	Cyclopropylpyrroloindole antibiotic	5′-CGCGTTGGGAG-3′
		Mithramycin A	Aureolic acid minor groove binder	
Adenine	*N3*	Duocarmycin A	Cyclopropylpyrroloindole antibiotic	
		CC-1065	Cyclopropylpyrroloindole antibiotic	5′-d(A/G)NTTA-3′
				5′-dAAAAA-3′
		Adozelesin, carzelesin, bizelesin	Minor groove binding antibiotic (A/T preference)	5′-(A/T)(A/T)A-3′
		Tallimustine	Minor groove binding antibiotic (A/T preference)	5′-TTTTGA-3′
Adenine	*N7*	Cisplatin	Platinum drug	
Adenine	*N1*	(Uncommon)		
Cytosine	*N3*	Fotemustine	Nitrosourea	
Cytosine	*N1*	(Uncommon)		

to perform the necessary animal experiments. Based on their successful research, Gustav Lindskog successfully treated a radio-resistant lymphosarcoma that compressed a patient's trachea with the injection of nitrogen mustard in December 1942. In 1943, Goodman and Gilman initiated the experimental treatment of Hodgkin disease and lymphosarcoma with nitrogen mustard. None of this was made public until 1946, when Goodman and Gilman reported their observation that exposure to mustard gas caused profound lymphoid and myeloid suppression, suggesting its utility for the treatment of lymphomata (Goodman et al. 1946; Gilman and Philips 1946). There was a parallel development: In World War II, General Eisenhower had ordered that a stockpile of mustard gas be kept near the front for possible use in a reprisal if the Nazis resorted to chemical warfare. During a military operation, allied ships in Bari Harbor, Italy[4], were sunk in an air assault by the German Luftwaffe on 2nd December 1943. At the center of the destruction was the vessel Liberty Ship S.S. John Harvey, laden with ammunition, supplies, and 2000 mustard gas bombs. A large number of military personnel were accidentally exposed to mustard gas and were later found by U.S. medical officer Lieutenant Colonel Stewart F. Alexander to have abnormally low white blood cell counts as a consequence of poisoning. It was implied that an agent, which damaged the rapidly growing white blood cells, might have a similar effect on cancer cells. Cornelius P. Rhoads served as chief of the medical division of the U.S. Army's chemical warfare unit during World War II. Based on his experience in the Bari incident, he investigated mustard gas as a tumor killing agent (Rhoads 1946). The research presaged classical chemotherapy[5]. Rhoads moved on to head one of the largest drug development programs at the Sloan-Kettering Institute in New York and pioneered the practice of contract research for pharmaceutical companies under confidentiality agreements.

Mustard gas is not derived from the mustard plant, it gets its name from its impurities. Impure mustard gas is yellow-brown and has an odor resembling mustard plants. Upon contact with the skin, it causes a burning sensation, which is similar to that caused by the oil from black mustard seeds. Sulfur mustards (bis(2-chloroethyl)-sulfide, 1,5-dichloro-3-thiapentane), which are related to mustard gas, are vesicants that have the ability to form large blisters on exposed skin. While sulfur mustards are too toxic for medical applications, nitrogen mustards[6] have found use as therapeutics.

[4] Allied ships were stationed in Bari under the assumption that the harbor was too far south to be reached by the Luftwaffe (the German airforce). The air raid was later called The Little Pearl Harbor.

[5] The recognition would have assured Rhoads' place in medical history had it not been revealed that he had likely committed serious ethics violations in unrelated assignments. In Puerto Rico, 1931, after Rhoads' car had been vandalized he wrote generally hateful comments on Puerto Ricans in a letter. He claimed that he had deliberately injected several Puerto Rican citizens with cancer cells.

[6] The characteristic bis(2-chloroethyl)amine- domain, which generates DNA cross-links, is contained in nitrogen mustards, phosphoramide mustards (ifosphamide is unique in its chain length that generates 7-membered cross-links), and selective minor groove DNA binding antibiotics (tallimustine and MEN 10710).

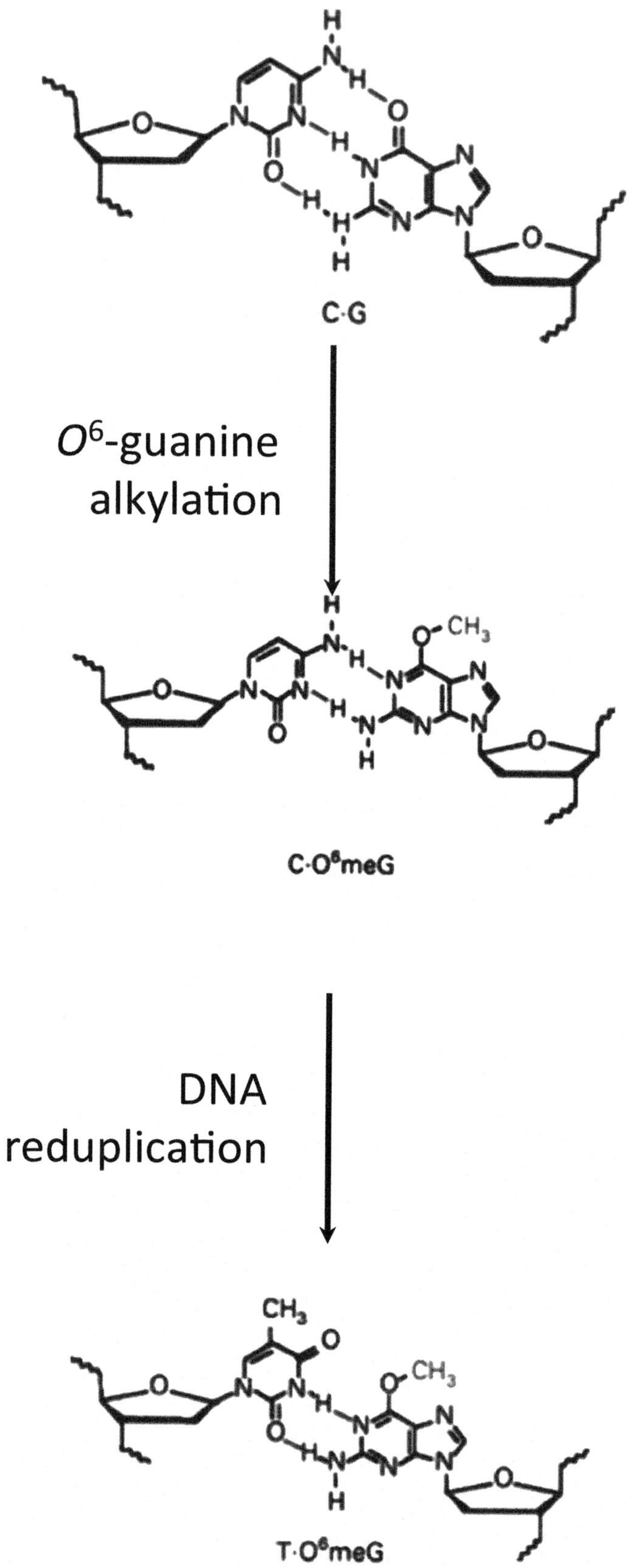

Fig. 2.2 DNA adducts caused by alkylating agents. The reaction scheme depicts the O^6 alkylation of guanine and the ensuing mispairing during DNA reduplication. (Adapted from Marra and Schär 1999)

After uptake, nitrogen mustard is metabolized to a highly reactive ethylene immonium derivative, which alkylates DNA (Papirmeister et al. 1985) and inhibits DNA reduplication (Fig. 2.3). In addition, increasing nitric oxide produced by Nitric Oxide Synthase may be responsible for some of the damage exerted by mustard drugs (Sawyer 1998). This toxicity probably comes from an over-production of reactive nitrogen species, in particular peroxynitrite ($ONOO^-$), by the reaction of nitric oxide and superoxide. There are several generations of nitrogen mustard drugs.

- In first generation nitrogen mustards, aliphatic radicals were attached to the mustard pharmacophore $–N(CH_2CH_2Cl)_2$.
- In second generation nitrogen mustards, electron withdrawing aromatic radicals were attached to reduce the reactivity and permit oral use.
- In third generation nitrogen mustards, the pyrimidine nucleus was chosen as a carrier for the mustard pharmacophore, which permits oral administration.
- More recent modifications include steroid-coupled nitrogen mustards and phosphoramide mustards

First generation nitrogen mustards The aliphatic alkylating agent mechlorethamine hydrochloride (2-chloro-*N*-(2-chloroethyl)-*N*-methyl-ethanamine, nitrogen mustard, chlormethine hydrochloride, mustine, chlorethazine hydrochloride, HN2 hydrochloride, N-Lost) (NSC-762) <Mustargen, Caryolysine, Cloramin, Erasol, Onco-Cloramin> is the salt of a synthetic nitrogen-containing sulfur mustard derivative (Fig. 2.4) with anti-neoplastic and lympholytic properties. Mechlorethamine hydrochloride is used because it induces a rapid response. It is primarily administered as part of the MOPP regimen. The agent may be indicated in treating Hodgkin disease (stages III and IV), lymphosarcoma, chronic myelocytic or chronic lymphocytic leukemia, polycythemia vera[7], mycosis fungoides[8], and bronchogenic carcinoma. It may also be included in the treatment of small cell lung cancer or medulloblastoma. The drug is not active in acute leukemias or chronic granulocytic leukemias (Knock 1967).

Mechlorethamine cannot be taken orally. It is given as an intravenous infusion over 20 min. The dosage varies with the clinical situation, the initial therapeutic response, and the magnitude of hematologic depression. Usually, a total dose of 0.4 mg/kg of body weight for each course is given either as a single dose or in divided doses of 0.1–0.2 mg/kg per day. Subsequent courses should not be given until the patient has recovered hematologically from the previous course. The drug administered intrapleurally, intraperitoneally, or

[7] A myeloproliferative disorder that results in the over-production of red blood cells.

[8] The most common form of cutaneous T-cell lymphoma.

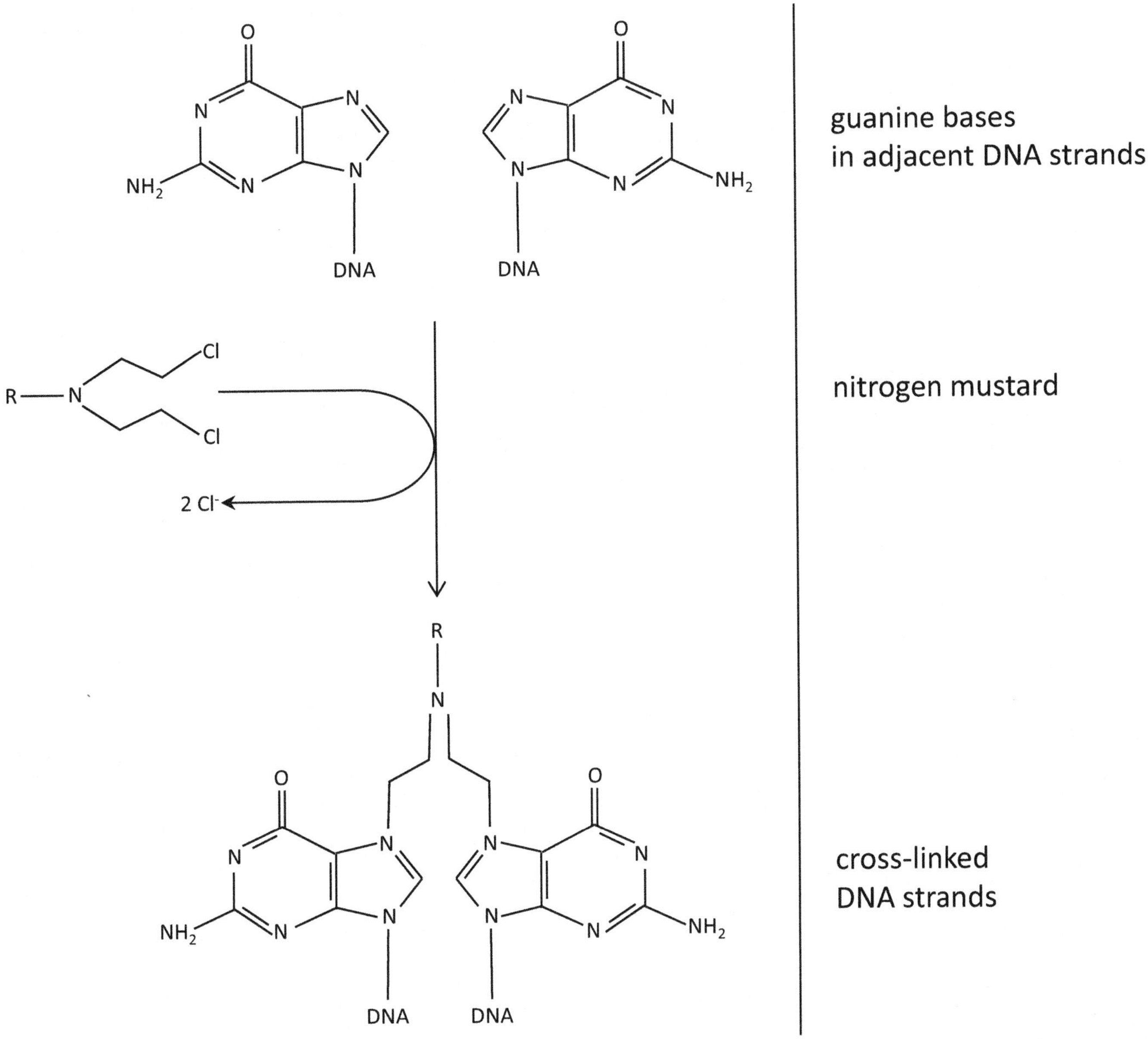

Fig. 2.3 Mechanism of action for nitrogen mustard. Alkylation of guanine bases in the DNA is partially responsible for the cytotoxic effect of nitrogen mustards. The alkylation of two guanines by the arms of the mustard leads to DNA cross-linking

intrapericardially is indicated for the palliative treatment of metastatic carcinoma resulting in effusion. Local therapy with nitrogen mustard is used only when malignant cells are present in the effusion. Intracavitary injection is not recommended when the accumulated fluid is chylous, because the results are likely to be poor. Paracentesis is first performed with most of the fluid being removed from the pleural or peritoneal cavity. The position of the patient should be changed every 5–10 min for an hour after injection to obtain more uniform distribution of the drug throughout the serous cavity.

- Mechlorethamine gel <Valchlor> is a topical gel for the second-line treatment of stage IA and IB mycosis fungoides cutaneous T-cell lymphoma

Pharmacokinetics Because of its extreme reactivity with water, nitrogen mustard is reconstituted immediately before use. In neutral or alkaline aqueous solution the drug is highly unstable and undergoes rapid chemical transformation. In body fluids, mechlorethamine combines with water or reactive compounds of cells within a few minutes after administration, so that the drug is no longer present in its active form.

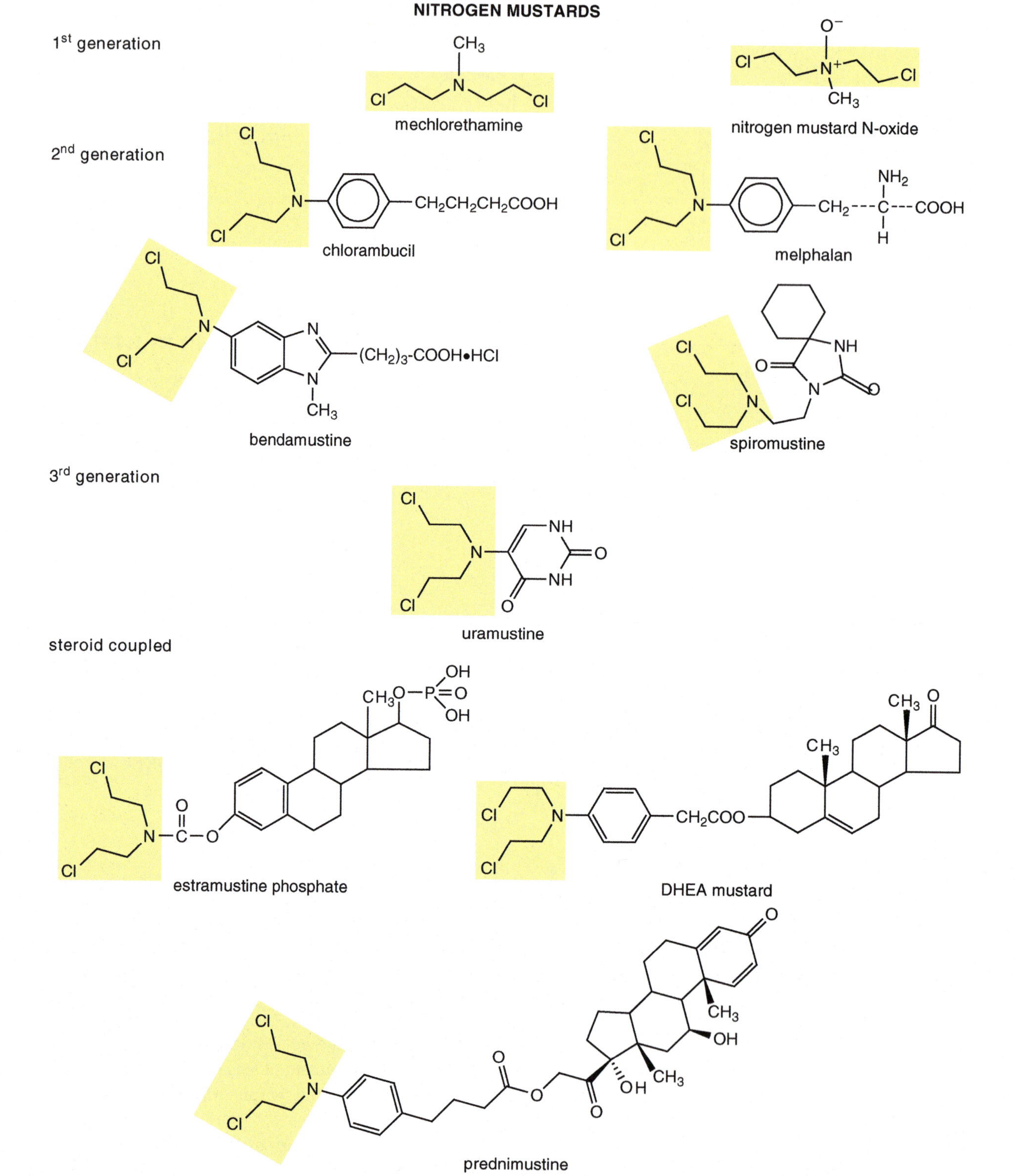

Fig. 2.4 Structures of nitrogen mustards. Three consecutive generations in this class of drugs have acquired increasing oral bioavailability. A 4th generation is coupled to steroids for bifunctionality. The common functional mustard moiety is highlighted in *yellow*

Adverse Effects For the comfort of the patient, nitrogen mustard may be given at bedtime, following administration of a barbiturate and an anti-emetic to minimize the adverse effects of nausea and vomiting, which usually occurs after 1–3 h. Emesis may disappear in the first 8 h, but nausea may persist for 24 h. Depression of the hematopoietic system may be present for up to 50 days (or more) after starting therapy. Mustard treatment generally produces lymphocytopenia within 24 h after the first injection. Substantial granulocytopenia occurs within 6–8 days and lasts for 10–21 days. Thrombocytopenia is variable but the time course of the appearance and recovery from reduced platelet counts generally parallels the granulocyte levels. Rarely, hemolytic anemia associated with such diseases as lymphomata and chronic lymphocytic leukemia may be precipitated by treatment with alkylating agents including mechlorethamine. Serious adverse effects can include anaphylactic reactions or bleeding (bloody urine, tar stools, bleeding gums). Other common adverse effects include hyperuricemia, fatigue, hair loss, maculopapular skin eruptions, and herpes zoster. Jaundice, vertigo, tinnitus and hearing loss occur infrequently. As nitrogen mustard therapy can contribute to the extensive and rapid development of amyloidosis, it should be used only if foci of acute or chronic suppurative inflammation are absent.

Alkylating agents are carcinogenic, mutagenic and teratogenic. Oligomenorrhea or azoospermia can be induced by mechlorethamine and may not recover for years after termination of therapy. During preganancy, the agent can cause damage to the fetus. It is in the U.S. FDA Pregnancy Category D.

After intravenous injection, a local rash, pain, or burning may occur. Extravasation into the tissue surrounding the injection site is a potentially serious problem. It causes severe painful induration. The area can be infiltrated with an isotonic solution of 0.11 M sodium thiosulfate as an antidote. The mustard also poses a risk for venous thromboses at the site of injection from direct sclerosing action. Transient cardiac irregularities may occur with intrapericardial injection.

A contraindication is hypersensitivity to mechlorethamine or any component of the formulation. The presence of known infectious diseases may be an indication against immunosuppressive agents, such as mechlorethamine. Because of the bone marrow suppression, vaccinations during or shortly before or shortly after chemotherapy with mechlorethamine should be avoided.

Drug Interactions Turmeric may decrease the effect of mechlorethamine. The use of this spice in the diet should be avoided while receiving treatment. Precautions must be observed with the use of mechlorethamine and radiation therapy in alternating courses. Both depress hematopoietic function and neither regimen should follow the other until bone marrow function has recovered. In particular, irradiation of such areas as sternum, ribs, and vertebrae shortly after a course of nitrogen mustard may lead to hematologic complications. The decrease in platelet count can increase the risk of bleeding. Therefore, any aspirin or salicylate containing medicines are to be avoided.

Nitrogen mustard *N*-oxide hydrochloride (2-chloro-*N*-(2-chloroethyl)-*N*-methyl-ethanamine-*N*-oxide hydrochloride, NMNO) (NSC-10107, SK-598) <Nitromin> is the chloride salt of the oxide of nitrogen mustard. It is closely related to mechlorethamine. Nitrogen mustard *N*-oxide has been used especially in Japan[9]. Nitrogen mustard *N*-oxide is usually administered intravenously at 1 mg/kg/day for 10 days. Its therapeutic spectrum resembles that of nitrogen mustard.

Adverse Effects As a DNA damaging agent, nitrogen mustard *N*-oxide hydrochloride is potentially carcinogenic.

Second generation nitrogen mustards Chlorambucil (4-[bis(2-chlorethyl)amino]benzenebutanoic acid) <Leukeran> was developed in 1953 at the Chester Beatty Research Institute, England. It is an orally active, bifunctional, aromatic nitrogen mustard that alkylates and cross-links DNA during all phases of the cell cycle, resulting in a disruption of DNA function, cell cycle arrest, and apoptosis. The electron withdrawing properties of the aromatic ring lead to slower reactions with serum and cellular constituents compared to first generation nitrogen mustards. Therefore, chlorambucil can be given orally in tablet form. Chlorambucil is indicated in the palliative treatment of chronic lymphocytic leukemia, malignant lymphoma, lymphosarcoma, giant follicular lymphoma, and Hodgkin disease. It has been used in the treatment of Waldenström macroglobulinemia[10], polycythemia vera, oat cell and undifferentiated carcinomata of the lungs, trophoblastic neoplasms, and ovarian carcinoma.

Chlorambucil is well tolerated by most patients, although for initial treatment it has been largely replaced by fludarabine (Rai 2000).

- Chlorambucil is usually given at 0.1–0.2 mg/kg/day for 3–6 weeks. The entire daily dose may be administered at one time. The dose is reduced when leukocyte counts drop or there are signs of clinical improvement. When lymphocytic infiltration of the bone marrow is present, or when the bone marrow is hypoplastic, the dose should not exceed 0.1 mg/kg/day. The maintenance dose is usually about 2 mg/day and can be extended over months or years.
- Alternate schedules for the treatment of chronic lymphocytic leukemia employ intermittent, bi-weekly, or once-monthly pulse doses of chlorambucil. Intermittent schedules begin with an initial single dose of 0.4 mg/kg, which is increased by 0.1 mg/kg until control of lymphocytosis or toxicity is observed. Subsequent doses are modified to produce mild hematologic toxicity.
- Continuous maintenance therapy is considered less safe than short courses of treatment. If a maintenance dosage is used, it should not exceed 0.1 mg/kg/day and may be as low as 0.03 mg/kg/day. It may be desirable to withdraw the drug after maximal control has been achieved, since intermittent therapy—reinstituted at the time of relapse—may be as effective as continuous treatment.

---

[9] Of note, in the U.K. Nitromin is a brand name for the unrelated agent glyceryl trinitrate.

[10] Waldenström macroglobulinemia (lymphoplasmacytic lymphoma) is a lymphoproliferative disease of IgM secreting B-lymphocytes.

Pharmacokinetics Oral chlorambucil undergoes rapid and complete gastrointestinal absorption and blood clearance. After single oral doses of 0.6–1.2 mg/kg, peak chlorambucil levels in the blood are reached within 1 h and the terminal elimination half-life of the parent drug is roughly 1.5 h. The agent is extensively metabolized in the liver, primarily to phenylacetic acid mustard, which has anti-neoplastic activity. Chlorambucil and its major metabolite spontaneously degrade, forming monohydroxyl and dihydroxyl derivatives. Both chlorambucil and its metabolites are extensively bound to plasma and tissue proteins (99 %), specifically to Albumin. Urinary excretion is below 1 % in 24 h.

Adverse Effects A prominent adverse effect is myelosuppression (anemia, neutropenia, thrombocytopenia). Severe neutropenia usually occurs only in patients who have received a total dosage of 6.5 mg/kg or more in one course of therapy with continuous dosing. Upon withdrawal from the drug, this effect may be reversible after about 10 days from the last dose, but bone marrow failure can arise in rare cases. Less commonly occurring adverse effects are gastrointestinal distress (nausea, vomiting, diarrhea, oral ulcerations) and central nervous system damage (tremors, muscular twitching, confusion, agitation, ataxia, hallucinations; increased risk of seizures in children with nephrotic syndrome and patients receiving high pulse doses of chlorambucil) that often resolves upon discontinuation of the drug, skin reactions (urticaria, angioneurotic edema, rarely skin rash progressing to erythema multiforme, toxic epidermal necrolysis, and Stevens-Johnson syndrome), and infertility (sterility when administered to prepubertal and pubertal males, induction of amenorrhea in females). Uncommon adverse reactions include pulmonary fibrosis, hepatotoxicity and jaundice, drug fever, peripheral neuropathy, interstitial pneumonia, and sterile cystitis. As all DNA damaging agents, chlorambucil is itself carcinogenic and bears a risk for secondary malignancies (specifically acute leukemia) with increasing cumulative dose.

Radiation and cytotoxic drugs render the bone marrow more vulnerable to damage, and chlorambucil should be used with particular caution within 4 weeks of a full course of radiation therapy or chemotherapy. If bone marrow is infiltrated by the tumor, the daily dosage of chlorambucil should not exceed 0.1 mg/kg. The drug crosses the placenta and is contraindicated during pregnancy (Category D), but it is not known whether it is excreted into breast milk.

Chlorambucil should not be used in patients whose disease has shown a prior resistance or known hypersensitivity to the agent. There may be cross-hypersensitivity between chlorambucil and other alkylating agents.

Melphalan A (2-amino-3-[4-[bis(2-chloroethyl)amino] phenyl]-propanoic acid, L-phenylalanine mustard, L-PAM, L-sarcolysin) <Alkeran> is a bifunctional phenylalanine derivative of nitrogen mustard[11]. Melphalan alkylates DNA at the *N*7 position of guanine and induces DNA inter-strand cross-linkages. This results in the inhibition of DNA and RNA synthesis and cytotoxicity against both dividing and non-dividing tumor cells.

Melphalan is indicated for the palliative treatment of multiple myeloma and for the palliation of non-resectable epithelial ovarian carcinoma. It is also used to treat breast cancer, neuroblastoma, and rhabdomyosarcoma. While it is occasionally applied to malignant melanoma, melphalan is not enriched in melanocytes, despite the role of phenylalanine as a precursor in the synthesis of Melanin. Administration is oral or intravenous. Dosing varies by purpose, route of administration, and patient weight. The entire daily dose may be given at one time.

- Orally, melphalan is usually given at 6–10 mg per day for 2–3 weeks, followed by a rest period of several weeks before initiation of the next cycle. When the white blood cell and platelet counts are rising, a maintenance dose of 2 mg daily may be instituted. In multiple myeloma, melphalan shows clinical effectiveness in 50 % of cases at 0.2 mg/kg/day orally.
- Alternatively, an initial course of 10 mg/day for 7–10 days is administered. The maximal suppression of the leukocyte and platelet counts occurs within 3–5 weeks and recovery within 4–8 weeks. Continuous maintenance therapy with 2 mg/day is instituted when the white blood cell count is greater than 4000 cells/μL and the platelet count is greater than 100,000 cells/μL. Dosage is adjusted to 1–3 mg/day depending upon the hematologic response. It is desirable to try to maintain a significant degree of bone marrow depression so as to keep the leukocyte count in the range of 3000–3500 cells/μL.
- A commonly employed regimen for the treatment of ovarian carcinoma is the administration of melphalan at a dose of 0.2 mg/kg daily for 5 days as a single course. Courses are repeated every 4–5 weeks, depending upon hematologic tolerance.

Melphalan has been used in combination with prednisone to boost effectiveness in the treatment of multiple myeloma. Early efforts to enhance chemotherapy with autologous bone marrow transplantation were performed with melphalan. For disseminated melanoma, bone marrow withdrawn from the sternum and stored cooled in citrate buffer plus dextrose was reinfused intravenously 6–8 h after administration of the chemotherapeutic (Ariel and Pack 1967).

[11] Melphalan is the active L-isomer of the D-isomer compound medphalan that was first synthesized in 1953 by Bergel and Stock. The L form is superior to the D form in anti-tumor activity.

Pharmacokinetics Blood melphalan levels are highly variable after oral dosing, possibly due to incomplete intestinal absorption, variable first-pass hepatic metabolism, or rapid hydrolysis. The time of the first appearance in the blood stream ranges approximately 0–6 h. The peak plasma concentration range is 70–4000 ng/mL, depending upon the dose. The extent of melphalan binding to plasma proteins ranges 60–90 %. Serum Albumin is the major binding protein, whileα_1-Acid Glycoprotein may account for about 20 % of the plasma protein binding. Approximately 30 % of melphalan is irreversibly bound to plasma proteins. Interactions with Immunoglobulins are negligible. Melphalan is eliminated from the circulation primarily by chemical hydrolysis to monohydroxymelphalan and dihydroxymelphalan. The terminal elimination half-life of the parent drug in the blood is about 1.5 h; its 24-h urinary excretion is about 10 %, indicating that renal clearance is not a major route of elimination. Penetration into cerebrospinal fluid is low.

Adverse Effects Myelosuppression with reduced white blood cell count, increased risk of infection, and decreased platelet count (causing an elevated risk of bleeding) is common. Although bone marrow suppression frequently occurs, it is usually reversible if melphalan is withdrawn early enough. However, irreversible bone marrow failure has occurred. Common adverse effects include nausea and vomiting. Less frequent adverse effects comprise pulmonary fibrosis after prolonged use, interstitial pneumonitis, compromised ovarian or testicular functions, and hair loss. Allergic reactions, including urticaria, edema, skin rashes, and rare anaphylaxis, have arisen after multiple courses of treatment. Cardiac arrest can rarely result in association with such events.

Secondary malignancies, including acute non-lymphocytic leukemia, myeloproliferative syndrome, and carcinoma can occur in patients treated with alkylating agents. At cumulative doses above 700 mg, the 10-year cumulative risk increases from about 2 % to about 20 %.

Melphalan should be used with extreme caution in patients whose bone marrow reserve may have been compromised by prior irradiation or chemotherapy, or whose marrow function is recovering from previous cytotoxic therapy. During treatment with melphalan A, the intake of salicylic acid <Aspirin> should be avoided as it could intensify any bleeding problems. Interactions with cimetidine, steroids, and cyclosporine are possible. The drug is Pregnancy Category D; it is not known whether this agent is excreted into breast milk.

In the 1960s, bendamustine hydrochloride (4-[5-[bis(2-chloroethyl)amino]-1-methylbenzimidazol-2-yl]butanoic acid) (SDX-105) <Treanda, Ribomustin, Treakisym, Levact> was designed with the aim of creating a bifunctional anti-cancer agent that possesses DNA damaging properties (by virtue of an alkylating group) and also potential anti-metabolite properties (associated with a purine-like benzimidazole ring). It was first marketed in Germany in the early 1970s. In 2008, bendamustine was approved by the U.S. Food and Drug Administration (FDA) for the treatment of chronic lymphocytic leukemia (CLL). The drug also has therapeutic activity against multiple myeloma, and indolent B-cell non-Hodgkin lymphoma that has progressed within 6 months of treatment with a rituximab containing regimen. For these conditions, bendamustine has strong efficacy as well as low cross-resistance with other alkylating agents and fludarabine. The agent causes DNA damage that leads to cell death via several pathways, including apoptosis and mitotic catastrophe. A standard dose is 100–120 mg/m^2 body surface area, administered intravenously over a period of 30–60 min, for chronic lymphocytic leukemia on days 1 and 2 of a 28-day cycle up to six cycles, for non-Hodgkin lymphoma on days 1 and 2 of a 21-day cycle up to eight cycles.

Pharmacokinetics The binding of bendamustine to plasma proteins is largely concentration independent and ranges 94–96 %. The drug distributes freely in red blood cells, rendering the mean steady state volume of distribution approximately 25 L. Bendamustine is primarily hydrolyzed to metabolites with low cytotoxic activity. Two active minor metabolites, γ-hydroxy bendamustine (M3) and N-desmethyl-bendamustine (M4), are primarily formed via CYP1A2. The parent drug does not induce or inhibit Cytochrome P450 enzymes. While the intermediate half-life of the parent compound is approximately 40 min, the mean apparent terminal elimination of the metabolites γ-hydroxy bendamustine and N-desmethyl-bendamustine are approximately 3 h and 30 min, respectively. 90 % of the drug is eliminated unmetabolized, mostly in the feces. Due to pharmacogenetic predisposition, Japanese patients may have higher exposure than non-Japanese subjects to identical doses.

Adverse Effects The most common hematologic abnormalities for both indications (indolent B-cell non-Hodgkin lymphoma and chronic lymphocytic leukemia) are lymphopenia, anemia, leukopenia, thrombocytopenia, and neutropenia. Most common non-hematologic adverse reactions in chronic lymphocytic leukemia are pyrexia, nausea and vomiting. Most common non-hematologic adverse reactions for non-Hodgkin lymphoma are nausea and vomiting, diarrhea or constipation, anorexia, headache, fatigue, pyrexia, cough, dyspnea, rash, and stomatitis. Dose reduction or delayed administration is required if grade 3 or grade 4 toxicities occur. Dose re-escalation in subsequent cycles may be considered. Tumor lysis syndrome can arise within the first treatment cycle. Without intervention it may lead to acute renal failure and death. Preventive measures include maintaining adequate volume status, and close monitoring of blood chemistry, particularly potassium and uric acid levels. Allopurinol may be used during the beginning of brendamustine therapy, however, it poses an increased risk of severe skin toxicity (Stevens-Johnson syndrome or the more severe manifestation of toxic epidermal necrolysis).

Contraindications are hypersensitivities to bendamustine or mannitol (in rare instances severe anaphylactic and anaphylactoid reactions can occur, particularly in the second and subsequent cycles of therapy), renal impairment with creatinine clearance below 40 mL/min, or moderate to severe hepatic impairment. The agent is Pregnancy Category D.

Drug Interactions Because the active bendamustine metabolites, γ-hydroxy bendamustine and N-desmethyl-bendamustine, are formed via Cytochrome P450 CYP1A2, the concomitant intake of CYP1A2 inhibitors (such as fluvoxamine <Luvox> or ciprofloxacin <Cipro>) has the potential to increase the exposure to bendamustine and decrease the exposure to the active metabolites. Conversely, inducers of CYP1A2 (including cigarette smoke and omeprazole <Losec, Antra, Gastroloc, Mopral, Omepral, Prilosec>) have the potential to decrease the concentration of bendamustine and increase the concentrations of its active metabolites in the body.

Spiromustine (spirohydantoin mustard) (NSC 172112) is a nitrogen alkylating agent that contains a lipophilic hydantoin group, which serves as a carrier to cross the blood-brain barrier. This lipophilicity may also enhance alkylating activity against tumors outside the brain. Spiromustine forms covalent linkages with nucleophilic centers in DNA, causing depurination, base pair miscoding, strand scission, and DNA cross-linking, which may result in cytotoxicity. The agent acts in a cell cycle non-specific manner.

Pharmacokinetics In an aqueous environment, spiromustine is rapidly hydrolyzed. The drug has a biphasic plasma decay curve, with hepatic metabolism and excretion, enterohepatic circulation of metabolites, and approximately 50 % renal excretion of the unmetabolized drug.

Third generation nitrogen mustards Uracil mustard (uramustine, 5-[bis(2-chloroethyl)amino]-1*H*-pyrimidine-2,4-dione) <Dopan> is a third generation nitrogen mustard that can be absorbed from the gastrointestinal tract. The drug is a bifunctional alkylating agent that acts in a cell cycle phase non-specific manner. Its activity is a result of the formation of an unstable ethylenimmonium ion. Uracil mustard has been administered to treat chronic lymphocytic leukemia (CLL), chronic myelogenous leukemia (CML), Hodgkin lymphoma, non-Hodgkin lymphomata of the histiocytic or lymphocytic type, lymphosarcoma, breast cancer, and ovarian cancer. It has generated response rates of 65–75 % in hematologic malignancies (Kennedy 1999), although its use has generally been replaced by that of other agents. The drug can be taken orally and is available as capsules. It is usually taken once a week for at least 4 weeks. The typical oral adult dose is 150 µg/kg; the typical oral pediatric dose is 300 µg/kg of body weight.

Pharmacokinetics The blood levels of uracil mustard drop to essentially undetectable levels within 2 h of administration. Less than 1 % of the dose is excreted unchanged in the urine.

Adverse Effects Uracil mustard is relatively well tolerated and does not cause alopecia. Adverse effects comprise nausea and vomiting, diarrhea, and dermatitis. They can also include nervousness, irritability, and depression. The bone marrow depressant effects of uracil mustard may result in an increased incidence of microbial infections, delayed healing, and bleeding. Dental work should be completed prior to initiation of therapy or deferred until the blood counts have returned to normal. Uracil mustard may rarely cause stomatitis, associated with considerable discomfort.

Drug Interactions Uracil mustard can raise the concentration of blood uric acid. Drug interactions may arise with antigout agents, such as allopurinol, colchicines, probenecid, or sulfinpyrazone. Dosage adjustment may be necessary. Allopurinol may be preferred to prevent or reverse uracil mustard induced hyperuricemia and the risk of uric acid nephropathy.

Steroid-coupled nitrogen mustards Estramustine phosphate sodium (estradiol 3-[bis(2-chloroethyl)carbamate] 17-(dihydrogen phosphate), disodium salt, monohydrate) <Emcyt> is an orally available synthetic drug that combines estradiol and mechlorethamine through a carbamate link. The molecule was designed with the intent that its estradiol portion would facilitate uptake of the alkylating agent into hormone sensitive prostate cancer cells. It is phosphorylated for better water solubility. This agent exhibits anti-androgenic effects and is used for the palliative treatment of metastatic or progressive prostate cancer. In the mid-1980s, the classification of estramustine as an alkylating agent was called into doubt as it may act as an anti-microtubule agent. Estramustine and its major metabolite bind covalently to microtubule-associated proteins (MAPs) and Tubulin, thereby causing their separation from the microtubules, inhibiting microtubule assembly, and eventually causing their disassembly.

Estramustine is taken orally, at least 1 h before or 2 h after meals. The recommended daily dose is 14 mg/kg body weight, given in three or four doses. Patients should be treated for 30–90 days before a determination is made of the possible benefits of continued therapy. Therapy should be continued as long as the favorable response lasts, and may extend for years.

Pharmacokinetics Estramustine phosphate taken orally is readily dephosphorylated during absorption, and the major metabolites in the blood are estramustine, its estrone analog, and estradiol. Prolonged treatment produces elevated total blood concentrations of estradiol. The metabolic urinary patterns of the estradiol moiety of estramustine phosphate and estradiol itself are very similar, although the metabolites derived from estramustine phosphate are excreted at a slower rate. Estramustine may be poorly metabolized in patients with impaired liver function.

Adverse Effects Adverse effects caused by estramustine include allergic reactions, with hives, difficulty breathing, and blood clots. Accordingly, contraindications for this agent are hypersensitivity to estradiol or nitrogen mustard. Hypertension may be a consequence and blood pressure should be checked periodically. Gynecomastia and impotence are possible estrogenic effects. Careful monitoring of treatment is required in specific risk groups:

- There is an increased risk of thrombosis, including fatal or non-fatal myocardial infarction, in men receiving estrogens for prostatic cancer. Estramustine capsules should be used with caution in patients with a history of thrombophlebitis, thrombosis, or thromboembolic disorders, especially if these events were associated with prior estrogen therapy. Active thrombophlebitis is a contraindication. Caution should also be used in patients with cerebral vascular disease or coronary artery disease. However, estramustine may be given in cases where the actual tumor mass is the cause of the thromboembolic phenomenon and the benefits of therapy may outweigh the risks.
- Exacerbation of preexisting or incipient peripheral edema or congestive heart disease can occur in some patients. Conditions that might be influenced by fluid retention, such as epilepsy, migraine, or renal dysfunction, require careful observation.
- Because estramustine may influence the metabolism of calcium and phosphate, it should be used with caution in patients with renal insufficiency or in patients with metabolic bone diseases that are associated with hypercalcemia. Patients with prostate cancer and osteoblastic metastases are at risk for hypocalcemia and should have calcium levels closely monitored.
- Because glucose tolerance may be decreased, diabetic patients should be carefully observed while receiving estramustine.

Drug Interactions The simultaneous ingestion of calcium-rich food with estramustine needs to be avoided because it may impair the absorption of the drug. Vaccination with a live vaccine should be avoided in patients receiving estramustine. Killed or inactivated vaccines may be administered. However, the response to such vaccines may be diminished due to immune suppression.

DHEA mustard is a steroidal alkylating agent. The natural steroid hormone (produced from cholesterol by the adrenal glands, gonads, adipose tissue, brain, and skin) and dietary supplement dehydroepiandrosterone (DHEA) is a precursor to both estrogen and testosterone. While dehydroepiandrosterone may have an anti-proliferative or pro-apoptotic effect on cancer cell lines (Schulz et al. 1992; Yang et al. 2002), the clinical significance of these effects may be low.

Adverse Effects Due to the estrogenic effects of dehydroepiandrosterone, high doses are associated with an increased risk for developing breast cancer (Tworoger et al. 2006).

Various esters of progestins and alkylating agents have been produced and studied. Prednimustine (Leo-1031) is a steroidal alkylating agent, in which a corticosteroid (pregnadiene-dione-triol) is linked to chlorambucil. The drug has both alkylating and corticosteroid effects (Harrap et al. 1977). It exerts effects in chronic lymphoid leukemia, lymphosarcoma, acute myeloid leukemia, mammary carcinoma, and melanoma.

Phosphoramide mustards The adverse effects of nitrogen mustard drugs are substantial. Phosphoramide mustards are generated by conversion of the base nitrogen mustard into nontoxic prodrugs (Fig. 2.5), which are actively transported into the cancer cells. Once taken up, these agents are enzymatically converted into their active, cytotoxic forms. Phosphoramide

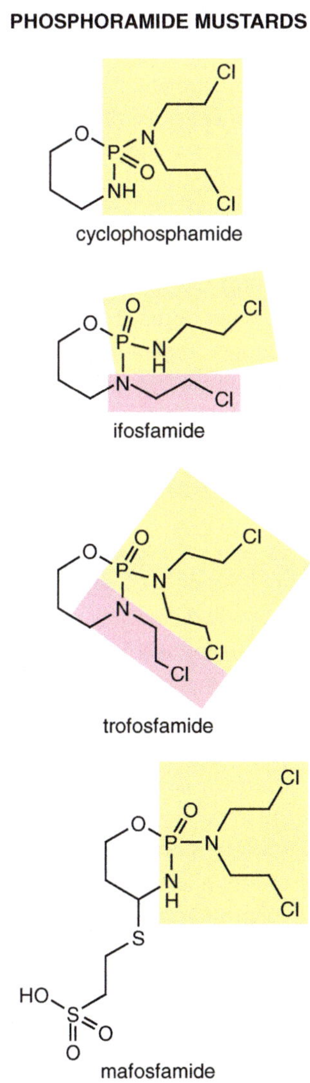

Fig. 2.5 Structures of phosphoramide mustards. The common phosphoramide mustard moiety is highlighted in *yellow*. In ifosfamide, one of the mustard chains is moved to a different nitrogen (shaded in *pink*); this leads to 7-member cross-links after DNA alkylation (the other phosphoramide mustards form 5-chain cross-links). Trofosfamide combines the two possible chain lengths

mustards form DNA inter-strand and intra-strand cross-links at guanine *N7* positions. This leads to cell death.

Cyclophosphamide was first synthesized in 1958 by Arnold, Bourseaux, and Brock at ASTA Werke (Arnold et al. 1958). The related ifosfamide followed. For these discoveries, Norbert Brock and his team synthesized and screened more than 800 candidate oxazaphosphorine compounds (Brock 1996).

Cyclophosphamide (*N*, *N*-bis(2-chloroethyl)-2-oxo-1-oxa-3-aza-2u{5}-phosphacyclohexan-2-amine, CPA) <Cytoxan, Endoxan, Neosar, Procytox, Revimmune> is a synthetic alkylating agent. Although cyclophosphamide was intended to be an inactive carrier for the alkylating moiety to be activated in neoplasms that are rich in Phosphamidases, the drug is mainly activated by blood and liver. The predominant use of cyclophosphamide is in combination chemotherapy. Malignancies that are often susceptible to cyclophosphamide treatment include lymphomata (stage III-IV malignant lymphomata, Hodgkin disease, nodular or diffuse lymphocytic lymphoma, mixed-cell type lymphoma, histiocytic lymphoma, Burkitt lymphoma, multiple myeloma) and some leukemias (chronic lymphocytic leukemia, chronic granulocytic leukemia except in acute blastic crisis, acute myelogenous and monocytic leukemia, advanced mycosis fungoides). Unlike other common alkylating agents, cyclophosphamide can occasionally induce remission in acute childhood leukemias, and it can be used to prolong remission. Solid tumors that may respond to the agent include bladder cancer, bone cancer, lung cancer, cervical cancer, endometrial cancer, ovarian adenocarcinoma, breast carcinoma, prostate cancer, testicular cancer, melanoma, cancer of the adrenal cortex, disseminated neuroblastoma, and retinoblastoma.

Cyclophosphamide can be administered orally or intravenously. Many regimens of intravenous and oral cyclophosphamide have been applied.

- When used as the only oncolytic drug therapy, the initial course of cyclophosphamide for patients with no hematologic deficiency usually consists of 40–50 mg/kg given intravenously in divided doses over a period of 2–5 days.
- A cyclophosphamide regimen for adults gives 200 mg per day intravenously for 5 days, followed by oral doses of 50–200 mg per day thereafter, depending on the extent of marrow depression.
- In recent years, cyclophosphamide has been studied as an agent of metronomic chemotherapy, which can be administered at a low dose on an every 6-day schedule or continuously.

The dosages must be adjusted in accord with evidence of anti-tumor activity and tolerable myelosuppression (transient decreases in the total white blood cell count to 2000 cells/mm^3 or more persistent reduction to 3000 cells/mm^3 are tolerated without serious risk of infection if there is no marked granulocytopenia).

Pharmacokinetics The oral bioavailability of cyclophosphamide is over 75 %. The blood concentrations of metabolites reach a maximum 2–3 h after an intravenous dose. Plasma protein binding of the unmodified drug is low, but some metabolites are bound to an extent greater than 60 %. The unchanged drug has an elimination half-life of 3–12 h with 5–25 % of the dose being excreted in the urine without having been altered.

Cyclophosphamide is metabolized in the liver by constitutive P450 enzymes of the CYP2C subfamily, and by drug-inducible enzymes belonging to the P450 subfamily CYP2B. CYP2B6 is the most active catalyst of 4-hydroxylation in the liver. The main active product is 4-hydroxy-cyclophosphamide, which exists in equilibrium with its tautomer, aldophosphamide. Most of the aldophosphamide is oxidized to the therapeutically inactive carboxyphosphamide by the enzyme Aldehyde Dehydrogenase (ALDH), while a small proportion is converted into phosphoramide mustard and acrolein. The active metabolites aldophosphamide and phosphoramide mustard bind to DNA. The mustard generates a highly electrophilic aziridinium species that forms DNA cross-links, which is the key cytotoxic lesion induced in tumors treated with oxazaphosphorines. The cross-links inhibit DNA reduplication and initiate cell death. There is no need for cyclophosphamide dosage modification in patients with renal function impairment.

Adverse Effects Leukopenia is common and increases the risk of infections. Thrombocytopenia or anemia develop occasionally, with high dosages causing pancytopenia. These hematologic effects usually can be reversed by reducing the drug dose or by interrupting treatment. Recovery from leukopenia usually begins 7–10 days after cessation of therapy.

Acrolein is toxic to the bladder epithelium and may lead to hemorrhagic cystitis, often diagnosed by the manifestation of hematuria. The cystitis can predispose to bladder cancer as a delayed adverse effect. It is preventable through the use of aggressive hydration or administration of mesna (sodium 2-sulfanylethanesulfonate) <Uromitexan>. When hemorrhagic cystitis occurs it requires the immediate discontinuation of cyclophosphamide.

Cyclophosphamide is itself carcinogenic, potentially causing transitional cell carcinoma of the bladder, myeloproliferative or lymphoproliferative disorders as long term complications. The agent also interferes with oogenesis and spermatogenesis. It may cause sterility in both sexes. Chemotherapy with cyclophosphamide, given to boys before or during puberty, results in a high rate of gonadal dysfunction. Amenorrhea associated with decreased estrogen and increased Gonadotropin secretion develops in a substantial proportion of women treated with cyclophosphamide. Affected patients generally resume regular menses within a few months after cessation of therapy. The drug is Pregnancy Category D.

Nausea and vomiting commonly occur with cyclophosphamide therapy. Anorexia, abdominal discomfort or pain, and diarrhea may arise. There are isolated incidents of hemorrhagic colitis, oral mucosal ulceration, and jaundice. Cyclophosphamide is a medication that causes dry eye. Remedies can include artificial tears, punctual plugs, and nutritional therapy, as well as adjustments in the patient's environment. Alopecia caused by cyclophosphamide is common, but usually temporary despite continued administration of the drug. Skin rashes occur occasionally in patients receiving the drug. Pigmentation of the skin and changes in nails can arise. Interstitial pneumonitis or interstitial pulmonary fibrosis can be associated with high doses of cyclophosphamide over a prolonged period. SIADH (syndrome of inappropriate Anti-Diuretic Hormone secretion)[12] is a rare adverse effect with the use of cyclophosphamide.

Drug Interactions The rate of metabolism and the leukopenic activity of cyclophosphamide are increased by chronic administration of high doses of phenobarbital. Cyclophosphamide treatment, which causes a marked and persistent inhibition of Cholinesterase activity, potentiates the effect of succinylcholine chloride. This is relevant for patients who need to undergo general anesthesia.

Ifosfamide (3-(2-chloroethyl)-2-[(2-chloroethyl)amino] tetrahydro-2H-1,3,2-oxazaphosphorine 2-oxide, isophosphamide, IFA) <Mitoxana, Ifex> is isomeric to cyclophosphamide. Ifosfamide generates 7-atom DNA cross-links, whereas cyclophosphamide generates 5-atom cross-links. Ifosfamide is used mainly in the treatment of germ cell testicular cancer, but also for breast cancer, non-Hodgkin lymphoma, soft tissue sarcoma, osteogenic sarcoma, lung cancer, cervical cancer, and ovarian cancer. Ifosfamide is administered intravenously at a dose of 1.2 g/m^2 body surface area per day for five consecutive days. Treatment is repeated every 3 weeks or after recovery from hematologic toxicity, which is reflected in platelet counts of at least 100,000/μL and white blood cell counts of at least 4000/μL.

Pharmacokinetics Ifosfamide exhibits dose dependent pharmacokinetics, which may reflect the saturation of relevant metabolic pathways at high concentrations. At single doses of 3.8–5.0 g/m^2, the plasma concentrations decay biphasically and the mean terminal elimination half-life is about 15 h. At doses of 1.6–2.4 g/m^2/day, the plasma decay is mono-exponential and the terminal elimination half-life is about 7 h. 4-carboxyifosfamide, thiodiacetic acid, and cysteine conjugates of chloroacetic acid are the major urinary metabolites of ifosfamide, with only small amounts of 4-hydroxyifosfamide and acrolein.

Ifosfamide is a prodrug alkylating agent that undergoes metabolic activation by the hepatic Cytochrome P450 monooxygenase system. 4-hydroxylation is primarily catalyzed by CYP3A enzymes, with minor contributions made by other CYP enzymes, including CYP2B6. Hydroxylation at C4 forms the unstable intermediate 4-hydroxyifosfamide. It initiates the metabolic pathway that ultimately results in fragmentation of the oxazaphosphorine to yield 2-propenal (acrolein) and an electrophilic phosphoramide mustard (Fig. 2.6). While acrolein can exhibit cytotoxic effects by binding covalently to proteins, the phosphoramide mustard possesses DNA alkylating activity (Weber and Waxman 1993a). Whereas both cyclophosphamide and ifosfamide are activated by Cytochromes P450 2B1 and 2C6/2C11, only ifosfamide is also activated by Cytochrome P450 3A.

N-dechloroethylation of the parent drug yields monofunctional metabolites that have lost their DNA cross-linking activity and therapeutic efficacy. In contrast to the metabolism of cyclophosphamide, the *N*-dechloroethylation pathway may consume up to 50 % of the administered ifosfamide. It is associated with the production of the neurotoxic metabolite chloroacetaldehyde.

Adverse Effects Dose fractionation and hydration aid substantially in limiting the toxicities of ifosfamide. Alopecia (over 80 %), nausea and vomiting (60 %), and temporary ridging of the nails may occur under therapy. Ifosfamide produces less myelotoxicity (mainly leukopenia) than cyclophosphamide and also exhibits little cross-resistance. The metabolic ifosfamide product acrolein can contribute to the hemorrhagic cystitis associated with oxazaphosphorine therapy. Hemorrhagic cystitis may require discontinuation of the drug. The adverse effect may be preventable with extensive hydration and co-administration of mesna <Uromitexan>. Ifosfamide is Pregnancy Category D. The drug is excreted into the breast milk and nursing should be avoided during treatment.

Some patients treated with ifosfamide develop severe neurotoxicity and urotoxicity, which may both be associated with the formation of chloroacetaldehyde via N-dechloroethylation, an alternative Cytochrome P450 catalyzed metabolic pathway, which deactivates the drug through side chain oxidation. It yields the inactive, mono-functional alkylating metabolites 2- and 3-dechloroethyl-ifosfamide and produces the toxic byproduct chloroacetaldehyde. This pathway, catalyzed mainly by CYP3A4 and CYP2B6, may consume up to 50 % of the therapeutic dose of ifosfamide. Encephalopathy (manifested in somnolence, confusion, depressive psychosis, hallucinations, dizziness, disorientation, cranial nerve dysfunction, seizures, or coma) is a serious, sometimes fatal,

[12] The syndrome of inappropriate antidiuretic hormone secretion (SIADH, Schwartz-Bartter syndrome) is characterized by an excessive release of Anti-Diuretic Hormone, typically from the posterior pituitary gland. The result is often dilutional hyponatremia, in which the sodium levels remain normal but the total body fluid increases.

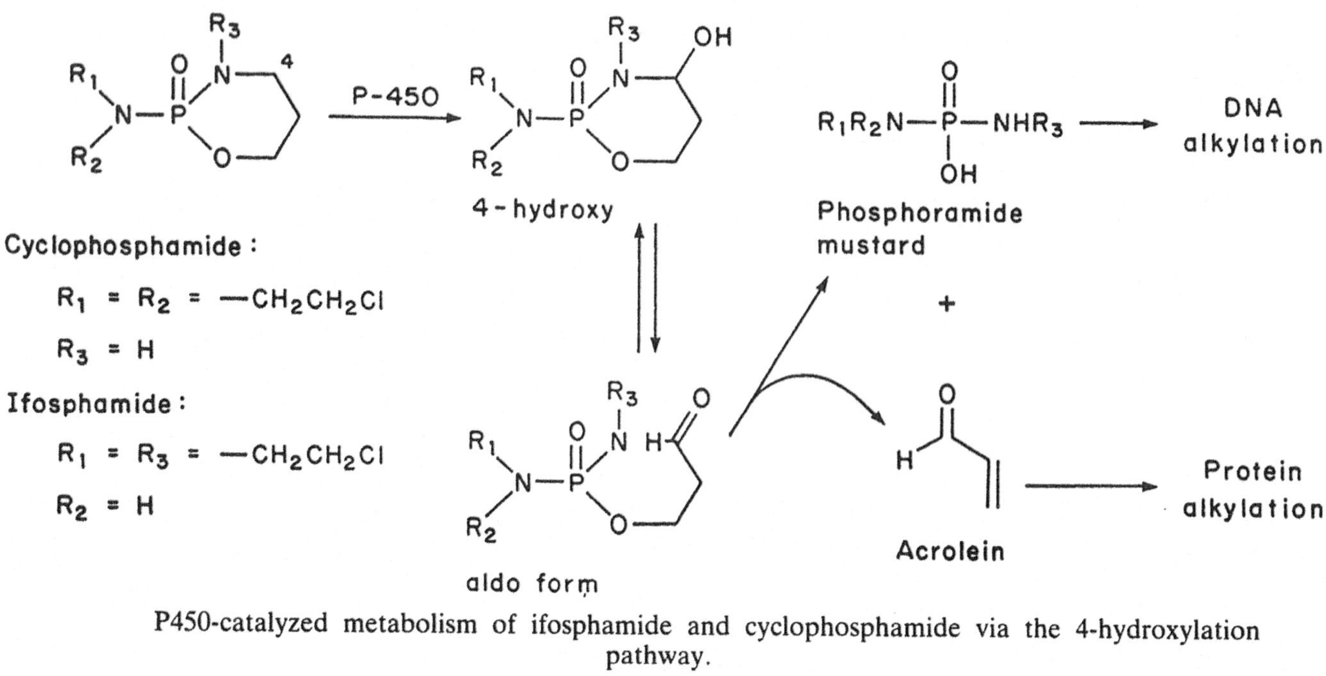

Fig. 2.6 CYP450 catalyzed metabolism of ifosfamide and cyclophosphamide via the 4-hydroxylation pathway. The prodrugs are converted by Cytochrome P450 enzymes into the active agents phosphoramide mustard and acrolein. (Weber and Waxman 1993a)

and limiting adverse effect. This adverse reaction is particularly associated with the oral administration of ifosfamide, where it may affect more than 30 % of patients. It is caused by drug metabolites that agonize AMPA/Kainate Receptors and induce cellular acidification in cortical neurons. The metabolite chloroacetaldehyde may lead to the formation of chloroacetic acid and then to S-carboxymethylcysteine (SCMC) after conjugation with the amino acid cysteine. S-carboxymethylcysteine can account for about 80 % of the administered dose of ifosfamide (Küpfer et al. 1996), which is then further degraded metabolically to thiodiglycolic acid (TDGA) (Hofmann et al. 1991). The S-carboxymethylcysteine chemical structure shares a close similarity with the excitatory neurotransmitter glutamic acid and may therefore affect glutamatergic neurons (Chatton et al. 2001).

Trofosfamide (*N*, *N*,3-tris(2-chloroethyl)-1,3,2-oxazaphosphinan-2-amide 2-oxide, TFF, TRO) (ASTA Z 4828) <Ixoten, Genoxal Trofosfamida> is an orally bioavailable oxazaphosphorine prodrug. The activation product, isophosphoramide mustard alkylates DNA to form DNA-DNA cross-links, which may cause inhibition of DNA, RNA, and protein synthesis, thus resulting in tumor cell death. Trofosfamide is used in first and second-line treatments of soft tissue sarcomata, and it may be effective as palliative treatment in non-Hodgkin lymphoma. Trofosfamide therapy has an overall response rate of 50–80 % at oral daily doses of 150 mg. In alternative regimens, remissions have been accomplished by administering trofosfamide metronomically at low dose.

Pharmacokinetics Trofosfamide is a substrate for Cytochrome P450s. After oral administration, the prodrug is mainly metabolized in the liver to its active 4-hydroxy derivative ifosfamide, which is then converted via hydroxylation at the cyclic C-4 position to the active isophosphoramide mustard. Compared with ifosfamide, trofosfamide is much more strongly hydroxylated to the tumoristatically active 4-OH derivatives with a 20–30 times higher mean area under the concentration-time curve[13]. Based on the lipid solubility, small molecular size, and minimal binding to plasma and tissue proteins, there is penetration by trofosfamide through the blood-brain barrier.

Adverse Effects Trofosfamide therapy is rather non-toxic. The maximum tolerated dose is around 125 mg/m^2. Adverse effects include dose dependent hematotoxicity and, rarely, hemorrhagic cystitis, nausea and vomiting.

Mafosfamide (2-{(2-[bis(2-chloroethyl)amino]-2-oxido-1,3,2-oxazaphosphinan-4-yl}thio)ethanesulfonic acid) is a synthetic oxazaphosphorine derivative that alkylates DNA, forming DNA cross-links and inhibiting DNA synthesis. Although closely related to cyclophosphamide, mafosfamide

[13] The area under the drug (plasma/serum/blood) concentration-time curve (AUC) reflects the actual body exposure to the drug after administration of one dose. It is typically visualized as a graph of the plasma drug concentration (on the y-axis) over time (on the x-axis) and is expressed in mg*h/L. The AUC is inversely proportional to the clearance of the drug. When a drug follows linear kinetics, the AUC is directly proportional to the dose.

NITROSOUREAS

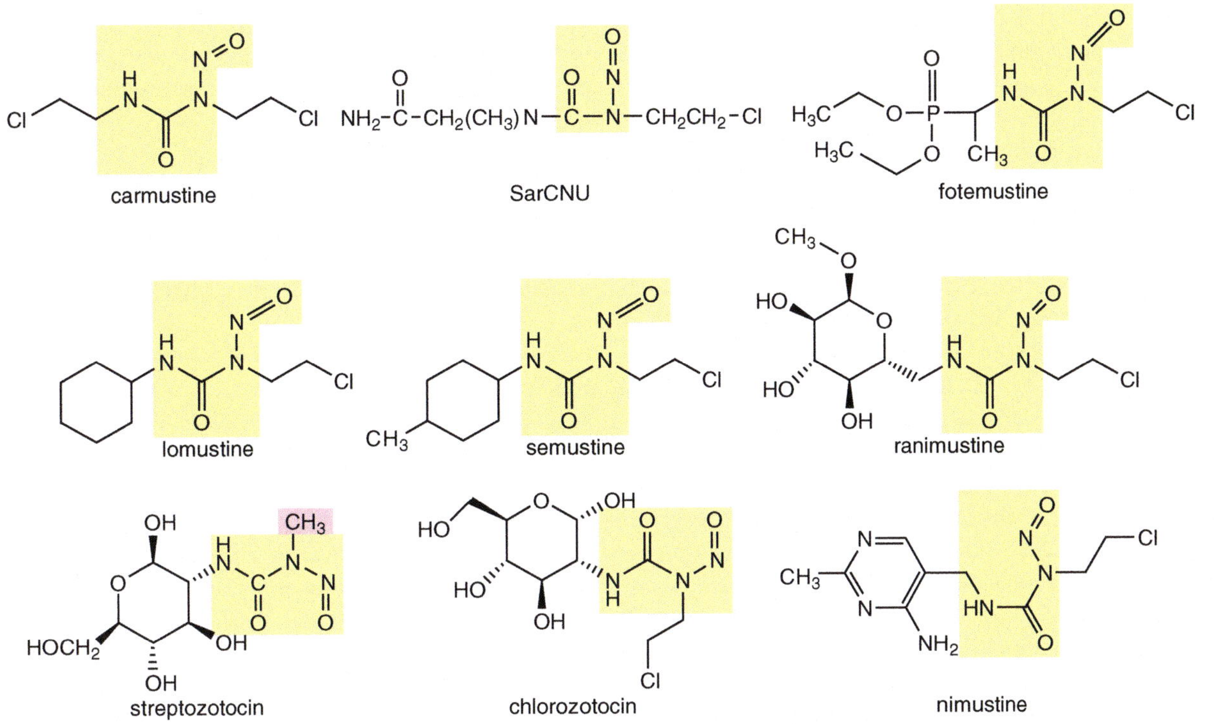

Fig. 2.7 Structures of nitrosoureas. All drugs in this class contain the nitrosoureea moiety (highlighted in *yellow*). With the exception of streptozotozin (*pink box*), all nitrosoureas have a chloroethyl side chain attached to the nitrogen adjacent to the N=O group

does not require hepatic activation to generate its active metabolite 4-hydroxy-cyclophosphamide. Accordingly, it is potentially useful in the intrathecal treatment of neoplastic meningitis.

The mustard pharmacophore is –N(CH$_2$CH$_2$Cl)$_2$.
The two arms of mustard drugs can cross-link DNA strands.
Nitrogen mustard also damages DNA through the production of reactive nitrogen species.

First generation nitrogen mustards cannot be taken orally.
In second generation nitrogen mustards, electron withdrawing aromatic radicals reduce the reactivity and permit oral use.
In third generation nitrogen mustards, the pyrimidine nucleus carrier for the mustard pharmacophore permits oral administration.
Steroid-coupled nitrogen mustards combine the effect of the alkylating agent with a steroid for selective uptake or combined anti-cancer action.
In phosphoramide mustards, the base nitrogen mustard is administered as non-toxic prodrug that is actively transported into the cancer cells and enzymatically converted into its cytotoxic forms.

2.1.2 Nitrosoureas

Under a contract with the U.S. National Cancer Institute (NCI), a group led by John Montgomery at the Southern Research Institute synthesized nitrosoureas, which contain a nitroso group and urea (Fig. 2.7). These are alkylating agents that cross-link DNA. Due to their lipophilicity, they cross the blood-brain barrier and can be applied to the treatment of brain tumors.

Adverse Effects Pulmonary toxicity is a common problem associated with nitrosoureas. Acute leukemia or bone marrow dysplasia can be complications in patients following long term nitrosourea therapy. Representatives of this drug class may affect the vision.

The alkylating agent carmustine (BCNU, 1,3-bis(2-chloroethyl)-1-nitrosourea) <BiCNU> cross-links DNA during all phases of the cell cycle, causing a disruption of DNA function, and resulting in cell cycle arrest and apoptosis. This agent also carbamoylates proteins, including DNA repair enzymes, which leads to an enhanced cytotoxic effect. As an irreversible Glutathione Reductase inhibitor, carmustine renders cells susceptible to oxidative stress[14]. Being highly lipophilic, carmustine is particularly useful for the treatment of brain tumors, owing to its ability to cross the blood-brain barrier. The drug is used as a single agent or in combination therapy in the palliative treatment of several types of brain cancer (including glioma and glioblastoma, medulloblastoma, astrocytoma, ependymoma, and metastatic brain

[14] Many alkylating agents readily react with thiol containing small molecules, such as cysteine and Glutathione. The resulting reduced cellular Glutathione levels can contribute to cytotoxicity.

cancers), multiple myeloma (in combination with prednisone), Hodgkin and non-Hodgkin lymphomata (as secondary combination chemotherapy in patients, who fail to respond to or relapse under primary therapy). The recommended dose of carmustine as a single agent in previously untreated patients is 150–200 mg/m^2 intravenously every 6 weeks. This may be given as a single dose or divided into daily injections of 75–100 mg/m^2 on two successive days. When administered in combination with other myelosuppressive drugs or in patients whose bone marrow reserve is depleted, dose reduction may be required. Doses subsequent to the initial one should be adjusted according to the hematologic response. A repeat course should not be given until the blood cell counts have recovered, which is usually after 6 weeks because the hematologic toxicity is delayed and cumulative.

Pharmacokinetics Intravenously administered carmustine is degraded within 15 min. About half of the drug given enters the cerebrospinal fluid. Its metabolism occurs in the liver prior to its excretion in the urine (60–70 %) and breath (about 10 %).

Adverse Effects Pulmonary and bone marrow toxicities are functions of lifetime cumulative dose. Pulmonary toxicity, characterized by infiltrates or fibrosis, occurs 1 week to 3.5 years after treatment. Risk factors include prolonged therapy with total doses reaching 1400 mg/m^2 and a past history of lung disease. Delayed onset progressive pulmonary fibrosis can occur up to 17 years after the treatment of adolescents with cumulative doses of 770–1800 mg/m^2 combined with cranial radio-therapy for intracranial tumors. Thrombocytopenia arises at about 4 weeks post administration and persists for 1–2 weeks. Leukopenia occurs at 5–6 weeks after a dose of carmustine and persists for 1–2 weeks. The thrombocytopenia is generally more severe than the leukopenia. Weekly monitoring of platelet and white blood cell counts is recommended as a basis for patient-specific adjustments to the dosage regimens.

Nausea and vomiting, appearing within 2 h and lasting 4–6 h, are frequent after intravenous infusion of carmustine. The prior administration of anti-emetics can alleviate, and sometimes prevent this adverse effect. Renal abnormalities (progressive azotemia, decrease in kidney size, renal failure) may arise in patients who have received large cumulative doses after prolonged therapy. Rapid infusion of carmustine may produce intensive flushing of the skin and suffusion of the conjunctiva within 2 h, lasting about 4 h. It is also associated with burning at the site of injection. Accidental contact of reconstituted carmustine with the skin can cause transient hyper-pigmentation of the affected areas. Rare adverse effects comprise neuroretinitis, chest pain, headache, allergic reaction, hypotension, and tachycardia. The drug is Pregnancy Category D.

Drug Interactions Drug interaction with cimetidine, amphotericin B, digoxin, or phenytoin may arise and require adjustment. There is no cross-resistance of carmustine with other alkylating agents.

Drug Resistance The emergence of carmustine resistant tumor cell populations is a common problem under treatment (Weber and Waxman 1993b). Resistance may be due to increased expression of Glutathione S-Transferase, activation of DNA repair mechanisms, or altered cellular transport of the agent. Specifically, carmustine anti-tumor efficacy is inversely correlated to the activity of the DNA repair enzyme MGMT (O^6-Methylguanine-DNA Methyltransferase).

SarCNU (sarcosinamide chloroethylnitrosourea, 2-chloroethyl-3-sarcosinamide-1-nitrosourea) (NSC364432) is an alkylating chloroethylnitrosourea that forms covalent linkages with nucleophilic centers in DNA, causing depurination, base pair miscoding, strand scission, and DNA cross-linking. It does not form an organic isocyanate because the *N*3 position is blocked with a methyl group. The carrier group of SarCNU is the amino acid derivative methylglycinamide. The compound was originally synthesized under the hypothesis that the carrier group would allow for uptake of the drug through amino acid transporters. SarCNU enters cells via transport through the Extraneuronal Transporter for Monoamine Transmitters (EMT, Extra-Neuronal Catecholamine Uptake-2 Carrier). Its cytotoxicity correlates positively with the expression levels of EMT as well as inversely with the DNA repair enzymes MGMT and ERCC2 (Chen et al. 1999). SarCNU is effective against gliomata.

Adverse Effects SarCNU has pulmonary toxicity (Webster et al. 2005). HIV patients have an increased risk of severe SarCNU toxicity.

Fotemustine (diethyl (1-{[(2-chloroethyl)(nitroso)carbamoyl]amino}ethyl)phosphonate) (S10036) <Muphoran> is a chloroethylating nitrosourea. It includes a bioisostere of alanine (1-amino ethylphosphonic acid) in order to facilitate cellular penetration and passage across the blood-brain barrier. Fotemustine alkylates guanine by forming chloroethyl adducts at the 6 position, resulting in *N*1 guanine-*N*3 cytosine cross-linkages. This leads to an inhibition of DNA synthesis, cell cycle arrest, and finally cell death. As a result of its alkylating and carbamoylating effect, the drug exerts a potent cytostatic activity on cells in cycle, inducing an accumulation of cells in G_2/M phase. Fotemustine is indicated for disseminated malignant melanoma. An interval of 8 weeks after the start of induction treatment and 3 weeks after each cycle of maintenance treatment is recommended. The agent should not be administered to patients who received chemotherapy in the previous 4 weeks (6 weeks if the treatment included nitrosoureas).

Pharmacokinetics Fotemustine is lipophilic and crosses the blood-brain barrier. After infusion, the blood levels decline to 0 within 3 h. The binding to plasma proteins is 25–30 %, mostly to Acid α-1-Glycoprotein and Albumin. 50–60 % of the dose administered is excreted in the urine, 5 % in the feces.

Adverse Effects Fotemustine may cause retinal atrophy or retinal detachment. Ophthalmoscopic examinations should be carried out routinely during treatment. Delayed hematologic toxicity is characterized by thrombocytopenia (nadir[15] 4–5 weeks after the first administration) and leukopenia (nadir 5–6 weeks). Moderate nausea and vomiting may occur during 2 h following the injection. The drug is Pregnancy Category D.

Lomustine (CCNU, 1-(2-chloroethyl)-3-cyclohexyl-1-nitroso-urea) <CeeNU> is a nitrosourea that carbamoylates, alkylates and cross-links DNA, thereby inhibiting DNA and RNA synthesis. This agent also carbamoylates amino acids in proteins, resulting in the disruption of RNA processing and protein function. Lomustine is lipophilic and crosses the blood-brain barrier. Malignancies for which lomustine is used include primary and metastatic brain tumors, Hodgkin lymphoma (as secondary combination chemotherapy in patients who fail to respond to or relapse under primary therapy), multiple myeloma, breast cancer, ovarian cancer, pancreatic cancer, lung cancer, and melanoma. The drug can be taken orally.

- As a single agent in previously untreated patients, the recommended oral dose every 6 weeks for adults and children is 100–150 mg/m^2.
- In individuals with compromised bone marrow function, the dose may need to be reduced to 100 mg/m^2 every 6 weeks.
- When lomustine is used in combination with other myelosuppressive drugs, dose reduction may be required.

Doses subsequent to the initial dose need to be adjusted according to the hematologic response of the patient to the preceding dose. A repeat course of lomustine should not be given until blood cell counts have returned to acceptable levels.

Pharmacokinetics The serum half-lives of the metabolites range from 16 h to 2 days. The tissue levels are comparable to the blood levels at 15 min after intravenous administration. About half of the drug given is excreted in the urine in the form of degradation products within 24 h.

Adverse Effects The most common and severe toxic effect of lomustine is bone marrow suppression 4–6 weeks after drug administration, notably thrombocytopenia (occurs at about 4 weeks post-administration and persists for 1–2 weeks) and leucopenia (occurs at 5–6 weeks and persists for 1–2 weeks), which may contribute to bleeding and overwhelming infections in already compromised patients. Anemia also occurs, but is less frequent and less severe than thrombocytopenia or leukopenia. The occurrence of acute leukemia and bone marrow dysplasia is possible in patients following long term nitrosourea therapy.

Pulmonary toxicity, characterized by pulmonary infiltrates or fibrosis can arise after an interval of 6 months or longer (up to 17 years) from the start of therapy, usually consecutive to cumulative doses greater than 1100 mg/m^2. Renal abnormalities consisting of progressive azotemia (elevated blood urea nitrogen), decrease in kidney size, and renal failure can occur in patients consecutive to large cumulative doses after prolonged therapy.

Nausea and vomiting may constitute acute adverse effects 3–6 h after an oral dose that usually last less than 24 h. Prior administration of anti-emetics is effective in diminishing and sometimes preventing this toxicity. Nausea and vomiting can also be reduced if lomustine is administered to fasting patients. Stomatitis, alopecia, optic atrophy, visual disturbances (possibly blindness), lethargy, ataxia, or dysarthria may arise infrequently. Lomustine is Pregnancy Category D.

Drug Resistance Lomustine does not encounter cross-resistance with other alkylators.

Semustine (methyl-CCNU, *N*-(2-chloroethyl)-*N′*-(4-methylcyclohexyl)-*N*-nitrosourea) is a methylated derivative of carmustine. As an alkylating agent, semustine forms covalent linkages with nucleophilic centers in DNA, causing depurination, base pair miscoding, strand scission, and DNA cross-linking. Together, these effects result in cytotoxicity. Semustine has been applied to the treatment of brain tumors, lymphomata, colorectal cancer, and stomach cancer. It is not widely in use because it has not proven clearly superior to other treatments for these diseases. Semustine is taken orally as a capsule at bedtime, 3–4 h after a meal.

Adverse Effects A common adverse effect of semustine is prolonged myelosuppression, which may result in infection and bleeding. Therefore, the required interval between courses of semustine is longer than with other agents. The drug causes nausea and vomiting. Sometimes anorexia or loss of appetite persists after nausea and vomiting have subsided. There is an increased risk for the development of secondary leukemia. Fetal abnormalities are likely if pregnancy occurs while taking this drug. Rare adverse effects include sores in the mouth or on the lips, hepatotoxicity, renal toxicity, disorientation, difficulty walking, blurred vision, and pulmonary fibrosis.

Ranimustine (methyl 6-({[(2-chloroethyl)(nitroso)amino] carbonyl}amino)-6-deoxy-α-D-glucopyranoside, MCNU)

[15] The nadir (from the Arabic term for opposite) is the point of the celestial sphere that is directly opposite the zenith and vertically downward from the observer. Its use has been broadened to indicate the lowest point of a state or a relationship. In chemotherapy, the nadir describes the lowest number in blood cell counts that occurs as a consequence of bone marrow suppression.

<Cymerin> is a chloroethylnitrosourea derivative that inhibits its proliferation and growth of tumor cells by alkylation and cross-linkage of DNA strands within tumor cells. It is approved in Japan for the treatment of chronic myelogenous leukemia and polycythemia vera.

Streptozotocin was discovered in the late 1950s as an antibiotic in a strain of the soil microbe Streptomyces achromogenes (Vavra et al. 1959). Streptozotocin (Streptozocin, STZ, 1-methyl-1-nitroso-3-[2,4,5-trihydroxy-6- (hydroxymethyl) oxan-3-yl]-urea) <Zanosar, Sicor, Teva> is a glucosamine-nitrosourea compound, which is sufficiently similar to glucose to be transported into the cell by the glucose transport protein GLUT2, but it is not recognized by other glucose transporters. This underlies its preferential toxicity to pancreatic β-cells, as these have relatively high levels of GLUT2. Accordingly, streptozotozin is used for the treatment of pancreatic islet cell cancer, but is generally limited to patients whose cancer cannot be resected surgically. Streptozotocin can reduce the tumor burden and ameliorate symptoms, such as hypoglycemia due to excessive Insulin secretion by insulinomata.

- A typical dose is 500 mg/m^2/day by intravenous injection or infusion for 5 days, repeated every 4–6 weeks. Dose escalation with this schedule is not recommended.
- An initial intravenous dose of 1000 mg/m^2 of body surface area can be given at weekly intervals for the first two courses. There is an option for dose escalation in subsequent courses for patients who have not achieved a therapeutic response and who have not experienced significant toxicity. On this schedule, the median time to onset of response is about 17 days (median total dose about 2000 mg/m^2) and the median time to maximum response is about 35 days (median total dose about 4000 mg/m^2).

Adverse Effects Because of its inherent renal toxicity, therapy with streptozotocin should be limited to patients with symptomatic or progressive metastatic disease. Many patients experience dose dependent renal toxicity, as manifested in azotemia, anuria, hypophosphatemia, glycosuria, and renal tubular acidosis. Such toxicity is cumulative and may be severe or fatal. Therefore, a single dose of 1500 mg/m^2 body surface area should not be exceeded.

Most patients experience severe nausea and vomiting, occasionally requiring discontinuation of the drug therapy. Some patients encounter diarrhea. Streptozotocin is generally non-myelosuppressive. However, rare cases of fatal hematologic toxicity are possible. Mild to moderate abnormalities of glucose tolerance arise in some patients. Local inflammation (edema, erythema, burning, tenderness) can be a consequence of extravasation of the product, possibly leading to tissue necrosis. The drug is Pregnancy Category D.

Drug Interactions Streptozotocin may demonstrate additive toxicity when used in combination with other cytotoxic agents. This drug should not be used concomitantly with other potential nephrotoxins. Streptozocin prolongs the elimination half-life of doxorubicin and thus can lead to severe bone marrow suppression. A reduction of the doxorubicin dosage may be required.

Chlorozotocin (1-(2-Chloroethyl)-1-nitroso-3-[(2R,3R,4S,5R)-3,4,5,6-tetrahydroxy-1-oxohexan-2-yl]urea, CZT) is a glucose linked chloroethylnitrosourea (Johnston et al. 1975). The glucose is intended to diminish bone marrow toxicity. The agent alkylates DNA and proteins, induces the formation of inter-strand DNA and DNA-protein cross-links, and causes DNA strand breakage, thereby damaging DNA and resulting in cell death.

Adverse Effects Chlorozotocin is a mutagen, but it is less myelotoxic than most other nitrosoureas.

Nimustine (ACNU) (CS 439) <Nidran> alkylates and cross-links DNA, thereby causing DNA fragmentation, inhibition of protein synthesis, and cell death. The drug is in use in China and Japan.

Nitrosoureas are alkylating agents that cross-link DNA.
Due to their lipophilicity, they cross the blood-brain barrier.
Pulmonary toxicity is a common adverse effect of nitrosoureas.
Acute leukemia or bone marrow dysplasia can be long term complications.

2.1.3 Triazenes and Hydrazines

Triazenes [3,3-bis(2-chloro ethyl)-l-triazeno] imidazole-carboxamides[16] constitute a series of prodrugs synthesized in the 1960s (Shealy et al. 1962; Shealy and Krauth 1966). They arose empirically out of the synthetic program at the U.S. National Cancer Institute for agents potentially useful in the inhibition of purine metabolism. Although these compounds had no such activity, they displayed anti-tumor effects in animal experiments prompting their further development. Triazene molecules have three adjacent nitrogen atoms, two of which are joined by a double bond, and the 3rd is affixed by a single bond (Fig. 2.8). Their activation occurs with the release of the single-bonded nitrogen, leaving the highly reactive double-bonded diazonium fragment exposed. Triazenes are anti-proliferative agents. When activated, they

[16] Carboxamide moieties are essential to the structures of triazenes, various small molecule kinase inhibitors (sunitinib, sorafenib, tandutinib, lonafarnib, veliparnib), the Topoisomerase inhibitor ascularine isethionate, the purine antagonist tiazofurin, the HSP90 inhibitor AUY922, and the hydroxamate MMP inhibitor prinomastat.

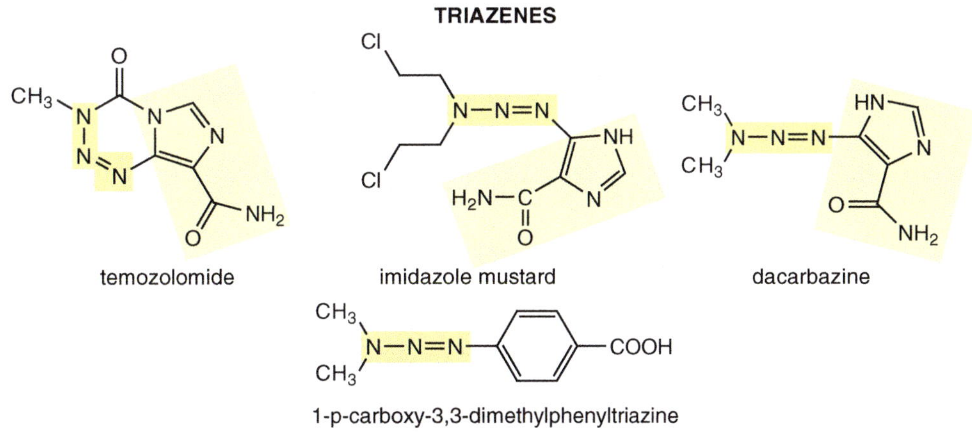

Fig. 2.8 Structures of triazene anti-cancer drugs. The common functional triazene moiety is highlighted in *yellow*. The *lighter shade* of *yellow* indicates the imidazole-4-carboxamide moiety that is common to three of the four representatives in this drug class

bind to cellular DNA and damage it. Both temozolomide and dacarbazine are prodrugs of the active monomethyl triazeno imidazole carboxamide (MTIC).

Temozolomide (methazolastone) (SCHS2.365, NSC 362856) <Temodar, Temodal> was first synthesized by Malcolm Stevens in Birmingham, Great Britain in the early 1980s and was approved for use in the U.S. in 1999. Temozolomide is an imidazotetrazine derivative of dacarbazine. Its indications are newly diagnosed glioblastoma multiforme in adult patients (concomitantly with radio-therapy and then as maintenance treatment) and refractory anaplastic astrocytoma (in patients who have experienced disease progression on a drug regimen containing nitrosourea and procarbazine). The drug may also be used in the treatment of metastatic melanoma and is effective against mycosis fungoides. Temozolomide is available in capsules and is taken orally. The initial dosage is determined based on body height and weight. The typical dose for the first treatment cycle is 150 mg per day taken for five consecutive days, with each treatment cycle lasting 28 days. The number of treatment cycles depends on patient tolerane for the drug and its effectiveness in treating the cancer. The maximum tolerated dose is 1000 mg/m^2/cycle in both children and adults. Dose adjustments may be required based on the nadir neutrophil and platelet counts in the previous cycle as well as the neutrophil and platelet counts at the time of initiating the next cycle.

Pharmacokinetics Temozolomide is nearly 100 % bioavailable when given on a completely empty stomach. Its absorption is affected by food. Peak plasma concentration is reached 1 h after intake. Bioequivalence exists between identical doses of the oral route and infusion over 90 min (infusion over a shorter or longer period of time may result in suboptimal dosing). The agent penetrates well into the central nervous system, and is therefore used primarily to treat refractory astrocytomata in adult patients. Temozolomide is metabolized by CYP450 enzymes to monomethyl triazeno imidazole carboxamide not only in the liver, but at all sites. The conversion is spontaneous, but pH dependent. The metabolic conversion yields the short-lived active compound monomethyl triazeno imidazole carboxamide (MTIC), the cytotoxicity of which is exerted primarily via DNA methylation at the O^6 and N^7 positions of guanine (Fig. 2.9). Inactive metabolites of temozolomide are amino imidazole carboxamide and temozolomide acid metabolite. Renal and hepatic excretions play a minor role in drug elimination.

Adverse Effects Women and patients over 70 years of age have about 5 % lower clearance than men under 70, resulting in a higher incidence of grade 4 neutropenia and thrombocytopenia in the first cycle of therapy. Patients may experience myelosuppression, including prolonged pancytopenia, which can result in aplastic anemia. Cases of myelodysplastic syndrome and secondary malignancies, including myeloid leukemia, can occur after temozolomide treatment. Prophylaxis against Pneumocystis carinii pneumonia is required for all newly diagnosed glioblastoma multiforme patients receiving concomitant temozolomide and radio-therapy for the 42 day regimen. Temozolomide is Pregnancy Category D. Although there is fetal risk, it may be acceptable in view of the benefits from temozolomide use in pregnant women.

Drug Interactions In astrocytoma therapy, temozolomide may be given in conjunction with irinotecan without pharmacokinetic interaction. Temozolomide clearance is not affected by CYP450 inducing drugs, nor does administration of temozolomide competitively inhibit the metabolism of those drugs. Temozolomide dosing may require interruption or discontinuation during concomitant radio-therapy (Table 2.2).

Imidazole mustard (5-[3,3-bis(2-chloroethyl)-1-triazeno] imidazole-4-carboxamide) (NSC 82196) alkylates DNA preferentially at guanine residues resulting in DNA interstrand cross-links, inhibition of DNA reduplication, and suppression of RNA and protein synthesis.

Pharmacokinetics Gastrointestinal absorption after oral administration is poor. The plasma half-life after intravenous administration is about 2 h. The drug has minimal penetration of the blood-brain barrier. The primary route of elimination is

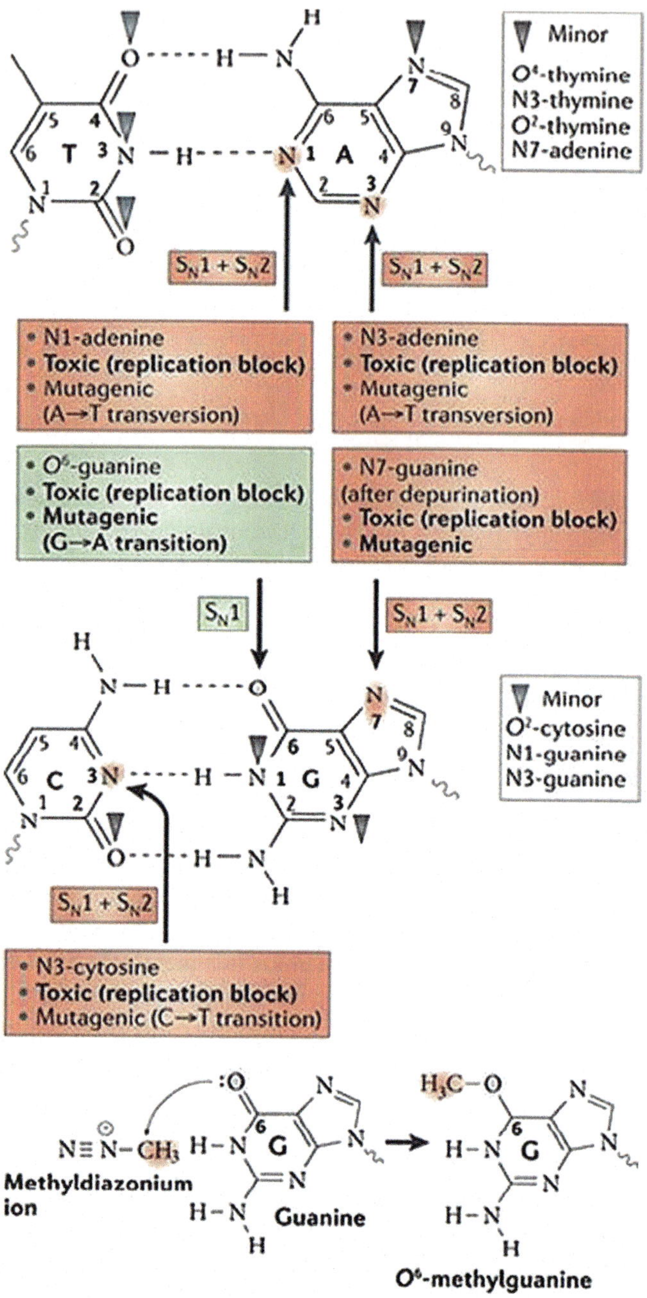

Fig. 2.9 Alkylation sites in DNA. **a** Alkylating agents react with the nitrogen and oxygen atoms of DNA bases to form covalent alkyl lesions. The major sites of alkylation on the DNA bases and biological effects of alkylation are shown in *red* and *green*, with minor lesions denoted by *grey arrow heads*. **b** An example of a DNA alkylation reaction between the methyldiazonium ion of the chemotherapeutic alkylating agent temozolomide with the O^6-position of guanine to form the O^6-methylguanine DNA lesion. (Fu et al. 2012)

renal, with greater than 60 % excreted in the urine within 6 h after i.v. administration. Approximately 2/3 of the excreted drug is metabolized to ionic transformation products.

Dacarbazine (5-(3,3-dimethyl-1-triazenyl)imidazole-4-carboxamide) (NSC 45388) <DTIC, DTIC-Dome, Imidazole Carboxamide> is a triazene derivative that alkylates and cross-links DNA during all phases of the cell cycle, resulting in a disruption of DNA function, cell cycle arrest, and apoptosis. Dacarbazine gained U.S. FDA approval in 1975. It is the first-line chemotherapy for metastatic malignant melanoma without cerebral metastasis and has a 15 % response rate. The drug is used in the ABVD (adriamycin, bleomycin, vinblastine, dacarbazine) regimen for Hodgkin lymphoma. It is administered by injection or intravenous infusion under immediate medical supervision.

- For malignant melanoma, the recommended dosage is 2–4.5 mg/kg/day for 10 days, which may be repeated at 4 week intervals.
- An alternative regimen uses 250 mg/m^2 for 5 days, which may be repeated every 3 weeks.
- For Hodgkin disease, the recommended dose is 150–375 mg/m^2 per day for 5 days, in combination with other effective drugs. Treatment may be repeated every 4 weeks.

Pharmacokinetics At therapeutic concentrations, dacarbazine is not appreciably bound to plasma proteins. Following injection, its clearance from the blood is biphasic with an initial half-life of 20 min and a terminal half-life of 5 h. In patients with renal and hepatic dysfunctions, these half-lives are prolonged. Dacarbazine is metabolized by CYP450 enzymes to monomethyl triazeno imidazole carboxamide (MTIC) only in the liver. The *N*-demethylation involved in MTIC formation is catalyzed by CYP1A1, CYP1A2, and CYP2E1 and is required for anti-tumor activity. The hydroxymethyl and the monomethyl intermediates derived from MTIC are unstable. The monomethyl species, or the methyl carbonium ion formed from it, is capable of methylating DNA and alkylating the O^6 position of guanine. The agent poorly penetrates the central nervous system. About 40 % of the unchanged drug is excreted into the urine.

Adverse Effects Symptoms of anorexia, nausea, and vomiting affect over 90 % of patients with the initial few doses. The vomiting lasts 1–12 h and is incompletely and unpredictably palliated with phenobarbital or prochlorperazine. Hematopoietic depression is one of the most common toxicities and involves primarily the leukocytes and platelets. Leukopenia and thrombocytopenia may be severe enough to cause death. Anemia can sometimes occur. Other serious adverse effects are sterility, which is possibly permanent, and anaphylactic reactions. Liver problems, headaches, fatigue, and diarrhea may arise. Dacarbazine is Pregnancy Category C (it is unknown whether the drug can harm a fetus). It is not known whether dacarbazine passes into breast milk.

Drug Resistance The principal mechanism of resistance arises via the DNA repair protein O^6-Alkylguanine DNA Alkyl Transferase (ATase). In an auto-inactivating reaction,

Table 2.2 Temozolomide dosing interruption or discontinuation during concomitant radiotherapy. (adapted from [http://www.temodar.com/temodar/application?origin=index.jsp...refresh&pageid=hp&__event=goto_support_pharmacyinformation])

Toxicity	TMZ interruption[a]	TMZ discontinuation
Absolute neutrophil count	$\geq$0.5 and <1.5 × 10^9/L	< 0.5 × 10^9/L
Platelet count	$\geq$10 and <100 × 10^9/L	<10 × 10^9/L
CTC non-hematologic toxicity (except for alopecia, nausea, vomiting)	CTC grade 2	CTC grade 3 or 4

TMZ temozolomide, *CTC* Common Toxicity Criteria

[a] Treatment with concomitant temozolomide may be continued when all of the following conditions are met: absolute neutrophil count $\geq$ 1.5 x 10^9 /L; platelet count $\geq$ 100 x 10^9 /L; common toxicity criteria = non-hematologic toxicity grade 1 (except for alopecia, nausea, vomiting)

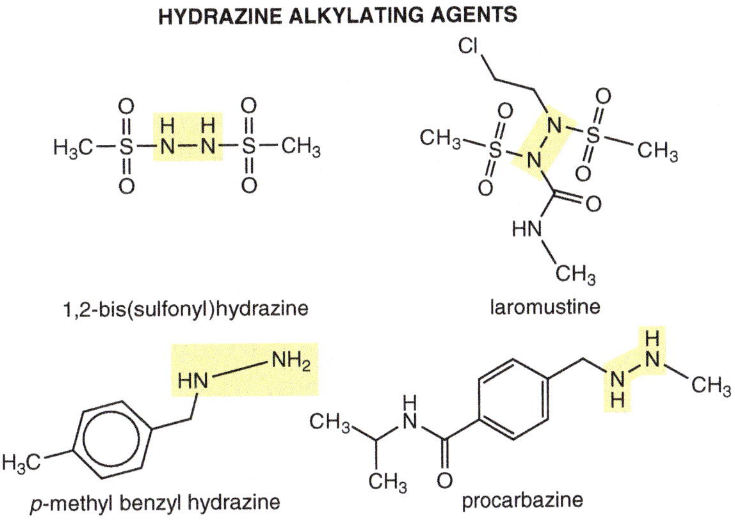

Fig. 2.10 Structures of hydrazine anti-cancer drugs. The basic structures of representatives in the sub-class are shown on the *left* (*top*: 1,2-bis(sulfonyl) hydrazine, *bottom*: methyl benzyl hydrazine), the major drug representatives of the sub-class are on the *right*. The common functional hydrazine moiety is highlighted in *yellow*

this enzyme mediates the stoichiometric transfer of the methyl group from the O^6 position of guanine in alkylated DNA to a cysteine residue in the protein itself.

1-*p*-carboxy-3,3-dimethylphenyltriazine (CB10–277) is a synthetic triazine derivative. It is soluble and stable in aqueous solutions at physiological pH. As a prodrug, 1-*p*-carboxy-3,3-dimethylphenyltriazine is metabolically converted to a monomethyl triazene form that alkylates DNA, resulting in the inhibition of DNA reduplication and repair. This agent may also act as a purine analog, thus causing the inhibition of DNA synthesis, and may interact with protein sulfhydryl groups.

Adverse Effects The dose limiting toxicity is nausea and vomiting which occurs in 80% of patients. A flushing or warm sensation occurs in over 75% of courses.

Hydrazines Hydrazine is an inorganic chemical compound with the formula N_2H_4 (Fig. 2.10).

- The 1,2-bis(sulfonyl)hydrazines are a class of alkylating agents that produce a chloroethylating species. Unlike other chloroethylating agents[17] they do not lead to vinylation or hydroxyethylation, which can produce toxicity in untransformed cells and damage healthy organs. The therapeutic index of bis(sulfonyl)hydrazine compounds may therefore be more favorable.
- Methyl benzyl hydrazine derivatives can suppress mitosis by prolonging interphase. These compounds act through slow auto-oxidation with the formation of hydrogen peroxide. The methyl group is important for biological activity.

The bifunctional sulfonyl hydrazine prodrug laromustine (1,2-bis(methylsulfonyl)-1-(2-choloroethyl)-2-(methylamino)carbonylhydrazine, 101M) (VNP40101M) <Cloretazine, Onrigin> releases the chloroethylating agent 1,2-bis(methylsulfonyl)-1-(2-chloroethyl)hydrazine (90CE), which alkylates the O^6 position of guanine, resulting in DNA cross-linking, strand breaks, chromosomal aberrations, and disruption of DNA synthesis. The parent compound also releases a thiophilic carbamoylating methyl isocyanate, which inhibits the DNA repair enzyme O^6-Alkyl-Guanine Transferase. The agent is under investigation for the treatment of relapsed or refractory acute myelogenous leukemia. Laromustine may be a suitable second-line treatment for cancers that have acquired resistance to melphalan, cytoxan, or BCNU. It is administered as an intravenous infusion at a dose of 600 mg/m^2.

[17] Chloroethylating agents include nitrogen mustards, phosphoramide mustards, nitrosoureas, many triazenes, and some antibiotics (MEN 10710).

Pharmacokinetics The cellular metabolism of laromustine releases the two short lived active species, 1,2-bis(methylsulfonyl)-1-(2-chloroethyl)hydrazine and methyl isocyanate.

The anti-cancer effects of the methyl benzyl hydrazine procarbazine were discovered by DeVita, Serpick, and Carbone (DeVita et al. 1966). Procarbazine hydrochloride (MBH, 1-methyl-2-(*p*-isopropylcarbamoyl) benzylhydrazine hydrochloride, ibenzmethyzin) (NSC 77213) <Matulane, Natulan, Indicarb> has shown most promise in patients with Hodgkin lymphoma, chronic granulocytic leukemia, glioblastoma, and polycythemia. The metabolism of procarbazine can result in the formation of formaldehyde, which acts as an alkylating agent. The common dosage is 2–4 mg/kg/day either in a single dose or divided, given for 7 days, then increased to 4–6 mg/kg/day until response is obtained or myelosuppression occurs. Procarbazine gained U.S. FDA approval in 1969.

Pharmacokinetics The drug is metabolized and activated in the liver.

Drug Interactions Procarbazine inhibits MAO thus increasing the effects of sympathomimetics, tricyclic anti-depressants, and tyramine (hypertensive crisis can be caused by the ingestion of tyramine-rich food). It also inhibits the hepatic CYP450 microsomal system, leading to an increased effect of barbiturates, phenothiazenes, and narcotics, which are normally inactivated by the CYP450 system. When combined with ethanol, procarbazine can cause adverse drug reactions in some patients. The dose may need to be adjusted for renal or hepatic disease.

Triazenes are prodrugs of their active monomethyl forms. Their activation occurs with the release of the single-bonded nitrogen, leaving the highly reactive double-bonded diazonium fragment exposed.
Oral availability and penetration of the blood-brain barrier vary among triazenes.
The bis(sulfonyl)hydrazines are alkylating agents that produce chloroethylating species.
Methyl benzyl hydrazine derivatives can suppress mitosis by prolonging interphase.

2.1.4 Ethylene Imines and Methylmelamines

ThioTEPA (*N, N′,N′*-triethylenethiophosphoramide) <Thioplex> was first developed by American Cyanamid in the early 1950s. As a synthetic agent related to nitrogen mustard, thioTEPA (Fig. 2.11) alkylates and cross-links DNA. It is mostly administered

- in the palliation of breast adenocarcinoma and ovarian adenocarcinoma,
- for controlling intracavitary effusions secondary to diffuse or localized neoplastic diseases of serosal cavities,
- for the treatment of superficial papillary carcinoma of the urinary bladder.
- ThioTEPA has been effective against lymphomata, such as lymphosarcoma and Hodgkin disease (it is now largely superseded by other treatments).
- ThioTEPA may be used as conditioning treatment for bone marrow transplantation.

ThioTEPA is typically given by rapid intravenous administration in doses of 0.3–0.4 mg/kg. These doses must be carefully individualized to minimize toxicity. After maximum benefit is obtained by initial therapy, it is necessary to continue the patient on maintenance therapy in 1–4 week intervals. ThioTEPA can be used for direct intra-tumor injection of accessible tumors to maximize the concentration within

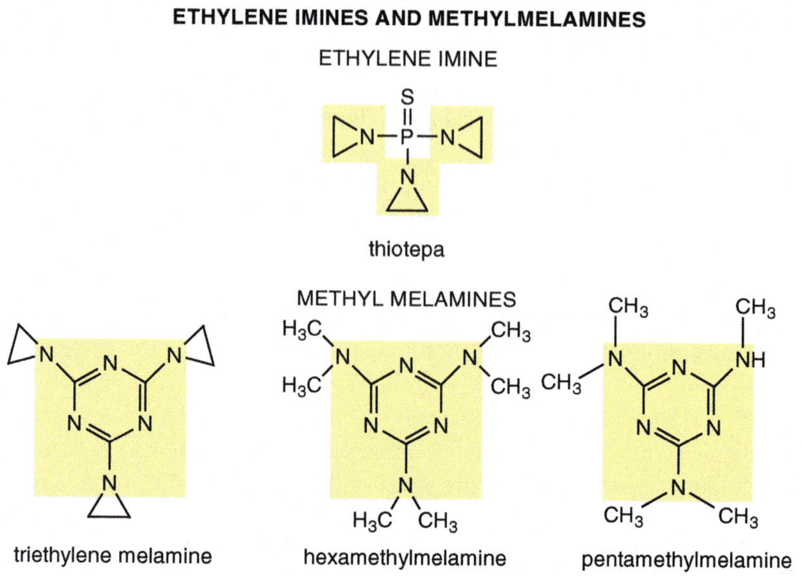

Fig. 2.11 Structures of ethylene imine and methylmelamine anti-cancer drugs. The functional moieties are highlighted in *yellow*

the tumor cells. This allows the application of about twice the dose compared to intravenous injection before comparable extents of bone marrow depression occur. For patients in good condition, 60 mg can be administered into the tumor. The maintenance weekly drug doses are adjusted to the leukocyte counts.

Pharmacokinetics Because absorption from the gastrointestinal tract is variable, thioTEPA should not be administered orally. After intravenous injection, the blood concentrations decline biexponentially with half-lives of 8 and 125 min. thioTEPA is activated by CYP3A4 and CYP2D6. TEPA, which possesses cytotoxic activity, is the major metabolite in the blood and urine.

Adverse Effects ThioTEPA is highly toxic to the hematopoietic system. The main adverse effect is myelosuppression, which can be fatal after intravesical administration. Dysuria and urinary retention are possible adverse effects. In rare cases, chemical cystitis or hemorrhagic cystitis may develop following intravesical, but not parenteral administration. Weight loss, fatigue, pain at the injection site, and tightness of the throat may occur. The drug is excreted onto the skin surface in the sweat, accumulates in covered areas (e.g. beneath adhesive bandages), and exerts a local toxic effect resulting in hyper-pigmentation. ThioTEPA causes amenorrhea and interferes with spermatogenesis. It is Pregnancy Category D.

Drug Interactions Following the combined use of thioTEPA with other anti-cancer agents, prolonged apnea can occur when succinylcholine is administered prior to surgery. This may be due to a decrease in Pseudocholinesterase activity induced by the anti-cancer treatment. It is generally not advisable to combine (simultaneously or sequentially) cancer chemotherapeutic modalities that have the same mechanism of action. Therefore, thioTEPA combined with other alkylating agents, such as nitrogen mustard or cyclophosphamide, or thioTEPA combined with irradiation would serve to intensify toxicity rather than to enhance therapeutic response.

Drug Resistance The aziridine moieties in thioTEPA are substrates for Glutathione S-Transferase (GST). The Glutathione conjugation may be a factor in the development of drug resistance.

The cytotoxic action of triethylenemelamine (TEM, tris-ethylene-imino-S-triazine) derives from the ethylene imine groups. The drug interacts primarily with phosphorylated DNA precursors, particularly with pyrimidines. Triethylenemelamine can be given orally and it rapidly distributes out of the blood stream. Because the reactivity of triethylenemelamine increases at low pH, its reliable resorption can be facilitated by formulation with a basic agent. However, its use has been restricted almost entirely to

- intraarterial infusion for the potentiation of radiation therapy of retinoblastoma
- treating diabetics with skin involvement by lymphosarcoma.

Due to the greater stability and shelf life of thioTEPA, triethylenemelamine has been largely replaced in clinical use.

Hexamethylmelamine (altretamine, HMM, N2,N2,N4,N4, N6,N6-hexamethyl-1,3,5-triazine-2,4,6-triamine) (ENT-50852, RB-1515, WR-95704) <Hexalen, Hexastat, Hexinawas> is a prodrug alkylating agent that may damage tumor cells through the production of the weakly alkylating species formaldehyde, which is a product of Cytochrome P450 mediated *N*-demethylation. The carbinolamine (methylol) intermediates of CYP450 metabolism also can generate electrophilic iminium species that are capable of reacting covalently with protein as well as guanine and cytosine residues in DNA. Hexamethylmelamine is not a first-line treatment but can be useful as salvage therapy. It is indicated for use as a single agent in the palliation of persistent or recurrent ovarian cancer following first-line therapy with a combination based on cisplatin or alkylating agents. It also has the advantage of being less toxic than other drugs used for treating refractory ovarian cancer. Hexamethylmelamine is active against various solid tumors including lung cancer and breast cancer. The drug was approved by the U.S. FDA in 1990. It is given orally as its sparing water solubility makes it unsuitable for parenteral administration. Capsules may be taken either for 14 or 21 consecutive days in a 28 day cycle at a dose of 260 $mg/m^2/day$. The total daily amount should be divided into four doses after meals and at bedtime.

Pharmacokinetics Administered orally, hexamethylmelamine is extensively metabolized on first pass, producing primarily mono- and di-demethylated metabolites. Additional demethylation reactions occur in the tumor cells, releasing formaldehyde. Excretion is mostly in the urine.

Adverse Effects Adverse effects include nausea, vomiting, diarrhea, renal toxicity, severe orthostatic hypotension, and neurotoxicity. The neurotoxicity can be reduced by intake of pyridoxine (vitamin B6), however, it adversely affects the response duration. Because of bone marrow suppression, peripheral blood counts should be monitored at least monthly, prior to the initiation of each course (temporary discontinuation of the drug is required if the white blood cell counts drop below $2000/mm^3$, granulocyte counts drop below $1000/mm^3$, or platelet counts drop below $5000/mm^3$). The drug is Pregnancy Category D.

Drug Interactions Concurrent administration of hexamethylmelamine and antidepressants of the MAO inhibitor class can cause severe orthostatic hypotension. Cimetidine is an inhibitor of microsomal drug metabolism that may increase the half-life and toxicity of hexamethylmelamine.

Water soluble analogs of hexamethylmelamine have been produced because of gastrointestinal adverse effects associated with the oral administration of the water insoluble preparation. Derivatives with greater intrinsic water solubility include pentamethylmelamine, N-methylether derivative, and N2,N4,N6-trimethylol-N2,N4,N6-trimethylmelamine.

Pentamethylmelamine is a principal metabolite of hexamethylmelamine. It alkylates DNA and other macro-molecules to form DNA intra-strand and DNA-protein cross-links, thereby preventing DNA reduplication.

Pharmacokinetics After administration, pentamethylmelamine is extensively demethylated by hepatic mixed-function oxidases. This leads to the formation of an intermediate hydroxymethyl product, which is cytotoxic, and can spontaneously degrade to result in the demethylated melamine and formaldehyde.

In patients with normal liver function, pentamethylmelamine is rapidly cleared from the plasma with a terminal half-life of 2.2 h. Compromised liver function correlates with an increased half-life and reduced total clearance.

Ethylene imines and methylmelamines are prodrugs that require metabolic activation.
Methylmelamines release the weakly alkylating formaldehyde upon demethylation.
Methylated melamines are extensively demethylated by hepatic mixed-function oxidases. Their anti-tumor activity decreases with a decreasing number of methyl groups.

2.1.5 Benzoquinone Containing Alkylating Agents

Quinones have traditionally represented a major source of anti-cancer compounds[18]. These agents are unique among cancer therapeutics insofar as they require enzyme catalyzed bioreduction of the quinine moiety before conversion to intermediates that can

- generate toxic free radical species
- bind to DNA and form covalent adducts.

3-membered ring compounds like aziridine are highly strained molecules because of the small bond angles[19]. This type of strain in an organic molecule is termed angle strain (Baeyer strain). Since the reaction of a nucleophile with an aziridine usually leads to an acyclic product, the ring strain is released, which highly favors the reaction. Chemical reduction facilitates the protonation of the aziridine (ethylene imine) ring[20], leading to the formation of the aziridinium ion, which is the required species for alkylation. Many one- and two-electron Reductases are capable of activating bioreductive drugs, including NADH:Cytochrome b_5 Reductase, Cytochrome P450 Reductase, and NAD(P)H:Quinone Oxidoreductase (NQO1). NQO1 is of specific importance in enzyme directed drug activation, because its activity and gene expression levels are elevated in various intrinsically drug resistant solid malignancies, including lung, colon, and liver cancer. Nevertheless, significant NQO1 expression is also present in untransformed tissues including the respiratory tract epithelium, kidney podocytes, and reproductive system, which may give rise to a potential mechanism of drug toxicity.

Triaziquone (2,3,5-tris-ethyleneimino-l,4-benzoquinone, 2,3,5-tris(1-aziridinyl)-2,5-cyclohexadiene-1,4-dione, tris-ethyleneiminoquinone) <Trenimon> (Fig. 2.12) was one of the first aziridinylbenzoquinone anti-cancer drugs synthesized at the Bayer scientific laboratories in Leverkusen, Germany (Gauss 1958). Triaziquone contains three ethylene imine rings linked to a quinone nucleus. This drug is a substrate for both one-electron and two-electron reducing agents and its cytotoxic activity may result from protein alkylation and oxidative stress. It is a polyfunctional compound, which combines the properties of a quinone, an α,β-unsaturated ketone, an enamine, and an aziridine (ethylene imine). Triaziquone exerts its anti-cancer effects through macromolecule alkylation of functional groups like –SH, –OH, and $-NH_2$. Since triaziquone has three aziridine groups with slightly different reactivity, it can react successively three times as an akylating reagent. By this mechanism, different parts of the DNA (even from different strands) can be connected. Cross-links may also be formed between DNA and other molecules, such as proteins (Rademacher 1995). Both the rate of reaction and the number of aziridine groups per molecule of trenimon that react are dependent on the acidity of the micro-environment. Therefore, the reactivity is increased in the acidic milieu of tumors. Triaziquone is especially efficacious for the treatment of polycythemias and carcinomatous effusions. The therapeutic dose is about 1 mg/kg body mass.

---

[18] Quinone is contained in the anti-cancer drug classes benzoquinones, anthracyclins, dynemicins, and anthracenediones. The photosensitizer perylenequinone also contains this functional group. The aminoquinone moiety is contained in the classical aminoquinones (mitomycin C, porfiromycin, KW-2149, streptonigrin), ansamycins (geldanamycin and derivatives, rafamycins, and maytansinoid agents), and actinomycin D.

[19] Alkylating anti-cancer drugs with 3-membered rings include ethylene imines, some methylmelamines (triethylenemelamine), benzoquinones, illudins and acylfulvenes, dianhydrogalactitol, and teroxirone.

[20] Aziridines (ethylene imines) include benzoquinones and thio-TEPA. Phosphoramide mustards and mitomycins may be metabolized to highly reactive aziridine derivatives. The Caspase activator imexon (see Sect. 3.3.4.) is a cyanoaziridine.

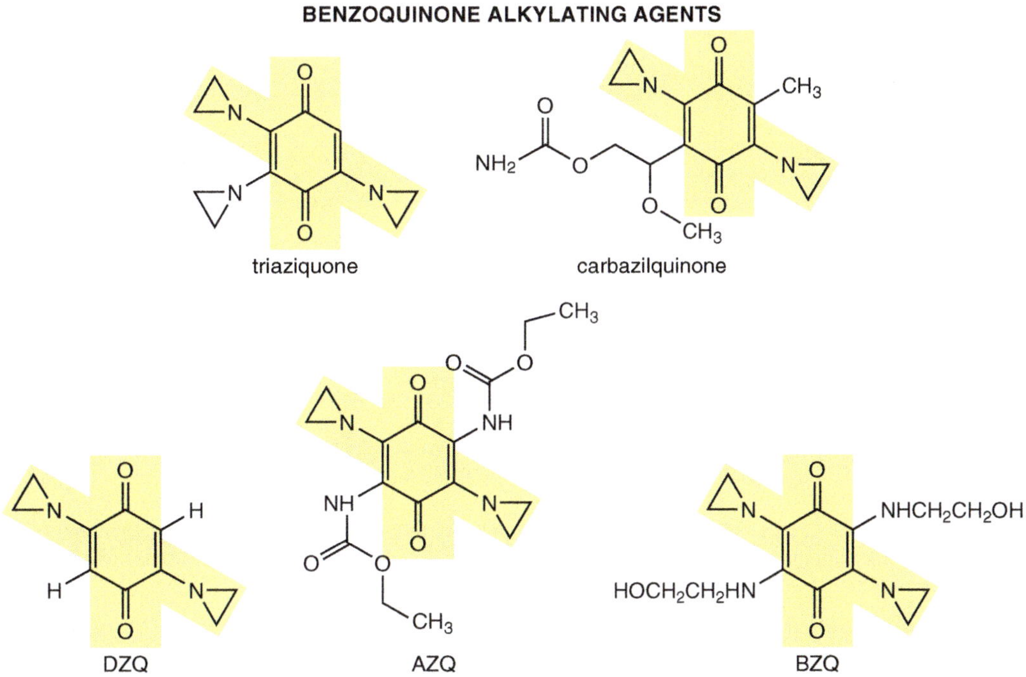

Fig. 2.12 Structures of benzoquinone alkylating anti-cancer drugs. The common aziridinyl benzoquinone moieties, shared by all compounds in this class, are highlighted in *yellow*

The agent was in more widespread use in Europe than in the United States. Because of its toxicity it has been replaced by other agents.

Pharmacokinetics Upon intravenous injection, triazoquinone is rapidly bound to blood proteins. The agent crosses the blood-brain-barrier. Detoxification of the drug involves its reduction by DT-Diaphorase (NAD(P)H:(Quinone Acceptor) Oxidoreductase).

Adverse Effects Triaziquone produces myelosclerotic reactions with low frequency.

P53 is a critical tumor suppressor protein that may arrest cell cycle progression or induce apoptosis. The cell cycle arresting function is exerted in part through $P21^{CIP1/WAF1}$. The P53→P21 signaling pathway may play a central role in mediating the gene regulatory and cytotoxic effects of aziridinylbenzoquinones (Wu et al. 1998). 3,6-diaziridinyl-1,4-benzoquinone (DZQ) causes the increased expression of $P21^{CIP1/WAF1}$, an inhibitor of Cyclin-Dependent Kinases. This induction is regulated at the transcriptional level and requires the activation of P53. In cancer cells that lack functional P53, DZQ mediated *p21* induction is greatly diminished. The drug is less effective.

Carbazilquinone ([2,5-bis(1-aziridine)-3-(1-methoxy-2-amino-formyl) ethyl]-6-methyl-1,4-benzoquinone) was first synthesized in 1970 as a mitomycin C analog having a quinone group and aziridine and carbamate alkylating groups (Arakawa et al. 1970). Carbazilquinone has been extensively studied in the clinic, primarily in Japan. It has activity as a single agent in gastric, ovarian and hematologic cancers.

Adverse Effects Leukopenia, thrombocytopenia, and anorexia are the major toxic effects of the drug.

Diaziquone (AZQ, 2,5-bis-(carboethoxyamino)-3,6-diaziridinyl-1,4-benzoquinone) (NSC 182986) is a synthetic bifunctional quinone derivative that alkylates and cross-links DNA during all phases of the cell cycle, resulting in a disruption of DNA function, cell cycle arrest, and apoptosis. This agent can also form free radicals, thereby initiating DNA damage via strand breaks. Due to its lipophilicity, diaziquone readily crosses the blood-brain barrier. It was first tested as a potential central nervous system anti-tumor agent in the early 1960s and displayed substantial activity in both intracerebral and intraperitoneal leukemias, as well as activity in solid tumors.

Adverse Effects Diaziquone is myelosuppressive with little non-hematopoietic toxicity. Its maximal tolerated dose is 30 mg/m^2 daily for 5 days.

2,5-bis-(2-hydroxyethylamino)-3,6-diaziridinyl-1,4-benzoquinone (BZQ) was first synthesized in 1976 (Chou 1976). The drug is not a substrate for DT-Diaphorase and does not produce DNA strand breaks. However, it produces DNA cross-links without reduction. The cytotoxicity of this agent may be due to its alkylating activity.

Quinones require enzymatic bioreduction of the quinine moiety to intermediates that generate free radicals and form covalent DNA adducts.

2.1.6 Alkyl Sulfonates

The sulfonic acid ester busulfan (1,4-butanediol dimethanesulfonate) <Busulfex, Myleran> is a dialkylating agent (Fig. 2.13), from which the methane sulfonate can be eliminated as a leaving group, resulting in a butylene cross-link

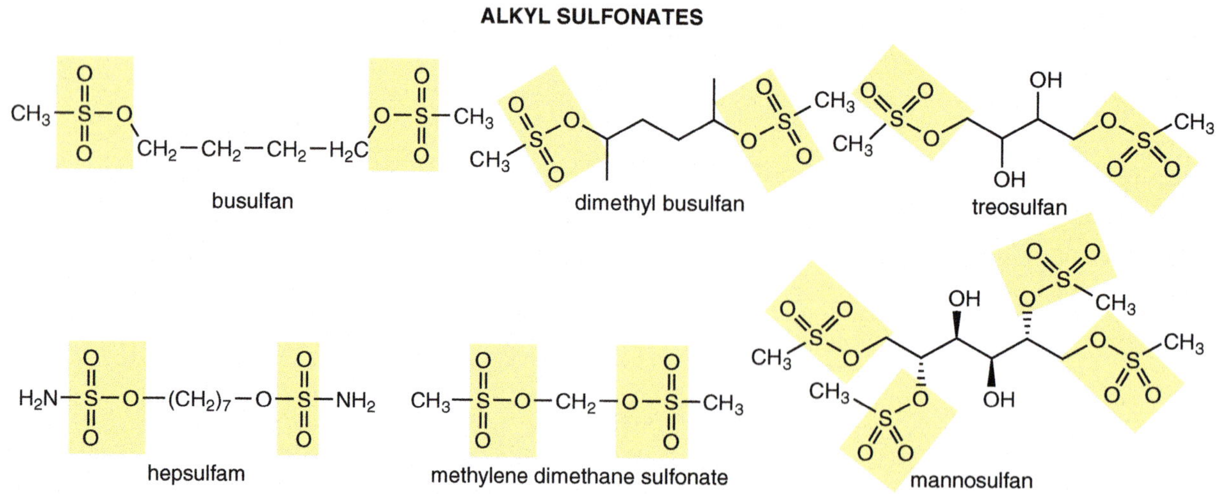

Fig. 2.13 Structures of alkyl sulfonates. The common pairs of sulfonate moieties are highlighted in *yellow*. In busufan, dimethyl busulfan, and treosulfan they are connected by a 4-member chain. The chain length varies in hepsulfam and methylene dimethane sulfonate. Mannosulfan has 4 sulfonate moieties

between biomolecule target groups. Busulfan attacks almost exclusively protein-sulfhydryl groups in the nucleus. In contrast to mustard drugs, it has little effect on DNA or RNA synthesis.

- Busulfan is relatively unique among conventional chemotherapy compounds in its ability to deplete non-cycling primitive stem cells in the host and consequently to allow for high levels of long-term, donor-type engraftment after bone marrow transplantation. It is therefore indicated in combination with cyclophosphamide as a conditioning regimen prior to allogeneic hematopoietic progenitor cell transplantation for chronic myelogenous leukemia (BuCy2 conditioning regimen).
- Chronic myelogenous leukemia (CML) frequently progresses through two phases. The chronic phase can be controlled for a number of years by busulfan. However, ultimately the majority of patients undergo blastic transformation (acute phase) and no longer respond to the antitumor effects of this drug.

Although busulfan is poorly soluble in water it is readily resorbed from the gastrointestinal tract and is therefore usually administered as an oral tablet. Initial doses of 4–12 mg are used and adjusted according to the response. Maintenance chemotherapy at 1–3 mg/day may be of benefit. Busulfan can also be administered as intravenous injection. The usual adult dose is 0.8 mg/kg of ideal body weight or actual body weight (whichever is lower) administered every 6 h for 4 days (at a total of 16 doses).

Pharmacokinetics Consistent with the reactive electrophilic properties of busulfan, the irreversible binding to plasma proteins (primarily Albumin) is around 30 %. The drug achieves concentrations in the cerebrospinal fluid approximately equal to those in the blood. It is predominantly metabolized by conjugation with Glutathione, both spontaneously and by Glutathione S-Transferase catalysis. The resulting conjugate undergoes further extensive oxidative metabolism in the liver. Approximately 30 % of the administered dose is excreted into the urine over 48 h, while negligible amounts are excreted in the feces.

Adverse Effects The most common adverse effect of busulfan is bone marrow depression, which requires frequent monitoring. Among the alkylating agents, busulfan is unique in affecting mainly the granulocytes (this has led to its clinical use for the treatment of chronic granulocytic leukemia. In chronic granulocytic leukemia, busulfan can induce remission in 90 % of patients after the initial course of therapy. It is not effective, however, in the blast crisis of chronic granulocytic leukemia or in acute leukemias). The rapid destruction of granulocytes can yield a dangerous rise in serum uric acid and consecutive kidney damage from urate stones. Preventive treatment with allopurine <Zyloprim> is available.

Neurological symptoms may comprise hallucinations (onset at 1 day post completion of administration, associated with EEG changes), somnolence, lethargy, and confusion. As with other alkylating agents, nausea and vomiting, diarrhea, impotence or sterility, and teratogenic effects can occur. Unusual complications from busulfan include skin pigmentation (especially in the creases of the hands), pulmonary fibrosis, gynecomastia, anhidrosis, cheilosis, and glossitis. Mild or moderate tachycardia or dyspnea are possible. Because busulfan is poorly water soluble the solvent used in the Busulfex preparation is dimethylacetamide (DMA), which has a maximum tolerated dose of 14.8 $g/m^2/d$ for 4 days. 16 doses of intravenous busulfan contain about 40 % of the maximum tolerated dose of dimethylacetamide. The drug is Pregnancy Category D.

Busulfan may be used in preconditioning prior to bone marrow transplantation. Hepatic veno-occlusive disease is a potential complication of this conditioning therapy. It may arise in 8% of patients treated with busulfan in the setting of allogeneic transplantation. Graft-versus-host disease can develop.

Busulfan is contraindicated in patients in whom a definitive diagnosis of chronic myelogenous leukemia has not been firmly established, and in patients who have previously suffered a hypersensitivity reaction to busulfan or any component of its preparation.

Drug Interactions Busulfan may cause additive myelosuppression when used with other myelosuppressive drugs. The anti-fungal itraconazole <Sporanox, Onmel> decreases busulfan clearance by up to 25%. The anti-convulsant phenytoin <Dilantin, Phenytek> increases the clearance of busulfan by 15% or more, possibly due to the induction of Glutathione-S-Transferase. A fraction of patients receiving continuous busulfan and thioguanine therapy for chronic myelogenous leukemia develop portal hypertension and esophageal varices associated with abnormal liver function. This condition is due to nodular regenerative hyperplasia.

Dimethylbusulfan (2,5-hexanediol dimethanesulfonate, 1,4-Bis(methylsulfonyloxy)-1,4-dimethylbutane) is an aliphatic analog of busulfan. It has been under investigation as a second-line treatment for various cancers.

Adverse Effects As an alkylating agent, dimethylbusulfan induces neutropenia.

Treosulfan (2,3-dihydroxybutane-1,4-diyl dimethanesulfonate) (NSC 39069) is the prodrug of a bifunctional sulfonate alkylating agent, which converts non-enzymatically via a monoepoxide intermediate to L-diepoxybutane. Both the monoepoxide intermediate and L-diepoxybutane can alkylate DNA at guanine residues. L-diepoxybutane can also produce DNA inter-strand cross-links. These DNA modifications lead to DNA fragmentation and cell death. Treosulfan also has myeloablative and immunosuppressive effects. Therefore, this agent may have applications in allogeneic stem cell transplantation conditioning regimens.

Hepsulfam (1,7-heptanediol disulfamate, sulfamic acid 1,7-heptanediyl ester) (NSC 329680) is a bisulfamic ester, which is similar in structure to busulfan but is more hydrophilic. Hepsulfam forms covalent linkages with nucleophilic centers in DNA, resulting in depurination, base miscoding, strand scission, DNA-DNA and DNA-protein crosslinking, and cytotoxicity. It has efficacy for the treatment of leukemias.

Pharmacokinetics Hepsulfam enters the cerebrospinal fluid following intravenous administration. The cerebrospinal fluid/plasma ratios are lower than those obtained following oral busulfan administration.

Adverse Effects Encephalopathy is the dose limiting toxicity of intravenous hepsulfam in patients with refractory leukemias. In patients with refractory solid tumors, the dose limiting toxicity is cumulative myelosuppression, resulting in prolonged leukopenia and thrombocytopenia. The symptoms are reversible upon discontinuation of therapy (because there is only minor non-hematologic toxicity, substantial dose escalation may be possible with hematopoietic stem cell support). Uncomfortable paresthesias can be avoided by slowing the infusion and administering it over 2 h.

Methylene dimethane sulfonate is a member of the homologous series of dimethane sulfonic acid esters with alkylating properties. Its anti-cancer properties are under study.

Mannosulfan ([(2R,3S,4S,5R)-3,4-dihydroxy-2,5,6-tris(methylsulfonyloxy)hexyl] methanesulfonate) <Zitostop> has been used, mostly in Hungary, in the treatment of chronic myeloid leukemia and polycythemia vera.

Alkyl sulfonates attack protein-sulfhydryl groups in the nucleus with little effect on DNA or RNA synthesis.
Busulfan is indicated in conditioning prior to allogeneic hematopoietic progenitor cell transplantation, because it depletes non-cycling stem cells.

2.1.7 Illudins

The illudins (Fig. 2.14) are a family of sesquiterpenes (terpenes that consist of three isoprene units and have the molecular formula $C_{15}H_{24}$), produced as antibiotic toxins by some mushrooms. They exert relatively selective cytotoxicity against some myelocytic leukemia cells and carcinoma cells. To the anti-cancer effects of this class of drugs may contribute

- their alkylating activity (Fig. 2.15),
- inhibition of DNA synthesis from thymidine,
- the depletion of the Glutathione and Thioredoxin systems.

At low pH, illudins act as bifunctional alkylating agents, but at physiological pH they do not react with oxygen or nitrogen nucleophiles. Rather, they react spontaneously with sulfur nucleotides. Acylfulvenes were derived from illudins to reduce the reactivity with thiol containing small molecules, and thus the non-specific toxicity.

Irofulven (6-hydroxymethylacylfulvene, HMAF) (MGI 114) is a semi-synthetic derivative of illudin S, which is synthesized by the mushroom Omphalotus illudens. While irofulven is less cytotoxic than illudin S, it exhibits much greater selectivity in damaging malignant cells compared to healthy cells. Besides alkylating DNA, the drug interferes with transcription-coupled DNA repair. Irofulven may undergo

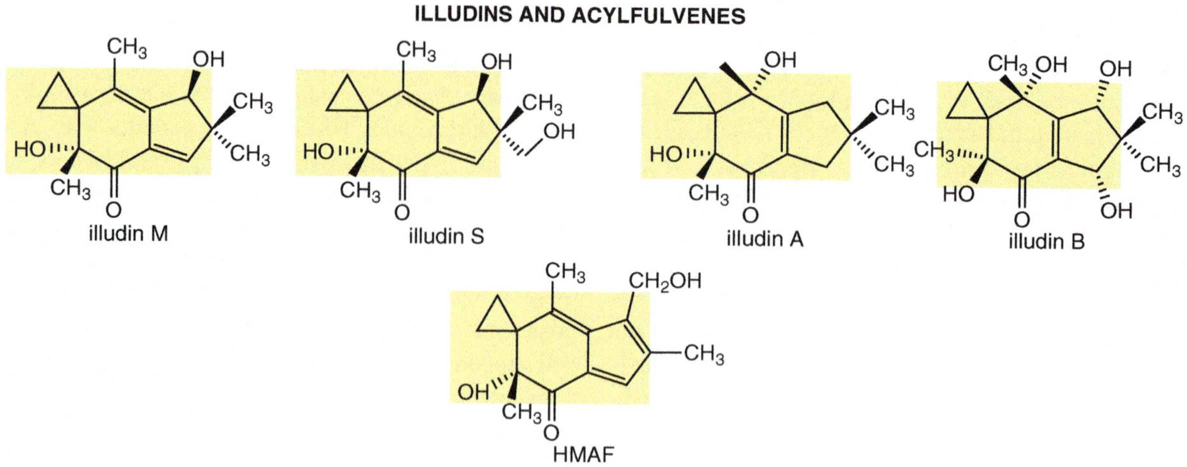

Fig. 2.14 Structures of illudins. The shared structural motif is highlighted in *yellow*. The molecule on the *bottom* represents the investigational drug 6-hydroxymethylacylfulvene (HMAF)

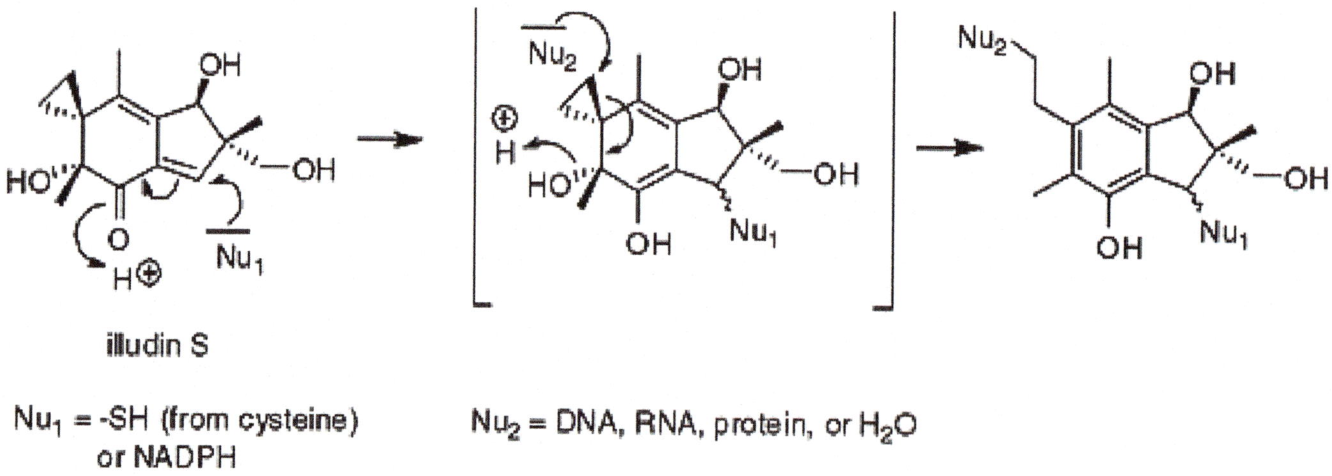

Fig. 2.15 Alkylation by illudins. The reaction scheme depicts the alkylation reaction of illudin S with the cellular nucleophiles Nu1 and Nu2. (Greve 2010)

bioreductive activation. The drug is under investigation as mono-therapy or in combination therapies for the treatment of refractory and relapsed ovarian, prostate, hepatocellular, pancreatic, breast, lung or colon cancers.

Adverse Effects Toxicity in the form of myelosuppression and fatigue are schedule dependent, with reduced toxicity under intermittent administration compared to continuous regimens.

Drug Interactions There is synergy between irofulven and Topoisomerase inhibitors. The repair of the irofulven induced DNA damage is dependent on functioning DNA Helicases (the double helical configuration, in which DNA strands naturally reside, requires their separation by Helicases for transcription or reduplication). Hence the drug efficacy can potentially be enhanced by Helicase inhibitors.

Illudins are sesquiterpenes.
Illudins and acylfulvenes alkylate DNA, inhibit DNA synthesis, and deplete thiol anti-oxidant defenses.

2.1.8 Platinum Drugs

In 1965, cisplatin was discovered by Barnett Rosenberg, who explored the effects of electric fields on the growth of Escherichia coli bacteria (Rosenberg 1965). He observed that the bacteria unexpectedly ceased to divide due to the exposure to an electrolysis product of the platinum electrodes. The discovery soon initiated studies into the effects of platinum compounds on cell division. Various platinum salts were synthesized, and cis-diamminetetrachloroplatinum, but not its trans-isomer, was identified to be the most effective inhibitor of tumor cell proliferation. Subsequently, Eve Wiltshaw and others at the Institute of Cancer Research, United Kingdom extended the clinical usefulness of the platinum compounds with the development of carboplatin, a cisplatin derivative with broad anti-tumor activity and comparatively less nephrotoxicity. Cisplatin proved pivotal in achieving full remission of testicular cancer, and most ovarian cancers initially respond well to platinum anti-cancer drugs.

There are two structural groups of platinum compounds,

- *cis*-[Pt(amine)$_2$X$_2$], including cisplatin <Platinol>, carboplatin <Paraplatin>, and oxaliplatin <Eloxatine>, for the treatment of testicular, ovarian, and colon cancers
- polynuclear Pt^{IV} species, including triplatin (BBR3464), satraplatin, and picoplatin, which are much more inert to ligand substitution reactions than their Pt^{II} counterparts. It is likely that Pt^{IV} complexes are reduced to Pt^{II} by extracellular and intracellular biomolecules prior to their reaction with DNA.

The compositions of platinum anti-tumor drugs mostly adhere to a set of consistent structure-activity relationships (Cleare and Hoeschele 1973). These entail that the Pt^{II} or Pt^{IV} complex should have a cis geometry with the general formulas of cis-[PtX$_2$(Am)$_2$] or cis-[PtX$_2$Y$_2$(Am)$_2$], where X is the leaving group[21] and Am is an inert amine with at least one N–H moiety. The leaving group should be an anion with intermediate binding strength to platinum and have a weak trans-effect to avoid labilizing the amine. Complexes with labile leaving groups such as ClO_4^- or NO_3^- are highly toxic, while complexes with inert leaving groups are generally inactive. Upon administration of platinum drugs, an integral ligand undergoes slow displacement with water molecules in a process termed aquation. The aqua ligand is highly reactive, allowing the platinum compounds to coordinate a base in DNA, forming a subsequent cross-link after loss of the second chlorine ligand. These linkages to DNA occur at the positions where the chloride ion (cisplatin, picoplatin), cyclobutane-1,1-dicarboxylate (carboplatin), or oxalate (oxaliplatin) ligands reside in the original platinum compound. The leaving group of carboplatin confers good aqueous solubility and stability because it forms a 6-membered ring with the platinum atom.

For some tumors (germ cell tumors, head and neck cancers, bladder cancers), cisplatin may be therapeutically more effective than carboplatin, whereas for lung cancer and ovarian cancer the effectiveness is comparable. The choice of the most appropriate analog is a function of the cancer being treated, the treatment goal (palliative or curative), and the other component drugs used in combination. The treatment of Estrogen Receptor-positive (ER$^+$) cells with estradiol sensitizes them to cisplatin. This has led to the design and synthesis of a series of estrogen tethered Pt^{IV} compounds (Barnes 2004).

[21] A leaving group is an atom or a group of atoms that is displaced as a stable species in heterolytic bond cleavage, taking with it the bonding electrons.

First generation platinum compound Cisplatin (cis-diamminedichloroplatinum^{II}, cis-DDP) (CS-310, NSC-134679) <Abiplatin, Biocisplatinum, Briplatin, Carboquone, Esquinon> is the prototypical first generation platinum anti-cancer drug (Fig. 2.16). It is an inorganic compound that forms highly reactive charged platinum complexes, which bind to nucleophilic groups, such as GC rich sites in the DNA. The intrastrand and inter-strand DNA cross-links, as well as DNA-protein cross-links caused in this manner result in the inhibition of cell growth and induction of apoptosis (Fig. 2.17). Although cisplatin often fails to cause G$_1$ arrest, the induction of G$_2$ arrest is essential to the process of engaging cell death following treatment (Sorenson and Eastman 1988). Cisplatin entered clinical trials in 1971 and proved effective against various cancers. It received approval for the treatment of testicular and ovarian cancers in 1978. The use of cisplatin, usually as a principal component of combination regimens, has rendered testicular cancer curable with a success rate in excess of 90 %, and is important in the treatment of bladder and ovarian cancers. Ovarian cancer initially responds well to platinum drugs[22]. Cisplatin is indicated in two regimens,

- in the initial treatment of advanced ovarian carcinoma, cisplatin is used in established combination chemotherapy; one established combination consists of cisplatin and cyclophosphamide.
- in the palliative treatment of patients with ovarian carcinoma recurrent after prior chemotherapy, including patients who have been previously treated with cisplatin.

The drug is also given to treat small cell lung cancers, sarcomata, lymphomata, germ cell tumors, and gestational trophoblastic tumors. Further, it is applied to the palliation of bladder, cervical, nasopharyngeal, esophageal, and head and neck cancers. Typical doses range 20–120 mg/m^2, usually for up to five consecutive days. The compound needs to be administered intravenously.

- Synthetic formulations, in which the anti-neoplastic agent cisplatin is encapsulated in lipids, generate cisplatin liposomal (liposome-encapsulated Carboquone) <CQ-liposome, Lipoplatin>. They consists of small aggregates of cisplatin (generated through the formation of reverse micelles between cisplatin and dipalmitoyl-phosphatidylglycerol under certain conditions) covered by a single lipid bilayer. The encasement in liposomes improves the tumor bioavailability and toxicity profile of cisplatin, while it does not directly affect the pharmacological properties of

[22] Although women with mutations in *brca1* or *brca2* have an increased lifetime risk of contracting ovarian cancer, mutations in *brca2* are associated with an increased response to platinum based drug treatment—and increased survival, because homologous recombination pathway deficiencies compromise DNA repair in response to chemotherapy.

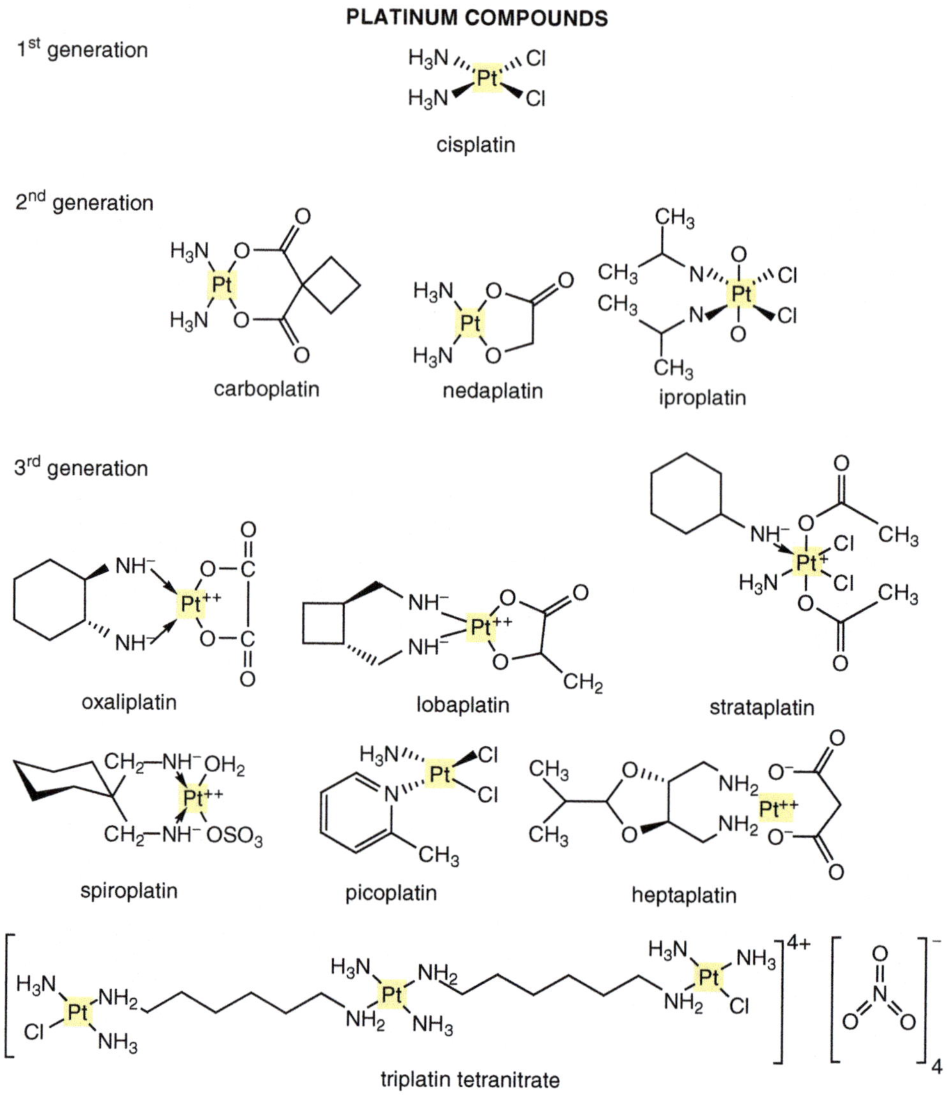

Fig. 2.16 Structures of platinum anti-cancer drugs. The agents are grouped by generations one through three. The essential platinum entity is highlighted in *yellow*

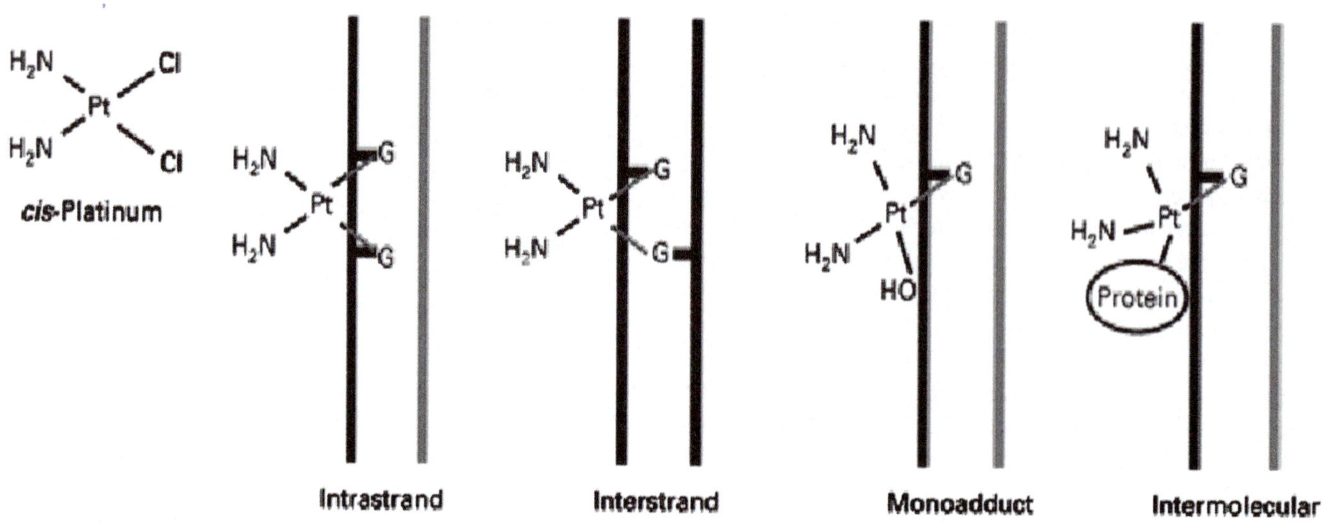

Fig. 2.17 DNA adducts generated by cisplatinum. Cisplatin produces inter-strand, intra-strand and mono-functional adduct cross-linking in DNA. The most prevalent form is the 1,2-intra-strand cross-link, where the platinum drug is covalently bound to the *N*7 position of adjacent purine bases (the inactive isomer of cisplatin, trans-DDP, cannot form this ubiquitous 1,2-intra-strand crosslink). In the 1,2-intra-strand cross-link, the DNA is unwound and bent towards the major grove. Other platinum-DNA adducts, including the mono-functional and the 1,3- and longer range intra-strand, inter-strand and protein-DNA cross-links, each form a distinct structural element that uniquely interferes with DNA function. ((http://bioweb.wku.edu/courses/Biol588/Bishopl.html; Marra and Schär 1999) with permission)

cisplatin. Cationic liposomes (cationic lipoplexes) have favorable interactions with negatively charged DNA and cell membranes. Further the encapsulation alters biodistribution, tumor uptake, and toxic exposure to healthy tissues. The negatively charged dipalmitoyl-phosphatidyl-glycerol (DPPG) on the particle surface conveys fusogenic properties for cell entry.

Pharmacokinetics Cisplatin enters the cells mainly by passive diffusion. Once inside the cell, it undergoes aquation to form $[Pt(NH_3)_2Cl(OH_2)]^+$ and $[Pt(NH_3)_2(OH_2)_2]^{2+}$. The aquated forms are more reactive to their cellular targets. Although many cellular components interact with cisplatin, DNA is the primary biological target of the drug. Most notable among the DNA changes are the 1,2 intra-strand cross-links with purine bases. These include 1,2 intra-strand d(GpG) adducts, which form nearly 90% of the adducts, and the less common 1,2 intra-strand d(ApG) adducts. 1,3 intra-strand d(GpXpG) adducts occur but are readily eliminated by the nucleotide excision repair mechanism (Farrell 2003). Cisplatin modifications distort the structure of the DNA duplex. The intra-strand 1,2 cross-links bend the DNA significantly towards the major groove, exposing a wide, shallow minor groove surface, to which HMG box proteins, repair proteins, transcription factors, and Histone H1 bind. The affinity of the high mobility group protein HMGB1 for cisplatin-damaged DNA is enhanced by P53. This can lead to cell cycle arrest or apoptosis. Further, HMG box proteins, such as HMGB1 (HMG Box Protein 1) and tsHMG (testes specific HMG Box Protein) shield the Pt-1,2-d(GpG) cross-link from nucleotide excision repair proteins.

Adverse Effects The adverse effects of cisplatin are severe. Its gastrointestinal and renal toxicity nearly led to the discontinuation of its use in the 1970s, until it was realized that they can be managed. Gastrointestinal events (nausea, vomiting, and diarrhea) can be softened by anti-emetic drugs (Serotonin Receptor antagonists). Although the kidney damage is cumulative and irreversible, the nephrotoxicity can be substantially managed by proactive hydration combined with the use of diuretics.

Angina pectoris and myocardial infarction have occurred during or shortly after cisplatin treatment, possibly due to direct endothelial damage or vasospasm. The vasospasm could be a consequence of magnesium wasting. Thromboembolic phenomena including arterial occlusion, deep venous thrombosis, pulmonary emboli, transient ischemic attack, stroke, and renal artery occlusion are possible with cisplatin treatment. Microalbuminuria, a marker of generalized endothelial dysfunction, is present in up to 20% of long-term testicular cancer survivors treated with cisplatin. Other indicators of endothelial cell activation (von Willebrandt Factor, Plasminogen Activator Inhibitor 1, carotid artery thickness) may also increase with cisplatin therapy, and could aid in monitoring the vascular risks of patients.

Peripheral neuropathies and hypomagnesemia with resulting tetany may be encountered (Von Hoff 1979). Ototoxicity (tinnitus and hearing loss) can lead to deafness. In rare cases, the administration of cisplatin is associated with anaphylactic reactions, myelosuppression, and occasional transient liver dysfunction. Due to the affinity of Pt^{II} for sulfur binding, sulfur compounds may be used as rescue agents in cisplatin toxicity (Reedijk 1999).

Drug Resistance If ovarian cancer recurs within less than 6 months after the completion of chemotherapy, the tumor is considered to be platinum resistant. Resistance to cisplatin can be caused by several mechanisms (Farrell 2003; Wang and Lippard 2005). It may be due to a combination of

- increased efflux of platinum from the cell. The transporter ATP7B (Copper Transporting P-Type Adenosine Triphosphate) has an important physiological role in regulating copper levels in the cell. It is associated with cisplatin resistance in various cancers. ABCC2 (ATP-Binding Cassette sub-family C 2, MRP2, cMOAT) also has a role in cisplatin resistance, presumably by promoting drug efflux.
- increased cytoplasmic detoxification through cellular thiols such as Glutathione (GSH). Due to the affinity of Pt^{II} for sulfur binding, platinum drugs can bind to Glutathione, Metallothionein, and serum Albumin. Therefore, the cellular thiol levels are associated with drug resistance.
- increased resistance to apoptosis. The kinase PKB (Protein Kinase B, AKT) promotes cell survival and down-regulates apoptosis. An elevated activity of PKB associated pathways protects cells from apoptotic death induced by cisplatin. c-ABL is a member of the SRC family of non-receptor tyrosine kinases, which also carries a DNA binding motif. Nuclear c-ABL activity can be stimulated by cisplatin and acts to transmit DNA damage signals. Because c-ABL tyrosine kinase has a role in cisplatin mediated activation of apoptosis, a reduction in its activity can confer cisplatin resistance. The P53 pathway can partially mediate cisplatin cytotoxicity. Many tumors harbor defective P53 and are deficient in this pathway.
- enhanced repair of platinum-DNA adducts. Cisplatin-DNA adducts are removed primarily by the nucleotide excision repair mechanism. High levels of nucleotide repair proteins in cancer cells can mediate resistance. The favorable clinical response of testicular cancer to cisplatin reflects, in part, its intrinsically low levels of the nucleotide excision repair proteins XPA and ERCC1/XPF. DNA Polymerase η is a lesion bypass polymerase that aids tumor cells to gain resistance against cisplatin based chemotherapy. It allows cells to reduplicate DNA across cross-link lesions such as 1,2-d(GpG) cisplatin adducts (Pt-GG).

Second generation platinum compounds The continuously improving understanding of the chemical properties and pharmacological actions of cisplatin guided the development of analogs that also have cis geometry but differ from cisplatin either in the ammine[23] carrier ligands or in the leaving chlorides. In general, modification of the chloride leaving groups of cisplatin results in compounds with different pharmacokinetic properties, whereas modification of the carrier ligands alters the efficacy or the spectrum of activity of the resulting complex (Coluccia and Natile 2007). The second generation compounds were developed in attempts to reduce toxicity or to expand the range of useful anti-cancer activity.

Carboplatin (cis-diammine(cyclobutane-1,1-dicarboxylate-*O, O'*)platinum^{II}) <Paraplatin, Blastocarb, Carbosin, Carbosol, Displata, Ercar, Nealorin, Novoplatinum, Ribocarbo> replaces the unidentate chloride ligands of cisplatin with a chelating cyclobutanedicarboxylate ligand. It has a lower rate of aquation and increased water solubility. Carboplatin entered the clinic in 1989 (U.S. FDA approval), principally in response to the necessity for reducing the toxic effects of the parent drug cisplatin. Carboplatin is essentially active in the same set of tumors as cisplatin, with no broader spectrum of activity indicated. The main uses include ovarian carcinoma, lung cancers, and head and neck cancers. The agent possesses tumoricidal activity similar to that of its parent compound, but is more stable and less toxic. Carboplatin is less effective than cisplatin to treat non-seminomatous germ cell tumors. It is not recommended for use except during a stem cell transplant.

Carboplatin contains a platinum atom complexed with two ammonia groups and a cyclobutane-dicarboxyl residue. The agent is activated intracellularly to form reactive platinum complexes that bind to nucleophilic groups, such as GC rich sites, in DNA, thereby inducing intra-strand and inter-strand DNA cross-links, as well as DNA-protein cross-links. These carboplatin induced DNA and protein effects result in apoptosis and cell growth inhibition. In keeping with the kinetic inertness of carboplatin, significantly higher doses, compared to cisplatin, are required for equivalent levels of DNA platination and to generate equitoxic and equivalent anti-tumor effects. The clinical doses are 800–900 mg/m^2. Carboplatin is usually given by intravenous infusion. It can also be administered intra-peritoneally.

- Experimental carboplatin formulations include nano-capsules and liposomes.

Pharmacokinetics The blood levels of intact carboplatin decay in a biphasic manner after a 30-minute intravenous infusion of carboplatin with an initial half-life of 1–2 h and a post-distribution half-life of 2.5–6 h. Carboplatin exhibits linear pharmacokinetics over a therapeutic dose range. The drug is not bound to plasma proteins. However, the platinum from carboplatin becomes irreversibly bound to plasma proteins and is slowly eliminated with a minimum half-life of 5 days. The major route of elimination for carboplatin is renal excretion.

Adverse Effects The benefit of carboplatin, compared to cisplatin, is reduced nephrotoxicity as the drug can be excreted essentially intact. Carboplatin is also substantially less emetogenic than cisplatin. Carboplatin causes thrombocytopenia with a nadir of 10–14 days. Neutropenia with granulocyte counts below 1000/mm^3 occurs in 15 % of patients; leukopenia with white blood cell counts below 2000/mm^3 arises in 15 %. Marrow suppression is usually more severe in patients with impaired kidney function. Patients with poor performance status also experience a higher incidence of severe leukopenia and thrombocytopenia.

Nausea and vomiting occur in 65 % of the patients (80 % of previously treated ovarian cancer patients) within 24 h of treatment, and in about 1/3 of these patients it is severe. Carboplatin also leads to alopecia, fatigue, and abnormal blood electrolyte levels (magnesium, sodium, potassium, calcium). With a frequency below 30 %, carboplatin injection can cause a burning sensation at the injection site, abdominal pain, diarrhea or constipation, mouth sores, taste changes, peripheral neuropathy (decreased sensation and paresthesia of the extremities), central neurotoxicity (patients over age 65 are at increased risk for dizziness, confusion, visual changes, tinnitus), ototoxicity (hearing loss of high pitched sounds), abnormal blood liver function, cardiovascular events (heart failure, blood clots, strokes), or allergic reaction. The adverse effects of carboplatin are almost always reversible. The drug is Pregnancy Category D.

Drug Interactions Aluminum reacts with carboplatin causing precipitate formation and loss of potency. Therefore, intravenous sets containing aluminum parts that may come in contact with the drug must not be employed. Very serious drug interactions may occur with nalidixic acid, a medication that is commonly used for the treatment of urinary tract infections. Drugs that may interact with carboplatin include, aminoglycoside antibiotics (gentamicin, neomycin), amphotericin B, hydantoin anti-seizure medications, loop diuretics (furosemide, bumetanide, ethacrynic acid).

Nedaplatin (cis-diammine-glycoloato-*O, O'*-platinum^{II}) <Aqupla> is a second generation cisplatin analog that initially received approval for use in Japan. Containing a ring structure, in which glycolate is bound to the platinum by a bidentate ligand, nedaplatin forms reactive complexes that bind to nucelophilic groups in the DNA. The agent is administered at 100 mg/m^2.

Adverse Effects Nedaplatin is less nephrotoxic and neurotoxic compared to both cisplatin and carboplatin. It causes myelosuppression with a late recovery of 6 weeks.

Iproplatin is a synthetic second generation platinum compound that is based on a Pt^{IV} complex. The agent binds to

[23] Metal ammine complexes contain one or more ammonia (NH_3) ligands.

and forms DNA cross-links and platinum-DNA adducts, resulting in failure of DNA reduplication and cell death.

Drug Resistance Although less prone to Glutathione inactivation compared to cisplatin, resistance to iproplatin may arise due to the repair of platination damage by tumor cells.

Third generation platinum compounds Oxaliplatin (ethanedioate platinum (2-aminocyclohexyl)amine, trans-L-diaminocyclohexane)oxalatoplatinum^{II}) <Eloxatin> was first synthesized in 1976. This third generation platinum analog received U.S. FDA approval in 2002. In this organoplatinum agent, the platinum atom is complexed with 1,2-diaminocyclohexane (DACH) and with an oxalate ligand as a leaving group. After displacement of the labile oxalate leaving group, active oxaliplatin derivatives (such as monoaquo- and diaquo- 1,2-diaminocyclohexane platinum) alkylate macro-molecules, forming both inter- and intra-strand platinum-DNA cross-links, which result in the inhibition of DNA reduplication and transcription, and in cell cycle non-specific cytotoxicity. The 1,2-diaminocyclohexane side chain may counteract alkylating agent resistance. Oxaliplatin is typically administered by infusion every 2 weeks in combination with fluorouracil and leucovorin for the treatment of advanced colorectal cancer (until the disease progresses or unacceptable toxicity sets in) or for the adjuvant treatment of stage III colon cancer in patients who have undergone complete resection of the primary tumor (12 cycles over 6 months). For this malignancy, oxaliplatin in combination with 5-fluorouracil/folinic acid (5-FU/FA) has increased the response rates from 15 % for 5-fluorouracil alone to over 40 %, although the increases in overall survival rates are modest. The FOLFOX regimen is the most common combination therapy use for oxaliplatin.

- Liposomal encapsulation of oxaliplatin generates lipoxal. Adverse effects are ameliorated to moderate myelotoxicity, nausea, peripheral neuropathy, and asthenia. Nausea can be controlled with ondansetron administration.
- Liposomally entrapped cis-bis-neodecanoato-trans-R, R-1,2-diaminocyclohexane platinum^{II} (L-NDDP) <Aroplatin> is a liposomal formulation of the structural oxaliplatinum analog cis-bis-neodecanoato-trans-R, R-1,2-diamino cyclohexane platinum^{II} (NDDP). This lipophilic, non-cross-resistant platinum compound is formulated in multi-lamellar liposomes of 1–3 mm diameter. The maximum tolerated dose after intravenous administration is 300 mg/m^2 with myelosuppression being dose limiting.

Pharmacokinetics At the end of a 2-h infusion, approximately 15 % of the administered platinum is present in the systemic circulation. The remaining 85 % is rapidly distributed into tissues or eliminated in the urine. The irreversible plasma protein binding of platinum is greater than 90 %, the main binding proteins being Albumin and γ-Globulins. The major route of platinum elimination is renal excretion, whereas only about 2 % of the drug are eliminated in the feces.

Adverse Effects Patients experience nausea and vomiting. Premedication with anti-emetics, including 5-HT$_3$ blockers (see Sect. 17.1.) with or without dexamethasone, is recommended. Other adverse effects may include diarrhea, neutropenia, or fatigue. Some patients experience an allergic reaction to platinum. Prolongation of the infusion time for oxaliplatin from 2–6 h may mitigate acute toxicities. Oxaliplatin has lower ototoxicity and nephrotoxicity than cisplatin and carboplatin. However, neuropathy (abnormal sensations around the mouth, possibly leading to an inability to swallow) may be dose limiting. Severe symptoms regress in most patients within 4–6 months. The drug is Pregnancy Category D.

Drug Resistance Oxaliplatin circumvents mismatch repair and reduplicative bypass (the ability of a cell to synthesize DNA past a site of DNA damage) (Fink et al. 1996; Raymond et al. 1998). In many types of tumor cells, it is not subject to cross-resistance with cisplatin. Although cisplatin and oxaliplatin form the same types of adducts at identical sites on DNA, their structures are distinct and are differentially recognized by mismatch repair proteins as well as some damage recognition proteins. They include HMGB1 (High Mobility Group Box Protein 1), TBP (TATA Box Binding Protein) and UBF (Upstream Binding Factor). DNA Polymerase η has a greater efficiency of error-free bypass of oxaliplatin adducts compared with cisplatin.

Lobaplatin (1,2-diammino-methyl-cyclobutaneplatinum^{II}-lactate) (D-19466) was developed by ASTA Medica (Degussa) for the treatment of cancer. ASTA Medica discontinued the development, and it subsequently became the responsibility of Zentaris AG, which had been formed in 2001 from the biopharmaceutical, inhalation technology and gene therapy activities of ASTA Medica. In 2002, Zentaris was acquired by AEterna Laboratories. Lobaplatin consists of a nearly equal mixture of two diastereoisomers, comprising the SSS configuration and the RRS configuration. Lobaplatin is approved in Japan and China for the treatment of chronic myelogenous leukemia (CML) and inoperable metastatic breast and small cell lung cancers. It is given at 50–70 mg/m^2 by intravenous bolus every 3–4 weeks.

Adverse Effects The limiting toxicity of lobaplatin is thrombocytopenia, with a nadir at approximately 2 weeks after drug administration. Leukopenia is less severe, and the drug does not induce nephrotoxicity, neurotoxicity, or ototoxicity. The pharmacokinetics and adverse effects of lobaplatin are strongly affected by the renal function, which determines total body clearance.

Drug Resistance Lobaplatin is not subject to cross-resistance with cisplatin.

Satraplatin is an orally administered third generation compound that forms highly reactive, charged platinum complexes, which bind to nucleophilic groups in the DNA. This binding induces intra-strand and inter-strand cross-links, as well as DNA-protein cross-links, resulting in cell growth inhibition and apoptosis. Satraplatin may be indicated for non-small cell lung cancer and for hormone refractory prostate cancer.

Spiroplatin (aqua-1,1-bis(aminomethyl)-cyclohexane-sulfatoplatinum^{II}) is a synthetic derivative of cyclohexane sulfatoplatinum that induces DNA cross-links. It is under study for the treatment of solid tumors. The recommended dose is 30 mg/m^2 by 4 h infusion every 3 weeks.

Adverse Effects Similar to other platinum compounds, this agent itself is mutagenic and carcinogenic. Myelosuppression and renal toxicity (glomerular and tubular damage) are dose limiting.

Picoplatin (cis-amminedichloro[2-methylpyridine]platinum^{II}) (ZD-0473, JM-473, AMD-473) is a cisplatin analog designed to sterically hinder the approach of Glutathione and other cellular thiols, which intercept and sequester platinum drugs before they can reach the genome, thus generating drug resistance. Compared to cisplatin, this third generation platinum drug has slower rates of hydrolysis, and the reactivities toward thiourea, pyridine, methionine, and GMP are lower. Picoplatin forms unique platinum-DNA adducts that differ from those of cisplatin or carboplatin. It displays improved safety and efficacy over earlier generations of platinum drugs. The agent is in clinical trials for mono-therapy as well as for combination with gemcitabine, navelbine, doxorubicin, docetaxel, paclitaxel, or topotecan. The compound is orally active.

Drug Resistance The drug contains a bulky methylpyridine ligand at its platinum center, which is responsible for its ability to overcome platinum resistance.

Cisplatin resistance is a major obstacle in the treatment of gastric cancer. Heptaplatin (cis-malonatol) (SKI-2053R) <Sunpla> is approved for the treatment of gastric cancers in South Korea.

Metallothioneins constitute a family of stress induced proteins that contain a substantial portion of cysteine residues. They have high affinity for heavy metals and free radical scavenging ability. Whereas the cellular Metallothionein levels may confer resistance to cisplatin, they have a lower involvement in heptaplatin resistance.

Multi-nuclear platinum complexes with bridging linkers have been designed to circumvent platinum resistance in tumor cells. Triplatin (trans-{bis[trans-diamminechloroplatinum^{II} (μ-1,6-hexanediamine)]} diammineplatinum^{II} tetranitrate) (BBR3463) is a trinuclear compound of the third generation. The agent contains two reactive platinum centers, each containing a single labile chloride.

Adverse Effects Adverse effects include nausea and vomiting, and neutropenia.

Drug Resistance Cisplatin resistant cells are not cross-resistant to BBR3463.

Emerging platinum drug derivatives According to the original empirical structure-activity relationships, the trans-platinum complexes were considered to be inactive due to

- the kinetic instability promoting their deactivation; trans-chloro species are more reactive than the corresponding cis-isomers, therefore undesired reactions could contribute to the lack of pharmacological activity
- the formation of DNA adducts characterized by a regioselectivity and a stereochemistry different from those of cisplatin; the major cytotoxic DNA lesion formed by cisplatin, the 1,2-intra-strand cross-link between adjacent purines, is stereochemically inaccessible to trans-isomers.

However, some newer trans compounds are under investigation for anti-tumor activity. Most of the active trans-platinum compounds fall into four classes. One class includes platinum^{IV} complexes of the general formula trans-[$PtCl_2X_2$(L)(L′)] (X = hydroxide, carbamate, or carboxylate; L, L′ = ammine or amine). The remaining three classes, all containing platinum^{II} species, have the general formula trans-[$PtCl_2$(L)(L′)] (with a) L = N-donor aromatic heterocycle and L′ = ammine, sulphoxide, or a second aromatic N-donor ligand; (b) L = sterically hindered aliphatic amine, including piperazine and L′ = ammine, a second aliphatic amine, or a pyridine-type ligand;(c) L = imino ligand and L′ = ammine or a second molecule of imino ligand) (Coluccia and Natile 2007). Both cisplatin and transplatin react preferentially at the *N*7 position of guanine and adenine residues of DNA to form a variety of mono-functional and bi-functional adducts. However, transplatin is characterized by a reduced capability to form bifunctional adducts in double helical DNA, and cannot produce DNA 1,2-intra-strand cross-links. Trans-platinum compounds may have value in the treatment of tumors that have developed resistance to cis-platinum compounds.

In the early development of analogs to the platinum compounds, complexes with windows of reactivity similar to the platinum complexes were examined extensively. Whereas direct Ni and Pd analogs of Pt complexes are too kinetically reactive to be of use as drugs, Ir and Os ammine compounds are in general too inert. Ruthenium and rhodium have produced compounds with the greatest promise, although no direct analogs have yet advanced to the clinic.

Upon aquation of a ligand, platinum drugs become highly reactive, allowing them to coordinate DNA bases.
Complexes with labile leaving groups are toxic, compounds with stable leaving groups are inactive. Modifications in the

chloride leaving group affect pharmacokinetics; modifications in the ligand affect efficacy and spectrum of activity.
Most platinum compounds cannot be taken orally.
Early generation platinum drugs have severe adverse effects.
Recent generation platinum drugs reduce toxicity and avoid cross-resistance.
Drug resistance may be caused by platinum efflux, detoxification through thiols, apoptosis resistance, or enhanced DNA repair.

2.1.9 Others

Ecteinascidins are isolated from marine organisms, ecteinascidin-743 (trabectedin, ET-743) <Yondelis> is produced by the Caribbean tunicate Ecteinascidia turbinate. The alkaloid is composed of three tetrahydroisoquinoline moieties, eight rings, and seven chiral centers (Fig. 2.18). It contains three fused tetrahydroisoquinoline subunits (A, B, and C). The A and B subunits provide the scaffold for DNA recognition and covalent bonding. The C subunit protrudes out and interacts with adjacent nuclear proteins. Ecteinascidin-743 binds to the minor groove of DNA, effects guanine *N*2 alkylation (via an intermediate iminium generated from an active carbinolamin functional group), and bends the duplex toward the major groove. This may sequester specific transcription factors, inhibit inducible gene transcription, and result in cytotoxicity. The alkylation at guanine 2–NH_2 positions is sequence selective and region specific to DNA triplets containing a central guanine (AGC, CGC, TGG). Ecteinascidin-743 also binds tightly to Topoisomerase 1, with which it produces cleavage complexes. The mechanism of action may also involve the production of superoxide via reduction of molecular oxygen near the DNA strand (through an unusual auto-redox reaction on a hydroxyquinone moiety), resulting in DNA backbone cleavage and cell apoptosis. The compound has activity against a variety of soft tissue sarcomata and is in clinical trials for breast, ovarian, and prostate cancers.

The pyrrolizidine alkaloids are distributed widely in nature as the tertiary bases of *N*-oxides and are typically generated in species of Compositae, Leguminosae, and Boraginaceae. Indicine-*N*-oxide (NSC 132319) is a natural pyrrolizidine alkaloid produced by Heliotropium indicum Linn. (family Boraginaceae). Indicine-*N*-oxide alkylates and cross-links DNA. It is under study as anti-cancer agent for use at 3.0 g/m^2 daily for 5 days, repeated every 5 weeks.

Pharmacokinetics The intravenous injection of indicine-*N*-oxide produces a dose dependent increase in blood levels. The blood concentrations then exhibit a biphasic decline (consistent with a 2-compartment open model). The gut flora as well as the liver are capable of reducing indicine-*N*-oxide to form indicine. Approximately 40 % of the administered dose is eliminated in the urine within 24 h as unmetabolized drug and below 5 % as the free base indicine.

Adverse Effects Dose limiting toxicities of indicine-*N*-oxide are reversible leukopenia and thrombocytopenia. Repetitive courses have a cumulative effect on the severity of myelosuppression. Other adverse effects include mild

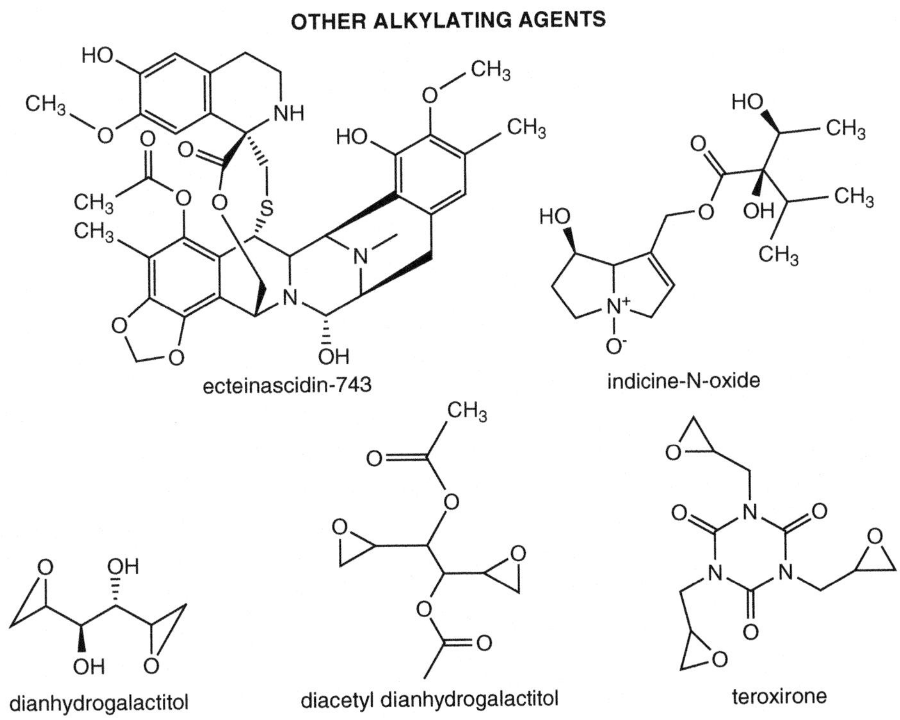

Fig. 2.18 Structures of various alkylating agents

nausea and vomiting during treatment, bone marrow hypoplasia, nephrosis, emesis, and bloody diarrhea.

Drug Interactions Prior treatment with a nitrosourea enhances the hematopoietic toxicity of indicine-*N*-oxide.

Dianhydrogalactitol (1,2:5,6-diepoxyhexane-3,4-diol, 1,2-di(oxiranyl)ethylene glycol, dulcitol diepoxide, DAG) (NSC 132313) is a bifunctional hexitol diepoxide that was developed in Budapest (Nemeth et al. 1972). It alkylates and cross-links DNA via an epoxide group during all phases of the cell cycle, resulting in a disruption of DNA function and cell cycle arrest. The drug has good penetration into the brain and can be applied to the treatment of brain tumors. It has been investigated in combination with radiation therapy.

- Diacetyl dianhydrogalactitol (DADAG) is a derivative of dianhydrogalactitol.

Pharmacokinetics The mean residence time for pharmacologically active dianhydrogalactitol in the body is 2 h. The drug is rapidly consumed by intracellular alkylation and degradation.

Adverse Effects Adverse effects comprise nausea and vomiting, bone marrow depression, immunosuppression, psychiatric and neurologic disturbances, and allergic eczema. With lesser incidence, kidney and liver damage or ulcerative stomatitis may arise.

Teroxirone (1,3,5-triglycidyl isocyanurate, Henkel's Compound) is a triazine triepoxide that alkylates and cross-links DNA, thereby inhibiting DNA reduplication (Atassi et al. 1980). An experimental regimen gives the drug intravenously on five consecutive days every 4 weeks.

Pharmacokinetics Following rapid intravenous administration, teroxirone has a rapid blood elimination half-life below 5 min, and total body clearance over 5 L/min. The drug is metabolized in the liver, and 70 % of the metabolites are excreted in the urine.

Adverse Effects Myelosuppression is the dose limiting toxicity. Local phlebitis and cutaneous flare reactions commonly arise at high doses. The maximal tolerated dose is 340 mg/m^2/day.

Treatment of Testicular Cancer

In the mid-1970s, following the work on acute leukemia, lymphoma and breast cancer, Lawrence Einhorn and his group, building on the initial work of M.C. Li at Memorial Hospital (Li 1969), began a series of studies that resulted in an improvement of the cure rate of metastatic testicular cancer. A landmark trial, reported in 1977, used a regimen of cisplatin, vinblastine, and bleomycin for four cycles, followed by 21 months of maintenance vinblastine to increase the complete response rates from 25 to 80 % (Einhorn and Donohue 1977). Today, chemotherapy is used for all stages of this tumor and testicular cancer is curable in most patients with rates of nearly 80 %, survival being primarily due to effective chemotherapy. Patients may initially present to a variety of practitioners, and delays in therapy are associated with more extensive disease, resulting in more intensive treatment and lower cure rates.

1. **Non-seminomatous cancers**

Testicular non-seminomatous cancers often respond well to cisplatin. By contrast, the substitution of the less toxic carboplatin for cisplatin results in poor relapse-free survival rates. Treatment decisions are made based on risk stratification into good, intermediate, and poor prognostic groups according to the universal classification scheme developed by the International Germ Cell Cancer Collaborative Group (IGCCG).

- Approximately 90 % of patients classified as having a good prognosis (primary site not mediastinum, no extrapulmonary visceral metastases, hCG below 5000 international units/L, AFP below 1000 units/L, LDH below 1.5-fold upper limits of normal) achieve a durable complete remission with either four cycles of etoposide and cisplatin (EP) or three cycles of bleomycin, etoposide, and cisplatin (BEP). The survival benefits of both regimens are comparable. Neutropenia is more common with EP, while neuropathy and adverse dermatologic effects occur more frequently with BEP.
- Complete responses are achieved less frequently for patients with intermediate and poor risk germ cell tumors, in whom four cycles of bleomycin, etoposide, and cisplatin (BEP) remains the standard of care. Attempts to improve outcomes by intensifying the BEP regimen (increased cisplatin dose, replacement of bleomycin with ifosfamide, high-dose chemotherapy with autologous stem cell support) have not demonstrated any advantage but have been associated with more intense toxicities.
- Fewer than 10 % of patients suffer relapses. For those, second- and third-line programs also have curative potential. They include standard doses of 3-drug combinations based on ifosfamide and cisplatin (plus either vinblastine or etoposide or paclitaxel). High-dose salvage chemotherapy has been used since the late 1980s, but was initially limited by high mortality rates. This prompted the addition of growth factor support or autologous stem cell support. At least two high dose cycles are con-

sidered necessary to achieve a benefit. Alternative options to provide disease control and palliation include the combination of gemcitabine with oxaliplatin or paclitaxel and the combination of cisplatin with epirubicin.

Adverse Effects The commonly used chemotherapeutic agents can all cause myelosuppression leading to anemia, bleeding, and febrile neutropenia (5–25 % risk with BEP or EP). Growth factor support and prophylactic fluoroquinolone may lower this risk. Acute cardiovascular and thromboembolic toxicities may be linked to germ cell tumor chemotherapy. Nephrotoxicity, ototoxicity, and neuropathy can occur and may persist in 20–40 % or patients. Azoospermia always arises during cisplatin therapy. However, approximately 50 % of patients regain normal sperm counts within 2 years from treatment, and this proportion increases to 80 % within 5 years. Testicular cancer survivors are at a 2–3-fold increased risk of secondary malignancies following chemotherapy, radiation, or a combination of these modalities. They include tumors of the pleura, pancreas, stomach, bladder, and connective tissue. Myelodysplastic syndrome and secondary leukemia (3–7 % risk) are also potential consequences of combination chemotherapy, in particular of etoposide.

Surgery may follow chemotherapy. Tumor marker normalization is a prerequisite for post-chemotherapy surgery because elevated markers predict a high likelihood of incomplete resection (Feldman et al. 2008).

Testicular cancer survivors have an elevated risk of serious co-morbidities. Of patients who survive at least a year from their initial diagnosis, more than 40 % of deaths are from non-malignant causes. These include gastrointestinal disorders (intestinal vascular lesions, hepatobiliary disease, ulcers), cardiovascular disease (angina pectoris, myocardial infarction), infections, and possibly respiratory illness. The metabolic syndrome, a constellation of three or more characteristics (abdominal obesity, hypertriglycerinemia, low levels of high-density lipoprotein, hypertension, Insulin resistance), may occur in 25–40 % of testicular cancer survivors compared to 3–4 % of the general population. Sarcoidosis is also more common in patients with germ cell tumors, although the causes underlying this association are unknown. Most relapses occur within the first 2 years after completion of treatment, but late relapses may also occur with an incidence of 2–5 %. Because of the generally poor outcome for late relapse testicular cancer with chemotherapy, surgery is the mainstay of management.

2. **Seminomatous cancers**

Almost all seminomata are curable with orchiectomy with or without radiation therapy. They rarely require chemotherapy. When chemotherapy is necessary, the same regimens are used as for other testicular germ cell tumors. Post-chemotherapy surgical resection of a seminoma carries a higher morbidity than other germ cell tumors due to the desmoplastic reaction frequently induced by the treatment.

Treatment of Astrocytoma

Chemotherapy The chemotherapy of brain cancers requires the administration of drugs that can penetrate the blood-brain barrier. Agents that commonly have efficacy in patients with high-grade gliomas include procarbazine, platinum analogs (cisplatin, carboplatin), the nitrosoureas, and temozolomide <Temodar>.

The oral alkylating agent temozolomide <Temodar> has become the standard therapy for glioblastoma. It is indicated for the treatment of

- adult patients with newly diagnosed glioblastoma multiforme concomitantly with radiotherapy and then as maintenance treatment
- adult patients with refractory anaplastic astrocytoma. These are patients who have experienced disease progression on a drug regimen containing nitrosourea and procarbazine.

The daily dose is calculated based on the body surface area and rounded off to the nearest 5 mg. The dosage must be adjusted according to nadir neutrophil and platelet counts in the previous cycle and neutrophil and platelet counts at the time of initiating the next cycle. Patients should take each day's dose with a full glass of water at the same time each day. Taking the medication on an empty stomach or at bedtime may help ease nausea.

Patients with newly diagnosed high grade glioma in the concomitant phase are treated with temozolomide at 75 mg/m^2 daily for 42 days concomitant with focal radiotherapy (60 Gy administered in 30 fractions). This is followed by maintenance temozolomide for six cycles. Although dose interruption or discontinuation may be inevitable if toxicity becomes substantial, no dose reductions are recommended during the concomitant phase. The dose should be continued throughout the 42-day concomitant period, if

- the absolute neutrophil count is at least 1500/µL
- the absolute platelet count is at least 100,000/µL
- common toxicity criteria do not exceed grade 1 (except for alopecia, nausea, and vomiting).

In the maintenance phase, temozolomide is administered for an additional six cycles of treatment. Dosage in cycle 1 is 150 mg/m^2 daily for 5 days followed by 23 days without treatment. At the start of cycle 2, the dose can be escalated to 200 mg/m^2 if the toxicity for cycle 1 is below grade 2 and the absolute neutrophil count and platelet count are in the acceptable range. The dose remains at 200 mg/m^2 per day for the first 5 days of each subsequent cycle except if toxicity occurs.

In 2009, the U.S. FDA approved an intravenous form of temozolomide. It is given by infusion over 90 min. Various dosing schedules are in use.

Adverse Effects The most common adverse effects are nausea and vomiting, constipation, anorexia, alopecia, headache, convulsions, fatigue, and thrombocytopenia. Patients may experience dose limiting myelosuppression, with grade 3–4 neutropenia occurring in 10% and grade 3–4 thrombocytopenia in 15% of cases. Prophylaxis against Pneumocystis carinii pneumonia is required for all patients receiving concomitant temozolomide and radiotherapy for the 42-day regimen. All patients receiving temozolomide, particularly patients who also receive steroids, should be observed closely for the development of Pneumocystis carinii pneumonia, regardless of the regimen applied. Temozolomide is contraindicated in patients who have hypersensitivity to any of its components or to dacarbazine (DTIC). The drug may cause fetal harm when administered to a pregnant woman; nursing should be discontinued in women during treatment. As temozolomide may affect testicular function, male patients should exercise adequate birth control measures.

Drug Resistance The DNA repair protein *O*^{6}-Alkylguanine DNA Alkyl Transferase (AGAT, MGMT), which removes methyl groups from *O*^{6}-methyl-guanine lesions that arise from temozolomide treatment, may confer dug resistance. MGMT is consumed stoichiometrically during the DNA repair reaction (it does not act as an enzyme). As DNA repair by MGMT is the primary mechanism of drug resistance to temozolomide, its expression level in the cancer cells determines the extent of the drug response.

BCNU (carmustine) <BiCNU> is a prodrug that has displayed efficacy against astrocytoma. It may be given systemically or topically. By applying it directly to the diseased area of the brain, adverse effects are limited and the drug has a more beneficial effect.

- The regimen BCNU-DAG entails 90 mg/m^2 carmustine and 70 mg/m^2 dianhydrogalactitol intravenously on day 1. Repetition of the cycle at 5 weeks, followed by subsequent cycles at 5–7 week intervals during the first year and 10–12 week intervals during the second year. It is used to treat primary brain tumor recurrence after irradiation.
- The regimen BCNU-FU entails 180 mg/m^2 carmustine intravenously on day 1 plus intravenous infusion of 1000 mg/m^2/day fluorouracil for 72 h beginning on day 15. The cycle is repeated every 6 weeks until there is evidence of tumor progression. The approach is a combination therapy for recurrent malignant brain tumors.
- A biodegradable polifeprosan 20 wafer impregnated with carmustine <Gliadel> may be used for topical postsurgical treatment preceding ionizing radiation. The wafers produce high local concentrations of carmustine for several weeks directly into the tumor bed after surgery when the tumor burden is low.

Molecularly targeted therapy The cells of glioblastomata and anaplastic gliomatas secrete glutamate and also express AMPA Glutamate Receptors, which contribute to proliferation, migration and neurotoxicity. Talampanel (GYKI 537773, LY300164) is a synthetic derivative of dioxolo-benzodiazepine, which non-competitively binds to the AMPA (α-amino-3-hydroxy-5-methyl-4-isoxazolepropionic acid) subtype of glutamate excitatory amino acid receptors and may inhibit the growth of gliomata by blocking a growth factor signal.

Adverse Effects The long-term effects of benzodiazepines include drug dependence as well as the possibility of adverse effects on cognitive function, physical health, and mental health. There is evidence that benzodiazepine use may lead to an increased risk for cancer.

Glioblastoma is a highly aggressive cancer, in which the PI 3-Kinase pathway is excessively activated via receptor tyrosine kinases. Activation of ERBB1 (EGFR) is a critical pathogenetic event. Other receptor tyrosine kinases, including PDGFR and MET may also be altered. Because these receptors can be co-activated, monotherapy with ERBB1 inhibitors or PDGFR inhibitors has a low rate of success. However, combined regimens that target multiple receptor tyrosine kinases may effectively suppress the PI 3-Kinase pathway, inhibit tumor growth, and lead to improvement (Stommel et al. 2007).

Supportive treatment Patients with malignant glioma may require anti-epileptic medicine. Often, their anti-cancer chemotherapy contains irinotecan. The plasma concentration of irinotecan and its active metabolite SN-38 is reduced and the clearance is increased in patients receiving anticonvulsants. This is likely based on the induction of hepatic Cytochrome P450 enzymes (CYPs) by anticonvulsant agents and needs to be considered in irinotecan dosing.

2.2 Antibiotics

Among the research programs related to World War II was a large scale screening of bacterial and fungal fermentation products by pharmaceutical companies to isolate and produce antibiotics suitable for treating wound infections. Some of the agents under investigation were also examined for their anti-tumor effects. The program was largely based on observations with penicillin, which had initially been thought to have tumor suppressing properties. In particular, Streptomyces species are a genus of soil bacteria, from which numerous antibiotic and antifungal compounds have been derived. The antibiotic actinomycin D, extracted from Streptomyces, was an early product of the large scale screening endeavor. Introduced by Sidney Farber into the clinic in 1954, actinomycin D[24] had substantial anti-cancer effects and therefore found considerable use in the treatment of pediatric tumors through the 1960s. This drug established feasibility and led to a continued search for more active anti-tumor antibiotics[25]. The effort has yielded a series of compounds that are in common use today (DeVita and Chu 2008).

Anti-neoplastic antibiotics fall into two broad functional classes. Cyclopropylpyrroloindoles, minor groove DNA binding antibiotics, and aminoquinones alkylate DNA. Polycyclic aromatic antibiotics (anthracyclins, anthracenediones, anthrapyrazoles) and enediynes generate free radicals through redox cycling by a mechanism that depends in part on cellular iron; the generated reactive oxygen species damage the DNA of cancer cells. In addition, polycyclic aromatic antibiotics inhibit Topoisomerase 2.

Adverse Effects The production of reactive oxygen species is in some measure responsible for the cardiotoxicity exerted by drugs in the class of redox cycling antibiotics. Specifically, the prolonged treatment with anthracyclins can lead to a distinctive and life threatening form of cardiomyopathy.

Cyclopropylpyrroloindoles, minor groove DNA binding antibiotics, and aminoquinones alkylate DNA.
Polycyclic aromatic antibiotics (anthracyclins, anthracenediones, anthrapyrazoles) and enediynes damage DNA through redox cycling.
Polycyclic aromatic antibiotics inhibit Topoisomerase 2.
Cardiotoxicity of redox cycling antibiotics is an adverse class effect.

2.2.1 Cyclopropylpyrroloindole Antibiotics

The cyclopropylpyrroloindole analogs (drug names ending on -zelesin) contain a cyclopropyl group, which mediates sequence selective *N*3 adenine covalent adduct formation. These DNA minor groove binding compounds do not react with single stranded DNA, RNA, or protein

Adverse Effects Myelosuppression, arising in a biphasic time course, is the dose limiting toxicity.

The prototypical cyclopropylpyrroloindole anti-cancer antibiotic CC-1065 (NSC 298223) (Fig. 2.19) was isolated from the fermentation products of the soil organism Streptomyces zelensis in the 1970s (Hanka et al. 1978). The drug had high potency and a novel mechanism of action. CC-1065 binds covalently, non-intercalatively to double stranded DNA within the minor groove with a sequence preference for 5′-d(A/G)NTTA-3′ and 5′-dAAAAA-3′ (N denotes any base). It alkylates the *N*3 position of the 3′-adenine with its left-hand cyclopropylpyrroloindole segment. It also inhibits gene transcription by interfering with the binding of TATA Box Binding Protein (TBP) to its target DNA.

Adverse Effects Despite the high potency and broad spectrum of anti-tumor activity, the clinical development of CC-1065 was precluded by irreversible hepatic and renal toxicities and delayed lethality.

CC-1065 analogs have been synthesized and tested to pursue compounds that retain the potent anti-cancer activity, but are devoid of the toxic effects of the parent compound. (+)-duocarmycin A and (+)-duocarmycin SA are derived from Streptomyces species. They exert their biological

[24] The suffix -mycin is conventionally used to describe a substance derived from a bacterium in the order Actinomycetales.

[25] The term antibiotic was coined by Selman Waksman, the discoverer of actinomycin D.

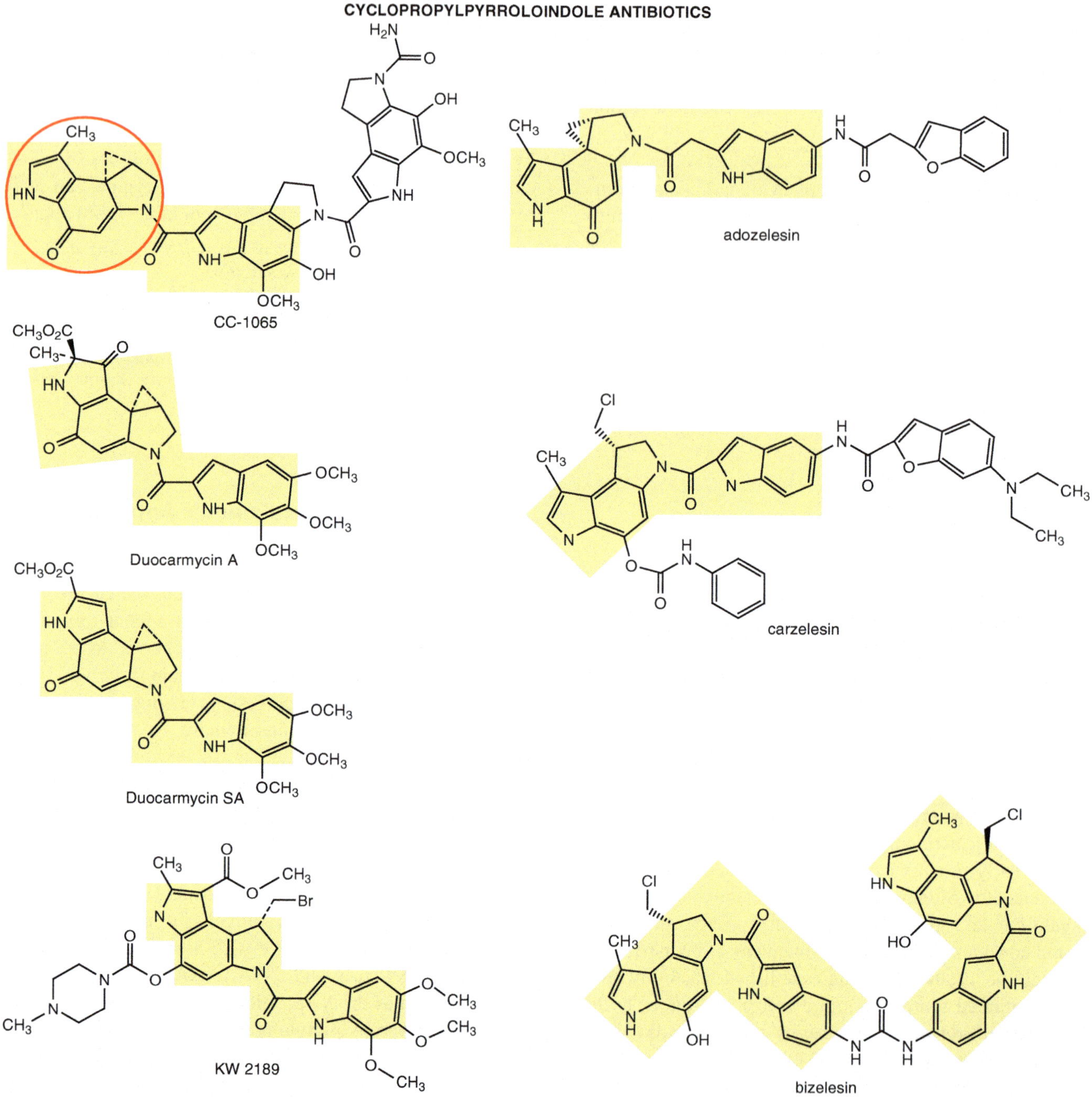

Fig. 2.19 Structures of cyclopropylpyrroloindole antibiotics. The common chemical components are highlighted in *yellow*. The alkylating unit of CC-1065 is circled in *red*.

effects through participation in a stereoelectronically controlled minor groove adenine *N*3 alkylation of duplex DNA. Duocarmycin A also alkylates a guanine in the recognition sequence 5′-CGCGTTGGGAG-3′.

KW 2189 (Methyl(1*S*)-1-bromomethyl-7-methyl-5-[(4-methylpiperazinyl)-carbonyloxy]-3-[(5,6,7-trimethoxy-2-indolyl)-carbonyl]-1,2-dihydro-3H-pyrrolo[3,2-e]indole-8-carboxylate 3 hydrobromide) (Kobayashi et al. 1994) is a semi-synthetic, water soluble derivative of duocarmycin B2. After activation by Carboxyl Esterase, KW 2189 alkylates DNA by binding to A/T-rich sequences in the minor groove of DNA, thereby inhibiting DNA reduplication and inducing apoptosis.

Adverse Effects Severe and prolonged hematologic toxicity is dose limiting and may prevent the further development of this agent for clinical use.

Adozelesin, carzelesin, and bizelesin were originally isolated from Streptomyces zelensis. They bind genomic DNA at the sequence motif 5′-(A/T)(A/T)A-3′ and alkylate the *N*3 position of adenine at the 3′ end of their binding sites. Adozelesin induces single strand DNA lesions, whereas bizelesin induces both single strand lesions and double strand DNA cross-links. At equivalent cytotoxic concentrations, these agents induce distinct biological responses. However, in cells lacking the tumor suppressor protein P21, bizelesin, as well as adozelesin, trigger apoptosis, reflecting a crucial role for P21 in sustained bizelesin induced G_2/M arrest (Cao 2003).

Adozelesin (U-73,975, NSC-615284) causes genomic lesions by alkylating DNA and introducing single strand breaks.

- The agent interacts with the minor groove of DNA and forms covalent adducts with the *N*3 of adenines. This results in the formation of adozelesin-DNA adducts, which leads to an inhibition of DNA reduplication. The S phase specific induction of DNA damage responses by adozelesin depends on active reduplication forks.
- The inhibition of DNA reduplication by adozelesin occurs in part through inactivation of the hetero-trimeric, trans-acting factor RPA (Replication Protein A). RPA is the major single strand DNA binding protein. It is essential for reduplication and plays critical roles in repair and recombination.
- Low adozelesin concentrations induce a transient S phase block and cell cycle arrest in G_2/M, as well as the induction of P53 and P21, whereas high drug concentrations cause apoptosis but no P21 induction.

Carzelesin (U-80,244, NSC-619029) is a prodrug cyclopropylpyrroloindole analog that contains a relatively non-reactive chloromethyl precursor to the cyclopropyl function. Activation of carzelesin requires two steps, the hydrolysis of a phenylurethane substituent followed by ring closure to form the cyclopropyl containing DNA reactive drug.

Adverse Effects Bone marrow suppression is the primary adverse effect. Fatal hepatotoxicity is possible.

Bizelesin (U-77,779, NSC-615291) is a cyclopropylpyrroloindole dimer with two reactive chloromethyl moieties that can form DNA adducts with adenines in either one or both DNA strands.

- Bizelesin binds to A/T-rich sequences in the minor groove of DNA and induces inter-strand cross-linking of DNA, thereby inhibiting DNA reduplication and RNA synthesis. The canonical 5′-T(A/T)$_4$A-3′ target motifs are on average scarce and scattered. However, they have higher local motif densities in distinct mini-satellite regions. These A/T islands exhibit the sequence attributes of matrix attachment regions, domains that organize DNA loops on the nuclear matrix. Bizelesin may interfere with that organization.
- Bizelesin enhances P53 and P21 induction and triggers G_2/M cell-cycle arrest, resulting in cell senescence without apoptosis.

Bizelesin has activity against colorectal cancer.

The cyclopropyl groups in cyclopropylpyrroloindole antibiotics mediate N3 adenine covalent adduct formation in a sequence selective fashion.
Myelosuppression is the dose limiting toxicity.
Adozelesin, bizelesin, and carzelesin alkylate the N3 of adenines at the 3′ end of the DNA sequence motif 5′-(A/T)(A/T)A-3′.
Low doses of adozelesin, bizelesin, or carzelesin induce cell cycle arrest, high doses induce apoptosis.
P21 is crucial to sustained bizelesin induced G2/M arrest.

2.2.2 Minor Groove DNA Binding Antibiotics

The minor groove of DNA represents a vulnerable site for attack that is normally unoccupied because most DNA interactive proteins bind to the major groove. Certain sequences in the minor groove are sites of highly specific, non-covalent, and reversible interactions with some antibiotics.

Binders to A/T-rich sites Minor groove binders to A/T-rich sequences are derived from distamycin A (Fig. 2.20), which is produced by Streptomyces distallicus. Distamycin A alters DNA conformation by forming strong reversible complexes preferentially at nucleotide sequences that consist of 4–5 adjacent A/T base pairs. Thus, the drug displaces essential transcription factors and interferes with gene expression. While distamycin A has anti-viral properties it exerts weak cytotoxicity and does not possess sufficient efficacy against cancer. Further, distamycin is cardiotoxic.

The pyrrole-amide backbone of distamycin A has been used as a sequence selective vehicle for the delivery of DNA alkylating functions, leading to a sharp gain in cytotoxicity. Several such derivatives are in testing for anti-cancer treatment.

Tallimustine (FCE-24517, PNU-152241) is a benzoyl nitrogen mustard derivative of distamycin. Tallimustine alkylates *N*3 adenines in the target sequence 5′-TTTTGA-3′. This may lead to an accumulation of cells in the G_2 phase of the cell cycle. The therapeutic dose is 750 μg/m^2, the maximally tolerable dose is 1250 μg/m^2. The agent is under study for anti-leukemia treatment.

Adverse Effects The dose limiting toxic effect is neutropenia, which may become febrile. Platelet counts may drop.

Drug Resistance Treatment with verapamil may reduce resistance to tallimustine.

MEN 10710 is a synthetic distamycin derivative that possesses four methyl-pyrrole rings and a bis-(2-chloroethyl) aminophenyl moiety linked to the oligopyrrole backbone by a flexible butanamido chain.

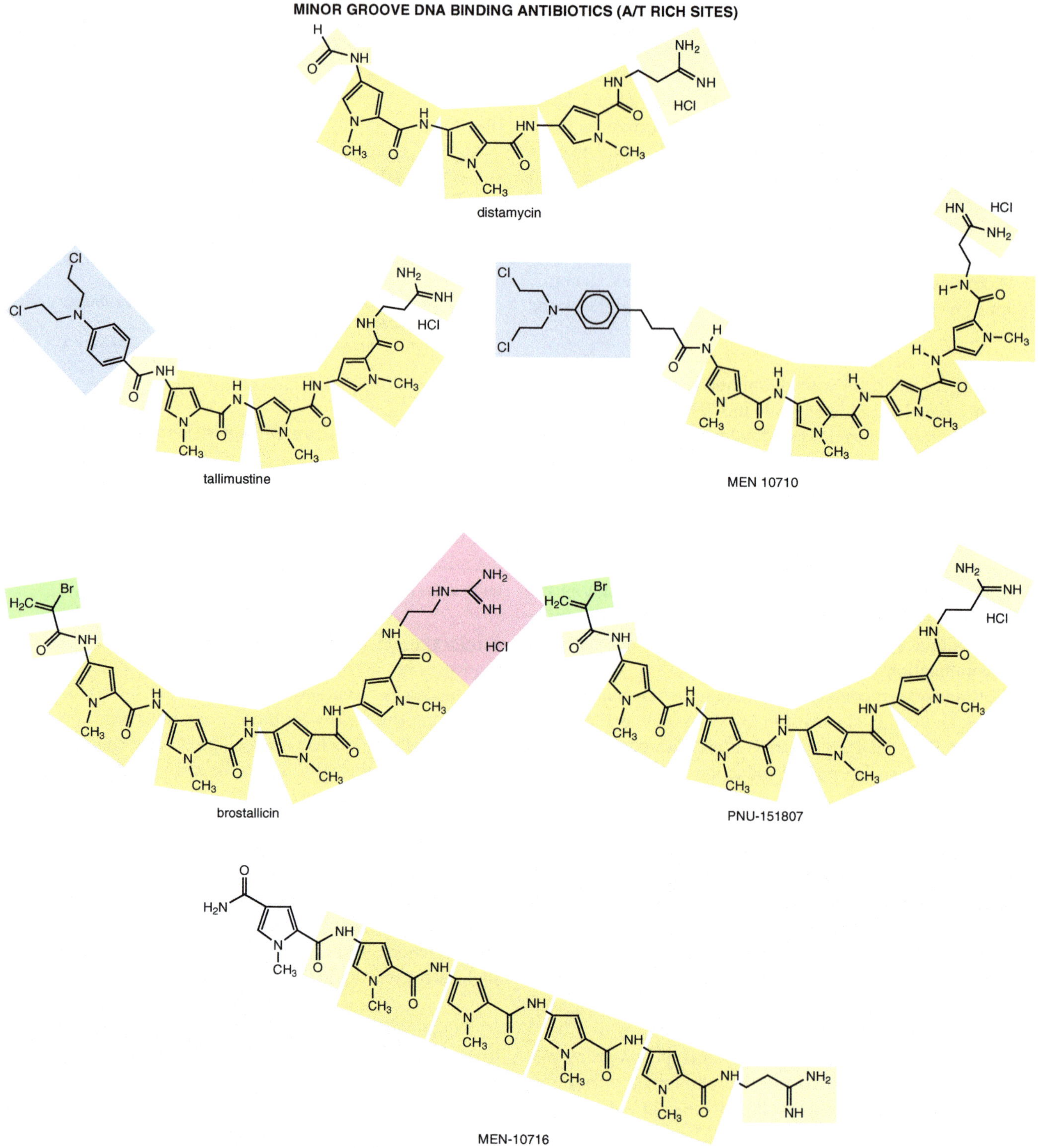

Fig. 2.20 Structures of minor groove DNA binding antibiotics with a preference for A/T rich sites. Bright *yellow* indicates the common methyl-pyrrole-carboxamide motif that repeats 3 (distamycin, tallimustine) or 4 (MEN 10710, brostallicin, PNU-151807, MEN 10716) times. The units are flanked by identical carboxamide and 3-amino-3-iminopropyl groups (light *yellow*), with only one modification within the drug class in brostallicin (pink). Tallimustine and MEN 10710 also have a bis-(2-chloroethyl)aminophenyl group (*blue*) that is similar to nitrogen mustards. Brostallicin and PNU-151807 contain a bromoacrylate functional group (*green*).

Brostallicin (PNU-166196) is a bromo-acrylamido tetra-pyrrole distamycin derivative with high cytotoxic potency. The action of the drug involves its activation upon binding to Glutathione, catalyzed by Glutathione-S-Transferase (GST). Therefore, cells with high GST and Glutathione levels (which is commonly the case in tumors) are susceptible to treatment with brostallicin. Activated brostallicin is capable of DNA minor groove attack, leading to alkylation of DNA nucleophilic functions. The agent is in clinical trials for the treatment of breast cancer, ovarian cancer, and soft tissue sarcomata.

Adverse Effects Brostallicin has reduced myelotoxicity compared with other minor groove DNA binding agents.

Drug Resistance Glutathione conjugation is a prevalent mechanism of resistance to various anti-cancer drugs. Therefore, brostallicin may be used to treat cells that are resistant to other forms of chemotherapy.

PNU-151807 is a synthetic α-bromoacryloyl derivative of distamycin A (Marchini et al. 1999) that interacts non-covalently with the same A/T-rich DNA regions. Unlike other drugs in this class, however, there is no evidence that it produces DNA alkylation. PNU-151807 abolishes the kinase activities of CDK2/Cyclin A, CDK2/Cyclin E, and CDC2/Cyclin B complexes. PNU-151807 triggers apoptosis via activation of Caspases. While it may induce the activation of P53, a disruption of P53 function does not substantially affect the cytotoxic activity of the drug. This may make it useful for treating tumors with inactivating *p53* mutations.

Drug Resistance Mismatch DNA repair deficiency is associated with resistance to certain anti-cancer drugs. It may occur as a consequence of loss of MLH1 expression. By contrast, loss of mismatch repair does not mediate resistance to PNU-151807.

The distamycin derivative MEN 10716 is a minor groove DNA binding antibiotic. After prolonged exposure, the drug also acts as a Telomerase inhibitor.

Binders to G/C-rich sites The aureolic acid anti-cancer antibiotics contain an identical tricyclic poly-ketide core moiety, with a unique dihydroxy-methoxy-oxo-pentyl side chain attached at *C3* (cyclized only in chromocyclomycin). These members are glycosylated compounds with 2 oligosaccharide chains of variable 2,6-dideoxy-sugar residue lengths. The *C7* residue can be either a H atom or a small alkyl side chain. Aureolic acid antibiotics non-intercalatively bind to the DNA minor groove in high-GC-content regions as dimers that form in the presence of divalent cations, such as Mg^{2+}. Upon binding to DNA, the chromophores form hydrogen bonds with NH_2 residues of guanines, thus determining the selectivity for C/G-rich sequences. A result is partial unwinding of the DNA.

These antibiotics are produced by various Streptomycete species. A common step in their biosynthesis is the formation of the tetracyclic intermediate pre-mithramycinone. Further steps (glycosylation, methylations, acylations) proceed through tetracyclic intermediates, which in the end are converted into tricyclic compounds by the action of a Monooxygenase, a key event for the biological activity.

Mithramycin A (MTA, aureolic acid, plicamycin) (LA-7017, PA-144) <Mithracin> (Fig. 2.21)is an anti-neoplastic antibiotic, produced by Streptomyces plicatus, that was first tested in cancer therapy in the 1960s. The drug binds to C/G-rich DNA tracts in the minor groove. Because of this sequence selectivity, mithramycin A blocks the binding of the SP-1 family of transcription factors to C/G-rich sequences in gene promoters and inhibits gene transcription, which in turn alters the regulation of cell proliferation and differentiation. Mithramycin A has been under study for the treatment of testicular cancer, Ewing sarcoma, and chronic myeloid leukemia. Mithramycin A also inhibits bone degradation, which in turn lowers blood calcium. Thus, it is used to treat hyper-calcemia and hyper-calciuria associated with a variety of advanced cancers. Plicamycin is given through intravenous infusion over a period of 4–6 h.

- Mithramycin SK is structurally related to mithramycin A.

Adverse Effects Mithramycin A has myelotoxicity, leading to leukopenia, neutropenia, anemia, and thrombocytopenia. Other adverse effects include nausea and vomiting, diarrhea, loss of appetite, mouth sores, and electrolyte imbalance.

Olivomycin A, a compound produced by Streptomyces olivoreticuli, causes apoptosis in transformed cells of the hematopoietic system, breast, colon, ovaries, and skin (melanoma). The drug suppresses the expression of genes coding for transcription factors, heat shock proteins, and DNA repair proteins. Among the transcription factors down-regulated by olivomycin A is c-MYC, a major regulator of DNA synthesis and cell survival.

Drug Resistance The drug effect is not dependent on P53, which implies efficacy in cancers with loss of function in P53.

Chromomycin A3 (toyomycin, aburamycin) is a fermentation product of Streptomyces griseus. Chromomycin binds to G/C sequences, usually at least three consecutive G/C, and inhibits transcription. The clinical use of chromomycin is limited because of its immunosuppressive properties and high cytotoxicity.

- Chromocyclomycin is a metabolite of Streptomyces LA-7017.

UCH9 is produced by Streptomyces species. It consists of one aglycone, three D-olivoses, one 4-*O*-methyl-D-olivose, and one D-oliose. In contrast to other aureolic acid derivatives, which have di- and trisaccharide moieties and a methyl or a hydrogen attached to the aglycone, in UCH9 there are mono- and tetra-saccharide moieties and a long hydrophobic side chain. UCH9 binds as a dimer to the minor groove of $d(TTGGCCAA)_2$. The agent exhibits cytotoxic activity against transformed cells.

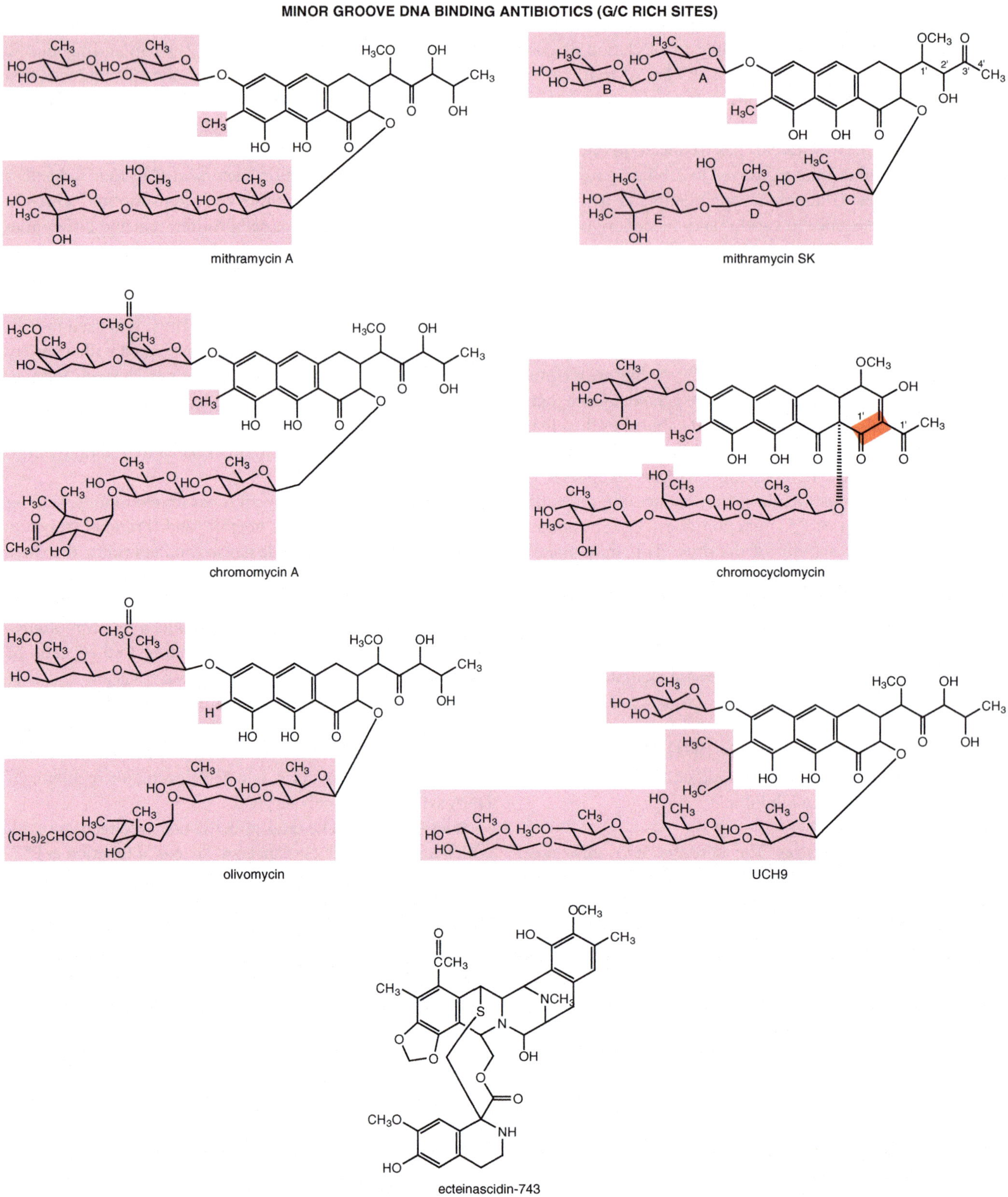

Fig. 2.21 Structures of minor groove DNA binding antibiotics with a preference for G/C rich sites. The aureolic acid antibiotics share a common tricyclic poly-ketide core motif but differ in their side chains in 3 positions (*pink*). Only chromocyclomycin also has a ring closure in the core structure (*red*). Ecteinascidin-743 is a non-aureolic acid minor groove binder.

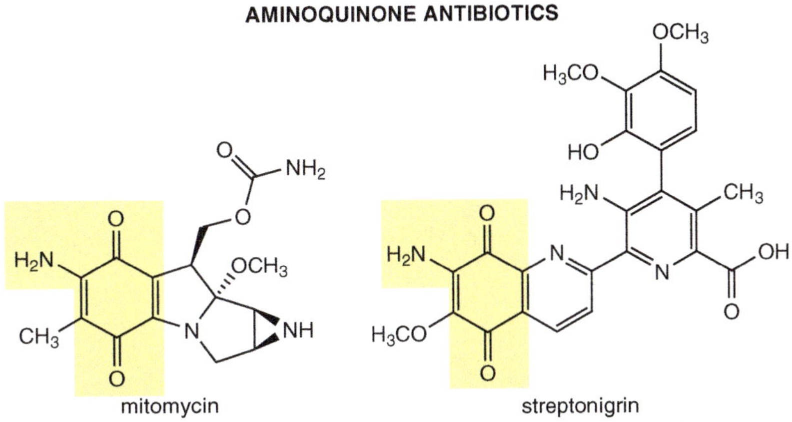

Fig. 2.22 Structures of aminoquinone antibiotics. The common aminoquinone functional unit is highlighted in *yellow*.

Ecteinascidins are isolated from marine organisms. Ecteinascidin-743 (ET-743) is produced by the Caribbean tunicate Ecteinascidia turbinate. The alkaloid is composed of three fused tetrahydroisoquinoline subunits (A, B, and C). The A subunit and the B subunit provide the scaffold for DNA recognition and covalent bonding. The C subunit protrudes out and interacts with adjacent nuclear proteins. Ecteinascidin-743 binds to the minor groove of DNA, effects guanine *N*2 alkylation (via an intermediate iminium generated from an active carbinolamin functional group), and bends the duplex toward the major groove. This may sequester specific transcription factors, inhibit inducible gene transcription, and result in cytotoxicity. The alkylation at guanine 2–NH_2 positions is sequence selective and region specific to DNA triplets containing a central guanine (AGC, CGC, TGG). Ecteinascidin-743 also binds tightly to Topoisomerase 1, with which it produces cleavage complexes. The compound has activity against a variety of soft tissue sarcomata and is in clinical trials for breast cancer.

Adverse Effects Prolonged infusion benefits efficacy, while hepatic toxicity and myelosuppression are ameliorated by low peak blood concentrations.

Drug Resistance Ecteinascidin-743 decreases the induced expression of ABCB1, the over-expression of which may account for multi-drug resistance in cancer cells.

The minor groove of DNA is frequently unoccupied and vulnerable for chemical attack.
Some minor groove binding antibiotics prefer A/T-rich sequences, others prefer G/C rich sequences.
Antibiotic binding may displace essential transcription factors and interfere with gene expression.
Antibiotics that bind sequence specifically, non-covalently, and reversibly to the minor groove may serve as carriers for alkylating moieties.

The pyrrole-amide backbone of distamycin A, which binds 4–5 adjacent A/T base pairs, serves as a sequence selective vehicle for the delivery of DNA alkylating functions.
Tallimustine alkylates N3 adenines in the target sequence 5'-TTTTGA-3'.
Brostallicin is activated upon binding to Glutathione, catalyzed by Glutathione-S-Transferase (GST). It may thus treat cancers that are resistant to other forms of chemotherapy.

PNU-151807 abolishes Cyclin/CDK kinase activity. Its cytotoxicity is not affected by disruption of P53 function or loss of DNA repair.

In the presence of divalent cations, aureolic acid antibiotics form dimers that non-intercalatively bind to the DNA minor groove in high-GC-content regions.
Upon binding to DNA, the aureolic acid chromophores form hydrogen bonds with NH2 residues of guanines.
Mithramycin A binds to C/G-rich tracts as a dimer and blocks SP-1 family transcription factors.
Ecteinascidin-743 effects guanine N2 alkylation.

2.2.3 Aminoquinone Antibiotics

Quinone containing alkylating drugs (Holzer 1958) have a quinone moiety, which can be reduced, and an alkylating group, which can form covalent bonds with a variety of cellular components (Fig. 2.22). The oxidation state of the quinone moiety modulates the activity of the alkylating element. In many of these agents, reduction of the quinone is required for induction of the alkylating activity. The quinone element may also contribute directly to cytotoxicity through the formation of reactive oxygen species during redox cycling.

The mitomycins were originally discovered by Hata and coworkers (Hata et al. 1956). As prodrugs, they require intracellular activation by 1-electron reducing enzymes like NADPH:Cytochrome P450 Reductase or NADH:Cytochrome b5 Reductase, or by 2-electron reducing enzymes like DT-Diaphorase or Xanthine Dehydrogenase. Reduction of the mitomycins activates the aziridine and carbamate alkylating groups and results in the formation of DNA cross-links, which is the primary mechanism for their anti-tumor effects. In the presence of sufficient levels of oxygen, the reduced mitomycin products can also redox cycle to form reactive oxygen species, which damage cellular components, including DNA.

The natural product mitomycin C <Mutamycin, Mitozytrex>(Wakakietal.1958)isamethylazirinopyrroloindoledione

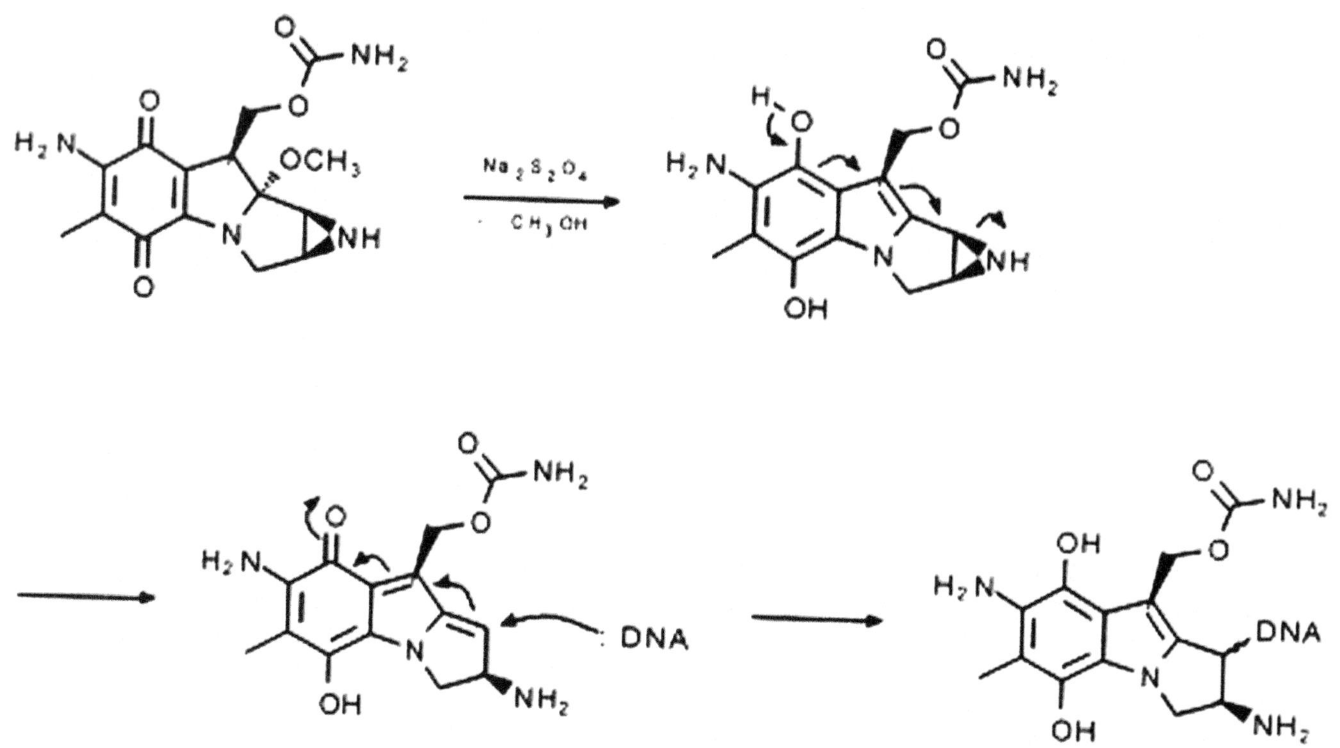

Fig. 2.23 DNA alkylation by mitomycin C. The quinone of mitomycin C is reduced, altering the azinidine group to be opened and set up a conjugated system to a susceptible carbon. Immediately, the nucleophilic DNA attacks the reactive carbon, and the DNA is successfully alkylated. [http://chemistry.creighton.edu/Opportunities/Baumann/WaetzigReport.html]

antibiotic[26] isolated from the bacterium Streptomyces caespitosus. It has been one of the most widely used quinine containing alkylating agents in the clinic (Begleiter 2000). Bioreduced mitomycin C alkylates DNA, produces inter-strand DNA cross-links, and generates oxygen radicals, thereby inhibiting DNA reduplication (Fig. 2.23). Mitomycin C at high concentrations also inhibits RNA and protein synthesis. There is effectiveness against hypoxic, radioresistant cells. The drug is most effective in the front line treatment of select solid tumors, including superficial bladder cancer, and gastric, pancreatic, anal, and esophageal carcinomata. Mitomycin C has been used extensively as a single agent in the treatment of gastric cancer, especially in Japan, with an overall objective response rate of 30 %. More recently, the drug has also been extensively applied in combination chemotherapy regimens. It is used in the palliative treatment of cancers that are advanced or have become resistant to other forms of therapy, generally in combination regimens with doxorubicin and 5-fluorouracil or with bleomycin and vincristine. Mitomycin C is normally administered intravenously at a single dose of 20 mg/m^2 or at 2 mg/m^2/day over 12 days. Other forms of drug delivery are used for specific tumors. Cycles are repeated every 6–8 weeks, provided the leucocyte and platelet counts have recovered sufficiently. The dose may need to be reduced if mitomycin C is combined with other myelosuppressive agents.

- Porfiromycin (methylmitomycin C) is a methyl derivative of mitomycin C, with the methyl group on the nitrogen of the aziridine ring. Porfiromycin was first isolated from Streptomyces ardus in 1960 (DeBoer et al. 1960). The agent is less toxic to tumor cells than mitomycin C under aerobic conditions, but shows similar or greater activity under hypoxic conditions. Thus, porfiromycin has a greater hypoxic:oxic ratio and has greater preferential toxicity to hypoxic cells than mitomycin C. This is likely due to poorer activation of porfiromycin by DT-Diaphorase and a greater dependence of this drug on activation by NADPH:Cytochrome P450 Reductase compared with mitomycin C (Begleiter 2000).
- KW-2149 (7-N-(2-((2-(γ-glutamylamino)ethyl)dithio)ethyl)mitomycin C) (KT6149) is a semi-synthetic, water soluble disulfide derivative of mitomycin C. Activated by blood components and Glutathione, KW-2149 causes inter-strand DNA cross-links and DNA-protein

[26] The pyrroloindole group is common between the mitomycins and cyclopropylpyrroloindole antibiotics.

cross-links, resulting in single strand DNA breaks and inhibition of DNA synthesis.

Pharmacokinetics After intravenous administration, mitomycin C is rapidly cleared from the blood with a half-life of about 15 min. Clearance occurs mostly through hepatic metabolism. Approximately 10% of the drug is excreted unchanged in the urine.

Adverse Effects The utility of mitomycin C is limited by substantial adverse effects. The dose limiting toxicity is myelosuppression, which occurs over 3–4 weeks after drug administration, and is followed by recovery within 8 weeks. This toxicity increases with doses in excess of 10–20 mg/m^2, but the effects are cumulative. Generally, thrombocytopenia or leukopenia are most severe, but anemia is also common. The appearance of thrombocytopenia after mitomycin C treatment is frequently delayed. Approximately 5% of patients receiving the drug develop pulmonary toxicity, including non-cardiogenic pulmonary edema, interstitial pneumonitis and pleural effusions, leading to progressive respiratory insufficiency and death. Corticosteroid therapy can improve the pulmonary symptoms. The risk for this toxicity may increase with exposure to high oxygen concentrations or when mitomycin C is combined with other anticancer drugs that cause pulmonary toxicity (like bleomycin). 5–15% of patients treated with mitomycin C develop cancer associated hemolytic-uremic syndrome, which comprises a complex of micro-angiopathic hemolytic anemia, thrombocytopenia, and renal failure that may lead to death. The syndrome is most common in patients who receive 6–12 months of mitomycin therapy or total doses over 60 mg. Other common toxicities include anorexia, nausea, vomiting and diarrhea.

Mitomycin C extravasation during administration can cause painful skin ulcerations. An important dermatological problem associated with the drug is the necrosis and consequent sloughing of tissue that results if the drug is extravasated during injection. Extravasation is not always immediately symptomatic through accompanying stinging or burning sensations.

Drug Interactions In some cases, severe congestive heart failure arises in patients previously treated with doxorubicin.

Streptonigrin (rufochromomycin, bruneomycin) (BA-163, PC-501) is a metal dependent aminoquinone antibiotic isolated from the bacterium Streptomyces flocculus. Streptonigrin forms complexes with DNA and Topoisomerase 2, resulting in DNA cleavage. This leads to inhibition of DNA reduplication and transcription. This agent also causes free radical mediated cellular damage. Metal-streptonigrin complexes can be reduced to their semiquinone forms by NADH to induce the cleavage of DNA in a manner that depends on superoxide and peroxides. At the chromosome level, this antibiotic causes chromosome damage and increases the frequency of sister chromatid exchanges. The clastogenic action of this compound is partially mediated by free radicals. Streptonigrin has been studied in the treatment of leukemias and lymphomata, breast and cervix carcinomata, gastrointestinal cancers, and head and neck cancers. Oral doses vary 0.2–0.4 mg/day, intravenous doses are 5–7 mg/kg/day for 6 days.

Adverse Effects The clinical potential has been limited by serious adverse effects.

The antibiotics in the class of ansamycins (ansa macrolides[27]), comprising geldanamycin and derivatives, rafamycins, and maytansinoid anti-tumor agents, contain aminoquinone moieties. However, their main mode of action is the inhibition of Heat Shock Protein 90 (HSP90) (see Sect. 4.2.2.).

Mitomycins and streptonigrins comprise the group of anticancer aminoquinone antibiotics.
In quinone containing alkylating drugs, the quinone moiety is subject to redox cycling, while the alkylating group can form covalent bonds with cellular components.
The mitomycins require intracellular activation of their alkylating groups by reducing enzymes (NADPH:Cytochrome P450 Reductase, NADH:Cytochrome b5 Reductase, DT-Diaphorase, or Xanthine Dehydrogenase).
Mitomycin C has effectiveness against hypoxic cells, which are resistant to radiation.
Streptonigrin forms complexes with DNA and Topoisomerase 2 and undergoes redox cycling, resulting in DNA damage.

2.2.4 Polycyclic Aromatic Antibiotics

The anti-tumor activity of polycyclic aromatic compounds is associated with their ability to intercalate into DNA. The planar 3-ring structure accounts for the biological characteristics of these molecules. Anthracyclines, anthracenediones and anthrapyrazoles are groups of agents in this class of drugs.

Classical anthracyclines The first anthracyclines were isolated from the pigment producing Streptomyces peucetius early in the 1960s and were named doxorubicin and daunorubicin. The only difference between these compounds is that the side chain of doxorubicin terminates with a primary alcohol, whereas that of daunorubicin terminates with a methyl group. While doxorubicin is an established component in the treatments of breast cancer, childhood solid tumors, soft tissue sarcomata, and aggressive lymphomata, daunorubicin shows activity in acute lymphoblastic or myeloblastic leu-

[27] The macrolides comprise drugs (typically antibiotics), whose activity stems from the presence of a large macrocyclic lactone ring (usually 14-, 15-, or 16-membered), to which one or more deoxy sugars (usually cladinose and desosamine) may be attached.

kemias. The anthracyclines (drug names end on -rubicin, except for the oligosaccharide anthracyclines which end on -mycin) share aglyconic and sugar moieties. Their two main modes of action comprise Topoisomerase inhibition and the generation of reactive oxygen species.

Topoisomerases modify the topology of DNA without altering the deoxynucleotide structure and sequence. Anthracyclines (Fig. 2.24) intercalate into the DNA. They act by stabilizing a reaction intermediate, in which DNA strands are cut and covalently linked to specific tyrosine residues of Topoisomerase 2, eventually impeding DNA resealing. The formation and stability of a ternary anthracycline-DNA-Topoisomerase 2 complex rely on defined structural determinants (Minotti et al. 2004):

- The planar ring system is important for the intercalation into DNA, as rings B and C overlap with adjacent base pairs and ring D passes through the intercalation site.
- The sugar residue and the cyclohexane ring A are non-intercalating moieties that may play an important role in the formation and stabilization of the ternary complex.
- The sugar moiety, located in the minor groove, is a critical determinant of the activity of anthracyclines as Topoisomerase 2 inhibitors, because inhibition increases in the absence of amino-substituents at C-3′ in the sugar or of the methoxy group at C-4 in ring D.

DNA damage through Topoisomerase 2 inhibition is followed by growth arrest in G_1 and G_2, suppression of RNA and protein synthesis, and ensuing programmed cell death.

Anthracyclines also produce toxic free radical intermediates (Fig. 2.25). A one-electron addition to the quinone moiety in ring C of anthracyclines results in the formation of a semiquinone that rapidly regenerates its parent quinone by reducing oxygen to superoxide anion (O_2^-) and hydrogen peroxide (H_2O_2). This redox cycle is supported by a number of NAD(P)H-Oxidoreductases.

- The redox cycling is accompanied by a release of iron from intracellular stores. Ligand binding interactions of anthracyclines with the released iron then result in the formation of 3:1 drug-iron complexes that convert O_2^- and H_2O_2 into more reactive hydroxyl radicals (OH). Iron mediated free radical reactions enable anthracyclines to produce formaldehyde (HCHO) from carbon cellular sources like spermine and lipids. The anthracy-

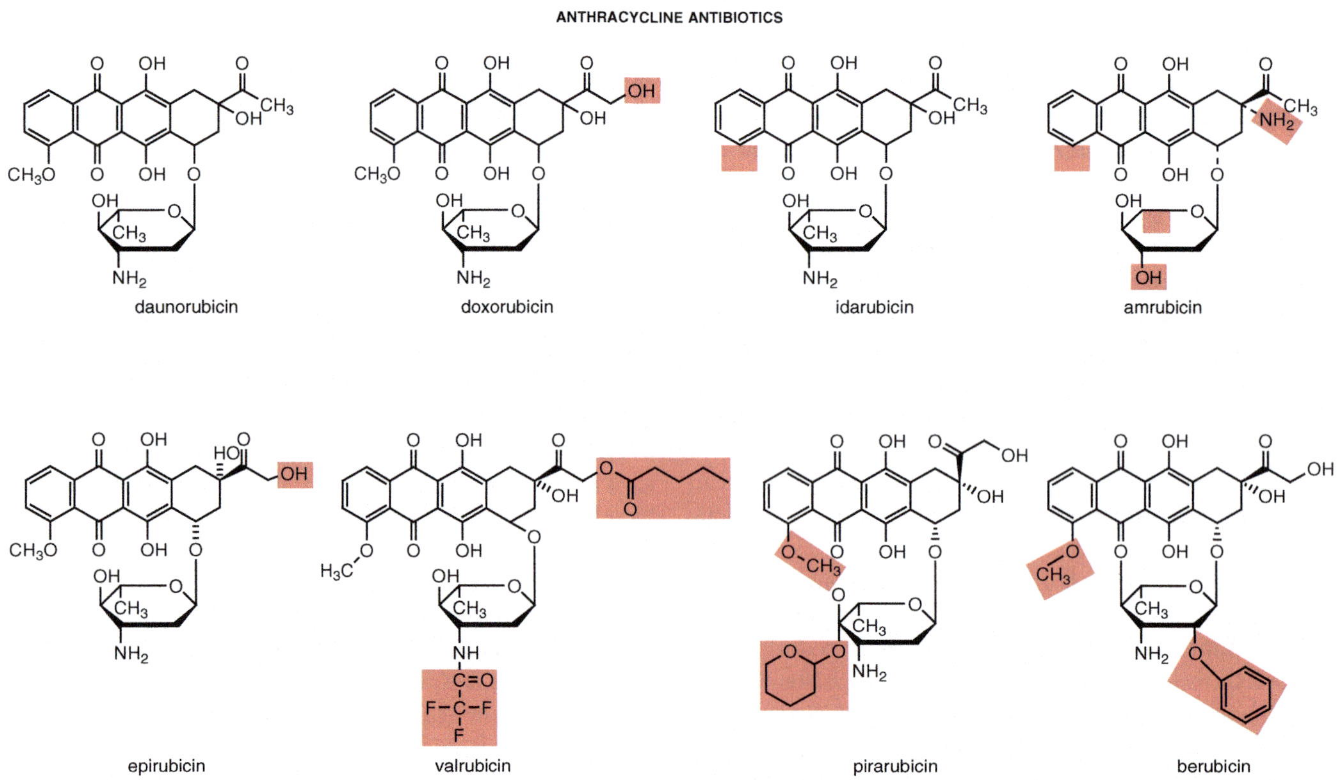

Fig. 2.24 Structures of anthracycline antibiotics. Functional groups that differ from the parent compound, daunorubicin, are highlighted in *pink*

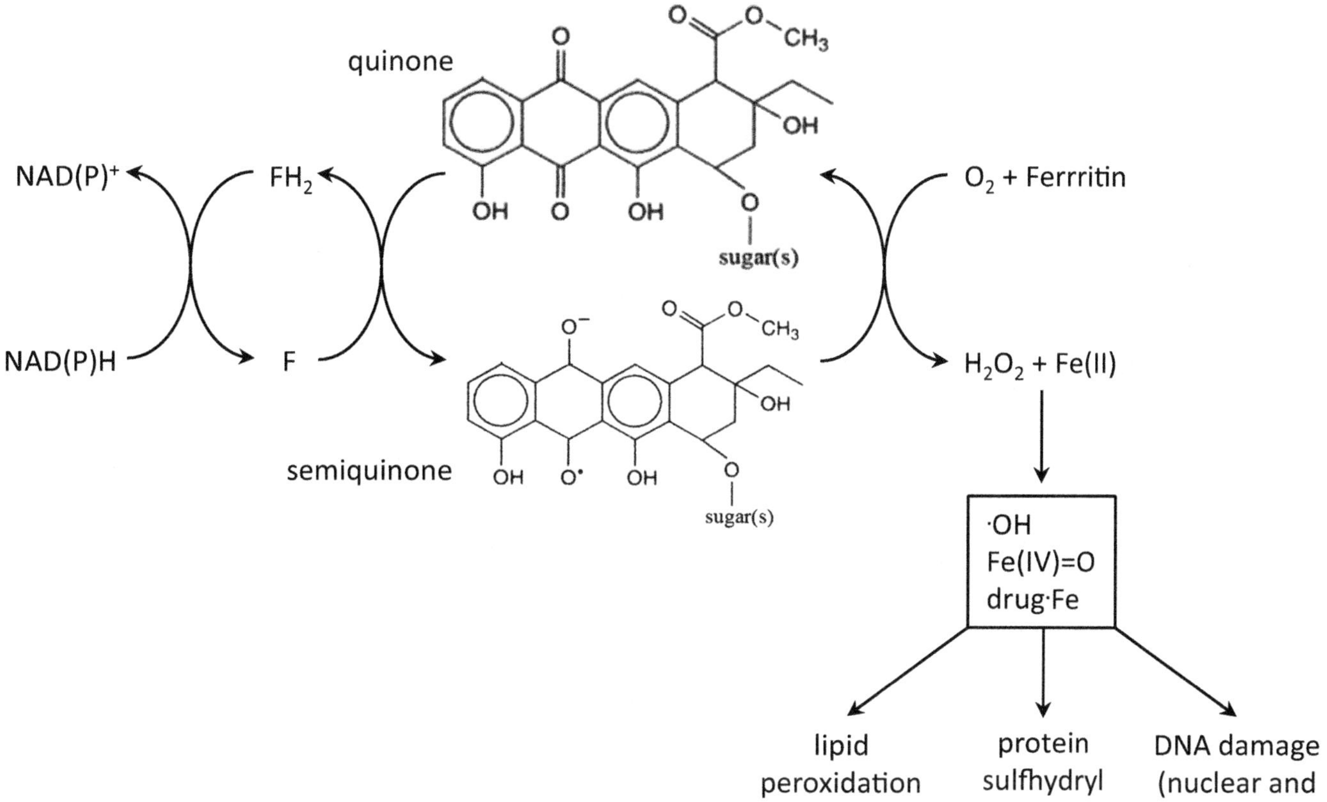

Fig. 2.25 The iron and free radical mechanism of anthracycline cytotoxicity. F/FH_2 represents oxidized/reduced flavoproteins (e.g. NADH Dehydrogenase, NADPH Cytochrome P450 Reductase); Fe(II) indicates low molecular weight Fe^{II}, OH stands for hydroxyl radical, Fe(IV)=O is ferryl ion; drug·Fe is a drug-iron complex. (Redrawn from Minotti et al. 1999)

cline and HCHO then react to form a conjugate, in which two anthracycline molecules bind together with three methylene groups, two forming oxazolidine rings and one binding the oxazolidines together at their 3′-amino nitrogens. The conjugate eventually hydrolyzes to give an active monomeric metabolite, in which the carbon of HCHO is recovered in the form of a Schiff base. Anthracycline-formaldehyde conjugates intercalate into DNA by covalent bonding of the Schiff base with the 2-amino group of a G in the minor groove of the DNA (Taatjes et al. 1997).

- Ceramide formation occurs after reactive oxygen activation of Neutral Sphingomyelinase. Anthracyclines interact with cell membrane lipids, causing lipid peroxidation. At clinically relevant concentrations, they trigger a cyclical cascade of sphingomyelin hydrolysis and formation of ceramide, which activates downstream cell death pathways.
- Anthracyclines can directly release Cytochrome *c* from the mitochondria, thereby inducing apoptosis regardless of DNA damage, active signaling pathways, or P53 status.

Like most anti-cancer drugs, the anthracyclines are used in combination chemotherapy. Because telomeres accumulate single strand breaks and shorten more rapidly after exposure to agents that induce oxidative stress and DNA damage, combining Telomerase inhibition with anthracycline treatment is under consideration as an option for cancer treatment (Minotti et al. 2004).

Pharmacokinetics The intracellular transport of anthracyclines follows a multi-step mechanism,

- they enter cancer cells by diffusion
- they bind with high affinity to the 20S proteasomal subunit in the cytoplasm, forming a complex that translocates into the nucleus via nuclear pores (an ATP-dependent process, facilitated by nuclear localization signals)
- due to their higher affinity for DNA, the anthracyclins dissociate from the proteasome and bind to DNA (Kiyomiya et al. 2001).

In an inactivation step, Carbonyl Reductase (AKR1B10) catalyzes the reduction of daunorubicin to the alcohol daunorubicinol.

Adverse Effects The clinical use of anthracycline antibiotics is hampered by toxicity in healthy tissues. Secondary acute myelogenous leukemia (AML) may arise in cancer patients after treatment. The occurrence of refractory secondary leukemia is more common when anthracyclines are given in combination with DNA damaging anti-neoplastic agents, when patients have been heavily pretreated with cytotoxic drugs, or when doses of anthracyclines have been escalated. Anthracyclines are Pregnancy Category D.

Anthracyclines can cause acute cardiotoxicity that consists of arrhythmias, hypotension, and a mild depression of contractile function—usually within a week of initiation of a regimen. With current treatment protocols, acute toxicity is infrequent, afflicting no more than 1 % of patients, and it is usually reversible. An even more rare acute complication may consist of myocarditis and pericardial effusion, occurring a few weeks after anthracycline administration (Zucchi and Danesi 2003). Chronic cardiac toxicity may develop any time after completion of anthracycline regimens. The prolonged administration induces cardiomyopathy—usually within a year, but very late forms of cardiac dysfunction can arise. Children may develop cardiotoxicity at longer intervals after treatment completion. Chronic cardiomyopathy can evolve into congestive heart failure, which is refractory to standard inotropic medications. The risk for cardiotoxicity is high in patients who have been given cumulative anthracycline doses above 550 mg/m^2. It may occur at lower cumulative doses if anthracyclines are given in combination with agents like taxanes or trastuzumab (anti-ERBB2), and possibly also in conjunction with COX-2 inhibitors. The adverse effects include the loss of myofibrils, dilation of the sarcoplasmic reticulum, cytoplasmic vacuolization, swelling of the mitochondria, and increased numbers of lysosomes. The main mechanism of anthracycline dependent cardiac toxicity is the induction of apoptosis. Cardiomyocytes are more susceptible than other tissues because they exhibit low levels of Catalase and readily undergo inactivation of GSH-PX1 (Selenium-Dependent GSH-Peroxidase-1) after drug exposure. Protection from the cardiotoxicity of anthracyclines can be achieved by slow infusion (48–96 h), provision of antioxidants (flavonoids), and administration of iron chelators such as dexrazoxane (ICRF-187, ADR 529) <Zinecard, Totect>. According to the American Society for Clinical Oncology (ASCO), the use of dexrazoxane is recommended in

- patients who have received more than 300 mg/m^2 for metastatic breast cancer and who may benefit from continued doxorubicin treatment
- patients who have received more than 300 mg/m^2 doxorubicin for the treatment of malignancies other than breast cancer
- patients who responded to previous anthracycline based chemotherapy for advanced breast cancer and who may benefit from continued therapy with epirubicin (Schuchter et al. 2002).

Dexrazoxane does not affect the pharmacokinetics of anthracyclines. Unrelated to cardiac protection, dexrazoxane may also be indicated as an emergency treatment of extravasation resulting from intravenous anthracycline chemotherapy[28].

Drug Resistance The clinical use of anthracycline antibiotics is hampered by the development of resistance in tumor cells, which may be due to an over-expression of ABCB1 (MDR1, PGP), increased levels of enzymes that protect form reactive oxygen damage, activation of the transcription factor NF-κB that exerts crucial functions in cellular resistance to oxidants, altered *topoisomerase 2* gene expression or activity, or enzymatic drug inactivation.

The anthracycline daunorubicin was originally isolated from bacteria in soil samples taken from the Italian castle Castel del Monte. A French research group also discovered the compound at about the same time. Jointly, the teams named it daunorubicin, combining the name Dauni (an ancient Roman tribe that once occupied the Italian area where the compound was isolated) with rubis (the French word for ruby describing the color of the compound). Based on the risk for adverse cardiac effects, the maximum recommended cumulative dose of daunorubicin is tentatively set at 500 mg/m^2.

- Daunorubicin hydrochloride <Cerubidine> for infusion is indicated in combination chemotherapy for remission induction in acute non-lymphocytic (myelogenous, monocytic, or erythroid) leukemia in adults and for remission induction in acute lymphocytic leukemia in children and adults. Profound myelosuppression is inevitable when used in therapeutic doses. Extravasation during administration results in severe local tissue necrosis.
- The use of liposomes as carriers is an approach to decrease anthracycline related cardiac toxicity. Liposomal PEGylated forms of daunorubicin have been designed to increase the amount of drug delivered to tumors and decrease the peak distribution to the heart and gastrointestinal mucosa. This formulation preferentially accumulates in the tumor vasculature, resulting in a sustained targeted release of free daunorubicin in the tumor micro-environment. Peglyation increases the half-life of the liposome through inhibiting its phagocytosis by the reticuloendothelial system. However, the polyethylene

[28] Dexrazoxane is administered over 3 days (1000 mg/m^2 within the first 6 h, 1000 mg/m^2 around 24 h, 500 mg/m^2 around 48 h). The dosages are reduced by half in patients with creatinine clearance values below 40 mL/min. Possible adverse effects include nausea and vomiting, diarrhea, sore mouth, decreased white blood cell count, decreased platelet count, and infusion site burning. Dexrazoxane may also compromise the anti-tumor effects of athracyclines.

glycol (PEG) in the formulation may cause hand-foot syndrome as an adverse effect[29].

- Liposomal daunorubicin <DaunoXome> is a liposome encapsulated preparation with a diameter of 45 nm that is free of polyethylene glycol. A bilayer of distearoylphosphatidylcholine and cholesterol encapsulates daunorubicin citrate (10:5:1 molar ratio). The half-life is shorter than that of PEGylated liposomes. Liposomal daunorubicin is under investigation for the treatment of AIDS-related Kaposi sarcoma, acute myeloblastic leukemia, multiple myeloma, non-Hodgkin lymphoma, and breast cancer.

Pharmacokinetics Carbonyl Reductase (CBR) catalyzes the reduction of daunorubicin to its corresponding alcohol, daunorubicinol, which changes the pharmacological properties of this cancer chemotherapeutic drug. The ratio of area under the concentration-time curve (AUC) for metabolite to parent drug is lower for liposomal daunorubicin than for free daunorubicin, mainly due to higher concentrations of the parent drug in the blood.

Researchers at the Italian pharmaceutical company Farmitalia mutated a strain of Streptomyces (Streptococcus peucetius var. caesius) using *N*-nitroso-*N*-methyl urethane to produce a red colored antibiotic different from daunorubicin. They originally named it adriamycin, after the Adriatic Sea. Doxorubicin (hydroxydaunorubicin, adriamycin) became available in 1968. The drug is an intercalator and a Topoisomerase 2 inhibitor that prevents DNA reduplication and ultimately inhibits protein synthesis. It also generates oxygen free radicals, resulting in the cytotoxic peroxidation of cell membrane lipids. Like many other genotoxic agents, doxorubicin activates the binding of P53 to DNA, likely inducing apoptosis in this manner. P53 activation also contributes to the induction of the $p21^{CIP1/WAF1}$ gene product, which is a strong inhibitor of Cyclin-Dependent Kinases (CDKs) involved in the G_1/S transition of the cell cycle. The maximum recommended cumulative dose of doxorubicin is tentatively set at 450–600 mg/m^2.

Pharmacokinetics Steady state plasma concentrations are 25–250 nM, with peak concentrations reaching 5 μM. Tissue uptake of doxorubicin is rapid, while its slow elimination from tissues is reflected by a terminal half-life of 20–48 h. Clearance occurs mostly through metabolism (mainly to doxorubicinol) and biliary excretion. The systemic clearance of doxorubicin is substantially reduced in obese women. The drug does not cross the blood brain barrier.

Formulations of doxorubicin include the salt, PEGylated liposomes, liposomes, coupling to HPMA, coupling to targeting peptides, conjugation to magnetic carriers, derivatization.

- The hydrochloride salt of doxorubicin <Adriamycin PFS, Adriamycin RDF, Rubex> is indicated for inducing regression in disseminated neoplastic conditions such as acute lymphoblastic leukemia, acute myeloblastic leukemia, Hodgkin lymphoma, Wilms tumor, neuroblastoma, soft tissue and bone sarcomata, ovarian carcinoma, transitional cell bladder carcinoma, thyroid carcinoma, gastric carcinoma, and small-cell bronchogenic carcinoma. Doxorubicin is also indicated as a component in the adjuvant therapy for women with axillary lymph node involvement of breast cancer.
- Liposomes are multi-lamellar lipid particles suitable for drug delivery. They improve doxorubicin penetration into tumors and decrease drug clearance, thereby increasing the duration of therapeutic drug effects. This form may exhibit an improved toxicity profile due to the lower concentrations of free doxorubicin to which non-transformed tissues are exposed. Liposomal PEGylated doxorubicin hydrochloride <Doxil, Dox-SL, Evacet, LipoDox, Caelyx, Doxilen> is a formulation, in which a doxorubicin containing liposome is surrounded by a layer of polyethylene glycol (PEG). Liposomal PEGylated forms of doxorubicin may be indicated for the second-line treatment of ovarian cancer (disease progression or recurrence after platinum based chemotherapy), multiple myeloma (in combination with bortezomib), AIDS-related Kaposi sarcoma (after failure of prior systemic chemotherapy), high grade glioma or glioblastoma or secondary brain tumors, and head and neck squamous cell carcinoma. An intermittent 3-weekly schedule is appropriate, and the maximum tolerated dose is 60–90 mg/m^2. Hypersensitivity may occur in up to 10 % of patients.
- Liposomal doxorubicin citrate (TLC D-99) <Myocet> is a liposome encapsulated form of the doxorubicin citrate salt that does not contain polyethylene glycol. The disposition of doxorubicin when administered as Myocet reflects that of the liposome and differs substantially from plain doxorubicin. The formulation improves the drug penetration into tumors and decreases drug clearance, thereby increasing the duration of therapeutic drug effects. It may have benefits in the treatment of breast cancer.
- Doxorubicin-HPMA conjugate is a co-polymer conjugate of doxorubicin and the water soluble polymer N-(2-hydroxypropyl) methacrylamide (HPMA). Conjugation with HPMA improves the therapeutic effects of doxorubicin, by promoting drug accumulation inside tumors, while decreasing systemic toxicity.

[29] Hand-foot syndrome (palmar-plantar erythrodysesthesia, acrauding erythema, Burgdof syndrome) manifests in painful bilateral swelling, erythema, and tenderness over the palms and soles that evolves into desquamation. The long-term circulation of the PEGylated daunorubicin allows protracted extravasation and underlies this form of hand-foot syndrome. Interactions between daunorubicin and metallic Cu^{II} ions abundant in skin tissue generate reactive oxygen species, which stimulate Chemokine secretion from keratinocytes and result in inflammation.

- An extracellularly tumor-activated prodrug (ETAP) incorporates both a tumor specific recognition site and a tumor selective enzymatic activation sequence. It is unable to enter healthy cells but is proteolytically activated by Peptidases that are rather selectively secreted by cancer cells. Doxocycline delivery to tumors can be improved by coupling it to ETAPs. The bicyclic peptide CDCRG-DCFC (RGD-4C) selectively binds to Integrins $\alpha_V\beta_3$ and $\alpha_V\beta_5$, which are highly over-expressed in invading tumor endothelial cells. A distinct tumor specific sequence is the tripeptide D-Ala-Phe-Lys that is recognized by the tumor associated protease Plasmin, an important factor of tumor invasion and metastasis. An aminocaproyl residue is incorporated as a spacer between the two peptide sequences, whereas a self-eliminating 4-aminobenzyl alcohol spacer is inserted between the Plasmin substrate and doxorubicin. This prodrug is designed to have Plasmin dependent cytotoxicity for endothelial cells and some tumor cells, but it requires improvements in water solubility and bioavailability (de Groot et al. 2002).
- L-377,202 is an extracellularly tumor-activated prodrug characterized by a covalent linkage of doxorubicin to N-glutaryl-[4-hydroxyprolyl]-Ala-Ser-cyclohexaglycyl -Glu-Ser-Leu. In the presence of prostate cancer cells that secrete the serine protease PSA (Prostate Specific Antigen), the peptide moiety of L-377,202 is hydrolyzed to release doxorubicin or Leu-doxorubicin, the latter being freely diffusible and activated to doxorubicin inside the target cells. L-377,202 is considerably more toxic to PSA expressing tumor cells than to PSA negative normal or tumor cells (Denmeade et al. 1998).
- The extracellularly tumor-activated prodrug N-succinyl-Ala-L-Leu-L-Ala-L-Leu- doxorubicin (CPI-0004Na) is a tetrapeptidic derivative of doxorubicin. CPI-0004Na does not undergo hydrolysis in the blood nor does it enter cells, but it is activated by tumor Peptidases to give N-(L-Leu- doxorubicin), which eventually diffuses inside the cells. CPI-0004Na is substantially less toxic than doxorubicin due to its lower accumulation in the heart and other untransformed tissues (Trouet et al. 2001).
- Doxorubicin-magnetic targeted carrier complex consists of doxorubicin bound to microscopic beads of activated carbon and iron (magnetic targeted carriers). With the placement of a magnet on the body surface overlying a tumor site, this carrier complex delivers doxorubicin preferentially to the tumor, thereby prolonging the duration of the therapeutic effects while decreasing its systemic toxicity.

Adverse Effects The occurrence of doxorubicin dependent cardiac toxicity is related to the total lifetime dose, and increases sharply in people who receive a cumulative dose of more than 400 mg/m^2. The combination of doxorubicin with cyclophosphamide causes a dramatic increase in the risk of secondary malignancies, most often acute myelomonocytic leukemia.

Second generation anthracyclines Idarubicin <Idamycin, Idamycin PFS> is a semi-synthetic anthracycline derived from daunorubicin. Due to its high lipophilicity (caused by the absence of a methoxyl group in position four), idarubicin penetrates cell membranes better than other anthracycline antibiotics. The hydrochloride salt is the therapeutic form of this drug, which is active against acute myelogenous leukemia (FAB classifications M1 through M7), multiple myeloma, non-Hodgkin lymphoma, and breast cancer (Borchmann et al. 1997). For adult AML, idarubicin is given at 12 mg/m^2 daily for 3 days by slow intravenous injection in combination with cytarabine for 12 days. A second course may be administered.

Pharmacokinetics Idarubicin may be administered orally with 10–30 % bioavailability. The tissue distribution of idarubicin is extensive. The elimination rate of idarubicin from the blood is slow with a mean terminal half-life around 22 h. The elimination of the metabolite idarubicinol is slower than that of the parent drug with a mean terminal half-life that exceeds 45 h. There is substantial hepatic metabolism, with idarubicinol being the primary active metabolite being formed. As idarubicinol has cytotoxic activity, it contributes to the effects of idarubicin. The drug is eliminated predominately by biliary excretion and to a lesser extent by renal excretion.

Adverse Effects Idarubicin is given slowly by intravenous infusion over 10–15 min. Local tissue necrosis can occur if there is extravasation. The agent is associated with a reduction in the left ventricular ejection fraction (LVEF) that may progress to congestive heart failure. The risk is increased in patients over 50 years of age. Severe myelosuppression occurs when idarubicin is used at effective therapeutic doses. Administration of the 2nd course should be delayed in patients who experience severe mucositis, until recovery from this toxicity has occurred, and a dose reduction of 25 % is recommended. Other adverse effects comprise infection, nausea and vomiting, hair loss, abdominal cramps and diarrhea, hemorrhage, alopecia, generalized rash, urticaria, and a bullous erythrodermatous rash of the palms and soles. The drug is Pregnancy Category D.

Amrubicin ((7S,9S)-9-acetyl-9-amino-7-[(2S,4S,5R)-4,5-dihydroxyoxan-2-yl]oxy-6,11-dihydroxy-8,10-dihydro-7*H*-tetracene-5,12-dione) (SM-5887) <Calced> is a synthetic anthracycline that exerts stronger anti-cancer activity than conventional anthracyclines, with reduced cumulative cardiotoxicity. Developed in Japan, it has been marketed there since 2002. Testing and use of this drug in the U.S. for small cell lung cancer and potentially for breast cancer has been expedited under the U.S. FDA orphan drug designation.

Adverse Effects Adverse events of grade 3 or worse occur in the majority of patients, with neutropenia (65 %) and thrombocytopenia (40 %) being the most common. The incidence is highest during the 1st or 2nd amrubicin cycle, and then decreases during subsequent cycles. There is no indication of cardiotoxicity.

Epirubicin hydrochloride <Pharmorubicin, Ellence> is a hydrochloride salt that intercalates into DNA and interacts with Topoisomerase 2, thereby inhibiting DNA reduplication and repair, as well as RNA and protein synthesis. This agent also produces toxic free radical intermediates and interacts with cell membrane lipids causing lipid peroxidation. The drug is a semi-synthetic derivative of doxorubicin obtained by an axial-to-equatorial epimerization of the hydroxyl group at C-4′ in daunosamine. This positional change has little effect on the spectrum of activity, but it introduces pharmacokinetic and metabolic effects, including an increased volume of distribution, 4-*O*-glucuronidation, and consequently enhanced total body clearance. It can therefore be used at high cumulative doses, resulting in anti-tumor activity without increased cardiotoxicity. Epirubicin is indicated as a component of adjuvant therapy following the resection of primary breast cancer with evidence of axillary node involvement. The recommended starting dose of epirubicin is 100–120 mg/m^2. The recommended maximum cumulative dose is 900 mg/m^2.

Pharmacokinetics Plasma clearance is not affected by the duration of infusion or administration schedule. The drug is rapidly and widely distributed into the tissues. About 75 % of the drug binds to plasma proteins. The blood concentration declines in a triphasic manner with mean half-lives for the α-, β-, and γ- phases of about 3 min, 3 h, and 33 h. Epirubicin is extensively and rapidly metabolized by the liver and by red blood cells. Four main metabolic inactivation pathways include

- reduction of the C-13 keto group to form the 13(S)-dihydro derivative epirubicinol
- conjugation of both the parent drug and epirubicinol with glucuronate
- hydrolytic removal of the amino sugar moiety to form epirubicin and epirubicinol aglycones
- loss of the amino sugar moiety through a redox process with the formation of the 7-deoxy-epirubicin aglycone and 7-deoxy-epirubicinol aglycone.

Epirubicin and its major metabolites are eliminated primarily through biliary excretion and, to a lesser extent, by urinary excretion. The dosage should be reduced in patients with impaired hepatic function. The clearance of epirubicin from the blood declines in older women.

Adverse Effects Substantial myelosuppression (predominantly leukopenia and neutropenia) is a common adverse effect. Generally, the white blood cell counts return to normal within 3 weeks after the end of treatment. Myocardial toxicity, potentially leading to fatal congestive heart failure, may occur either during therapy with epirubicin or months to years after the termination of therapy. Amenorrhea and hot flashes (hot flushes) can arise in female patients. Lethargy, nausea and vomiting (can be limited with prophylactic antiemetics), and alopecia are common. Mucositis of the mouth or esophagus is possible. Extravasation may cause severe local tissue necrosis. Contraindications are

- baseline neutrophil count below 1500 cells/mm^3
- severe myocardial insufficiency, recent myocardial infarction, severe arrhythmias
- previous treatment with anthracyclines up to the maximum cumulative dose
- hypersensitivity to epirubicin, other anthracyclines, or anthracenediones
- severe hepatic dysfunction.

The drug is Pregnancy Category D.

Drug Interactions The concomitant use of epirubicin with compounds that can cause heart failure requires close constant monitoring of cardiac function. The administration of paclitaxel prior to epirubicin or cimetidine with epirubicin results in an increase in the epirubicin drug exposure.

Valrubicin (*N*-trifluoroacetyladriamycin-14-valerate) <Valstar> is a semi-synthetic analog of the anthracycline doxorubicin. Valrubicin causes DNA damage, inhibits Topoisomerase 2, and leads to cell cycle arrest in G_2. It is administered by infusion directly into the bladder to treat BCG-refractory bladder cancer[30]. It penetrates into the bladder wall. The drug is given at a dose of 800 mg, administered intravesically once a week for 6 weeks. The success rate of valrubicin for remission of bladder carcinoma in situ is about 20 %. If there is not a complete response to treatment within 3 months or if there is a recurrence, cystectomy must be considered to avoid the development of metastatic bladder cancer.

Pharmacokinetics During a 2 h dose-retention period in the bladder wall, conversion to the major metabolites *N*-trifluoroacetyladriamycin and *N*-trifluoroacetyladriamycinol is negligible. The drug is essentially completely excreted by voiding the instillate.

Adverse Effects Over 80 % of patients experience local adverse events. They are typically reversible within 1 week.

---

[30] Immunotherapy in the form of Bacillus Calmette-Guerin (BCG) instillation is used to treat and prevent the recurrence of superficial bladder tumors. Patients at highest risk for recurrence after transurethral resection may receive adjuvant intravesical immunotherapy with BCG. It is effective in up to 2/3 of the cases at this stage.

Urinary tract infections can arise. Most systemic adverse events associated with the use of valrubicin are mild, resolving within 24 h after drug administration. To avoid systemic exposure, valrubicin should not be administered if the integrity of the bladder mucosa is compromised. It is contraindicated in patients with known hypersensitivity to anthracyclines or polyoxyl castor oil. Valrubicin is Pregnancy Category C, the drug is secreted into the milk.

Pirarubicin (4′-O-tetrahydropyranyl doxorubicin) <Pinorubicin, Theprubicine, Therarubicin, THP-Doxorubicin> is a 4-tetrahydropyranyl doxorubicin.

Pharmacokinetics Pirarubicin has a triphasic elimination α, β, and γ half-lives of 0.1, 1.4, and 34 h, respectively. The cumulative 24-h urinary excretion is less than 10 % of the administered dose. Pirarubicin has a higher hepatic extraction than doxorubicin. It may therefore be suited for intraportal injection to treat liver metastases.

Adverse Effects Pirarubicin may cause a significant decrease in the left ventricular ejection fraction at cumulative doses over 460 mg/m^2. In elderly patients with non-Hodgkin lymphoma, pirarubicin may cause severe cardiac dysfunction at cumulative doses as low as 360 mg/m^2 (Dhingra et al. 1995; Niitsu et al. 1998).

Berubicin hydrochloride (RTA 744) is an anthracycline derivative that intercalates into DNA and interrupts Topoisomerase 2 activity. It has U.S. FDA approval as an orphan drug for the treatment of malignant gliomata.

Pharmacokinetics Unlike other anthracycline derivatives, berubicin crosses the blood-brain barrier and reaches therapeutic levels in the brain. It is therefore used for the treatment of primary and secondary (breast or lung cancer metastases) brain cancers.

Drug Resistance The drug is not subject to efflux via ABC transporters.

Carubicin (carminomycin) is an anthracycline cytostatic antibiotic, initially isolated from Actinomadura carminata and developed in the former USSR. Carubicin intercalates into DNA and interacts with Topoisomerase 2, thereby inhibiting DNA reduplication and repair, as well as RNA and protein synthesis. The agent is used to treat patients with advanced breast cancer or leukemia. Carubicin may be given at 20 mg/m^2 every 3 weeks.

Adverse Effects There is no substantial risk for cardiotoxicity at a cumulative dose of up to 150 mg/kg. The drug has similar hematotoxicity to doxorubicin. Other adverse effects include nausea, vomiting, anorexia, and diarrhea.

Esorubicin (4′-deoxydoxorubicin) (NSC 267469) is a synthetic derivative of doxorubicin which differs by the lack of a hydroxyl group in the 4′ position of the amino sugar. The recommended dose is 30 mg/m^2 intravenously every 3 weeks

Adverse Effects The mucosal injury, which has deterred advocacy for doxorubicin in the treatment of acute leukemia, is not induced by esorubicin. However, the drug causes dose limiting bone marrow suppression in solid tumor patients, leading to a higher incidence of neutropenia (and resulting risk of sepsis). Esorubicin may offer slightly less cardiotoxicity than doxorubicin. A 5 % drop in the left ventricular ejection fraction (LVEF) arises following approximately 240 mg/m^2, a 10 % drop arises after approximately 480 mg/m^2. Nausea and vomiting are severe in 15 % of patients, total alopecia arises in about 5 % of all cases.

Detorubicin (14-Diethoxyacetoxydaunorubicin) is the semi-synthetic 14-diethoxyacetoxy ester of daunorubicin. Detorubicin remains stable in acidic environments while it is very quickly hydrolyzed into doxorubicin under neutral pH conditions, and therefore acts as a prodrug. Although hydrolysis occurs within minutes after injection in the blood stream the tissue distribution of detorubicin is unique. The drug is administered in a dose range of 120–180 mg/m^2 and repeated at 3-week intervals.

Adverse Effects The cardiotoxicity is similar to daunorubicin. The general myelosuppressive and gastrointestinal toxicities were acceptable and short in duration.

Duborimycin (daunorubicinol, 13-dihydrodaunorubicin) (KST-1A3492, AC1Q6JIZ, CID83845, LS-94072) is an anthracycline that represents the main metabolite of daunorubicin.

Adverse Effects In rare cases, grade 3–4 mucositis can arise. Cardiac toxicity may arise in close to 20 % of patients and can be serious.

Zorubicin (rubidazone, benzoyl hydrazone daunorubicin) (RP-22050) is a benzoyl-hydrazone derivative of daunorubicin. It has limited activity against breast cancer and hairy cell leukemia.

New generation anthracyclines New generation anthracyclines include

- anthracyclines with morpholinyl or alkyl substituents at the amino group at C-3 and disaccharide anthracyclines, in which the amino group is displaced to the second sugar. Like the first generation anthracyclines, these are nuclear targeted compounds that intercalate into DNA
- anthracyclines that combine modifications at C-14 with modifications of the aminosugar. These non-nuclear targeted analogs no longer intercalate into DNA, but potentiate apoptotic events modulated by Protein Kinase C (PKC)

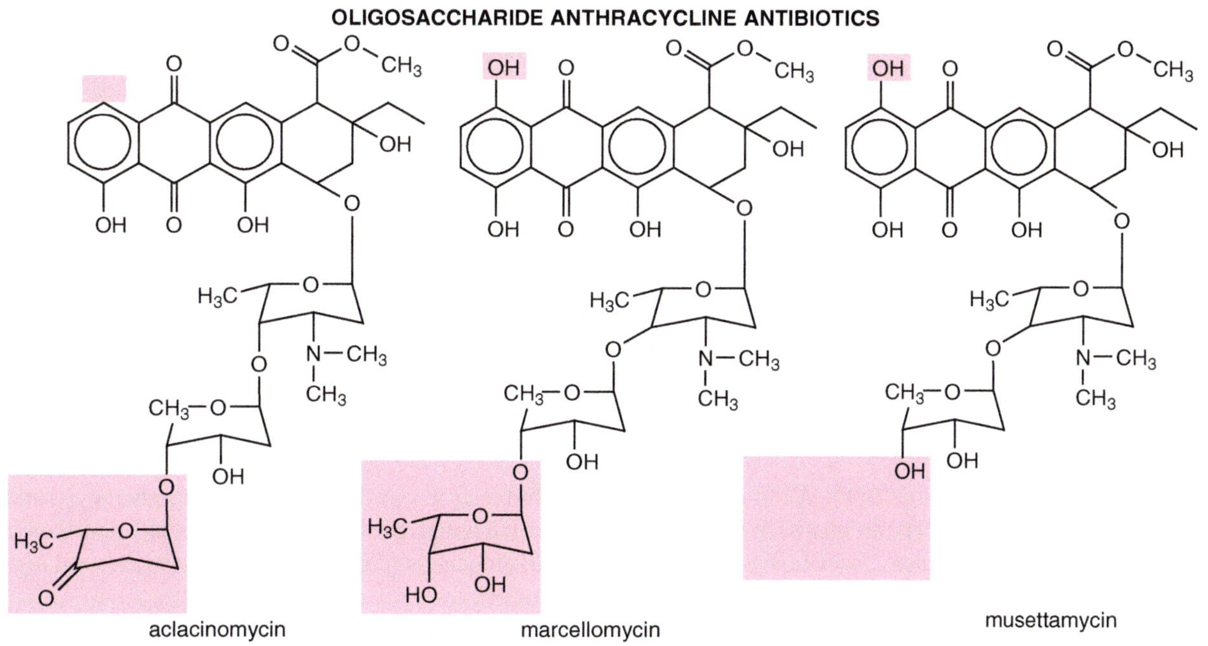

Fig. 2.26 Structures of oligosaccharide anthracycline antibiotics. The agents in this sub-group differ predominantly in the lengths of the sugar chains. Domains of structural variation are highlighted in *pink*

- Oligosaccharide anthracyclines constitute a class of inducers of hematopoietic differentiation.

Aclarubicin (aclacinomycin A) (NSC-208734, MA144-A1) <Aclacin, Aclacinomycine, Aclacinon, Aclaplastin, Jaclacin, Klasinomycin> is a trisaccharide anthracycline isolated form the bacterium Streptomyces galilaeus (Fig. 2.26). It is active in adult patients with acute myeloblastic leukemia. However, it is inactive in women with metastatic breast cancer (Natale et al. 1993). The drug is administered by intravenous infusion. In adults, the initial dose is 175–300 mg/m^2, divided over 3–7 consecutive days, followed by maintenance at 25–100 mg/m^2 every 3–4 weeks.

Adverse Effects Aclarubicin is contraindicated in patients with severe heart disease, bone marrow depression, or hypersensitivity. It is generally cardially tolerable but may induce late cardiac events in adult patients with refractory acute myelogenous or lymphoblastic leukemia (Dabich et al. 1986). The agent has no known mutagenicity or carcinogenicity. The drug is Pregnancy Category D.

Drug Resistance Aclarubicin is non-cross-resistant to the first line anthracyclines daunorubicin and doxorubicin.

The oligosaccharide anthracyclines marcellomycin, musettamycin, and rudolfomycin were isolated from the bacterium Actinosporangium bohemicum and are poetically named after characters in Puccini's opera La Boheme.

The trisaccharide marcellomycin intercalates into DNA and induces DNA cross-links. This agent may induce differentiation in promyelocytic leukemia cells by interfering with glycoprotein synthesis. Marcellomycin induces little myelosuppression and is less cardiotoxic than doxorubicin.

Musettamycin, collinemycin, and schaunardimycin are disaccharides.

Anthracenedione antibiotics The anthracenediones (anthraquinones, dioxoanthracenes) (drug names end on -antrone) were developed to reduce the frequency and severity of anthracycline induced adverse effects on the heart by substituting the cardiotoxic aminoglycone with aminoalkylamino side chains (Fig. 2.27). The diaminoalkyl groups are crucial for the biological activity of these compounds. However, while the anthracenedione mitoxantrone is less cardiotoxic than the anthracyclines, it is also somewhat less effective. Ametantrone and mitoxantrone are structurally similar members of the class. While both drugs are strong intercalators, their cytostatic, cytotoxic, and anti-tumor activities differ, with mitoxantrone being 10–100 times more potent on a molar basis. There is a correlation between their potency and their ability to condense nucleic acids inasmuch as mitoxantrone condenses nucleic acids at concentrations that are 5–40-fold lower than those of ametantrone. The condensation is base- and sugar-specific, with the long purine sequences of single stranded RNA being the most sensitive

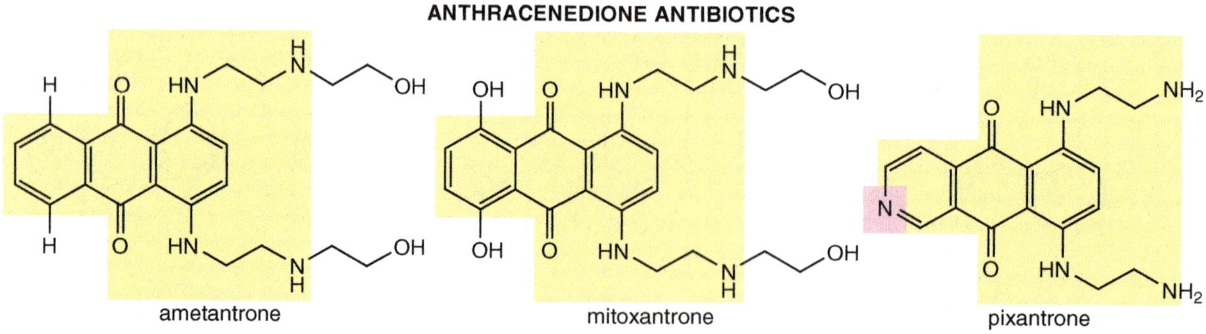

Fig. 2.27 Structures of anthracenedione antibiotics. The common functional unit is highlighted in *yellow*. The divergent nitrogen in the triple ring structure of pixantrone is highlighted in *pink*

(Kapuscinski and Darzynkiewicz 1986). Anthracenediones may also act as anti-oxidants. These agents concentration-dependently inhibit conjugated diene formation from linoleic acid.

Pharmacokinetics Anthracenediones may require metabolic activation before effectively intercalating into DNA. They are substrates for UDP-Glucuronosyl Transferase 1–8 (UGT1A8).

Random screening at the U.S. National Cancer Institute of a large number of compounds provided by the Allied Chemical Company identified the anti-cancer activity of ametantrone acetate (1,4-bis((2-((2-hydroxyethyl)amino)ethyl) amino)-9,10-anthracenedione diacetate) (NSC 287513, NSC-196473).

Pharmacokinetics The blood levels of ametantrone decline in a triexponential fashion, with a mean terminal half-life of 25 h. The steady state volume of distribution is large. About 5 % of the total dose is excreted unchanged in the urine, indicating that there is another major route of elimination.

Adverse Effects Reversible leukopenia is the dose limiting toxic effect. Non-hematologic toxicity includes a marked cumulative blue discoloration of the skin that occurs in patients who have received more than three courses of the drug. The agent is teratogenic.

Mitoxantrone was synthesized in an attempt to develop agents with comparable anti-tumor activity to doxorubicin, but with an improved safety profile. It was designed as a deliberate modification of the parent 1,4-dehydroxyl analog, ametantrone. Mitoxantrone hydrochloride (DHAD, 1,4-dihydroxy-5,8-bis[[2-[(2-hydroxyethyl) amino]ethyl] amino]-9,10-anthracenedione dihydrochloride) (NSC-29919) <Novantrone> intercalates into and cross-links DNA, thereby disrupting DNA reduplication and RNA synthesis. This agent also binds to Topoisomerase 2, resulting in DNA strand breaks and inhibition of DNA repair. The mechanism of action of mitoxanthrone is similar to that of the anthracyclines.

- Mitoxantrone in combination chemotherapy is indicated in the initial treatment of adult acute non-lymphocytic (myelogenous, promyelocytic, monocytic, and erythroid) leukemias.
- Mitoxantrone in combination with corticosteroids is indicated as a palliative treatment for advanced hormone refractory prostate cancer.
- Because mitoxantrone is somewhat less effective than the anthracyclines it has not received U.S. FDA approval for the treatment of breast cancer.

The recommended individual dose is 12–14 mg/m^2 with the timing being determined by the combination therapy regimen used.

Pharmacokinetics The pharmacokinetics of mitoxantrone is characterized by a three compartment distribution, with the mean α half-life of mitoxantrone being 5–15 min, the mean β half-life 1–3 h, and the mean γ (terminal or elimination) half-life 1–10 days (median approximately 75 h). The distribution to tissues is extensive with the steady-state volume of distribution exceeding 1,000 L/m^2. In patients administered 15–90 mg/m^2 of mitoxantrone intravenously, there is a linear relationship between dose and the area under the concentration-time curve. In the concentration range of 25–450 ng/mL, mitoxantrone is 80 % bound to plasma proteins. The metabolites are composed of monocarboxylic and dicarboxylic acid derivatives and their glucuronide conjugates. The drug is excreted in urine and feces, either unchanged or in the form of inactive metabolites.

Adverse Effects Mitoxantrone is administered slowly by infusion. Severe local tissue damage can occur if there is extravasation during this process. Except for the treatment of acute non-lymphocytic leukemia, mitoxantrone therapy generally should not be given to patients with baseline neutrophil counts of fewer than 1500 cells/mm^3. The occurrence of bone marrow suppression can cause neutropenia, which may lead to infections. Although mitoxantrone is less cardiotoxic than doxorubicin, the monitoring of the left ventricular ejection fraction is important during therapy. Secondary acute myelogenous leukemia (AML) may arise in cancer patients treated with mitoxantrone.

Pixantrone was originally synthesized by Miles P. Hacker and Paul A. Krapcho. It was developed to reduce the heart damage resulting from anthracycline treatment while retaining efficacy. The drug was structurally designed so that it cannot bind iron and perpetuate oxygen radical production or form a long-lived hydroxyl metabolite, both of which are mechanisms for anthracycline induced acute and chronic cardiotoxicity.

Pixantrone dimaleate (6,9-bis[(2-aminoethyl)amino] benzo[*g*]isoquinoline-5,10-dione) (BBR 2778) <Pixuvri> acts as a Topoisomerase 2 inhibitor and intercalating agent. It is under study for the treatment of various solid and hematologic malignancies. It received fast track designation by the U.S. FDA for patients who have previously been treated two or more times for relapsed or refractory aggressive non-Hodgkin lymphoma. In Europe it is available on a Named-Patient basis (a compassionate use designation). The drug is administered through intravenous infusion.

Anthrapyrazole antibiotics Chromophore modification of the anthracenediones in an attempt to provide agents with diminished or no cardiotoxicity has resulted in the anthrapyrazole class of DNA binders. The anthrapyrazoles maintain the planar conformation and cationic nature of the anthracyclines, essential for DNA intercalation. Anthrapyrazole analogs show a broad range of activity for inhibiting Topoisomerase 2. Several anthrapyrazoles have been developed (Fig. 2.28). A tertiary amine in the basic side chain at N2 increases the cytotoxic activity compared with a secondary amine in this side chain (unless there is a basic side chain at the C5 position). A chlorine substituent on the basic side chain at N2 does not have a consistent effect on activity, neither does moving a chlorine substituent from C5 to C7 or introducing a basic side chain at C5 (Begleiter et al. 2006).

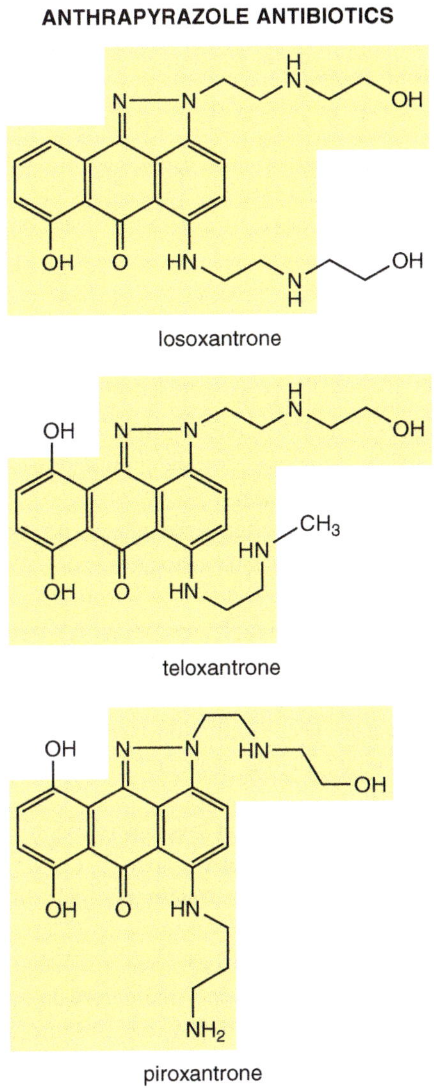

Fig. 2.28 Structures of anthrapyrazole antibiotics. The major portion of the molecule is common to all members of the class (highlighted in *yellow*)

Losoxantrone (biantrazole, 7-hydroxy-2-[2-[(2-hydroxyethyl)amino]ethyl]-5-[[2-[(2-hydroxyethyl)amino]ethyl] amino]anthra[1,9-cd]pyrazol-6(2H)-one dihydrochloride) (DuP-941, CI-941) is an anthrapyrazole that induces both single and double strand breaks in DNA and is a potent inhibitor of DNA synthesis. The drug is in clinical trials for the treatment of breast cancer and of prostate cancer that is refractory to androgen ablation. It is used at a total dose of 50 mg/m^2 per course of losoxantrone therapy.

Pharmacokinetics 60 % of the administered dose is excreted in the feces unmetabolized, presumably via biliary excretion. 10 % is excreted in the urine, primarily during the first 24 h. The remainder is metabolized,

- mono-hydroxylation of the phenolic sub-structure of the chromophore occurs via Cytochrome P450 catalysis, resulting in metabolites that have ortho- and para-hydroquinonoid sub-structures, respectively
- the ortho-hydroxylated losoxantrone metabolite undergoes Glutathione conjugation or forms covalent bonds with intracellular nucleophilic targets.

Adverse Effects Acute toxicity is negligible. Losoxantrone may be less cardiotoxic than doxorubicin. When the drug is administered in an intermittent single-dose schedule, the maximum tolerated dose is 55 mg/m^2, the dose limiting toxicities being leukopenia and neutropenia. Up to 40 % of patients encounter alopecia. 3 % of patients develop congestive heart failure.

Teloxantrone hydrochloride (moxantrazole hydrochloride) (CI-937, DuP-937) is the salt of an anthrapyrazole. The

Fig. 2.29 Structure of bisantrene

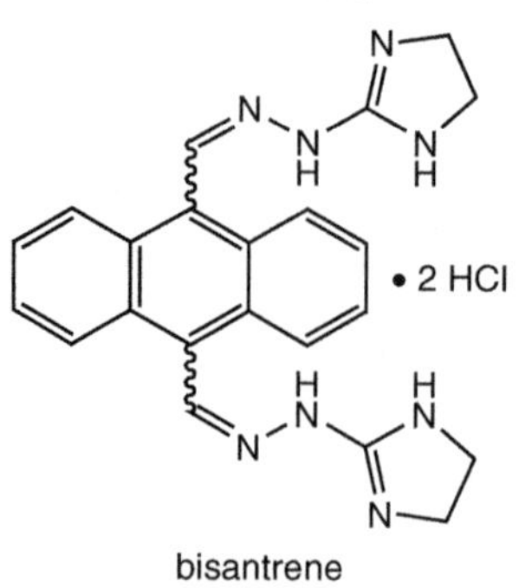

drug intercalates into DNA and interacts with Topoisomerase 2, thereby inhibiting DNA reduplication and repair, as well as RNA and protein synthesis.

Adverse Effects The pattern, frequency, and severity of toxicity are similar to those of losoxantrone.

Piroxantrone (oxanthrazole, oxantrazole) (CI-942, PD-111815) is an anthrapyrazole that intercalates into DNA and interacts with Topoisomerase 2.

Pharmacokinetics The elimination from the blood is biexponential with an α half-life of around 3 min and a β half-life of around 80 min.

Adverse Effects While being less cardiotoxic than doxorubicin, this agent exhibits a narrow spectrum of anti-neoplastic activity. The dose limiting toxicity is myelosuppression.

Related compounds Bisantrene (NSC-33776) (Fig. 2.29) is an anthracenyl bishydrazone that intercalates with and disrupts the configuration of DNA, resulting in DNA single strand breaks, DNA-protein cross-linking, and inhibition of DNA reduplication. This agent is similar to doxorubicin in activity, but unlike doxorubicin, does not exhibit cardiotoxicity. Bisantrene has low anti-tumor activity and needs to be taken at a high dose to be effective.

Anthracyclines, anthracenediones and anthrapyrazoles are related anti-neoplastic antibiotics. They share a polycyclic aromatic core structure.

The 2 main modes of anthracycline action comprise Topoisomerase inhibition and generation of reactive oxygen species.
Because first generation anthracyclines are associated with myocardial dysfunction and alopecia, second generation drugs attempt to reduce these adverse effects.
Because of enhanced total body clearance, epirubicin can be used at high cumulative doses without increased cardiotoxicity.
Oligosaccharide anthracyclines induce hematopoietic differentiation.

The diaminoalkyl groups are crucial for the biological activity of anthracenediones. Anthracenediones may require metabolic activation before effectively intercalating into DNA.
Anthracenediones may act as anti-oxidants by inhibiting conjugated diene formation from linoleic acid.

2.2.5 Enediyne Antibiotics

Enediyne antibiotics are a class of anti-tumor antibiotics, which are produced by Actinomadura verrucosospora, Micromonospora echinospora, and Streptomyces species. The structures of the calicheamicins and esperamicins were described in 1987, the dynemicins in 1989, kedarcidin in 1992, and lidamycin and maduropeptin in 1993. The unique structures of antibiotics in this class (Fig. 2.30) contribute to their very high potency as anti-tumor agents (Sugiura et al. 1989). The heart of these molecules is a bicyclo [7.3.1] tridecane system that combines a methyl trisulfide and double and triple bonds in a 3-ene-1,5-diyne formation. The enediyne group readily undergoes cyclo-aromatization via a diradical intermediate. The highly reactive radical is capable of abstracting hydrogen atoms from the DNA backbone, resulting in DNA damage at specific sites (Table 2.3) and giving rise to a powerful anti-proliferative activity. Enediyenes bind at specific sites to the minor groove of double-helical DNA and inflict primarily sequence specific DNA double-strand breaks. These drugs have three important functional domains,

- an assemblage that consists of an enediyne moiety
- a delivery system that conveys the enediyne moiety to its DNA target
- a triggering device that, when activated, initiates a cascade of reactions that generate the reactive chemical species (Shao and Zhen 2008).

Enediynes are characterized by a 9- or 10-membered ring containing two triple bonds separated by a double bond (called the warhead). The sub-family of 10-membered cyclic enediynes includes calicheamicins, esperamicins, dynemicins, and shishijimicins A-C. The subfamily of 9-membered cyclic enediynes includes neocarzinostatin, kedarcidin, lidamycin, maduropeptin, and N1999A2.

A major challenge to clinical applications of the enediyne antibiotics is their inadequate selectivity. This has stimulated efforts to conjugate members of this class of drugs to tumor targeting entities, such as monoclonal antibodies.

10-membered cyclic enediynes The enediyne core is essential for biological activity. Calicheamicins, esperamicins, and dynemicins have potent DNA breakage activity in the presence of thiol compounds. They cleave DNA via free radical damage after activation by Cytochrome P450 Reductase and NADPH[31]. The 10-membered cyclic enediynes (drug names

[31] Cytochrome P450 Reductase and NADPH can generate superoxide anion (O_2^-) from quinone containing anti-tumor agents, heterocyclic amines, or enediynes.

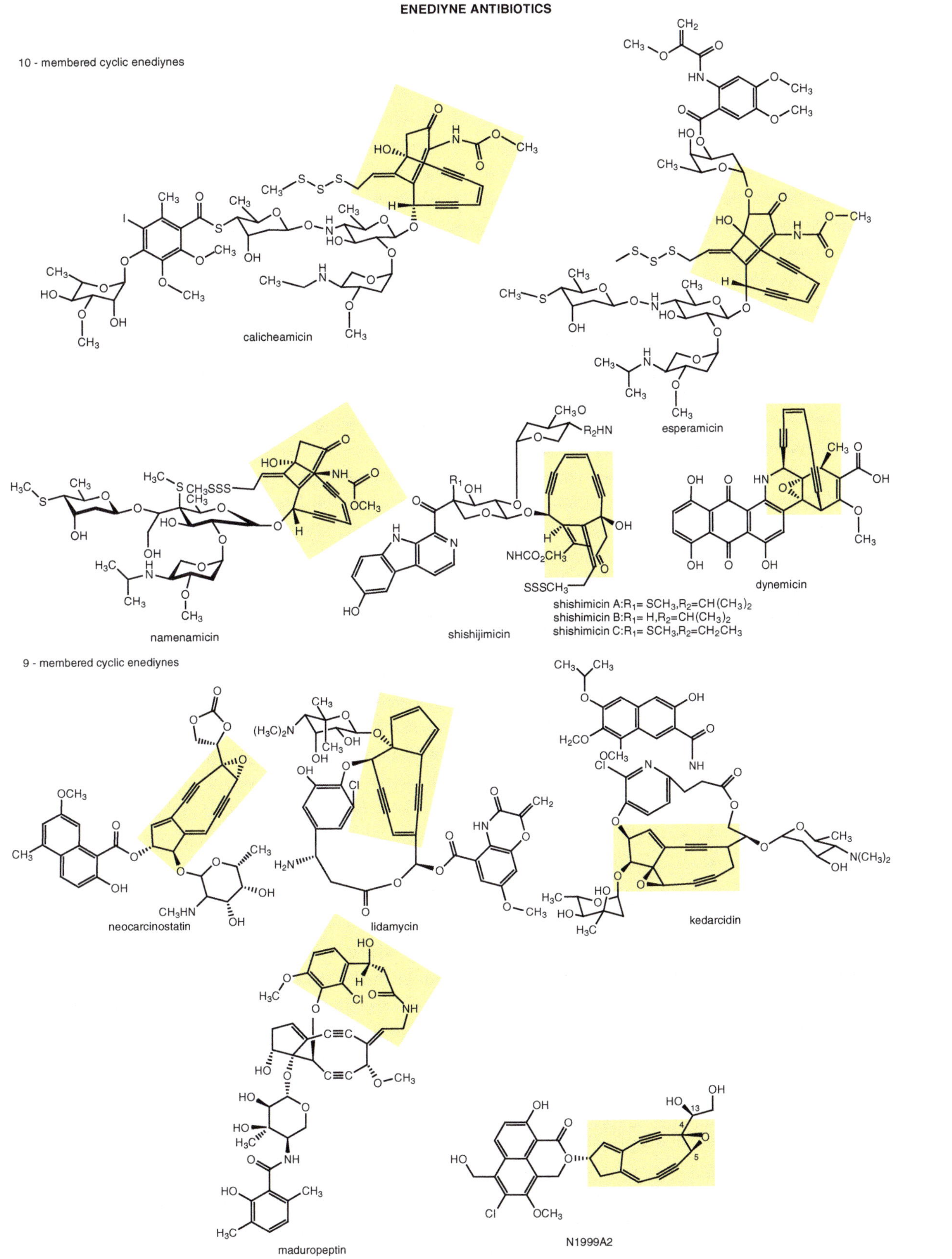

Fig. 2.30 Structures of cyclic enediyne antibiotics. For each group, 9-membered and 10-membered enediynes, the shared portion of the molecule is highlighted in *yellow*. In addition to the chromophor, the 9-membered enediynes also contain an apoprotein portion, which is not shown

Table 2.3 Preferred DNA binding sites for endiyne antibiotics

Drug	Recognition sequence	DNA domain
Chalicheamicins	5′-TCCT-3′, 5′-TTGT-3′, 5′-ATCT-3′	Minor groove
Esperamicins	5′-CTC-3′, 5′-TTC-3′, 5′-TTT-3′	Minor groove
Dynemicins	5′-CTACTACTGG-3′, 5′-AG-3′, 5′-AT-3′,5′-GC-3′	Minor groove
Neocarcinostatin	5′-GGAGCGC-3′	Minor groove
Lidamycin	5′-CTTTT-3′, 5′-ATAAT-3′, 5′-CTTTA-3′, 5′-CTCTT-3′, 5′-GTTAT-3′	Minor groove
Kedarcidin	5′-TCCT-3′	Minor groove
N1999A2	5′-GGT-3′	Minor groove

ending on -micin) do not contain apoproteins. They tend to be more stable than the 9-membered cyclic enediynes.

The chalicheamicins were discovered at the Medical Research Division of American Cynamid in the 1980s through the use of a biochemical induction assay. They were isolated from the fermentation broth of the bacterium Mocromonospora echinospora species calichensis. Several components of the calicheamicins (at least 15 are known) are assigned Greek letters based on their HPLC retention times. Calicheamicin is one of the most complex natural products to have been developed into an anti-cancer drug. After binding to the minor groove of DNA, preferentially to the sequences 5′-TCCT-3′, 5′-TTGT-3′, or 5′-ATCT-3′, calicheamicin is reduced by cellular thiols. The resultant product undergoes a rearrangement to generate 1,4-dehydrobenzene diradical that abstracts hydrogen atoms from DNA, thereby initiating double strand breaks.

- Calicheamicin exhibits a very narrow therapeutic window and delayed toxicities. The agent can be modified by reaction with a thiol hydrazide to contain a hydrazine disulfide linker, which can be reacted with the oxidized carbohydrates of a monoclonal antibody. Thus, the drug has been improved by conjugation to tumor specific antibodies, such as gemtuzumab (anti-CD33) for the treatment of AML. This combination gemtuzumab ozogamicin (CMA-676) <Mylotarg> was approved by the U.S. FDA in 2000 for patients 60 years and older in first relapse with CD33-positive acute myeloid leukemia (AML), who are not candidates for cytotoxic chemotherapy. After infusion, near complete saturation of CD33 antigenic sites is reached for AML blasts, monocytes, and granulocytes. Gemtuzumab ozogamicin does not bind to lymphocytes. The mechanism of action involves the drug binding to CD33 antigen on the AML cell membrane, then being internalized. Calicheamicin (ozogamicin) is released from the antibody inside the lysosomes of cells. It enters the cell nucleus and binds to DNA, causing breaks in the double helix resulting in cell death.

Adverse Effects Gemtuzumab ozogamicin therapy does not result in hair loss, severe oral mucositis, or damage to the intestinal mucosa. An acute infusion related symptom complex of fever and chills, and less commonly hypotension and dyspnea, may occur within 24 h of treatment. Hypertension, hyperglycemia, and hypoxia may also arise. The drug was withdrawn in 2010, when a clinical trial indicated that it increased patient death and added no benefit over conventional cancer therapies.

The esperamicins were discovered in the 1980s at Bristol-Myers Squibb. Esperamicin A1 is a bacterial chromoprotein enediyne antibiotic produced by Actinomadura verrucosospora. The esperamicins (A, B, C, and D) are extremely toxic DNA splicing compounds. The favored DNA binding sites are 5′-CTC-3′, 5′-TTC-3′, and 5′-TTT-3′ sequences. The preferential cutting sites of esperamicin are adjacent to thymidylate residues.

Shishijimicins A-C were isolated from the tunicate Didemnum proliferum Kott (Oku et al. 2003). They encompass a unique sugar component, which is a conjugation product of a hexose and a β-carboline, attached to the calicheamicinone aglycone. Shishijimicins A-C are highly cytotoxic.

Namenamicin was isolated from the tunicate Polysynchraton lithostrotum off the coast of the Fiji island of Namenalala (McDonald et al. 1996). It is the first enediyne natural product of marine origin. The trisaccharide domain contains an isopropyl aminosugar (C ring) and two unusual 6-deoxysugars (A and B rings), with an unusual linkage between the A and B rings, in which C-4 of the A ring is disubstituted with a methyl thioether and a two carbon fragment to which the B ring is appended at the C-7 oxygen.

Dynemicins are synthesized by Micromonospora chersina M956-1. Dynemicin A binds DNA at 5′-CTACTACTGG-3′, 5′-AG-3′, 5′-AT-3′, or 5′-GC-3′ sequences. It intercalates into the DNA base stack with its anthraquinone functional group, while the (*Z*)-enediyne bridge is positioned in the minor groove. Dynemicin A cleaves double stranded DNA in the presence of reducing cofactors, such as GSH or NADPH. The ID_{50} is around 30–60 μg/kg.

9-membered cyclic enediynes 9-membered cyclic enediynes are composed of non-covalently bound chromophore and apoprotein. The anti-cancer activity lies in the chromophore, while the apoprotein has a stabilizing function. Major binding interactions between the apoprotein and the chromophore are the hydrophobic contacts between the core of the chromophore and the hydrophobic side chains of the pocket forming residues.

Neocarzinostatin (zinostatin, vinostatin), discovered in 1964, was the first enediyne antibiotic used clinically and has become a prototypical anti-cancer agent for the treatments of leukemia, gastric carcinoma and pancreatic adenocarcinoma. The agent is produced by the bacterium Streptomyces carzinostaticus. It is an enediyne antibiotic hybrid containing an aminoglycoside chromophore. Neocarcinostatin consists of a non-protein chromophor, which is complexed with a protein carrier and stabilizer. The aminoglycoside component intercalates into DNA, and the benzene diradical intermediate of the enediyne core binds to the minor groove of double-helical DNA at 5′-GGAGCGC-3′ sites. Neocarzinostatin requires sulfhydryl activation. It is converted to a diradical that directly attacks the deoxyribose of residues in DNA, resulting in single and double strand breaks in DNA and consecutive apoptosis.

- Styrene maleic acid neocarzinostatin (SMANCS) is a chemical conjugate of a synthetic co-polymer of styrene maleic acid (SMA) and neocarzinostatin (NCS). The drug is soluble in organic solvents, such as pyridine, acetone, and Lipiodol[32]. The coupling to a styrene maleic acid based polymer reduces the immunogenicity of neocarzinostatin. A principal advantage is the tumor targeting mechanism through an enhanced permeability and retention effect, and the potential for a reduction of toxicity, such as a marked reduction in bone marrow toxicity. SMANCS was approved in Japan in 1993 for the treatment of hepatoma, gastric carcinoma, and lung cancer. SMANCS may also be beneficial in the treatment of renal cell carcinoma. Hepatic arterial infusion of a SMANCS/Lipiodol emulsion has been used as a treatment for advanced or recurrent hepatocellular carcinoma. SMANCS is used most successfully when it is administered as a treatment of dose per tumor size and follow-up treatments are given on an as needed basis (Duncan 2006).

Adverse Effects Anorexia, nausea, and vomiting are the most frequent adverse effects of neocarcinostatin. Dose limiting toxicity is myelosuppression, which tends to occur late. Myelosuppression is more pronounced in patients who have received prior chemotherapy. Acute administration of neocarcinostatin is associated with fever, chills, and cyanosis (rigors) in approximately half of the patients. Severe allergic reactions are possible.

In 1988, Otani and coworkers isolated and characterized lidamycin (C-1027) from the broth filtrate of Streptomyces globisporus C-1027 (the strain was isolated from a soil sample collected in the Qianjiang area of China to serve antibiotic production) (Hu et al. 1988). Lidamycin is water soluble and has a molecular weight of 15 kD. The apoprotein consists of a single polypeptide chain cross-linked by two disulfide bonds and contains a total of 110 amino acid residues. The chromophore possesses a highly strained 9-membered 1,5-diyn-3-ene core structure together with a 16-membered macrocyclic ring. Functionally important domains of the chromophore include the benzoxazine moiety that is necessary for DNA intercalation and the 9-membered enediyne moiety that is necessary for DNA cleavage. Lidamycin acts through

- inducing DNA double strand breaks at target sequences 5′-CTTTT-3′, 5′-ATAAT-3′, 5′-CTTTA-3′, 5′-CTCTT-3′, and especially 5′-GTTAT-3′
- directly causing DNA single strand breaks without the need for reducing agents
- inhibiting DNA and RNA synthesis and subsequently delaying the progression through the cell cycle (lidamycin induces G_1 arrest in cells with wild-type P53 and G_2/M arrest in cells with mutant P53)
- inducing apoptosis and mitotic cell death (lidamycin induced apoptosis is likely more effective in cancers with wild type P53 than those with mutant or deleted P53) (Shao and Zhen 2008).

Besides inhibiting tumor growth, lidamycin suppresses angiogenesis by blocking the binding of FGF-2 to its receptor and inhibiting the formation of the FGF-2/Receptor immune complex (Zhen et al. 2005).

- Efforts are in progress to generate conjugates with targeting moieties, such as monoclonal antibodies. This is more difficult for 9-membered cyclic enediynes than for 10-membered cyclic enediynes because the apoprotein is important for function. Instead of linking the chromophor directly to the antibody, an assembled conjugate is synthesized, which links the apoprotein to the antibody and then reconstitutes the complex by adding the chromophore.

Kedarcidin is an enediyene natural product produced by Actinomycete strain L585-6. It is water-soluble and acidic with a molecular weight of 12.4 kD. The holoprotein is 10-fold more potent than the chromophore itself. It binds the minor groove of DNA at 5′-TCCT-3′ sequences. The apoprotein has activity as a Peptidase and may cleave Histones.

Maduropeptin, produced by Actinomadura madurae, has the ability to cleave DNA by undergoing a Bergman cyclization and forming a *p*-benzyne biradical, which abstracts hydrogens from DNA and initiates a cascade of DNA breakage, ultimately leading to cell death. Beside the enediyne core, maduropeptin also contains a 3,6-dimethylsalicylic acid moiety, an aminosugar (previously named madurose),

[32] Lidipol is an ethyl ester of iodinated poppy seed oil, in which most of the unsaturated double bonds in oleic, linoleic and linolenic acid are almost completely iodinated.

and an (S)-3-(2-chloro-3-hydroxy-4-methoxyphenyl)-3-hydroxypropionic acid moiety.

Only N1999A2 is a non-protein 9-membered cyclic enediyne antibiotic that lacks an aminoglycoside residue (which is present in neocarcinostatin). It is epimeric with the neocarzinostatin chromophore at positions 4, 5, and 13. N1999A2 binds DNA at sites containing 5′-GGT-3′.

Enediyenes bind at specific sites to the minor groove of double-helical DNA and inflict primarily sequence specific DNA double strand breaks.
The 9-membered, but not the 10-membered cyclic enediynes contain apoproteins. The anti-cancer activity of the 9-membered cyclic enediynes lies in the chromophore, while the apoprotein has a stabilizing function.
The 10-membered cyclic enediynes tend to be more stable than the 9-membered cyclic enediynes.
The 10-membered cyclic enediynes cause DNA double strand breaks in the presence of thiol compounds, the characteristic of DNA cleavage is the induction by NADPH.
The 9-membered cyclic enediynes may also cause DNA single strand breaks, cell cycle arrest, or apoptosis.

2.2.6 Others

Actinomycins were first described by Selman Waksman and H.B. Woodruff in 1940 (Waksman and Woodruff 1940). Actinomycin D <Dactinomycin, Cosmegen, Oncostatin K, Actinomycin IV, Actinomycin C1> was isolated from the soil bacterium Streptomyces parvulus. It is a polypeptide antibiotic containing an aminoquinone chromophore.

- Actinomycin D specifically intercalates to GC-rich sites of DNA. It inhibits transcription by binding to the DNA at transcription initiation complexes and preventing elongation by RNA Polymerase.
- As actinomycin D can bind DNA duplexes, it can interfere with DNA reduplication. The agent acts in a cell cycle non-specific manner.
- Actinomycin D causes single strand DNA breaks, possibly via a free radical intermediate or an interaction with Topoisomerase 2.

The potential of Actinomycin D to act as a radio-sensitizer is under debate.

Actinomycin D (Fig. 2.31) was approved by the U.S. FDA in 1964. The drug is administered intravenously for the treatment of gestational trophoblastic neoplasia, germ cell tumor, choriocarcinoma, testicular cancer, melanoma, neuroblastoma, retinoblastoma, Wilms tumor, rhabdomyosarcoma, Ewing sarcoma, uterine sarcoma, Kaposi sarcoma, sarcoma botryoides, or soft tissue sarcoma. It may be a component of regional perfusion for the palliative or adjunctive treatment of locally recurrent or locoregional solid malignancies. While actinomycin D can produce a response, the duration of remission varies among patients. The usual dose is 15 mg/kg/day, repeated for 5 days as a course. A 2nd course can be started after 2–4 weeks. Dosage reduction may be necessary when additional chemotherapy or radiation therapy is used concomitantly or has been applied previously.

Pharmacokinetics Actinomycin D is minimally metabolized. The drug does not cross the blood-brain barrier. The terminal plasma half-life is 35 h. Approximately 30 % of the dose is excreted in urine and feces within 1 week.

Adverse Effects The drug solution is extremely irritating and extravasation produces severe tissue damage (intermittent application of ice to the site for 15 min four times per day for 3 days may be useful). Blistering, ulceration, or persistent pain are indications for wide excision surgery, followed by split-thickness skin grafting. Nausea and vomiting may occur several hours after administration of actinomycin D and can be alleviated through anti-emetics. Toxic effects on bone marrow, kidneys, and liver may not become manifest until several days after completion of the course of treatment, and reach their maximum for 1–2 weeks. Liver toxicity may manifest in ascites, hepatomegaly, hepatitis, or hepatic veno-occlusive disease associated with intravascular clotting disorder and the risk for multi-organ failure. Other adverse reactions include glossitis, cheilitis, ulcerations of the oral mucosa, and proctitis. Actinomycin is Pregnancy Category D.

Bleomycin was discovered in 1962 in Japan, when Hamao Umezawa found anti-cancer activity while screening culture filtrates of Streptomyces verticullus. The findings were published in 1966. Bleomycin refers to a family of structurally related, glycosylated linear peptide antibiotics produced by Streptomyces verticillus. When used as anti-cancer agents, the chemotherapeutic forms are primarily bleomycin A_2 and B_2. Bleomycin is toxic to cells in the G_2 and early M phase of the cell cycle. The main damaging action is DNA strand scission. It depends on binding of a bleomycin/iron complex to DNA, which then reduces molecular oxygen to free oxygen radicals that cause primarily single strand breaks.

Bleomycin sulfate <Blenoxane, Teva> is used in the treatment of Hodgkin and non-Hodgkin lymphoma as a component of the ABVD (adriamycin, bleomycin, vinblastine, dacarbazine) regimen, of squamous cell carcinoma, and of testicular cancer. The drug may be given by intramuscular, intravenous, subcutaneous, or intrapleural routes. It is effective as a sclerosing agent for the treatment of malignant pleural effusions and for the prevention of recurrent pleural effusions (60 units administered as a single dose, intrapleural bolus injection). Bleomycin was launched in Japan in 1969. It gained U.S. FDA approval in 1973.

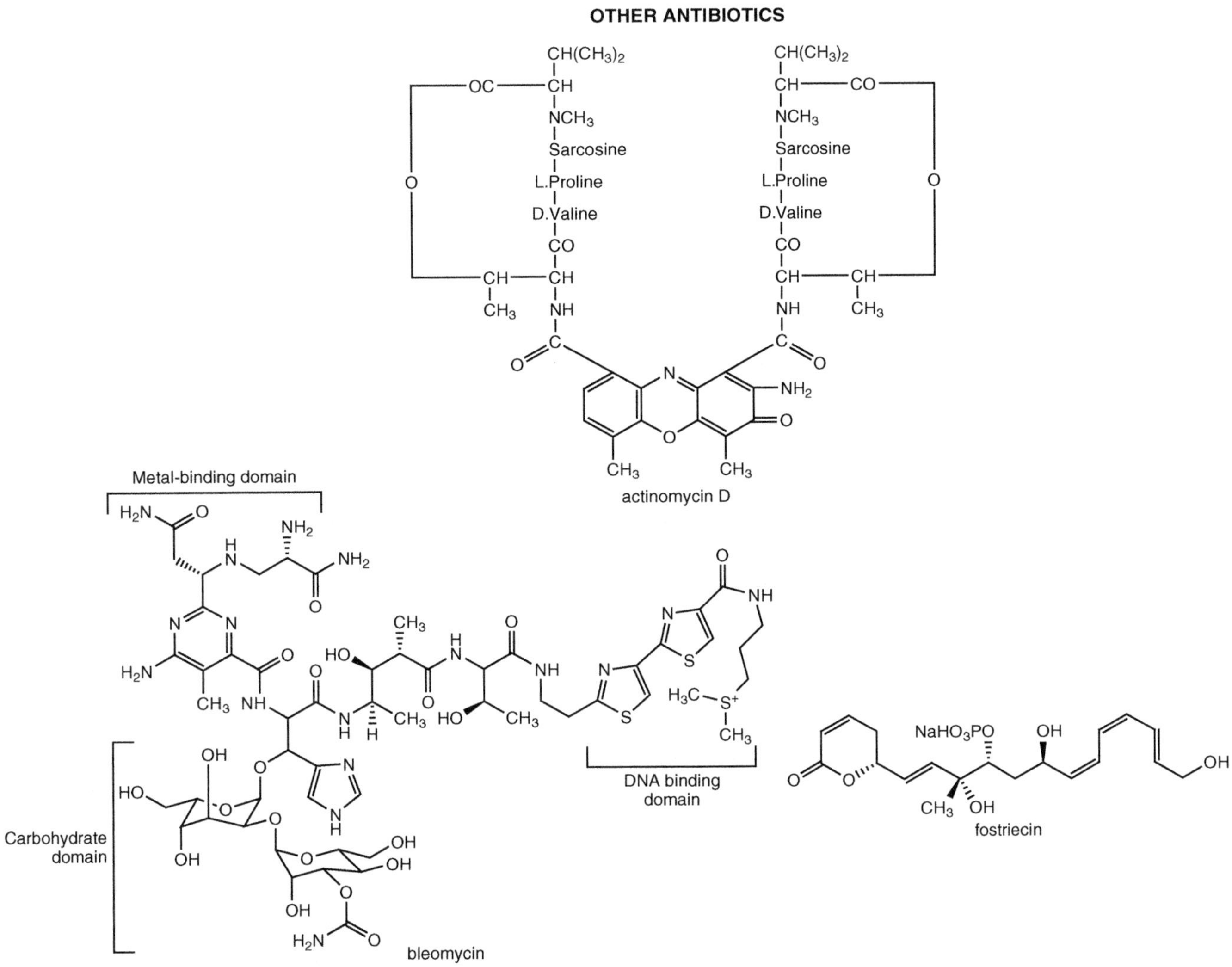

Fig. 2.31 Structures of other antibiotics. Antibiotics with very diverse chemical structures may exert anti-cancer effects

Pharmacokinetics Bleomycin is rapidly absorbed following intravenous (100 % systemic bioavailability), intramuscular (100 % bioavailability), subcutaneous (70 % bioavailability), intraperitoneal (45 % bioavailability), or intrapleural (45 % bioavailability) administration, reaching peak blood concentrations in 30–60 min. As the main route of elimination is through the kidneys, dose reduction may be necessary for patients with renal insufficiency. Systemic elimination of the drug by enzymatic degradation is probably only important in patients with severely compromised renal function. Bleomycin is inactivated by the cytosolic Aminohydrolase (Bleomycin Hydrolase). The enzyme is widely distributed in healthy tissues with the exception of the low expression in skin and lungs, both of which are susceptible to bleomycin toxicity.

Adverse Effects Toxic pulmonary effects may manifest as interstitial pneumonitis or as bronchiolitis obliterans with organizing pneumonia. There is a risk of pulmonary fibrosis at large doses. The incidence of pulmonary toxicity is elevated in patients over 70 years of age and is proportionate to the cumulative bleomycin dose, occurring in about 10 % of patients treated with more than 300 units, and causing death in up to 3 %. Cases of pulmonary toxicity may resolve with the administration of corticosteroids. Adverse reactions of the skin and mucous membranes consist of erythema, rash, striae, vesiculation, hyper-pigmentation, hyperkeratosis, nail changes, alopecia, pruritus, and stomatitis. They arise in 50 % of patients, usually in the 2nd–3rd week of treatment, after 150–200 units have been administered. The incidence of the Raynaud phenomenon (transient vasoconstriction of the digital arteries causing pallor or cyanosis) may reach 35 %, occurring most commonly 4–12 months after completion of chemotherapy. In 25 % of afflicted patients, the symptoms may persist for 10–20 years after treatment. Other adverse effects include fever, alopecia, vascular toxicities, and ototoxicity. However, no significant myelosuppression is associated with the drug. The drug is Pregnancy Category D.

As a natural product, bleomycin may be the cause of anaphylactic reactions, immediate or delayed for several hours. Such adverse events occur in approximately 1 % of lymphoma patients, usually after the 1st or 2nd dose. They manifest in hypotension, confusion, fever, chills, wheezing, shortness of breath, or low blood pressure. They require the drug to be stopped for treatment with dexamethasone, diphenhydramine, and if necessary epinephrine. Therefore, lymphomata should be treated with ≤2 units for the first two doses; if no acute reaction occurs, regular dosage schedule is followed.

Drug Resistance The presence of Hydrolases in tumor cells is the primary mechanism of resistance to bleomycin. Cells can also become resistant by repairing the DNA breaks produced by bleomycin.

Drug Interactions The response to bleomycin is compromised in patients with previously irradiated head and neck cancer. Because bleomycin is eliminated predominantly through renal excretion, the administration of nephrotoxic drugs with bleomycin may affect its renal clearance.

Fostriecin (2H-Pyran-2-one,5,6-dihydro-6-[3,6,13-trihydroxy-3-methyl-4-(phosphonooxy)-1,7,9,11-tridecatetraenyl) (CI-920, NSC 339638, PD 110 161) was isolated from the bacterium Streptomyces pulveraceus subspecies fostreus. It is a phosphate monoester anti-tumor antibiotic containing an unsaturated lactone and a conjugated triene system.

- Fostriecin inhibits Topoisomerase 2 catalytic activity, resulting in protein associated strand breaks and impaired DNA and RNA synthesis in various malignant cell types.
- This agent inhibits serine/threonine Protein Phosphatase type 2A (and to a lesser extent type 1) and Protein Phosphatase 4 (PP4), which leads to phosphorylation and reorganization of Vimentin filaments, thereby interfering with cellular proliferation.
- Fostriecin activates the mitotic entry checkpoint, leading to G_2/M arrest.

Adverse Effects Renal tubular damage, reflected in a rise in serum creatinine after 1–2 doses, is reversible and not dose limiting.

Actinomycin D suppresses transcription, interferes with DNA reduplication, and inhibits Topoisomerase 2.
Bleomycin is inactivated by Aminohydrolase (widely expressed except in skin and lungs, both of which are targets of bleomycin toxicity). The presence of Hydrolases in tumor cells is the primary mechanism of resistance to bleomycin.
Fostriecin is a Topoisomerase 2 inhibitor and acts as an inhibitor of several Protein Phosphatases.

2.3 Topoisomerase Inhibitors

Otherwise identical loops of DNA having different numbers of twists are topoisomers (Gr. τόπος= place, ἰσομερής= equal parts). They cannot be interconverted by any process that does not involve the breaking of DNA strands. Topoisomerases (Gyrases) (type 1: EC 5.99.1.2, type 2: EC 5.99.1.3) are enzymes that catalyze and guide the unknotting of DNA. They can cause transient single strand (Topoisomerase 1) or double strand (Topoisomerase 2) DNA breaks that are resealed after changing the twisting status of the double helix. Topoisomerases wrap around the DNA and make cuts permitting the helix to spin. Once the DNA is relaxed, the enzymes reconnect the broken strands. Thus, Topoisomerase activity releases the tension generated by the winding of DNA and facilitates transcription and reduplication. Topoisomerase inhibitors interfere with this process.

2.3.1 Topoisomerase 1 Inhibitors

Topoisomerase 1 is a 100 kD monomeric protein that makes a single cut in the DNA duplex and relieves transcription-associated torsional strain. No energy cofactor is required to carry out this reaction. Drugs may stabilize the Topoisomerase 1/DNA complex (referred to as the "cleavable complex"), thus blocking DNA relegation and converting the enzyme into a DNA damaging agent. Topoisomerase 1 inhibitors exhibit S phase cytotoxicity and G_2/M cell cycle arrest.

In 1956, C. Gordon Zubrod, who had formerly led the development of anti-malarial agents for the United States Army, took over the Division of Cancer Treatment of the National Cancer Institute and guided the development of new drugs. In the two decades that followed the establishment of the NCCSC (National Cancer Chemotherapy Service Center), a large network of cooperative clinical trial groups evolved under its auspices to test anti-cancer agents. Zubrod had a particular interest in natural products, and established a broad program for collecting and testing plant and marine sources. Although this was a controversial project, it led to the discovery of the camptothecins in 1966.

Camptothecins Camptothecin (4-ethyl-4-hydroxy-1*H*-pyrano[3′,4′:6,7]indolizino[1,2-b]quinoline-3,14-(4*H*,12*H*)-dione) is a cytotoxic, quinoline based, non-terpenoid alkaloid that was extracted from the Asian tree Camptotheca acuminata in 1966 (Wall et al. 1966) (Fig. 2.32). The drug was isolated and characterized by the laboratory of Monroe Wall at the Research Triangle Institute in the U.S. During the S phase of the cell cycle, camptothecin inhibits Topoisomerase 1 activity by stabilizing the cleavable complex between Topoisomerase 1 and DNA, resulting in DNA T-G/A single

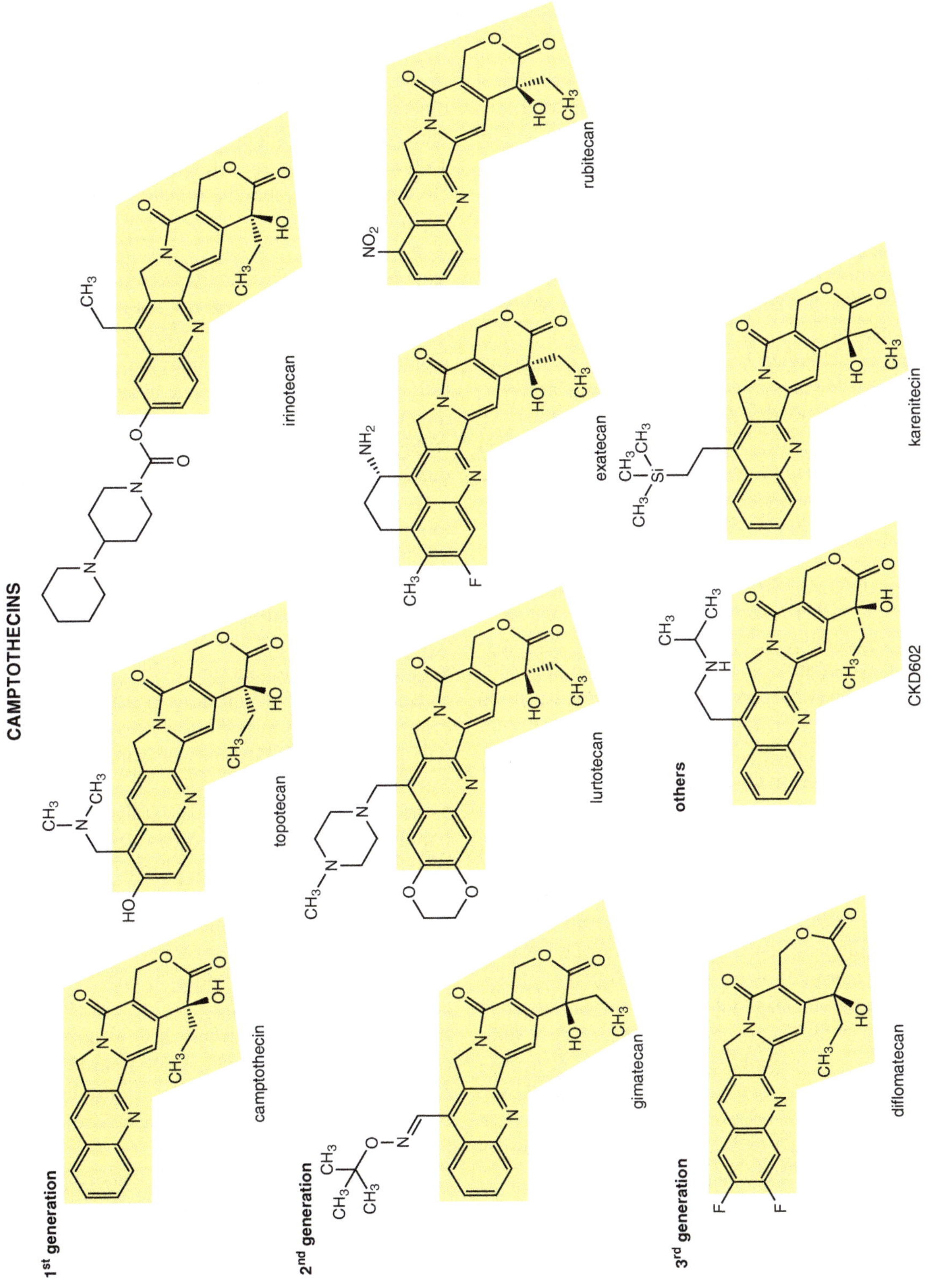

Fig. 2.32 Structures of camptothecins. The core structure, common to all camptothecins in all generations is highlighted in *yellow*

strand breaks that cannot be religated. Camptothecin/Topoisomerase 1/DNA cleavable complexes are rapidly conjugated with SUMO by SUMO-Protein Ligase (UBE2I, UBC9). This inhibits reduplication and triggers apoptotic cell death. Camptothecin also blocks RNA synthesis through Topoisomerase 1 mediated effects.

Pharmacokinetics Because camptothecin exists in equilibrium between the lactone and the ring-opened conformations its drug action is limited. The E ring-opened carboxylate form has less than 10% potency of the lactone form. The stability of the lactone ring at physiological pH is a determinant of activity for all camptothecin analogs.

Adverse Effects Despite showing promise in preclinical studies, camptothecin had poor bioavailability and little antitumor activity in early clinical trials. Dosing was limited by severe diarrhea and urinary tract toxicity (the unstable lactone ring at neutral pH is activated in the acidic environment of the kidneys, exerting damage to the renal tubules). Because Camptothecin manifests a life threatening adverse reaction in the form of severe cystitis, chemically related analogs with less toxicity and enhanced therapeutic potency have been developed.

Drug Resistance Although camptothecin and its analogs can freely enter cells via passive diffusion, their intracellular concentrations are greatly reduced by efflux pumps. All camptothecins are substrates for the efflux pump ABCG2 (Breast Cancer Resistance Protein, BCRP, MRX). Leukemia cells may develop the Topoisomerase 1 mutations Asn722Ser or Arg364His and become resistant to camptothecins.

Topotecan hydrochloride ((S)-10-[(dimethylamino) methyl]-4-ethyl-4,9-dihydroxy-1*H*-pyrano[3′,4′:6,7] indolizino[1,2-b]quinoline-3,14(4*H*,12*H*)-dione monohydrochloride) <Hycamptin> is the water soluble salt of a semi-synthetic derivative of camptothecin. Approved in 1996 for treating ovarian cancer, topotecan was the first Topoisomerase inhibitor in clinical use. During the S phase of the cell cycle, the agent selectively stabilizes Topoisomerase 1/ DNA covalent complexes, thereby inhibiting the religation of the single strand DNA breaks mediated by Topoisomerase 1. This constellation may produce potentially lethal double strand DNA breaks when encountered by the DNA reduplication machinery. Topotecan is indicated for small cell lung cancer after the failure of first-line chemotherapy, metastatic carcinoma of the ovary following failure of initial or subsequent chemotherapy, and stage IV-B, recurrent, or persistent cervical carcinoma which is not amenable to surgery or radiation therapy. The drug is sometimes used to treat acute myelogenous leukemia (AML) and renal cell carcinoma (RCC). Topotecan is given at 0.75–1.5 mg/m^2 by infusion daily for 5 days at the beginning of a 3 week cycle. Topotecan capsules can be taken orally over five dosings a day.

- ^{11}C-topotecan is a semi-synthetic derivative, radio-labeled with carbon 11. It has therapeutic and radio-tracer properties. Quantitation of ^{11}C-topotecan accumulated in tumor tissues by positron emission tomography (PET) may help predict the responses to topotecan therapy.

Pharmacokinetics Topotecan exhibits multi-exponential pharmacokinetics with a terminal half-life of 2–3 h. Binding to plasma proteins is about 35 %. Like camptothecin, topotecan undergoes a reversible, pH dependent hydrolysis of its pharmacologically active lactone moiety. Renal clearance is an important determinant of topotecan elimination (50 % of the administered dose as parent drug, 3 % as desmethyl topotecan, 2 % as topotecan-*O*glucuronide and *N*-desmethyl topotecan-*O*-glucuronide). Fecal elimination accounts for 15 % of the parent drug and 1.5 % of *N*-desmethyl topotecan. Dose adjustments may be required in patients with renal or hepatic impairment.

Adverse Effects The dose limiting toxicity of topotecan is leucopenia, which results in lowered resistance to infections. Adverse effects include bruising or bleeding, anemia, nausea or vomiting (70 %), hair loss (60 %), asthenia or fatigue, sore mouth and ulcers (30 %), diarrhea (40 %), loss of appetite (20 %), and a reversible change in taste. Topotecan is contraindicated in patients who have a history of severe hypersensitivity reactions to the drug or to any of its ingredients. The drug is Pregnancy Category D, it is secreted into the milk.

Drug Interactions Myelosuppression is more severe when topotecan is given in combination with cisplatin or other cytotoxic agents, thereby necessitating a dose reduction. Concomitant treatment with G-CSF and topotecan can prolong the duration of neutropenia. Therefore, G-CSF should not be initiated until day 6, 24 h after completion of the administration of topotecan.

Drug Resistance Multi-drug resistance can result from drug efflux via transporters. Topotecan is a substrate for ABCB1 (MDR1, P-Glycoprotein) and ABCG2.

Irinotecan hydrochloride ((*S*)-4,11-diethyl-3,4,12,14-tetrahydro-4-hydroxy-3,14-dioxo1*H*-pyrano[3′,4′:6,7]-indol izino[1,2-b]quinolin-9-yl-[1,4′bipiperidine]-1′-carboxylate) (CPT-11) <Campto, Camptosar> is the water soluble salt of a semi-synthetic camptothecin derivative. Because ongoing DNA synthesis is necessary for irinotecan to exert its cytotoxic effects, it is classified as S phase specific agent. The drug was approved by the U.S. FDA in 1994. It is indicated for colorectal cancers, where it is usually a component of combination chemotherapy, such as in FOLFIRI, and confers a survival benefit. This agent is also used to treat (small cell and non-small cell) lung cancers, ovarian cancers, leukemias, and lymphomata.

Pharmacokinetics As a prodrug, irinotecan is converted to the 1000-fold more active metabolite 7-ethyl-10-hydroxy-camptothecin (SN-38) by a Carboxylesterase, primarily in the liver. 95 % of SN-38 is bound to plasma proteins, compared to approximately 50 % of irinotecan. Both irinotecan and SN-38 exist in an active lactone form and an inactive hydroxy acid anion form. Acidic pH promotes the formation of the lactone, while a more basic pH favors the hydroxy acid anion form. Irinotecan blood concentrations decline in a multi-exponential manner, with a mean terminal elimination half-life of 6–12 h. The mean terminal elimination half-life of the active metabolite SN-38 is 10–20 h. SN-38 is inactivated via glucuronidation by UGT1A1 (Uridine Diphosphate Glucoronosyltransferase 1A1) into the non-toxic SN-38-glucuronide (SN-38G) and is excreted into the gastrointestinal tract.

Adverse Effects The most substantial adverse effects of irinotecan are grade 2 or higher nausea and vomiting, alopecia, asthenia, fever, and abdominal pain. Extensive suppression of the immune system due to neutropenia is likely. A new cycle of therapy should not begin until the granulocyte count has recovered to at least 1500/mm^3 and the platelet count has recovered to at least 100,000/mm^3. Hypersensitivity reactions including severe anaphylactic or anaphylactoid reactions may arise. Interstitial pulmonary disease-like events, including fatalities, are possible. The drug is Pregnancy Category D. It is secreted in the milk.

Irinotecan can induce both early and late forms of diarrhea, which may be severe.

- Early diarrhea can be accompanied by cholinergic symptoms of rhinitis, increased salivation, miosis, lacrimation, diaphoresis, flushing, and intestinal hyperperistalsis that can cause abdominal cramping. It may be prevented or ameliorated by 0.25–1.0 mg atropine (i.v. or s.c.).
- β-Glucuronidases expressed by intestinal commensal bacteria can hydrolyze SN-38-glucuronide to generate SN-38. SN-38 amounts in the intestinal lumen play an essential role in the delayed severe diarrhea that prevents dose intensification and efficacy in up to 40% of treated patients. Late diarrhea (generally occurring more than 24 h after administration) can be life threatening as it may be prolonged and may lead to dehydration, electrolyte imbalance, or sepsis. Late diarrhea should be treated promptly with loperamide. Before the next ensuing chemotherapy administration, patients should return to pre-treatment bowel function without requiring anti-diarrhea medications for at least 24 h. Intestinal biota play essential roles in carbohydrate metabolism, vitamin production, and the processing of bile acids, sterols, and xenobiotics. Thus, the removal of gastrointerstinal bacteria is not recommended for patients already challenged by neoplastic growths and chemotherapy. In addition, elimination of symbiotic gastrointestinal flora increases the chances of infections by pathogenic bacteria, including enterohemorrhagic Escherichia coli and Clostridium difficile. Inhibitors of β-Glucuronidases prevent this conversion and diminish irinotecan gut toxicity.

The Glucuronyltransferase UGT1A1, which conjugates bilirubin and renders it water-soluble, is largely responsible for the metabolism of irinotecan. The allele TA_7 (*28 variant) is expressed at lower levels than other alleles. Gilbert syndrome (Gilbert-Meulengracht syndrome), is the most common hereditary form of increased unconjugated blood bilirubin, based on the autosomal recessive inheritance of the reduced activity allele of UGT1A1. During chemotherapy, homozygous patients effectively receive a larger than expected dose of irinotecan because the drug is not cleared as fast as in non-carriers of this allele. Hence, Gilbert syndrome is associated with a high incidence of severe diarrhea and neutropenia in patients who are treated with irinotecan. Genetic testing can predict this toxicity before chemotherapy administration and can allow dose adjustment. Irinotecan is one of the first widely used chemotherapy agents to be dosed for each patient according to the underlying genotype.

Drug Interactions Ketoconazole (a strong inhibitor of CYP3A4 enzymes), CYP3A4 enzyme-inducing anticonvulsants (including phenytoin, phenobarbital, carbamazepine), and St. John's Wort (an inducer of CYP3A4 enzymes) have drug-drug interactions with irinotecan.

Drug Resistance Multi-drug resistance results from drug efflux via ABCB1 (MDR1, P-Glycoprotein). Irinotecan is a substrate for ABCB1.

Gimatecan (7-t-butoxyiminomethylcamptothecin) (ST1481) is a second generation, 7-position modified lipophilic camptothecin that was developed to provide rapid uptake and accumulation in cells and to achieve a stable Topoisomerase 1/DNA/drug ternary complex.

Pharmacokinetics Gimatecan is orally rapidly absorbed. Its plasma levels are related to the plasma concentrations of α_1-Acid Glycoprotein (AGP). Gimatecan has a long elimination phase (mean half-life of 90 h) with a clearance of 0.6 L/h. Fecal excretion is the main elimination pathway. Gimatecan is not a substrate for ABCB1 or ABCG2.

Adverse Effects Bone marrow suppression is the main dose limiting toxicity. Diarrhea is less severe than with camptothecin.

The second generation camptothecin derivative lurtotecan is a semi-synthetic analog of camptothecin, which selectively stabilizes the Topoisomerase 1/DNA covalent complex and forms an enzyme/drug/DNA ternary complex. As a consequence of the formation of this complex, both the initial cleavage reaction and the religation step are inhibited. Subsequently, collision of the reduplication fork with the cleaved strand of DNA results in inhibition of DNA reduplication, double strand DNA breakage, and triggering of apoptosis. Through additional mechanisms of action, lurtotecan also inhibits RNA synthesis, multi-ubiquitination and degradation of Topoisomerase 1, and chromatin reorganization.

The second generation camptothecin derivative exatecan mesylate[33] is a semi-synthetic water soluble drug. It inhibits

[33] Mesylate is a salt or ester of methanesulfonic acid, which may be used to to obtain crystalline salts of amine containing drug substances. Mesylate is a suitable leaving group in nucleophilic substitution reactions.

Topoisomerase 1 activity by stabilizing the cleavable complex between Topoisomerase 1 and DNA, thus blocking the religation of DNA breaks. Thereby exatecan inhibits DNA reduplication and triggers apoptotic cell death. This agent does not require enzymatic activation and exhibits greater potency than other camptothecin analogs.

The second generation camptothecin derivative rubitecan (9-NC, 9-Nitro-20(S)-Camptothecin, 9-Nitro-Camptothecin, 9-Nitrocamptothecin) (RFS 2000, RFS2000) <Orathecin> is a semi-synthetic agent that binds to and inhibits Topoisomerase 1. It is extracted from the bark and leaves of the Camptotheca acuminata tree, which is native to China. Rubitecan is under investigation for the treatment of advanced pancreatic cancer, as well as for prostate, breast, lung, and ovarian cancers.

Pharmacokinetics Rubitecan is an orally available camptothecin analog that also has potential for delivery transdermally or by inhalation. The drug exists in equilibrium between 9-nitro-camptothecin (9-NC) and 9-amino-camptothecin (9-AC). Both contain a lactone ring that is required for activity. The open ring, carboxylic acid forms are substantially less active or inactive. An acidic environment favors the lactone ring structure, whereas neutral or basic conditions favor the conversion to the carboxylic acid structure.

Homocamptothecins, in which the metabolically labile 6-membered α-hydroxylactone of camptothecin is replaced with a more stable 7-membered β-hydroxylactone, are potent anti-cancer agents. Diflomotecan (10,11-difluoro-homocamptothecin) (BN80915) is a third generation camptothecin derivative. The drug may be given intravenously or orally (Kroep and Gelderblom 2009). The recommended dose is 4 mg/m^2 for intravenous administration.

Pharmacokinetics Diflomotecan has enhanced plasma stability and superior anti-tumor activity as compared to the established camptothecins, irinotecan and topotecan. It has an oral bioavailability of 70–95 %.

Adverse Effects In contrast to other Topoisomerase 1 inhibitors, there is no severe gastrointestinal toxicity. The adverse effects are primarily hematologic, with severe neutropenia occurring in some patients.

Drug Resistance The homocamptothecins, like the camptothecins, are substrates for cellular efflux pumps, such as ABCG2. Cancer cells that are resistant to camptothecins due to over-expression of multi-drug resistance efflux pumps or mutations in Topoisomerase 1 are also resistant to homocamptothecins.

Derivatives of camptothecins have been synthesized to improve the pharmacokinetic properties. S-CKD602 (STEALTH-CKD602) is a sterically stabilized, polyethylene glycol coated (PEGylated) liposomal formulation containing CKD602, a semi-synthetic analog of campthotecin. The agent stabilizes the Topoisomerase 1/DNA complex, thereby preventing religation of DNA breaks. This leads to an inhibition of DNA reduplication and triggers apoptosis.

Pharmacokinetics The polyethylene glycol coating of S-CKD602 allows for greater plasma circulation time, thus enhancing the concentration of CKD602 at the tumor site. Encapsulation of CKD602 also preserves the active lactone form, leading to an increased cytotoxic effect of CKD602.

Karenitecin is a synthetic silicon containing agent related to camptothecin. It stabilizes the cleavable complex between Topoisomerase 1 and DNA, resulting in DNA breaks, and consequently triggering apoptosis.

Pharmacokinetics Because it is lipophilic, karenitecin exhibits enhanced tissue penetration and bio-availability compared to water soluble camptothecins.

Indolocarbazoles The indolocarbazole family of natural products was discovered in 1977. Its members are defined by their characteristic structure containing either indolo[2,3-a]pyrrolo[3,4-c]carbazole, indolo[2,3-a]carbazole, or bis-indolyl-maleimide[34]. The chemical structures (Fig. 2.33), pharmacokinetics, and pharmacodynamics of indolocarbazoles differ from many other Topoisomerase 1 inhibitors, including camptothecin derived agents.

Rebeccamycin (Bush et al. 1987), the first anti-cancer active indolocarbazole, was described in 1987 by Bristol-Myers scientists and named after the daughter of the group leader. Rebeccamycin is a secondary metabolite originally isolated from cultures of the actinobacterium Lechevalieria aerocolonigenes in 1985. The compound is halogenated and possesses a maleimide indolo[2,3-a]carbazole framework with a carbohydrate moiety attached to one of the indole nitrogens. As a sugar derivative, it has increased (albeit still poor) water solubility compared to the parent indolocarbazole. Rebeccamycin acts as a potent stabilizer of the Topoisomerase 1/DNA complex.

NB-506 (L-753 000) is a synthetic Topoisomerase 1 inhibitor with an indolocarbazole structure. Edotecarin (J-107088, ED-749, PHA-782615) is a derivative of NB-506 that more effectively induces DNA cleavage. It also targets

[34] Indolocarbazole antibiotics with a single glycosidic linkage are often strong inhibitors of Topoisomerases, whereas indolocarbazoles with two bonds between the glycoside and indolocarbazole heterocycle act as inhibitors of Protein Kinases. The staurosporine sub-class is characterized by two bonds between the glycoside and indolocarbazole heterocycle. These fused structures exhibit potent inhibition of protein kinases, such as Protein Kinase C (PKC), FLT3, and RET (see Sect. 4.1.3., 4.1.5., and 4.1.7.).

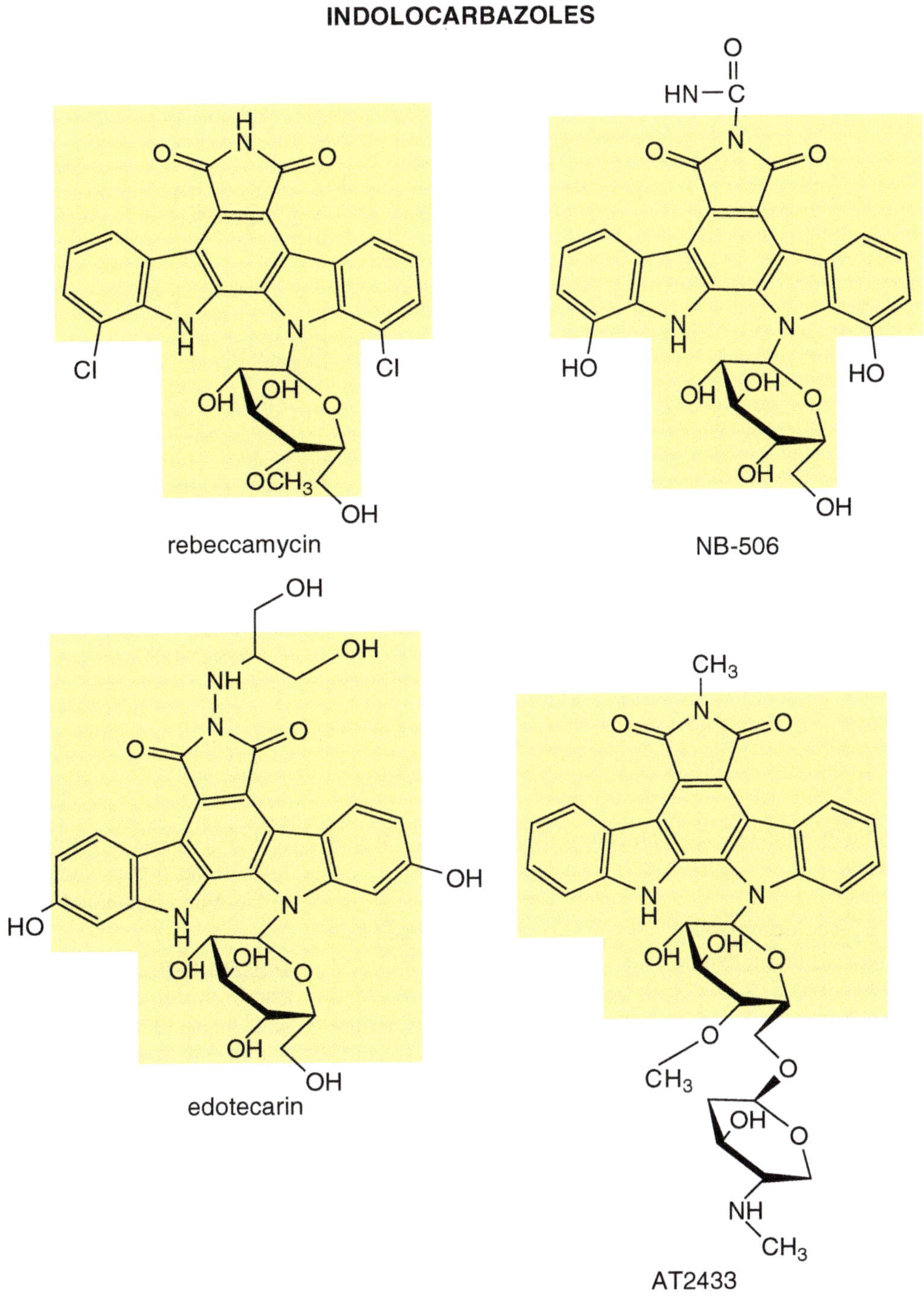

Fig. 2.33 Structures of indolocarbazoles. The common core structure, comprising the bulk of the drug molecules in this class, is highlighted in *yellow*

different DNA sequences than camptothecin or NB-506. The drug stabilizes the enzyme/DNA complex and enhances single strand DNA cleavage at C/T-G sites, resulting in inhibition of DNA reduplication and suppression of tumor cell proliferation. Endotecarin may have potent anti-tumor activity in the mono-therapy of colorectal cancer, and it is under study for the treatment of locally advanced breast cancer and glioblastoma. A recommended dose is 13 mg/m^2 intravenously every 3 weeks.

Pharmacokinetics Edotecarin has a moderate plasma clearance (45–53 L/h/m^2) and a large volume of distribution (650–850 L/m^2). It is largely eliminated as unchanged parent molecule via biliary excretion (Yin et al. 2005).

Adverse Effects The dose limiting toxicity is hematologic, comprising neutropenia, leukopenia and anemia.

Drug Resistance Edotecarin is subject to efflux from cells via ATP-binding cassette transporters (ABC transporters). Drug resistance may be acquired by over-expression of

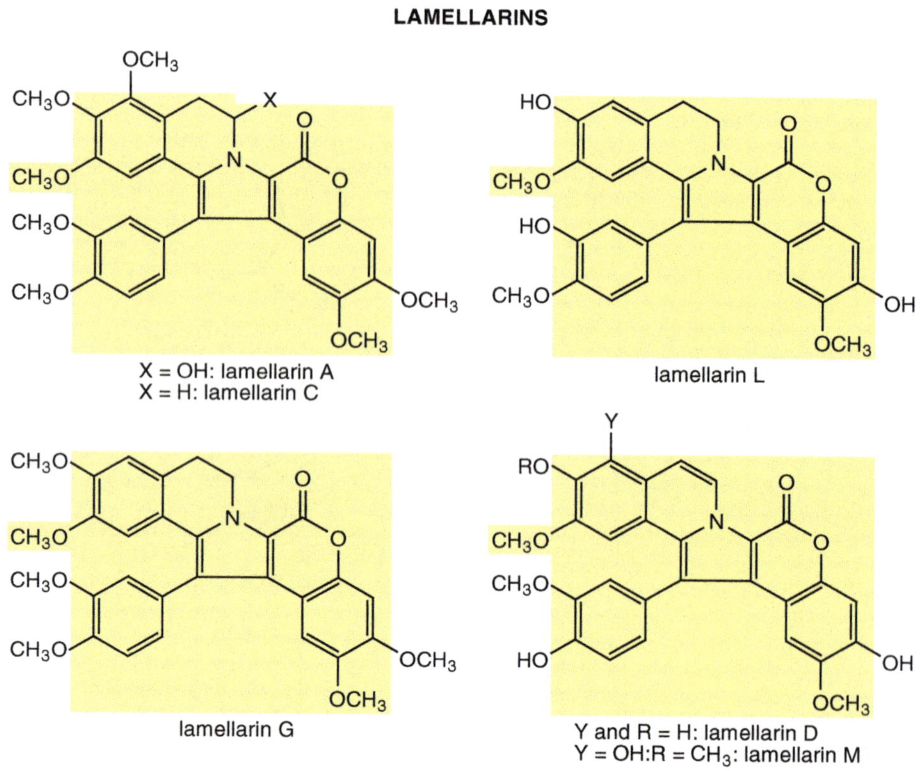

Fig. 2.34 Structures of lamellarins. The common core structure, highlighted in *yellow*, comprises the bulk of the molecules

ABCP (BCRP/MXR), which pumps the drug out of the cancer cells.

The indolocarbazole AT2433 was originally isolated from Actinomadura melliaura. There are five forms, AT2433-A1, AT2433-A2, AT2433-B1, its diastereoisomer iso-AT2433-B1, and AT2433-B2. It contains a unique disaccharide (aminodideoxypentose disaccharide, consisting of a methoxyglucose and the amino sugar subunit 2,4-dideoxy-4-methylamino-l-xylose) and an asymmetrically halogenated *N*-methylated aglycon.

Lamellarins Lamellarins were isolated from the marine mollusk Lamellaria in 1985, and have subsequently been identified in various ascidians (Fig. 2.34). More than 30 lamellarins have been produced since, some of which display equally potent cytotoxic activities against both multidrug resistant tumor cells and their corresponding non-resistant cells.

Lamellarin-D (LAM-D) is a hexacyclic marine alkaloid initially isolated from a prosobranch mollusk of the genus Lamellaria (Facompré et al. 2003). It bears a 6H-[1]benzopyrano[4′,3′:4,5]pyrrolo[2,1-a]isoquinolin-one pentacyclic planar chromophore. Lamellarin-D recognizes structural elements of the Topoisomerase 1/DNA covalent complex different from those recognized by camptothecin.

LAM-501 is a synthetic 5,6-dehydro analog of lamellarin-D. It has a non-planar structure. LAM-501 does not bind to DNA and fails to inhibit Topoisomerase 1.

Indenoisoquinolines The indenoisoquinolines selectively trap Topoisomerase 1/DNA cleavage complexes (Cushman and Cheng 1978) in a manner that is more persistent than the complexes induced by camptothecins. The indenoisoquinolines target different genomic sites (break DNA at different sequences) than camptothecins and therefore may potentially exhibit a different spectrum of anti-cancer activity. Unlike camptothecins, indenoisoquinolines are not subject to inactivation by lactone hydrolysis at physiological pH. They are seldom substrates for the ABCG2 multi-drug efflux pump that confers resistance to irinotecan and topotecan.

The indenoisoquinoline NSC314622 (Fig. 2.35) was identified in 1978 as a potential Topoisomerase 1 inhibitor by analysis from 48-h cytotoxicity screening of the NCI panel of 60 cell lines, where it had moderate activity. The second lead compound, MJIII-65 (NSC 706744) reversibly traps Topoisomerase 1/DNA cleavage complexes. It is not a DNA intercalator by itself, as it does not unwind DNA in the absence of Topoisomerase 1. MJ-III-65 remains active against the camptothecin resistant Topoisomerase 1 mutants Asn722Ser and Arg364His. However, the poor solubility of MJ-III-65 impaired its further development.

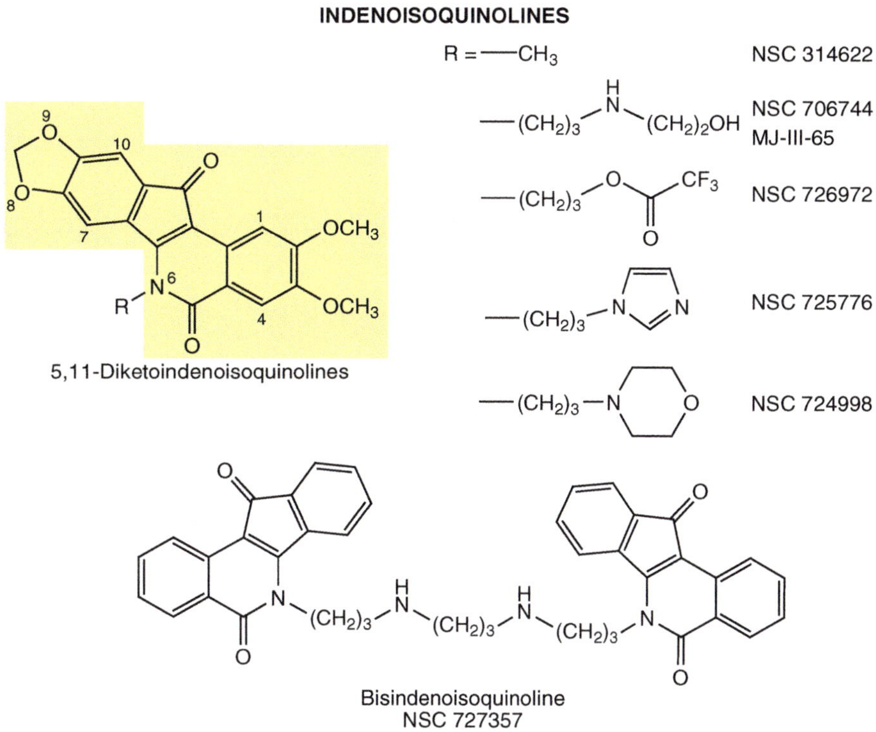

Fig. 2.35 Structures of indenoisoquinolines. The common core structure for various lead compounds is highlighted in *yellow*. Bisindenoisoquinoline comprises two indenoisoquinoline moieties bridged by a linker

Lead compounds under investigation are indimitecan (NSC 725776) and indotecan (NSC 724998). The agents achieve concentration dependent foci formation of the Histone γ-H2A.X, which is a biochemical indicator of DNA double strand breaks, at pharmacologically relevant doses.

The dimeric indenoisoquinoline NSC 727357 induces Topoisomerase 1 cleavage complexes at specific DNA sites. NSC 727357 also induces a limited number of Topoisomerase 2/DNA cleavage complexes. In contrast to the effect of other Topoisomerase 1 inhibitors, cells treated with NSC 727357 display arrest of cell cycle progression in G_1 with no significant inhibition of DNA synthesis following a short exposure to the drug. The cytotoxicity of NSC 727357 is only partially dependent on Topoisomerase 1 and P53, indicating that this drug has additional targets.

Others Ecteinascidin-743 (trabectedin, ET-743) <Yondelis> is produced by the Caribbean tunicate Ecteinascidia turbinate. The drug binds tightly to Topoisomerase 1, with which it produces cleavage complexes. It also alkylates DNA and may induce the production of superoxide near the DNA strand, resulting in DNA backbone cleavage and cell apoptosis. The compound has activity against a variety of soft tissue sarcomata and is in clinical trials for breast, ovarian, and prostate cancers.

Camptothecin/Topoisomerase 1/DNA complexes inhibit reduplication and trigger apoptosis. Camptothecin also inhibits RNA synthesis.

Irinotecan is an S phase specific agent.
Camptothecins exist in a pH dependent equilibrium between their active lactone and inactive ring-opened conformations.
The stability of the lactone ring at physiological pH is a determinant of activity for all camptothecin analogs.
Topotecan and irinotecan are substrates for the efflux pump ABCB1. Camptothecins are substrates for ABCG2.
Indolocarbazoles with one glycosidic linkage are Topoisomerase inhibitors, indolocarbazoles with two glycosidic bonds are Protein Kinase inhibitors.
The sugar moieties of indolocarbazoles increase their water solubility.
Indolocarbazoles are substrates for efflux pumps, which may constitute a mechanism of drug resistance.

Lamellarins may be second-line-of-defense drugs for multi-drug resistant tumor cells.

Indenoisoquinolines trap Topoisomerase 1-DNA cleavage complexes in unique genomic sites.
Indenoisoquinolines are seldom substrates for the multi-drug resistance efflux pumps.
Bisindenoisoquinolines induce Topoisomerase 1-DNA cleavage complexes and Topoisomerase 2-DNA cleavage complexes. They lead to cell cycle arrest in G1.

2.3.2 Topoisomerase 2 Inhibitors

Type 2 Topoisomerases are enzymes that change the topology of DNA by introducing transient double strand breaks to from a cleavage complex, through which other DNA strands are passed. These 2-fold symmetric enzymes cleave a pair of opposing phosphodiester bonds four base pairs apart.

PODOPHYLLOTOXINS

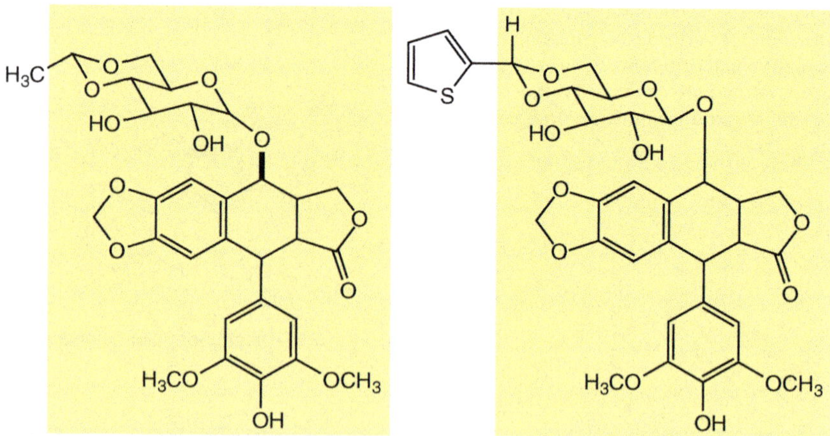

etoposide teniposide

Fig. 2.36 Structures of podophyllotoxins. The common core is highlighted in *yellow*. The drug structures differ in one position

Topoisomerase 2 inhibitors promote the formation of DNA lesions by increasing the steady state level of the cleavage complex.

Podophyllotoxins Podophyllotoxin (5,8,8a,9-Tetrahydro-9-hydroxy-5-(3,4,5-trimethoxylphenyl) furo[3′,4′:6,7] naphtho[2,3,d]-1,3-dioxol-6(5aH)-one, podofilox) is a plant derived lignin that is present in the mandrake roots of the American mayapple (podophyllum peltatum) and in the Indian podophyllum hexandrum royle. Podophyllum plants were used as cathartics for centuries. Podophyllotoxin <Oclassen's Condylox, Condyline, Warticon> is used for the treatment of genital warts[35]. It constitutes the parent molecule for the cytostatic drugs etoposide and teniposide (Fig. 2.36).

Etoposide (4′-Demethylepipodophyllotoxin 9-[4,6-O-(R)-ethylidene-β-D-glucopyranoside]) <Etopophos, Vepesid, VP-16> is a semi-synthetic derivative of podophyllotoxin. The drug exerts its anti-neoplastic properties by binding to and inhibiting Topoisomerase 2, which prevents the religation of cleaved DNA molecules, resulting in the accumulation of strand breaks, the inhibition of DNA reduplication, and apoptotic cell death. It acts primarily in the G_2 and M phases of the cell cycle. Etoposide is used in combination chemotherapy, mainly to treat refractory testicular cancer following unsuccessful standard treatment and in first-line treatment for small cell lung cancers. It also has use in the treatment of chorionic carcinoma, Kaposi sarcoma, malignant melanoma, and lymphomata. A phosphate salt improves the drug properties because the water solubility of etoposide phosphate lessens the potential for precipitation following dilution and during intravenous administration. Etoposide is administered intravenously or orally as liquid capsules. Standard dosing covers the range of 5–100 mg/m^2/day.

Pharmacokinetics On intravenous administration, the disposition of etoposide follows a biphasic process with a distribution half-life of about 1.5 h and a terminal elimination half-life of 4–11 h. In the blood, etoposide is 97 % protein bound. The cytotoxicity of the prodrug etoposide phosphate is lower than that of etoposide, which may be due to the necessity for conversion to the active moiety by dephosphorylation. *O*-demethylation of the etoposide dimethoxyphenol ring occurs through the CYP450 3A4 pathway to produce the corresponding catechol. The hydroxy acid metabolite 4′-demethylepipodophyllic acid-9-(4,6-*O*-(R)-ethylidene-β-D-gluco-pyranoside) is formed by opening of the lactone ring. It enters the blood, likely as the trans isomer. Within 5 days, 55 % of the injected dose is excreted in the urine and 45 % in the feces. The hydroxy acid metabolite, as well as glucuronide or sulfate conjugates of etoposide are excreted renally.

Individuals with low Albumin have an elevated fraction of free drug, which may represent an increased risk for etoposide associated toxicities or may lead to accelerated renal excretion. In patients with impaired renal function, initial dose modification should be considered based on creatinine clearance.

Adverse Effects The most frequent adverse effects is leukopenia. The occurrence of a platelet count below 50,000/mm^3 or an absolute neutrophil count below 500/mm^3 is an indication to withhold further therapy until the blood counts have sufficiently recovered. Nausea and vomiting are the major gastrointestinal toxicities. Their severity is generally mild to moderate with treatment discontinuation required in 1 % of patients. Nausea and vomiting can usually be controlled with standard anti-emetic therapy. Major additional adverse effects include reversible hair loss (45 % of patients), anorexia, and diarrhea. Due to its mechanisms of action through genetic damage, etoposide may increase the

[35] Genital warts, which are caused by the human papillomavirus (HPV), are associated with an increased risk for squamous cell carcinomata of the genitals.

risk of developing leukemia. The drug causes fetal damage and birth defects, and hence should not be used by pregnant or nursing women.

Hypersensitivity reactions can occur in 0.5–2 % of patients and manifest as chills, fever, shortness of breath, wheezing, or low blood pressure. In such cases, the drug needs be stopped and the reaction treated with dexamethasone, diphenhydramine, and if necessary epinephrine. For mild reactions, the infusion may be restarted at a slower rate along with intravenous fluids and gradually increased with blood pressure monitoring.

Drug Interactions In combination regimens, the etoposide dosage needs to be modified to take into account the myelosuppressive effects of other drugs. Similarly, the effects of prior radiation or chemotherapy, which may have compromised the bone marrow reserve, can mandate dose reduction. Caution must be exercised when administering etoposide phosphate with drugs that inhibit Phosphatase activities (such as levamisole hydrochloride). High-dose cyclosporin A, resulting in concentrations above 2000 ng/mL, administered with oral etoposide leads to an 80 % increase in etoposide exposure with a 40 % decrease in total body clearance compared to etoposide alone. Phenylbutazone, sodium salicylate, and aspirin can displace Albumin bound etoposide. The use of cisplatin therapy is associated with reduced total body clearance of etoposide. Prior use of cisplatin may also result in a decrease of etoposide total body clearance in children.

Teniposide <Vumon, VM-26, EPT> is a semi-synthetic derivative of podophyllotoxin. It forms a ternary complex with Topoisomerase 2 and DNA, resulting in dose dependent single and double stranded breaks, as well as DNA/protein cross-links. This agent acts in the late S or early G_2 phase of the cell cycle. Teniposide is used to treat lymphomata and leukemias, mainly childhood acute lymphocytic leukemia.

Adverse Effects Common adverse effects include nausea, vomiting, diarrhea, and thinned or brittle hair. A major problem with teniposide is the lowered count of white blood cells 1–2 weeks after treatment. Although they mostly return to normal after 3–4 weeks, the decreased count puts the patient at risk for infections. The time course for platelets is similar. When given as an intravenous infusion over 30–60 min, teniposide causes a burning sensation if it leaks under the skin.

Quinoxalines Chloroquinoxaline sulfonamide (chlorosulfaquinoxaline, CQS) (NSC 339004) is a chlorinated heterocyclic sulfanilamide (Fig. 2.37). It inhibits Topoisomerase 2α and Topoisomerase 2β, thereby causing DNA double strand breaks and accumulation of unrepaired DNA, which result in apoptosis (Gao et al. 2000).

Adverse Effects This agent exerts lymphotoxicity by inhibiting lymphocyte activation in a cell cycle specific manner.

The synthetic quinoxaline phenoxypropionic acid derivative XK469 has structural similarity to chloroquinoxaline sulfonamide. The agent selectively inhibits Topoisomerase 2β (Gao et al. 1999) by stabilizing the enzyme/DNA intermediates, in which Topoisomerase subunits are covalently linked to DNA through 5-phospho-tyrosyl linkages. The formed complexes interfere with DNA repair and reduplication, as well as with RNA synthesis. XK469 possesses solid tumor selectivity and activity against multi-drug resistant cancer cells. The racemic form XK469R is more water soluble and active than either of the pure isomers R(+)XK469 and S(−)XK469.

Antibiotics Some of the anti-neoplastic antibiotics also inhibit Topoisomerase 2. They include several anthracyclines (daunorubicin, doxorubicin, epirubicin, detorubicin, carubicin, idarubicin, RTA 744), anthracenediones (mitoxantrone), anthrapyrazoles (teloxantrone, piroxantrone), dactinomycin, fostriecin, and streptonigrin (see Sect. 2.2.).

Others Asulacrine isethionate (amsalog, 9-[2-Methoxy-4-(methylsulfonylamino)phenylamino]-N,5-dimethyl-4-acridinecarboxamide 2-hydroxyethanesulfonate) (NSC-343499, CI-921) (Fig. 2.38)is a synthetic derivative of acridine carboxamide and an amphiphilic analog of amsacrine. It inhibits Topoisomerase 2, thereby blocking DNA reduplication and RNA synthesis.

Razoxane (ICRF 159, ICI 59118) <Razoxin> is a bisdioxopiperazine and a derivative of the chelating agent EDTA. It constitutes a racemic mixture, of which dexrazoxane (used for cardioprotection in anthracyclin treatment)

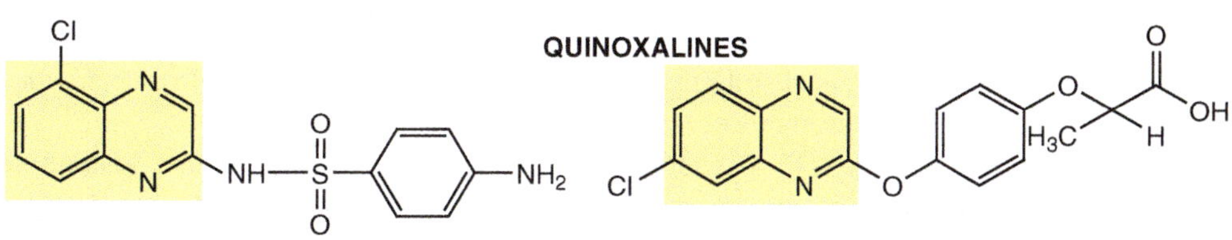

chloroquinoxaline sulfonamide

XK469

Fig. 2.37 Structures of quinoxalines. The quinoxaline structure is highlighted in *yellow*

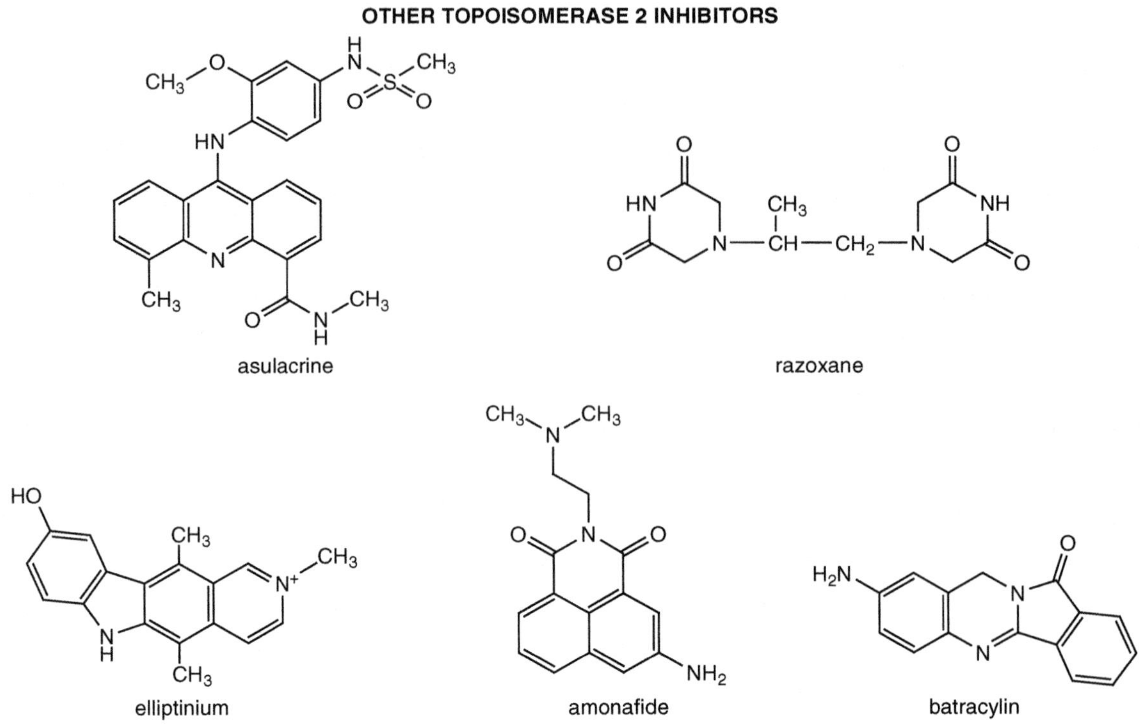

Fig. 2.38 Structures of other Topoisomerase 2 inhibitors

is the S(+)-enantiomer. Razoxane inhibits Topoisomerase 2 without inducing DNA strand breaks, thereby inhibiting DNA synthesis and inducing cytotoxicity. The drug also exhibits anti-angiogenic activity.

Adverse Effects Secondary malignancies, primarily acute myeloid leukemia, may arise in patients treated chronically with oral razoxane. The risk is high in patients, whose total cumulative dose of razoxane ranges 25–500 g over 40–320 weeks.

Drug Interactions The use of dexrazoxane concurrently with the initiation of fluorouracil, doxorubicin, and cyclophosohamide (FAC) therapy of breast cancers interferes with the anti-tumor efficacy of the regimen. Dexrazoxane should only be used in those patients who have received a cumulative doxorubicin dose of 300 mg/m^2 and are continuing with doxorubicin therapy, not at the onset of FAC treatment.

Elliptinium acetate (9-hydroxy-2,5,11-trimethyl-6H-pyrido[4,3-b]carbazolium acetate, 9-HME) <Celiptium> was developed in the 1970s. It is a derivative of the alkaloid ellipticine, isolated from species of the plant family Apocynaceae, including Bleekeria vitensis. As a Topoisomerase 2 inhibitor and intercalating agent, elliptinium stabilizes the cleavable complex of Topoisomerase 2 and induces DNA breakages, thereby inhibiting DNA reduplication and RNA synthesis. The agent has anti-tumor activity against breast, kidney, and other cancers (Buzdar et al. 1990).

Adverse Effects Although the drug lacks myelosuppressive toxicity, other adverse effects, including hemolytic anemia and renal failure, limit its clinical use. Hence, semi-synthetic analogs with molecular modifications have been developed to reduce the severe dose limiting toxicities of the parent compound.

Amonafide dihydrochloride (benzisoquinolinedione, nafidimide) (AS1413) <Quinamed> , an imide derivative of naphthalic acid, is a Topoisomerase 2 inhibitor and intercalating agent that is in clinical trials for the treatment of cancer. It also affects a number of targets in the EGFR pathway. The drug has modest anti-tumor activity against prostate and small cell lung cancer.

Pharmacokinetics Amonafide is acetylated to N-acetyl-amonafide. Therefore, the rate of metabolism of the drug is strongly determined by the genotype of NAT2. Fast acetylators have a much higher overall response rate than slow acetylators. Dosing should account for the genotype of the patient.

Adverse Effects The dose limiting toxicity is reversible myelosuppression. Non-hematologic toxicity is mild, consisting mostly of nausea and vomiting, which is easily controlled with anti-emetics.

Batracylin (isoindolo[1,2-b]quinazolin-12(10*H*)-one) (NSC 320846) was developed at the U.S. National Cancer Institute as an anti-cancer agent, but was dropped in 1989 and resumed much later. Topoisomerase 2 inhibition by the compound is not dependent on ATP, which implies a favorable characteristic for treating hypoxic tumors.

Pharmacokinetics Oral absorption is variable. Drug activation to the highly toxic acetylated form, *N*-acetyl-batracylin is catalyzed by *N*-Acetyl Transferase 2 (NAT2). In patients with the fast-metabolizing NAT2 allele dose reduction may be required to avoid toxicity.

Drug Resistance Batracylin is not a substrate for ABCB1, thus eliminating this mechanism for resistance.

Topoisomerase 2 inhibitors promote the formation of DNA lesions by increasing the steady state level of the cleavage complex.
Podophyllotoxins (etoposide and teniposide) arrest cells in G2/M phase. They may cause DNA single and double strand breaks.
Quinoxalines may be active in multi-drug resistant cancers.
Other Topoisomerase 2 inhibitors include asulacrine isethionate, razoxane, elliptinium, amonafide, and batracyclin.

Treatment of Embryonic Tumors

1. **Seminomatous tumors**

The therapy regimen depends on the stage of the tumor. External beam radiation is used for stage I and non-bulky stage 2 disease. Over a 3-week period, 2500 cGy are administered in a "hockey-stick field", including the para-aortic, para-caval, bilateral common iliac, and external iliac nodal regions. In some cases, the radiation field can be reduced only to the para-aortic area. As an alternative to radiotherapy or as a follow-up to radiation, single agent carboplatin protocols are under study. The long-term success of carboplatin therapy is unknown and should be considered experimental (Oliver et al. 2005).

For stage 2 bulky or stage 3 disease, radical orchiectomy and metastatic workup, are followed by administration of four cycles of chemotherapy without radiation therapy. The combination of bleomycin, etoposide, and cisplatin (BEP) is standard. Ongoing clinical trials are evaluating the omission of the 4th cycle, or of bleomycin, in patients with favorable prognosis. For high risk and salvage cases, alternative regimens may use ifosfamide and vinblastine with dose escalation.

2. **Non-seminomatous tumors**

Metastatic non-seminomatous germ cell tumors (NSGCT) are highly sensitive to cisplatin based chemotherapy, with cure rates of approximately 80% for advanced disease and nearly 100% for early stage disease. Risk-adapted protocols are available to tailor treatment regimens toward patients with good, moderate, or poor risk factors.

Despite a high cure rate in men with testicular cancer, some in the poor prognosis group require aggressive treatment. Poor prognosis non-seminomatous germ cell tumors are defined as those with high tumor markers, non-pulmonary visceral metastases, or a mediastinal primary site at presentation. When treated with standard chemotherapy regimens, such as bleomycin, etoposide and cisplatin (BEP), cure rates below 50% are achieved. Some strategies aimed at improving results include the use of multi-agent regimens (e.g. POMB/ACE: cisplatin, vincristine <Oncovin>, methotrexate, bleomycin, actinomycin D, cyclophosphamide, etoposide) and intensive-induction chemotherapy (e.g. CBOP/BEP: carboplatin, bleomycin, vincristine <Oncovin>, cisplatin followed by BEP). Other drugs, such as ifosfamide, gemcitabine, oxaliplatin, and paclitaxel have been added to therapeutic strategies in first-line and salvage treatment of poor-prognosis non-seminomatous germ cell tumors (Sirohi and Huddart 2005).

Choriocarcinoma Historically, methotrexate <Trexall> was the first drug treatment to force a cancer into remission when it was used for treating choriocarcinoma.

Choriocarcinoma is highly sensitive to chemotherapy, which is therefore the main type of treatment. The cure rate, even for metastatic choriocarcinoma, is around 90–95%. However metastatic disease to the kidneys or the brain is usually fatal. Hysterectomy and radiation therapy are rarely needed. In the case of a molar pregnancy (gestational trophoblastic disease, hydatiform mole), prophylactic chemotherapy (methotrexate and actinomycin D) at the time of molar evacuation reduces the frequency of postmolar tumors.

- Single agent chemotherapy with either methotrexate (MTX-FA: intramuscular methotrexate 1.0 mg/kg days 1, 3, 5, and 7, intramuscular or oral folinic acid 0.1 mg/kg on days 2, 4, 6, and 8; 5-day MTX: intravenous or intramuscular methotrexate 0.4 mg/kg/day for 5 days; Pulse MTX: intramuscular methotrexate 50 mg/m^2 weekly) or actinomycin D (5-Day Act-D: intravenous actinomycin D 12 µg/kg/day for 5 days; Pulse Act-D: intravenous actinomycin D 1.25 mg/m^2 every 2 weeks) is the preferred treatment in patients with stage 1 gestational trophoblastic tumors, who desire to retain fertility.
- Patients with resistance to single agent chemotherapy are treated with combination chemotherapy of methotrexate, actinomycin D, and cyclophosphamide (MAC), or etoposide, methotrexate, actinomycin D, cyclophosphamide, and vincristine <Oncovin> (EMA-CO), or surgical therapy. MAC is pre-

ferred as the initial combination chemotherapy in these patients because etoposide is associated with an increased risk for secondary tumors.

- While patients with low-risk stages 2 and 3 are treated with primary single agent chemotherapy with methotrexate or actinomycin D, patients with high-risk disease are managed with primary combination chemotherapy with EMA-CO. Patients with disease resistant to single agent chemotherapy are then treated with EMA-CO. Patients with disease resistant to EMA-CO may be treated by modifying that regimen by substituting cisplatin and etoposide on day 8, and escalating the dose of methotrexate infusion to 1 g/m^2 (EMA-CE).
- All patients with stage 4 disease are managed with primary EMA-CO combination chemotherapy. In the presence of cerebral metastases, the methotrexate dosage in the infusion is increased to 1 g/m^2. Patients with disease resistant to EMA-CO may then be treated with EMA-CE (Kufe et al. 2003).
- Choriocarcinoma in primary locations other than the placenta is rare. Very rarely it arises in testicles. These tumors are aggressive and highly resistant to chemotherapy. The same is true of choriocarcinoma of the ovaries.

Yolk sac tumor Primary chemotherapy may be initiated with VAC (vincristine, actinomycin D, cyclophosphamide), PVB (cisplatin, vinblastine, bleomycin), or BEP (bleomycin, etoposide, cisplatin). Therapeutic effect can be monitored with the levels of α-Fetoprotein (AFP) in the blood.

Teratoma The treatment of choice is complete resection. Teratomata are normally well encapsulated and non-invasive, hence they are relatively easy to remove from surrounding tissues. For malignant teratomata, surgery is followed by chemotherapy.

Desmoplastic small round cell tumor is a form of teratoma. Although there is no standard protocol for the disease, some patients respond to high dose chemotherapy (P6 Protocol) (Donadio et al. 2003), maintenance chemotherapy, surgery, and radiation therapy. Other treatment options include hematopoietic stem cell transplantation or intraperitoneal hyperthermic chemoperfusion. The tumor may be responsive to irinotecan.

2.4 Anti-Metabolites

Folic acid (folacin, vitamin B9) was discovered and synthesized by Lucy Wills in 1937. Previously, nutritional research in the early part of the twentieth century had identified a factor present in green leafy vegetables that was important for bone marrow function. It turned out to be folic acid, a vitamin crucial for DNA metabolism. However, the same compound administered to children with acute lymphoblastic leukemia (ALL) seemed to exacerbate their cancer (Farber 1949). Sidney Farber (1903–1973) in Boston recognized that folic acid stimulated the proliferation of leukemia cells. In one of the first examples of rational anti-cancer drug design, he collaborated with Harriett Kilte and Lederle Laboratories of the American Cyanamid Company to devise folate analogs. In November 1947, when a sufficient amount of aminopterin became available[36], Farber administered it to 16 children with acute leukemia and achieved remissions in ten of them. He demonstrated that aminopterin blocked a critical chemical reaction needed for DNA reduplication (Farber et al. 1948). Aminopterin was the predecessor of methotrexate (developed by Seeger and colleagues at Lederle Laboratories in 1948 and called amethopterin), which in 1956 became the first compound cure of metastatic cancer, when it was used by Roy Hertz (1909–2002) and Min Chiu Li (-1980) to treat two cases of choriocarcinoma. The principal architect of the treatment, using methotrexate in an unusual way for the time, was Min Chiu Li. As a sign of the times, after the first two patients went into remission, they were presented at National Cancer Institute Grand Rounds under the title "the spontaneous regression of cancer" with the speaker being Gordon Zubrod (Li's superior and at that time a detractor of chemotherapy). Li was told if he persisted in using his radical treatment, he would have to forfeit his position at the newly opened clinical center. He continued and was asked to leave. After his initial success with methotrexate, Li went on to develop the first effective combination chemotherapy programs for metastatic testicular cancer (DeVita and Chu 2008). In 1972, when the Lasker Prize was awarded to investigators who had contributed to studies of

[36] Aminopterin was synthesized by Yellapragada Subbarao at Lederle Laboratories. Subbarao had been denied tenure at Harvard, despite his discovery of the roles of phosphocreatine and adenosine triphosphate (ATP) in muscular activity. He joined Lederle, where he developed a method to synthesize folic acid, and with considerable input from Farber, he produced anti-folates. Subbarao remained obscure because he did not actively publicize his work or himself. It was said that some of the nucleotides isolated by him at Harvard Medical School had to be rediscovered years later by other workers because his superior, Cyrus Fiske, apparently out of jealousy, had not let Subbarao's contributions see the light of the day.

the cure of gestational choriocarcinoma, Li had to share his part of the prize with the person who had discharged him.[37]

The development of anti-purines was based on the hypothesis that nucleic acid synthesis in cells might be stopped by nucleic acid base analogs. In the early 1940s, very few chemists were interested synthesizing nucleic acid bases, so that relevant references dated back to the manuscripts of Emil Fischer (1852–1919) in the old German literature. Gertrude Belle Elion (1918–1999) was a medicinal chemist interested in the pharmacology of anti-purines. She had enrolled in City College of New York at the age of 15 (importantly, it was tuition-free as her father had been bankrupted by the stock market crash), and earned her chemistry degree from Hunter College at age 19. Unable to obtain a graduate research position due to gender discrimination during the great depression, she worked as a laboratory assistant and a high school chemistry teacher. During that period, her fiancé died from endocarditis. Elion never married and it seems that her love was entirely devoted to medicinal chemistry. She finally took a position as an assistant to George H. Hitchings (1905–1998) at the pharmaceutical company Burroughs Wellcome & Company. From 1942 on, research by Hitchings and Elion tested many purine analogs and corroborated that it was possible to treat cancer with anti-metabolite compounds. By 1951, they had synthesized and tested over 100 purine analogs. Using one of them, 6-mercaptopurine, Joseph N. Burchenal (1912–2006) achieved a high percentage of complete remissions in childhood leukemias. Later, Sullivan and co-workers improved on the efficacy by infusing methotrexate intra-arterially into solid tumors with systemic protection by intramuscular citrovorum factor.

Anti-metabolites have affinity to the enzymes of nucleic acid biosynthesis. They may be incorporated into cellular polymers and act as false building blocks. Alternatively, they may compete with the normal monomeric components of nucleic acids for essential synthetic enzymes and inhibit them. Because this group of drugs compromises the synthesis of DNA and RNA in healthy and transformed cells alike, they are more effectively used in localized therapy than in systemic therapy. However, only a few types of cancer are accessibly for this treatment modality.

Anti-metabolites may act as false building blocks for nucleic acids.
Anti-metabolites may inhibit essential synthetic enzymes for nucleic acids.

[37] The clinical use of the anti-metabolite parent drug aminopterin discontinued in favor of the successor drug methotrexate. In some parts of the world, aminopterin is still used as a rodent poison in farming. It is a suspect in a 2007 pet poisoning incident that led to a massive recall of pet food by Menu Foods, U.S. The wheat gluten used as a base for the preparation of these foods had been imported from China. It was likely contaminated.

Due to their mechanism of action, anti-metabolites inhibit cell proliferation in S phase.

2.4.1 Anti-Folates

Folic acid (pteroylglutamic acid) dependent oxidation or reduction reactions of single carbons are important in biosynthetic pathways leading to the production of DNA, RNA, and membrane lipids. Dietary folates must be chemically reduced to their tetrahydro-forms, bearing four hydrogens on the pteridine ring, to be active. The enzyme responsible for this reduction is Dihydrofolate Reductase (DHFR). Folic acid in its fully reduced form serves as a carbon carrier for transfer reactions that are required in purine and thymidylate synthesis, and consecutively in the formation of DNA and cell division. The folic acid cycle also supports the synthesis of certain amino acids, such as methionine (Fig. 2.39). Natural folates circulating in the blood have a single glutamic acid group, but within cells they are converted to poly-glutamates, which are more efficient cofactors and are preferentially retained inside the cells. Hence, folate is an important biosynthetic component for proliferating cells.

The cytotoxic activity of anti-folates is mainly due to their ability to inhibit several folate dependent enzymes involved in DNA synthesis. Old generation anti-folates comprise Dihydrofolate Reductase inhibitors and Thymidylate Synthase inhibitors. The new generation of anti-folates includes Glycinamide Ribonucleotide Formyl Transferase inhibitors and Dihydropteroate Synthase inhibitors (Fig. 2.40).

The intracellular antifolate concentration is important for the inhibition of specific target enzymes. It depends on

- uptake: antifolate membrane transport into cells, typically via the Reduced Folate Carrier (RFC)
- retention: the conversion to poly-L-γ-glutamate forms catalyzed by Folylpoly-γ-Glutamate Synthetase (FPGS)
- elimination: cellular hydrolysis of antifolate poly- L-γ-glutamates to mono-glutamates and the extrusion of the mono-glutamates through the cell membrane.

Recent synthetic efforts have focused on developing antifolates that are selectively delivered to cancer cells, but not to normal proliferating cells, exploiting differences in the properties of their folate transporters. In another approach, drugs structurally and mechanistically unrelated to folates are linked to and use folic acid as a carrier to be endocytosed by folate receptors, which are abundant on cancer cells, and then released to inhibit their cellular targets (Goldman et al. 2010).

Dihydrofolate Reductase inhibitors Dihydrofolates must be reduced to tetrahydrofolates by Dihydrofolate Reductase

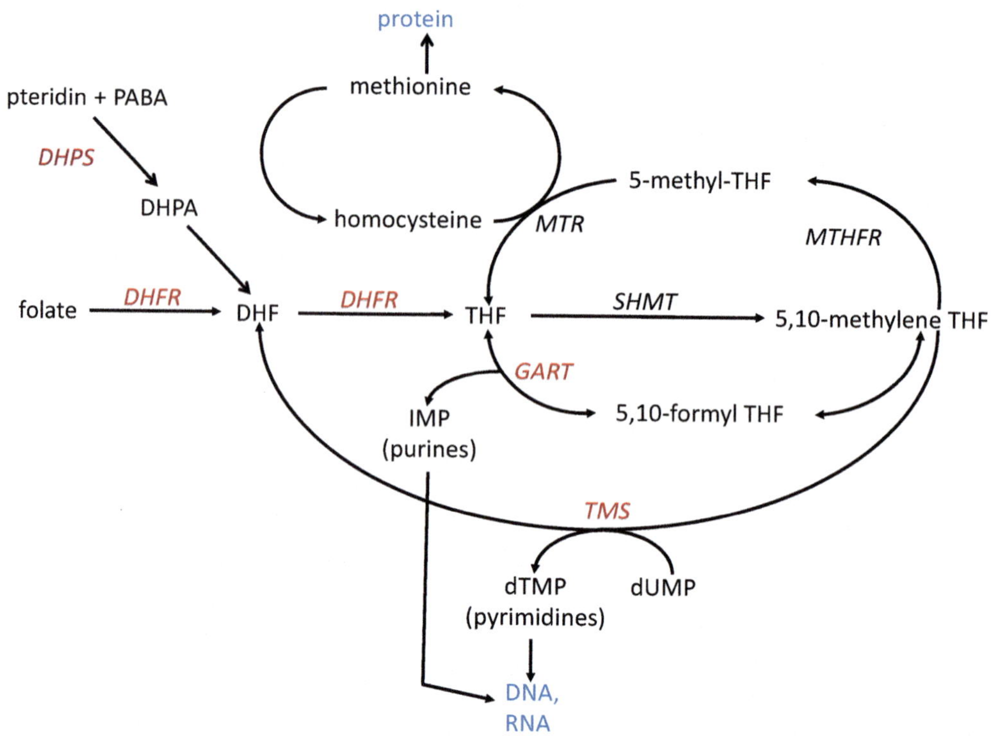

Fig. 2.39 The folate pathway. The synthetic end products DNA, RNA, and protein are shown in *blue*. The enzymes that serve as drug targets for anti-folates are depicted in *dark red*. Enzyme names are written in italics. *PABA* para-aminobenzoate, *DHPS* Dihydropteroate Synthase, *DHPA* dihydropteroate, *DHFR* Dihydrofolate Reductase, *DHF* dihydrofolate, *THF* tetrahydrofolate, *TMS* Thymidylate Synthase, *GART* Glycinamide Ribonucleotide Formyl Transferase, *SHMT* Serine Hydroxyl Methyl Transferase, *MTR* 5-Methyltetrahydrofolate-Homocysteine S-Methyltransferase (Methionine Synthase), *MTHFR* Methylene Tetrahydrofolate Reductase

before they can be utilized as carriers of one-carbon groups in the synthesis of purine nucleotides and thymidylate.

Aminopterin, the first antifolate drug, was used in the United States from 1953 through 1964 for pediatric leukemia. Due to manufacturing difficulties it was discontinued in favor of methotrexate. Aminopterin (4-aminofolic acid, 4-aminopteroylglutamic acid) is a synthetic derivative of pterin. The agent acts as an enzyme inhibitor by competing for the folate binding site of Dihydrofolate Reductase. Its affinity for this enzyme effectively blocks tetrahydrofolate synthesis, resulting in the depletion of nucleotide precursors and inhibition of DNA, RNA, and protein synthesis.

Adverse Effects Adverse effects include nausea and vomiting, weight loss, chills or fever, stomatitis (inflammation of the oral mucosa), pharyngitis, erythematous rashes, gastrointestinal hemorrhage, and renal failure. Exposure to aminopterin during pregnancy is associated with congenital malformations, collectively described as the fetal aminopterin syndrome. It includes short stature, skull anomalies (delayed calvarial ossification, craniosynostosis, clover-leaf skull), hydrocephalus, abnormal auricles, ocular hypertelorism, micrognathia, and cleft palate. The risk of malformation associated with aminopterin exposure is estimated at 50%.

Methotrexate ((S)-2-(4-(((2,4-diaminopteridin-6-yl)methyl)methylamino)benzamido) pentanedioic acid, mtx, amethopterin, MTX) <Trexall> binds to, and competitively and reversibly inhibits the enzyme Dihydrofolate Reductase. The affinity of methotrexate for Dihydrofolate Reductase is about 1000-fold that of folate. This results in the suppression of purine nucleotide and thymidylate synthesis, and subsequently in the inhibition of DNA, RNA, and protein synthesis (Fig. 2.41). The drug is cytotoxic during the S phase of the cell cycle.

- Methotrexate is used for the treatment of acute leukemia in children. In adult leukemias, it is applied in the VAMP (vincristine, amethopterine, 6-mercaptopurine, prednisone) combination. Methotrexate is also administered in combination with other chemotherapeutic agents in the treatment of advanced stage non-Hodgkin lymphomata and advanced mycosis fungoides (cutaneous T-cell lymphoma).
- Regression of solid tumors can be achieved with methotrexate. Indications include gestational choriocarcinoma, chorioadenoma destruens, and hydatidiform mole. This drug is used alone or in combination with other anti-cancer agents in the treatment of breast cancer, epidermoid cancers of the head and neck, and lung cancer (particularly the squamous cell and small cell types).

The agent gained U.S. FDA approval as an oncology drug in 1953. Various preparations and modifications of methotrexate are in use.

- Methotrexate-e therapeutic implant (methotrexate/epi, MTX/epi gel) is an injectable Collagen matrix gel containing the anti-metabolite methotrexate and the

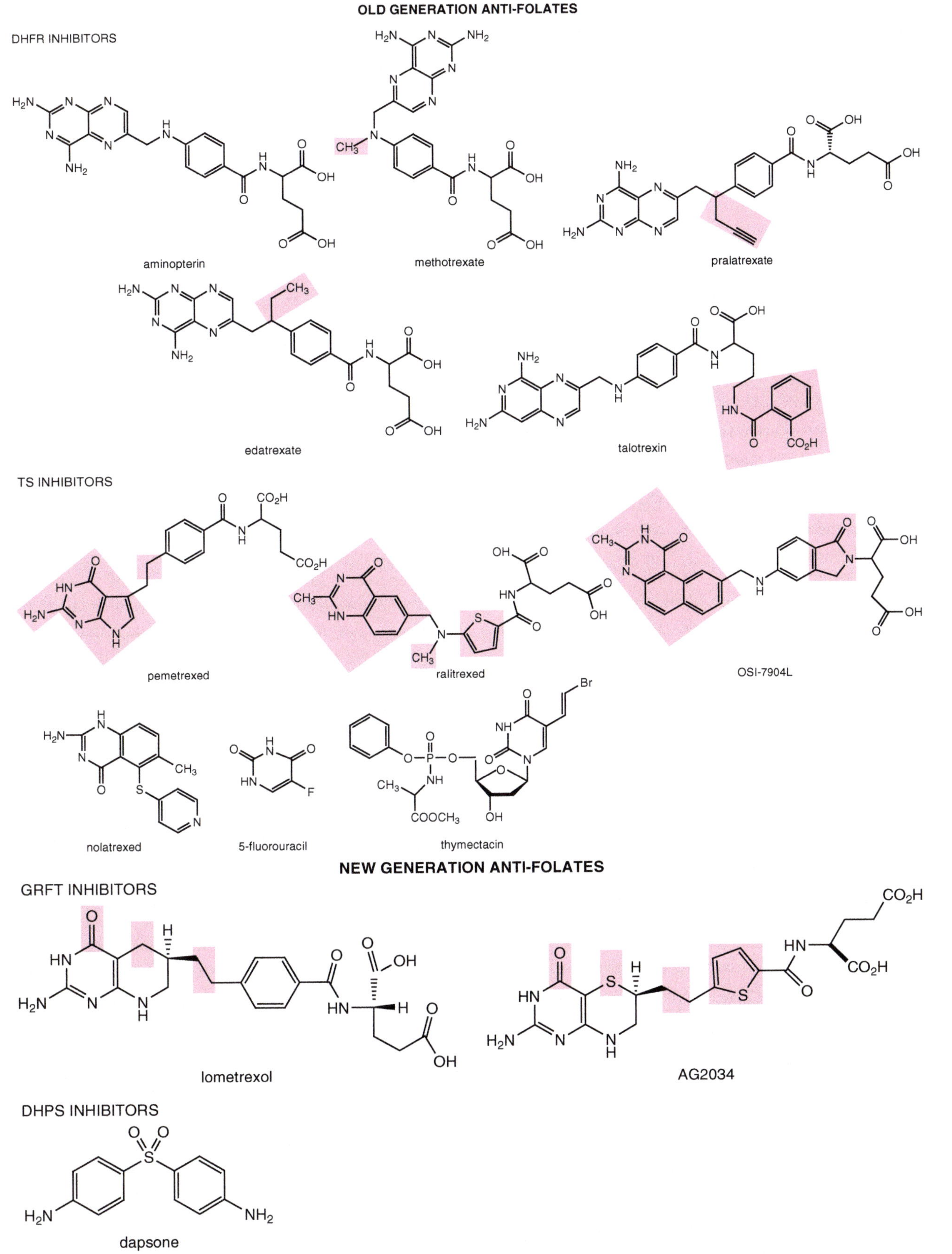

Fig. 2.40 Structures of anti-folates. Old generation drugs inhibit Dihydrofolate Reductase (*DHFR*) or Thymidylate Synthase (*TS*). New generation agents comprise inhibitors of Glycinamide Ribonucleotide Formy7ltransferase (*GRFT*) and Dihydropteroate Synthase (*DHPS*). Many anti-folate drugs are analogs of folate. Within this subgroup, differences in structure from the parent compound aminopterin are shaded in *pink*

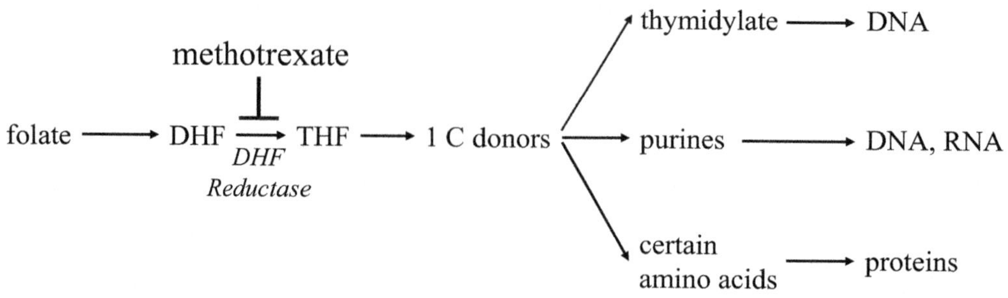

Fig. 2.41 Mechanism of action of methotrexate. The drug (*large font*) inhibits the enzyme Dihydrofolate Reductase (*DHF* Reductase, italics). Consequently, downstream steps of the synthetic pathway are blocked, comprising the synthesis of tetrahydrofolate (*THF*), 1-carbon donors (1 C donors), and the production of essential molecules for cell proliferation

sympathicomimetic agent epinephrine. After intra-tumoral injection, methotrexate inhibits DNA and RNA syntheses. The vasoconstrictor epinephrine in the gel enhances the penetration of methotrexate into the tumor tissue and reduces the dispersion to the surrounding tissues, thereby increasing the local concentration of methotrexate and improving its anti-tumor activity. Intra-tumoral injection of methotrexate combined with epinephrine may increase the chemotherapeutic efficacy and reduce systemic adverse effects compared to systemic administration.

- 3′,5′-Dichloromethotrexate (DCM, *N*-[3,5-dichloro-4-[(2,4-diamino-6-pteridinylmethyl)methylamino]benzoyl] glutamic acid) (NSC 29630) is a chlorinated methotrexate derivative that is inactivated by the liver to the primary metabolic product 4-deamino-4,7-dihydroxy dichloromethotrexate. Most tumors do not metabolize dichloromethotrexate thus allowing the active drug to accumulate. Frequently occurring toxicities include leukopenia, thrombocytopenia, and mucositis. Nausea, vomiting, diarrhea, and an elevation of hepatic enzymes and bilirubin occur less often.
- Trimetrexate glucuronate (TMQ, 2,4-diamino-5-methyl-6-[(3,4,5-trimethoxyanilino)methyl] quinazoline mono-D-glucuronate) <Neutrexin> is a lipid soluble methotrexate derivative that inhibits Dihydrofolate Reductase. Trimetrexate glucuronate is administered by injection, and must be given with concurrent leucovorin protection to avoid potentially serious toxicities.
- Triazinate is a synthetic dihydrotriazine derivative of methotrexate. It inhibits Dihydrofolate Reductase as well as the transport of folates. Unlike methotrexate, this agent is not converted to polyglutamate forms and may be selectively toxic to methotrexate resistant tumor cells.

Methotrexate can be taken orally or administered by injection (subcutaneous, intramuscular, intravenous, or intrathecal). Although daily preparations are occasionally used, most patients take weekly doses. Numerous treatment protocols involving methotrexate have been applied. For choriocarcinoma and similar trophoblastic diseases, methotrexate is administered orally or intramuscularly in doses of 15–30 mg daily for a 5-day course. Courses are usually repeated 3–5 times as required, with rest periods of 1 or more weeks interposed between courses, until any manifesting toxic symptoms subside. In Burkitt lymphoma, a recommended dosage for stage I-II disease is 10–25 mg/day orally for 4–8 days; for stage III-IV disease, methotrexate is commonly given concomitantly with other anti-tumor agents with methotrexate given in doses of 0.625–2.5 mg/kg daily.

Pharmacokinetics The oral absorption of methotrexate is dose dependent. At doses below 30 mg/m^2, methotrexate is generally well absorbed with a mean bioavailability of about 60%. The absorption of doses greater than 80 mg/m^2 is significantly less, possibly due to a saturation effect. Peak blood levels are reached within 1–2 h. In leukemic pediatric patients, there is substantial interindividual variability in both, oral bioavailability and time to peak concentration. Factors that decrease the absorption of the drug and reduce its peak concentration include food, oral non-absorbable antibiotics, and rapid transit through the gastrointestinal tract as it occurs in diarrhea, while slower transit time in the gastrointestinal tract from constipation will increase the absorption. Oral methotrexate is metabolized by intestinal bacteria to the inactive 4-amino-4-deoxy-*N*-methylpteroic acid (DAMPA), which accounts for less than 5% loss of the dose. In contrast, the drug is generally completely absorbed from parenteral routes of administration. After intramuscular injection, peak blood concentrations occur in 30–60 min. In pediatric patients receiving methotrexate for acute lymphocytic leukemia, the terminal half-life ranges 0.5–6 h. Methotrexate does not penetrate the blood-brain barrier in therapeutic amounts, however, high cerebrospinal fluid concentrations of the agent may be attained by intrathecal administration.

At low concentrations, methotrexate competes with reduced folates for the active transport across cell membranes by means of a single carrier mediated process. At concentrations greater than 100 μM, passive diffusion becomes a major pathway, by which effective intracellular concentrations can be achieved. After uptake, methotrexate undergoes hepatic and cancer cell metabolism to polyglutamated forms.

The formation of poly-γ-glutamyl metabolites, catalyzed by Folylpolyglutamate Synthase (FPGS), allows the prolonged retention of methotrexate in various tissues. These metabolites also have very high affinity to Thymidylate Synthase and potentiated inhibitory activity, and they are likely to exert a substantial portion of the drug action. The polyglutamated forms can be converted back to methotrexate by Hydrolases. At therapeutic doses, a small fraction of the drug may be metabolized to 7-hydroxymethotrexate. The aqueous solubility of 7-hydroxymethotrexate is 3–5 fold lower than the parent compound.

Methotrexate clearance rates vary widely and are generally decreased at higher doses. The terminal half-life for methotrexate is approximately 3–10 h for patients receiving low dose anti-neoplastic therapy (less than 30 mg/m^2). For patients receiving high doses of methotrexate, the terminal half-life is 8–15 h. Renal excretion by glomerular filtration and active tubular secretion is the primary mode of elimination, and is dependent on dosage and route of administration (with intravenous administration, 80–90 % of the dose is excreted unchanged in the urine within 24 h). There is limited biliary excretion, amounting to 10 % or less of the administered dose. Enterohepatic recirculation of methotrexate may occur. Delayed drug clearance is one of the major factors responsible for methotrexate toxicity. When a patient has delayed drug elimination due to compromised renal function, third-space effusion, or other causes, the methotrexate blood concentrations may remain elevated for prolonged periods. The extent of adverse effects exerted on healthy tissues may be more dependent on the duration of exposure to the drug than on the peak level achieved.

Adverse Effects In general, the incidence and severity of acute adverse effects are related to dose and frequency of methotrexate administration. There are assays available for the measurement of serum methotrexate levels that allow therapeutic drug monitoring, which also enables individualized dosing based on target levels. The threshold for cytotoxic effects of the agent is approximately 50 nM. Toxicity and efficacy are determined by the time span for which the concentrations remain above this threshold level.

The high doses of methotrexate often used in cancer chemotherapy can cause toxic effects to the rapidly dividing cells of the bone marrow and the gastrointestinal mucosa, resulting in myelosuppression (leukopenia, anemia) and mucositis (gingivitis, pharyngitis, ulcerative stomatitis). The myelosuppression can lead to potentially fatal opportunistic infections (Pneumocystis carinii pneumonia, nocardiosis, histoplasmosis, cryptococcosis, Herpes zoster, Herpes simplex hepatitis, disseminated Herpes simplex). Pericarditis, pericardial effusion, hypotension, and thromboembolic events are possible. Respiratory fibrosis, interstitial pneumonitis, or chronic interstitial obstructive pulmonary disease can occasionally occur. There have been occurrences of central nervous system reactions to methotrexate, including myelopathies and leukoencephalopathies, especially when the agent was given via the intrathecal route. Methotrexate causes ocular adverse effects in up to 25 % of patients[38]. They may include blepharitis, periorbital edema, conjunctival hyperemia, increased tearing, or photophobia. Methotrexate is secreted into breast milk. Methotrexate exposure during pregnancy can lead to congenital malformations. It is Pregnancy Category X.

Anorexia, nausea and vomiting, diarrhea, hematemesis, melena, or pancreatitis can arise. These symptoms may be preventable by rescue therapy with folinic acid (leukovorin) supplements. High doses of methotrexate (generally doses greater than 1000 mg/m^2) require leucovorin rescue. Leucovorin must be administered until the levels fall below 50 nM.

Although methotrexate competes with folate for Dihydrofolate Reductase, the enzyme inhibition caused by methotrexate is sometimes referred to as pseudo-irreversible because it cannot be displaced substantially by any physiologically attainable concentration of folate. Thus, an overdose of methotrexate cannot be corrected by administering folate. It requires folinic acid as an antidote.

Drug Interactions Vitamin preparations containing folic acid or its derivatives decrease the responses to systemically administered methotrexate. Vitamin C supplements can increase the adverse effects of methotrexate. Oral antibiotics, such as tetracycline, chloramphenicol, and non-absorbable broad spectrum antibiotics, may decrease the intestinal absorption of methotrexate or interfere with the enterohepatic circulation by inhibiting bowel flora and suppressing the metabolism of the drug by bacteria. There is a risk of a severe adverse reaction if penicillin is prescribed alongside methotrexate. Methotrexate in the blood is approximately 50 % protein bound. It may be displaced by various compounds including sulfonamides, salicylates, phenylbutazone, tetracyclines, chloramphenicol, and phenytoin. The concurrent use of drugs that also undergo tubular secretion can markedly increase the methotrexate blood levels. Non-steroidal anti-inflammatory drugs (NSAIDs) and probenecid reduce the tubular secretion of methotrexate. Concomitant administration of some NSAIDs with high dose methotrexate therapy can elevate and prolong the blood methotrexate levels, resulting in deaths from severe hematologic and gastrointestinal toxicity.

Drug Resistance The efflux transporter ABCG2 (Breast Cancer Resistance Protein, BCRP) exports polyglutamates out of cells, and mutations within the *abcg2* gene may confer resistance to various antifolates. Polymorphisms of the gene *slc19A1* (*reduced folate carrier*, *rfc*), such as A80G, which encodes the uptake transporter for methotrexate, or its

[38] The drug is excreted in the tears and may cause ocular irritation, thus interfering with corneal and conjunctival epithelial metabolism.

regulatory elements are associated with clinical outcome in the treatment of osteosarcoma or childhood acute lymphoblastic leukemia (ALL). In high doses, passive diffusion of the drug can to some degree overcome tumor cell resistance caused by saturated active transport systems. Cancers can become resistant to antifolates by amplification of *dihydrofolate reductase* or decreased affinity of Dihydrofolate Reductase for methotrexate. Other potential causes of resistance are slow rates of thymidylate synthesis and lack of polyglutamation within tumor cells.

Pralatrexate (PDX, *N*-(4-{1-[(2,4-diaminopteridin-6-yl) methyl]but-3-yn-1-yl}benzoyl)-L-glutamic acid) <Folotyn> is a folate analog metabolic inhibitor. It is the first drug to have been approved (in 2009 by the U.S. FDA) as a treatment for patients with relapsed or refractory peripheral T-cell lymphoma (PTCL), a biologically diverse group of aggressive blood cancers with a poor prognosis.

Pharmacokinetics Pralatrexate preferentially enters cancer cells through the transporter SLC19A1 (Reduced Folate Carrier type 1, RFC-1).

Adverse Effects Common adverse effects include mucositis (70 %, grade 2 or higher requires dose adjustment or discontinuation), myelosuppression (40 % thrombocytopenia), nausea (40 %), fatigue (35 %), skin reactions, vomiting, and diarrhea. Other adverse effects may include dizziness or fainting spells, rash or itching, loss of appetite and weight loss, joint and muscle pain. Patients should be instructed to take folic acid and receive vitamin B12 to potentially reduce treatment related hematologic toxicity and mucositis. The drug is Pregnancy Category D.

Drug Interactions The co-administration of drugs subject to renal elimination may result in delayed renal clearance of pralatrexate.

Edatrexate (10-ethyl-10-deaza-aminopterin, 10-EDAM, EDX) (CGP-30694) is a water soluble, polyglutamatable analog of methotrexate. Edatrexate inhibits Thymidylate Synthase and Glycinamide Ribonucleotide Formyl Transferase, impairing the synthesis of purine nucleotides and amino acids, and resulting in tumor cell death. Advantages over methotrexate include better transport across cancer cell membranes and increased selectivity for tumor cells, resulting in greater anti-tumor effect. Edatrexate may be suitable for treating lung cancer, head and neck cancer, breast cancer, and non-Hodgkin lymphoma. The dosage is 40–80 mg/m^2 by infusion once a week.

Adverse Effects The adverse effects have a profile similar to methotrexate, but are tolerable. Mouth ulcers are the dose limiting toxicity, followed by myelosuppression with decreased formation of all blood elements, diarrhea, skin rash, nausea and vomiting, pneumonitis, and a mild impact on liver function.

Drug Resistance Edatrexate may overcome tumor resistance to methotrexate. Unlike methotrexate, edatrexate has additive activity when used with cisplatin.

Talotrexin ammonium (*N*(α)-(4-amino-4-deoxypteroyl)-*N*(δ)-hemiphthaloyl-L-ornithine) (PT523) <Talvesta> is a non-polyglutamable anti-metabolite analog of aminopterin that binds to and inhibits the function of Dihydrofolate Reductase. Talotrexin is water soluble and is actively transported into cells by SLC19A1 (RFC, Reduced Folate Carrier). In 2006, the U.S. FDA granted orphan drug designation for talotrexin use in patients with ALL. The agent is also under study for the treatment of solid tumors, including non-small cell lung cancer.

As folylpolyglutamates are essential for cell survival and proliferation, the synthesis of poly(γ-glutamate) metabolites of natural folates is a critical process. Polyglutamates of antifolates are formed as long half-life metabolites (Baugh et al. 1973; Nair and Baugh 1973), and they are often critical for their cytotoxic action. The poly-glutamylation of anti-folates has been attempted to stabilize the compounds.

Thymidylate Synthase inhibitors Thymidylate Synthase catalyzes the methylation of 2′-deoxyuridine-5′-monophosphate (dUMP) to 2′-deoxythymidine-5′-monophosphate (dTMP), which is subsequently phosphorylated to thymidine triphosphate, an essential precursor in DNA synthesis (Fig. 2.42). Over-expression of Thymidylate Synthase is associated with many solid tumors.

Pemetrexed disodium (*N*-[4-[2-(2-amino-4,7-dihydro-4-oxo-1H-pyrrolo[2,3-d]pyrimidin-5-yl)ethyl]benzoyl]-L-glutamic acid disodium salt) <Alimta> is a synthetic pyrimidine based antifolate that binds to and inhibits Thymidylate Synthase. It also is an inhibitor of Dihydrofolate Reductase (DHFR), and Glycinamide Ribonucleotide Formyl Transferase (GARFT). The agent is taken up into cells by membrane carriers, such as SLC19A1 (Reduced Folate Carrier) and membraneous folate binding protein transport systems. Once in the cell, pemetrexed is converted to polyglutamate forms by the enzyme Folylpolyglutamate Synthase. The drug is indicated

- as a single agent for the treatment of patients with locally advanced or metastatic non-squamous, non-small cell lung cancer after prior chemotherapy
- for the maintenance treatment of patients with locally advanced or metastatic non-squamous, non-small cell lung cancer whose disease has not progressed after four cycles of platinum based first-line chemotherapy

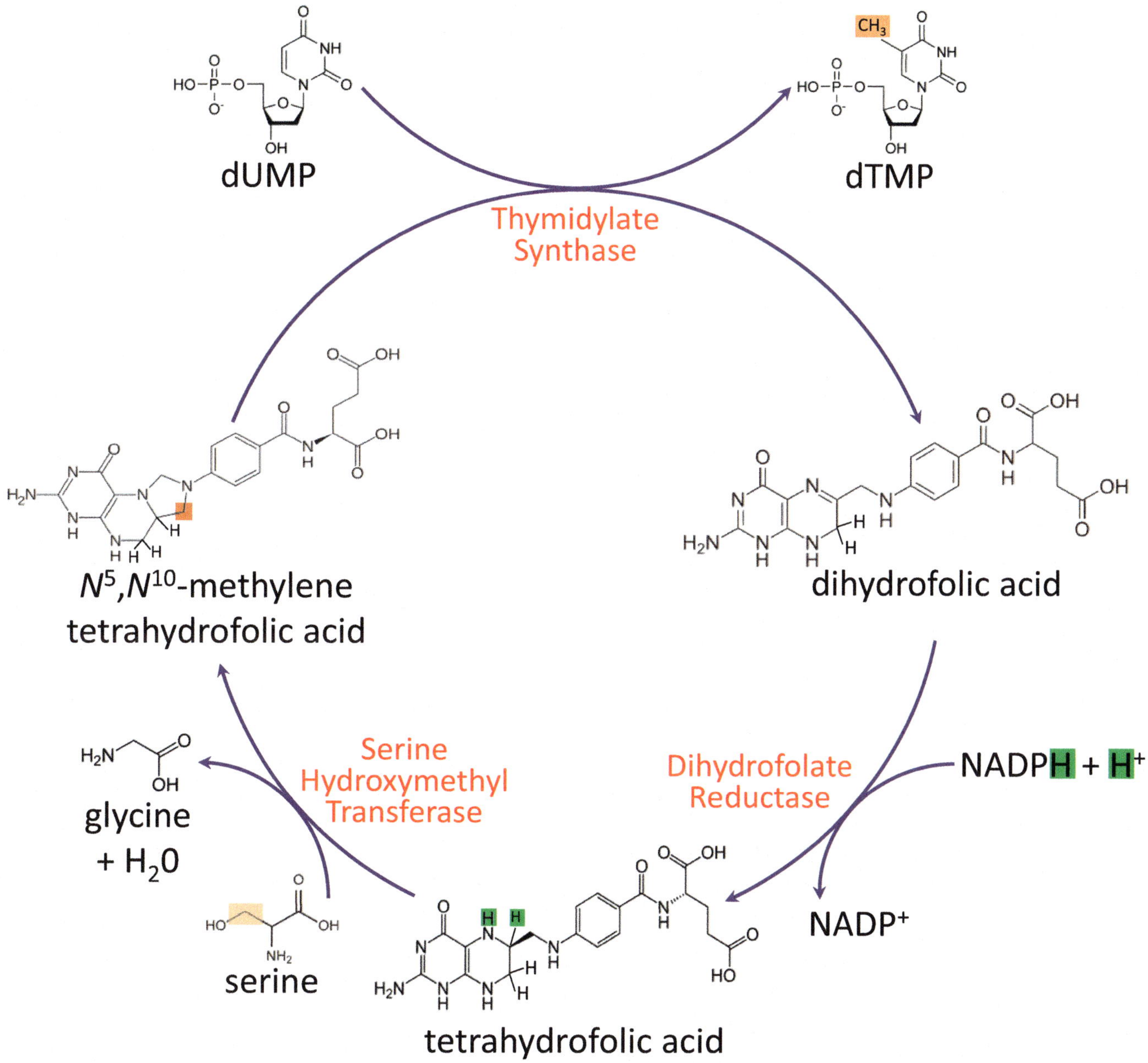

Fig. 2.42 The Thymidylate Synthase cycle. Thymidylate Synthase is embedded in a cycle that supplies the co-substrate methylene-tetrahydrofolate and yields dihydrofolate, which then regenerates methylene-tetrahydrofolate via tetrahydrofolate. In the process, glycine is synthesized from serine and *dTMP* (deoxythymidine monophosphate, thymidylate) is synthesized from *dUMP* (deoxyuridine monophosphate). Transferred functional groups are tracked by color (*green, orange*)

- in combination with cisplatin therapy for the initial treatment of patients with locally advanced or metastatic non-squamous, non-small cell lung cancer
- in combination with cisplatin for the treatment of patients with malignant pleural mesothelioma, whose disease is unresectable or who are otherwise not candidates for curative surgery.

The recommended dose for single agent use is 500 mg/m^2 administered as an intravenous infusion over 10 min on day 1 of each 21-day cycle. If used in combination, the recommended dose of cisplatin is 75 mg/m^2 infused over 2 h beginning approximately 30 min after the end of the pemetrexed administration (appropriate hydration of patients under cisplatin treatment is important).

Pharmacokinetics Pemetrexed total systemic exposure and maximum blood concentration increase proportionally with the dose. Approximately 80 % of taken up drug is bound to plasma proteins (this binding is not affected by the degree of renal impairment). Pemetrexed is not metabolized to any appreciable extent and does not affect Cytochrome P450 enzymes. The agent is primarily eliminated in the urine, with 70–90 % of the dose excreted unchanged within the first 24 h following administration. The drug should not be given to patients with a creatinine clearance below 45 mL/min. While the effect of third-space fluid, such as pleural effusion or ascites, is unknown, in affected patients consideration should be given to draining the effusion prior to pemetrexed administration. The pharmacokinetics does not change over multiple treatment cycles.

Adverse Effects In single-agent therapy, the most common adverse effects are fatigue, nausea, and anorexia. Myelosuppression is usually the dose limiting toxicity of pemetrexed. Complete blood cell counts, including platelets, and periodic chemistry tests should be performed on all patients receiving the drug. Dose adjustments at the start of a subsequent cycle are to be based on nadir hematologic counts or maximum non-hematologic toxicity from the preceding cycle of therapy. Pemetrexed therapy should be discontinued if a patient experiences any hematologic or non-hematologic grade 3–4 toxicity after two dose reductions or immediately if grade 3–4 neurotoxicity is observed. The drug is contraindicated in patients who have a history of severe hypersensitivity reactions to pemetrexed or to any ingredient used in the formulation. Pemetrexed is Pregnancy Category D.

Patients must be instructed to take folic acid and vitamin B_{12} during treatment as a prophylaxis to reduce hematologic and gastrointestinal adverse effects. The toxicity of pemetrexed is reduced by daily intake of a low dose oral folic acid preparation (commonly 400 µg) or multi-vitamin with folic acid. Supplementation should continue for 21 days after the last dose of pemetrexed. Patients must also receive one intra-muscular injection of vitamin B_{12} during the week preceding the first dose of pemetrexed and every three cycles thereafter[39].

Drug Interactions In combination with cisplatin, common adverse reactions include vomiting, neutropenia, leukopenia, anemia, stomatitis or pharyngitis, thrombocytopenia, and constipation. Patients with mild to moderate renal insufficiency should avoid taking non-steroidal anti-inflammatory drugs (NSAIDs) with short elimination half-lives for a period of 2-days-before through 2-days-following the administration of pemetrexed. Although ibuprofen (400 mg four times a day) can decrease the clearance of pemetrexed, it may be given to patients with normal renal function (creatinine clearance 80 mL/min or higher). The concomitant administration of nephrotoxic drugs or substances that are tubularly secreted could result in delayed clearance of pemetrexed.

Raltitrexed (*N*-(5-[*N*-(3,4-dihydro-2-methyl-4-oxoquinazolin-6-ylmethyl)-*N*-methylamino]-2-thenoyl)-L-glutamic acid) <Tomudex> is a quinazoline folate analog. It has been used in the treatment of colorectal cancer since 1998. After transport into cells via SLC19A1 (Reduced Folate Carrier 1, Folate Transporter), raltitrexed undergoes intracellular polyglutamation and blocks the folate binding site of Thymidylate Synthase. Thereby it inhibits tetrahydrofolate activity and DNA reduplication and repair, thus resulting in cytotoxicity.

OSI-7904 ((S)-2-(5-(((3-methyl-1-oxo-1,2-dihydrobenzo[f]quinazolin-9-yl)methyl)amino)-1-oxoisoindolin-2-yl) pentanedioic acid) (GW1843, OVI-237, GS7904L) is a 3-methyl substituted benzoquinazoline folate analog. It non-competitively binds to Thymidylate Synthase and acts as an inhibitor, resulting in the suppression of thymine nucleotide synthesis and DNA reduplication.

- OSI-7904L (GS7904L) is a liposome encapsulated formulation of the drug. Liposome encapsulation improves the efficacy and increases the half-life of OSI-7904.

Nolatrexed dihydrochloride (3,4-dihydro-2-amino-6-methyl-4-oxy-5-(4-pyridylthio)-quinazoline dihydrochloride) (AG337) <Thymitaq> is a quinazoline folate analog that occupies the folate binding site of Thymidylate Synthase, resulting in the inhibition of enzymatic activity and thymine nucleotide synthesis with subsequent blocking of DNA reduplication. This leads to DNA damage, S phase cell cycle arrest, and Caspase mediated apoptosis. Nolatrexed also exhibits radio-sensitizing activity.

Originally synthesized in the late 1950s, 5-fluorouracil (5-FU) is a fluorinated analog of the naturally occurring pyrimidine uracil. It is a prodrug and must be metabolized to the nucleotide form, fluorodeoxyuridine monophosphate, to be active. In the presence of folates, fluorodeoxyuridine monophosphate binds tightly to and interferes with the function of Thymidylate Synthase, resulting in decreased thymidine synthesis and consecutively reduced DNA synthesis. Another metabolite of 5-fluorouracil, the triphosphate nucleotide, is incorporated into RNA as a false base, and interferes with RNA function. Various forms of 5-fluorouracil are in use (see Sect. 2.4.2. pyrimidine analogs).

- 5-(trifluoromethyl)-2′-deoxyuridine (F_3TDR) was synthesized by Heidelberger as a trifluoromethyl analog of 5-fluorouridine deoxyribose (5-FUDR, floxuridine). The

[39] The pretreatment causes skin rashes, more commonly in men than in women. Dexamethasone (4 mg orally twice daily the day before, the day of, and the day after pemetrexed administration) or its equivalent may reduce the incidence and severity of the skin rash.

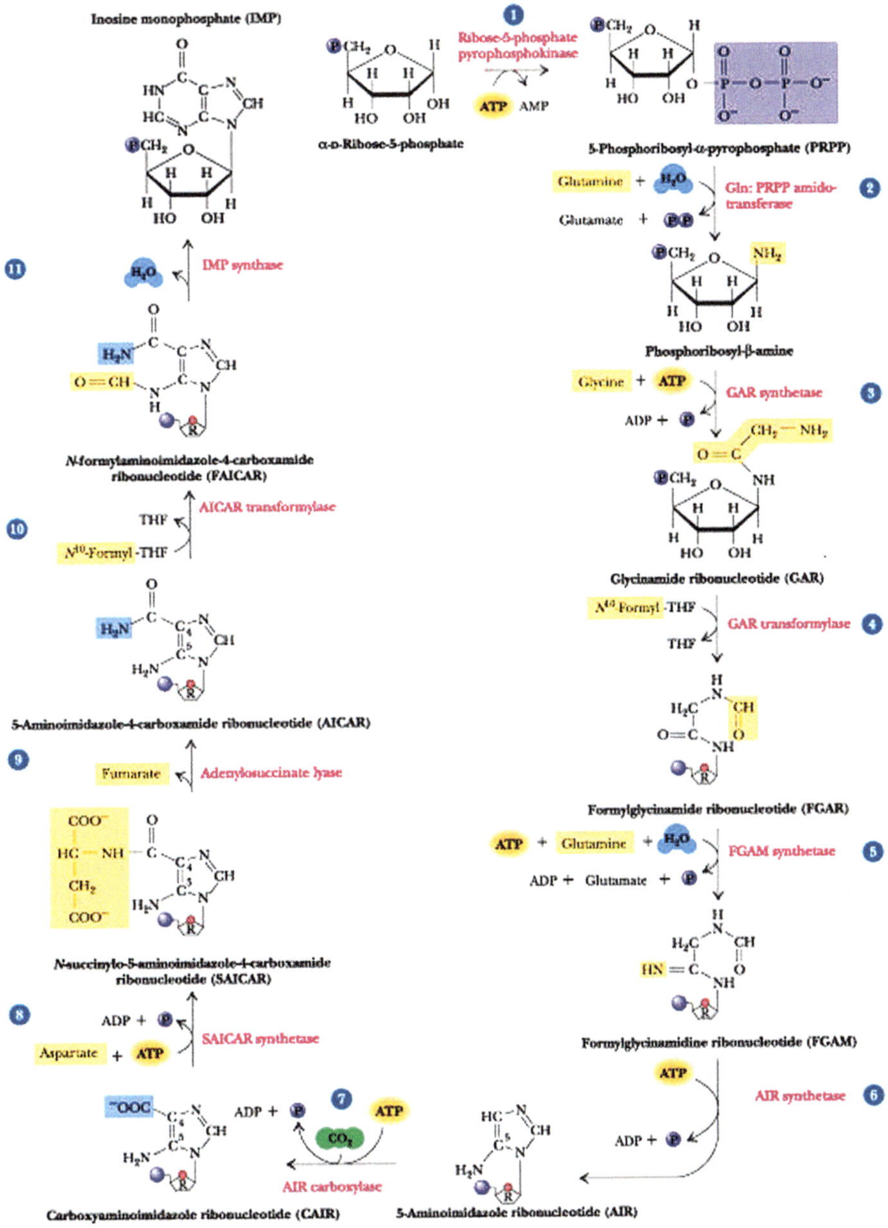

Fig. 2.43 De novo purine biosynthetic pathway. The pathway synthesizes inosine monophosphate from ribose-5-phosphate, the ribonucleotide of hypoxanthine and the first nucleotide formed during the synthesis of purine. Step 4 is catalyzed by Glycinamide Ribonucleotide Formyl Transferase. [http://images.google.com/imgres?imgurl=http://web.virginia.edu/Heidi/chapter27/Images/8883n27_29.jpg&imgrefurl= http://web.virginia.edu/Heidi/chapter27/chp27.htm&usg=__pQ-tPnCfgUt4p7CCSR1gLMpFd7k=&h=319&w=338&sz=21&hl=en&start=3&sig2=OqPAmXXgOx6sEqnhNQ35Bw&tbnid=fGhtr2vXFFlvSM:&tbnh=112&tbnw=119&prev=/images%3Fq%3Dthymidylate%2Bsynthase%26gbv%3D2%26hl%3Den&ei=cDqySu6OB4qo8AbGtd3FDQ] There are instances where we have been unable to trace or contact the copyright holder. If notified the publisher will be pleased to rectify any errors or omissions at the earliest opportunity

drug undergoes metabolic phosphorylation to become a Thymidylate Synthase inhibitor. It may also be incorporated into DNA in place of thymidine.

Thymectacin (NB1011) is a small molecule phosphoramidate derivative of (E)-5-(2-bromovinyl)-2′-deoxyuridine. It is selectively active against tumor cells that express high levels of Thymidylate Synthase, a critical enzyme in DNA biosynthesis, the over-expression of which is associated with many solid tumors. In contrast to other Thymidylate Synthase targeting drugs, which are effective through inhibition of the enzyme, the cytotoxicity of thymectacin depends on its activation by Thymidylate Synthase. While it is independent of the tumor suppressor P53, it may induce the expression of *bax* (encodes a pro-apoptotic BCL-2 family member), *p21* (encodes a cell cycle checkpoint protein), and *gadd45* (encodes a DNA damage response protein). The activation of these genes results in a deregulation of the cell cycle and leads to apoptosis (Neuteboom et al. 2002).

Glycinamide Ribonucleotide Formyl Transferase inhibitors Purine depletion causes slow cell death in cells that have passed the G_1 checkpoint (many cancer cells), but cytostasis in cells that reside in G_0 or are arrested at the G_1 checkpoint (most differentiated cells). Therefore, Glycinamide Ribonucleotide Formyl Transferase inhibitors, at physiological folate concentrations, cause selective cytotoxicity to cells lacking a functional G_1 checkpoint (Zhang et al. 1998).

In the late 1980s, Gerald B. Grindey demonstrated anti-tumor activity for lometrexol, the first selective inhibitor of Glycinamide Ribonucleotide Formyl Transferase (GARFT), the enzyme that catalyzes a key step of the de novo purine biosynthetic pathway (Fig. 2.43). The agent showed efficacy against tumors that were unresponsive to methotrexate, and it had enhanced adverse effects in conjunction with a folate depleted diet[40].

Lometrexol (6R-5,10-dideazatetrahydrofolate, (6R)-DDATHF, LMTX) is a folate analog anti-metabolite. As the 6R diastereomer of 5,10-dideazatetrahydrofolate, lometrexol inhibits Glycinamide Ribonucleotide Formyl Transferase, thereby inhibiting DNA synthesis, arresting cells in the S phase of the cell cycle, and inhibiting tumor cell proliferation.

Pharmacokinetics Since lometrexol is extensively polyglutamylated, it is cleared from cells slowly, and the extensive accumulation that occurs in low folate conditions causes delayed toxicity.

Adverse Effects Repetitive administration of the drug is compromised by cumulative myelosuppression and gastrointestinal toxicities. Weekly administration of lometrexol is feasible and well tolerated when co-administered with daily oral folic acid (Roberts et al. 2000).

Drug Resistance Lometrexol is active against tumors that are resistant to the folate antagonist methotrexate.

4-[2-(2-amino-4-oxo-4,6,7,8-tetrahydro-3H-pyrimidino[5,4–6] [1,4]thiazin-6-yl)-(S)-ethyl]-2,5-thienoyl-L-glutamic acid (AG2034) is an inhibitor of Glycinamide Ribonucleotide Formyl Transferase (Boritzki et al. 1996). AG2034 also has a high affinity for the Folate Receptor, and is a substrate for Folylpolyglutamate Synthetase. This compound can enter cells by utilizing the Reduced Folate Carrier. The recommended dose is 5.0 mg/m^2.

Adverse Effects Dose limiting toxicities are anemia, thrombocytopenia, mucositis, diarrhea, hyperbilirubinemia, fatigue, and insomnia. They are modestly cumulative over three courses.

Dihydropteroate Synthase inhibitors Dihydropteroate Synthase (DHPS) catalyzes the condensation of *p*-aminobenzoate and 6-hydroxymethyl-7,8-dihydropterin pyrophosphate to form 7,8-dihydropteroate, which is an essential precursor to the cofactor tetrahydrofolate. Sulfa drugs are blockers of folate synthesis, acting as competitive inhibitors of *p*-aminobenzoate.

Dapsone (4,4′-sulfonyldianiline) <Croysulfone, Diphenasone, Dumitone, Novophone, Sulfona-Mae, Sulphadione> is a synthetic derivative of diamino-sulfone. A structural analog of *p*-aminobenzoic acid (PABA), dapsone inhibits Dihydropteroate Synthase, resulting in a depletion of the folate pool and a reduction in the amount of thymidylate available for DNA synthesis. Dapsone has been used to treat Kaposi sarcoma.

Adverse Effects Adverse effects include hemolysis, which may lead to hemolytic anemia, and methemoglobinemia. Agranulocytosis occurs rarely in mono-therapy, but is more frequent in combination regimens. Abnormalities in white blood cell formation (including aplastic anemia) are rare, but are the major cause of death due to dapsone therapy. Toxic hepatitis and cholestatic jaundice may occur.

Dapsone reaction is a form of hypersensitivity that is more frequent in patients receiving multiple drug therapy. It always involves a rash and may also include fever, jaundice, and eosinophilia. These symptoms will generally occur within the first 6 weeks of therapy or not at all, and may be ameliorated by corticosteroid therapy.

Drug therapy supportive of anti-folates Agents are available to enhance the therapeutic effects or ameliorate the adverse effects caused by anti-folates.

Folinic acid (citrovorum factor, levoleucovorin, (6-S)-leucovorin) <Leucovorin> is the active l-isomer of the 5-formyl derivative of tetrahydrofolic acid. As an active metabolite of folic acid, it does not require activation by Dihydrofolate Reductase. Folinate calcium (leucovorin calcium) counteracts the toxic effects of anti-metabolite medications, rescuing the patient while permitting the anti-tumor activity of the folate antagonist. This agent may also enhance the effects of fluoropyrimidines by stabilizing their binding to the enzyme Thymidylate Synthase, thus prolonging drug activity. The drug is indicated

- after high dose methotrexate therapy in osteosarcoma,
- to diminish the toxicity and counteract the effects of impaired methotrexate elimination and of inadvertent overdosage of folic acid antagonists,
- in combination with 5-fluorouracil to prolong survival in the palliative treatment of patients with advanced colorectal cancer.

The agent is given by intravenous injection. There are multiple distinct regimens that combine 5-fluorouracil and folinic acid. The de Gramont regimen is initiated by infusion of folinic acid over 2 h, followed by 5-fluorouracil over 22 h. This is repeated over day 2. A rest period of 12 days completes the cycle. In the modified de Gramont protocol, the infusions are administered through a portable pump, allowing outpatient treatment. In the case of treating a methotrexate overdose, folinic acid needs to be given within 4 h to avoid irreversible damage.

[40] Lometrexol is transported by Folic Acid Binding Protein (FBP), the expression of which is unregulated under folate restriction, with the result that some healthy tissues accumulate much greater amounts of lometrexol when dietary folate is limited.

Serum creatinine levels should be determined daily. In the case of high dose methotrexate therapy, hydration and urinary alkalinization need to be continued. Folinic acid can enhance the toxicity of 5-fluorouracil; in elderly patients, deaths from severe enterocolitis, diarrhea, and dehydration can result. The drug is Pregnancy Category C.

Folic acid in large amounts may counteract the anti-epileptic effect of phenobarbital, phenytoin and primidone, and increase the frequency of seizures in susceptible children. It is not known whether folinic acid has the same effects.

5-fluorouracil causes myelosuppression. Uridine is a nucleoside consisting of uracil and D-ribose, which is incorporated into RNA. Uridine may serve as a rescue agent to reduce the toxicities associated with 5-fluorouracil, thereby allowing the administration of higher doses of 5-fluorouracil in chemotherapy regimens.

Old generation anti-folates comprise Dihydrofolate Reductase inhibitors and Thymidylate Synthase inhibitors.
New generation anti-folates include Glycinamide Ribonucleotide Formyl Transferase inhibitors and Dihydropteroate Synthase inhibitors.
Within cells, anti-folates are converted to polyglutamates, which typically are more efficient enzyme inhibitors.
Agents are available to enhance the efficacy and ameliorate the toxicity of anti-folates (folinic acid and uridine).

2.4.2 Anti-Pyrimidines

Anti-pyrimidines were developed in attempts to synthesize analogs that inhibit uracil utilization by tumors (Fig. 2.44). In 1954, Abraham Cantarow and Karl Paschkis had found that liver tumors absorbed uracil more readily than healthy liver cells. Because tumors tend to use more uracil than orotic acid for nucleic acid synthesis, Charles Heidelberger reasoned that an anti-metabolite resembling uracil would show some selectivity for inhibiting tumors over normal tissues. He hypothesized "because acetic acid is vinegar and fluoroacetic acid is rat poison" a fluorine-substituted compound might be active. Such substitution in position five of the uracil ring was feasible and stable. The substitution also interfered with the synthesis of thymine nucleotides from uracil nucleotides. This rationale resulted in the anti-cancer drug 5-fluorouracil. It was synthesized in 1957 in a collaboration of Duschinsky, Pleven, and Heidelberger (Duschinsky et al. 1957; Heidelberger et al. 1957).

Uracil analogs Thymine (5-methyl uracil) is the base that distinguishes DNA from RNA (which uses uracil instead). The class of halogenated uracil drugs carries a halogen on uracil or its derivatives. The replacement of the 5-methyl group with a halogen interferes with DNA synthesis. As the van der Waals radii are similar for hydrogen and fluoride, 5-fluorouracil behaves like uracil with hydrogen in the five position. For the heavier halogenated analogs (containing chlorine, bromine, or iodine), the radius of the methyl group of thymine is more closely approximated.

5-fluorouracil (5-fluoro-1*H*-pyrimidine-2,4-dione, 5-FU) is a fluoropyrimidine nucleoside analog that was introduced into the clinic in 1958. This agent has broad activity against a range of solid tumors. Fluorouracil and its metabolites possess a various mechanisms of action that lead to S phase specific anti-proliferation:

- Fluoruracil is converted to the active metabolite 5-fluoroxyuridine monophosphate (F-UMP). FUMP is further metabolized to FUTP, which inhibits RNA and protein synthesis by competing with uridine triphosphate for incorporation into the RNA strand, thereby suppressing cell growth.
- The active metabolite 5-fluoro-2′-deoxyuridine-5′-*O*-monophosphate (F-dUMP), inhibits Thymidylate Synthase, resulting in the depletion of thymidine triphosphate (TTP), a necessary constituent of DNA. FdUMP inhibits DNA synthesis and cell division by reducing thymidine production.
- Several fluorouracil metabolites incorporate into both RNA and DNA. Incorporation into RNA results in major effects on both RNA processing and functions. When 5-fluorouracil is incorporated into DNA it is removed by Uracil N-Glycosylase, leaving an apyrimidinic sugar for the process of DNA repair. Errors in this process provide a basis for cytotoxicity.

Safety and efficacy of 5-fluorouracil administration are higher with continuous intravenous infusion than with a bolus injection. Intra-arterial infusion into the tumor may be beneficial. Tumors that have previously been irradiated respond poorly to fluorinated pyrimidines. 5-fluorouracil is not radiosensitizing, but is a potentially phototoxic drug.

Diverse preparations and various pro-forms of 5-fluorouracil are in use for cancer chemotherapy.

- 5-Fluorouracil <Adrucil, Fluoroplex, Fluorouracil> has its principal use is in colorectal cancer and pancreatic cancer, in which it is the established form of chemotherapy. For good-risk patients, 5-fluorouracil is usually given intravenously (infusion is superior to bolus injection) at 15 mg/kg for 5 days. After rest for 1 day, 7.5 mg/kg are then given every other day for 4–5 doses. A new course of treatment is repeated after an interval of 4 weeks. For poor-risk patients, the dose of 5-fluorouracil is reduced or 4 doses of 15 mg/kg/day are given as a course, whereafter treatment is stopped.
- Cream preparations of 5-fluorouracil <Efudex, Fluoroplex, Carac> are used for the topical treatment of multiple

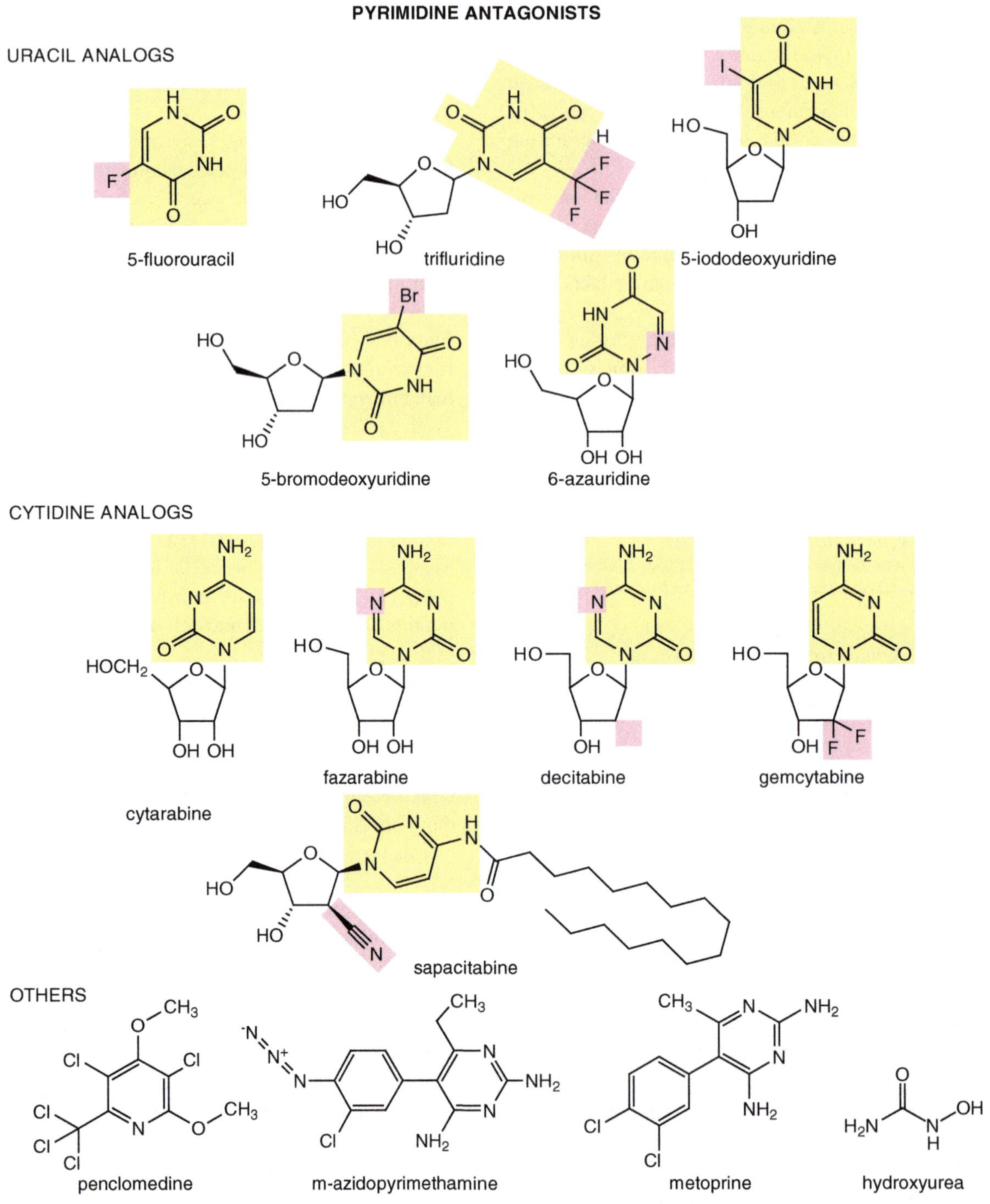

Fig. 2.44 Structures of anti-pyrimidines. Three groups comprise uracil analogs, cytidine analogs, and others. The common uracil-related or cytosine-related functional groups are highlighted in *yellow*. Differences among the uracil analogs are shaded in *pink*. They pertain mostly to various halogen substitutes (in one case to a nitrogen substitution in the ring structure). All cytidine analogs contain a sugar, analogous to the DNA building block. In this group, changes in the sugar moiety are shaded in *pink*. Also shaded in *pink* are the nitrogen substitutions of the base in fazarabine and decitabine

actinic or solar keratoses. Efudex 5 % strength is administered to treat superficial basal cell carcinomata. The most common adverse effects include reversible pain, itching, burning, soreness, scaling, rash, irritation, dryness, swelling, inflammation, tenderness at the injection site. Less commonly (10–30 % of patients), increased sensitivity to sunlight, discoloration of the skin, or scarring can arise.

- Floxuridine (5-fluoro-2′-deoxyuridine-5′-phosphate, 5-FUDR monophosphate) <FUDR, FUDR-MP> is a fluorinated pyrimidine monophosphate analog of 5-fluorouracil that was synthesized by Duschinsky. The goal was a reduction in the toxicity of 5-fluorouracil that arises when the drug is converted to a ribonucleotide. It competes with 2′-deoxyuridylate for Thymidylate Synthase and thereby blocks thymidylate synthesis. The resulting lack of thymidylate consecutively impairs DNA synthesis. This agent is metabolized to fluorouracil and other derivatives that can be incorporated into RNA and inhibit the utilization of preformed uracil in RNA synthesis. 5-FUDR, but not 5-fluorouracil, is incorporated preferentially into colon carcinoma compared to normal colon (Mukherjee et al. 1963). Floxuridine is usually given rapidly at twice the dose of 5-fluorouracil. It first gained U.S. FDA approval in 1970.

- Dihydropyrimidine Dehydrogenase represents the initial rate-limiting step in the catabolism of the pyrimidines uracil, thymine, and 5-fluorouracil. Doxifluridine (5′-deoxy-5-fluorouridine) is a fluoropyrimidine derivative and oral prodrug of 5-fluorouracil, designed to circumvent the rapid degradation of 5-fluorouracil by Dihydropyrimidine Dehydrogenase in the gut wall and liver. The agent is converted into 5-fluorouracil by Pyrimidine Nucleoside Phosphorylase.
- 5,10-methylenetetrahydrofolate (MTHF) is a folate based biomodulator that stabilizes the covalent binding of the fluorouracil metabolite 5–5-fluoro-2′-deoxyuridine-5′-O-monophosphate (FdUMP) to its target enzyme, Thymidylate Synthase. The binding results in enzyme inhibition and depletion of the essential DNA constituent thymidine triphosphate (TTP). Tumor cell death ensues. 5,10-methylenetetrahydrofolate, as the active form of folate, does not require metabolic activation and may exceed the chemotherapeutic effects of fluorouracil with lower toxicity.
- Tegafur (5-fluoro-1-(oxolan-2-yl)pyrimidine-2,4-dione, tetrahydrofuranyl-5-fluorouracil) is a prodrug that is gradually converted to fluorouracil by Cytochrome P450 in the liver. Tegafur competes with uridine triphosphate, thus inhibiting RNA and protein synthesis.
- Tegafur-uracil (UFT) <Ftorafur, Tefudex, Ufur, Uftoral> is a formulated oral agent consisting of a combination of the 5-fluorouracil prodrug, tetrahydrofuranyl-5-fluorouracil, and uracil (1:4). Because of its higher concentration in the combination, uracil saturates the uracil reducing enzymatic activity of Ddihydropyrimidine Ddehydrogenase, thereby inhibiting first pass hepatic metabolism of 5-fluorouracil and permitting its administration as the orally bioavailable prodrug tetrahydrofuranyl-5-fluorouracil. Tegafur-uracil was developed in Japan during the 1980s. The drug has been administered on a continuous daily basis for 6–65 months at 300–400 mg per day in divided doses (metronomic dosing), in cycles of 5 days dosed at 300 mg/m^2 per day followed by the weekend off, or in cycles of 28 days dosed at 300–600 mg/m^2 per day followed by a week off.
- S-1 was developed in Japan. It is an anti-pyrimidine preparation composed of tegafur combined with two modulators of 5-flurouracil activity, 5-chloro-2,4-dihydroxypyridine (CDHP) and potassium oxonate, in a molar ratio of 1:0.4:1. 5-chloro-2,4-dihydroxypyridine is a reversible inhibitor of Dihydropyrimidine Dehydrogenase, the liver enzyme responsible for rapid catabolism of 5-fluorouracil into inactive metabolites. Potassium oxonate preferentially localizes in the gut and inhibits the enzyme Orotate Phosphoribosyl Transferase, which is the major enzyme responsible for 5-fluorouracil activation. Thus it decreases the activation of 5-fluorouracil in the gut and the associated gastrointestinal toxicity. S-1 is orally more active than 5- fluorouracil.
- Capecitabine (5′-deoxy-5-fluoro-*N*-[(pentyloxy) carbonyl]-cytidine) <Xeloda> is a fluoropyrimidine carbamate with nearly 100% oral bioavailability. As a prodrug, capecitabine is metabolized by the liver to 5′-deoxy-5-fluorocytidine and subsequently to 5′-deoxy-5-fluorouridine (5′-dFUR). 5′-deoxy-5-fluorouridine is converted to 5-fluorouracil by Thymidine Phosphorylase, which is present in amounts 3–10-fold higher in neoplastic tissue compared with untransformed tissue. A typical daily oral dose is 1250–2000 mg/m^2. It is split into morning and evening intake (within 30 min after a meal) for 2 weeks, followed by 1 week of rest to complete a cycle. Capecitabine may be used in mono-therapy or combination chemotherapy. It is indicated for the adjuvant treatment of Dukes C colon cancer[41] following the complete resection of the primary tumor, as first-line treatment of metastatic colorectal carcinoma, for metastatic breast cancer after failure of prior anthracycline containing chemotherapy (combination with docetaxel), for metastatic breast cancer resistant to both paclitaxel and anthracycline containing chemotherapy or resistant to paclitaxel and contraindicated for anthracycline therapy. The safety profile of capecitabine is superior to that of 5-fluorouracil, with less diarrhea, stomatitis, nausea, alopecia, and grade 3–4 neutropenia, but a higher incidence of hand and foot syndrome and hyperbilirubinemia (typically unconjugated bilirubin). Care needs to be exercised when capecitabine is co-administered with CYP2C9 substrates. Patients receiving concomitant oral coumarin derivatives should have their anticoagulant response closely monitored. The phenytoin dose may need to be reduced when given simultaneously with capecitabine.

Pharmacokinetics 5-fluorouracil is limited by poor oral absorption, its administration therefore requires a permanent venous access and a portable pump. The drug has a volume of distribution of 0.20–0.25 L/kg, which reflects distribution

[41] Dukes classification of colorectal cancer: Dukes A means the cancer is only in the lining of the colon or rectum. Dukes B means the cancer has grown through the muscle layer of the colon or rectum. Dukes C means the cancer has spread to at least one lymph node in the area close to the bowel. Dukes D means the cancer has spread to distant sites, such as the liver or lung.

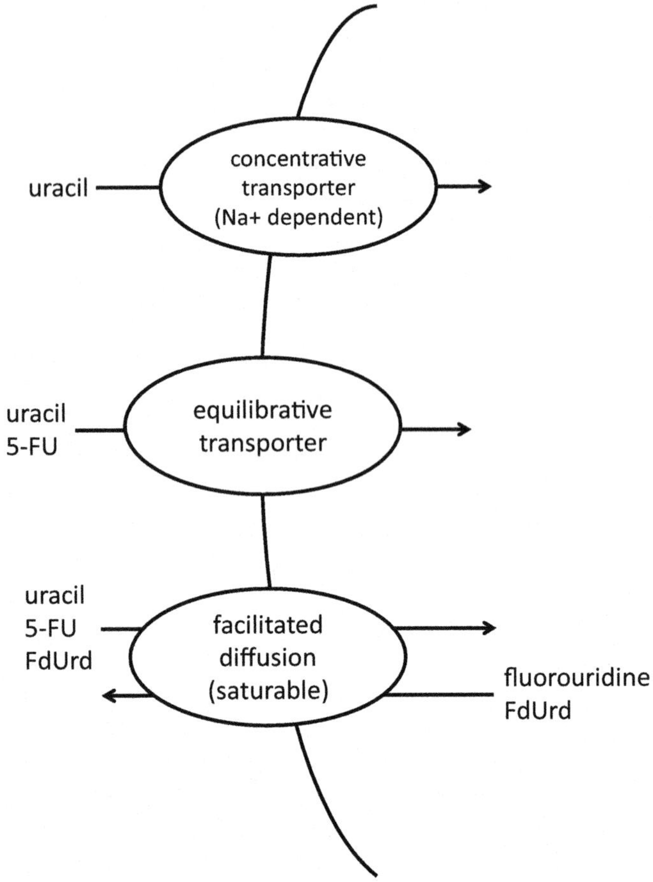

Fig. 2.45 Pyrimidine uptake and excretion. Three transport mechanisms differentially shuttle pyrimidines between the extracellular space (*left*) and the intracellular space (*right*). *5-FU* 5-fluorouracil, *FUdR* fluorouridine deoxyribose

into the extracellular space. There is good penetration into the cerebrospinal fluid, lymph, and neoplastic effusions. The rate of blood clearance generally is 1st order with a half-life of 10–20 min and ranges between 500 and 1500 mL/min. 5-fluorouracil enters cells by a carrier mediated transport mechanism and by facilitated diffusion (however, alterations of 5-fluorouracil entry into cells are not responsible for either natural or acquired resistance). In contrast to 5-fluorouracil, the entry of fluorodeoxyuridine (FdUrd) into most neoplastic cells involves the saturable but non-concentrative mechanism for the facilitated diffusion of nucleosides. Fluorouridine and FdUrd, released from 5-fluorouridylic acid and 5-fluorodeoxyuridylate by Phosphatase action, exit the cells via this same facilitated diffusion transporter (Fig. 2.45). Thus, agents that affect this transporter may affect 5-fluorouracil cytotoxicity[42].

The route of administration of anti-pyrimidine drugs influences the mechanism of action, with thymidylate synthesis inhibition playing a greater role in continuous infusion regimens, and incorporation into RNA being more important for intermittent bolus schedules. Intraarterial infusion of 5-fluorouracil can be used in patients with isolated hepatic metastases. 5-fluorouracil is metabolized to the 2 active moieties 5-fluoro-2-deoxyuridine mono-phosphate (FdUMP) and 5-fluorouridine mono-phosphate (FUMP) by both tumor cells and untransformed cells. The anabolic path, in which 5-fluorouracil is incorporated into nucleotides, is the mechanism of carcinostatic action. Catabolism via the degradation pathway for uracil is the immediate fate of the bulk of an administered dose of 5-fluorouracil and leads to drug inactivation (Fig. 2.46). α-fluoro-β-alanine is the major urinary excretion product of 5-fluorouracil. In patients with cancer, it is conjugated with bile acids and constitutes the primary biliary secretion product. There are marked circadian variations in the metabolism of 5-fluorouracil related to 24-h cyclic fluctuations in Dihydrouracil Dehydrogenase activity, which are reflected in inverse variations of 5-fluorouracil blood concentrations during infusions.

Adverse Effects Gastrointestinal toxicity and myelosuppression are the most common adverse reactions to 5-fluorouracil. Specifically, they include anemia, thrombocytopenia, leukopenia, neutropenia, nausea and vomiting, and diarrhea (4–5 liquid stools per day). Also, stomatitis, mucositis, and hand-foot syndrome (palmar-plantar erythrodysesthesia; drug leakage through capillaries results in redness, tenderness, and possibly peeling of the palms and soles) may arise. Cardiotoxicity can occur due to supraventricular arrhythmia.

Dihydropyrimidine Dehydrogenase, involved in the metabolism of uracil and thymine, is responsible for much of the intra-individual and inter-individual variability in clinical pharmacokinetics of 5-fluorouracil. An autosomal recessive deficiency of Dihydropyrimidine Dehydrogenase constitutes a metabolic disorder that affects over 5 % of the population. Individuals with this condition may develop life threatening toxicity following exposure to 5-fluorouracil or capecitabine.

Drug Resistance Reduced anabolism of 5-fluorouracil to the nucleotide form can lead to drug resistance. This may reflect altered condensation with pyrophosphorylribose-5-phosphate (PRPP) or activation via the salvage pathway that involves ribose-1-phosphate or deoxyribose-1-phosphate and the appropriate Nucleoside Phosphorylase, with subsequent phosphorylation of the resultant nucleoside by Uridine Kinase or Thymidine Kinase. Alternatively, lack of drug sensitivity may be correlated with enhanced Nucleotide Phosphatase activity. Increases in the catabolism of 5-fluorouracil, mainly dependent on the rate limiting enzyme

[42] The facilitated diffusion mechanism may play a secondary role in the modulation of 5-fluorouracil action by uridine because this natural nucleoside, but not 5-fluorouridine (5-FUrd) or fluorodeoxyuridine, is actively concentrated by a Na^+dependent system. Neoplastic cells are less capable of this transport and are not protected by the added uridine.

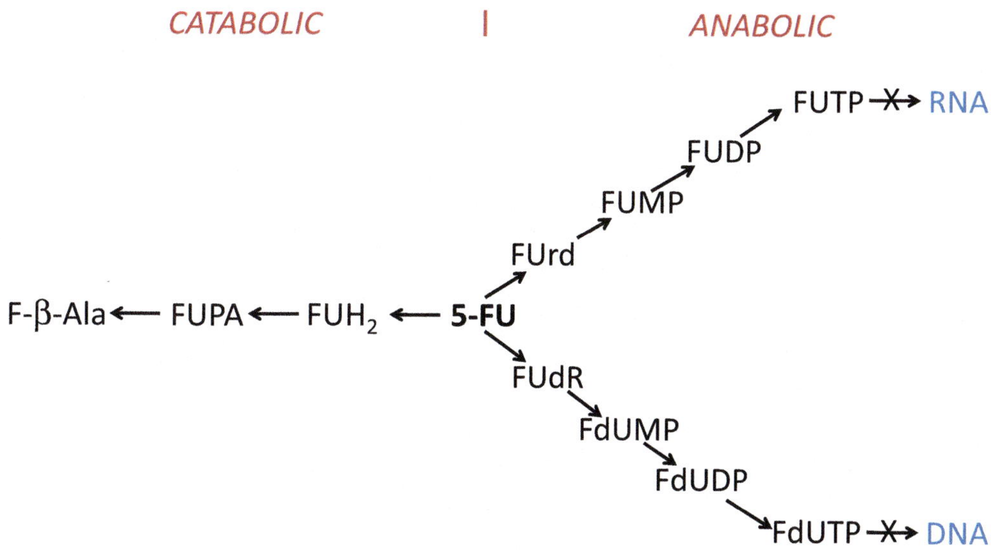

Fig. 2.46 Pathways of 5-fluorouracil metabolism. Two anabolic pathways convert the drug 5-fluorouracil (*5-FU*) into false building blocks for RNA or DNA. Their incorporation terminates the synthesis of these biopolymers. A catabolic pathway incorporates the drug into alanine (*Ala*) to inactivate it. *FUdR* fluorouridine deoxyribose, *F(d)UMP* flouro-(deoxy)uridine-monophosphate, *F(d)UDP* flouro-(deoxy)uridine-diphosphate, *F(d)UTP* flouro-(deoxy) uridine-trisphosphate, *FUH_2* 5,6-dihydro-5-fluorouracil, *FUPA* α-fluoro-β-ureidopropionic acid

Dihydropyrimidine Dehydrogenase, can cause resistance to fluoropyrimidine based chemotherapy. Another mechanism of resistance includes changes in Thymidylate Synthase, with reduced affinity for FdUMP, or increases in the rate of synthesis and activity of the enzyme, possibly associated with gene amplification or altered enzyme turnover rates.

Trifluridine (5-(trifluoromethyl)-2′-deoxyuridine, trifluorothymine deoxyriboside, 1-[4-hydroxy-5-(hydroxymethyl) oxolan-2-yl]-5-(trifluoromethyl) pyrimidine-2,4-dione) was synthesized by Heidelberger as a trifluoromethyl derivative of 5-FUDR[43]. It represents a fluorinated thymidine analog that undergoes metabolic phosphorylation to become a Thymidylate Synthase inhibitor. It may also be incorporated into DNA in place of thymidine. These effects result in the suppression of DNA and protein synthesis, and in the induction of apoptosis.

5-Iododeoxyuridine (IUDR) <Idoxuridine> is an analog of deoxyuridine, which has an iodine atom substituted for the fluorine atom of 5-fluorodeoxyuridine (FUDR). The agent can undergo metabolic phosphorylation and incorporation of the resulting nucleotide into DNA instead of thymidylate, because the van der Waals radius of iodine is similar to that of the methyl group in thymine. In contrast to the generally immunosuppressive actions of most conventional anti-cancer drugs, iododeoxyuridine does not interfere with some components of the immune system. The incorporation of iodine conveys radio-sensitizing properties to the drug that depend on the incorporation of this molecule into DNA during S phase. When this agent contains a radioactive isomer of iodine, the radioactive drug kills cancer cells directly after preferential incorporation into the DNA of rapidly dividing tumor cells.

Pharmacokinetics Iododeoxyuridine differs from fluorodeoxyuridine in metabolic disposition.

5-Bromodeoxyuridine (BrUDR) substitutes a bromine for fluorine in 5-FUDR. After incorporation into DNA, it causes increased susceptibility to breakage of the phospho-ester bond to the adjacent nucleotides. The drug also acts as an immunosuppressive agent and has radio-sensitizing properties.

6-Azauridine (AzUR) is a triazine analog of uridine. It acts at an essential step along the de novo path of pyrimidine biosynthesis by inhibiting Orotidylate Decarboxylase, which suppresses the formation of uridylic acid from its carboxylated precursor, orotidylic acid. Although the drug can produce remissions in some acute adult leukemias, results are mostly only temporary. The triacetylated derivative 6-azauridine 2′,3′,5′-triacetate (6-AzUrd-TA) can be absorbed from the gastrointestinal tract.

Adverse Effects Anemia is a common and moderate adverse effect. 6-Azauridine causes a metabolic disturbance similar to congenital orotic aciduria. Large amounts of orotic acid and orotidine are excreted by patients. Hypercholesterolemia may arise (Knock 1967).

Cytidine analogs Cytarabine (cytosine arabinoside, 1-β-D-arabinofuranosylcytosine, ara-C) <Cytosar-U> was discovered in Europe in the 1960s; it was approved by the U.S. FDA in 1969. The compound of arabinose and cytosine is metabolized by Deoxycytidine Kinase and other nucleotide kinases to a nucleotide triphosphate, which is an effective inhibitor of DNA Polymerase A and competes with

[43] While used as an antiviral drug mainly in the treatment of primary keratoconjunctivitis and recurrent epithelial keratitis due to herpes simplex virus <Trifluridine, Viroptic>, trifluridine has also been tested as an anti-cancer agent in clinical trials.

thymidine for incorporation into DNA. The agent also interferes with DNA synthesis by inhibiting the conversion of cytidylic acid to deoxycytidylic acid, leading to a deficiency of deoxycytidine. Cytarabine therefore kills cells primarily during S phase. Best results are achieved when contact of the drug with the tumor is ensured while the largest possible fraction of cells is in the susceptible S phase.

The introduction of this drug constituted a major advance in the treatment of leukemia, as it achieved 25–40 % complete remission in adults with acute myelogenous leukemia (AML) or acute lymphocytic leukemia (ALL). The agent is also useful for remission induction in acute non-lymphocytic leukemia of pediatric patients and the treatment of acute lymphocytic leukemia and the blast phase of chronic myelocytic leukemia. Intrathecal administration is indicated in the prophylaxis and treatment of meningeal leukemia. Cytarabine can effect some improvement of reticulum cell sarcoma, melanoma, and metastasizing cancers of bladder or testicles. Total doses of 20–100 mg/kg per course can be used. The pharmacological effect is dependent on the treatment schedule. Courses of therapy need to be separated by intervals sufficient to permit adequate host recovery. The drug is not effective orally as only 20 % of the administered dose is absorbed from the gastrointestinal tract.

- Liposomal cytarabine is an intrathecal formulation of cytarabine. The liposomal composition allows more effective delivery to the brain.

Pharmacokinetics The therapeutic efficacy and toxicity of cytarabine are sensitively dependent on the schedule of administration. Following intravenous injection, clearance from the blood is biphasic with an initial distributive phase of 10 min half-life, followed by an elimination phase of 1–3 h half-life. By the end of the distributive phase, more than 80 % of the drug in circulation is converted by a Pyrimidine Nucleoside Deaminase to the inactive metabolite 1-β-D-arabinofuranosyluracil (ara-U). After intrathecal administration, the levels of cytarabine in the cerebrospinal fluid decline with a first order half-life of about 2 h. Because cerebrospinal fluid levels of Deaminase are low, there is little conversion to ara-U. Within 24 h, about 80 % of the administered drug is excreted into the urine.

Adverse Effects Cytarabine is contraindicated in patients who have hypersensitivity to the drug or any of its components. Adverse effects include leukopenia, thrombocytopenia, megaloblastosis, nausea, and vomiting. The cytarabine syndrome is characterized by fever, myalgia, bone pain, occasionally chest pain, maculopapular rash, conjunctivitis and malaise, which usually occurs 6–12 h following drug administration. Corticosteroids are beneficial in treating or preventing this syndrome, and cytarabine therapy may be continued (Castleberry et al. 1981).

The toxicity of cytarabine is dose dependent. Experimental high dose regimens of cytarabine may induce toxicities not commonly associated with standard cytarabine therapies. They include reversible corneal toxicity and hemorrhagic conjunctivitis (preventable or treatable with corticosteroid eye drops), cerebral dysfunctions (personality changes, somnolence, coma), severe gastrointestinal ulceration (pneumatosis cystoides intestinalis, leading to peritonitis, sepsis, liver abscess) or bowel necrosis and necrotizing colitis, pulmonary edema, rare skin rashes leading to desquamation, and sudden respiratory distress (rapidly progressing to pulmonary edema, cardiomegaly). The most characteristic toxicity of high-dose (more than 1 g/m^2 per dose) cytarabine regimens is a cerebellar syndrome of dysarthria, nystagmus, and ataxia. The risk is strongly correlated with advanced age and renal dysfunction. Hepatic dysfunction, high cumulative doses, and bolus dosing may also increase the risks of neurotoxicity. The drug is Pregnancy Category D.

Drug Interactions Acute pancreatitis can occur in patients who have had prior treatment with L-asparaginase. The risk for cardiomyopathy is high when cytarabine is used in combination with cyclophosphamide for bone marrow transplant preparation.

Fazarabine (arabinosyl-5-azacytidine, Ara-AC) is an orally active pyrimidine analog of an aza-substituted cytidine, in which the ribose moiety is replaced by an arabinose sugar. Similar in action to cytarabine, fazarabine is phosphorylated by Deoxycytidine Kinase to a triphosphate form, which competes with thymidine for incorporation into the DNA. Once incorporated, it inhibits DNA synthesis, resulting in tumor cell death.

Drug Resistance The presence of Deoxycytidine Kinase in a tumor is a determinant of its sensitivity to fazarabine.

5,6-dihydro-5-azacytidine (NSC-264880) is a synthetic nucleoside analog of deoxycytidine. Dihydro-5-azacytidine inhibits DNA Methyl Transferase, thereby interfering with the DNA methylation patterns that are associated with genetic instability in some tumor cells. Inhibition of this enzyme may restore the expression of tumor suppressor genes and result in anti-tumor activity.

Decitabine (5-aza-2′-deoxycytidine; 5-AzaC) (NSC-127716) <Dacogen> is a cytidine anti-metabolite that incorporates into DNA, resulting in intra-S phase arrest of DNA reduplication. The agent also inhibits DNA Methyltransferase and exerts anti-cancer activity via the hypo-methylation of DNA (see Sect. 3.2.5.). Decitabine is used for the treatment of myelodysplastic syndrome, acute myelogenous leukemia (AML), and chronic myelogenous leukemia (CML). It was approved by the U.S. FDA in 2004.

Adverse Effects The dose limiting toxicity is bone marrow suppression. Neutropenia occurs in 90 % of patients.

It requires a recovery phase of 30–50 days and may need growth factor support. While worsening neutropenia is common in the first two treatment cycles, it may not correlate with progression of an underlying myelodysplastic syndrome. Febrile neutropenia arises in 30 % of patients. Also common are thrombocytopenia (90 %), anemia (80 %), leukopenia (30 %), and lymphadenopathy (10 %).

Gemcitabine hydrochloride (2′-deoxy-2′,2′-difluorocytidine hydrochloride, 4-amino-1-[3,3-difluoro-4-hydroxy-5-(hydroxymethyl) tetrahydrofuran-2-yl]-1H-pyrimidin-2-one hydrochloride) <Gemzar> is an analog of the antimetabolite nucleoside deoxycytidine. Gemcitabine exhibits cell cycle specificity, primarily killing cells in S phase and blocking their progression through the G_1/S boundary. The agent was approved by the U.S. FDA in 1998 after a clinical trial reported improvements in the quality of life in patients with advanced prostate cancer. This marked the first U.S. FDA approval of a chemotherapy drug for a non-survival endpoint. Gemcitabine is indicated

- in combination with cisplatin for the first-line treatment of patients with inoperable, locally advanced (stage IIIA or IIIB), or metastatic (stage IV) non-small cell lung cancer,
- in combination with paclitaxel for the first-line treatment of patients with metastatic breast cancer after failure of prior anthracycline containing chemotherapy, unless anthracyclines were contraindicated.
- as first-line treatment for patients with locally advanced (non-resectable stage II or stage III) or metastatic (stage IV) pancreas adenocarcinoma, also for patients previously treated with 5-fluorouracil,
- in combination with carboplatin for the treatment of patients with advanced ovarian cancer that has relapsed at least 6 months after completion of platinum based therapy.

Gemcitabine is administered by injection over a period of 30 min. The dosage and number of administrations depend on a variety of factors, including the type of cancer, body size, gender, and other concurrent treatments. A common regimen is 1000 mg/m^2 on days 1 and 8 of a 21-day cycle. Dosage adjustment is based on the degree of hematologic toxicity experienced by the patient.

Pharmacokinetics Gemcitabine plasma protein binding is negligible. Compared with cytarabine, gemcitabine achieves intracellular concentrations about 20-fold higher, secondary to an increased penetration of cell membranes via equilibrative and concentrative nucleoside transporters, and a greater affinity for the activating enzyme Deoxycytidine Kinase. The drug is converted intracellularly to the active metabolites difluorodeoxycytidine di- and triphosphate (dFdCDP and dFdCTP).

- dFdCDP inhibits Ribonucleotide Reductase[44], thereby decreasing the deoxynucleotide pool available for DNA synthesis
- dFdCTP is incorporated into DNA, resulting in DNA strand termination and apoptosis.

After incorporation into DNA, gemcitabine has a prolonged intracellular half-life. Drug inactivation to 2′-deoxy-2′,2′-difluorouridine (dFdU) is catalyzed by Cytidine Deaminase. Polymorphisms in this enzyme, in particular homozygous Ala70Thr (CDA*3), are major determinants of drug clearance. The administered dose is almost entirely excreted in the urine as the parent drug (10 %) and its inactive uracil metabolite 2′-deoxy-2′,2′-difluorouridine (90 %). Gemcitabine clearance in women and the elderly is compromised. Therefore, women tend to be somewhat less able to progress to subsequent cycles.

Adverse Effects Gemcitabine may temporarily reduce the number of white blood cells, particularly during the first 10–14 days after administration. Treatment can cause chicken pox or shingles (herpes zoster) to become very severe and spread to various parts of the body. Immunizations or contact with individuals who have recently taken oral polio vaccines should be avoided during or after gemcitabine administration. Flu-like symptoms are common following the first treatment cycle. The drug can also lower the blood platelet count. The risk of bleeding may be reduced by using caution when cleaning teeth, avoiding dental work, and avoiding cuts, bruises, or other injuries.

Non-hematologic adverse effects of gemcitabine may include nausea, vomiting, chills and fever. Gemcitabine induced severe pulmonary toxicity (GISPT) is an inflammatory reaction in the lungs following treatment with gemcitabine. The incidence ranges 0.5–5 % of patients. A potentially fatal adverse event is vasculitis. The hemolytic uremic syndrome is very rare but potentially fatal. The drug is Pregnancy Category D.

Drug Resistance Failure of gemcitabine therapy in pancreatic cancer is often due to chemoresistance after initial response. Resistance is typically mediated by the down-regulation of Equilibrative Nucleoside Transporter 1 (hENT1) and Concentrative Nucleoside Transporter 1 (hCNT1), which are required for the cellular entry of gemcitabine.

Sapacitabine (CYC682) is an orally available 2′-deoxycytidine analog. It synergizes with inhibitors of Histone Deacetylase or DNA Methyl Transferases. The agent can be effectively combined with other nucleoside analogs, particularly clofarabine and gemcitabine, which inhibit Ribonucleotide Reductase.

[44] Inhibitors of Ribonucleotide Reductase include gemcitabine (via its metabolite dFdCDP), clofarabine, fludarabine, inosine dialdehyde, triapine, 5-azacytidine, zebularine, and GTI-2040 (a phosphorothioate oligonucleotide that suppresses gene expression).

Other pyrimidine antagonists Penclomedine (3,5-dichloro -2,4-dimethoxy-6 trichloromethyl pyridine) (NSC338720) is a synthetic derivative of pyrimidine that alkylates and cross-links DNA, resulting in DNA strand breaks and inhibition of DNA and RNA synthesis. This agent is more active against tumor cells that are defective in P53 function than in cells with intact P53. Neurotoxicity (ataxia, vertigo, nystagmus, motor aphasia) may be dose limiting.

m-Azidopyrimethamine is an anti-metabolite derived from diaminopyrimidine. With a mechanism of action similar to that of antifolates, m-azidopyrimethamine blocks tetrahydrofolate synthesis, resulting in the depletion of nucleotide precursors and inhibition of DNA, RNA and protein synthesis. The agent is lipophilic.

Metoprine (DDMP, 2,4-diamino-5-(3′,4′-dichlorophenyl)-6-methylpyrimidine) (BW 197U) is a diaminopyrimidine folate antagonist that inhibits Dihydrofolate Reductase, resulting in decreased cellular folate metabolism and cell growth. It also inhibits Histamine-N-Methyltransferase, resulting in decreased histamine catabolism. Due to its lipid solubility, metoprine is capable of crossing the blood-brain barrier.

Adverse Effects The drug has a long duration of action, leading to adverse effects related to its blood levels. The usual dose limiting toxicity is thrombocytopenia. Other possible adverse effects include skin rashes, headaches, nausea, and dyspepsia.

Hydroxyurea (hydroxycarbamide, carbamyl hydroxamate) <Hydrea, Droxia, Biosupressin, Litalir, Myelostat> was first synthesized in 1869 by W.F.C. Dresler and R. Stein in Heidelberg, Germany, and was investigated as an antineoplastic agent in the 1960s. It is a monohydroxyl-substituted urea anti-metabolite. Hydroxyurea selectively inhibits Ribonucleoside Diphosphate Reductase, an enzyme required to convert ribonucleoside diphosphates into deoxyribonucleoside diphosphates[45]. Thereby the drug prevents cells from leaving the G_1/S phase of the cell cycle. Hydroxyurea also exhibits radio-sensitizing activity by maintaining cells in the radiation sensitive G_1 phase and interfering with DNA repair. The agent is used to treat hematologic malignancies, such as chronic myelogenous leukemia (CML) and myeloproliferative disease, specifically polycythemia vera, essential thrombocytosis, and hypereosinophilic syndrome. It also has had positive results in the treatment of chronic granulocytic leukemia. Responses by melanomata, epidermoid carcinomata, teratocarcinomata, or cervical carcinomata can be achieved.

Hydroxyurea is readily absorbed from the gastrointestinal tract. It can be given orally or intravenously. Numerous dosing schedules exist and depend on underlying disease, initial response, and concomitant therapy. For treating solid tumors in adults, intermittent therapy may comprise 80 mg/kg administered orally as a single dose every 3rd day, while continuous therapy may be 20–30 mg/kg as a single dose daily. Accumulation occurs with daily dosing. For hematologic malignancies, continuous treatment is typically given. The dosage may be reduced or delayed in patients with bone marrow depression due to prior myelotoxic therapy.

Pharmacokinetics Peak blood levels are reached in 1–4 h after an oral dose. The drug is distributed throughout the body and crosses the blood-brain barrier. It concentrates in leukocytes and erythrocytes. Hydroxyurea is converted to the free radical nitroxide (NO) and transported into cells by diffusion. 50–60 % of the agent is metabolized in the liver, resulting in the inactive products carbon dioxide and urea. The major route of elimination with first order kinetics is renal (55 %), the CO_2 metabolite is exhaled. A minor pathway of breakdown may be the degradation by Urease in intestinal bacteria.

Adverse Effects There are marked adverse effects. They include a rapid fall in white cell and platelet counts, nausea and vomiting, diarrhea, stomatitis, alopecia, and impaired renal function[46]. If taken for the long term, hydroxyurea is potentially leukemogenic. Patients who have received irradiation therapy prior to hydroxyurea may have an exacerbation of post-irradiation erythema. Additional, possibly fatal toxicities, including pancreatitis, hepatic failure, or peripheral neuropathy may occur in HIV infected patients during combination therapy that includes hydroxyurea. Hydroxyurea is Pregnancy Category D, the drug is secreted in the milk.

Drug Resistance Resistance to hydroxyurea can arise. It may be caused by elevated synthesis of the Ribonucleoside Diphosphate Reductase component R_2 or by elevated levels of Ferritin.

Anti-pyrimidines inhibit uracil utilization by tumors.
Anti-pyrimidines may radio-sensitize by maintaining cells in the radiation sensitive G1 phase and interfering with DNA repair. However, tumors that have previously been irradiated respond poorly to fluorinated pyrimidines.
Halogenated uracil drugs carry a halogen on uracil or its derivatives.
Cytidine drugs interfere with DNA synthesis by inhibiting the conversion of cytidylic acid to deoxycytidylic acid.
Other anti-pyrimidine drugs have various modes of action.

2.4.3 Anti-Purines

In 1948, Gertrude Elion and George Hitchings discovered diaminopurine, an adenine antagonist, which inhibited

[45] Ribonucleoside Diphosphate Reductase consists of two proteins, R_1 and R_2. Hydroxyurea destroys a tyrosyl free radical that is formed in the catalytic center of the enzyme. This results in the destabilization of the iron center in protein R_2, rendering the enzyme inactive.

[46] Due to the effect of hydroxyurea on the bone marrow, regular monitoring of the full blood count is vital, as well as swift responses to possible infections. In addition, renal function, uric acid and electrolytes, as well as liver enzymes, are commonly checked.

experimentally induced leukemia. Clinical trials in patients were initially promising but had to be terminated due to toxic effects. By 1951, Elion and Hitchings had developed 6-thioguanine and 6-mercaptopurine as a part of a comprehensive chemical program to generate analogs for the purine constituents of nucleic acids. The substitution of sulfur for oxygen in position six of guanine and hypoxanthine produces compounds with substantial anti-tumor activity (Fig. 2.47). These drugs inhibited adenine metabolism and later played an important role in the treatment of acute leukemia. In collaboration with the Sloan-Kettering Institute, 6-mercaptopurine was tested in leukemic patients who were resistant to methotrexate. About 1/3 of the patients responded with complete remission. In part for this work, Elion and Hitchings received the Nobel Prize in Physiology or Medicine in 1988.

One limitation of anti-purines is a relative lack of specificity because purines are required for multiple biochemical pathways in addition to nucleic acid synthesis. These pathways are vital to tumor cells and host cells alike.

First generation purine antagonists 6-Mercaptopurine (6-MP,3,7-dihydropurine-6-thione) <Purinethol> is a prodrug, the free base form of which is converted by sensitive tumor cells via 6-thioinosine 5′-monophosphate (timp) to the ribonucleotide 6-mercaptopurin-9-yl (mprp). 6-Mercaptopurine competes with hypoxanthine and guanine for the enzyme Hypoxanthine-Guanine Phosphoribosyltransferase (HGPRT), and is converted by it to thioinosinate. Further, 6-methylthioinosinate is formed by the methylation of thioinosinate. The intracellular nucleotide thioinosinate inhibits the conversion of inosinate to xanthylate and the conversion of inosinate to adenylate. Both thioinosinate and 6-methylthioinosinate inhibit Glutamine-5-Phosphoribosylpyrophosphate Amidotransferase, the first enzyme unique to the de novo pathway for purine ribonucleotide synthesis.

6-Mercaptopurine is indicated in combination regimens for the maintenance therapy of acute lymphatic (lymphocytic, lymphoblastic) leukemia. However, the response depends on the particular sub-classification of the disease and the age of the patient. The drug is also used for treating pediatric non-Hodgkin lymphomata and sometimes choriocarcinomata. 6-Mercaptopurine may be beneficial for treating the pre-cancerous condition polycythemia vera. The drug is not effective for prophylaxis or treatment of central nervous system leukemia, or for treatment of acute myelogenous leukemia, chronic lymphatic leukemia, and solid tumors.

Derivatives of 6-mercaptopurine have been synthesized with the goal to improve its pharmacological properties:

- The guanosine analog 6-thioguanine (6-TG, 2-amino-6-mercaptopurine) <Tabloid> was synthesized and developed by Hitchings, Elion and associates at the Wellcome Research Laboratories. It is one of a large series of purine analogs, which interfere with nucleic acid biosynthesis. After phosphorylation by Hypoxanthine-Guanine Phosphoribosyltransferase, thioguanine incorporates into DNA and RNA, resulting in the inhibition of DNA and RNA synthesis and cell death. This agent also inhibits Glutamine-5-Phosphoribosylpyrophosphate Amidotransferase, thereby suppressing purine synthesis. Thioguanine is used for the treatment of acute non-lymphocytic leukemia.

  Adverse Effects Serious adverse effects resulting from the exposure to thioguanine include allergic reactions (difficulty breathing, closing of the throat, swelling of the lips, tongue, or face, hives), decreased bone marrow function (extreme fatigue, easy bruising or bleeding, tarry stools, fever or chills, sore throat), impaired liver function (jaundice, abdominal pain), severe nausea, vomiting, diarrhea, loss of appetite, or sores in the mouth. Symptoms of a thioguanine overdose tend to be similar to the adverse effects caused by the medication, although often more severe. Thioguanine causes birth defects if taken during pregnancy.

  Drug Interactions Administration of a live vaccine can be dangerous during treatment with thioguanine. Dose adjustments may be required for patients on balsalazide <Colazal> , mesalamine <Asacol, Pentasa, Rowasa>, olsalazine <Dipentum>, or sulfasalazine <Azulfidine>.

- Azathioprine (6-[(1-methyl-4-nitro-γ-imidazolyl)thio] purine) (BW57–322) <Azasan, Imuran> was synthesized by Ellion and coworkers to provide a 6-mercaptopurine derivative, in which the 6-mercapto group is substituted to limit oxidative degradation. Azathioprine has become one of the most commonly used anti-purine drugs. It is non-enzymatically cleaved to 6-mercaptopurine, the active agent that acts as a purine analog and an inhibitor of DNA synthesis.

  Adverse Effects The principal and potentially serious toxic effects are hematologic and gastrointestinal. There are also risks of secondary infection and neoplasia. The frequency and severity of adverse reactions depend on the dose and duration of azathioprine treatment as well as on the underlying disease or concomitant therapies. Adverse effects of low frequency include skin rashes, alopecia, fever, arthralgias, diarrhea, steatorrhea, and reversible interstitial pneumonitis. Patients with low or absent Thiopurine S-Methyltransferase (TPMT) activity are at an increased risk of developing severe, life threatening myelotoxicity. The drug is Pregnancy Category D.

Pharmacokinetics 6-Mercaptopurine is given orally at 2.5 mg/kg. However, the absorption of an oral dose is incomplete and variable, averaging approximately 50%. Plasma protein binding is around 20%. Variability in 6-mercaptopurine metabolism is one of the major causes of

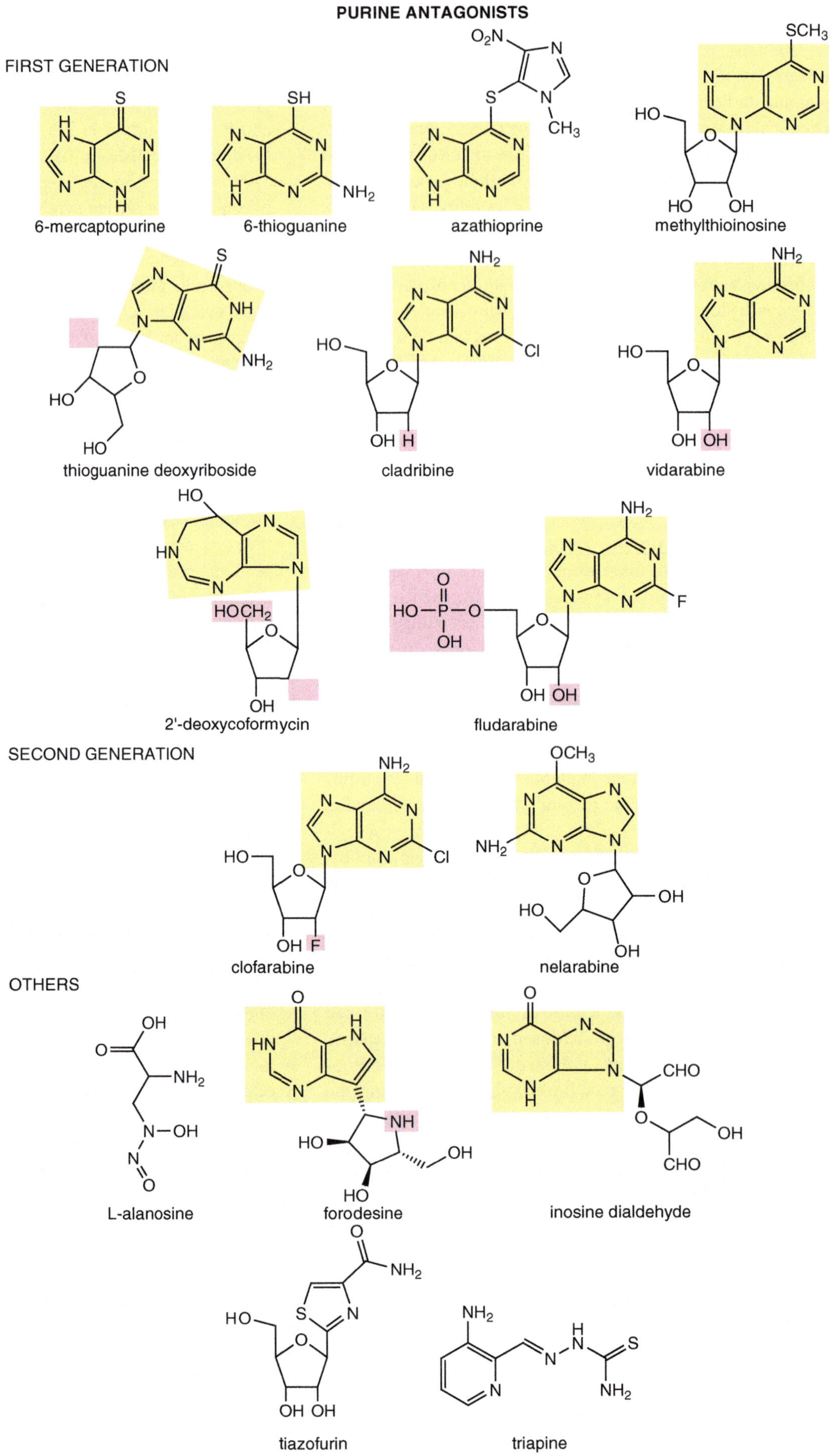

Fig. 2.47 Structures of anti-purines. The common purine moiety is highlighted in *yellow*. Among the first generation anti-purines, the *top row* contains drugs without a sugar moiety, the *second row* depicts ribose containing drugs, and the *third row* shows drugs with arabinose as the sugar. Variations in the structure of the nucleoside sugar are depicted in *pink*

interindividual differences in systemic exposure to the drug and its active metabolites. The half-life of 6-mercaptopurine in the blood is shorter in pediatric patients than in adult patients. It ranges about 0.75–1.5 h, reflecting a combination of cellular uptake and degradation. 6-Mercaptopurine is inactivated via two major pathways,

- thiol methylation is catalyzed by the highly polymorphic enzyme Thiopurine S-Methyltransferase (TPMT), to form methyl-6-mercaptopurine.
- oxidation is catalyzed by Xanthine Oxidase and forms 6-thiouric acid.

The metabolic products are rapidly eliminated by the kidneys, with close to 50% of the administered dose being excreted in the first 24 h.

Adverse Effects Bone marrow depression is the main toxic effect. The induction of complete remission of acute lymphatic leukemia is frequently associated with marrow hypoplasia. This may be manifest as anemia, leukopenia, thrombocytopenia, or any combination of these. The marrow depression is usually reversible upon termination of the drug treatment. Other adverse effects include anorexia, nausea, vomiting, and less frequently alopecia, stomatitis, diarrhea, intestinal ulceration, and dermatologic disorders (skin rashes, hyper-pigmentation). Rare cases of drug fever can arise, but differential diagnosis needs to exclude more common causes of pyrexia in acute leukemia patients, such as sepsis. The drug is Pregnancy Category D.

As a consequence of the rapid death of neoplastic cells, hyperuricemia or hyperuricosuria may occur. The ensuing renal adverse effects can be limited by hydration, urine alkalinization, and the prophylactic administration of a Xanthine Oxidase inhibitor, such as allopurinol. Allopurinol may diminish the rate of 6-mercaptopurine degradation by competing for the oxidizing enzymes that are part of the inactivating pathway, specifically the Xanthine Oxidase mediated degradation to thiouric acid. Therefore, when allopurinol and 6-mercaptopurine are administered concomitantly, the dose of mercaptopurine must be reduced to 1/4–1/3 of the usual dose to avoid severe toxicity. Patients with inherited low Thiopurine S-Methyltransferase activity are at increased risk for severe toxicity from conventional doses of 6-mercaptopurine and generally require substantial dose reduction. In patients with impaired renal or hepatic function the starting doses of 6-mercaptopurine should be reduced. Clinically detectable jaundice can be an adverse effect. It usually appears within the first 1–2 months in the course of treatment. Hepatic injury can occur with any dosage, but seems have higher frequency when doses of 2.5 mg/kg/day are exceeded. In rare cases, fatal hepatic necrosis may be a consequence of 6-mercaptopurine therapy. Hepatic encephalopathy has occurred.

Drug Resistance 6-Mercaptopurine should not be used in patients whose disease has demonstrated prior resistance to this drug. There is usually complete cross-resistance between mercaptopurine and thioguanine. Drug resistance can arise through several mechanisms. Some tumors that are resistant have lost the ability to convert 6-mercaptopurine to 6-thioinosine 5′-monophosphate. A loss of 5-Phosphoribosyl Transferase in the tumor cells may lead to the inability to convert the free base form of 6-mercaptopurine to the active ribonucleotide 6-mercaptopurin-9-yl.

Drug Interactions Enhanced marrow suppression may occur in some patients who also receive trimethoprim-sulfamethoxazole. 6-Mercaptopurine can inhibit the anti-coagulant effect of warfarin, when given simultaneously. Because aminosalicylate derivatives may inhibit the enzyme Thiopurine S-Methyltransferase (TPMT) they should be administered with caution to patients on 6-mercaptopurine therapy.

The mercaptopurine derivative methylthioinosine (6-(methylmercapto)purine riboside, 6-MMPR) inhibits Amidophosphoribosyl Transferase, the first committed step in de novo purine synthesis, and inhibits cell proliferation induced by Fibroblast Growth Factor-2 (FGF-2).

β-Thioguanine deoxyriboside is a thiopurine nucleoside derivative. After conversion to a triphosphate, β-thioguanine deoxyriboside is incorporated into DNA, resulting in inhibition of DNA reduplication. This agent is cytotoxic against leukemia cells. It demonstrates anti-neoplastic activity against 6-thioguanine resistant tumor cells.

Cladribine (2-chlorodeoxyadenosine, 2-CDA) <Leustatin, Litak> is an adenosine analog. Cladribine triphosphate, a phosphorylated metabolite of cladribine, incorporates into DNA, resulting in single strand breaks, and depletion of nicotinamide adenine dinucleotide (NAD) and adenosine triphosphate (ATP). These events lead to apoptosis. Because the agent is resistant to Adenosine Deaminase (ADA), an enzyme that inactivates some anti-neoplastic agents, it is selectively toxic to lymphocytes and monocytes, which exhibit little Deoxynucleotide Deaminase activity. Cladribine is mostly used for the treatment of hairy cell leukemia. It is also a second-line treatment for patients with chronic lymphocytic leukemia (CLL) who have not responded to alkylating agents. The drug is administered by injection or infusion. The recommended dose and schedule for active hairy cell leukemia is as a single course given by continuous infusion for seven consecutive days at 0.09 mg/kg/day.

Adverse Effects Treatment should be delayed or discontinued if renal toxicity or neurotoxicity occurs. Common adverse effects include fatigue, bone marrow depression (neutropenia predisposing to infections), and fever. Less common adverse effects comprise dizziness, insomnia, abdominal cramps and constipation, diarrhea, skin reaction at the infusion side (swelling, pain, redness), tachycardia, swollen ankles (arthralgia), cough, or loss of fertility. The drug is Pregnancy Category D.

The two nucleosides spongothymidine and spongouridine, isolated in the 1950s from the Caribbean sponge Tethya crypta, provided the structural basis for the exploration of the sugar-modified nucleoside analog vidarabine (2-amino-2-deoxy-β-arabinofuranosyladenine, adenine arabinoside, Ara-A). The drug was first synthesized in 1960 by Bernard Randall Baker at the Stanford Research Institute. In 1969, it was isolated from the fermentation beers of Streptomyces antibioticus.

Vidarabine contains an arabinoside sugar rather than a ribose. The agent inhibits DNA Polymerase, resulting in the inhibition of DNA reduplication. Due to this mechanism, cytotoxicity is S phase specific. Vidarabine has been administered as an anti-leukemic drug. However, it has limited clinical usefulness because of its rapid inactivation by Adenosine Deaminase.

A product of the fermentation by Streptomyces antibioticus is 2′-deoxycoformycin (co-vidarabine, dCF) (NSC-218321, CL-825) <Premarin, Pentostatin, Nipent>. Co-vidarabine is a 6-thiopurine analog of the naturally occurring purine bases hypoxanthine and guanine. The agent is an inhibitor of Adenosine Deaminase (ADA), an enzyme that is critical in purine base metabolism and has its highest activity in cells of the lymphoid system. T-lymphocytes have higher Adenosine Deaminase activity than B-lymphocytes, and T-cell malignancies have higher activity than B-cell malignancies. The inhibition of Adenosine Deaminase by deoxycoformycin leads to an intracellular accumulation of deoxy-ATP, which causes apoptosis. The drug is effective in the treatment of several lymphoproliferative conditions, particularly acute non-lymphocytic leukemia, hairy-cell leukemia that is refractory to Interferon-α, and relapsed chronic lymphocytic leukemia (CLL). It is not suitable for the treatment of acute lymphocytic leukemia because the transformed cells contain such high levels of Adenosine Deaminase that their suppression would require toxic doses of 2′-deoxycoformycin. Deoxycoformycin is given by intravenous bolus injection or diluted in a larger volume for infusion over 20–30 min once every 2 weeks for 3–6 months until a complete response is achieved, then two additional cycles are administered. The standard dosage is 4 mg/m^2.

Pharmacokinetics Deoxycoformycin is not absorbed orally. Plasma protein binding after injection is 5 % and the half life is 5–6 h. The agent crosses the blood-brain barrier. Biotransformation occurs primarily in the liver, but only small amounts are metabolized. 90 % of the drug is eliminated in the urine unchanged or as metabolites. Patients should receive hydration with 0.5–1 L of 5 % dextrose in saline before administration. An additional 0.5 L should be administered after deoxycoformycin is given.

Adverse Effects Common adverse effects (occurring in more than 30 % of patients) include nausea and vomiting, low blood counts, skin rashes, fever, and fatigue. Less common adverse effects comprise itching, muscle aches, chills, headache, diarrhea, abdominal pain, anorexia, weakness, upper respiratory infections, mouth sores, cough, and shortness of breath. Patients with severe pre-existing infections should not receive deoxycoformycin. It is contraindicated in patients with severe renal impairment. The drug is Pregnancy Category D.

Drug Interactions Simultaneous treatment of deoxycoformycin with clozapine or carbamazepine is to be avoided. The combined use with fludarabine may lead to severe, even fatal, pulmonary toxicity.

Fludarabine phosphate ([(2R,3R,4S,5R)-5-(6-amino-2-fluoro-purin-9-yl)-3,4-dihydroxy-oxolan-2-yl]methoxyphosphonic acid, 2-fluoro-ara-AMP) <Fludara, Oforta> is a fluorinated analog of vidarabine.

- Fludarabine phosphate is susceptible to glycosidic bond cleavage, which results in the formation of 2-fluoro-adenine, and is further converted to the highly toxic 2-fluoro-ATP.
- Fludarabine phosphate may be rapidly dephosphorylated by Phosphorylase cleavage to 2-fluoro-arabinosyladenine and then phosphorylated intracellularly by Deoxycytidine Kinase to the active triphosphate, 2-fluoro-arabinosyl-ATP. This metabolite inhibits DNA Polymerase α, Ribonucleotide Reductase, and DNA Primase, thereby interrupting DNA synthesis and inhibiting tumor cell growth.

Fludarabine is used in the treatment of hematologic malignancies. Specifically, it is indicated for patients with B-cell chronic lymphocytic leukemia after an initial treatment with alkylating agents has failed. The recommended adult dose of the intravenous drug is 25 mg/m^2, administered over a period of approximately 30 min daily for five consecutive days. The recommended adult dose of the tablet form (to be swallowed with water) is 40 mg/m^2 daily for five consecutive days. Cycles should commence every 28 days. The dosage may be decreased or delayed based on hematologic, neurologic, or other toxicity.

Adverse Effects Fludarabine causes anemia, thrombocytopenia and neutropenia. Severe pancytopenia can arise and sometimes lead to death. The association with profound lymphopenia is a substantial risk factor for opportunistic infections. Patients on fludarabine are often treated with co-trimoxazole or monthly nebulized pentamidine to prevent Pneumocystis jiroveci pneumonia. Ractivations of latent viral infections, such as varicella zoster virus (Herpes zoster), Epstein-Barr virus (lymphoproliferative disorders), or JC virus (progressive multifocal leukoencephalopathy) have occurred. Because the lymphopenia also renders patients susceptible to potentially fatal transfusion associated graft-versus-host disease, all patients who have ever received fludarabine should only be given irradiated blood components.

Fludarabine is associated with the development of severe autoimmune hemolytic anemia or autoimmune thrombocytopenia in a proportion of patients. Other common adverse events include fever and chills, infection, nausea and vomiting, malaise, fatigue, and anorexia. Less common are confusion, seizures, optic neuritis or optic neuropathy, adult respiratory distress syndrome (ARDS), pulmonary fibrosis, and skin rashes. Advanced age, renal insufficiency, or bone marrow impairment constitute predispositions to increased fludarabine toxicity. The drug is Pregnancy Category D.

Drug Interactions The use of fludarabine in combination with deoxycoformycin is not recommended due to the risk of severe pulmonary toxicity.

Second generation purine antagonists Clofarabine (2-Chloro-9-(2-deoxy-2-fluoroarabinofuranosyl)adenine) <Clolar, Clofarex, Evoltra> is a second generation nucleoside analog, which was developed to reduce the glycosidic cleavage that its predecessor drugs are susceptible to. The agent is activated to its triphosphate inside the tumor cells.

- Clofarabine acts by terminating DNA chain elongation and inhibiting DNA repair through incorporation into the DNA. When the ratio of clofarabine triphosphate to dATP is >1, clofarabine monophosphate is preferentially inserted into the end of the DNA chain, resulting in the termination of chain elongation. A ratio of clofarabine triphosphate to dATP <1 results in the insertion of clofarabine monophosphate into the middle of the DNA structure and inhibits DNA repair.
- Clofarabine triphosphate inhibits Ribonucleotide Reductase, leading to a depletion of the deoxyribonucleotide triphosphate (dNTP) pools.
- Clofarabine induces apoptosis through direct and indirect action on mitochondria by releasing Cytochrome *c* and other pro-apoptotic factors, including AIF (Apoptosis Inducing Factor), APAF-1 (Apoptotic Protease Activating Factor-1), and Caspase-9.

The agent received accelerated approval from the U.S. FDA in 2004. Clofarabine is used for the treatment of pediatric patients (up to 21 years), with relapsed or refractory acute lymphoblastic leukemia, consecutive to at least two prior regimens.

Pharmacokinetics Except for tissues with specialized barriers, such as eyes, brain, and testes, clofarabine distribution is fairly widespread, with the highest concentrations occurring in the metabolic and excretory organs (kidneys and liver) and in the gastrointestinal tract (small and large intestine). Clofarabine is a prodrug that gains entry into cells primarily by nucleoside transporter mechanisms. Nucleoside transporters are specialized proteins located in the cell membrane that mediate the uptake and release of nucleosides and nucleoside analogs. Clofarabine is efficiently taken up via the equilibrative transporters hENT1 and hENT2, and the concentrative transporter hCNT2[47]. The abundance of nucleoside transporters on a tumor or host cell may be a major determinant of the amount of nucleoside or nucleoside analog that is taken up into a particular tissue type. At higher concentrations and longer exposure times, the slightly lipophilic agent clofarabine also enters cells by passive diffusion across lipid membranes.

Clofarabine is phosphorylated by cytosolic kinases, including Deoxycytidine Kinase (DCK) and a Purine Nucleoside Monophosphate Kinase, to yield the active form clofarabine triphosphate. Transformed cells have higher DCK concentrations than their healthy counterparts.

Because of the natural lipophilicity of the parent drug and the need to de-phosphorylate the active clofarabine nucleotides prior to their export out of the cell, the tissue-to-blood concentration ratios in organs without special barriers are almost always larger than two (Bonate et al. 2006). Removal of the phosphates by 5′-Nucleotidase is a prerequisite for the cellular export of clofarabine. Hence, the ratio of DCK to 5′-Nucleotidase activities may be an indicator of tumor cell sensitivity to this drug. Even though clofarabine has a short half-life of 4–6 h its active metabolite remains in the cells much longer, having a half-life of at least 24 h (Gandhi et al. 2003).

Adverse Effects The adverse effects of the drug, involving bone marrow, lymphoid tissue, heart, and liver, are not the result of unique tissue uptake. The predominant toxicities are reversible liver dysfunction (reflected in elevated Transaminases and hyperbilirubinemia), skin rashes, palmoplantar erythrodysesthesia (hand-foot syndrome), and mucositis. Clofarabine can produce systemic inflammatory response syndrome (SIRS) and capillary leak syndrome, manifested by the rapid development of tachypnea, tachycardia, hypo-

[47] The ENT transporters work bi-directionally, driven by the nucleoside concentration gradient between the inside and the outside of the cell membrane. The CNT channels transport purine nucleosides inward, coupled to the inward movement of sodium along its concentration gradient.

tension, shock, and multi-organ failure. Cardiac toxicity may cause tachycardia or left ventricular systolic dysfunction.

Nelarabine (506U78) <Arranon, Atriance> is an arabinonucleoside anti-metabolite prodrug. After uptake, it is *O*-demethylated by Adenosine Deaminase to ara-G, monophosphorylated by Deoxyguanosine Kinase and Deoxycytidine Kinase, and subsequently converted to the biologically active 9-β-D-arabinosylguanine 5′-triphosphate (ara-GTP). Arabinosylguanine incorporates into DNA, thereby inhibiting DNA synthesis and inducing the apoptosis of tumor cells during S phase. Nelarabine is indicated as a chemotherapy drug for T-cell acute lymphoblastic leukemia and T-cell lymphoblastic lymphoma that has not responded to or has relapsed following treatment with at least two chemotherapy regimens. It was approved in the U.S. in October 2005 and in the European Union in 2007. The recommended adult dose is 1500 mg/m^2 (650 mg/m^2 for pediatric patients) administered intravenously over 2 h on days 1, 3, and 5. This cycle is repeated every 21 days. Treatment is generally continued until there is evidence of disease progression, until the patient experiences unacceptable toxicity, until the patient becomes a candidate for bone marrow transplantation, or until the patient no longer benefits from treatment.

Pharmacokinetics Conversion of nelarabine to arabinosylguanine occurs rapidly and extensively after injection. Less than 25% of nelarabine or its metabolite are bound to plasma proteins. Both are partially eliminated by the kidneys (5–25% over 24 h). Age and gender have no effect on the pharmacokinetics of nelarabine or arabinosylguanine.

Adverse Effects Adverse events associated with the use of nelarabine may include

- in the pediatric population, hematologic toxicities (anemia, neutropenia, leukopenia, thrombocyopenia), infections, asthenia, liver damage (elevation of hepatic enzymes), vomiting, deficiencies of potassium, calcium, or magnesium
- in the adult population, hematologic toxicities (anemia, neutropenia, thrombocyopenia), febrile neutropenia, fatigue, asthenia, nausea, cough, dyspnea, edema, and petechiae.

Neurological adverse events arise in over 60% of subjects. Most are mild to moderate (grade 1–2), including headache, somnolence, neuropathy, hypoesthesia. Grade 4 and grade 5 (fatal) adverse neurological events (including 3rd and 6th nerve paralysis, progressive multifocal leukoencephalopathy, demyelination similar to Guillain-Barré syndrome, cerebral and intracranial hemorrhage, coma, and metabolic encephalopathy) are possible. Close monitoring of such events is recommended. The appearance of grade 2 or higher neurological toxicities may require the discontinuation of treatment. Appropriate measures must be taken to prevent hyperuricemia. They may include hydration, urine alkalinization, and prophylaxis with allopurinol. The drug is Pregnancy Category D.

Drug Interactions 2′-deoxycoformycin is an inhibitor of Adenosine Deaminase, which may cause a reduction in the activation of the prodrug nelarabine. Co-administration can lead to a reduction in nelarabine efficacy or changes in the adverse reaction profile of either drug.

Other purine antagonists Purine Nucleoside Phosphorylase (PNP) is an enzyme in the purine salvage pathway that mediates the phosphorolysis of (deoxy)nucleoside analogs to their respective bases and (deoxy)ribose phosphate. Forodesine hydrochloride (BCX-1777) <Immucillin-H> is a salt of the synthetic high affinity transition state analog forodesine[48]. Forodesine binds preferentially to and inhibits Purine Nucleotide Phosphorylase, resulting in the accumulation of deoxyguanosine triphosphate, the subsequent inhibition of the enzyme Ribonucleoside Diphosphate Reductase[49], and the abrogation of DNA synthesis. This agent selectively causes apoptosis in stimulated or transformed T-lymphocytes. It is orally available. Forodesine has been granted orphan drug status by the U.S. FDA for T-cell non-Hodgkin lymphoma, chronic lymphocytic leukemia (CLL) and related leukemias, and for treatment of B-cell acute lymphocytic leukemia (ALL).

Inosine dialdehyde (NSC 118994) <Inox> is a toxic purine analog that inhibits Ribonucleotide Reductase, resulting in the decreased synthesis of DNA, RNA, and proteins, and leading to cell cycle arrest at the G_2/M transition. This agent also forms stable covalent cross-links in proteins, thereby inhibiting the activity of enzymes involved in nucleic acid synthesis. Thus, the effects of inosine dialdehyde are different from those caused by typical inhibitors of Ribonucleotide Reductase, which rapidly suppress DNA synthesis and cause arrest of the cells in G_1, with minimal effects on RNA and protein synthesis.

In salvage pathways, nucleotides are synthesized from intermediates of canonical degradative pathways. These salvage pathways recover nucleosides (nucleobases bound to sugars) and nucleotides (composed of nucleobase, sugar, and at least one phosphate) that are formed during the degradation of RNA and DNA. They are particularly important in tissues that cannot undergo de novo synthesis. Most healthy cells utilize both de novo purine synthesis and the adenine

[48] A transition state analog is a substrate designed to mimic the properties or the geometry of the transition state of a reaction.

[49] Ribonucleoside Diphosphate Reductase is also inhibited by hydroxyurea.

salvage pathway to produce ATP. Methylthioadenosine Phosphorylase (MTAP) plays a major role in polyamine metabolism and is important for the salvage of both adenine and methionine. Its encoding gene is located in the same 9p21 chromosomal region as the gene for the tumor suppressor $P16^{INK4A}$. *mtap* and *p16*, along with other genes in that region, are frequently co-deleted in select cancers. Tumors deficient in Methylthioadenosine Phosphorylase are dependent on the de novo purine synthesis pathway, making them potential targets for selective chemotherapy with inhibitors of adenine synthesis.

L-alanosine (L-2-amino-3-(N-hydroxy-N-nitrosamino) propionic acid) (NSC153353, SDX-102) is an amino acid analog derived from Streptomyces alanosinicus, a purine antagonist, and an Adenylosuccinate Synthetase inhibitor. L-alanosine deprives Methylthioadenosine Phosphorylase deficient tumor cells of de novo synthesized adenosine and is responsible for diminished DNA synthesis.

Adverse Effects The clinical use of L-alanosine may be narrow due to its toxicity profile. Mucositis, fatigue, nausea, or renal failure can be dose limiting. In several clinical trials, tolerable doses of L-alanosine have not shown efficacy.

Tiazofurin (2-β-D-ribofuranosyl-4-thiazolecarboxamide) (NSC 286193) <Riboxamide> is a synthetic nucleoside analog. It is anabolized intracellularly to tiazole-4-carboxamide adenine dinucleotide (TAD), an analog of nicotinamide adenine dinucleotide (NAD) and a potent inhibitor of Inositol Monophosphate Dehydrogenase (IMPDH). Inositol Monophosphate Dehydrogenase is the rate limiting enzyme for de novo purine synthesis, the inhibition of which leads to reduced levels of guanylates, resulting in the suppression of tumor cell growth.

Triapine (3-aminopyridine-2-carboxaldehyde thiosemicarbazone) (OCX-191) is a synthetic heterocyclic carboxaldehyde thiosemicarbazone. Triapine acts as an iron chelator and suppresses the enzyme Ribonucleotide Reductase. This inhibits the conversion of ribonucleoside diphosphates to deoxyribonucleotides necessary for DNA synthesis. Triapine is administered at a dose of 95 mg/m^2 by intravenous infusion daily for 5 days, on a biweekly schedule. It displays an acceptable safety profile.

Sensitive tumor cells convert the prodrug 6-mercaptopurine to thioinosinate and 6-methylthioinosinate, which inhibit Glutamine-5-Phosphoribosylpyrophosphate Amidotransferase, the first enzyme unique to the de novo synthesis pathway for purine ribonucleotides.

The Adenosine Deaminase (ADA) inhibitor co-vidarabine is effective against several lymphoproliferative conditions, but not acute lymphocytic leukemia because the transformed cells contain too high levels of Adenosine Deaminase.

After uptake, nelarabine is O-demethylated by Adenosine Deaminase to ara-G, mono-phosphorylated by Deoxyguanosine Kinase and Deoxycytidine Kinase, and subsequently converted to the biologically active 9-β-D-arabinosylguanine 5'-triphosphate (ara-GTP).

Because cladribine is resistant to Adenosine Deaminase it is selectively toxic to lymphocytes and monocytes, which exhibit little Deoxynucleotide Deaminase activity.

Methylthioadenosine Phosphorylase-deficient tumors depend on the de novo purine synthesis pathway, making them targets for inhibitors of de novo adenine synthesis, such as L-alanosine.

References

Arakawa M, Aoki T, Nakao H (1970) Effect of carbazilquinone on lymphoid leukemia L-1210. Gann 61:485–493

Ariel IM, Pack GT (1967) Treatment of disseminated melanoma by systemic melphalan, methotrexate and autogenous bone marrow transplants. Experience with 114 patients. Cancer 20:77–85

Arnold H, Bourseaux F, Brock N (1958) Chemotherapeutic action of a cyclic nitrogen mustard phosphamide ester (B 518-Asta). Nature 8:1–9

Atassi G, Spreafico F, Dumont P, Nayer P, Klatersky J (1980) Antitumoral effect in mice of a new triepoxide derivative: 1,3,5-triglycidyl-S-triazinetrione (NSC 296934). Eur J Cancer 16:1561–1567

Barnes KR, Kutikov A, Lippard SJ (2004) Synthesis, characterization, and cytotoxicity of a series of estrogen-tethered platinum(IV) complexes. Chem Biol 11:557–564

Baugh CM, Krumdieck CL, Nair MG (1973) Polygammaglutamyl metabolites of methotrexate. Biochem Biophys Res Commun 52:27–34

Begleiter A (2000) Clinical applications of quinine-containing alkylating agents. Front Biosci 5:e153–e171

Begleiter A, Lin D, Larson KK, Lang J, Wu X, Cabral T, Taylor H, Guziec LJ, Kerr PD, Hasinoff BB, Guziec FS Jr (2006) Structure-activity studies with cytotoxic anthrapyrazoles. Oncol Rep 15:1575–1580

Bonate PL, Arthaud L, Cantrell, Jr. WR, Stephenson K, Secrist JA III, Weitman S (2006) Discovery and development of clofarabine: a nucleoside analogue for treating cancer. Nat Rev Drug Discov 5:855–863

Borchmann P, Hubel K, Schnell R, Engert A (1997) Idarubicin: a brief overview on pharmacology and clinical use. Int J Clin Pharmacol Ther 35:80–83

Boritzki TJ, Barlett CA, Zhang C, Howland EF (1996) AG2034: a novel inhibitor of glycinamide ribonucleotide formyltransferase. Invest New Drugs 14:295–303

Brink A, Lutz U, Völkel W, Lutz WK (2006) Simultaneous determination of O^6-methyl-2′-deoxyguanosine, 8-oxo-7,8-dihydro-2′-deoxyguanosine, and 1,N^6-etheno-2′-deoxyadenosine in DNA using on-line sample preparation by HPLC column switching coupled to ESI-MS/MS. J Chromatogr B Anslyt Technol Biomed Life Sci 830:255–261

Brock N (1996) The history of the oxazaphosphorine cytostatics. Cancer 78:542–547

Bush JA, Long BH, Catino JJ, Bradner WT, Tomita K (1987) Production and biological activity of rebeccamycin, a novel antitumor agent. J Antibiot (Tokyo) 40:668–678

Buzdar AU, Hortobagyi GN, Esparza LT, Holmes FA, Ro JS, Fraschini G, Lichtiger B (1990) Elliptinium acetate in metastatic breast cancer-a phase II study. Oncology 47:101–104

Cao P-R, McHugh MM, Melendy T, Beerman T (2003) The DNA minor groove-alkylating cyclopropylpyrroloindole drugs adozelesin and bizelesin induce different DNA damage response pathways in human colon carcinoma HCT116 cells. Mol Cancer Ther 2:651–659

Castleberry RP, Crist WM, Holbrook T, Malluh A, Gaddy D (1981) The cytosine arabinoside (Ara-C) syndrome. Med Pediatr Oncol 9:257–264
Chatton J-Y, Idle JR, Vågbø BC, Magistretti PJ (2001) Insights into the mechanisms of ifosfamide encephalopathy: drug metabolites have agonistic effects on a-Amino-3-hydroxy-5-methyl-4-isoxazolepropionic acid (AMPA)/kainate receptors and induce cellular acidification in mouse cortical neurons. J Pharmacol Exp Ther 299:1161–1168
Chen Z-P, Remack J, Brent TP, Mohr G, Panasci LC (1999) Extraneuronal monoamine transporter expression and DNA repair Vis-à-Vis 2-Chloroethyl-3-sarcosinamide-1-nitrosourea cytotoxicity in human tumor cell lines. Clin Cancer Res 5:4186–4190
Chou F, Khan AH, Driscoll JS (1976) Potential central nervous system antitumor agents. Aziridinylbenzoquinones. 2. J Med Chem 19:1302–1308
Cleare MJ, Hoeschele JD (1973) Anti-tumour platinum compounds. Relationship between structure and activity. Platin Met Rev 17:2–13
Coluccia M, Natile G (2007) Trans-platinum complexes in cancer therapy. Anticancer Agents Med Chem 7:111–123
Cushman M, Cheng L (1978) Stereoselective oxidation by thionyl chloride leading to the indeno[1,2-c]isoquinoline system. J Org Chem 43:3781–3783
Dabich L, Bull FE, Beltran G, Athens JW, Coltman CA Jr, Weick JK, Van Slyck EJ, Amare M (1986) Phase II evaluation of aclarubicin in refractory adult acute leukemia: a Southwest Oncology Group Study. Cancer Treat Rep 70:967–969
DeBoer C, Dietz A, Lummis NE, Savage GM (1960) Porfiromycin, a new antibiotic. I. Discovery and biological activities. In: Antimicrobial agents annual. Plenum Press, New York, pp 17–22
de Groot FM, Broxterman HJ, Adams HP, van Vliet A, Tesser GI, Elderkamp YW, Schraa AJ, Kok RJ, Molema G, Pinedo HM, Scheeren HW (2002) Design, synthesis and biological evaluation of a dual tumor-specific motive containing integrin-targeted plasmin-cleavable doxorubicin prodrug. Mol Cancer Ther 1:901–911
Denmeade SR, Nagy A, Gao J, Lilja H, Schally AV, Isaacs JT (1998) Enzymatic activation of a doxorubicin-peptide prodrug by prostate-specific antigen. Cancer Res 58:2537–2540
DeVita VT Jr, Chu E (2008) A history of cancer chemotherapy. Cancer Res 68:8643–8653
DeVita VT, Serpick A, Carbone PP (1966) Preliminary clinical studies with ibenzmethyzin. Clin Pharmacol Ther 7:542–546
Dhingra K, Frye D, Newman RA, Walters R, Theriault R, Fraschini G, Smith T, Buzdar A, Hortobagyi GN (1995) Phase II clinical and pharmacological study of pirarubicin in combination with 5-fluorouracil and cyclophosphamide in metastatic breast cancer. Clin Cancer Res 1:691–697
Donadio AC, Motzer RJ, Bajorin DF, Kantoff PW, Sheinfeld J, Houldsworth J, Chaganti RSK, Bosl GJ (2003) Chemotherapy for teratoma with malignant transformation. J Clin Oncol 21:4285–4291
Duncan R (2006) Polymer conjugates as anticancer nanomedicines. Nat Rev Cancer 6:688–701
Duschinsky R, Pleven E, Heidelberger C (1957) The synthesis of 5-fluoro pyrimidines. J Am Chem Soc 79:4559–4560
Einhorn LH, Donohue J (1977) Cis-diamminedichloroplatinum, vinblastine, and bleomycin combination chemotherapy in disseminated testicular cancer. Ann Intern Med 87:293–298
Facompré M, Tardy C, Bal-Mahieu C, Colson P, Perez C, Manzanares I, Cuevas C, Bailly C (2003) Lamellarin D. a novel potent inhibitor of topoisomerase I. Cancer Res 63:7392–7399
Farber S (1949) Some observations on the effect of folic acid antagonists on acute leukemia and other forms of incurable cancer. Blood 4:160–167
Farber S, Diamond LK, Mercer RD, Sylvester RF, Wolff JA (1948) Temporary remissions in acute leukemia in children produced by folic antagonist, 4-aminopteroylglutamic acid (aminopterin). N Engl J Med 238:787–793
Farrell N (2003) 9.18 metal complexes as drugs and chemotherapeutic agents. In Meyer TJ, McCleverty JA (eds) Comprehensive coordination chemistry II. Elsevier, pp 809–840
Feldman DR, Bosl GJ, Sheinfeld J, Motzer RJ (2008) Medical treatment of advanced testicular cancer. JAMA 299:672–684
Fink D, Nebel S, Aebi S, Zheng H, Cenni B, Nehme A, Christen RD, Howell SB (1996) The role of DNA mismatch repair in platinum drug resistance. Cancer Res 56:4881–4886
Fu D, Calvo JA, Samson LD (2012) Balancing repair and tolerance of DNA damage caused by alkylating agents. Nat Rev Cancer 12:104–120
Gandhi V, Kantarjian H, Faderl S, Bonate P, Du M, Ayres M, Rios MB, Keating MJ, Plunkett W (2003) Pharmacokinetics and pharmacodynamics of plasma clofarabine and cellular clofarabine triphosphate in patients with acute leukemias. Clin Cancer Res 9:6335–6342
Gao H, Huang KC, Yamasaki EF, Chan KK, Chohan L, Snapka RM (1999) XK469, a selective topoisomerase IIb poison. Proc Natl Acad Sci U S A 96:12168–12173
Gao H, Yamasaki EF, Chan KK, Shen LL, Snapka RM (2000) Chloroquinoxaline sulfonamide (NSC 339004) is a topoisomerase IIa/b poison. Cancer Res 60:5937–5940
Gauss W (1958) Über die Umsetzung einiger Alkoxy-p-Benzochinone mit äthylenimin. Chemische Berichte 91:2216–2222
Gilman A, Philips FS (1946) The biological actions and therapeutic applications of the β-chloroethylamines and sulfides. Science 103:409–415
Goldman ID, Chattopadhyay S, Zhao R, Moran R (2010) The antifolates: evolution, new agents in the clinic, and how targeting delivery via specific membrane transporters is driving the development of a next generation of folate analogs. Curr Opin Invest Drugs 11:1409–1423
Goodman LS, Wintrobe MM, Dameshek W, Goodman MJ, Gilman A, McLennan MT (1946) Nitrogen mustard therapy. Use of methyl-bis(beta-chloroethyl)amine hydrochloride and tris(beta-chloroethyl) amine hydrochloride for Hodgkin's disease, lymphosarcoma, leukemia, and certain allied and miscellaneous disorders. JAMA 132:126–132
Greve H, Mohamed IE, Pontius A, Kehraus S, Gross H, König GM (2010) Fungal metabolites: structural diversity as incentive for anticancer drug development. Phytochem Rev 9:537–545
Hanka LJ, Dietz A, Gerpheide SA, Kuentzel SL, Martin DG (1978) CC-1065 (NSC-298223), a new antitumor antibiotic. Production, in vitro biological activity, microbiological assays and taxonomy of the producing microorganism. J Antibiot (Tokyo) 31:1211–1217
Harrap KR, Riches PG, Gilby ED, Sellwood SM, Wilkinson R, Koenyves I (1977) Studies on the toxicity and antitumour activity of predimustine, a prednisolone ester of chlorambucil. Eur J Cancer 13:873–881
Hata T, Sano Y, Sugawara R, Matsumae A, Kanamori K, Shima T, Hoshi T (1956) Mitomycin, a new antibiotic from Streptomyces. J Antibiot 9:141–146
Heidelberger C, Chaudhuri NK, Danneberg P, Mooren D, Griesbach L, Dushinsky R, Schnitzer RJ, Pleven E, Scheiner J (1957) Fluorinated pyrimidines, a new class of tumour-inhibitory compounds. Nature 179:663–666
Hofmann U, Eichelbaum M, Seefried S, Meese CO (1991) Identification of thiodiglycolic acid, thiodiglycolic acid sulfoxide, and (3-carboxymethylthio)lactic acid as major human biotransformation products of S-carboxymethyl-L-cysteine. Drug Metab Dispos 19:222–226
Holzer H (1958) Zum Mechanismus der Glykolysehemmung durch Karzinostatisch wirkende äthylenimin Verbindungen. Biochemische Zeitschrift 330:59–72
Hu JL, Xue YC, Xie MY, Zhang R, Otani T, Minami Y, Yamada Y, Marunaka TJ (1988) A new macromolecular antitumor antibiotic, C-1027. I. Discovery, taxonomy of producing organism, fermentation and biological activity. J Antibiot 41:1575–1579

Johnston TP, McCaleb GS, Montgomery JA (1975) Synthesis of chlorozotocin, the 2-chloroethyl analog of the anticancer antibiotic streptozotocin. J Med Chem 18:104–106

Kapuscinski J, Darzynkiewicz Z (1986) Relationship between the pharmacological activity of antitumor drugs Ametantrone and mitoxantrone (Novatrone) and their ability to condense nucleic acids. Proc Natl Acad Sci U S A 83:6302–6306

Kennedy BJ, Torkelson JL, Torlakovic E (1999) Uracil mustard revisited. Cancer 85:2265–2272

Kiyomiya K, Matsuo S, Kurebe M (2001) Mechanism of specific nuclear transport of adriamycin: the mode of nuclear translocation of adriamycin-proteasome complex. Cancer Res 61:2467–2471

Knock FE (1967) Anticancer agents. Charles C. Thomas, Springfield

Kobayashi E, Okamoto A, Asada M, Okabe M, Nagamura S, Asai A, Saito H, Gomi K, Hirata T (1994) Characteristics of antitumor activity of KW-2189, a novel water-soluble derivative of duocarmycin, against murine and human tumors. Cancer Res 54:2404–2410

Kroep JR, Gelderblom H (2009) Diflomotecan, a promising homocamptothecin for cancer therapy. Expert Opin Investig Drugs 18:69–75

Krumbhaar EB (1919) Role of the blood and the bone marrow in certain forms of gas poisoning. JAMA 72:39–41

Krumbhaar EB, Krumbhaar HD (1919) The blood and bone marrow in yellow gas (mustard gas) poisoning. Changes produced in bone marrow in fatal cases. J Med Res 40:497–508

Kufe DW, Pollock RE, Weichselbaum RR, Bast RC, Gansler TS, Holland JF, Frei E III (2003) Cancer medicine, 6 edn. BC Decker, Hamilton

Küpfer A, Aeschlimann C, Cerny T (1996) Methylene blue and the neurotoxic mechanisms of ifosfamide encephalopathy. Eur J Clin Pharmacol 50:249–252

Li MC, Whitmore WF, Goldbey RB, Grabstald H (1969) Effects of combined drug therapy on metastatic cancer of the testis. JAMA 74:1291

Marchini S, Cirò M, Gallinari F, Geroni C, Cozzi P, D'Incalci M, Broggini M (1999) Alpha-bromoacryloyl derivative of distamycin A (PNU 151807): a new non-covalent minor groove DNA binder with antineoplastic activity. Br J Cancer 80:991–997

Marra G, Schär P (1999) Recognition of DNA alterations by the mismatch repair system. Biochem J 338:1–13

McDonald LA, Capson TL, Krishnamurthy G, Ding W-D, Ellestad GA, Bernan VS, Maiese WM, Lassota P, Discafani C, Kramer RA, Ireland CM (1996) Namenamicin, a new enediyne antitumor antibiotic from the marine ascidian polysyncraton lithostrotum. J Am Chem Soc 118:10898–10899

Minotti G, Cairo G, Monti E (1999) Role of iron in anthracycline cardiotoxicity: new tunes for an old song? FASEB J 13:199–212

Minotti G, Menna P, Salvatorelli E, Cairo G, Gianni L (2004) Anthracyclines: molecular advances and pharmacologic developments in antitumor activity and cardiotoxicity. Pharmacol Rev 56:185–229

Mukherjee KL, Boohar J, Wentland D, Ansfield FJ, Heidelberger C (1963) Studies on fluorinated pyrimidines XVII. Tissue distribution of 5-fluorouracil-2-C14 and 5-fluoro-2′-deoxyuridine in cancer patients. Cancer Res 23:67–77

Nair MG, Baugh CM (1973) Synthesis and biological evaluation of poly-gamma-glutamyl derivatives of methotrexate. Biochemistry 12:3923–2927

Natale RB, Cody RL, Simon MS, Wheeler RH (1993) An in vivo and in vitro trial of aclarubicin in metastatic breast cancer: a novel approach to the study of analogs. Cancer Chemother Pharmacol 31:485–488

Nemeth L, Institoris L, Somfai S, Ghal F, Sugar J, Csuka O, Szentirmay Z, Kellner B (1972) Pharmacologic and antitumor effect of 1,2:5,6-dianhydrogalactitol (NSC-132313). Cancer Chemother Rep 56:593–602

Neuteboom ST, Karjian PL, Boyer CR, Beryt M, Pegram M, Wahl GM, Shepard HM (2002) Inhibition of cell growth by NB1011 requires high thymidylate synthase levels and correlates with p53, p21, bax, and GADD45 induction. Mol Cancer Ther 1 :377–384

Niitsu N, Yamazaki J, Nakayama M, Umeda M (1998) Pirarubicin-induced myocardial damage in elderly patients with non-Hodgkin's lymphoma. Nihon Ronen Igakkai Zasshi 35:358–362

Oku N, Matsunaga S, Fusetani N (2003) Shishijimicins A-C, novel enediyne antitumor antibiotics from the ascidian Didemnum proliferum. J Am Chem Soc 125:2044–2045

Oliver RT, Mason MD, Mead GM (2005) Radiotherapy versus single-dose carboplatin in adjuvant treatment of stageI seminoma: a randomised trial. The Lancet 366:293–300

Papirmeister B, Gross CL, Meier HL, Petrali JP, Johnson JB (1985) Molecular basis of mustard-induced vesication. Fundam Appl Toxicol 5:S134–S149

Rademacher P, Obe G (1995) Trenimon: structure and reactivity of a versatile chemical agent. Mutat Res 340:37–49

Rai KR, Peterson BL, Appelbaum FR, Kolitz J, Elias L, Shepherd L, Hines J, Threatte GA, Larson RA, Cheson BD, Schiffer CA (2000) Fludarabine compared with chlorambucil as primary therapy for chronic lymphocytic leukemia. N Engl J Med 343:1750–1757

Raymond E, Faivre S, Woynarowski JM, Chaney SG (1998) Oxaliplatin: mechanism of action and antineoplastic activity. Semin Oncol 25(Supp 5):4–12

Reedijk J (1999) Why does Cisplatin reach Guanine-n7 with competing s-donor ligands available in the cell? Chem Rev 99 :2499–2510

Rhoads CP (1946) The Edward Gemaliel Janeway lecture: the sword and the ploughshare. J Mount Sinai Hosp 13:299–309

Roberts JD, Poplin EA, Tombes MB, Kyle B, Spicer DV, Grant S, Synold T, Moran R (2000) Weekly lometrexol with daily oral folic acid is appropriate for phase II evaluation. Cancer Chemother Pharmacol 45:103–110

Rosenberg B, VanCamp L, Krigas T (1965) Inhibition of cell division in Escherichia coli by electolysis products from a platinum electrode. Nature 205:698–699

Sawyer TW (1998) Characterization of the protective effects of l-nitroarginine methyl ester (L-NAME) against the toxicity of sulphur mustard in vitro. Toxicology 131:21–32

Schuchter LM, Hensley ML, Meropol NJ, Winer EP (2002) American society of clinical oncology chemotherapy and radiotherapy expert panel. 2002 update of recommendations for the use of chemotherapy and radiotherapy protectants: clinical practice guidelines of the American Society of Clinical Oncology. J Clin Oncol 20:2895–2903

Schulz S, Klann RC, Schönfeld S, Nyce JW (1992) Mechanisms of cell growth inhibition and cell cycle arrest in human colonic adenocarcinoma cells by dehydroepiandrosterone: role of isoprenoid biosynthesis. Cancer Res 52:1372–1376

Shao RG, Zhen YS (2008) Enediyne anticancer antibiotic lidamycin: chemistry, biology and pharmacology. Anticancer Agents Med Chem 8:123–131

Shealy YF, Krauth CA (1966) Complete inhibition of mouse leukaemia L1210 by 5(or 4)-[3,3-bis(2-chloroethyl)-1-triazeno]imidazole-4(or 5)-carboxamide (NSC-82196). Nature 210:208–209

Shealy YF, Krauth CA, Montgomery JA (1962) Imidazoles. I. Coupling reactions of 5-Diazoimidazole-4-carboxamide. J Org Chem 27:2150–2154

Sirohi B, Huddart R (2005) The management of poor-prognosis, non-seminomatous germ-cell tumours. Clin Oncol (R Coll Radiol) 17:543–552

Sorenson CM, Eastman A (1988) Influence of cis-diamminedichloroplatinum(II) on DNA synthesis and cell cycle progression in excision repair proficient and deficient Chinese hamster ovary cells. Cancer Res 48:6703–6707

Stommel JM, Kimmelman AC, Ying H, Nabioullin R, Ponugoti AH, Wiedemeyer R, Stegh AH, Bradner JE, Ligon KL, Brennan C, Chin L, DePinho RA (2007) Coactivation of receptor tyrosine kinases affects the response of tumor cells to targeted therapies. Science 318:287–290

Sugiura Y, Uesawa Y, Takahashi Y, Kuwahara J, Golik J, Doyle TW (1989) Nucleotide-specific cleavage and minor-groove interaction of

DNA with esperamicin antitumor antibiotics. Proc Natl Acad Sci U S A 86:7672–7676
Taatjes DJ, Gaudiano G, Resing K, Koch TH (1997) Redox pathway leading to the alkylation of DNA by the anthracycline, antitumor drugs adriamycin and daunomycin. J Med Chem 40:1276–1286
Trouet A, Passioukov A, Van derpoorten K, Fernandez AM, Abarca-Quinones J, Baurain R, Lobl TJ, Oliyai C, Shochat D, Dubois V (2001) Extracellularly tumor-activated prodrugs for the selective chemotherapy of cancer: application to doxorubicin and preliminary in vitro and in vivo studies. Cancer Res 61:2843–2846
Tworoger SS, Missmer SA, Eliassen AH, Spiegelman D, Folkerd E, Dowsett M, Barbieri RL, Hankinson SE (2006) The association of plasma DHEA and DHEA sulfate with breast cancer risk in predominantly premenopausal women. Cancer Epidemiol Biomarkers Prev 15:967–971
Vavra JJ, Deboer C, Dietz A, Hanka LJ, Sokolski WT (1959) Streptozotocin, a new antibacterial antibiotic. Antibiot Annu 7:230–235
Von Hoff DD Schilsky R Reichert CM Reddick RL Rozencweig M Young RC Muggia FM (1979) Toxic effects of cis-dichlorodiammineplatinum(II) in man. Cancer Treat Rep 63:1527–1531
Wakaki S, Marumo H, Tomioka K, Shimizu G, Kato E, Kamada H, Kudo S, Fujimoto Y (1958) Isolation of new fractions of antitumor mitomycins. Antibiot Chemother 8:228–240
Waksman SA, Woodruff HB (1940) Bacteriostatic and bacteriocidal substances produced by soil actinomycetes. Proc Soc Exp Biol 45:609–614
Wall M E, Wani MC, Cook CE, Palmer KH, McPhail AT, Sim GA (1966) Plant antitumor agents. 1. The isolation and structure of camptothecin, a novel alkaloidal leukemia and tumor inhibitor from Camptotheca acuminata. J Am Chem Soc 88:3888–3890
Wang D, Lippard SL (2005) Cellular processing of platinum anticancer drugs. Nat Rev Drug Discov 4:307–320
Weber GF, Waxman DJ (1993a) Activation of the anti-cancer drug ifosphamide by rat liver microsomal P450 enzymes. Biochem Pharmacol 45:1685–1694
Weber GF, Waxman DJ (1993b) Denitrosation of BCNU by glutathione transferase and P-450 monooxygenases. Arch Biochem Biophys 307:369–378
Webster M, Cairncross G, Gertler S, Perry J, Wainman N, Eisenhauer E (2005) Phase II trial of SarCNU in malignant glioma: unexpected pulmonary toxicity with a novel nitrosourea. A phase II trial of the national cancer institute of canada clinical trials group. Invest New Drugs 23:591–596
Wu RC, Hohenstein A, Park JM, Qiu X, Mueller S, Cadenas E, Schönthal AH (1998) Role of p53 in aziridinylbenzoquinone-induced p21waf1 expression. Oncogene 17:357–365
Yang NC, Jeng KC, Ho WM, Hu ML (2002) ATP depletion is an important factor in DHEA-induced growth inhibition and apoptosis in BV-2 cells. Life Sci 70:1979–1988
Yin D, Toler S, Guo F, Duncan B, Sharma A (2005) Pharmacokinetics (PK) of edotecarin (J-107088), a topoisomerase I inhibitor, in patients with metastatic breast cancer (mBC) or glioblastoma (GBM). J Clin Soc 23(Suppl.):2073
Zhang CC, Boritzki TJ, Jackson RC (1998) An inhibitor of glycinamide ribonucleotide formyltransferase is selectively cytotoxic to cells that lack a functional G1 checkpoint. Cancer Chemother Pharmacol 41:223–228
Zhen HY, Huang YH, Zhen YS (2005) Lidamycin inhibits the cancer cell PKC activity induced by basic fibroblast growth factor. Yao Xue Xue Bao 40:1110–1115
Zucchi R, Danesi R (2003) Cardiac toxicity of antineoplastic anthracyclines. Curr Med Chem 3:151–171

Drugs that Suppress Proliferation

3

3.1 Anti-Mitotic Agents

Microtubules are polymeric filaments composed of α-Tubulin/β-Tubulin hetero-dimers. Their complex polymerization dynamics are crucial to their key role in cell division. Microtubules are also a major component of the mitotic spindle that separates chromosomes during mitosis. Hence, the inhibition of microtubules can slow the proliferation of cancer cells. Several families of compounds that interact with the Tubulin subunits, thereby disrupting the microtubule dynamics involved in mitosis, have potent anti-cancer activity. These anti-mitotic compounds (Fig. 3.1) are typically classified into two main groups:

- microtubule-stabilizing agents (including taxanes and epothilones)
- microtubule-destabilizing agents (including alkaloids, benzoylphenylureas, and peptide drugs).

Both, microtubule-stabilizing and -destabilizing agents are named spindle poisons or mitosis poisons, but they act by distinct mechanisms.

Adverse Effects The Tubulin binding agents do not distinguish between mitosis and microtubule dependent sub-cellular transport in synaptic vesicles or Golgi apparatus. The disruption of microtubule dynamics in cellular processes not involved in proliferation leads to neurotoxicity, which can be dose limiting.

The partial success of the Tubulin binding agents in cancer treatment has stimulated the development of additional anti-mitotic compounds, growing this class of anti-cancer drugs. A new mechanism of action was introduced with inhibitors of mitotic Kinesins. Cell Cycle Kinase inhibitors (discussed in Sect. 4.1.6) also have anti-mitotic effects, however, they do not directly act on the machinery of cytokinesis.

Inhibition of microtubules can slow cancer cell proliferation. Anti-mitotic compounds comprise microtubule-stabilizing agents (including taxanes and epothilones) and microtubule-destabilizing agents (including alkaloids, benzoylphenylureas, and peptide drugs).
Tubulin binding agents may be neurotoxic.
Inhibition of mitotic Kinesins suppresses cell division without interfering with Tubulin turnover.

3.1.1 Taxanes

The Cancer Chemotherapy National Service Center (CCNSC), set up by the U.S. National Cancer Institute in 1955, initially screened mostly synthetic compounds for anti-cancer activity. A plant screening operation was launched by Jonathan Hartwell in 1958. Two years later, it led to the commissioning of U.S. Department of Agriculture botanists to collect samples from about 1000 plant species per year. In this program, Arthur Barclay collected bark from a Pacific yew tree, Taxus brevifolia, in a forest north of Packwood, Washington in 1962. Screening tests identified promising cytotoxic activity in Taxus extracts from the bark. Other yew species did not show the same activity, and tests for other parts of the tree were inconclusive. Fractionation done by Monroe E. Wall and Mansukh C. Wani in Research Triangle Park, North Carolina isolated the active ingredient and initially called it taxol (later renamed paclitaxel). The finding was announced at the 1967 American Chemical Society meeting.

Before the availability of synthetic protocols, the extraction of taxol required large amounts of tree bark, because 1200 kg of bark ultimately yielded only 10 g of pure taxol material. The unfavorable yield conditions posed procedural problems and they led to disputes over priorities with environmentalists (Goodman and Walsh 2001). To manage production with the help of commercial partners, the National Cancer Institute published a Cooperative Research and Development Agreement (CRADA) in 1989, offering its existing supplies, data, and cost sharing. Within a few months, Bristol-Myers Squibb was selected from only four respondent companies. The terms of the arrangement were later questioned and became the subject of congressional hearings in 1991. In 2003, a report by the General Accounting Office concluded that the financial benefits to the National Institute of Health had not been in proportion to its substantial investments.

Originally, paclitaxel proved difficult to synthesize. In 1993 it was discovered that paclitaxel was produced in a fun-

G. F. Weber, *Molecular Therapies of Cancer*, DOI 10.1007/978-3-319-13278-5_3,

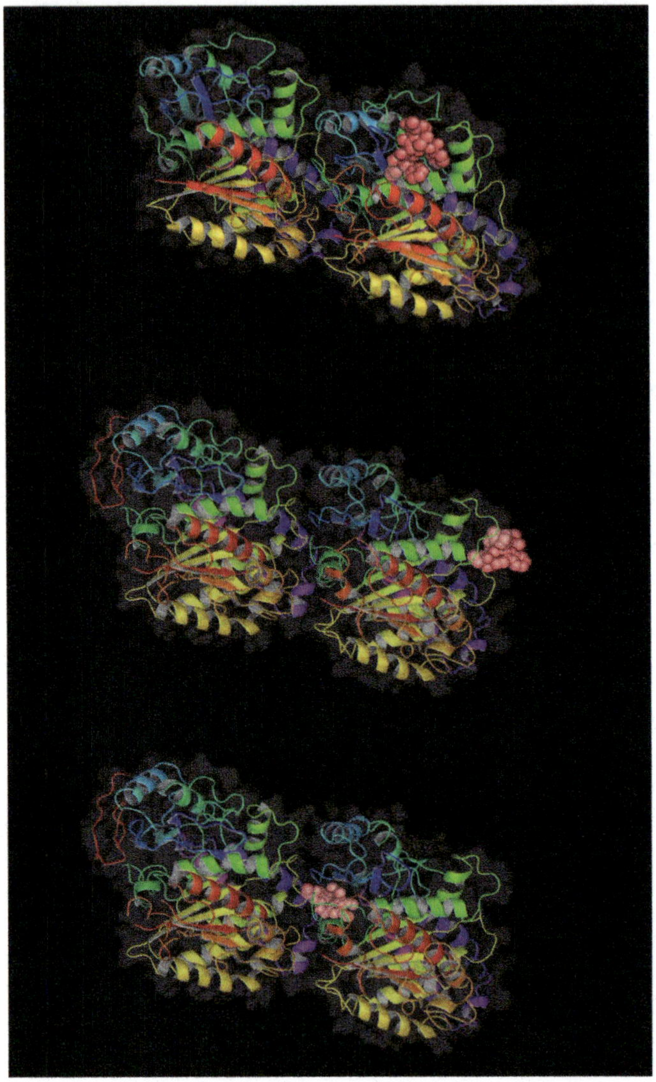

Fig. 3.1 Tubulin binding drugs. Tubulin binding molecules act as carcinostatic agents by targeting the mitotic spindle. Shown are the binding sites of drugs (*pink filled models*) to the Tubulin molecule; *top*—taxol, *middle*—vinblastine, *bottom*—colchicine. (http://en.wikipedia.org/wiki/Discovery_and_development_of_tubulin_inhibitors)

gus living in the yew tree, opening the possibility of its production by culturing fungal species. Paclitaxel total synthesis was reported by Robert A. Holton only in 1994. With this announcement the raison d'etre for some of the environmental groups disappeared and the Pacific Yew Act was ended as a consequence of a sunset clause[1].

Taxanes (Fig. 3.2) are diterpenes. The taxane binding site in β-Tubulin is located along the protofilament direction in a pocket that is lined by several hydrophobic residues and is situated on the luminal side of the microtubule wall. It is near the boundary between the nucleotide binding domain and the middle domain and in contact with the M-loop. The principal mechanism of taxane action is the stabilization of GDP-bound Tubulin, which disrupts microtubule function through the promotion of microtubule assembly and the interference with microtubule disassembly. As microtubule dynamics is essential to cell division, taxanes stop this process. Additionally, this class of drugs may also be radio-sensitizing.

Loss of function of P53, which is common in many types of cancer, may confer hypersensitivity to taxanes as a result of an altered expression of *p53* target genes. Loss of P53 function results in up-regulation of Microtubule Associated Protein 4 (MAP-4), which enhances microtubule polymerization and allows for increased intracellular concentrations of taxanes under treatment.

Drug Resistance Microtubule-Associated Protein τ (MAPT) is a microtubule binding protein important for the assembly and stabilization of microtubules. Alternative splicing may generate up to six forms of the gene product. The level of MAPT expression is negatively correlated with cancer cell sensitivity to both paclitaxel and docetaxel.

Resistance to the anti-tumor effects of the taxanes is often caused by

- alterations in Tubulin or Tubulin binding sites
- ABCB1 (MDR, P-Glycoprotein) mediated drug export (the C-7 to C-10 region of paclitaxel is important in the binding of this drug to ABCB1).

Although paclitaxel and docetaxel have very similar mechanisms of action, cross-resistance between these agents is limited.

Paclitaxel (5β,20-Epoxy-1,2α,4,7β,10β,13α-hexahydroxytax-11-en-9-one 4,10-diacetate 2-benzoate 13-ester with (2R,3S)-*N*-benzoyl-3-phenylisoserine) <Taxol, Oncol> binds to Tubulin and inhibits the disassembly of microtubules, thereby preventing their depolymerization. The molecular result is the formation of microtubule bundles in interphase cells and spindle asters in mitotic cells. Regions directly interacting with Tubulin are the side chain, the C-2 benzoate, and the C-4 acetate. The agent inhibits cellular motility and mitosis. It also induces apoptosis by binding to and blocking the function of the apoptosis inhibitor protein BCL-2 (B-Cell Leukemia 2). After 4 years of clinical testing in solid tumors, paclitaxel was found in 1987 to be effective in ovarian cancer therapy, and received U.S. FDA approval in 1992. Paclitaxel is now used to treat patients with lung cancer (first-line treatment), advanced ovarian cancer, node-positive breast cancer (second-line treatment), head and neck cancer, and advanced forms of Kaposi sarcoma (second-line treatment). There are diverse formulations:

- Paclitaxel poliglumex (CT-2103) <Opaxio, Xyotax> is paclitaxel linked to a biodegradable, water soluble poly-

[1] In public policy, a sunset clause specifies that a law or regulation shall cease to have effect after a specific date, unless legislative action is taken to extend the law.

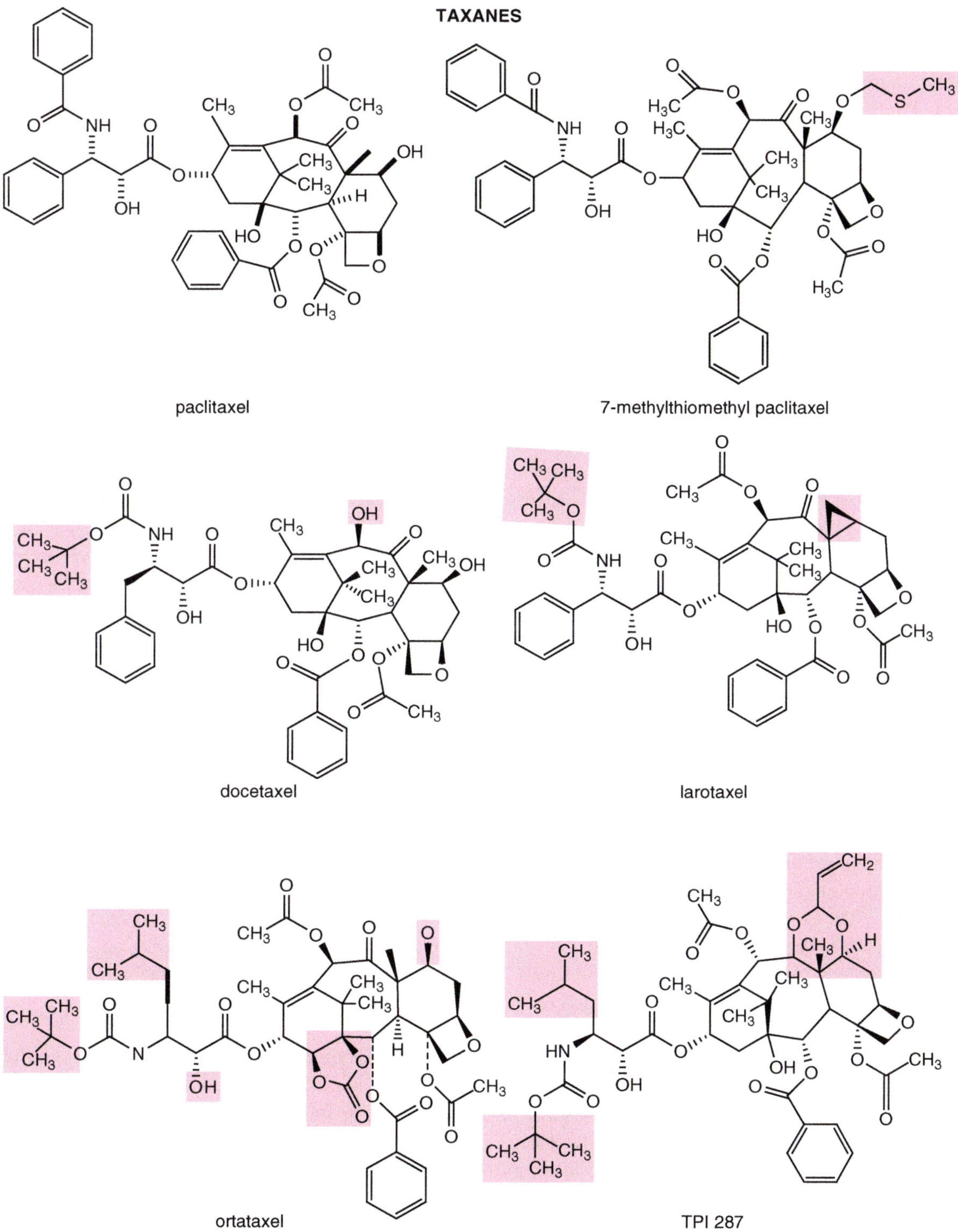

Fig. 3.2 Structures of taxanes. Differences in structure from the parent compound paclitaxel (*top left*) are shaded in *pink*

glutamate polymer. The polyglutamate residue increases the water solubility of the drug and allows delivery of higher doses than those achievable with paclitaxel alone.

- Paclitaxel-loaded polymeric micelle <Genexol-PM> is a biodegradable poly(ethylene glycol)-poly(D, L-lactide) co-polymer micelle, nano-particle entrapped formulation of paclitaxel. The co-polymer residue increases the water solubility of paclitaxel and allows delivery of higher doses than those achievable with paclitaxel alone.
- DHA-paclitaxel <Taxoprexin> is a prodrug comprised of the naturally occurring ω-3 fatty acid docosahexaenoic acid (DHA) covalently conjugated to the anti-microtubule agent paclitaxel. Because tumor cells take up docosahexaenoic acid, DHA-paclitaxel is delivered preferentially to tumor tissue, and exhibits improved pharmaco-

kinetic and toxicity profiles when compared to conventional paclitaxel.

- Paclitaxel vitamin E based emulsion formulation (S-8184) <Tocosol Paclitaxel> is a cremophor-free emulsion particle formulation of paclitaxel. The vitamin E based emulsion may diminish hypersensitivity reactions and allows bolus infusion without steroid premedication. Tumor tissue may be passively targeted due to a preferential deposition of emulsion particles. An emulsion formulation component inhibits the ABCB1 drug efflux pump, facilitating the retention of the drug inside cancer cells.
- Paclitaxel albumin-stabilized nano-particle formulation <Abraxane> is a cremophor ELP-free, albumin-stabilized nano-particle formulation of paclitaxel, which solubilizes the drug without the use of cremophor ELP. The absence of the cremophor is intended to reduce the risks of hypersensitivity reactions and myelosuppression, thus permitting the safe administration of larger doses of this agent.
- 7-Methylthiomethyl paclitaxel (BMS-184476) is a paclitaxel derivative that has enhanced potency (Altstadt et al. 2001). It also inhibits the growth of paclitaxel resistant cancer cells with either up-regulated ABCB1 (because of the ether modification in position C-7) or mutated Tubulin.

Pharmacokinetics Following intravenous administration, the plasma concentration of paclitaxel declines in a biphasic manner. The initial rapid decline represents the distribution to peripheral compartments and elimination of the drug. The later phase is due, in part, to a relatively slow efflux of paclitaxel from the peripheral compartments. More than 90 % of the drug in the blood stream is bound to plasma proteins. Excretion is over 70 % in the feces. Paclitaxel is metabolized primarily to 6α-hydroxypaclitaxel by CYP2C8, and to the minor metabolites 3'-*p*-hydroxypaclitaxel and 6α,3'-*p*-dihydroxypaclitaxel by CYP3A4. Patients with hepatic impairment may be at increased risk of toxicity, particularly grade 3–4 myelosuppression.

Adverse Effects Bone marrow suppression, predominantly with leukopenia and neutropenia, is a common adverse effect. Nausea and vomiting, diarrhea, and peripheral neuropathy can arise. Paclitaxel can trigger hypersensitivity reactions, often caused by its formulation (due to its lipophilicity, paclitaxel needs to be given in polyoxyethylated castor oil <Cremophor EL>), Severe cases manifest with shortness of breath, wheezing, generalized urticaria, angioedema, and low blood pressure, which occur within minutes after treatment—usually following the 1st or 2nd dose. Most reactions resolve completely after stopping treatment and providing fluids. The drug may be restarted at a slower infusion rate and gradually increased after the administration of premedications. The frequency of hypersensitivity reactions with premedication is 2–3 %. The hypersensitivity reactions are pretreated with

- dexamethasone <Decadron, Ozurdex, Maxidex, Baycadron> 20 mg orally 12 and 6 h before treatment and 20 mg intravenously just before administration
- ranitidine <Zantac> 150 mg or cimetidine <Tagamet> 300 mg intravenously 30 min prior to administration
- diphenhydramine <Benadryl> 50 mg orally and intravenously in the same schedule as dexamethasone.

Drug Interactions The pharmacokinetics of paclitaxel may be altered as a result of its interactions with compounds that are substrates, inducers, or inhibitors of CYP2C8 or CYP3A4.

Drug Resistance Up-regulation of the efflux transporter ABCB1 (MDR, P-Glycoprotein) may confer drug resistance to cancer cells. Drug resistance to taxanes may arise due to alterations in Tubulin, such as the β-Tubulin mutations A231T, T274I, R282Q, or A364T. Over-expression of Aurora Kinases disrupts the spindle checkpoint activated by paclitaxel treatment, thus inducing the affected cancer cells to become resistant to paclitaxel.

Docetaxel <Taxotere> is a semi-synthetic, second generation taxane derived from a compound present in the European yew tree, Taxus baccata. It binds to and stabilizes Tubulin, thereby inhibiting microtubule disassembly, which results in cell cycle arrest at the G_2/M transition and consecutive cell death. This agent also inhibits pro-angiogenic factors such as Vascular Endothelial Growth Factor (VEGF) and displays immunomodulatory and pro-inflammatory properties by inducing various mediators of the inflammatory response. Docetaxel may have use as a radiation sensitizing agent. Displaying potent and broad anti-neoplastic properties, the drug is indicated for

- locally advanced or metastatic breast cancer after failure of prior chemotherapy
- adjuvant treatment of patients with operable node-positive breast cancer (in combination with doxorubicin and cyclophosphamide)
- locally advanced or metastatic non-small cell lung cancer after failure of prior platinum-based chemotherapy
- unresectable, locally advanced or metastatic non-small cell lung cancer in patients who have not previously received chemotherapy
- androgen independent (hormone refractory) metastatic prostate cancer (in combination with prednisone)
- advanced gastric adenocarcinoma, including adenocarcinoma of the gastroesophageal junction (in combination with cisplatin and fluorouracil) in patients who have not received prior chemotherapy

- the induction treatment of locally advanced squamous cell carcinoma of the head and neck (in combination with cisplatin and fluorouracil).

Adverse Effects The incidence of treatment related mortality is elevated in patients with abnormal liver function, in patients receiving high doses, and in patients with non-small cell lung carcinoma and a history of prior treatment with platinum-based chemotherapy who receive docetaxel as a single agent at a dose of 100 mg/m^2.

Despite premedication, docetaxel may induce hypersensitivity reactions to the active ingredient or to the polysorbate formulation. Most of these hypersensitivity reactions are minor and characterized by flushing, chest tightness, and low back pain. All patients should be premedicated with two times daily 8 mg dexamethasone orally for 5 days starting 1 day prior to docetaxel in order to reduce the incidence and severity of fluid retention as well as the severity of hypersensitivity reactions.

Drug Resistance Taxanes may be subject to drug resistance due to alterations in Tubulin or up-regulation of ABCB1 (MDR, P-Glycoprotein).

Larotaxel (RPR 109881) is a semi-synthetic derivative of the taxane 10-deacetylbaccatin III. Larotaxel binds to Tubulin, promoting microtubule assembly and stabilization while preventing microtubule depolymerization, thereby inhibiting cell proliferation.

Pharmacokinetics Larotaxel penetrates the blood-brain barrier.

Drug Resistance As larotaxel represents a poor substrate for ABCB1 (P-Glycoprotein) related drug resistance mechanisms, this agent may be useful for treating multi-drug resistant tumors.

Ortataxel (IDN-5109, BAY 59–8862) is effective against cells expressing ATP-binding cassette (ABC) transport proteins by virtue of evading efflux of through ABCB1, ABCC1 (MRP-1), and ABCG2 (BCRP).

TPI 287 is a synthetic, 3rd generation taxane. Its binding to Tubulin results in the inhibition of microtubule assembly/disassembly dynamics, cell cycle arrest at the G_2/M transition, and ensuing cell death.

Taxanes stabilize GDP-bound Tubulin and interfere with microtubule disassembly.
Taxanes may be radio-sensitizing.
Taxanes may induce hypersensitivity reactions.
The limited water solubility of the taxanes may pose difficulties with regard to formulation.
Resistance to taxanes is often attributable to alterations in Tubulin or up-regulation of ABCB1.
Although paclitaxel and docetaxel have very similar mechanisms of action, cross-resistance between these agents is limited.

3.1.2 Epothilones

The epothilones, which are macrolides produced by the myxobacterium Sorangium cellulosum, were first isolated in 1987 by Höfle and Reichenbach. Their total synthesis was accomplished in 1996 (Balog et al. 1996). In the same year, the structure of epothilone A was determined by X-ray crystallography. The name epothilone is combined from epoxide, thiazole and ketone, which describe three characteristic functional groups of these molecules. Epothilones A through F have been characterized.

Epothilones (drug names ending on -ilone) act as microtubule stabilizing agents (Bollag et al. 1995). Early studies in cell lines suggested that they have superior efficacy to taxanes and prompted their development as anti-cancer drugs. Supporting their pharmacological use is their good water solubility, which allows them to be administered without cremophors (unlike taxanes).

In the epothilone structure (Fig. 3.3), the ring size and the C12 substituent are important for anti-cancer activity. Although characteristic for the class of molecules, the epoxide is not considered to be functionally critical. It is replaceable with episulfide, alkene, cyclopropane or aziridine. The large side chain off position C15 may be a thiazole, oxazole or pyridyl.

Epothilone B (patupilone) (EPO906) causes cell cycle arrest at the G_2/M transition phase, thus leading to cytotoxicity. It binds to the αβ-Tubulin hetero-dimer at the same binding site, and with similar binding affinity as paclitaxel. Similar to taxanes, epothilone B induces microtubule polymerization and microtubule stabilization against depolymerization conditions, which causes the rate of αβ-Tubulin dissociation to decrease. Clinical studies involve the administration of EPO906 intravenously over 5 min at a dose of 2.5 mg/m^2 weekly for 3 weeks, followed by a rest period of 1 week.

Pharmacokinetics After intravenous infusion, the blood levels of epothilone B follow a three compartment model with 0 order input and 1st order elimination. The half-life of epothilone B is 5 days.

Adverse Effects Diarrhea is dose limiting. Less common toxicities include nausea, vomiting, and fatigue.

Drug Resistance Mutations in β-Tubulin, such as T274I or R282Q, may lead to drug resistance. However, epothilone cytotoxicity is unaffected by the A364T substitution in β-Tubulin that confers resistance to paclitaxel.

Epothilone B is cytotoxic for cells that over-express ABCB1 (P-Glycoprotein), a characteristic that distinguishes it from the taxanes. Hence, epothilone B may be active against cancers that do not respond to paclitaxel.

Various derivatives of epothilone B have favorable pharmacological properties, such as solubility, while maintaining

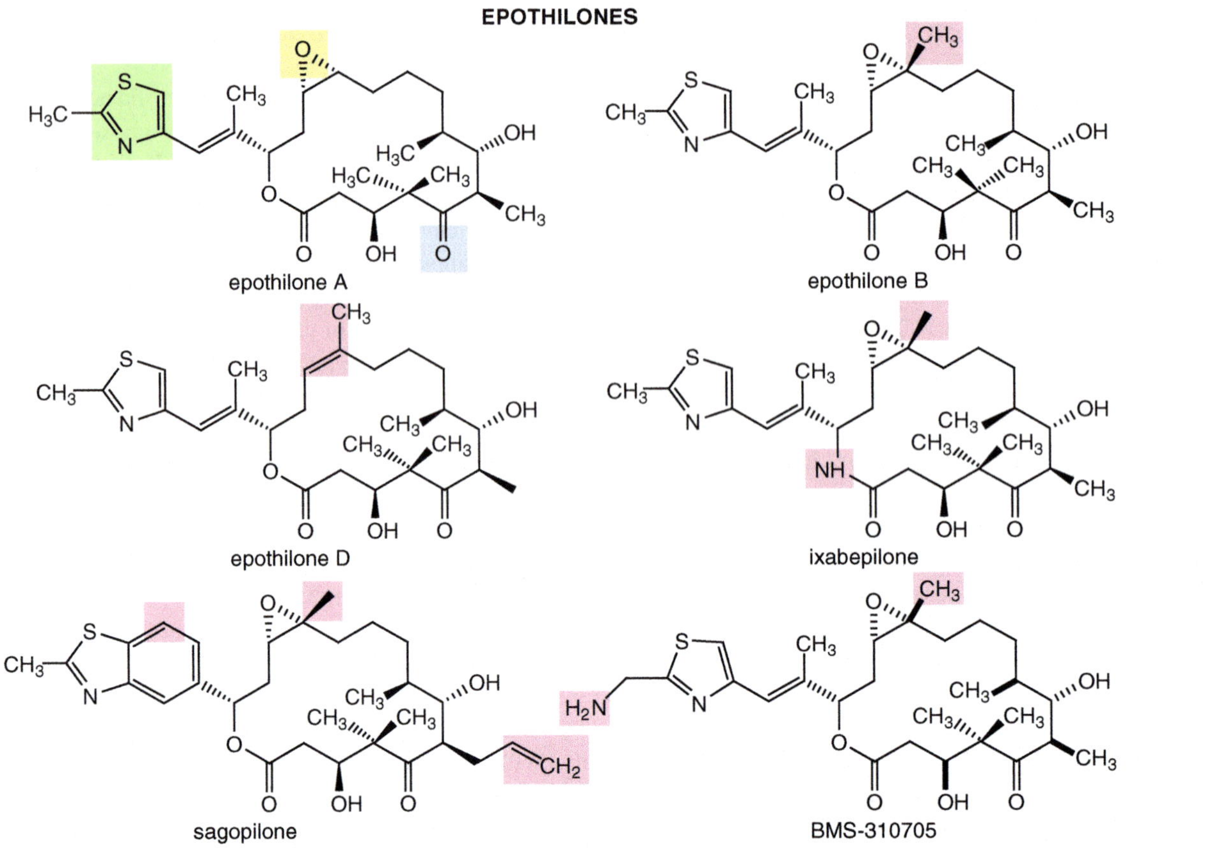

Fig. 3.3 Structures of epothilones. The three characteristic functional groups, epoxide (*yellow*), thiazole (*green*), and ketone (*blue*), are highlighted in epothilone A (*top left*). For each of the other agents, differences in structure from the parent compound are shaded in *pink*

anti-mitotic activity. Epothilone D (desoxy-epothilone B) (KOS-862) lacks the epoxide moiety.

Pharmacokinetics Epothilone D crosses the blood-brain barrier. The half-life in the blood is approximately 10 h.

Drug Resistance The β-Tubulin mutation A231T may lead to resistance to epothilone D.

Synthesis and testing of more than 300 semi-synthetic epothilone analogs with the aim of addressing the poor metabolic stability and unfavorable pharmacokinetics of the parent epothilones led to the identification of ixabepilone (Lee et al. 2001). Ixabepilone (16-aza-epothilone B, (1S,3S,7S,10R,11S,12S,16R)-7,11 dihydroxy-8,8,10,12,16-pentamethyl-3-[(1E)-1-methyl-2-(2-methyl-4-thiazolyl)ethenyl]-17-oxa-4-azabicyclo[14.1.0] heptadecane-5,9-dione) (BMS-247550, NSC-710428) <Ixempra> contains a chemically modified lactam substitution for the naturally existing lactone oxygen. The drug binds directly to the β-Tubulin subunit of microtubules. It prevents microtubule disassembly, thereby leading to cell cycle arrest in the G_2/M phase and apoptosis. Ixabepilone received U.S. FDA approval in 2007.

- The drug is administered as a mono-therapy for the treatment of metastatic or locally advanced breast cancer in patients whose tumors are resistant or refractory to anthracyclines, taxanes, and capecitabine.
- The agent may act synergistically with capecitabine, and this combination is indicated for patients with metastatic or locally advanced breast cancer after the failure of anthracycline and taxane.

Ixabepilone, formulated with Cremophor EL, is infused intravenously at 40 mg/m^2 over 3 h every 3 weeks. Dose adjustments at the start of a cycle should be based on non-hematologic toxicity or blood counts from the preceding cycle.

Pharmacokinetics Epothilones with a lactone are subject to cleavage by Esterases in blood plasma and tissues. The lactam in ixabepilone is intended to increase the stability of the compound. In the blood, ixabepilone follows a linear pharmacokinetic with the maximal plasma concentration at the end of a 3 h infusion. The binding to plasma proteins is about 60 %. Ixabepilone is extensively metabolized in the liver, the main route being via CYP3A4. The drug is eliminated primarily as metabolized drug in the feces (65 % of the dose) and in the urine (20 % of the dose).

Adverse Effects As a single agent in metastatic breast cancer, ixabepilone is well tolerated with peripheral sensory neuropathy (burning sensation, hyper- or hypo-esthesia, paresthesia, discomfort or pain) (15 %), fatigue (10 %), and myalgia/arthralgia (5 %) being the most common grade 3–4 toxicities. Hepatic impairment, fatigue, and hand-foot syndrome may arise. Patients should not drive or operate machinery immediately after infusions as the formulation contains alcohol. The drug is Pregnancy Category D.

Myelosuppression (neutropenia) may occur. The drug is contraindicated in patients who have a neutrophil count below 1500 cells/mm^3 or a platelet count below 100,000 cells/mm^3. Among patients with grade 2 liver dysfunction at baseline, there is a high risk of death from toxicity related to neutropenia (due to high levels of exposure to the active drug). In particular, the combination of ixabepilone with capecitabine is recommended only for patients with grade 1 or less liver dysfunction. Tests for liver function should be conducted before the initiation of therapy.

To reduce the risk of hypersensitivity reactions, all patients need to be premedicated approximately 1 h before the infusion with a histamine H_1 receptor antagonist (diphenhydramine 50 mg orally or equivalent) and a histamine H_2 receptor antagonist (ranitidine 150–300 mg orally or equivalent). Patients who had a prior hypersensitivity reaction also require corticosteroids (dexamethasone 20 mg intravenously, 30 min before infusion or orally, 60 min before infusion). Patients with a history of allergic reactions to Cremophor cannot receive ixabepilone infusions.

Drug Interactions Required precautions include avoiding grapefruit juice while receiving this medication as it could interfere with metabolism and cause unsafe blood levels of the drug. Inducers of CYP3A4 may reduce the drug concentration, while inhibitors of this enzyme may increase the drug levels. Therefore, the dose must be adjusted if taken simultaneously with strong modulators of CYP3A4.

Drug Resistance Ixabepilone has a low susceptibility to various drug resistance mechanisms, including the up-regulation of efflux transporters.

Sagopilone (Epothilone ZK219477) (SH-Y03757A, ZK-EPO) was developed under Ulrich Klar at Bayer Schering Pharma. It was the first fully synthetic epothilone to enter clinical trials. Because sagopilone penetrates the blood-brain barrier it is under consideration for the treatment of primary and metastatic brain cancers.

Adverse Effects Peripheral neuropathy can become dose limiting. The administration of acetyl-L-carnitine is under study as a prophylactic agent against this adverse effect.

BMS-310705 is a water soluble semi-synthetic, C-21-substituted derivative of epothilone B. The compound was selected for clinical development because of anti-cancer activity similar to that of optimally dosed ixabepilone. It has substantial resistance to inactivation by blood Esterases. The drug is in clinical trials for the treatment of ovarian, renal, bladder, and lung carcinomata.

Pharmacokinetics BMS-310705 has a linear dose-response curve. The elimination half-life is 42 h.

Adverse Effects Neuropathy or grade 3 diarrhea can become dose limiting. Hypersensitivity may occur.

Epothilones are a class of microtubule stabilizing agents, which cause cell cycle arrest in G_2/M.
Epothilones are active against cells that over-express ABCB1.
Epothilones have better water solubility than taxanes.
Sensory neuropathy, diarrhea, myelosuppression and hypersensitivity may be dose limiting for epothilones. Their intensity varies among compounds.

3.1.3 Other Microtubule Stabilizers

Microtubule stabilizing drugs have overlapping binding sites on Tubulin. Five distinct chemotypes that induce Tubulin polymerization and microtubule bundling in the absence of GTP comprise natural products, including

- taxanes and rhazinilam (from tree bark)
- the epothilones (from a myxobacterium)
- discodermolide and eleutherobin (from a marine sponge and soft coral, respectively).

Discodermolide was isolated in 1990 from the Caribbean marine sponge Discodermia dissoluta by Sarath Gunasekera and Ross Longley. The carbon skeleton of the molecule is composed of eight polypropionate units and four acetate units with 13 stereocenters. (+)-Discodermolide is a polyketide natural product that acts as an inhibitor of cell division. It binds to microtubules at the same site as paclitaxel, but has higher affinity. The drug hyper-stabilizes microtubules and leads to cell cycle arrest in G_2/M.

Adverse Effects In clinical trials, patient accrual was halted due to toxicity.

Drug Resistance Discodermolide is effective against cells that are resistant to paclitaxel and epothilone due to ABCB1 over-expression.

Rhazinilam (Fig. 3.4) is an alkaloid produced by Aspidosperma quebracho-blanco leaves and tree bark. First isolated from Melodinus australis in 1965, the structure of rhazinilam was established in 1972, and its anti-Tubulin activity was reported in 1987. The main active isomer is (-)-rhazinilam. The mode of action of rhazinilam is different from the mode of action of paclitaxel, even though both compounds induce Tubulin spiralization and microtubule stabilization. Rhazinilam may also have analgesic activity.

Eleutherobin is a diterpene glycoside initially isolated from the Western Australian soft coral Eleutherobia species. It is a mitosis inhibitor that competes with paclitaxel for Tubulin binding and has an effectiveness similar to that of paclitaxel.

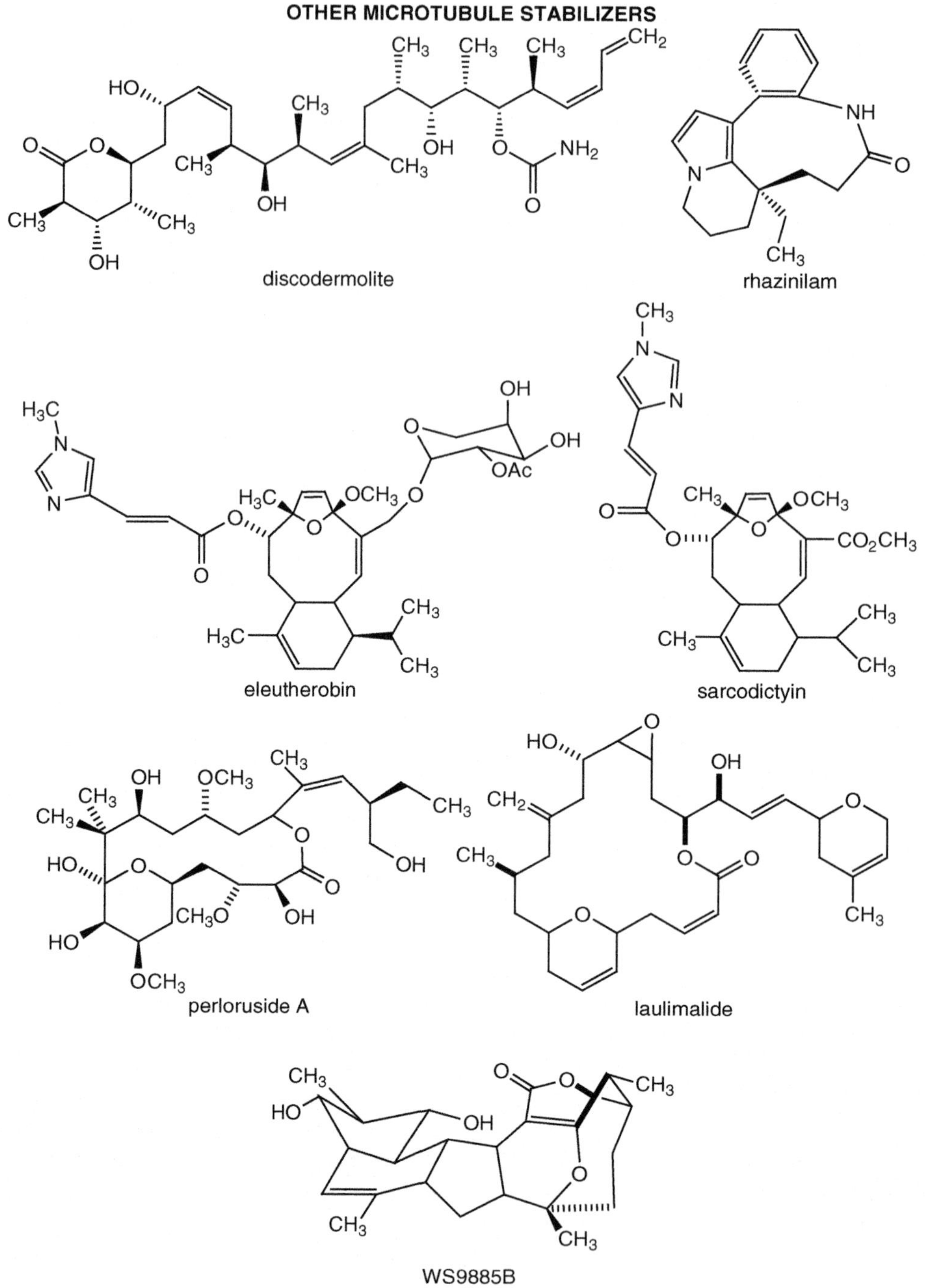

Fig. 3.4 Structures of other microtubule stabilizing agents

- Sarcodictyins represent a class of cytotoxic agents that are structurally related to eleutherobin in that they contain the same eunicellan carbon skeleton, a *N*-methylurocanic acid ester at the C8 position, and a unique C4-C7 oxygen bridge, but eleutherobin differs from the sarcodictyins by the presence of a 2-acetylarabinose glycoside side chain extending from the C3 of the 4,7-oxoeunicellan core. Sarcodictyins are about 100-fold less cytotoxic than eleutherobin.

Drug Resistance Eleutherobin is subject to cross-resistance in paclitaxel resistant cells.

Peloruside A is a secondary metabolite isolated from the New Zealand marine sponge Mycale hentscheli. It has paclitaxel-like microtubule stabilizing activity and is cytotoxic at nanomolar concentrations. Its 16-membered macrolide ring is similar to that of epothilone. The 6-membered pyranose ring of peloruside is essential for both its cytotoxicity and microtubule-stabilizing effects. Like paclitaxel, peloruside A arrests cells in the G_2/M phase of the cell cycle and induces apoptosis.

Laulimalide (figianolide B) and isolaulimalide, isolated from the marine sponge Cacospongia mycofijiensis, are microtubule stabilizing agents. The laulimalides are 18-membered macrocyclic lactones. Because naturally occurring laulimalide is intrinsically unstable, synthetic variants have been studied. Laulimalide may synergize with paclitaxel in sensitive cells and shows effectiveness against paclitaxel resistant cells.

Drug Resistance Laulimalides are poor substrates for ABCB1.

The bacterial metabolite WS9885B acts as a microtubule stabilizing agent. It has a hexacyclic architecture, a reactive bridgehead alkene, and 12 stereocenters.

3.1.4 Alkaloids

The word alkaloid was initially drawn from the term vegetable alkali, which was used to express the alkalinity of a various plant extracts. Alkaloids are produced as abundant secondary metabolites in plants (also in bacteria, fungi, and animals), and many alkaloids are derived from the amino acid ornithine. Alkaloids represent a widespread class of compounds with varied pharmacological properties. The majority of the alkaloids are heterocyclic (containing a closed ring of atoms, of which at least one is not a carbon atom), incorporating nitrogen. Alkaloids can be grouped into indoles (including vinca alkaloids), quinolones and isoquinolines (including anti-mitotic drugs), pyrrolidines, pyridines and piperidines, pyrrolizidines and quinolizidines, purines, and terpenoids.

Vinca alkaloids In 1952, Clark Noble sent leaves from the Madagascar periwinkle plant to his brother Robert at the University of Western Ontario. Tea from Madagascar periwinkle (Vinca rosea, Catharanthus roseus, Lochnera rosea, Ammocallis rosea) leaves was used by Jamaicans to treat diabetes. Moreover, the plant had a long history of being applied as a medicine in China, Central and South America, and the Caribbean as a remedy for colds, insect stings, and eye infections. Although no activity was found to suggest it could be beneficial to treat diabetes, the plant induced granulocytopenia and bone marrow suppression, suggesting a potential application to the treatment of leukemia. In 1958, Noble and Charles C. Beer identified vinblastine (initially named vincaleukoblastine, VLB) as the active extract. They then joined forces with Gordon Svoboda from the Eli Lilly natural products group for clinical tests. The trials were carried out in the Princess Margaret Hospital in Toronto on patients with lymphoid cancers. When the test showed positive results, Eli Lilly started producing the drug. The success spurred broader interest in plants as potential sources of anticancer drugs.

The anti-tumor effect of the vinca alkaloids (names beginning with vin-) (Fig. 3.5) is due to their ability to inhibit microtubule polymerization, and consecutively cell division. Tubulin has a vinca domain, the binding of which inhibits Tubulin polymerization and the assembly of microtubules. The vinca alkaloids therefore affect all rapidly dividing cell types including cancer cells, but also intestinal epithelium, bone marrow, and hair follicles.

Vincristine (leurocristine, LCR, VCR) <Oncovin, Oncovorin, Vincasar PFS, Vincrex> is a natural alkaloid isolated from the plant Vinca rosea Linn. This agent binds irreversibly to microtubules and depolymerizes them. Vincristine also binds irreversibly to spindle proteins and interferes with the formation of the mitotic spindle. Spindle fibers are responsible for the alignment and separation of chromosomes in anaphase. Preventing their formation arrests tumor cells in metaphase. Vincristine was approved by the U.S. FDA in 1963. Its main uses are in acute lymphoblastic leukemia, in non-Hodgkin lymphoma as part of the chemotherapy regimen CHOP (cyclophosphamide, hydroxydaunorubin, oncovin, prednisone), and in Hodgkin lymphoma as part of MOPP (mechlorethamine, oncovin, procarbazine, prednisone) or COPP (cyclophosphamide, oncovin, procarbazine, prednisone) or BEACOPP (bleomycin, etoposide, adriamycin, cyclophosphamide, oncovin, procarbazine, prednisone) or VAMP (vincristine, amethopterin, mercaptopurine, prednisone) or Stanford V. In contrast to vinblastine, vincristine can induce remission of acute leukemias in children. It may also be of value against Wilms tumor, neuroblastoma, ovarian dysgerminoma, reticulum cell sarcoma, rhabdomyosarcoma, and Ewing sarcoma. However, vincristine does not prevent the development of leukemia in the central nervous system in patients who are otherwise responding. Because of its toxicity, the agent cannot be given intrathecally.

- Vincristine <Vincristine Sulfate Injection> is administered by intravenous injection at weekly intervals.
- Vincristine is a cell cycle specific agent, the activity of which is dependent on the duration of drug exposure. Its activity is limited by its short half-life, and the impossibility to dose escalate beyond 2 mg due to neurotoxicity. Vincristine sulfate liposomes <Marqibo> utilize vincristine encapsulated in a rigid lipid bilayer of sphingomyelin for injection. The active agent leaks out of the liposome slowly and drug levels are maintained for prolonged periods of time. The formulation is under investigation for the treatment of lymphoproliferative diseases, such as acute lymphoblastic leukemia (ALL), Hodgkin and non-Hodgkin lymphomata.

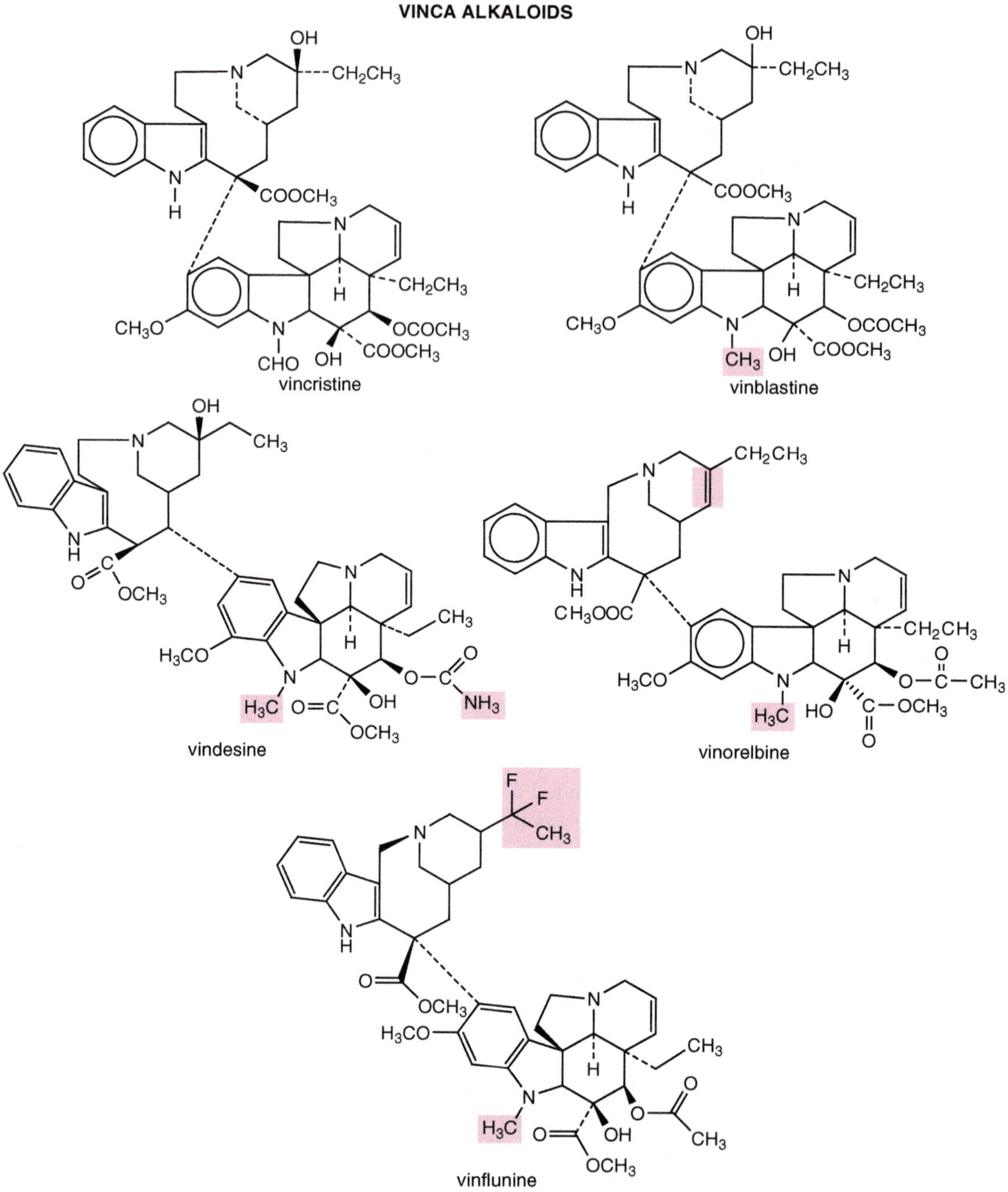

Fig. 3.5 Structures of vinca alkaloids. Differences in structure from vincristine (*top left*) are shaded in *pink*

Pharmacokinetics Following rapid intravenous injection, the serum decay curve is triphasic with half-lives of about 5 min, 2 h, and 85 h. The drug does not penetrate well into the cerebrospinal fluid. The liver is the major excretory organ. The metabolism of vinca alkaloids is mediated by CYP3A enzymes. About 80 % of the drug is eliminated into the feces and 10–20 % in the urine.

Adverse Effects Because of the possibly rapid action of vincristine against some tumors, prophylactic allopurinol may be given to avoid high uric acid blood levels consecutive to tumor lysis. Unlike some of the other vinca alkaloids, vincristine does not cause severe bone marrow suppression. The main associated adverse effects are hyponatremia, hypertension, alopecia, constipation, vomiting, and oral ulcerations. Paralytic ileus may occur, particularly in young pediatric patients. It is reversible with discontinuation of the drug and symptomatic care. Hepatic veno-occlusive disease can arise in patients, particularly children, who receive vincristine as part of standard combination chemotherapy regimens. Therefore, vincristine should not be given while patients receive radiation therapy through ports that include the liver. The drug is Pregnancy Category D.

Peripheral neuropathy may manifest in paresthesias, loss of deep tendon reflexes, tingling and pain of the extremities, occasional slapping gait, or ataxia. Paresis or paralysis and atrophy of extensor muscles may occur late. Paralysis of cranial nerves, especially abducens paralysis, and visual effects can arise. Generalized sensorimotor dysfunction may become progressively more severe with continued treatment, and can persist for a prolonged time after treatment termination. Patients with the demyelinating form of Charcot-Marie-Tooth syndrome should not be given vincristine.

Drug Interactions Other chemotherapy drugs, including mitomycin and doxorubicin, may raise the risk of subsets of adverse effects from vincristine if used concomitantly. When vincristine is administered in combination with L-Asparaginase (see Sect. 4.2.2.), it should be given 12–24 h before given of the enzyme. Administering L-Asparaginase before vincristine may reduce the hepatic clearance of vincristine. Because vincristine may cause dysuria and bladder atony, other drugs that cause urinary retention should be discontinued for the first few days following treatment initiation. The simultaneous administration of phenytoin and vincristine can reduce the blood levels of the anticonvulsant and increase seizure activity. Dosage adjustment should be based on serial blood level monitoring. Due to the metabolism by CYP3A, grapefruit or grapefruit juice may change the blood levels of vincristine.

Vinblastine <Velbe, Velban, Velsar> is a natural alkaloid produced by the plant Vinca rosea Linn. Except for the replacement of a formyl group in vincristine with methyl in vinblastine, the chemical structures of the two compounds are identical. Vinblastine binds to Tubulin and inhibits microtubule formation, resulting in a disruption of mitotic spindle assembly and arrest in the M phase of the cell cycle. This agent may also interfere with cyclic AMP function, ATPase activity, Glutathione metabolism, Calmodulin dependent Ca^{2+} transport, cellular respiration, and amino acid, nucleic acid and lipid biosynthesis. Vinblastine is used in the treatment of breast cancer, testicular cancer, Hodgkin lymphoma, choriocarcinoma, and various forms of leukemia (but not acute leukemias in children). It is given intravenously at weekly intervals, usually starting at 0.1 mg/kg and increasing by 0.05 mg/kg. The dose is not increased if the leukocyte count drops below 3000/mm^3.

Pharmacokinetics The drug enters cells through passive uptake, without a requirement for ATP. The metabolism of vinca alkaloids is mediated by CYP3A enzymes.

Adverse Effects The dose limiting toxicity is a suppression of the white blood cell count, with leukopenia being worse than thrombocytopenia. Other common adverse effects include constipation or ileus, bone or muscle pain, nausea and vomiting, sores in mouth and on lips, alopecia, and swelling of the feet or lower legs. Urinary retention, gastrointestinal bleeding, phlebitis at the site of injection, and SIADH (syndrome of inappropriate Anti-Diuretic Hormone) may occur.

Adverse neurological effects include transient mental depression, paresthesias, loss of deep tendon reflexes, peripheral neuritis, occasional convulsions, and hallucinatory psychoses. The neurological manifestations may be caused by the nature of vinblastine as an indole derivative (Knock 1967).

Vinblastine is a potentially phototoxic drug. Redness typically occurs within 24 h of exposure to the sun in the uncovered areas of the body (forehead, nose, lips, hands, forearms). In severe cases, the protected areas of skin may be also be involved. The skin changes usually resolve within several days by sloughing off (desquamation) of the affected areas. Hyper-pigmentation of the affected area of the skin may develop after the resolution of a phototoxicity reaction, but it is rare in a photoallergic reaction.

Vindesine <Eldisine, Fildesin> is a synthetic derivative of vinblastine that binds to and stabilizes Tubulin, thereby interrupting Tubulin polymerization and preventing the formation of the mitotic spindle. Treated cells are unable to undergo mitosis and are arrested in metaphase. This agent also disrupts the synthesis of macro-molecules. Malignancies against which vindesine is used include acute lymphocytic leukemia, lung carcinomata, breast cancer, chronic myelogenous leukemia, and colorectal cancer.

Adverse Effects Common adverse effects include, hair loss, nausea and vomiting, constipation, stomach cramps, jaw pain, rash, phlebitis, and decreased blood cell counts.

Vinorelbine was developed in the mid-1990s at the Pierre Fabre Company. Vinorelbine ditartrate <Navelbine> is a salt of the semi-synthetic vinca alkaloid derived from the leaves of the periwinkle plant Vinca rosea. Vinorelbine binds to Tubulin, thereby inhibiting Tubulin polymerization and spindle formation, which results in the apoptosis of susceptible cells. This agent is also radiation sensitizing. Malignancies in which vinorelbine is used include breast cancers, testicular cancers, epithelial ovarian cancers, and non-small cell lung cancers. The agent is administered intravenously.

Adverse Effects The adverse effects and toxicity of vinorelbine are generally milder than those of other vinca alkaloids. However, adverse effects that frequently occur with treatment include myelosuppression, shortness of breath, constipation or loose bowels, alopecia, and numbness in the hands or feet. Because of the lowered number of white blood cells during treatment it is critical that no immunizations are administered while taking vinorelbine. Likewise, it is important to avoid interaction with individuals who have recently received an oral polio vaccination.

The inhibition of mitotic microtubules correlates with anti-tumor activity, whereas the inhibition of axonal microtubules may correlate with vinorelbine neurotoxicity. Compared to related vinca alkaloids, vinorelbine is more selective against mitotic microtubules than axonal microtubules, which may account for its decreased neurotoxicity.

Vinflunine is a semi-synthetic, bi-fluorinated Vinca alkaloid that has anti-proliferative and anti-angiogenic activities. This agent inhibits Tubulin polymerization without affecting assembled microtubules. It arrests the cell cycle in mitosis and induces apoptosis. Vinflunine binds Tubulin at the vinca binding site but has a lower affinity for the site than vinorelbine, vinblastine, or vincristine. Vinflunine has enhanced anti-tumor activity than vinorelbine against a variety of human tumor types. It is under investigation for the treatment of bladder cancer.

Colchicine alkaloids The tricyclic alkaloid colchicine (Fig. 3.6) was isolated in 1820 by the French chemists P.S. Pelletier and J. Caventon. Its plant source is the autumn crocus Colchicum autumnale. Colchicine (colchecine) is a spindle poison that causes metaphase arrest. Although the drug shows some activity against chronic granulocytic leukemia and Hodgkin disease it has been replaced with less toxic agents.

Demecolcine (*N*-deacetyl-*N*-methylcolchicine, colcemid) is a colchicine derivative that may have an enhanced metaphase inhibiting effect, but it is less toxic to the gastrointestinal tract than colchicine. It has been used for the treatment of chronic granulocytic leukemia, but is less reliable than myleran.

Adverse Effects Adverse effects include myelosuppression, dermatitis, alopecia, and gastrointestinal ulcers.

Trimethylcolchicinic acid (deacetylcolchiceine) is a colchicine analog that binds to Tubulin, inhibiting its polymerization into microtubules and preventing cell division. It is in clinical trials for cancer treatment.

Other alkaloids Quinoline and isoquinoline alkaloids are benzopyridines, which are composed of a benzene ring fused to a pyridine ring comprising 1 nitrogen atom.

- The aporphinoids constitute a broad subgroup of benzylisoquinoline alkaloids. Thalicarpine (thaliblastine) (NSC 68075) is a natural member of this class. The agent (Fig. 3.7) induces single strand breaks in DNA and arrests cancer cells at the G_1 phase and G_2/M phase of the cell cycle. Thalicarpine inhibits ABCB1.
- Trabectedin is a tetrahydroisoquinoline alkaloid isolated from the marine tunicate Ecteinascidia turbinate. Trabectedin (ecteinascidin 743) (ET743) exhibits cytotoxicity by prolonging the G_2/M transition of the cell cycle. This agent interacts with the transcription coupled DNA repair machinery to induce DNA strand breaks that lead to cell death.

Ukrain (NSC-631570) is a semi-synthetic compound of thiophosphoric acid and the alkaloid chelidonine derived from the plant Chelidonium majus (a common weed in Europe and Western Asia). For many centuries, the plant has been used in the therapy of warts and skin cancers. It has been a component of alternative herbal medicine without knowledge of its mechanism of action. Ukrain inhibits pancreatic cell cycle progression in the M phase by stabilizing monomeric Tubulin.

Alkaloids are nitrogen containing secondary metabolites in plants.

Vinca alkaloids exert anti-tumor effects by inhibiting microtubule polymerization and consecutively cell division.
Neurotoxicity is a common adverse effect of vinca alkaloids.
Vincristine, in contrast to vinblastine, can induce remission of acute leukemias in children.
Vincristine does not prevent the development of leukemia in the central nervous system in patients who are otherwise responding.

Vinblastine is potentially phototoxic.
Colchicine derivatives cause metaphase arrest.
Quinoline and isoquinoline alkaloids are benzopyridines.

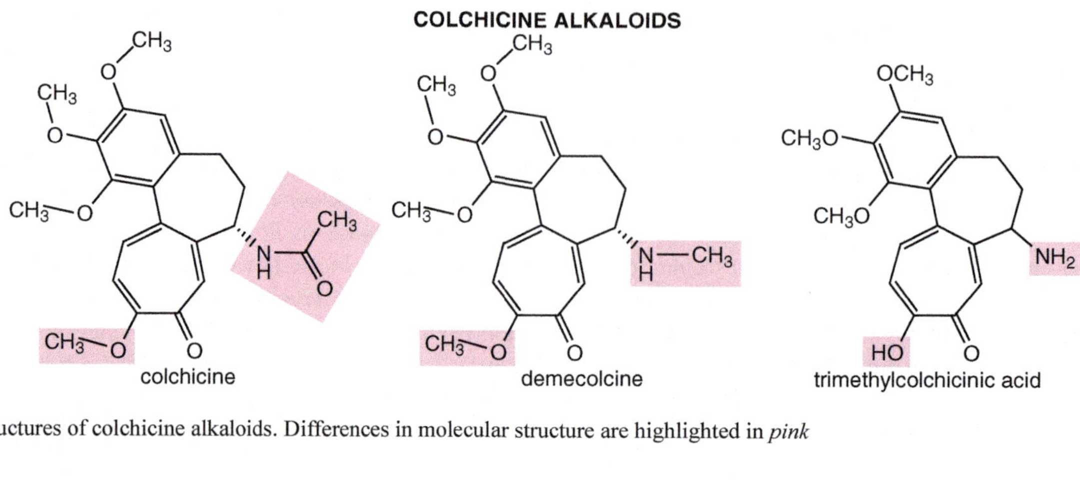

Fig. 3.6 Structures of colchicine alkaloids. Differences in molecular structure are highlighted in *pink*

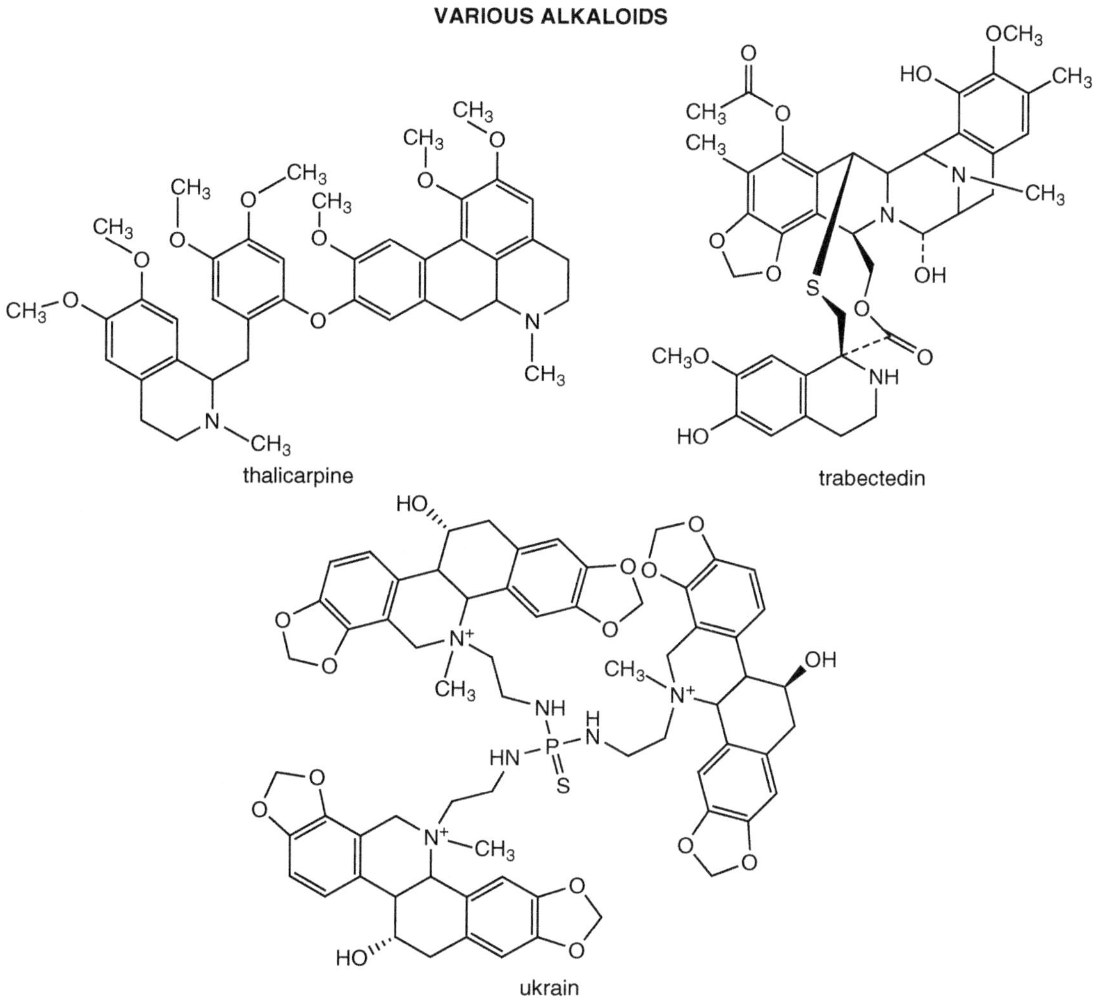

Fig. 3.7 Structures of various alkaloids

Besides inducing G2/M arrest, isoquinoline alkaloids may arrest cells in G1 and interfere with DNA repair.

3.1.5 Benzoylphenylureas

Benzoylphenylureas (BPUs) are low molecular weight agents that were initially developed as insecticides, but were found during random screening to possess anti-tumor activity (Okada et al. 1991). Benzoylphenylureas interact with the colchicine binding site on Tubulin, thereby blocking Tubulin polymerization and disrupting mitotic function. These agents also inhibit DNA Polymerase, which may contribute to their anti-cancer effects.

Dimethylamino-benzoylphenylurea (*N*-4-(5-bromo-2-pyrimidyloxy)-3-methylphenyl-(dimemethylamino)-benzoylphenylurea) (NSC-639829) (Fig. 3.8) blocks cell cycle progression in S or G_2/M phase. The drug is under clinical development. Due to its low solubility, it is administered in liposome formulation. Dimethylamino-benzoylphenylurea may act as a radiation sensitizer.

A family of sulfur containing derivatives is in testing for prostate, breast, and pancreas cancer. Two of these compounds, SG410 and SG430, have promise. The sensitivity is increased in tumors that are deficient in Microtubule Associated Protein τ.

N-[4-(5-bromo-2-pyrimidinyloxy)-3-chlorophenyl]-*N*'-(2-nitrobenzoyl) urea (HO-221) is a derivative of benzoylphenylurea that is under study as an anti-cancer agent.

3.1.6 Other Microtubule Destabilizers

Indanocine (Fig. 3.9) is a synthetic indanone that was identified by the Developmental Therapeutics Program of the U.S. National Cancer Institute as having anti-proliferative activity by acting as a microtubule disrupting drug. It has a flex-

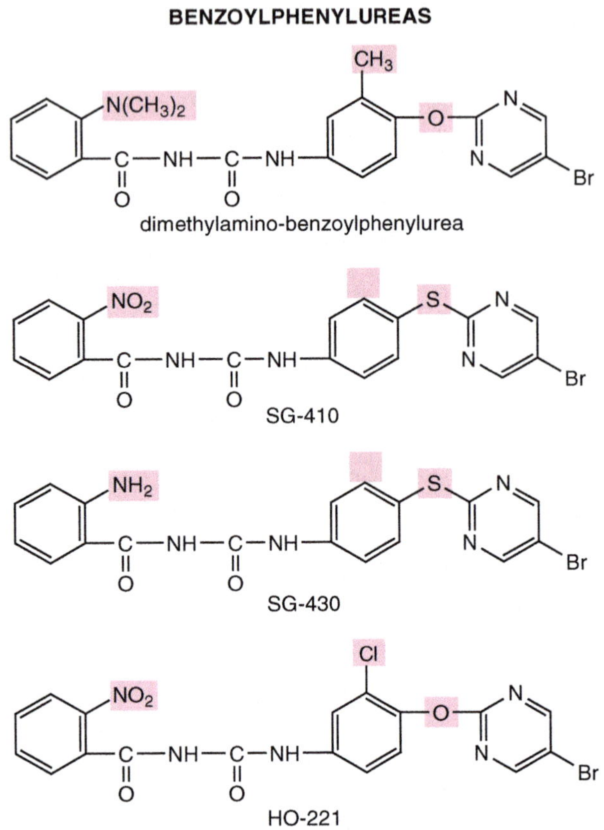

Fig. 3.8 Structures of benzoylphenylureas. Differences in structure among the compounds in this class are shaded in *pink*

ible structure, in which two halves of the molecule are connected through a single bond. Although it bears no structural similarity with colchicine, indanocine reversibly binds to the colchicine site of Tubulin. The association process follows biphasic kinetics similar to that of the colchicine/Tubulin interaction.

Drug Resistance Indanocine displays toxicity toward multi-drug resistant cells. There is cross-resistance with colchicine and vinblastine in cells that encounter mutations in β-Tubulin.

The combretastatins are a class of natural stilbenoid phenols. Diverse natural combretastatin molecules are present in the bark of Combretum caffrum (South African Bush Willow). Molecules of the combretastatin family contain a trimethoxy ring, a ring containing substituents (often at C3 and C4), and an ethene bridge between the two rings. Combretastatin binds to the β subunit of Tubulin at the colchicine site. The drug exerts part of its anti-mitotic action on tumor vascular cells. Endothelial cells treated with combretastatin rapidly balloon in shape, causing necrosis of the tumor core.

Nocodazole interferes with the polymerization of microtubules. Treated cells enter mitosis but cannot form metaphase spindles because the microtubules cannot polymerize. The absence of microtubule attachment to kinetochores activates the spindle assembly checkpoint, causing the cell to arrest in prometaphase with a G_2 phase DNA content.

Pentafluorophenylsulfonamides can have anti-mitotic effects.

- The sodium salt of 2-fluoro-1-methoxy-4-pentafluorophenylsulfonamidobenzene (T138067) is a synthetic pentafluorophenylsulfonamide that covalently binds to and selectively modifies the β1, β2, β3, and β4 isotypes of Tubulin at a conserved cysteine residue, resulting in a disruption of microtubule polymerization, a collapse of the cytoskeleton, an increase in chromosomal ploidy, and tumor cell death.
  Pharmacokinetics Pentafluorophenylsulfonamides are not substrates for drug efflux pumps that confer resistance to other anti-mitotic agents, however, glutathione conjugation mediated by Glutathione-S-Transferase plays a major role in their metabolism.
  Drug Resistance 2-fluoro-1-methoxy-4-pentafluorophenylsulfonamidobenzene has cytotoxicity against tumor cells that exhibit substantial resistance to vinblastine, paclitaxel, doxorubicin, and actinomycin D.
- T900607 is a pentafluorophenylsulfonamide compound that inhibits Tubulin polymerization by binding irreversibly to colchicine binding sites, resulting in cell cycle arrest and cell death.
  Adverse Effects The most frequent adverse events include rigors (40 %), pyrexia (30 %), nausea (30 %), vomiting (20 %), anemia (20 %), fatigue (15 %), and anorexia (10 %).

Eribulin mesylate (E7389) <Halaven> is a synthetic form of halichondrin B, derived from the sea sponge Halichondria okadai. Eribulin engages microtubule plus ends with high affinity. Its binding site is located on β-Tubulin, at a heterodimer interface, and overlaps the GTP-binding site. Eribulin sequesters Tubulin into non-productive aggregates. This causes an inhibition of microtubule dynamics that arrests the cell cycle in G_2/M through suppression of the growth of microtubules, without interfering with microtubule shortening. The disruption of mitotic spindles ultimately leads to apoptotic cell death after prolonged mitotic blockage.

Based on a survival benefit of about 3 months, the dug received U.S. FDA approval in 2008 for the treatment of patients with metastatic breast cancer who have received at least two prior chemotherapy regimens for late stage disease. Before treatment with eribulin, patients should have received prior anthracycline- and taxane-based chemotherapy for early or late stage breast cancer. The drug is administered at 1.4 mg/m^2 intravenously over 2–5 min on days 1 and 8 every 21 days.

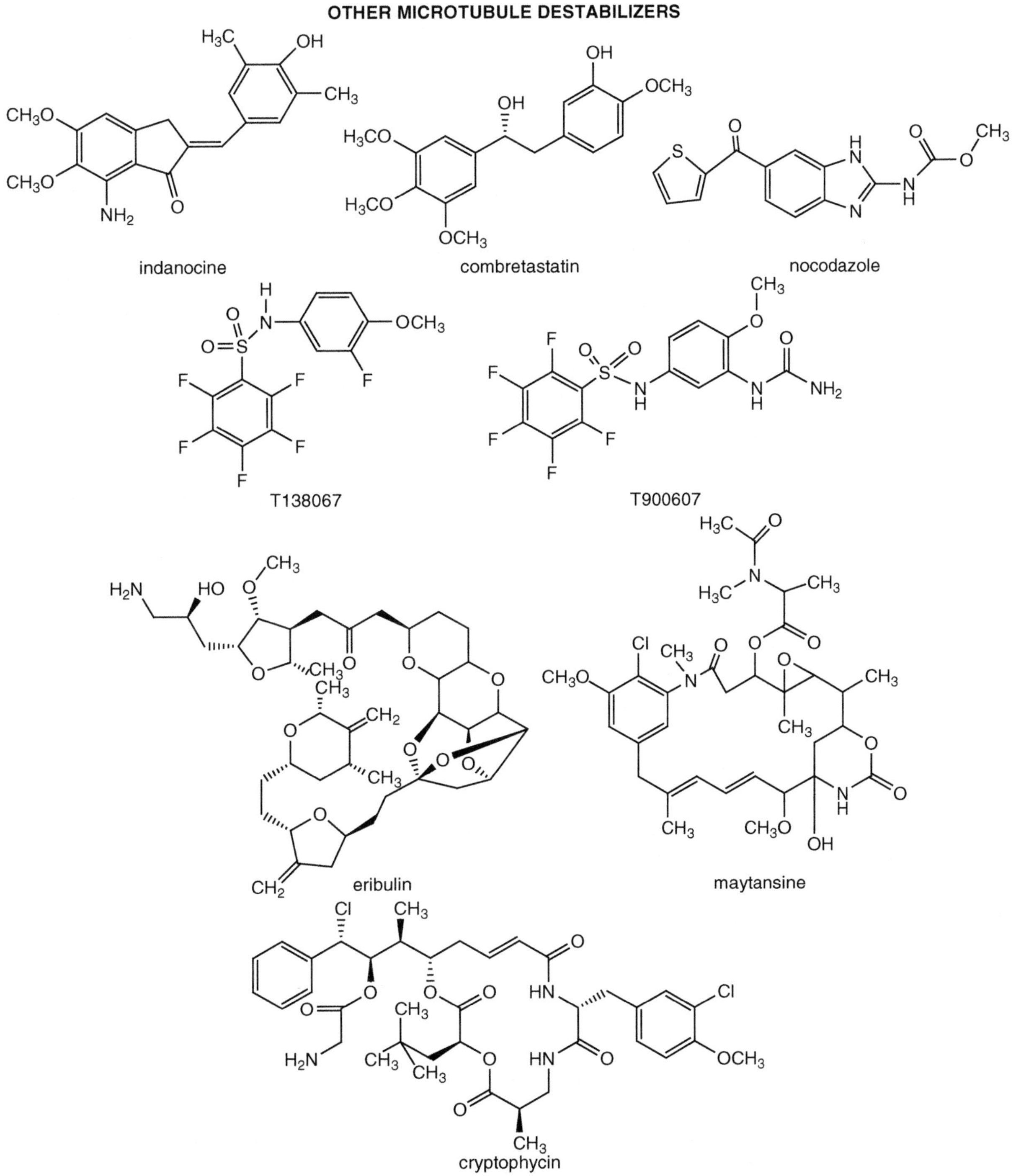

Fig. 3.9 Structures of other microtubule destabilizers

Pharmacokinetics Eribulin is not substantially metabolized and is primarily eliminated unchanged in the feces. Hepatic or renal impairment require dose reduction.

Adverse Effects The most common adverse event of eribulin treatment is myelosuppression, most prominently neutropenia. Febrile neutropenia or grade 4 neutropenia, lasting more than 7 days, requires delay or reduction of subsequent doses. In addition, anemia, asthenia or fatigue, alopecia, peripheral neuropathy, nausea, or constipation may arise. The drug can cause possible QT prolongation. Caution and monitoring may be required if given together with class IA and III anti-arrhythmics.

Maytansine (maitansine, maysanine) is an ansamycin antibiotic originally isolated from the Ethiopian shrub Maytenus serrate. The agent binds to Tubulin at the rhizoxin binding site, distinct from the binding site of vinblastine. It inhibits microtubule assembly, induces microtubule disassembly, and disrupts mitosis. Maytansine exhibits cytotoxicity against rapidly dividing cells and may inhibit tumor growth.

Cryptophycin is a cytotoxin produced by cyanobacteria of the genus Nostoc. It works by attacking the Tubulin microfilaments in eukaryotic cells and thereby preventing cell division. Cryptophycin may be active against cancers of the brain, colon, ovarian, prostate, pancreas, lung and breast. It can destroy the cells of multi-drug resistant tumors (Smith et al. 1994).

3.1.7 Anti-Mitotic Peptide Drugs

Originally identified as natural products from marine sponges (Hemiasterella minor, as well as Cymbastela, Siphonochalina, and Auletta species), hemiasterlins comprise a small family of tripeptides containing highly modified amino acids. Hemiasterlin (Fig. 3.10) binds at stoichiometric amounts to the vinca domain in Tubulin, disrupts the microtubule dynamics and depolymerizes the microtubules.

- The hemiasterlin analog E7974 may have affinity predominantly for the β3 subunit of Tubulin.
- The synthetic hemiasterlin analog HTI-286 inhibits Tubulin polymerization, and remains active against cells that over-express the efflux transporters ABCB1, ABCC1 or ABCG2.

Dolastatin 10 (NSC376128, AC1L2OAS) is a pentapeptide originally isolated from the marine mollusk Dolabella auricularia. It consists of four amino acid residues (dolavaline, valine, dolaisoleuine, dolaproine) linked to a complex primary amine (dolaphenine). The compound binds to Tubulin at a distinct site for peptide anti-mitotic agents, near the exchangeable GTP and vinca alkaloid sites. It inhibits microtubule assembly, resulting in the formation of Tubulin aggregates and inhibition of mitosis. Dolastatin 10 also induces tumor cell apoptosis through a mechanism that involves BCL-2, an oncoprotein that is over-expressed in some cancers.

- Soblidotin (TZT-1027, NSC-654663) is a dolastatin 10 derivative, which inhibits Tubulin polymerization, resulting in cell cycle arrest and induction of apoptosis (Kobayashi et al. 1997).

Pharmacokinetics Dolastatin 10 enters cells through passive uptake, without a requirement for ATP. It is retained intracellularly for several hours.

Cemadotin (*N*, *N*-dimethyl-L-valyl-L-valyl-*N*-methyl-L-valyl-L-prolyl-L-prolinebenzylamide) (LU103793, NSC D-669356) is a water soluble synthetic analog of dolastatin 15 (an anti-proliferative compound that was isolated from the mollusk Dolabella auricularia). The drug blocks cells at mitosis by strongly suppressing microtubule dynamics. Cemadotin is in clinical trials as a cancer chemotherapeutic agent.

Tubulysin A is a natural product isolated from the myxobacterial strain Archangium geophyra. Although it has a peptide backbone, it contains mostly atypical amino acids, a central thiazole heterocycle, a basic *N*-terminal tertiary amine and an aromatic and acidic *C*-terminal end. Tubulysin A depolymerizes microtubules and induces mitotic arrest. The drug may have anti-angiogenic properties.

Drug Resistance Tubulysin A has efficacy irrespective of the multidrug resistance properties of the targeted cancer cells. It is a substrate neither for CYP enzymes nor for efflux pumps.

Phomopsin A is a mycotoxin and anti-mitotic compound. It binds selectively to dimeric Tubulin at a site overlapping that of vinblastine and maytansine, inhibiting the formation of the microtubule spindle required for cell division. Phomopsin A stabilizes Tubulin.

Diverse peptidic compounds can bind to Tubulin and interfere with mitosis.

3.1.8 Kinesin Spindle Protein Inactivating Drugs

Mitotic Kinesins are microtubule associated motor proteins that utilize the energy from ATP hydrolysis for bipolar spindle assembly, as well as for chromosome alignment and segregation during cell division. The mitotic motor protein Kinesin Spindle Protein (KSP, Kinesin Family Member 11, Kinesin-5, Eg5) is importantly involved in the early stages of mitosis, as it is essential for the formation of bipolar spindles during mitosis (Fig. 3.11). With energy from the hydrolysis of ATP, Kinesin Spindle Protein moves along anti-parallel microtubules toward the plus end, thereby separating the centrosomes. It is selectively expressed in proliferating cells. Inhibition of Kinesin Spindle Protein causes the formation of monopolar mitotic spindles, activates the spindle assembly checkpoint, and arrests cells at mitosis in pro-metaphase, which leads to subsequent cell death. The prolonged inhibition of Kinesin Spindle Protein activates BAX and Caspase-3, which requires a competent spindle checkpoint and couples with mitotic slippage.

Because anti-mitotic drugs that target Tubulin suffer from limitations in solubility, neurotoxicity, and resistance profile, small molecule inhibitors of Kinesin Spindle Protein have promise for the treatment of cancer without these adverse effects. The first Kinesin Spindle Protein inhibitor identified was monastrol (named because it causes the formation of monostral spindles), which allosterically inhibits its ATPase activity (Mayer et al. 1999). Certain quinazolinone deriva-

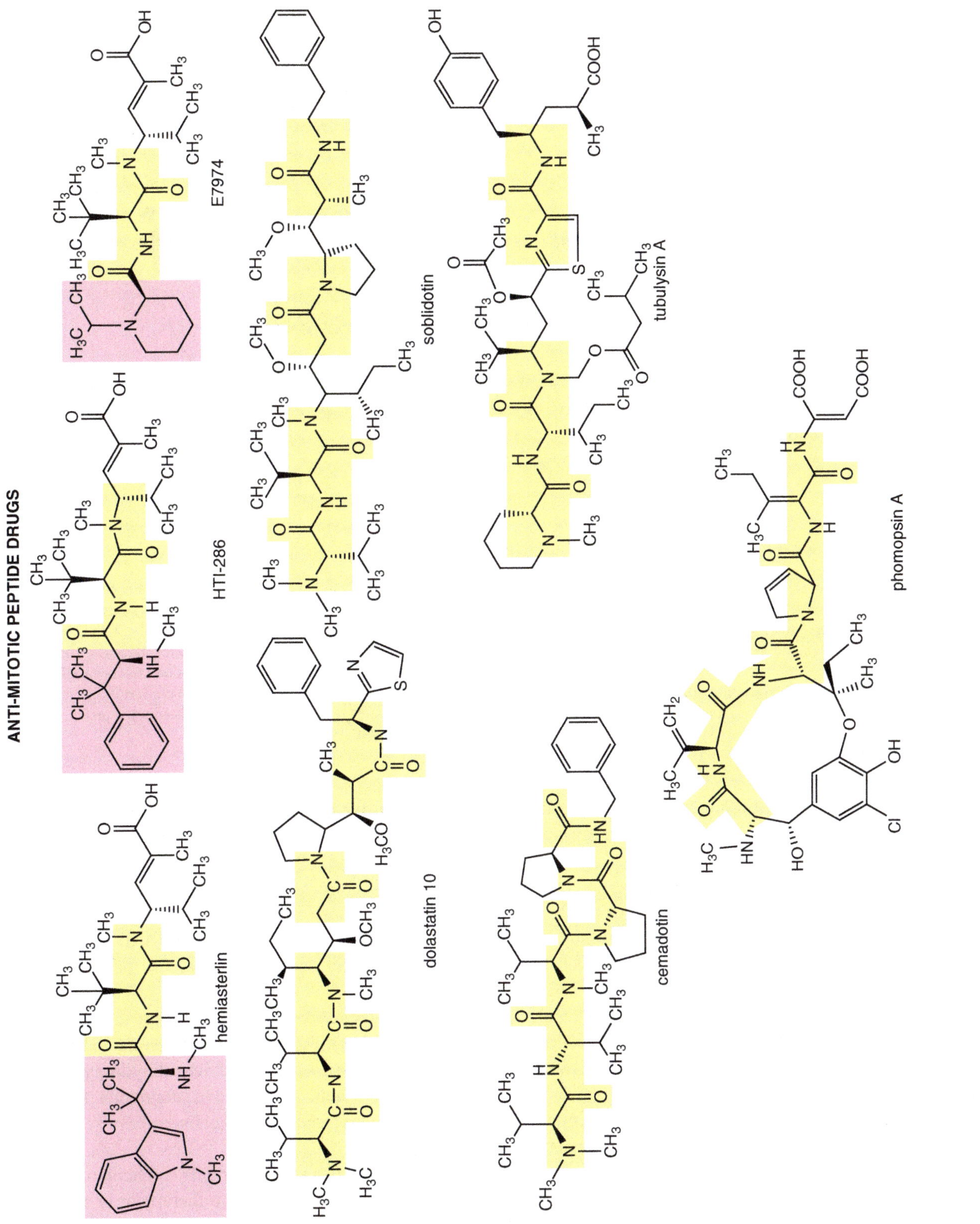

Fig. 3.10 Structures of anti-mitotic peptide drugs. The common peptide bond backbone is highlighted in *yellow*. The different N-terminal cyclic residues that distinguish the hemiasterlin derivatives (*left panel*) are shaded in *pink*

tives, dihydropyrazoles and dihydropyrroles, fused indoles and carbazoles, and pyrazolobenzoxazines act as selective Kinesin Spindle Protein inhibitors.

Quinazolinones and Derivatives Since the 1950s, quinazolinones have been studied as potential anti-malarial drugs. Later, the derivative methaqualone was used as a hypnotic.

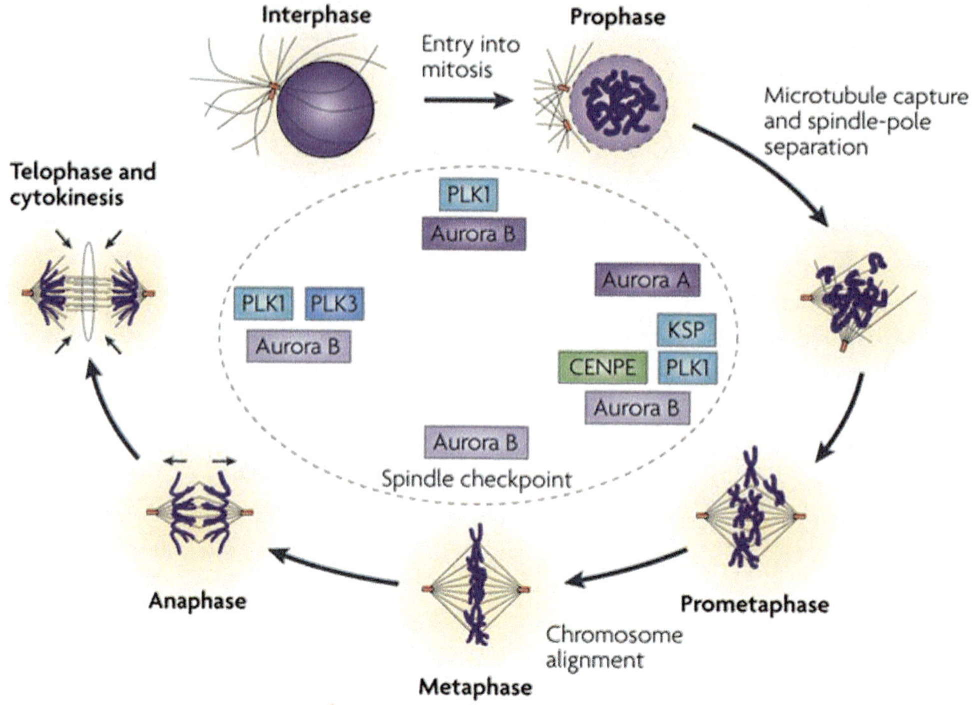

Fig. 3.11 Progression through mitosis. The progression of mitosis through the canonical morphological stages is shown. Kinesin Spindle Protein (*KSP*) is required to establish mitotic spindle bipolarity through driving centrosome separation. Centromeric Protein E (*CENPE*) is required for accurate chromosome congression at metaphase during mitosis. *Aurora A* is crucial for centrosome maturation and separation during early prophase. *Aurora B* is a member of the chromosomal passenger complex (*CPC*) and is involved in Histone H3 phosphorylation, chromosomal condensation, chromosomal alignment on the metaphase plate, bi-polar centromere-microtubule attachments, spindle checkpoint and cytokinesis. During mitosis, Polo-Like Kinase 1 (*PLK1*) is involved in centrosome maturation and formation of the mitotic spindle. It is also required for exit from mitosis and the separation of sister chromatids during anaphase. PLK1 may have a role in cytokinesis through the phosphorylation of the Kinesin-like motor protein MKLP1. (Jackson 2007 with permission)

Due to their ability to inhibit Kinesin Spindle Protein, quinazolinones can serve to treat cell proliferative disorders including cancer.

Ispinesib (SB-715992, CK0238273) (Fig. 3.12) is a synthetic small molecule derived from quinazolinone. Loop 5 within the Kinesin Spindle Protein motor domain forms an essential portion of the binding pocket for the drug, which allosterically inhibits the ATPase activity. Ispinesib effects the inhibition of mitotic spindle assembly, induction of cell cycle arrest during M phase, and cell death in actively dividing tumor cells.

Adverse Effects Because Kinesin Spindle Protein is not involved in non-mitotic processes, such as neuronal transport, ispinesib entails a low risk of causing the peripheral neuropathy that is often associated with Tubulin targeting agents.

Drug Resistance Point mutations in the ispinesib binding site of Kinesin Spindle Protein can lead to drug resistance.

The second generation Kinesin Spindle Protein inhibitor SB-743921 is a synthetic small molecule. SB-743921 is 5-fold more potent against the ATPase activity of Kinesin Spindle Protein than ispinesib.

Dihydropyrazoles and thiazoles MK0731 is a synthetic 3,5-diaryl-4,5-dihydropyrazole that selectively inhibits Kinesin Spindle Protein. This may result in the inhibition of mitotic spindle assembly, the induction of cell cycle arrest during M phase, and apoptosis in tumor cells that express high levels of the target protein. MK0731 is compromised by poor water solubility, caused in part by its difluorination.

Drug Resistance ABCB1 transport correlates with amine basicity for dihydropyrrole inhibitors. The incorporation of β,β-difluoro substituents into dihydropyrrole derivatives moderates their basicity and maintains their potency in multi-drug resistant cancer cells.

ARRY-520 acts preferentially on hematopoietic cells and is in clinical trials—as mono-therapy or in combination regimens—for the treatment of multiple myeloma. Blood cancers frequently depend on the myeloid cell leukemia protein MCL-1 (a member of the BCL-2 family) as a key survival protein. Besides inhibiting Kinesin Spindle Protein, ARRY-520 also induces a rapid onset of apoptosis in tumor cells that depend on MCL-1.

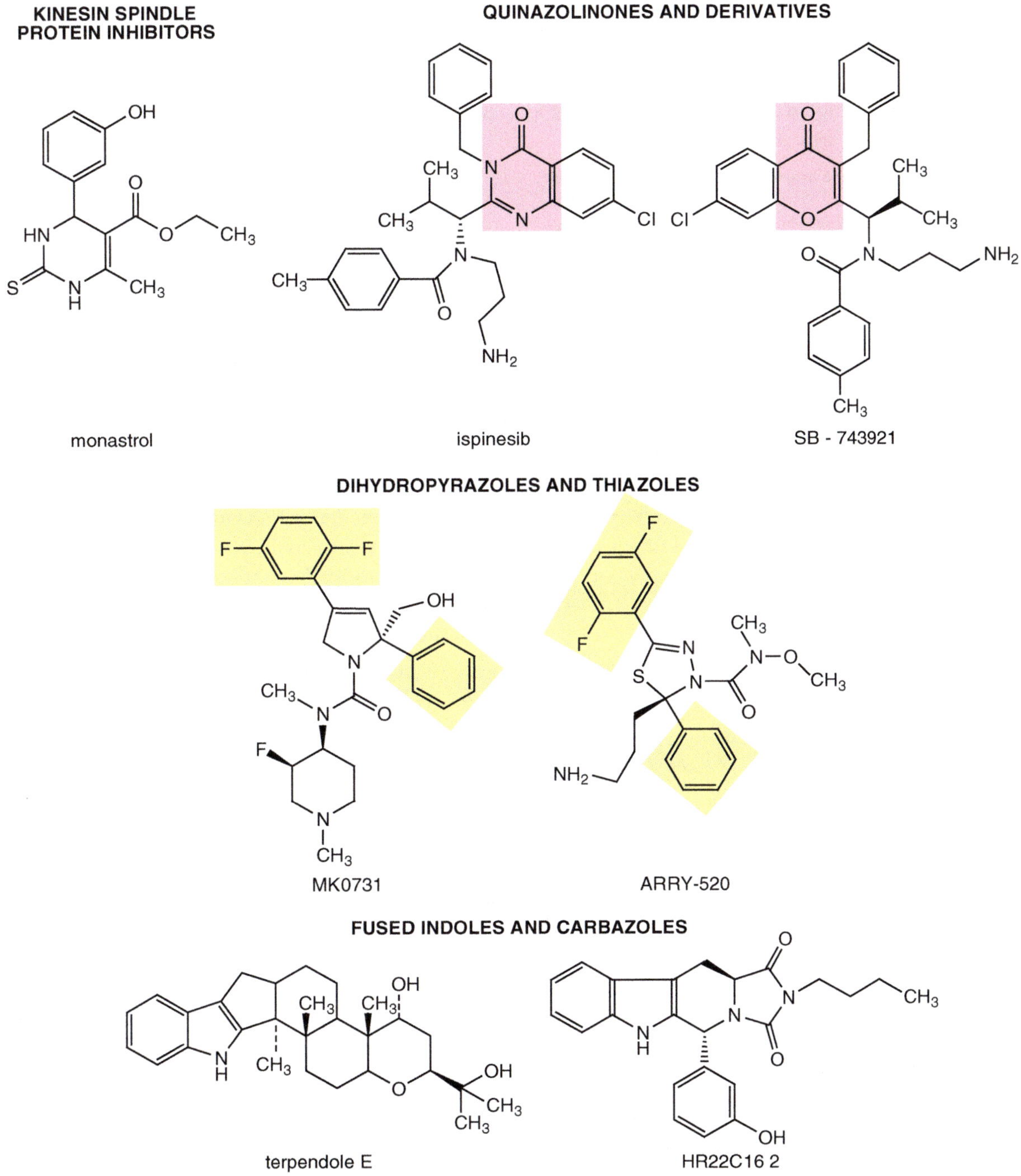

Fig. 3.12 Structures of Kinesin Spindle Protein inhibitors. In addition to the parent compound monasterol, the class of drugs comprises three chemical groups, quinazolinones and derivatives, dihydropyrazoles and thiazoles, and fused indoles and carbazoles. The moiety that is distinct between the quinazolinones is highlighted in *pink*, while the common structures of dihydropyrazoles and thiazoles are shaded in *yellow*

Adverse Effects Because Kinesin Spindle Protein is not involved in post-mitotic processes, such as neuronal transport, ARRY-520 does not cause the peripheral neuropathy that is often associated with Tubulin targeting agents. The drug is associated with minor non-hematologic adverse events, including gastrointestinal and skin toxicities.

Fused indoles and carbazoles 2,3-fused indoles constitute a common minimal scaffold for Kinesin Spindle Protein inhibitory activity. Terpendole E (1'α-hydroxy-paspaline) is a fungal derived Kinesin Spindle Protein inhibitor with a 2,3-fused indole (carbazole) scaffold. Its core structure consists of indole and diterpene moieties.

Derivatives of carboline and carbazole are ATP-competitive Kinesin Spindle Protein inhibitors. HR22C16 is a cell permeable Kinesin Spindle Protein inhibitor with a tetrahydro-β-carboline structure. The agent induces apoptotic cell death via the intrinsic pathway.

The suppression of mitotic Kinesins arrests cells in pro-metaphase.
Kinesin Spindle Protein inhibitors do not display the neurotoxicity that is associated with Tubulin binding anti-mitotic drugs.

3.2 Differentiating Agents

Differentiation and proliferation are mutually exclusive. The proliferative potential of cells decreases with their increasing level of differentiation. Terminally differentiated cells are in a form of irreversible cell cycle arrest, referred to as senescence. Hence, the induced differentiation of tumor cells is a potential anti-cancer strategy. Further, differentiating agents are under study as chemopreventives in high risk individuals and in patients with premalignant lesions.

Differentiation and proliferation are mutually exclusive.
The induced differentiation of tumor cells is a potential anti-cancer strategy.
Differentiating agents may serve as chemopreventives in high risk individuals and in patients with premalignant lesions.

3.2.1 Retinoids

Vitamins are organic compounds that are essential for an adequate diet, as they are required by various biochemical processes of the body. Vitamins are divided into fat-soluble (A, D, E, and K) and water-soluble (C and vitamin B complex). Retinoids are formed from dietary vitamin A or the pro-vitamin β-carotene. The basic structure of the retinoid molecule consists of a cyclic end group, a polyene side chain and a polar end group. Many different geometric isomers of retinol, retinal and retinoic acid are possible as a result of either a trans or cis configuration in four of the five double bonds within the polyene chain. Although the cis isomers are less stable and can readily convert to the all-trans configuration, some cis isomers occur naturally and carry out essential functions.

The pool of stem cells and progenitor cells, which are potentially susceptible to malignant transformation, is restricted by retinoic acid signaling. Retinoids induce cell differentiation, inhibit cell proliferation, and may mediate apoptosis. During retinoid deficiency, stem cells fail to mature, which is accompanied by enhanced cellular proliferation and the formation of premalignant lesions. Retinoids are under study as chemopreventives in high risk individuals and in patients with premalignant lesions.

Retinoids (agonists of Retinoid A Receptor (RAR)) and rexinoids (agonists of Retinoid X Receptor (RXR)) bind to their cognate receptors, which then hetero-dimerize and act as transcriptional regulators in retinoic acid response elements (RAREs). Predominantly, retinoids activate genes that limit proliferation and support differentiation.

- Actions of retinoids are usually associated with cell cycle arrest in G_1 and ensuing growth suppression. This is due to the increased expression of $p21^{CIP1/WAF1}$, a direct target gene of ligated Retinoid Receptors.
- The chemopreventive activity of retinoids is mediated, in part, by a decline in the expression of G_1 Cyclin proteins, specifically Cyclin D1, which undergoes Ubiquitin dependent proteolysis.
- Retinoids down-regulate Survivin in cancer cells.

Adverse Effects The class of retinoids has been associated with photosensitivity. Patients should minimize the exposure of treated areas to sunlight and sunlamps during the use of retinoids. Vitamin A associated toxicities limit the extended administration of retinoids to individuals who are at high risk for cancer development.

First generation retinoids In 1913, Elmer McCollum and Marguerite Davis identified a fat soluble nutrient in butter and cod liver oil, confirming an independent observation by Thomas Osborne and Lafayette Mendel. The agent turned out to be retinol (vitamin A) (Fig. 3.13). In 1925, Wolbach and Howe reported that retinoid functions are essential for the proper regulation of differentiation and proliferation in all the epithelia that are the common sites of carcinogenesis (Wolbach and Howe 1925). Retinol was synthesized in 1947 by the Dutch chemists David Adriaan van Dorp and Jozef Ferdinand Arens.

Obtained from certain fruits and vegetables, β-carotene is a naturally occurring retinal precursor that is composed of 2 retinyl groups. It is broken down to retinal in the mucosa of the small intestine by β-Carotene 15,15'-Monooxygenase. As an anti-oxidant, β-carotene inhibits free radical damage to DNA. This agent also induces cell differentiation and apoptosis in some tumor cell types, particularly at early stages of tumorigenesis, and enhances immune system activity by stimulating the release of natural killer cells, lymphocytes, and monocytes. Retinal (retinaldehyde, vitamin A aldehyde) has been under study for the prevention of lung cancer.

Retinyl acetate (all-trans Vitamin A acetate) is a naturally occurring fatty acid ester form of vitamin A. Retinyl acetate binds to and activates Retinoid Receptors, inducing cell differentiation and decreasing cell proliferation. This agent also inhibits the carcinogen induced neoplastic transformation in some cell types and exhibits immunomodulatory properties.

The fat soluble tretinoin (vitamin A acid, all-trans retinoic acid, ATRA) <Retin-A, Vesanoid> was introduced into cancer therapy in 1985. It is a naturally occurring acid of retinol that binds to and activates Retinoic Acid Receptors (RARs), thereby inducing changes in gene expression that lead to cell differentiation, decreased cell proliferation, and inhibition of tumorigenesis. This agent also inhibits Telomerase, resulting in telomere shortening and eventual apoptosis of some tumor cell types. Retinoic acid also inhibits the growth of breast cancer cells, in which the tumor suppressor gene *p53* is inactivated.

- Tretinoin liposomal (L-ATRA) (AR-623) <Atragen> is an intravenous formulation of tretinoin encased in liposomes. Liposome encapsulation extends the half-life of intravenously administered tretinoin. The formulation is under study for promyelocytic leukemia and soft tissue sarcomata.

Retinoate induces differentiation in lymphoid and myeloid cells via transcriptional activation. In myeloid differentiation, the absence of retinoate causes the nuclear receptor hetero-dimer RXR/RARα complex to be bound to Histone Deacetylase and to be transcriptionally inactive. Physiological doses of retinoate induce the release of Histone Deacetylase, followed by expression of RXR/RARα target genes and ensuing differentiation. Chimeric transcription factors (resulting from chromosome translocations) can be the cause for cellular transformation in various leukemias. PML-RARα and PLZF-RARα are chimeric leukemogenic transcriptional repressors, which cause acute promyelocytic leukemia. They are unresponsive to physiological doses of retinoate. However, pharmacological doses of tretinoin induce the dissociation of Histone Deacetylase from PML-RARα. This allows the induction of retinoate dependent genes and differentiation of the leukemic cells. In contrast, even at pharmacological doses of tretinoin, PLZF-RARα represses transcription because the PLZF moiety causes retinoate insensitive interactions with Histone Deacetylase (Fig. 3.14).

Adverse Effects Adverse effects include arthralgia, headaches, and dry skin. High doses can lead to chemical hepatitis.

Isotretinoin (13-cis retinoic acid) <Accutane, Roaccutane> is a naturally occurring retinoic acid, which binds

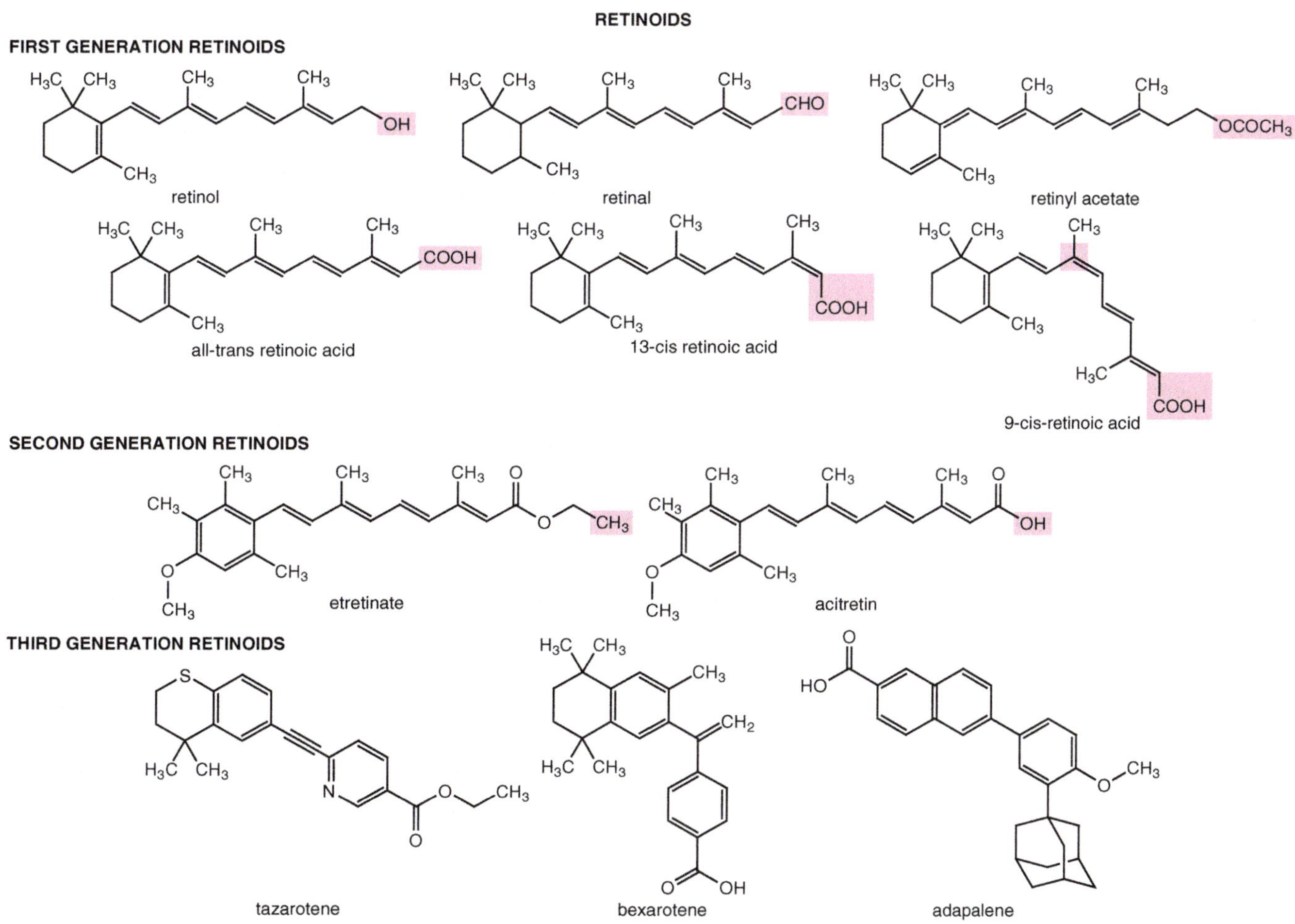

Fig. 3.13 Structures of retinoids. With the exception of third generation retinoids, the representatives within a subgroup have similar structures. Chemical groups that differ among the compounds within the same subgroup are shaded in *pink*

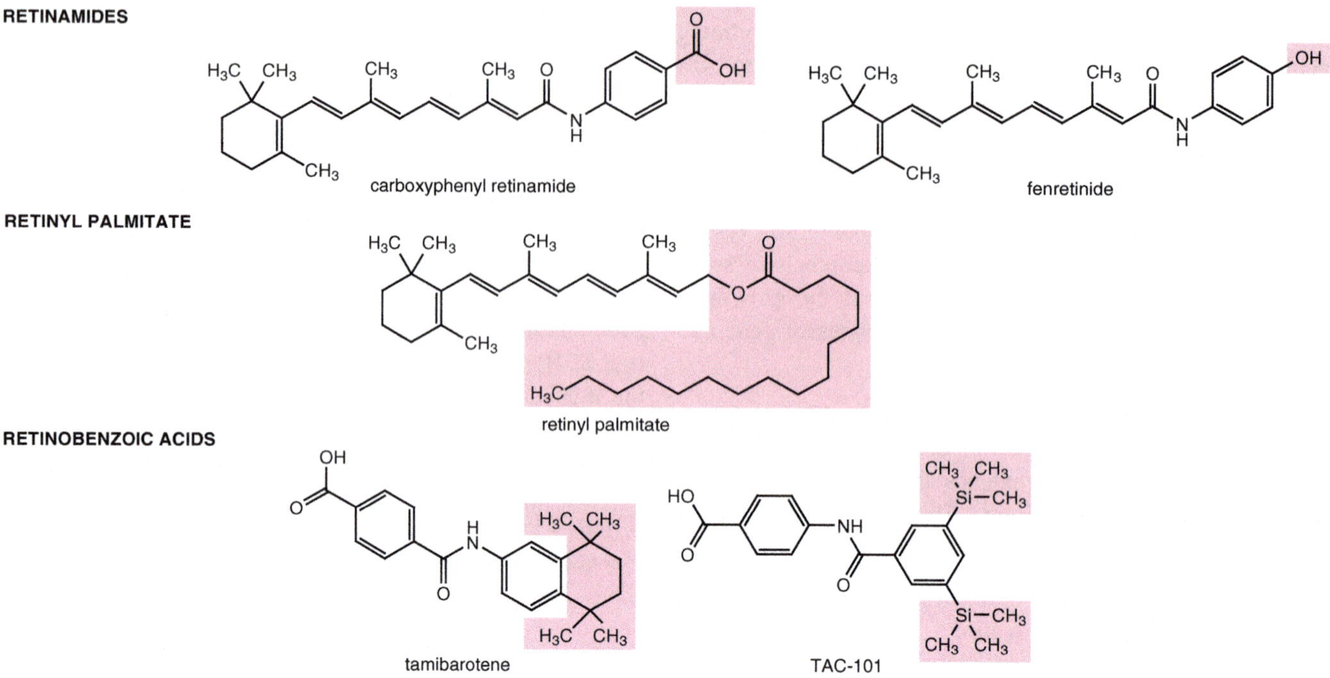

Fig. 3.13 (continued)

to and activates nuclear Retinoic Acid Receptors (RARs), thereby regulating cell proliferation and differentiation. This agent also exhibits immunomodulatory and anti-inflammatory responses and inhibits Ornithine Decarboxylase, thereby decreasing polyamine synthesis and keratinization. Isoretinoin has been used in the treatment of leukemia, neuroblastoma, and genital warts. In oral leukoplakia, a clinical response is associated with isoretinoin-induced RARβ expression and clinical response.

Adverse Effects Patients receiving isotretinoin can experience redness and dryness of the skin, itching and increased sensitivity to sunlight (adequate precautions should be taken). There may be a relationship between administration of the drug and the onset of psychological symptoms including depression, suicidal ideation, and psychosis. Isotretinoin is a possible cause of Crohn disease and ulcerative colitis in some individuals. The agent acts as a severe teratogen.

Alitretinoin (9-cis-retinoic acid) <Panretin> is the drug form of an endogenous retinoid that binds to and activates all intracellular retinoid receptor subtypes (RARα, RARβ, RARγ, RXRα, RXRβ, RXRγ). In their activated state, these receptors transcribe genes that control differentiation and proliferation in both healthy and neoplastic cells. While altitretinoin is indicated for the topical treatment of cutaneous lesions in patients with AIDS-related Kaposi sarcoma, it cannot treat visceral Kaposi sarcoma. The drug is initially applied two times a day to the cutaneous lesions. The application frequency can be gradually increased to 3–4 times a day, according to individual lesion tolerance. If application site toxicity occurs, the application frequency needs to be reduced. Treatment should be continued as long as there is benefit.

Adverse Effects Adverse events occur almost exclusively at the site of application. The dermal toxicity begins as erythema, which may progress and edema may develop. In rare cases, intense erythema, edema, and vesiculation may become treatment limiting. 9-cis-retinoic acid is contraindicated in patients with a known hypersensitivity to retinoids or to any of the ingredients of the product. The drug is Pregnancy Category D.

Drug Interactions Patients who apply alitretinoin gel should not concurrently use products that contain *N, N*-diethyl-m-toluamide (DEET, a common component of insect repellent products), as *N, N*-diethyl-m-toluamide toxicity is increased.

Second generation retinoids Second generation retinoids have been used predominantly for the treatment of psoriasis. They have limited applications in cancer.

Etretinate <Tegison> was developed at Hoffmann-La Roche and was approved by the U.S. FDA in 1986. The drug has a therapeutic effect on existing basal cell carcinomata and a prophylactic effect in inhibiting new tumor formation. It may reduce the risk of leukoplakia (a premalignant lesion in the mouth) and oral cancer.

Adverse Effects Etretinate has a low therapeutic index and a long elimination half-life of 120 days, which make dosing difficult. Due to the high lipophilicity of the aromatic retinoid, etretinate is stored in and slowly released from adipose

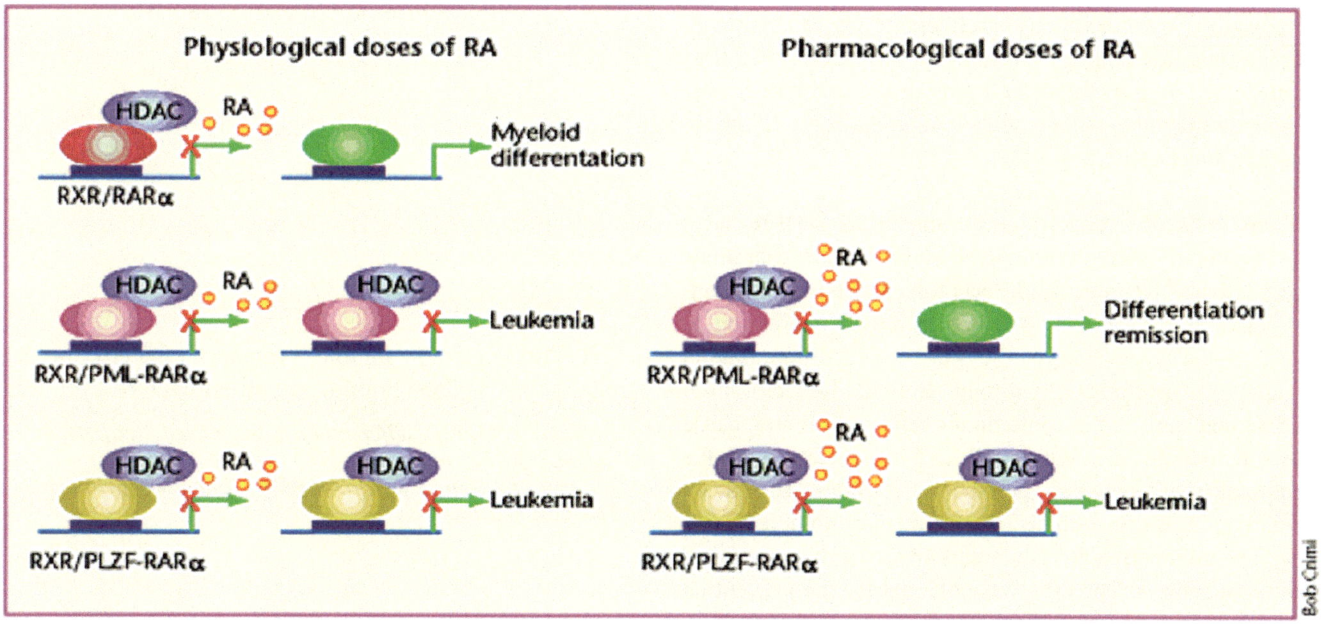

Fig. 3.14 Mechanisms by which chimeric transcription factors can lead to cellular transformation. In the absence of retinoic acid, the retinoic acid receptor complex RXR-RARα is bound to Histone Deacetylase (*HDAC*) and is therefore transcriptionally inactive. Physiological doses of retinoic acid (*RA*, *left*) induce the release of HDAC from the RXR-RARα complex, thus allowing the expression of the target genes and the onset of differentiation. Both *PML-RARα* and *PLZF-RARα* are unresponsive to physiological doses of retinoic acid, and act as leukemogenic transcriptional repressors. In contrast, pharmacological doses of retinoic acid (*right*) induce the dissociation of Histone Deacetylase from the PML-RARα complex, allowing the induction of retinoic acid dependent genes and differentiation of the acute promyelocytic leukemia (APL) blasts. However, even at pharmacological doses of retinoic acid, PLZF-RARα is still able to repress transcription because the PLZF moiety engages in retinoic acid insensitive interactions with co-repressors and Histone Deacetylase. Inhibitors of Histone Deacetylase could be developed as anti-leukemic drugs. (Salomoni 2000 with permission)

tissue, causing prolonged effects. In children, the drug may interfere with bone growth. Etretinate was removed from the market in Canada in 1996 and in the U.S. in 1998, in part due to the high risk of birth defects.

Acitretin <Soriatane> is a metabolite of etretinate. It is under study for the treatment or prevention of skin cancer. A therapeutic effect occurs after 2–4 weeks or longer.

Pharmacokinetics Acitretin is readily absorbed and widely distributed after oral administration. It has a half-life of approximately 2 days.

Adverse Effects Because acitretin can be metabolized into etretinate, there is a risk for delayed teratogenicity (potentially in pregnancies as late as 3 years after discontinuation of acitretin).

Third generation retinoids Third generation retinoids have higher specificity than their predecessors and bind to select subsets of Retinoid or Rexinoid Receptors.

Tazarotene <Tazorac, Avage, Zorac> binds to RARα, RARβ, and RARγ with a relative selectivity for RARβ, and RARγ. It constitutes a topical retinoid for the treatment of skin damage and is under study for basalioma and basal cell nevus syndrome.

Adverse Effects Common adverse effects include acne, dry skin, pruritus, and redness. For most patients these discomforts are mild and decrease markedly after 2–4 weeks of use.

Bexarotene (LGD1069) <Targretin> is an orally active, synthetic retinoic acid agent that selectively binds to and activates Retinoid X Receptors (RXRs), thereby inducing changes in gene expression that lead to cell differentiation and decreased cell proliferation, and in some cancer cell types to apoptosis. In 2000, bexarotene was indicated by the U.S. FDA for cutaneous T-cell lymphoma. It has been used off-label for lung cancer, breast cancer, and Kaposi sarcoma. The drug may have chemopreventive properties.

Adverse Effects Bexarotene may be teratogenic and embryotoxic.

Adapalene does not bind to the cytosolic retinoic acid binding proteins but instead selectively engages RARβ and RARγ. The agent is active as a topical retinoid, primarily used in the treatment of skin conditions. Adapalene in small concentrations is a moderator of cellular differentiation, keratinization, and inflammatory processes. It has both exfoliating and anti-inflammatory effects.

Retinamides Carboxyphenyl retinamide is a synthetic phenylretinamide analog of retinol that induces cell differentiation and inhibits tumor cell growth and carcinogenesis. This agent may also induce cell cycle arrest in the G_1 phase in some cancer cell types.

Fenretinide (4-hydroxy(phenyl)retinamide, 4-HPR) (RT-101) is an orally active synthetic phenylretinamide that binds to and activates Retinoic Acid Receptors. It also transcriptionally activates RARγ and up-regulates RARβ expression in several tissue types. Fenretinide induces cell differentiation and apoptosis (preferentially through Retinoid Receptor independent mechanisms) in some tumor cell types. It may cause ceramide to build up in tumor cells and is associated with the accumulation of reactive oxygen species, resulting in cell death through apoptosis or necrosis. Fenretinide also inhibits tumor growth by modulating growth factors and receptors associated with angiogenesis. The drug has potential for the prevention of bladder cancer or secondary breast cancer. It accumulates preferentially in fatty tissue, such as the breast, which may contribute to its effectiveness against breast cancer.

Adverse Effects Common adverse effects associated with fenretinide include dry skin and night blindness, which are reversible upon cessation of treatment.

Retinyl palmitate Retinyl palmitate (vitamin A palmitate) is the ester of vitamin A and palmitic acid. It constitutes a synthetic alternate for retinyl acetate in vitamin A supplements, and is available in both oral (dry) and injectable (oily) forms for the treatment of vitamin A deficiency.

Retinobenzoic acids TAC-101 is a retinobenzoic acid that inhibits Retinoblastoma (RB) phosphorylation and increases the presence of Cyclin-Dependent Kinase Inhibitors (CDKIs), resulting in cell cycle arrest. This agent also causes a cytotoxic decline in Cyclin A and Thymidylate Synthase expression.

Retinobenzoic acid (tamibarotene) (AM 80) <Amnoid, Tamibaro> is a synthetic retinoid in development as a treatment for acute promyelocytic leukemia (APL). Originally developed by Shionogi with involvement from the University of Tokyo, tamibarotene has been licensed to Nippon Shinyaku. The compound is pending approval in Japan.

Modulators of retinoid metabolism Liarozole (Fig. 3.15) inhibits the Cytochrome P450 dependent metabolism of all-trans-retinoic acid. The orally active, imidazole containing liarozole fumarate (R85246) acts as a retinoic acid metabolism blocking agent (RAMBA) by inhibiting All-Trans-Retinoic Acid-4-Hydroxylase (ATRA-4-Hydroxylase), resulting in an increase in endogenous all-trans retinoate production, inhibition of cell proliferation, and induction of cell differentiation. This agent also inhibits Aromatase, the enzyme that catalyzes the final, rate limiting step in estrogen biosynthesis.

MODULATOR OF RETINOID METABOLISM

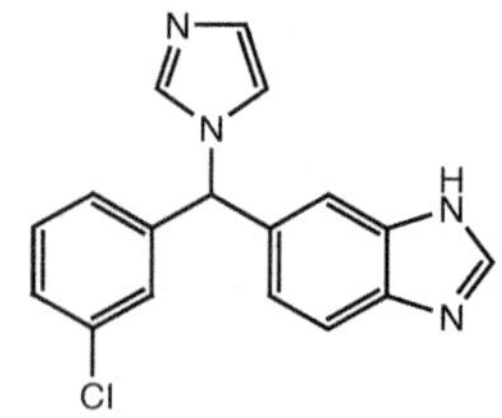

liarozole

Fig. 3.15 Structure of a modulator of retinoid metabolism

Retinoids induce cell differentiation, inhibit cell proliferation, and may mediate apoptosis.
Adverse effects include teratogenicity, photosensitivity, and chemical hepatitis.

3.2.2 Vitamin D

Vitamin D describes a group of fat soluble secosteroids[2] that comprise 5 forms, vitamin D_1 through D_5. They may function as pro-hormones. Calcitriol (1,25-dihydroxycholecalciferol, 1,25$(OH)_2$ vitamin D_3, 1,25-dihydroxyvitamin D_3) is the hormonally active form of vitamin D. As a nutrition supplement, the recommended dosing of vitamin D is 400–800 IU per day. Vitamin D_3 can also be endogenously synthesized when sun exposure is adequate. Vitamin D

- maintains homeostatic blood levels of calcium, magnesium, zinc, and phosphorus
- aids in regulating bone mineralization (in conjunction with Parathyroid Hormone, calcitriol regulates bone growth)
- facilitates the absorption of calcium (calcitriol regulates calcium by promoting its absorption in the intestine and reabsorption in the kidneys).

Vitamin D binds to the Vitamin D Receptor (VDR, 1,25-α-Dihydroxy-Vitamin D_3 Receptor, Vitamin D Hormone Receptor, Calcitriol Receptor, NR1I1). Upon engagement, the Vitamin D Receptor forms a hetero-dimer with the Retinoid X Receptor and binds to hormone response elements in DNA promoter regions, resulting in the expression or repression of specific genes. Downstream targets of this nuclear hormone receptor complex are principally involved in mineral metabolism.

[2] Secosteroids (Latin: secare = to cut) are structurally similar to steroids, but the B-ring carbon atoms C9 and C10 are not joined, constituting a 3-ring structure (as opposed to four rings in steroids).

Calcitriol has pro-differentiative and growth inhibitory effects, which underlie its potential anti-cancer actions. The expression of the tumor suppressor gene $p21^{CIP1/WAF1}$ can be induced by low concentrations of vitamin D and correlates with the induction of a differentiated phenotype.

- In the prostate, vitamin D induces the expression of IGF-BP, which counteracts IGF induced proliferation.
- Polymorphisms of the Vitamin D Receptor are associated with an increased risk of breast cancer. Low levels of vitamin D in the blood are correlated with breast cancer progression and bone metastases.
- High vitamin D intake may reduce the risk for colon cancer, pancreatic cancer, and ovarian cancer.
- Vitamin D compounds induce the differentiation of some leukemic cells.

Calcitriol (1,25-Dihydroxycholecalciferol, 1,25-dihydroxyvitamin D_3) <Rocaltrol, Calcijex, Decostriol> (Fig. 3.16) induces cell cycle arrest at the G_0/G_1 transition of the cell cycle and differentiation, resulting in an inhibition of proliferation of some tumor cell types. It also down-regulates Survivin in cancer cells, which can result in apoptosis. Many of the effects of calcitriol are mediated by its interaction with the Vitamin D Receptor (VDR, Calcitriol Receptor). This agent may be chemopreventive for colon and prostate cancers. For the prevention of colon cancer, 1000–2000 IU/day have been used. Calcitriol blood levels of 30–60 ng/ml are considered to be protective.

Adverse Effects The main adverse drug reaction associated with calcitriol therapy is hypercalcemia (reflected in nausea and vomiting, constipation, anorexia, apathy, headache, thirst, sweating, polyuria).

Doxercalciferol (1-α-hydroxyvitamin D_2) <Hectorol> is a synthetic analog of vitamin D. In the liver, doxercalciferol is converted to its biologically active vitamin D metabolites, which control the intestinal absorption of dietary calcium and the tubular reabsorption of calcium by the kidney. In conjunction with Parathyroid Hormone (PTH), the active vitamin D metabolites induce the mobilization of calcium from the skeleton. Through interactions with specific receptor proteins in target tissues, these vitamin D metabolites act directly on osteoblasts to stimulate skeletal growth, and on the parathyroid glands to suppress PTH synthesis and secretion. Doxercalciferol inhibits the growth of retinoblastomas, and may exhibit anti-proliferative activity against prostate cancer cells.

Paricalcitol (19-nor-1α,25-dihydroxyvitamin D_2) <Zemplar> is a synthetic non-calcemic, non-phosphatemic vitamin D analog. Paricalcitol increases the expression of the tumor suppressor gene *pten* in leukemic cells, resulting in tumor cell differentiation into normal phenotypes. The agent binds to the Vitamin D Receptor and reduces Parathyroid Hormone levels. It is under study for the treatment of advanced breast and prostate cancers, both of which have a high propensity to metastasize to bones.

Pharmacokinetics Most of the administered paricalcitol is metabolized by enzymes in the liver. The half-life of the drug is 5–7 h, but is doubled by severe kidney impairment. A large fraction of the metabolized drug is eliminated in the feces.

Vitamin D derivatives induce cell cycle arrest and support cell differentiation.

3.2.3 COX Inhibitors

There are two genes for Cyclooxygenase enzymes (COX, Prostaglandin Endoperoxide Synthase), *cox-1* and *cox-2*. COX-1 (PTGS-1) is constitutively expressed, while COX-2 (PTGS-2) is inducible. The two gene products also differ in their tissue distribution. Cyclooxygenases catalyze the rate limiting step in the conversion of arachidonate to prostaglandins, which act as mediators of inflammation. Cyclooxygenase related metabolic pathways can affect cell proliferation and differentiation as well as angiogenesis, which may underlie their roles in cancer. Specifically, COX-1 and COX-2 contribute importantly to limiting epidermal differentiation. Like WNT signaling, which occurs normally in developing cells, prostaglandin E_2 (PGE2) down-regulates the formation of an Axin/GSK3β/APC complex and hence stabilizes β-Catenin accumulation in the cytoplasm. This allows the up-regulation of several key transcription factors, including TCF-4, that maintain cells in a progenitor-like state. Targets of prostaglandin E_2 induced TCF-4 transcription include the mediators of cell growth and proliferation c-MYC, Cyclin D_1, PPARδ, and c-JUN. A deficiency of the *cox-1* or *cox-2* genes leads to abundant Keratin-1 and Keratin-10 expression in the epidermal basal cells and to premature onset of keratinocyte terminal differentiation (Tiano et al. 2002). By contrast, Cyclooxygenases are produced by pre-cancerous tissues, and some epithelial tumor cell types (esophageal, gastrointestinal, pancreatic, lung, head and neck, and prostatic cancers) as well as gliomata over-express COX-2. There is a role for COX-2 early in the progression of prostatic intraepithelial neoplasia lesions to prostate carcinoma.

Cyclooxygenase inhibitors (Fig. 3.17) either suppress the activities of both COX enzymes or act inhibitory preferentially on COX-2. The most substantial difference between the two forms of the enzyme, which allows for selective inhibition, is at position 523 the substitution of isoleucine in COX-1 with valine in COX-2. The smaller valine residue allows access to a hydrophobic side-pocket in the enzyme, which isoleucine sterically hinders.

Adverse Effects COX-1 promotes the production of the mucus lining in the stomach, contributes to reduced acid

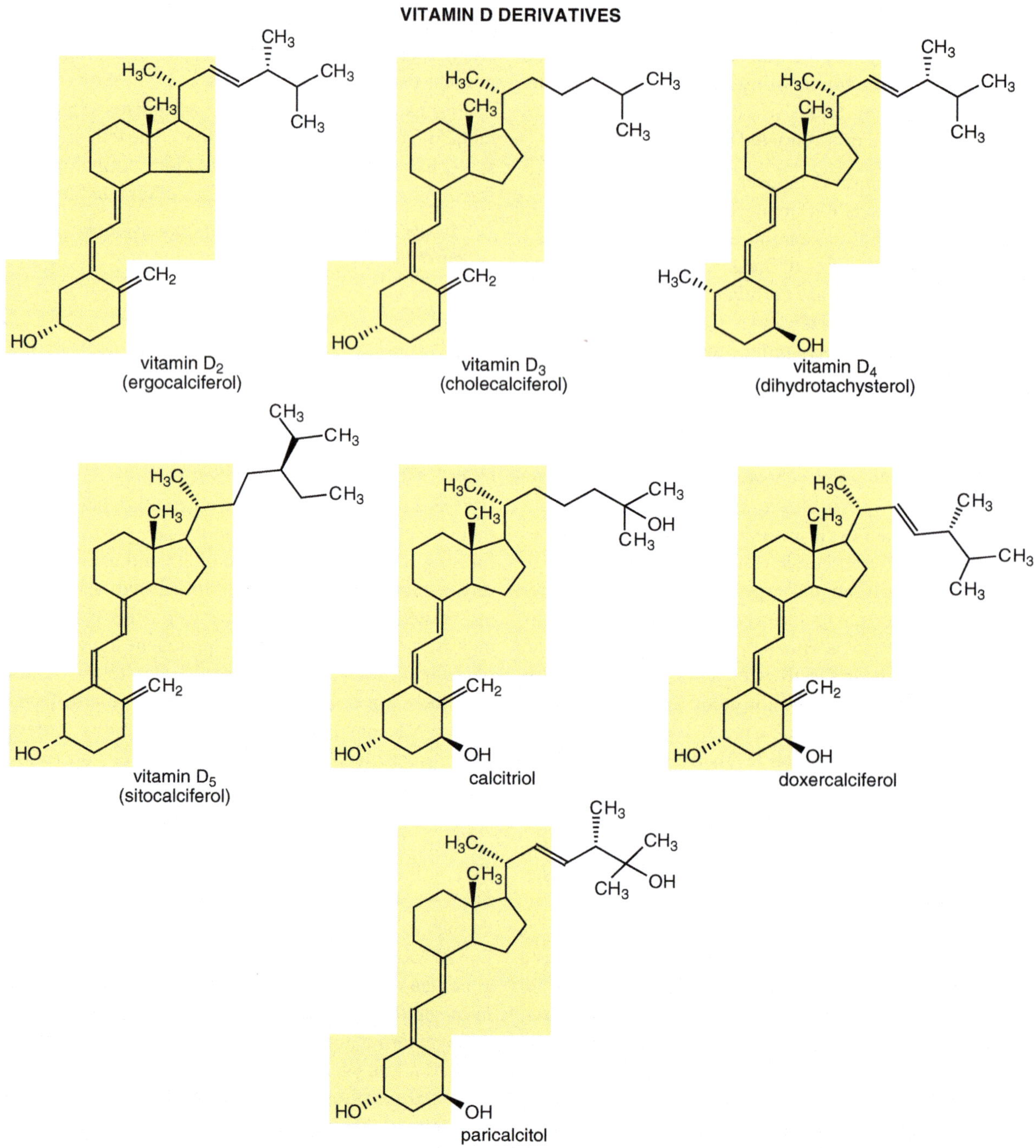

Fig. 3.16 Structures of vitamin D derivatives. Members of the vitamin D complex are shown in the top row. Vitamin D_1 is a molecular compound of ergocalciferol with lumisterol, and therefore does not have one structure. The common core structure of vitamin D derivatives is highlighted in *yellow*

secretion, and reduced Pepsin content. Therefore, the effectiveness of non-selective COX inhibitors, taken regularly for long period of time, is limited by the risk of serious—potentially life-threatening—gastrointestinal bleeding. Non-steroidal anti-inflammatory drugs (NSAIDs) that inhibit only COX-2 enzymes were created to allow patients to have relief from pain and inflammation while avoiding stomach bleeding. Selective COX-2 inhibition decreases inflammation with minimal gastroduodenal erosions and nephrotoxicity. However, prostaglandins act as regulators of coagulation and selective COX-2 inhibition may disturb the homeostasis of this mechanism. Adverse effects of selective COX-2 inhibitors include increased coagulation and an elevated risk for serious adverse cardiovascular events.

Non-selective COX inhibitors The daily intake of non-steroidal anti-inflammatory drugs, such as acetyl salicylate <Aspirin>, can reduce the risk for some skin cancers, breast

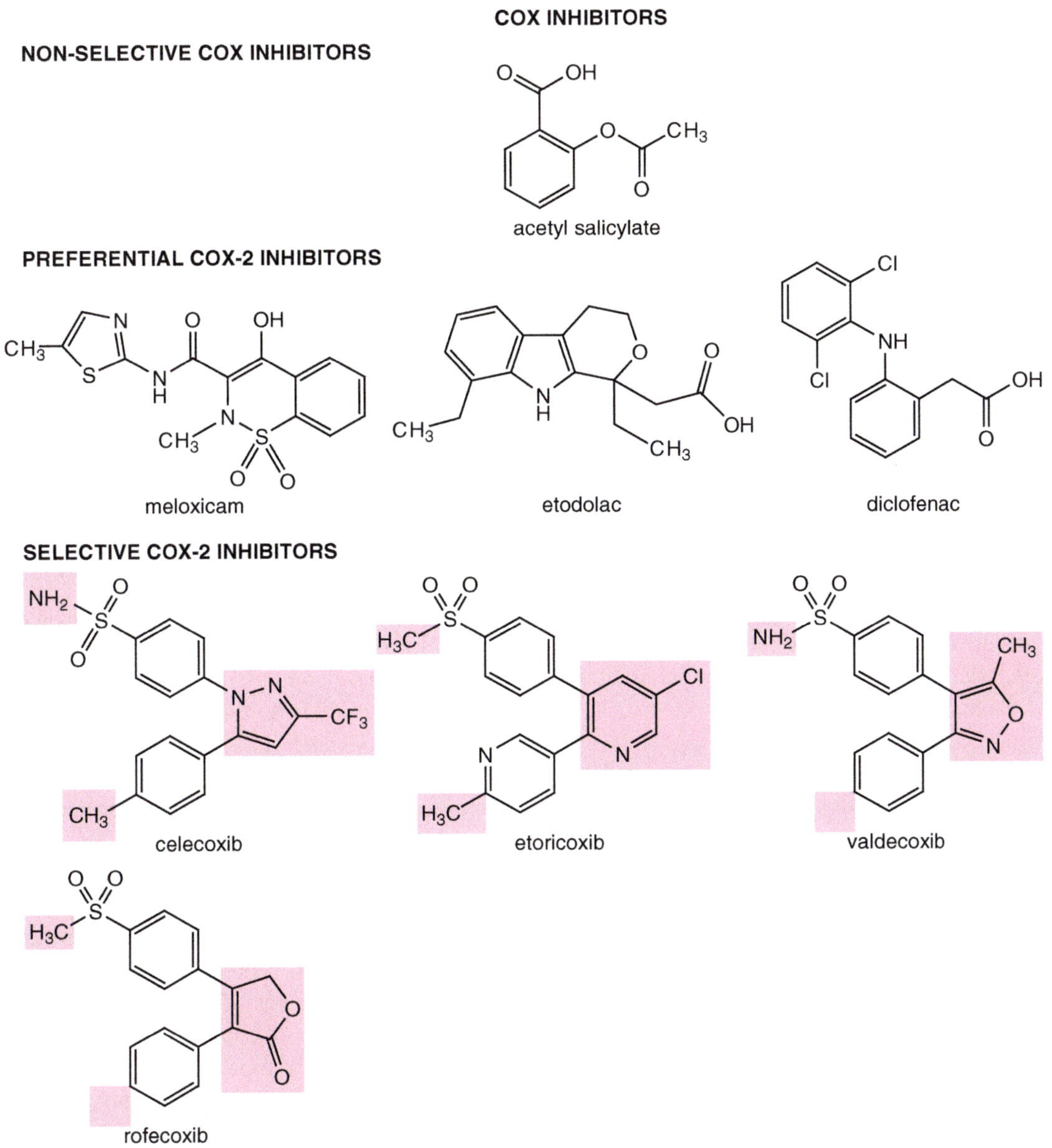

Fig. 3.17 Structures of *COX* inhibitors. Structural differences among the *COX-2* selective inhibitors are highlighted in *pink*

cancer, ovarian cancer, and prostate cancer, and may offer similar benefit in the prevention of colon and lung cancers. Further, the drug may be beneficial in the treatment of neoplastic disease in conjunction with conventional therapeutics. Salicylate decreases inflammation, which plays a role in cancer development. It also blocks platelet function. Platelets carry growth factors that may contribute to tumor growth in areas of tissue injury.

Preferential COX-2 inhibitors Meloxicam <Mobic> is an oxicam derivative and a non-steroidal anti-inflammatory drug with anti-pyretic and analgesic activities. Unlike non-selective drugs in this class, meloxicam preferentially inhibits the activity of COX-2, but does not have the specificity of the selective COX-2 inhibitors. The resulting decrease in prostaglandin synthesis is responsible for the therapeutic effects. Meloxicam is under investigation for the prevention or treatment of various cancers, including lung, colorectal, and prostate cancers, and extra-abdominal desmoid tumors.

Etodolac <Lodine> inhibition of Cyclooxygenase is preferentially active against COX-2. Through the regulation of protein and promoter activities, etodolac also increases the β-Catenin/E-Cadherin complexes in the cell membrane, which has an anti-metastasis effect. While generic versions may be available, the brand name <Lodine> has been discontinued in the U.S. Etodolac may suppress the expression of *thymidylate synthase*, thus sensitizing cancer cells to the effects of 5-fluorouracil.

Diclofenac (2-(2-(2,6-dichlorophenylamino)phenyl)acetic acid) <Aclonac, Cataflam, Voltaren> has a low to moderate preference to block COX-2 over COX-1. While the drug is commonly used to treat inflammatory disorders and dysmenorrhea, fever due to malignant lymphogranulomatosis (Hodgkin lymphoma) often responds to diclofenac, it has benefit in treating chronic pain associated with cancer, and the COX-2 suppressive effect may impact the process of transformation.

Selective COX-2 inhibitors COX-2 inhibitors (drug names ending on -coxib) are synthetic, non-steroidal derivatives of phenyl-furanone with anti-pyretic and analgesic properties that may induce apoptosis, inhibit tumor cell proliferation, and suppress angiogenesis. Inhibition of COX-2 may be particularly beneficial in the treatment of colon cancer.

Adverse Effects Non-steroidal anti-inflammatory drugs selective for the inhibition of COX-2 are less likely than non-selective non-steroidal anti-inflammatory drugs to cause gastrointenstinal adverse effects, but they can cause cardiovascular events, such as heart failure, myocardial infarction, and stroke, with a higher incidence.

Celecoxib (4-(5-(4-methylphenyl)-3-(trifluoromethyl)-1H-pyrazol-1-yl)benzenesulfonamide) <Celebrex> can reduce the risk of colon adenomata. In 1999, the U.S. FDA approved celecoxib for polyp prevention in patients with familial adenomatous polyposis (FAP). A 35–45 % polyp recurrence reduction may be achieved in people taking 400–800 mg per day. Celecoxib may induce apoptosis independently from its COX-2 inhibitory action via a mitochondrial apoptosis pathway that is not inhibited by over-expression of BCL-2. In addition, the drug exerts antagonistic effects on the anti-apoptotic proteins MCL-1 and Survivin. Consequently, the use of Celecoxib as single drug or in combination with radiotherapy, chemotherapy, or targeted pro-apoptotic drugs, may be of specific value for the treatment of apoptosis resistant tumors with over-expression of BCL-2, MCL-1, or Survivin.

A 2005 meta-analysis found that the addition of a COX-2 inhibitor may provide a survival benefit when used in combination with an Aromatase inhibitor in the neoadjuvant setting. In post-menopausal women with early breast cancer, etoricoxib <Arcoxia> plus anastrozole achieves a modest improvement in progression-free survival. Etoricoxib is also under study for the treatment or prevention of colorectal cancer, prostate cancer, and glioma.

Valdecoxib <Bextra> is about 300-fold more potent at inhibiting COX-2 than COX-1. It may suppress the proliferation of colon cancer cells.

- The drug has been formulated in microspheres (film coating with the pH sensitive polymer Eudragit S100, sodium alginate or chitosan as mucoadhesive polymer in the core) for the targeted delivery to colorectal cancer.

The addition of rofecoxib <Vioxx> to standard chemotherapy of colon cancer has not yielded a beneficial outcome. The drug has been withdrawn from the market due to its adverse effects.

Cyclooxygenase related metabolic pathways can affect cell proliferation and angiogenesis.
COX inhibitors (non-steroidal anti-inflammatory drugs, NSAIDs) have an anti-proliferative, pro-differentiating effect.
Non-selective COX inhibitors may cause gastro-duodenal ulcers, selective COX-2 inhibitors convey an increased risk for adverse cardiovascular events (myocardial infarction, stroke).

3.2.4 HDAC Inhibitors

Histone proteins organize the DNA into nucleosomes, which are regular repeating structures of chromatin. Nucleosomes contain 146 base pairs of DNA wrapped around a core Histone octamer, which is composed of two copies of each of H2A, H2B, H3, and H4. The linker Histone H1 stabilizes the assembly of the octameric core to higher order structures of chromatin. Because the chromatin structure limits the access of DNA binding proteins to the DNA, the regulation of gene transcription is controlled, in part, by distinct modifications to Histones that result in the opening or closing of the nucleosomes. In general terms, condensed chromatin mediates transcriptional repression, whereas transcriptionally active genes are in areas of open chromatin. The chromatin mediated repression is counteracted by acetylation, methylation, or phosphorylation of the NH_2-terminal tails of the Histones, which then interact with DNA regulatory proteins. Specifically, Histone Acetyl Transferases (HATs) and Histone Deacetylases (HDACs) (Table 3.1) determine Histone conformation, and thus the access of the transcriptional machinery to DNA. In addition to regulating access, Histone Acetyl Transferases function as transcriptional co-activators, and are recruited to chromatin by interacting with sequence specific DNA binding proteins.

The opposing actions of Histone Acetyl Transferases and Histone Deacetylases allow gene expression to be tightly regulated through chromatin remodeling. Aberrant transcription due to altered expression or mutation of genes that encode Histone Acetyl Transferases, Histone Deacetylases or their binding partners, may be a critical component in the onset and progression of cancer. In particular, loss of Histone Acetyl Transferase activity is associated with certain cancers. Histone Deacetylase inhibitors (HDAC inhibitors) (Fig. 3.18) can restore a balance, reactivating the expression of less than 10 % of all genes, including several that inhibit the growth and survival of tumor cells. These compounds induce Histone hyperacetylation, reactivate

Table 3.1 Classes of histone deacetylases. (Adapted from Wikipedia)

Class	Members	Catalytic sites	Subcellular localization	Tissue distribution	Substrates	Binding partners
I	*HDAC1*	1	Nucleus	Ubiquitous	Androgen Receptor, SHP, P53, MyoD, E2F1, STAT3	
	HDAC2	1	Nucleus	Ubiquitous	Glucocorticoid Receptor, YY1, BCL6, STAT3	
	HDAC3	1	Nucleus	Ubiquitous	SHP, YY1, GATA1, RELA, STAT3, MEF2D	
	HDAC8	1	Nucleus/cytoplasm			EST1B
IIA	*HDAC4*	1	Nucleus/cytoplasm	Heart, skeletal muscle, brain	GCMA, GATA1, HP1	RFXANK
	HDAC5	1	Nucleus/cytoplasm	Heart, skeletal muscle, brain	GCMA, SMAD7, HP1	REA, Estrogen Receptor
	HDAC7	1	Nucleus/cytoplasm/mitochondria	Heart, skeletal muscle, pancreas, placenta	PLAG1, PLAG2	HIF1A, BCL6, Endothelin Receptor, ACTN1, ACTN4, Androgen Receptor, TIP60
	HDAC9	1	Nucleus/cytoplasm	Brain, skeletal muscle		FOXP3
IIB	*HDAC6*	2	Mostly cytoplasm	Heart, liver, kidney, placenta	α-Tubulin, HSP90, SHP, SMAD7	RUNX2
	HDAC10	1	Mostly cytoplasm	Liver, spleen, kidney		
III	*sirtuins SIRT1, SIRT2, SIRT3, SIRT4, SIRT5, SIRT6, SIRT7*		Various	Various		
IV	*HDAC11*	2	Nucleus/cytoplasm	Brain, heart, skeletal muscle, kidney		

suppressed genes and have pleiotropic cellular effects that inhibit tumor cell growth and survival. All Histone Deacetylase inhibitors, in clinical use or in development, target the zinc molecule in the active site of the enzymes. Almost all inhibitors activate the transcription of the Cyclin-Dependent Kinase inhibitor *cdkn1A* ($P21^{CIP1/WAF1}$), which can inhibit Cyclin E/CDK2 and Cyclin A/CDK2 complexes. Many Histone Deacetylase inhibitors also down-regulate the Cyclins A and D. This results in hypo-phosphorylation of the tumor suppressor protein RB, and inhibition of S phase progression (G_1 arrest). The arrest of cells in G_1 is often associated with differentiation. Treatment with Histone Deacetylase inhibitors of cells deficient in CDKN1A (P21) (many cancers) results in an accumulation of cells with a polyploid DNA content and sensitization to apoptosis (Johnstone 2002). Histone Deacetylase inhibitors acetylate Histones in untransformed and tumor cells to the same extent. In response to treatment, untransformed cells activate a G_2 checkpoint and survive.

Drug Resistance The intrinsic pathway to apoptosis is important for the function of Histone Deacetylase inhibitors. Elevated levels of the anti-apoptosis protein BCL-2, which can block the intrinsic cell death pathway while leaving the death receptor pathway intact, suppress Histone Deacetylase inhibitor mediated apoptosis and convey resistance.

Hydroxamate-type HDAC inhibitors The essential structural characteristics of hydroxamic acid-based, hybrid polar compounds entail a polar site, the hydroxamic group, a 6-carbon hydrophobic methylene spacer, a second polar site, and a terminal hydrophobic group[3]. The catalytic sites of Histone Deacetylases have a tubular structure with a zinc atom at their base. Hydroxamate HDAC inhibitors fit into this structure with the hydroxamic moiety of the inhibitor binding to the zinc of the enzyme.

Vorinostat (suberoylanilide hydroxamic acid, SAHA) <Zolinza> is a synthetic agent that induces differentiation in some cell types. In contrast to other HDAC inhibitors, which act through the activation of Caspases, vorinostat can induce

[3] Compounds with substitution of the hydroxamic acid by a carboxylic acid or an amide oxime group are inactive, as are compounds with modification of the hydroxamic acid by introduction of a methyl group on an adjacent carbon or *N*-methylation. Although the benzene ring in the hydrophobic moiety may be modified in the meta and para positions, larger substituents are generally associated with loss of activity. The optimal methylene spacer has a chain length of 6, 5- and 7-carbon spacers being less active.

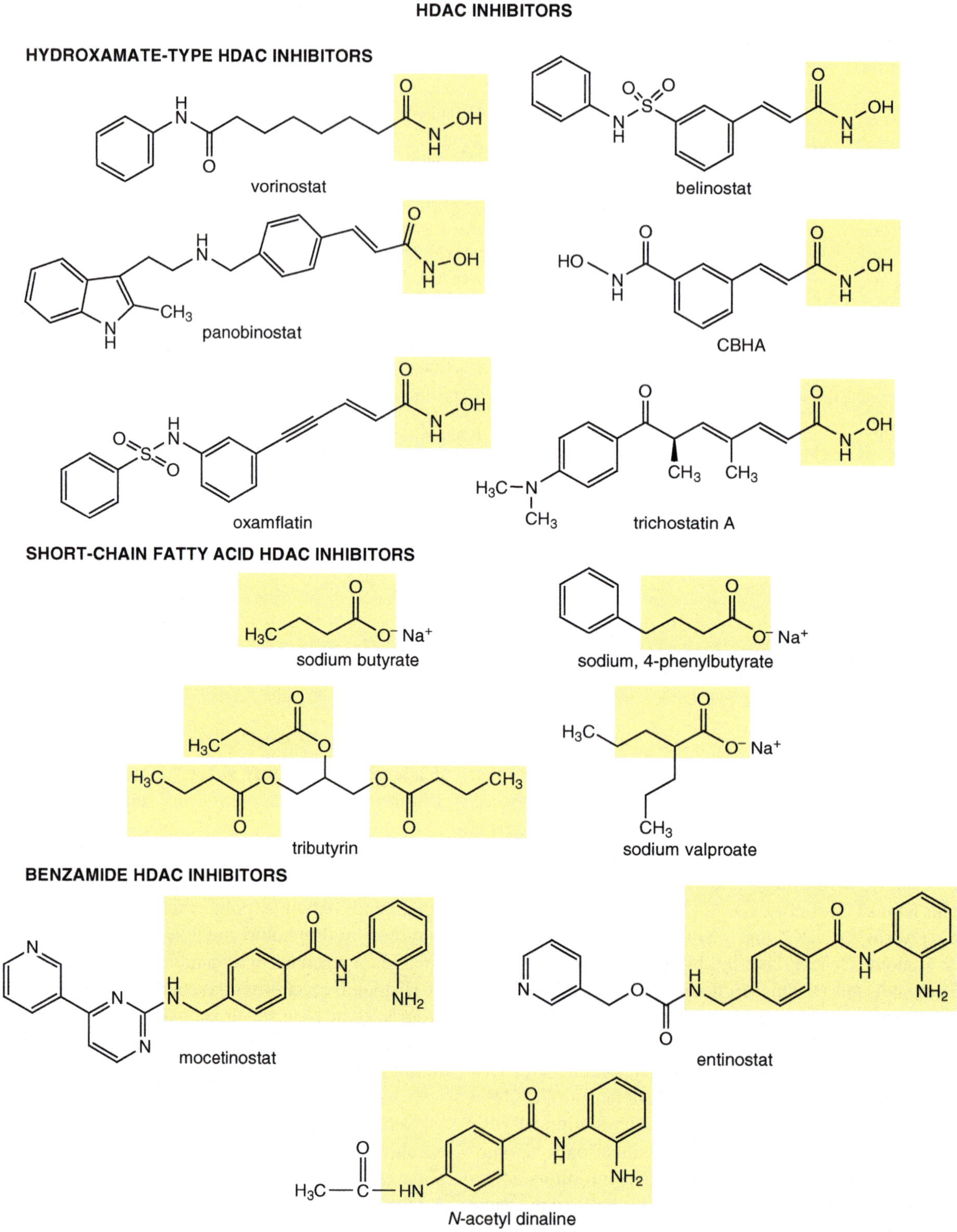

Fig. 3.18 Structures of *HDAC* inhibitors. There are four structural groups in the class. Highlighted in *yellow* are common moieties within the members of a group (hydroxamate in the hydroxamate-type *HDAC* inhibitors, butyrate in the short-chain fatty acid *HDAC* inhibitors, dinaline in the benzamide *HDAC* inhibitors, the peptide bonds in peptide *HDAC* inhibitors)

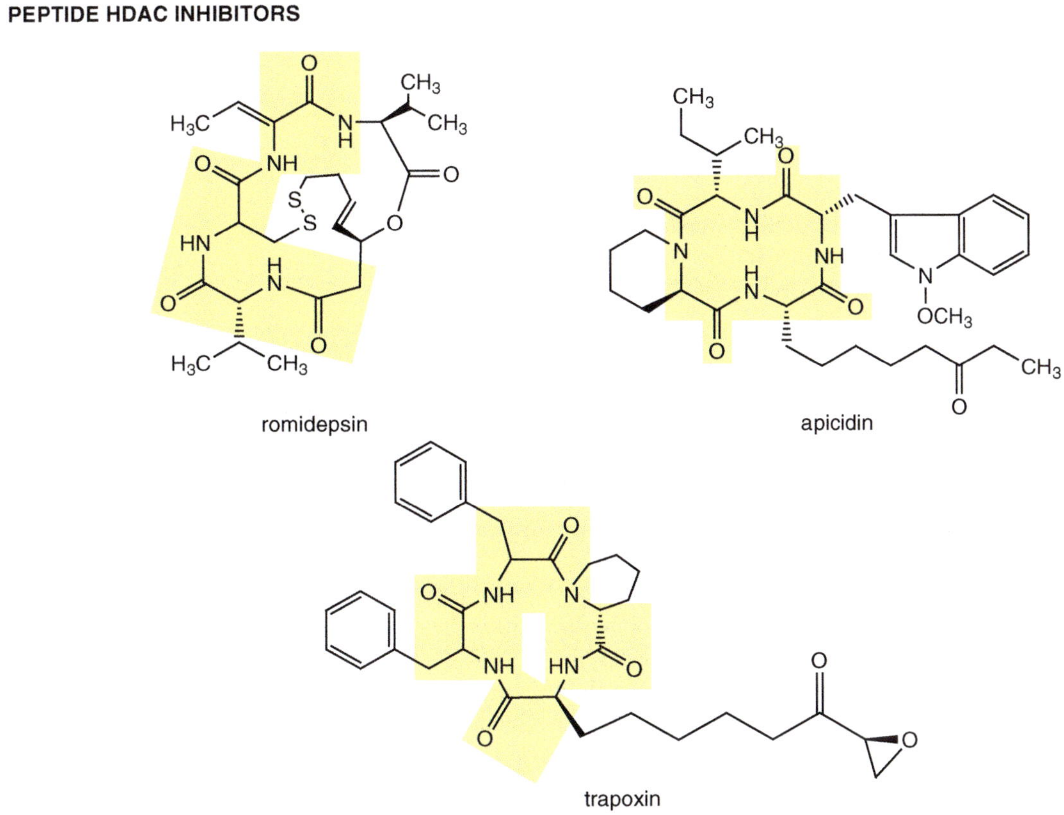

Fig. 3.18 (continued)

cell death in the absence of Caspase activation and independently of P53. The drug activates the intrinsic apoptotic pathway by inducing cleavage and activation of BID, resulting in mitochondrial membrane disruption and the production of reactive oxygen species (Ruefli et al. 2001). Vorinostat activates the expression of *cdkn1A* and represses *myb* and *myc*. In 2006, vorinostat became the first Histone Deacetylase inhibitor to be approved by the U.S. FDA. It is used to treat cutaneous T-cell lymphoma (CTCL) in patients whose disease has not improved, has worsened, or has relapsed after conventional treatment. The maximum tolerated dose is 250 mg when given 3 times daily for 14 days in a 21-day cycle.

Pharmacokinetics Vorinostat is orally bioavailable and crosses the blood-brain barrier. While the drug is not metabolized by and does not inhibit the Cytochrome P450 system, it is metabolized and excreted after glucuronidation by Uridine Diphosphate Glucuronosyl Transferase (UGT). Polymorphisms in the gene *ugt1A1*, which encodes for this enzyme, may be an important predictor of vorinostat toxicity and response levels in individual patients. However, hepatic dysfunction does not affect the pharmacokinetics of the drug.

Adverse Effects The most common adverse events are diarrhea, anorexia, fatigue, and nausea. Thrombocytopenia occurs in 25 %, anemia in 15 % of patients, and pulmonary embolism in rare cases. 5 % of patients experience grade 3–5 adverse events. The drug is Pregnancy Category D.

Because a high rate of adverse effects limits vorinostat as a single agent therapeutic, its combination with bortezomib <Velcade> has been tested with some success in experimental treatments.

Drug Interactions Patients also taking warfarin derivatives have a higher risk of bleeding due to prolonged prothrombin time. Patients also taking valproic acid or other HDAC inhibitors may develop severe thrombocytopenia and bleeding of the gastrointestinal tract.

Belinostat ((2*E*)-*N*-Hydroxy-3-[3-(phenylsulfamoyl)phenyl]prop-2-enamide) (PXD101) is in clinical trials for the treatments of T-cell lymphoma, liver cancer, and thymoma. The agent also inhibits angiogenesis. The recommended dose for hematologic neoplasia is 1000 mg/m^2/d intravenously on days 1–5 of a 21-day cycle. For solid tumors, the dose may reach 1200 mg/m^2/d over a 5-day cycle.

Adverse Effects Common adverse events comprise nausea, vomiting, diarrhea or constipation, loss of appetite and weight loss, fatigue, headaches, muscle aches, abnormal taste and dry mouth, hair loss, fever and chills, upper respiratory tract infection, cough, swelling in the lower extremities, and itching. Serious adverse effects may include deep vein thrombosis, pulmonary embolus, dehydration (particularly in conjunction with vomiting or diarrhea), low erythrocyte or platelet counts, and high blood sugar.

Drug Interactions Belinostat may sensitize drug resistant tumor cells to other anti-neoplastic agents, possibly through a mechanism involving the down-regulation of Thymidylate Synthase. Drug interactions are possible with valproate or warfarin.

Panobinostat (LBH589) <Faridak> is a cinnamic hydroxamic acid analog that induces the hyper-acetylation of core Histone proteins, which may result in a modulation of cell cycle protein expression, cell cycle arrest in the G_2/M phase, and apoptosis. In addition, this agent may modulate the expression of angiogenesis related genes, including *hypoxia inducible factor-1α* (*hif-1α*) and *vascular endothelial growth factor* (*vegf*), thus impairing endothelial cell migration. Panobinostat is in clinical trials for the treatments of cutaneous T-cell lymphoma, Hodgkin lymphoma, multiple myeloma, acute myeloid leukemia, and myelodysplastic syndromes. Its efficacy against breast and prostate cancers is under investigation. The drug is administrered orally or by intravenous infusion.

Adverse Effects Common toxicities include nausea, vomiting, diarrhea, loss of appetite, hypokalemia (muscle cramps, muscle aches, heart palpitations), and thrombocytopenia.

m-Carboxy cinnamic acid bishydroxamic acid (CBHA) may cause apoptosis by inducing the expression of the cell death triggering receptor/ligand pair *cd95* and *cd95L*. It is under investigation as an anti-cancer agent.

Oxamflatin ((2E)-5-[3-[(phenylsufonyl) aminol phenyl]-pent-2-en-4-ynohydroxamic acid) (Sonoda et al. 1996) is an aromatic sulfonamide derivative with a hydroxamic acid group. Through the HDAC inhibitory effect of oxamflatin, *gelsolin* and genes for CDK inhibitors such as *cdkn1A* are highly up-regulated. Oxamflatin suppresses *cyclin A* and *cyclin D*. It induces the transcriptional activation of *junD*, which enhances *fibronectin* expression via the cyclic AMP-responsive element (CRE) in the promoter of the *fibronectin* gene and competing for AP-1 sites of other growth associated genes.

Trichostatin A (TSA) is an organic compound that selectively and reversibly inhibits class I and II Histone Deacetylases (Fig. 3.19), but not class III Histone Deacetylases (Sirtuins). Trichostatin A inhibits the cell cycle during the beginning of the growth stage and alters gene expression. This compromises the ability of transcription factors to access the DNA molecules inside chromatin. Trichostatin A suppresses the expression of *cyclin-A*, *bcl-x_L*, *hif-1α*, and *vegf*.

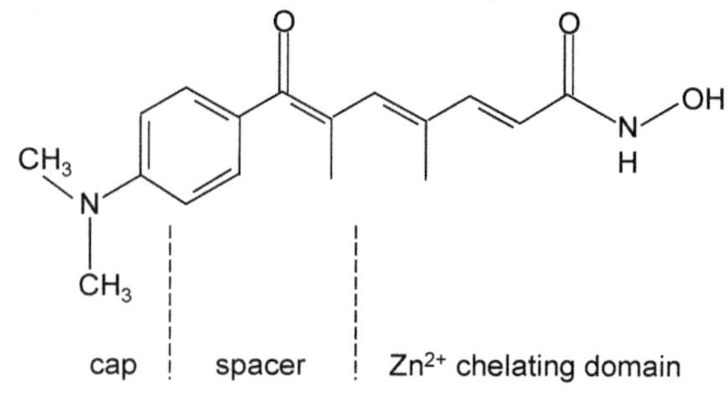

Fig. 3.19 Functional domains of trichostatin A. Trichostatin A chelates the Zn^{2+} in the catalytic pocket of Histone Deacetylase, which is crucial to the enzymatic activity. Its structure includes a cap group, a spacer, and a chelating motif. (redrawn from Zhou 2009)

Drug Resistance Resistance to trichostatin A may be caused by alterations in the target Histone Deacetylases.

Short-chain fatty acid HDAC inhibitors Butyrates induce the expression of *cdkn1A*, *bak*, *rar-β*, and *icam1*. They repress *cyclin-D1*, *cyclin-A*, *bcl2*, and *bcl-x_L*. Sodium butyrate is the prototype HDAC inhibitor (Riggs et al. 1977). It acts non-competitively, reversibly and specifically for Histone Deacetylase activity. This agent is compromised by a short plasma half-life and the requirement for millimolar concentrations for its action. Therefore, butyrates with more favorable pharmacodynamic and pharmacokinetic properties have been developed to form the class of short-chain fatty acid HDAC inhibitors.

Sodium phenylbutyrate is an orally active derivative of the short-chain fatty acid butyrate. 4-Phenylbutyrate inhibits Histone Deacetylase, resulting in the modulated expression of cell cycle genes, reduced cell proliferation, increased cell differentiation, and apoptosis. This agent also initiates the fragmentation of genomic DNA, resulting in decreased DNA synthesis. It is in development for the treatment of AML, CML, myelodysplastic syndrome, and advanced solid tumors.

Adverse Effects A biologically active dose of 0.5 mM can be attained with low grade fatigue, dyspepsia, hyperuricemia, or hypocalcemia. Other adverse reactions include neurocortical disturbances (somnolence, confusion, and tremor).

Tributyrin is a triglyceride prodrug of butyrate. The active metabolite inhibits Histone Deacetylase, resulting in increased differentiation, decreased proliferation, cell cycle arrest, and apoptosis in some tumor cell types.

Valproic acid was first synthesized by B.S. Burton in 1882. In 1962, Pierre Eymard discovered its anticonvulsant properties. Valproate (2-propylpentanoate) <Depakene, Depakote, Valparin, Stavzor, Myproate> also acts as HDAC inhibitor with some specificity for Histone Deacetylase-1. It activates *β-catenin* gene expression. By itself, valproate is a weak inducer of apoptosis. However, when combined with the NF-κB inhibitor parthenolide or the PKC inhibitor staurosporine it is a promising targeted therapeutic for cancer. Valproate has also been studied in combination with all-trans retinoic acid. With intravenous administration, the maximum tolerated dose is 60 mg/kg/d.

Adverse Effects Valproate is in clinical use as an anti-convulsant and anti-depressant. Accordingly, adverse effects in the treatment of cancer include neurocortical disturbances (somnolence, confusion, and tremor), which may be dose limiting. The exposure to valproate during pregnancy causes birth defects.

Benzamide HDAC inhibitors Mocetinostat (mecetinostat) (MGCD0103) is a class I specific HDAC inhibitor (mainly acting on Histone Deacetylase 1, but also on Histone Deacetylases 2, 3, and 11) in clinical trials for follicular lymphoma, Hodgkin lymphoma, and acute myelogenous leukemia. The drug is orally bioavailable.

Adverse Effects Dose limiting adverse effects comprise fatigue, nausea, vomiting, and diarrhea. Grade 3 toxicities may also include myelosuppression (neutropenia, thrombocytopenia, and anemia).

Entinostat (SNDX-275, MS-275) inhibits the class I Histone Deacetylases -1 and -3. This agent exerts growth arrest and differentiation through CDKN1A ($P21^{CIP1/WAF1}$). Entinostat in combination with the Aromatase inhibitor exemestane <Aromasin> has received breakthrough therapy designation[4] from the U.S. FDA for its potential to reverse resistance to hormonal therapies in advanced Estrogen Receptor-positive breast cancer. The maximum tolerated dose is 6 mg/m^2.

Adverse Effects Dose limiting toxicities are hypophophatemia, hyponatremia, hypocalcemia, hyperglycemia, and hypoalbuminemia, which are all reversible upon discontinuation of treatment. Common toxicities include injection site reactions, nausea and vomiting, constipation, fatigue, and cytopenias.

N-acetyl dinaline (tacedinaline) (CI994) is an orally active compound that inhibits Histone Deacetylases -1 and -2 and results in inhibition of cellular proliferation. The drug has a wide spectrum of potential anti-cancer activity. It is under investigation for combination therapy with conventional chemotherapeutics.

Peptide HDAC inhibitors Cyclic tetrapeptides containing a 2-amino-8-oxo-9,10-epoxy-decanoyl moiety (AOE moiety), as does as trapoxin A, can inhibit Histone Deacetylase activity. Some cyclic peptides, such as depsipeptide and apicidin, may also be HDAC inhibitors without containing the AOE moiety.

Depsipeptide[5] was first reported in the literature in 1994, by a team from Fujisawa Pharmaceutical Company in Tsukuba, Japan.

Depsipeptide (romidepsin) (FK228, FR901228) <Istodax> is a bicyclic tetrapeptide antibiotic isolated from Chromobacterium violaceum. It represents a highly stable prodrug, which has no catalytic activity until it is activated by Glutathione-mediated reduction within the cell. The reduction of its disulfide bond releases a thiol (Fig. 3.20) that binds to the zinc in the catalytic center of class I Histone Deacetylase enzymes and inhibits their activity. Thereby, the drug affects the regulation of gene expression and induces cell differentiation, cell cycle arrest, and apoptosis. As an anti-RAS agent, depsipeptide selectively decreases the expression of the *c-myc* proto-oncogene. It can induce HSP90 acetylation and inhibit the HSP90 interacting oncoproteins RAF-1, PKB (AKT), CDK4, and SRC. Depsipeptide also inhibits hypoxia-induced angiogenesis. In 2009, it was approved by the U.S. FDA for the treatment of CTCL, after 5 years in the agency's fast track development program. The maximum tolerated dose is 15 mg/m^2.

Pharmacokinetics The blood concentration time profile fits a 2-compartment model with a distribution phase half-time of 0.35 h, and a clearance phase half-time of 3.5–8 h.

Adverse Effects Adverse effects are generally mild (Piekarz et al. 2001). Commonly, they include nausea (65 %), fatigue (65 %), vomiting (40 %), and anorexia (40 %). Anemia, leucopenia, neutropenia, or thrombocytopenia may arise. Cardiotoxicity is possible.

Drug Resistance As depsipeptide is activated by Glutathione, it has strong potential for the treatment of cancers that are resistant to other drugs because of elevated Glutathione. Depsipeptide is a substrate for ABCB1 and ABCC1.

Apicidin is a fungal metabolite that exhibits potent broad-spectrum antiprotozoal activity and inhibits Histone Deacetylase activity at nanomolar concentrations. Apicidin induces *cdkn1A*, *cd95*, *cd95L*, and *gelsolin*.

The cyclic tetrapeptide trapoxin (cyclo-(L-phenylalanyl-L-phenylalanyl-D-pipecolinyl-L-2-amino-8-oxo-9,10-epoxy-decanoyl)) is a fungal product from Helicoma ambiens. It acts as a covalently binding, irreversible inhibitor of Histone Deacetylases. Trapoxin induces cell cycle arrest in the G_1 and G_2 phases. Two variants, trapoxin A and trapoxin B, are under study.

[4] The breakthrough therapy designation is intended to expedite the development and review of drugs for serious or life threatening conditions. The criteria for breakthrough therapy designation require preliminary clinical evidence that demonstrates the drug may have substantial improvement on at least one clinically significant endpoint over available therapy.

[5] Depsipeptides are peptides, in which some peptide bonds are replaced by ester bonds. Other members of the class of depsipeptides are kahalalide F, which affects mitochondria (see Sect. 3.3.1.) and didemnins, which inhibit protein turnover (see Sect.4.2.2.).

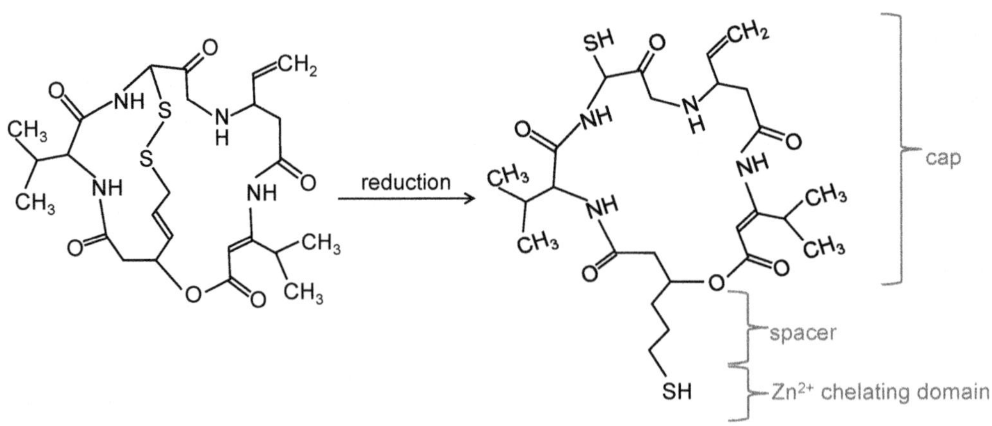

Fig. 3.20 Metabolic model for the activation of depsipeptide. Depsipeptide is inherently stable and devoid of catalytic activity, until it is taken up into cells and activated by Glutathione mediated reduction. It then is capable of inhibiting class I Histone Deacetylases. The active, reduced form of depsipeptide possesses a functional sulfhydryl group that fits inside the catalytic pocket of class I Histone Deacetylases, with resultant zinc chelation, and inhibition of the enzymatic activity. (redrawn from Zhou 2009)

Experimental HDAC inhibitors Chimeric proteins that contain Histone Acetyl Transferase or Histone Deacetylase recruitment domains fused to hairpin polyamides or zinc finger proteins that can be engineered to specifically target virtually any DNA sequence, have been employed experimentally to activate or silence specific genes. The successful use of these synthetic transcription factors in research settings raises the prospect that such agents might be therapeutically useful in the future (Dervan 1999; Mapp 2000; Liu et al. 2001).

Loss of Histone Acetyl Transferase activity is associated with certain cancers.
HDAC inhibitors can reactivate gene expression for growth inhibition and apoptosis.
HDAC inhibitors arrest untransformed cells at the G_2 checkpoint.
HDAC inhibitors activate the transcription of cdkn1A, leading to G_1 arrest and differentiation.
Suitable targets are cancers with lacking or altered Histone Acetyl Transferase activity, but not cancers with elevated BCL-2.
The main adverse effects of HDAC inhibitors are fatigue (cause for drug discontinuation in 30 %) and gastrointestinal toxicities (anorexia, nausea, vomiting, diarrhea).
Reversible disturbances of blood biochemicals and thrombocytopenia are common.

3.2.5 DNA Methyl Transferase Inhibitors

After the completion of S phase, DNA is covalently modified by methylation at the C5 positions of select cytosine bases, predominantly within CpG dinucleotides. The 4 DNA Methyl Transferases, DNMT1, DNMT2, DNMT3A, and DNMT3B, that catalyze this modification use a highly conserved catalytic mechanism. Further, these enzymes can directly recruit Histone Deacetylases, resulting in Histone deacetylation and transcriptional repression. In addition, methylated CpG islands are targeted by methyl-CpG binding proteins, such as MECP2, MBD1, MBD2, and MBD3, which can recruit HDACs and ATP-dependent chromatin-remodeling proteins to form a tightly condensed chromatin structure. DNA methylation and Histone modification are intricately interrelated, working together to determine the status of gene expression and cell fate.

In cancer, the silencing of key genes that are involved in controlling cell proliferation, survival, and tumor architecture often shows a strong causal relationship to aberrant DNA methylation. Global DNA hypo-methylation is closely linked to chromatin restructuring and nuclear disorganization in cancer cells, leading to chromosomal instability. Therefore, the treatment of cancer cells with demethylating agents can reactivate sets of genes, such as *p16*, *mlh1* (*mutL homolog-1*) and *rb* (*retinoblastoma*), that are often crucial in regulating cell proliferation, differentiation, apoptosis, and other key homeostatic mechanisms. In general, nucleoside inhibitors are more effective than non-nucleoside inhibitors in their inhibition of DNA methylation and in their reactivation of methylation-silenced genes. As there is an association between DNA methylation and Histone deacetylation, HDAC inhibitors (see Sect. 3.2.4.) display enhanced antitumor potential when acting synergistically with DNMT inhibitors (Fig. 3.21).

Nucleoside analog inhibitors Nucleoside analog DNMT inhibitors have a modified cytosine ring that is attached to either a deoxyribose or a ribose moiety[6]. They are metabolized by kinases that convert the nucleosides into nucleotides for

[6] They are structurally closely related to the cytidine analog anti-metabolites (see Sect. 2.4.2.).

incorporation into DNA or RNA. DNA methylation is inhibited when the drug compounds are incorporated into DNA.

During DNA reduplication, the DNA Methyl Transferases flip out cytosine rings from the double helix to form an intermediate complex, into which S-adenosyl-L-methionine is incorporated. In a normal cytosine ring, a methyl group is transferred from S-adenosyl-L-methionine to the C5 of the base and the enzyme is released in a β-elimination reaction. In the case of cytosine analogs, the modification at C5 of the ring prevents the release of the enzyme and results in the formation of a covalent complex. This prevents further methylation of the genome and, as a result, the DNA of the progeny cells is not methylated.

Oligodeoxynucleotides (including 5-azadeoxycytidine and 5-fluorodeoxycytidine) inhibit cytosine-C5 specific DNA Methyl Transferases (C5 Methyl Transferases). Ribonucleoside analogs (such as 5-azacytidine and zebularine) are phosphorylated by Uridine/Cytidine Kinase and other kinases into corresponding mono-, di- and triphosphates, which ultimately get incorporated into RNA.

The DNA hypo-methylating agent 5-aza-2'-deoxycytidine (AzadC, 5-AzaC) (NSC-127716) <Decitabine, Dacogen> is a cytidine anti-metabolite that incorporates into DNA and inhibits DNA Methyltransferase. The U.S. FDA has approved the drug for the treatment of elevated risk myelodysplastic syndrome. 5-aza-2'-deoxycytidine also has anti-pyrimidine properties, resulting in the hypo-methylation of DNA and intra-S phase arrest of DNA reduplication (see Sect. 2.4.2.).

Pharmacokinetics The drug is subject to deamination by Deoxycytidine Deaminase, and is thereby rendered inactive.

Adverse Effects Deoxycytidine analogs, such as 5-aza-2-deoxycytidine, are carcinogenic. Their dose limiting toxicity is neutropenia.

The deoxyribonucleoside analog 5-fluoro-2'-deoxycytidine (5-F-CdR, FdCyd) is phosphorylated by Deoxycytidine Kinase and other kinases, is incorporated into DNA, and inhibits DNA Methyl Transferase activity. However, it must be administered in combination with the Cytidine Deaminase inhibitor 3,4,5,6-tetrahydrouridine to prevent its rapid metabolism to the pharmacologically active, yet mechanistically different, metabolites 5-fluoro-2'-deoxyuridine (FdUrd), 5-fluorouracil (FU), and 5-fluorouridine (FUrd).

Substantial challenges to the clinical use of 5-azacytidine derivatives stem from the instability of these compounds in aqueous solutions as well as in their deamination by Cytidine Deaminase. Efforts to circumvent the problems of metabolic instability have yielded the dinucleotide SGI-110 (S110). The drug includes a deoxyguanosine in its structure, which makes it largely resistant to Cytidine Deaminase. SGI-110 exhibits DNA hypomethylation activity, thereby causing genome-wide non-specific hypomethylation and inducing cell cycle arrest in S phase. The agent is in clinical trials for the treatment of myelodysplastic syndromes and acute myelogenous leukemia.

Zebularine (1-β-d-ribofuranosyl-2(1*H*)-pyrimidinone) was synthesized in 1961 and characterized as an inhibitor of Cytidine Deaminase. Its demethylating activity was not recognized until 2003. Zebularine forms a covalent complex with DNA Methyl Transferase. Its deoxy form is not a good substrate for Deoxycytidine Kinase, so that zebularine is only incorporated into DNA via the Ribonucleotide Reductase pathway, which constitutes a rate liming step for the drug action. Zebularine is stable at acidic to neutral pH and in aqueous solution, and is less toxic than the 5-aza-nucleosides, making oral administration possible. However, the near millimolar dose requirement, mutagenicity, and limited bioavailability have been barriers to clinical use.

5-azacytidine (5-Aza-CR, azacitidine) <Vidaza> is a nucleoside analog with a ribose structure that gets incorporated into RNA and DNA via Ribonucleotide Reductase catalysis. It utilizes a covalent trapping mechanism, mediated by the nitrogen at position 5 of the nucleobase, for the inhibition of DNA Methyl Transferases. This triggers the proteasome mediated degradation of DNMT1. The compound possesses a hydrolytically unstable 5,6-imino bond, which limits its stability in aqueous solution and puts constraints on drug delivery. In 2004, the U.S. FDA approved 5-azacytidine for the treatment of elevated risk myelodysplastic syndrome.

Pharmacokinetics Subcutaneous administration has about 90 % bioavailability compared to intravenous injection. 5-azacytidine is subject to deamination by Cytidine Deaminase, and is thereby rendered inactive. Urinary excretion is the primary route of elimination of azacytidine and its metabolites.

Adverse Effects The most commonly occurring adverse reactions are leukopenia, anemia, thrombocytopenia, nausea and vomiting, pyrexia, injection site erythema, diarrhea or constipation, and ecchymosis. As a DNA damaging agent, 5-azacytidine has potentially carcinogenic properties.

5,6-dihydro-5-azacytidine (dihydro-5-azacytidine, DHAC) (NSC 264880) was developed to overcome the low stability of 5-azacytidine in water. It is hydrolytically more stable than 5-azacytidine and may be administered by prolonged intravenous infusion, potentially avoiding acute toxicities associated with the bolus administration of 5-azacytidine. However, 5,6-dihydro-5-azacytidine is about 10-fold less cytotoxic than 5-azacytidine. This may reflect the lack if inhibition of polysomal RNA synthesis by 5,6-Dihydro-5-azacytidine.

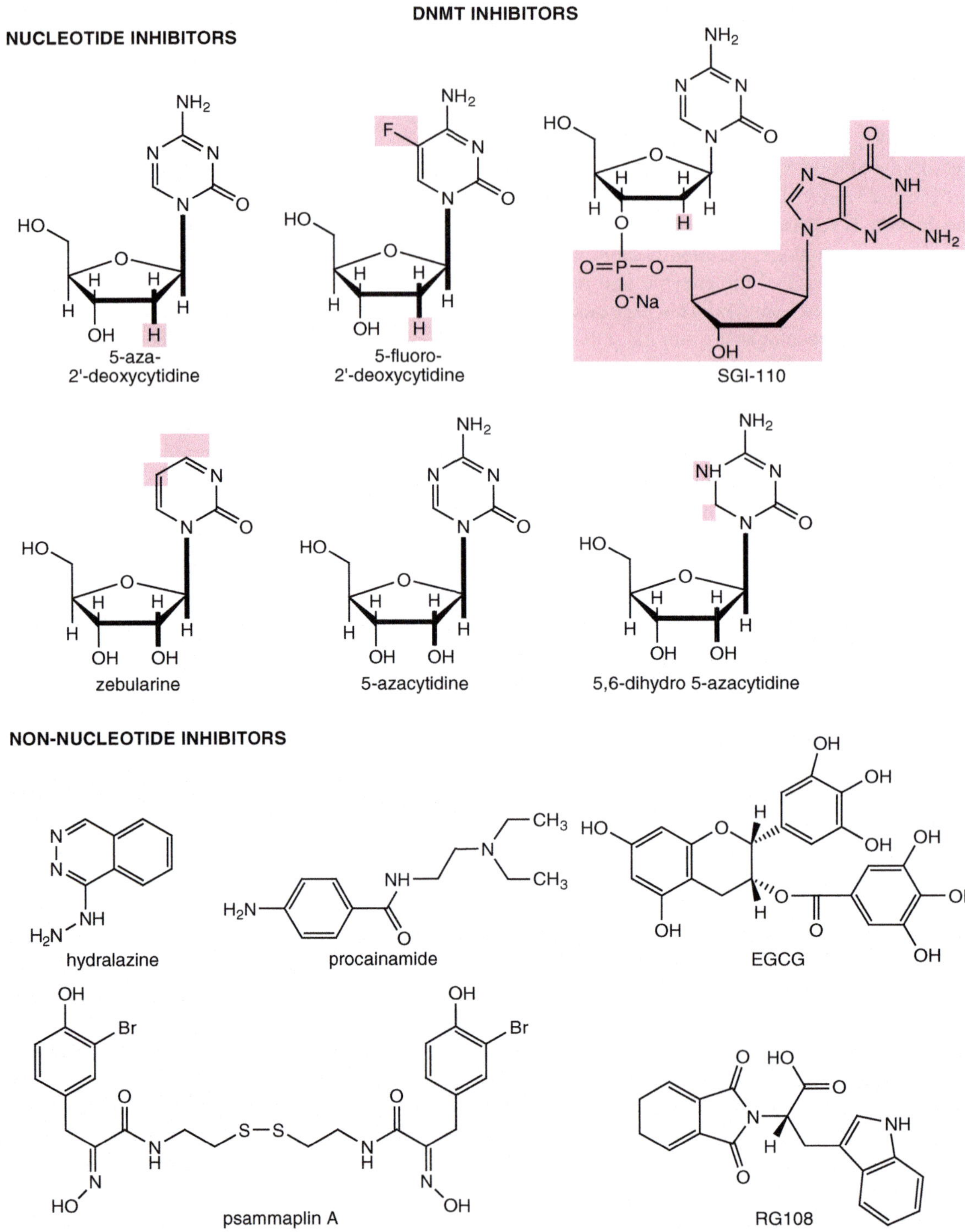

Fig. 3.21 Structures of DNMT inhibitors. Among the nucleotide inhibitors, structural differences from the parent compound 5-azacytidine are highlighted in *pink*. The non-nucleoside inhibitors are structurally diverse with no striking similarities

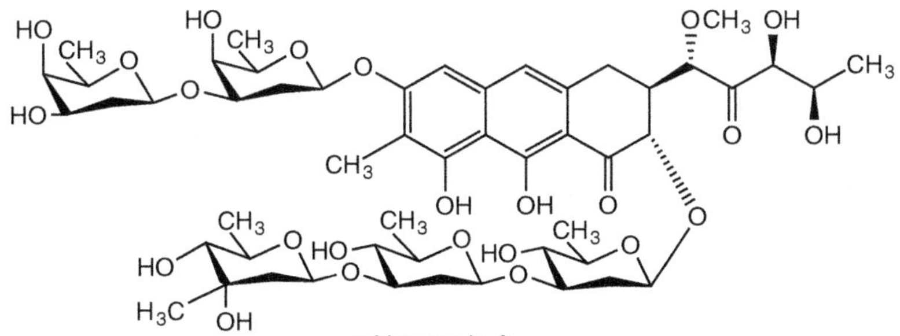

mithramycin A

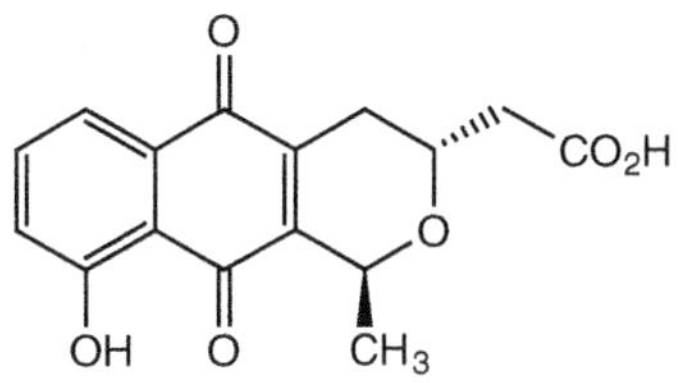

nanaomycin A

Fig. 3.21 (continued)

Pharmacokinetics Up to 20% of the administered dose is excreted unchanged in the urine.

Adverse Effects The maximum tolerated dose is 7 g/m^2, at which the limiting toxicity is pleuritic chest pain. Adverse effects include nausea and vomiting, which are not dose limiting.

Non-nucleoside analog inhibitors There are small molecules that inhibit DNA methylation. These non-nucleoside inhibitors may have advantages over nucleoside inhibitors because they suppress DNA methylation by binding directly to the catalytic region of the DNA Methyl Transferase enzyme, without being incorporated into DNA.

Hydralazine is a vasodilator that serves clinically as an anti-hypertensive drug. It was first reported in 1988 (Cornacchia et al. 1988) to inhibit DNA methylation, which results from an interaction between its nitrogen atoms and residues lysine 162 and arginine 240 of the DNA Methyl Transferase active site. Hydralazine also decreases the expression of the DNA Methyl Transferases DNMT1 and DNMT3A.

Adverse Effects Hydralazine toxicities are mild, most commonly entailing nausea, dizziness, fatigue, headache, and palpitations. It induces autoimmunity. The hypotensive effects of the drug may limit its use.

Procainamide <Pronestyl, Procan, Procanbid> is in clinical use as an anti-arrhythmic. It was first reported in 1988 to have inhibitory properties for DNA methylation. Procainamide is a partially competitive, specific inhibitor of DNMT1, reducing the affinity of the enzyme for its substrates, hemi-methylated DNA and S-adenosyl-L-methionine. Procainamide is administered intravenously or orally.

Adverse Effects Adverse effects include rash, hypersensitivity reactions with fever and agranulocytosis, myalgia, and (rarely fatal) proarrhythmic events. After long-term use, drug induced lupus erythematosus can arise (particularly in slow acetylators) because of anti-nuclear antibody production. After parenteral administration, there may be pain, swelling, or redness at the injection site.

EGCG ((–)-Epigallocatechin-3-gallate), the major polyphenol in green tea, has chemopreventive activity. It directly inhibits DNA Methyl Transferase enzymes and reactivates methylation-silenced genes such as *rarβ* and *p16*. The drug binds and inhibits the anti-apoptotic protein BCL-x_L, which contributes to cell survival. EGCG suppresses the expression of the heat shock proteins HSP70 and HSP90. It also modifies the association of HSP90 with several co-chaperones such as P23 and HSC70. It functionally inhibits Glucose-Regulated Protein 78 (GRP78), a member of HSP70 family, by competing with ATP for binding to the GRP78 active site. EGCG—along with other flavonoids—can be beneficial in treating brain, prostate, cervical, and bladder cancers.

Drug Interactions The consumption of green tea and EGCG should be strongly contraindicated for patients undergoing treatment for multiple myeloma and mantle cell lymphoma. EGCG binds to the anti-cancer drug bortezomib <Velcade>, significantly reducing its bioavailability and thereby rendering it therapeutically useless. EGCG may reduce the bioavailabilty of sunitinib <Sutent> when they are taken together.

Psammaplins comprise a family of bromotyrosine derivatives extracted from marine sponges, such as Pseudoceratina purpurea. They can inhibit both DNA Methyl Transferases and Histone Deacetylases. Psammaplin A (bisprasin) (NSC-614495) was originally isolated in 1987 from the Psammaplysilla sponge. It is a symmetrical disulfide dimer. In addition to suppressing DNA Methyl Transferases and Histone Deacetylases, psammaplin A may exhibit inhibition of Topoisomerase 2, Farnesyl Protein Transferase, and Leucine Aminopeptidase, all of which enhance its anti-tumor activity. The agent is active against cells that over-express ABCB1. However, its insolubility in water poses limitations.

RG108 (2-(1,3-dioxo-1,3-dihydro-2*H*-isoindol-2-yl)-3-(1*H*-indol-3-yl)propanoic acid) is a small molecule inhibitor that was rationally designed based on molecular modeling. It specifically fits into the catalytic pocket of DNMT1 and renders the enzyme inactive. RG108 causes demethylation and reactivation of tumor suppressor genes, but it does not affect the methylation of centromeric satellite sequences.

The antibiotic mithramycin A reduces DNA methylation at tumor suppressor gene CpG islands, resulting in tumor suppressor gene reactivation. Exposure to the drug leads to DNMT1 depletion as well as decreased mobility of cancer cells. Mithramycin A also acts by binding to C/G-rich DNA tracts in the minor groove (see Sect. 2.2.2.).

Pyranoquinone antibiotics are produced by various Streptomycin species. Nanaomycin A is a pyranonaphthoquinone antibiotic from strain OS-3966 of Streptomyces rosa var. notoensis. It selectively inhibits DNMT3B, substantially inhibits cytosine methylation in cells, and result in the re-expression of the tumor suppressor gene product RASSF1A.

MG98 is a second generation, mixed-backbone, phosphorothioate antisense oligodeoxynucleotide directed to the 3' untranslated region of the *DNA methyl transferase-1* (*(cytosine-5)-methyl transferase 1*) mRNA. The agent prevents the mRNA translation to DNMT1. This silencing may result in the prevention or reversal of the abnormal methylation of tumor suppressor genes and ultimately in tumor growth inhibition or tumor regression. MG98 is in clinical trials.

Aberrant DNA methylation is associated with tumor suppressor gene silencing in cancers.
Treatment with demethylating agents can reactivate crucial genes for regulating cell proliferation, differentiation, and apoptosis.
HDAC inhibitors display enhanced anti-tumor potential when they act synergistically with DNMT inhibitors.
Nucleoside analogs have a modified cytosine ring attached to a ribose or a deoxyribose moiety.
Deoxycytidine analogs are potentially carcinogenic. Their dose limiting toxicity is neutropenia.

3.2.6 PPAR Activators

Peroxisome Proliferator-Activated Receptors (PPARs) belong to the nuclear hormone receptor super family. They function as receptors for extracellular signals and also as transcription factors that activate specific genetic programs. There are three sub-types, PPARα, PPARβ, and PPARγ. PPARs bind to DNA in hetero-dimers with Retinoid X Receptors (RXRs) and bind to PPREs (Peroxisome Proliferator hormone response elements) on the DNA of target genes. PPARs play a role in the regulation of cancer cell growth.

Activators of PPAR in the class of thiazolidinediones (drug names ending on -glitazone) are in use for the treatment of type 2 diabetes because they facilitate the transcription of Insulin response genes. These agents are under study for cancer therapy because they suppress the expression of Cyclin D1 via transcriptional repression. They may be beneficial in chemoprevention and in increasing the effectiveness of chemotherapy drugs, such as platinum compounds, when administered together.

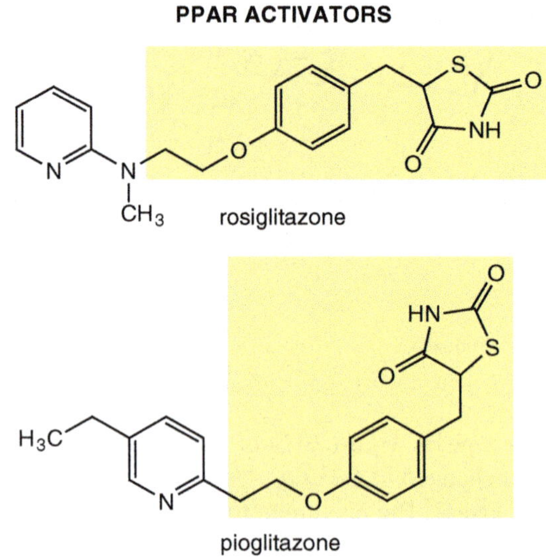

Fig. 3.22 Structures of *PPAR* activators. The drug names end in -glitazone. The common structural motif is highlighted in *yellow*

Rosiglitazone maleate <Avandia> is a salt of an orally active thiazolidinedione (Fig. 3.22). Rosiglitazone engages the ligand activated transcription factor PPARγ (Peroxisone Proliferator-Activated Receptor γ), thereby inducing cell differentiation and suppressing cell growth. This agent also inhibits macrophage and monocyte activation, and it acts as an Insulin sensitizer that is used to treat type 2 diabetes.

Adverse Effects Rosiglitazone bears an elevated risk of cardiovascular events, stroke, macular edema, and bone fractures of the upper arms, hands and feet.

Pioglitazone <Actos, Glustin> is a thiazolidinedione that selectively stimulates the nuclear receptor PPARγ. It modulates the transcription of Insulin ensitive genes involved in the control of glucose and lipid metabolism in the lipidic tissues, the muscular tissues, and the liver.

Adverse Effects Pioglitazone may be associated with and increased risk of bladder cancer.

PPAR activators have potential in chemoprevention and in enhancement of chemotherapy effectiveness.
They induce cell differentiation and suppress cell proliferation.

3.3 Inducers of Apoptosis

Proto-oncogene products promote cell survival and proliferation. Tumor suppressor gene products antagonize the proto-oncogene effects either by activating cell cycle checkpoints or by inducing apoptosis. The abnormal growth rate of cancerous cells is mediated by the activation of genetic programs that promote cell cycle progression and overcome the otherwise dominant control mechanisms of cell cycle arrest and apoptosis.

3.3.1 Modulators of Mitochondrial Function

Mitochondria constitute general integrators of various pro-apoptotic signals. They respond to apoptosis inducing events with the release of the mediator molecules (Cytochrome *c*, AIF, or SMAC/DIABLO) and converge on common apoptotic pathways consisting of effector molecules (P53, Caspases, Nucleases). Mitochondria may also procure cell death through the alteration of cellular reduction-oxidation potential (redox potential), the disruption of electron transport and ATP generation (Fig. 2.23). In various cancers, mitochondrial mechanisms of apoptosis induction are impaired and their re-establishment is a potential treatment strategy.

During programmed cell death, various cellular proteins translocate to or from the mitochondria. BCL2 normally blocks mitochondrial pores and prevents Cytochrome *c* release. In apoptosis, it is removed from the mitochondria. P53 may mediate its apoptosis inducing function not only through transcriptional regulation, but also through translocation into the mitochondria.

S-dimethylarsino-Glutathione (darinaparsin) (ZIO-101) is an organic arsenic compound composed of the antioxidant Glutathione combined with dimethylarsenic. The drug targets the mitochondria, where it disrupts electron transport and induces intracellular reactive oxygen species. The resulting changes in mitochondrial membrane potential induce G_2/M arrest and lead to Caspase dependent apoptosis. S-dimethylarsino-Glutathione has a more favorable therapeutic index than inorganic arsenic compounds. The agent is orally bioavailable. It is in clinical trials for multiple myeloma, leukemias, and solid tumors.

Mitochondria harbor a robust transmembrane potential. The low conductance state of the permeability transition pore complex may regulate the exchange of small metabolites between the cytosol and the mitochondrial matrix. Within the permeability transition pore complex, ANT1 and ANT3 are pro-apoptotic, whereas ANT2 (which is often over-expressed in proliferating cells) is anti-apoptotic.

Adenine Nucleotide Translocase (ANT) ligands may induce apoptosis through mitochondrial disruption. 4-(*N*-(S-glutathionylacetyl)amino)phenylarsonous acid (GSAO), a Glutathione coupled trivalent arsenical compound, cross-links the critical cysteine residues 160 and 257 of ANT, resulting in the inhibition of its ATP/ADP antiporter activity, reactive oxygen species over-production, cytosolic ATP depletion, mitochondrial depolarization and apoptosis. GSAO may preferentially target proliferating cells due to their high mitochondrial Ca^{2+} levels and elevated respiration rates, which renders them more susceptible to permeability transition pore complex opening than normal cells. The relative selectivity of GSAO for the endothelial component of tumors may be related to their higher amounts of mitochondria compared to tumor cells and may have a reduced capacity to buffer the arsenical moiety of GSAO.

Thioredoxin Reductase, over-expressed in many cancer cell types, inhibits apoptosis, promotes cell growth, and plays a role in resistance to chemotherapy. The enzyme catalyzes the reduction of oxidized thioredoxin and plays an essential role in regulating cellular redox homeostasis. Auranofin <Ridaura> is an orally available, lipophilic, organogold compound. It interacts with a selenocysteine residue within the redox-active domain of mitochondrial Thioredoxin Reductase, thereby blocking its activity. The resulting mitochondrial oxidative stress leads to the induction of apoptosis. Auranofin also inhibits the JAK1/STAT3 signal transduction pathway. While the agent is used to treat rheumatoid arthritis, its potential anti-neoplastic activity is under study.

Lonidamine, an indazole carboxylate, is a putative ANT ligand that triggers apoptosis. The drug may also suppress aerobic glycolysis in cancer cells, but enhance it in untransformed cells, likely through the inhibition of the mitochondrial Hexokinase. This causes a decrease in cellular ATP. The addition of lonidamine to the anthracycline epirubicin increases the response rate of patients with solid tumors, but the agent has no additional effects when combined with an epirubicin/cyclophosphamide regimen. Lonidamine is in clinical trials for the treatment of brain and prostate cancers.

Zalcitabine (Fig. 3.24) was first synthetized in the 1960s by Jerome Horwitz. Zalcitabine (2'3'-dideoxycytidine, ddC) <Hivid> is a synthetic nucleoside analog of pyrimidine, in which the 3' hydroxyl group on the sugar moiety is replaced by a hydrogen. This modification prevents the formation of phosphodiester linkages which are needed for the completion of nucleic acid chains. After intracellular phosphorylation to its active metabolite, zalcitabine preferentially inhibits the γ form of DNA Polymerase that is present in mitochondria, resulting in the inhibition of mitochondrial DNA reduplication and tumor cell death. Zalcitabine is in clinical use as an anti-retroviral drug.

Pharmacokinetics The oral bioavailability is over 80%, but is reduced when administered with food. The maximum plasma concentration is reached after 0.8 h (fasting) to 1.6 h (with food). The agent penetrates the blood-brain barrier. The mean elimination half-life of zalcitabine is 2 h. Only about 15% of the administered drug undergoes metabolism to dideoxyuridine (ddU) in the liver. Renal excretion of

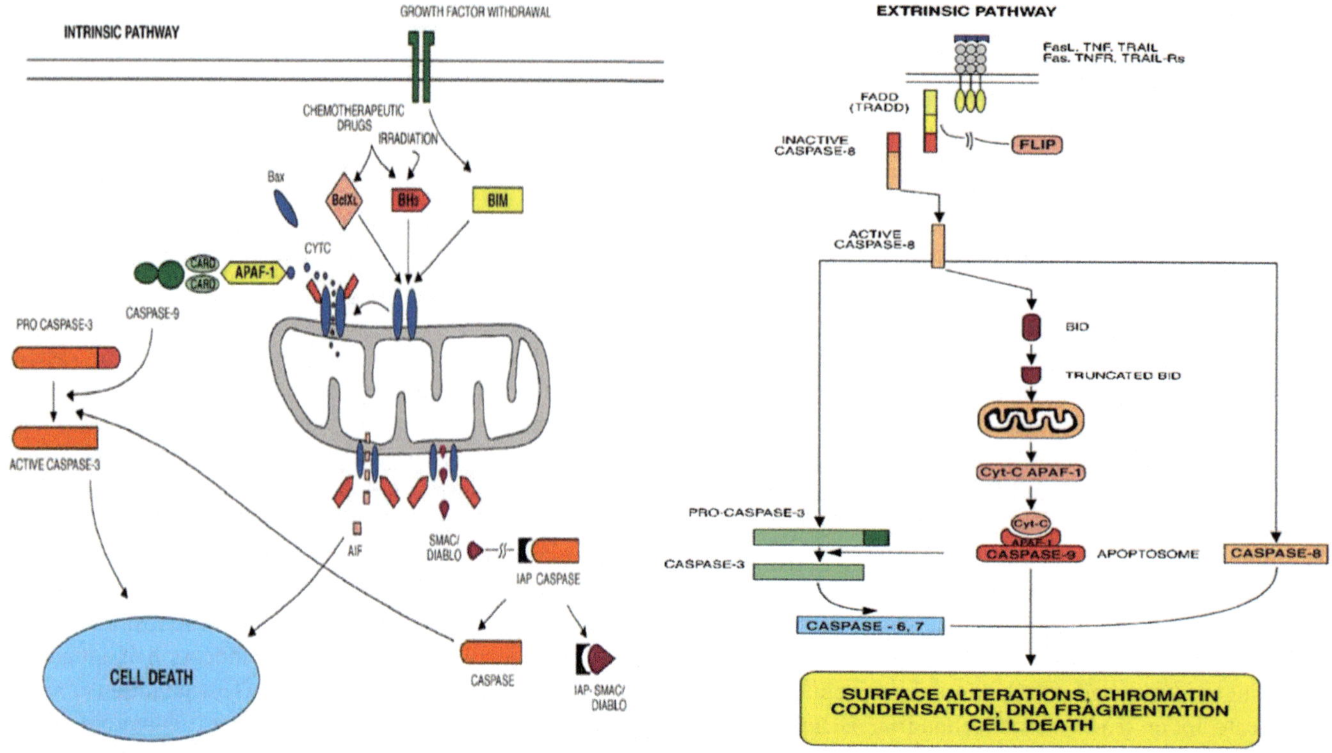

Fig. 2.23 Extrinsic and intrinsic pathways to apoptosis. (*Left*) the intrinsic pathway is induced by stimuli such as DNA damage or endoplasmic reticulum stress. It activates BH3-only proteins, leading to mitochondrial outer membrane permeabilization. (*Right*) the extrinsic pathway is triggered by the engagement of death receptors on the cell surface by their cognate ligands. Apoptosis proceeds via permeabilization of the mitochondria. Both pathways converge on the release of Cytochrome *c* into the cytoplasm. Cytochrome *c* then recruits a multiprotein complex in the apoptosome and initiates activation of the Caspase cascade through Caspase 9. (Testa 2004 with permission)

unchanged drug is the primary route of elimination, accounting for approximately 80 % of an intravenous dose and 60 % of an oral dose. Renal clearance exceeds the glomerular filtration rate, suggesting that tubular secretion contributes to the elimination of zalcitabine by the kidneys. Approximately 10 % of an orally administered dose of zalcitabine appears in the feces, comprised primarily of unchanged drug and dideoxyuridine.

Adverse Effects The most common adverse events at the beginning of treatment comprise nausea and headache. More serious adverse events are oral or esophageal ulcers. The drug can cause serious peripheral neuropathy. In rare cases, pancreatitis may arise. Lactic acidosis or severe hepatomegaly with steatosis are possible with the use of nucleoside analogs. High doses of zalcitabine induce an increased incidence of thymic lymphoma. The drug is Pregnancy Category C.

Drug Interactions Zalcitabine should not be used with other drugs that can cause peripheral neuropathy, such as cisplatin, vincristine, certain anti-infective drugs (aminoglycosides, amphotericin, chloramphenicol, nitrofurantoin, dapsone, isoniazid, ethionamide, metronidazole, iodoquinol), the anti-alcoholism drug disulfiram, gold, the smooth muscle relaxant hydralazine, the sedative glutethimide, the anti-epileptic phenytoin, or anti-retroviral nucleoside analogs. Death due to fulminant pancreatitis is possible if intravenous pentamidine is given with zalcitabine. Concomitant administration of probenecid or cimetidine decreases the elimination of zalcitabine, most likely by inhibiting the renal tubular secretion of zalcitabine. Because lamivudine inhibits the intracellular phosphorylation of zalcitabine to its active form it should not be administered simultaneously.

Kahalalide F is a natural depsipeptide isolated from the Hawaiian herbivorous marine mollusk Elysia rufescens. Like other Kahalalides, it is likely a secondary metabolite synthesized by the mollusk from peptides produced by a diet of the green alga Bryopsis pennata. Kahalalide F induces a loss of mitochondrial membrane potential and of lysosomal integrity. The agent has cytotoxic activity against solid tumor cells, including prostate, breast and colon carcinomas, chondro- and osteosarcomata, and neuroblastoma, with untransformed cells being severalfold less sensitive.

Adverse Effects The dose limiting toxicity is transaminitis.

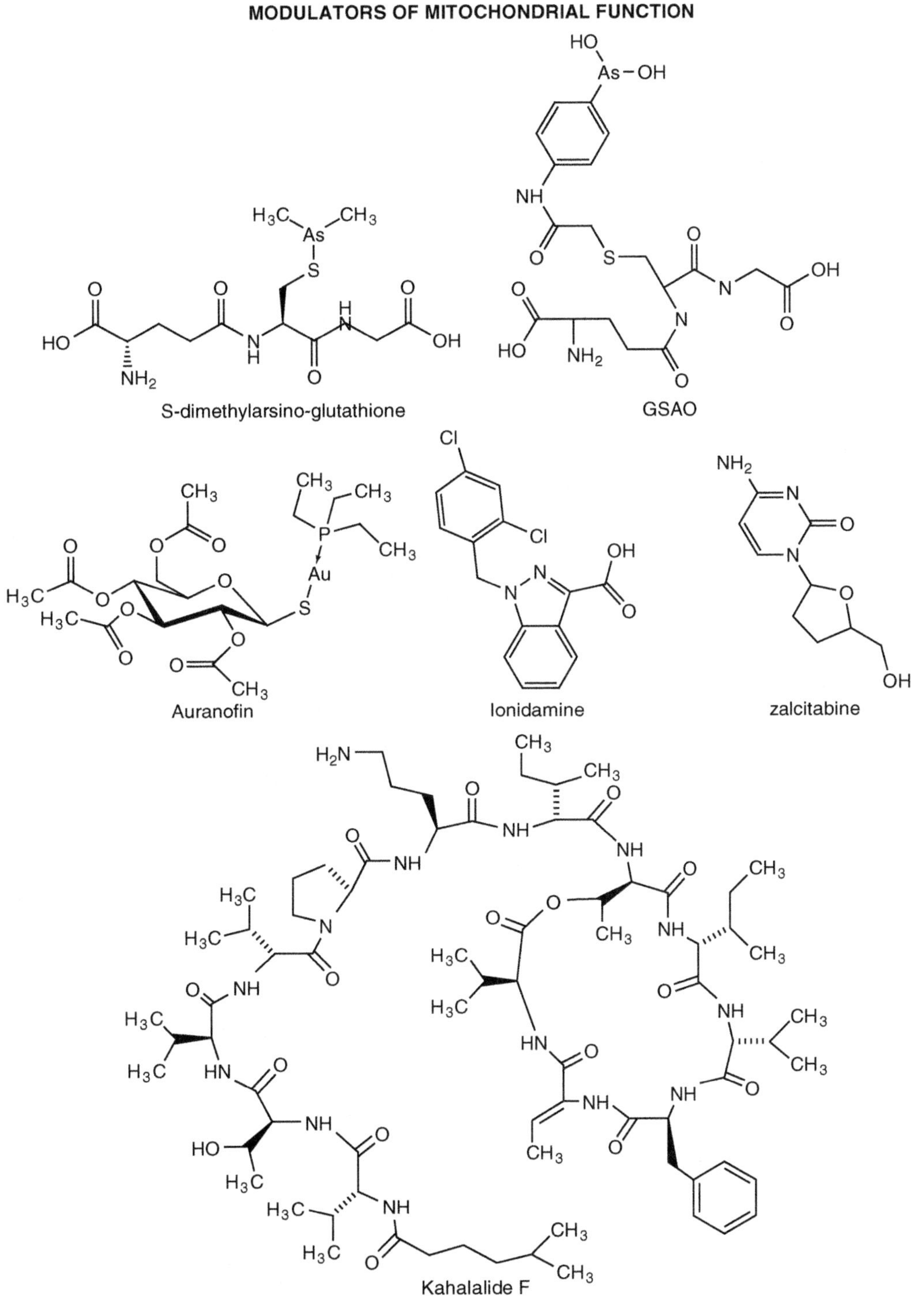

Fig. 3.24 Structures of modulators of mitochondrial function. The drugs act in a pro-apoptotic manner through various mechanisms

3.3.2 BCL-2 Family Inhibitors

The cellular pathways to apoptosis are controlled by regulatory molecules, including BCL family members. The ratio of anti-apoptotic to pro-apoptotic representatives in this protein family is important in determining whether programmed cell death proceeds. Excess death antagonists promote survival, whereas excess death agonists promote apoptosis. The BCL-2 subfamily regulates pore formation in the mitochondria. The release of pro-apoptotic substances into the cytoplasm is facilitated by opening of the permeability transition pore, which is normally blocked by BCL-2. BCL-2 can maintain organelle integrity by preventing the pore formation induced by the death agonist BAX, thus blocking the release of Cytochrome *c* from mitochondria. The over-expression of the pro-survival protein BCL-2 in cancer cells prevents the permeability transition and protects from apoptosis. This underlies the development of BCL-2 antagonists as anti-cancer agents.

Oblimersen sodium (G3139) <Genasense, Augmerosen> was the first antisense agent targeting *bcl-2* mRNA to enter clinical trials. Oblimersen is a 18-mer phosphothioate oligodeoxynucleotide that targets the first 6 codons of the *bcl-2* open reading frame. It is under investigation in combination with conventional chemotherapy (O'Brien et al. 2009) for the treatment of patients with relapsed or refractory chronic lymphocytic leukemia (CLL) or patients with metastatic melanoma.

L-gossypol (AT-101) (Fig. 3.25) is an orally bioavailable polyphenolic aldehyde, derived from unrefined cottonseed oil. It binds to BCL-2, Bcl-x_L, BCL-W, and MCL-1 and mimics the inhibitory BH3 domain. This leads to the induction of apoptosis. A derivative of L-gossypol, apogossypol, is in preclinical development.

Adverse Effects The gastrointestinal toxicity of L-gossypol is dose limiting.

Obatoclax mesylate (GX15-070) is a small-molecule indole bipyrrole compound that antagonizes BCL-2, BCL-x_L, BCL-W, and MCL1, which can rapidly accumulate in cells treated with anti-cancer agents (Nguyen M 2007). Obatoclax has modest activity as a single agent, but is under evaluation in combination regimens. The agent restores sensitivity to several anti-cancer drugs. It is in clinical trials for leukemia, lymphoma, myelofibrosis, and mastocytosis. The drug is orally bioavailable.

Drug Resistance Obatoclax efficiently disrupts the interaction between BAK and MCL1, thereby overcoming the MCL1 dependent resistance to ABT-737 and to the proteasome inhibitor bortezomib in multiple myeloma patients.

Drug Interactions Obatoclax synergizes with ABT-737 and cytarabine to induce apoptosis in leukemic cells.

Navitoclax (ABT-263) is an inhibitor of BCL-X_L, BCL-2 and BCL-w. It disrupts their interactions with pro-apoptotic proteins. This exerts an anti-tumor effect. The agent is orally bioavailable. In aggressive B-cell lymphoma and multiple myeloma navitoclax displays modest or no single agent activity, but may act synergistically with other chemotherapeutics. It is in clinical trials for the treatment of chronic lymphocytic leukemia.

Pharmacokinetics The oral bioavailability of navitoclax is 20–50%.

BH3 domains in anti-apoptotic proteins contain an essential α-helix that engages and regulates BCL-2 family members. ABT-737 (4-[4-[(4'-chloro[1,1'-biphenyl]-2-yl) methyl]-1-piperazinyl]-*N*-[[4-[[(1R)-3-(dimethylamino)-1-[(phenylthio)methyl]propyl]amino]-3-nitrophenyl]sulfonyl] benzamide) is a relatively selective inhibitor of BCL-2, BCL-x_L, and BCL-w, which sequester BH-3 domain pro-apoptotic proteins, thus promoting BAX and BAK oligomerization and leading to apoptosis. ABT-737 does not inhibit MCL-1.

Drug Resistance High levels of the anti-apoptotic protein and BCL-2 binding partner MCL-1 in cancer cells are associated with resistance to ABT-737.

A-385358 ((R)-4-(3-dimethylamino-1-phenylsulfanylmethyl-propylamino)-*N*-[4-(4,4-dimethyl-piperidin-1-yl)-benzoyl]-3-nitro-benzenesulfonamide) is a small molecule that binds avidly to BCL-x_L. A-385358 enhances cell death induced by various chemotherapeutic agents, including paclitaxel, etoposide, cisplatin and doxorubicin. Clinical trials with A-385358 have not yet been initiated.

HA14-1 (2-amino-6-bromo-4-(1-cyano-2-ethoxy-2-oxoethyl)-4*H*-chromene-3-carboxylate) is an organic compound that acts as a BCl-2 inhibitor. HA14-1 enhances the sensitivity of glioblastoma cells to chemotherapy or radiotherapy. The development of HA14-1 is still preclinical.

Dideoxypetrosynol A ((3S,4E,15Z,26E,28S)-4,15,26-triacontatriene-1,12,18,29-tetrayne-3,28-diol), a polyacetylene from the sponge Petrosia, has selective cytotoxic activity against some solid tumor cells by inhibiting DNA reduplication and causing apoptotic cell death. Exposure of transformed cells to dideoxypetrosynol A can result in dose dependent growth inhibition and induction of apoptosis. Programmed cell death is mediated by an up-regulation in BAX expression and down-regulation of BCL-2, leading to Caspase-3 and Caspase-9 activation.

3.3.3 P53 Activators

When activated by damage to the DNA, P53 may induce cell cycle arrest, apoptosis, or senescence[7]. The gene product is defective in 50% of human cancers. Mutant P53 is unable to affect the downstream genes necessary for DNA repair, cell cycle regulation, and apoptosis. Therefore, successful anti-cancer drugs targeting P53 need to activate or stabilize the defective protein. Although P53 was discovered in 1979, small molecule drugs to stabilize P53 functions are only now in preclinical and clinical development. The reason for

[7] Due to its critical roles in controlling cell proliferation, P53 is commonly referred to as "the guardian of the genome".

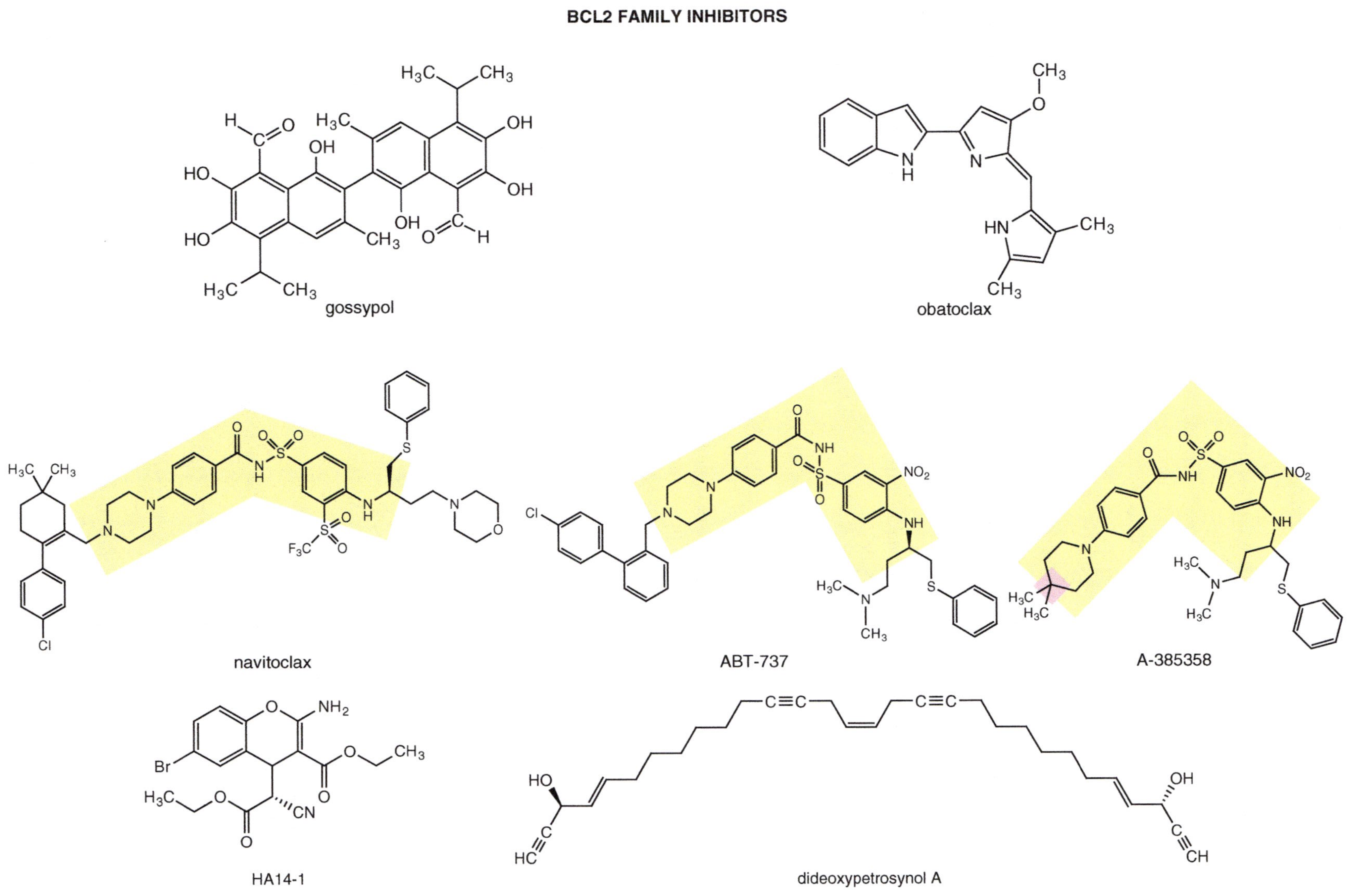

Fig. 3.25 Structures of *BCL-2* family inhibitors. The core structure shared among navitoclax, *ABT-737*, and *A-385358* is highlighted in *yellow*, with the replacement of a nitrogen within that core structure in *A-385358* being marked in *pink*

this lag period is likely the relative difficulty of rescuing the function of a tumor suppressor protein as compared to inhibiting the excessive function of an oncoprotein.

A number of amino acids in the central DNA binding domain of P53 contribute to structural stability. Mutations frequently reduce the thermodynamic stability of this domain. Library screening retrieved multiple classes of small molecules that promote the conformational stabilization of wild-type P53. This led to the identification of the styrylquinazoline CP-31398 (Foster 1999). CP-31398 has no effect on the DNA binding activity of the P53 homologs P63 and P73.

High throughput screening of chemical libraries identified the small molecule PRIMA-1 (2,2-bis(hydroxymethyl)-1-azabicyclo[2,2,2]octan-3-one), which can restore function by stabilizing the active conformation of P53 that is destabilized in many mutants. Distinct from most anti-cancer drugs, PRIMA-1 selectively inhibits the growth of tumor cells that harbor mutant P53 (Bykov et al. 2002).

MDM2 binds to P53 with high affinity and negatively modulates its transcriptional activity and stability. Overexpression of MDM2 by various tumors effectively impairs P53 function. Inhibition of the MDM2-P53 interaction can stabilize P53. Selective small molecule antagonists of MDM2 bind MDM2 in the P53 binding pocket and activate the P53 pathway in cancer cells, leading to cell cycle arrest, apoptosis, and growth inhibition (Vassilev et al. 2004).

Penicillamine is a β dimethyl analog of the amino acid cysteine. The anti-neoplastic properties of penicillamine are based on the induction of apoptosis by a P53 mediated mechanism. As a degradation product of penicillin antibiotics, penicillamine chelates heavy metals and increases their urinary excretion. The compound also inhibits blood vessel formation by chelating copper, a cofactor for angiogenesis.

3.3.4 Caspase Pathway Activators

Caspases are a family of intracellular Cysteine Proteases that play a central role in the initiation and execution of programmed cell death. Caspases share similarity in their amino acid sequence, structure, and substrate specificity. A variety of death signals to cells proceed in a cascade that converges on the activation of initiator Caspases (Caspases -2, -8, -9, and -12), which in turn activate effector Caspases (Caspases -3, -6, and -7) as a final common pathway to apoptosis. The initiator Caspases may respond to the ligation of death receptors ("extrinsic pathway", Caspase-8), cytotoxicity ("intrinsic pathway", Caspases -2 and -9), or endoplasmic reticulum stress ("endoplasmic pathway", Caspase-12).

Inhibitors of Apoptosis (IAP) counteract programmed cell death through the negative regulation of Caspases (Cysteine Containing Aspartate Specific Proteases). Their over-expression leads to diminished Caspase activity and increased resistance to a variety of apoptotic stimuli. XIAP (X-linked Inhibitor of Apoptosis) binds directly to (pro-)Caspase-9 and prevents the proteolytic processing of the pro-Caspases-3, -6 and -7 through blockage of the Cytochrome *c* induced activation of pro-Caspase-9 (Fig. 3.26). Survivin and XIAP protect from BAX induced and CD95 induced apoptosis by inhibiting the processing of pro-Caspase-7. Survivin and XIAP bind to active Caspase-3 and Caspase-7, but not their inactive pro-forms. Therefore, they act on the level of the effector Caspases, but do not act on the level of initiator Caspases.

Cancer cells often over-express and can use XIAP to evade extrinsic (death receptor mediated) and intrinsic (mitochondria mediated) apoptotic cues, including chemotherapy. The effectiveness of death receptor agonists, such as TRAIL, CD95 (FAS), and Tumor Necrosis Factor-α (TNF-α), to evoke apoptosis is substantially influenced by the cellular status of XIAP.

AEG35156 (GEM640) is a second generation synthetic antisense agent. It represents a 19-mer, fully phosphorothioated (replacement of a non-bridging oxygen in the normal phosphate backbone with sulfur) oligonucleotide in which the core 11 DNA bases are flanked by 4 2'-*O*-methyl-modified RNA residues at the 3' and 5' ends. AEG35156 selectively blocks the cellular expression of XIAP. This suppression sensitizes tumor cells to conventional chemotherapy.

Imexon (4-imino-1,3-diazabicyclo[3.1.0]hexan-2-one) <Amplimexon> is a 2-cyanoaziridine derivative, which may induce apoptosis via a pathway that involves cleaved Caspase-3, Caspase-9, or Caspase-8. Other cytotoxic mechanisms of action of this agent may engross thiol depletion, generation of reactive oxygen species, and decreases in the mitochondrial membrane potential. The drug is under study for the treatment of pancreatic, lung, breast, and prostate cancers, multiple myeloma, and melanoma.

3.3.5 Others

The engagement of death receptors is sufficient for the initiation of apoptosis. TNF (Tumor Necrosis Factor) and TRAIL (TNF-Related Apoptosis Inducing Ligand, TNFSF10, APO-2 Ligand) are members of the TNF super-family. They induce apoptosis upon binding to the cell surface death receptors TNFR1, TNFR2, CD95 (FAS), and TRAIL Receptors 1 and 2. Apoptosis induction by TRAIL requires the transduction of a signal that includes Caspase activity within the death inducing signaling complex. Activating antibodies that bind to death receptors can induce signals that promote programmed cell death.

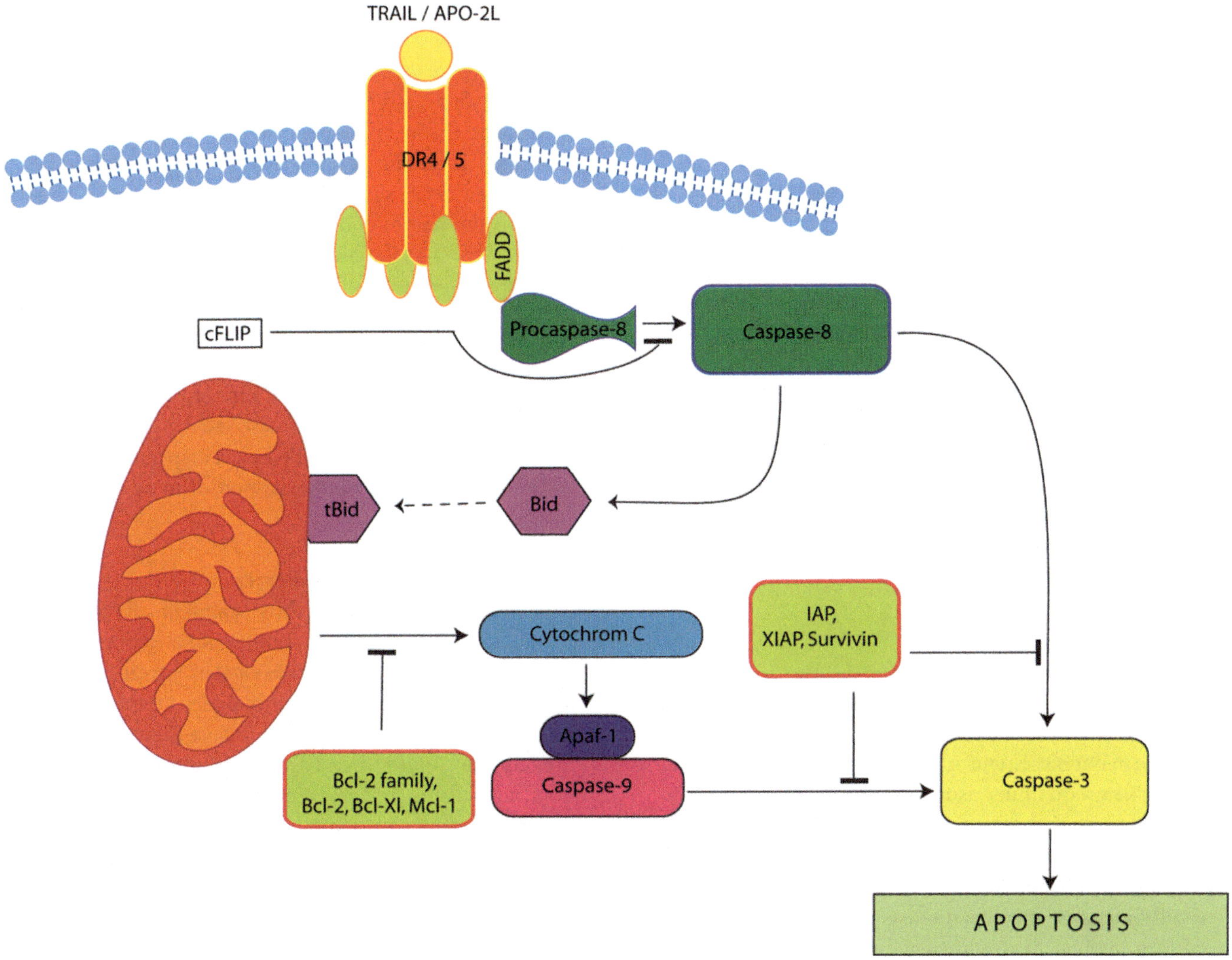

Fig. 3.26 Regulation of apoptosis. The death receptor ligand *TRAIL* interacts with its membrane bound receptors, *DR4/DR5*, leading to the activation of *Caspase-8*, which can either directly activate *Caspase-3* to induce apoptotic cell death (extrinsic pathway) or cleave *BID*, leading to the release of Cytochrome-*c* from the mitochondria with subsequent formation of the apoptosome and activation of *Caspase-9*. *Caspase-9*, in turn, activates *Caspase-3* (intrinsic pathway). (Siegelin 2011)

Several therapeutic agonist monoclonal antibodies with modest anti-tumor activity but good safety profile target death receptors. LBY135, AMG 665, lexatumumab, HGS-TR2J, and Apomab are TRAIL-R2 (DR5) agonists.

TRAIL-R1 (Tumor Necrosis Factor Related Apoptosis Inducing Ligand Receptor-1, DR4) is a cell surface death receptor expressed on many malignant cell types. Mapatumumab (HGS-ETR1) is a fully human agonistic monoclonal antibody to TRAIL-R1, with apoptosis promoting activities. Mapatumumab selectively binds to and activates TRAIL-Rl, thereby inducing programmed cell death and reducing tumor growth. The agent is in clinical trials. CS-1008 is a TRAIL-R1 agonist in development.

Hexamethylene bisacetamide (HMBA) is a hybrid polar-planar compound that induces terminal differentiation, inhibits cell growth, and may cause apoptosis in tumor cells. Hexamethylene bisacetamide mediates inhibition of the AKT and ERK/MAPK cascades, both of which are critical for cell survival and proliferation via regulation of NF-κB activation. Within about 1 day after exposure, hexamethylene bisacetamide decreases BCL-2 protein expression in cancer cells and sensitizes them to apoptosis.

Pharmacokinetics Metabolites include the major product, 6-acetamidohexanoic acid, the monodeacetylated product, N-acetyl-1,6-diaminohexane, the bis-deacetylated diamine, 1,6-diaminohexane, as well as the amino acid, 6-aminohexanoic acid and its lactam, caprolactam.

The intracellular pH is important for drug responses by tumor cells, especially with regard to apoptosis inducing drugs. The intracellular pH is regulated mainly by Na^+/H^+-antiporters, ATP dependent H^+ pumps, lactate/H^+ symporters, and bicarbonate based mechanisms (Cl^-/HCO_3^- exchange, Na^+/HCO_3^- symport). The acidic extracellular environment in advanced tumors traps weakly basic drugs and enhances the influx of weakly acidic drugs into cells. In addition, intracellular pH may affect the molecular interactions between drugs and their targets.

Exisulind (2-[(1Z)-5-fluoro-1-[(4-methanesulfonylphenyl)methylidene]-2-methyl-1*H*-inden-3-yl]acetic acid) <Aptosyn, Prevatac> is the sulfone derivative of sulindac. It acts by inhibiting the enzyme Cyclic Guanosine Monophosphate Phosphodiesterase, which is over-expressed in transformed colorectal cells. This inhibition down-regulates β-Catenin via PKG signaling and leads to cancer cell apoptosis.

Cancer cells activate genetic programs that promote cell cycle progression and overcome the otherwise dominant control mechanisms of cell cycle arrest and apoptosis.
Pro-apoptotic agents provide a very effective anti-cancer treatment strategy.

Treatment of Myelodysplastic Syndromes

Myelodysplastic syndromes are a heterogeneous group of bone marrow disorders characterized by ineffective hematopoiesis and a tendency to develop leukemia. The group of diseases is characterized by anemia, neutropenia, and thrombocytopenia. These disorders may arise de novo or appear years after exposure to mutagenic chemotherapy. De novo myelodysplastic syndrome is primarily a disease of elderly individuals, with a median age at presentation of 75 years and a slight male predominance.

The availability of growth factors has improved the management of ineffective hematopoiesis. Granulocyte Colony-Stimulating Factor (G-CSF) can increase the neutrophil count.

The U.S. FDA has approved 2 DNA hypo-methylating agents, 5-azacytidine <Vidaza> and decitabine (5-aza-2'-deoxycytidine) <Dacogen> for the treatment of elevated risk myelodysplastic syndrome. Both drugs convey a survival benefit. 5-Azacytidine is a nucleoside analog with a ribose structure that gets incorporated into RNA and DNA via Ribonucleotide Reductase, it can also induce DNA demethylation. Azacitidine is delivered either through an intravenous infusion or as a subcutaneous injection. Typically, a treatment cycle is a 28 day period, in which treatment is given daily for 7 days, followed by 21 days without treatment. Individual treatment cycles can vary based on blood counts and other factors that may require an increase in the cycle time.

In some patients, the immune system plays a role in the pathogenesis of early myelodysplastic syndromes. Immunosuppressive therapy can produce hematologic responses in those patients, it may improve survival and halt leukemic progression. Younger individuals with a low IPSS score (International Prognostic Scoring System score) and those who are positive for the HLA locus DR15 are most likely to respond to immunosuppression (Olnes 2011).

- After treatment with the anti-CD52 antibody alemtuzumab, blood cell counts may return to normal.
- Immune thrombocytopenic purpura may be treated with courses of systemic steroids.
- Anti-Thymocyte Globulin or cyclosporine, alone or in combination, generate responses in up to 30 % of patients.

1. Acute myelogenous leukemia

Chemotherapy Successful treatment of pediatric AML involves intensive, multi-cyclic therapy with drug combinations that have various mechanisms of action and dosing regimens. It includes DNA and RNA alkylation (cyclophosphamide), anti-folates (methotrexate), anti-purines and anti-pyrimidines (6-mercaptopurine, 6-thioguanine), incorporation into DNA or RNA (cytarabine), microtubule inhibition (vincristine), membrane stabilization (prednisone), and inhibition of Topoisomerase 1 (topotecan) and 2 (anthracycline) (Bonate et al. 2006).

- Induction: vincristine, prednisone, L-Asparaginase, possibly including anthracyclines, depending on whether the patient is at high or low risk.
- Consolidation: 5 weeks of prednisone, cyclophosphamide, 6-mercaptopurine, vincristine, cytarabine, and methotrexate, plus radiotherapy.
- Interim maintenance: 8 weeks of mercaptopurine and methotrexate.
- Delayed intensification: re-induction with 4 weeks of dexamethasone, vincristine, doxorubicin, L-Asparaginase; or re-consolidation with 3 weeks of vincristine, cyclophosphamide, 6-thioguanine, cytarabine, and methotrexate.
- Maintenance: 12 weeks of vincristine, prednisone, mercaptopurine, and methotrexate.

In general, approximately 50 % of leukemic pediatric patients will experience disease recurrence. Once a pediatric patient relapses, the primary therapeutic alternatives include further chemotherapy, bone marrow transplant, or hematopoietic stem cell transplant, with the timing of patient relapse being an important prognostic indicator and determinant of the type of treatment to be considered. Treatment outcomes for patients who relapse in their 2nd or 3rd remission are characterized by substantially decreased long term probability for a complete cure.

The majority of elderly patients are not considered for standard induction therapies that incorporate cytarabine (araC) plus anthracycline, and complete remission rates, leukemia-free and overall survival are significantly lower than in younger patients.

Chemotherapy resistance A partial tandem duplication (PTD), in which a genomic fragment containing several exons of *mll* becomes duplicated, is common in patients with acute myelogenous leukemia. The MLL-PDT mutation underlies a cytgenetically normal form of the disease. The presence of this mutation predicts a poor response to chemotherapy alone, but a good response to chemotherapy plus autologous stem cell transplantation.

High levels of $P21^{CIP1/WAF1}$ correlate with chemoresistance in acute myelogenous leukemia. P21 expression may protect the transformed cells from chemotherapeutic DNA damage because the G_1 block facilitates repair before the cells undergo DNA reduplication.

The leukemic cells from about 1/3 of patients with acute myelogenous leukemia at the time of diagnosis, and more than ½ of patients at relapse express the efflux transporter ABCB1. Elevated levels occur in certain subtypes, including secondary leukemias. ABCB1 expression is correlated with a reduced complete remission rate and a higher incidence of refractory disease. Common treatment regimens for acute myelogenous leukemia include the ABCB1 substrate daunorubicin, which has reduced efficacy in high ABCB1 expressors.

2. Acute Promyelocytic leukemia

Acute promyelocytic leukemia (APL) is a unique subtype of acute myeloid leukemia that is curable with targeted therapies and potentially without exposure to conventional DNA-damaging chemotherapy. Cure rates may be further increased by adopting management strategies to reduce early hemorrhagic deaths, which now are among the major causes for treatment failure.

Retinoic acid induces myeloid differentiation. The absence of retinoic acid causes the nuclear receptor hetero-dimer RXR/RARα complex to be bound to Histone Deacetylase and to be transcriptionally inactive. Physiologic doses of retinoic acid induce the release of Histone Deacetylase, followed by the expression of RXR/RARα target genes and ensuing differentiation.

Chimeric transcription factors can be the cause for cellular transformation in various leukemias. PML-RARα and PLZF-RARα are chimeric leukemogenic transcriptional repressors, which cause acute promyelocytic leukemia. They are unresponsive to physiologic doses of retinoic acid. However, pharmacologic doses of retinoic acid induce the dissociation of Histone Deacetylase from PML-RARα. This allows the induction of retinoic acid dependent genes and differentiation of the leukemic cells. In contrast, even at pharmacologic doses of retinoic acid, PLZF-RARα represses transcription because the PLZF moiety causes retinoic acid insensitive interactions with Histone Deacetylase.

Acute promyelocytic leukemia may be curable with all-trans retinoic acid (ATRA) combined with anthracycline based chemotherapy. Over 90 % of responsive patients achieve complete remission, and cure rates approximate 80 %.

About ¼ of cases of acute promyelocytic leukemia do not respond to or will relapse from first line therapy. Arsenic trioxide (As_2O_3) (NSC-706363) <Trisenox> is in use for the treatment of patients who have relapsed or are refractory to retinoid and anthracycline chemotherapy (approved by the U.S. FDA in 2000). The recommended dose is 0.15 mg/kg/d until remission. Arsenic trioxide[8] may affect numerous intracellular signal transduction pathways and cause many alterations in cellular function. Thus, the anti-cancer mechanisms of action by arsenic trioxide include the induction of apoptosis, the inhibition of proliferation, and the inhibition of angiogenesis. Arsenic trioxide inhibits Glutathione Peroxidase, possibly through the generation of arsenic-GSH conjugates, and consecutively increases the cellular hydrogen peroxide levels. Consistently, ascorbic acid, which may increase the

[8] The roots of this agent go back to the treatment of syphilis by Ehrlich, which is one of the foundation stones for the science of chemotherapy. Arsenic has been used therapeutically for more than 2000 years and was applied in the 1930s for the treatment of chronic myelogenous leukemia until supplanted by newer chemotherapies. Recent interest in arsenic trioxide initially arose through Chinese reports of its efficacy and use. The introduction of arsenic trioxide for the treatment of acute promyelocytic leukemia in 1994 has provided the opportunity to minimize standard cytotoxic chemotherapy in initial regimens without compromising outcomes.

cellular hydrogen peroxide content, enhances the arsenic trioxide induced apoptosis of lymphoma cells, but not of healthy bone marrow cells. Apoptosis is associated with the collapse of mitochondrial transmembrane potentials in a thiol dependent manner. This classifies arsenic trioxide as a mitochondriotoxic anti-cancer agent.

Adverse Effects Adverse effects entail cardiotoxicity, skin rashes, and hyperglycemia.

The traditional Chinese medicinal formula Realgar-Indigo naturalis may be an effective treatment for promyelocytic leukemia. It intensifies the ubiquitination and degradation of the chimeric oncoprotein PML-RARα. This improves the reprogramming of myeloid differentiation regulators and enhanced cell-cycle arrest.

3. Chronic myelogenous leukemia

Chronic myelogenous leukemia is a disease that evolves through three successive stages, from the chronic phase via the accelerated phase to the end stage of blast crisis that resembles acute leukemia. A treatment agenda that has evolved for the disease includes cytotoxic chemotherapy, Interferon-α, first generation tyrosine kinase inhibitors (imatinib mesylate), second generation tyrosine kinase inhibitors (dasatinib and nilotinib), and allogeneic hematopoietic stem cell transplantation.

Among the alkylating agents, bone marrow suppression by busulfan <Busulfex, Myleran> is unique in affecting mainly the granulocytes. Therefore, busulfan is the drug of choice for chronic granulocytic leukemias. It can induce remission in 90% of patients after the initial course of treatment. Reduction in peripheral counts usually occurs in the 2nd or 3rd week of therapy, with a decrease in the size of the spleen thereafter. The rapid destruction of granulocytes can yield a dangerous rise in serum uric acid and consecutive kidney damage from urate stones. Preventive treatment with allopurinol <Zyloprim> is available.

Whereas the chronic phase of chronic myelogenous leukemia can be controlled for a number of years by busulfan, ultimately the majority of patients undergo blastic transformation (acute phase) and no longer respond to the anti-tumor effects of this drug. In the blast crisis (often the terminal event in the disease), 6-mercaptopurine is the drug of choice.

Before kinase inhibitors became available, therapy with the cytokine Interferon-α was considered the best therapy. Interferon-α was often used for treating chronic myeloid leukemia because it reduces the growth and division of leukemia cells. This drug was most often given as daily subcutaneous (less commonly intramuscular) injections. To treat chronic myeloid leukemia, Interferon was administered for several years; it is now rarely used. Overall, the median survival time of newly diagnosed patients is approximately 5–6 years on an Interferon-based treatment regimen.

Adverse Effects Substantial adverse effects comprise flu-like symptoms (including muscle aches, bone pain, fever, headaches, fatigue, nausea and vomiting). Patients taking this drug may have problems thinking and concentrating. Interferon can also lower blood cell counts. These effects continue as long as the drug is used, but can become easier to tolerate over time and tend to improve after the treatment ends. In some cases, early discontinuation of the treatment may be necessary.

Tyrosine kinase inhibitors are the mainstay of treatment. Patients with chronic myelogenous leukemia in chronic phase who receive imatinib from the time of diagnosis have a very good prognosis. Their projected overall survival rate approaches 90% by 60 months and freedom from progression to accelerated phase or blast crisis is over 90%. There is evidence that high-dose imatinib (800 mg daily) compared with standard dose (400 mg daily) produces superior progression-free survival. However, if imatinib is discontinued, recurrence is the rule.

The second-line ABL inhibitors dasatinib and nilotinib are emerging as effective salvage therapies for imatinib failure. However, T315I mutations in the oncogenic tyrosine kinase BCR-ABL lead to a form of chronic myeloid leukemia that is resistant to all ABL kinase inhibitors that are in clinical use, including imatinib, nilotinib, and dasatinib. The inhibitor SGX393 blocks the growth of hematopoietic cells which harbor BCR-ABL^{T315I}. Combining SGX393 with nilotinib or dasatinib may preempt the emergence of resistant subclones of chronic myelogenous leukemia cells.

4. Premalignant myeloproliferative conditions

Myeloproliferative disorders are clonal hematopoietic disorders, in which a hypersensitivity of progenitor cells to growth factors results in an excessive production of terminally differentiated cells. Due to the over-production of erythrocytes in polycythemia vera and thrombocytes in essential thrombocythemia, patients are at risk of major thrombotic events and bleeding complications, and at risk of progressing to acute myelogenous leukemia. Polycythemia vera and essential thrombocythemia can also progress to myelofibrosis, in which the bone marrow is replaced by scar tissue, commonly leading to death within 12 months.

- Polycythemia vera is associated with a particular mutation in the tyrosine kinase JAK2, which is present in almost all patients. The same mutation, JAK2^{V617F}, is also associated with about ½ of the patients with essential thrombocythemia and myelofibrosis. Hence, JAK2 is a primary target for therapeutic intervention. TG101348 is a specific ATP-competitive JAK2 inhibitor in development for this application. Also under investigation for this application is the JAK1/JAK2 inhibitor ruxolitinib ((INC424, INCB18424) <Jakafi, Jakavi>
- Several mustards, including uracil mustard, chlorambucil, and mannosulfan have been used in the palliative treatment of polycythemia vera, before the development of leukemia or myelofibrosis.
- Mannosulfan and mitobromitol are effective in treating polycythemia vera. They are available in some countries (not in the U.S.).

Adverse Effects Transformation to acute leukemia occurs in polycythemia vera and essential thrombocythemia. Myelosuppressive therapy with alkylating agents increases this risk in both disorders. Therefore, unsymptomatic patients should not receive this treatment.

References

Altstadt TJ, Fairchild CR, Golik J, Johnston KA, Kadow JF, Lee FY, Long BH, Rose WC, Vyas DM, Wong H, Wu MJ, Wittman MD (2001) Synthesis and antitumor activity of novel C-7 paclitaxel ethers: discovery of BMS-184476. J Med Chem 44:4577–4583

Balog DM, Meng D, Kamanecka T, Bertinato P, Su D-S, Sorensen EJ, Danishefsky SJ (1996) Totalsynthese von (-)-Epothilon A. Angew Chem 108:2976

Bollag DM, McQueney PA, Zhu J, Hensens O, Koupal L, Liesch J, Goetz M, Lazarides E, Woods CM (1995) Epothilones, a new class of microtubule-stabilizing agents with a taxol-like mechanism of action. Cancer Res 55:2325–2333

Bonate PL, Arthaud L, Cantrell, Jr. WR, Stephenson K, Secrist JA III, Weitman S (2006) Discovery and development of clofarabine: a nucleoside analogue for treating cancer. Nat Rev Drug Discov 5:855–863

Bonnet S, Archer SL, Allalunis-Turner J, Haromy A, Beaulieu C, Thompson R, Lee CT, Lopaschuk GD, Puttagunta L, Bonnet S, Harry G, Hashimoto K, Porter CJ, Andrade MA, Thebaud B, Michelakis ED (2007) A mitochondria-K+ channel axis is suppressed in cancer and its normalization promotes apoptosis and inhibits cancer growth. Cancer Cell 11:37–51

Bykov VJ, Issaeva N, Shilov A, Hultcrantz M, Pugacheva E, Chumakov P, Bergman J, Wiman KG, Selivanova G (2002) Restoration of the tumor suppressor function to mutant p53 by a low-molecular-weight compound. Nat Med 8:282–288

Cooper G (1997) The cell. A molecular approach. ASM, Washington, DC

Cornacchia E, Golbus J, Maybaum J, Strahler J, Hanash S, Richardson B (1988) Hydralazine and procainamide inhibit T cell DNA methylation and induce autoreactivity. J Immunol 140:2197–2200

Dervan PB, Bürli RW (1999) W. Sequence-specific DNA recognition by polyamides. Curr Opin Chem Bi;ol 3:688–693

Foster BA, Coffey HA, Morin MJ, Rastinejad F (1999) Pharmacological rescue of mutant p53 conformation and function. Science 286:2507–2510

Goodman J, Walsh V (2001) The story of taxol: nature and politics in the pursuit of an anti-cancer drug. Cambridge University Press, Cambridge

Jackson JR, Patrick DR, Dar MM, Huang PS (2007) Targeted antimitotic therapies: can we im;prove on tubulin agents? Nat Rev Cancer 7:107–117

Johnstone RW (2002) Histone-deacetylase inhibitors: novel drugs for the treatment of cancer. Nat Rev Drug Discov 1:287–299

Knock FE (1967) Anticancer agents. Springfield, IL: Charles C. Thomas

Kobayashi M, Natsume T, Tamaoki S, Watanabe J, Asano H, Mikami T, Miyasaka K, Miyazaki K, Gondo M, Sakakibara K, Tsukagoshi S (1997) Antitumor activity of TZT-1027, a novel dolastatin 10 derivative. Jpn J Cancer Res 88:316–327

Lee FY, Borzilleri R, Fairchild CR, Kim SH, Long BH, Reventos-Suarez C, Vite GD, Rose WC, Kramer RA (2001) BMS-247550: a novel epothilone analog with a mode of action similar to paclitaxel but possessing superior antitumor efficacy. Clin Cancer Res 7:1429–1437

Liu PQ, Rebar EJ, Zhang L, Liu Q, Jamieson AC, Liang Y, Qi H, Li PX, Chen B, Mendel MC, Zhong X, Lee YL, Eisenberg SP, Spratt SK, Case CC, Wolffe AP (2001) Regulation of an endogenous locus using a panel of designed zinc finger proteins targeted to accessible chromatin regions. Activation of vascular endothelial growth factor A. J Biol Chem 276:11323–11334

Mapp AK, Ansari AZ, Ptashne M, Dervan PB (2000) Activation of gene expression by small molecule transcription factors. Proc Natl Acad Sci U S A 97:3930–3935

Mayer TU, Kapoor TM, Haggarty SJ, King RW, Schreiber SL, Mitchison TJ (1999) Small molecule inhibitor of mitotic spindle bipolarity identified in a phenotype-based screen. Science 286:971–974

O'Brien S, Moore JO, Boyd TE, Larratt LM, Skotnicki AB, Koziner B, Chanan-Khan AA, Seymour JF, Gribben J, Itri LM, Rai KR (2009) 5-year survival in patients with relapsed or refractory chronic lymphocytic leukemia in a randomized, phase III trial of fludarabine plus cyclophosphamide with or without oblimersen. J Clin Oncol 27:5208–5212

Okada H, Koyanagi T, Yamada N, Haga T (1991) Synthesis and antitumor activities of novel benzoylphenylurea derivatives. Chem Pharm Bull (Tokyo) 39:2308–2315

Olnes MJ, Sloand EM (2011) Targeting immune dysregulation in myelodysplastic syndromes. J Am Med Assoc 305:814–819

Piekarz RL, Robey R, Sandor V, Bakke S, Wilson WH, Dahmoush L, Kingma DM, Turner ML, Altemus R, Bates SE (2001) Inhibitor of histone deacetylation, depsipeptide (FR901228), in the treatment of peripheral and cutaneous T-cell lymphoma: a case report. Blood 98:2865–2868

Riggs MG, Whittaker RG, Neumann JR, Ingram VM (1977) n-Butyrate causes histone modification in HeLa and Friend erythroleukaemia cells. Nature 268:462–464

Ruefli AA, Ausserlechner MJ, Bernhard D, Sutton VR, Tainton KM, Kofler R, Smyth MJ, Johnstone RW (2001) The histone deacetylase inhibitor and chemotherapeutic agent suberoylanilide hydroxamic acid (SAHA) induces a cell-death pathway characterized by cleavage of BID and production of reactive oxygen species. Proc Natl Acad Sci U S A 98:10833–10838

Salomoni P, Pandolfi PP (2000) Transcriptional regulation of cellular transformation. Nat Med 6:742–744

Siegelin MD, Siegelin Y (2011) Novel therapeutic venues for glioblastoma: novel rising preclinical treatment opportunities. In: Abujamra AL (ed) Brain tumors—current and emerging therapeutic strategies. Intech, Rijeka

Smith CD, Zhang X, Mooberry SL, Patterson GM, Moore RE (1994) Cryptophycin: a new antimicrotubule agent active against drug-resistant cells. Cancer Res 54:3779–3784

Sonoda H, Nishida K, Yoshioka T, Ohtani M, Sugita K (1996) Oxamflatin: a novel compound which reverses malignant phenotype to normal one via induction of JunD. Oncogene 13:143–149

Testa U (2004) Apoptotic mechanisms in the control of erythropoiesis. Leukemia 18:1176–1199

Tiano HF, Loftin CD, Akunda J, Lee CA, Spalding J, Sessoms A, Dunson DB, Rogan EG, Morham SG, Smart RC, Langenbach R (2002) Deficiency of either cyclooxygenase (COX)-1 or COX-2 alters epidermal differentiation and reduces mouse skin tumorigenesis. Cancer Res 62:3395–3401

Vassilev LT, Vu BT, Graves B, Carvajal D, Podlaski F, Filipovic Z, Kong N, Kammlott U, Lukacs C, Klein C, Fotouhi N, Liu EA (2004) In vivo activation of the p53 pathway by small-molecule antagonists of MDM2. Science 303:844–848

Wolbach SB, Howe PR (1925) Tissue changes following deprivation of fat soluble A vitamin. J Exp Med 42:753–777

Zhou W, Zhu W-G (2009) The changing face of HDAC inhibitor depsipeptide. Curr Cancer Drug Targets 9:91–100

Molecular Inhibitors of Growth Signals

4

Signal transduction associated with growth factor receptors typically mediates the activation of cell cycle promoting gene products or the inactivation of cell cycle checkpoints. These signals are frequently transduced through G-Protein pathways, kinase receptor pathways, or nuclear receptor pathways (Fig. 4.1), are dependent on proto-oncogenic transcription factors, and lead to the expression of Cyclins and Cyclin-Dependent Kinases (CDKs), which are drivers of the cell cycle (Fig. 4.2). Physiologically, growth signals are transient and entirely depend on the engagement of a growth factor receptor by its cognate ligand. Upon termination of this interaction, the growth signal ceases. Gain-of-function mutations in cancer keep the growth signal active, regardless of the presence of the transient growth factor-receptor interaction. Such deregulated signaling cascades are appropriate drug targets in the treatment of cancer.

- Inhibitors of gene products with gain-of-function mutations may suppress the growth of cancer. Except in familial cancer syndromes, cancer causing mutations are somatic. Inhibitors of the mutant gene products selectively affect the cancer cells.
- Downstream signaling molecules are suitable drug targets, while inhibitors that act upstream of gain-of-function defects are ineffective. Drugs acting on immediate downstream molecules are more efficacious than drugs acting on far downstream molecules.
- Due to their specificity, molecular inhibitors of growth signals avoid the severe adverse effects of conventional chemotherapeutics on proliferating tissues (gastrointestinal, hematopoietic, hair).

The discovery that the genomes of some oncogenic viruses encode tyrosine kinases initiated research to identify drugs that suppress tyrosine kinase enzymes. Anti-proliferation activity was identified in herbimycin and staurosporine, but these compounds were insufficiently specific for individual kinases and exerted extensive toxicity. Intensive screening of chemical libraries for narrowly focused kinase inhibitors was initially viewed with scepticism, because the activity of these reagents relied on the competitive inhibition of ATP binding and the ATP binding domain was seen as a highly conserved motif in all kinases. The discovery of imatinib mesylate, which specifically inhibits BCR-ABL, the causative kinase for chronic myelogenous leukemia (CML), was a breakthrough to overcome this bias.

Drug Resistance Characteristically, molecularly targeted drugs are initially very successful but often loose efficacy after several months. It is likely that cells that are sensitive to the targeted drugs are eliminated, but the genetic instability of cancers leads to the presence of cells with mutations that confer drug resistance. Under the selective pressure of the drug treatment, the resistant cells preferentially proliferate.

Cancer cells exhibit a mutator phenotype, because defects in their DNA repair make their genomes instable. Therefore, considerable variation occurs in the spectrum of DNA alterations. Some of these genetic changes are "driver" mutations that play a causative role in transformation and constitute unique drug targets that are absent from normal cells (Table 4.1). However, most of the somatic mutations inside tumor cells are likely "passenger" mutations that are not involved in cancer formation. Their targeting with anti-cancer drugs has a low likelihood of success.

Inhibitors of gene products with gain-of-function mutations (or their downstream signaling targets) may suppress the growth of cancer.
Due to the genetic instability of cancer cells, molecularly targeted drugs often loose efficacy after several months.

4.1 Small Molecule Kinase Inhibitors

The coalescence of increasing insights into the molecular pathways associated with growth signals—specifically kinase cascades—with efforts to replace cancer therapy compounds that have intrinsic mutagenic potential have resulted in the development of small molecule kinase inhibitors. Most of their drug names end on -nib or -tinib.

- The majority of these agents block the ATP (adenosine triphosphate) binding site in their kinase drug target

G. F. Weber, *Molecular Therapies of Cancer*, DOI 10.1007/978-3-319-13278-5_4,

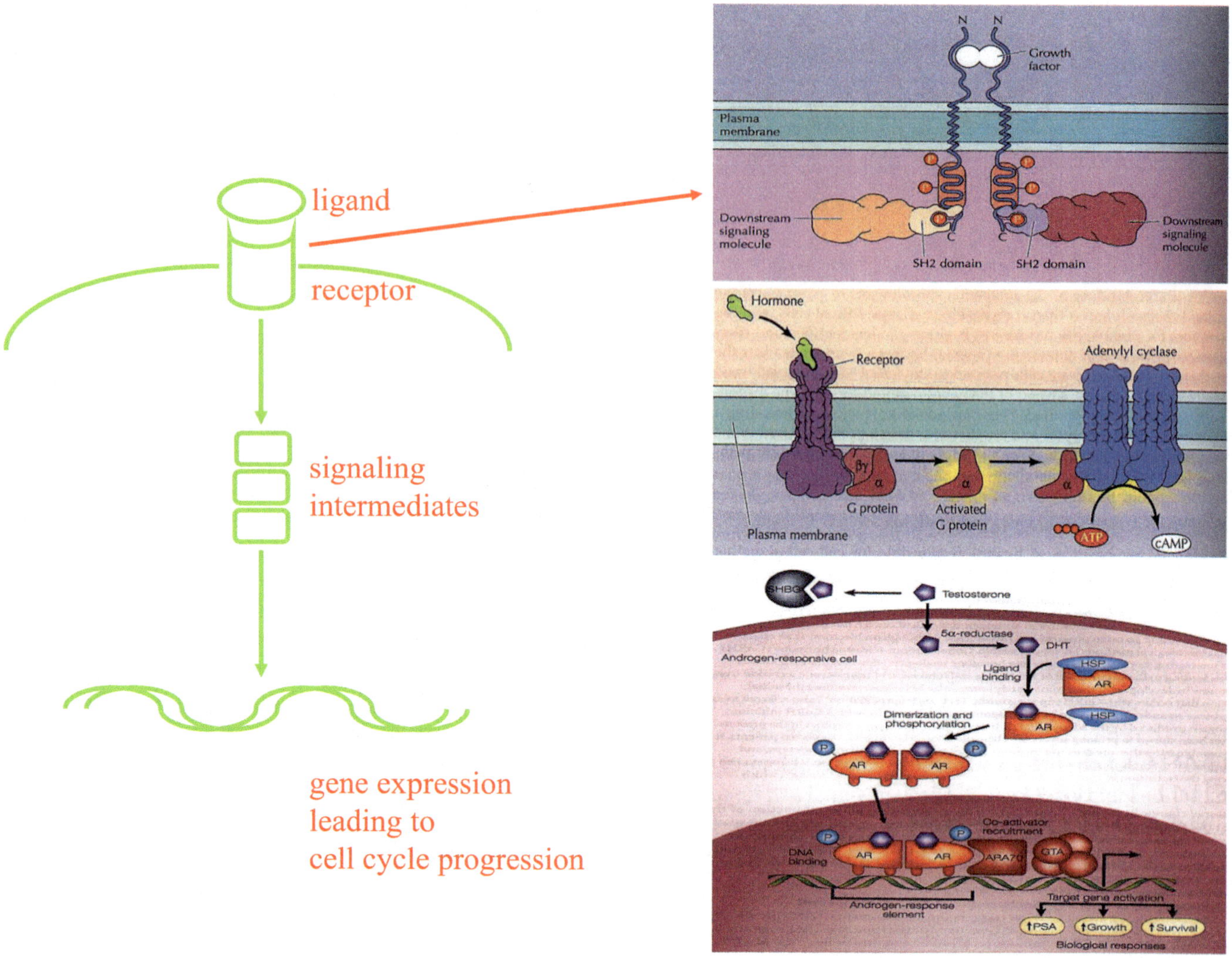

Fig. 4.1 Cellular growth pathways. (*Left*) the engagement of a growth factor receptor by its cognate ligand activates a pathway of signaling intermediates that causes changes in gene expression, which lead to cell cycle progression. (*Right*) most growth factor receptors belong to three families, comprising G-Protein Coupled Receptors (*top panel*), Receptor Tyrosine Kinases (*middle panel*), and Nuclear Hormone Receptors (*bottom panel*). (Parts adapted from Cooper 1997)

(type I inhibitors). Because all protein kinases have an ATP binding site that serves as the phosphate donor, there is potential for cross-reactivity and off-target effects. The close structural similarities among protein kinases can make achieving specificity for a particular kinase challenging, potentially leading to unwanted adverse effects. In clinical practice, this has not been a major problem. Despite the generic nature of the co-substrate ATP, the shapes of the binding pockets in various kinases are still sufficiently specific to allow for the development of unique kinase inhibitors.

- Type II inhibitors recognize the inactive conformation of the kinase.
- Some drugs are allosteric modulators that bind outside the ATP binding site.
- Covalent inhibitors are capable of forming irreversible, covalent bonds to the kinase active site, most frequently by reacting with a nucleophilic cysteine residue.

Drug Resistance Mechanisms of resistance to tyrosine kinase blockers include tyrosine kinase gene amplification and point mutations in the drug binding domain. Oncogenic switching is frequently induced as a resistance mechanism to tyrosine kinase inhibitors. The oncogenic switch allows cancer cells to signal through other receptor tyrosine kinases when one is blocked.

Most kinase inhibitors block the ATP binding site.
Mechanisms of resistance to tyrosine kinase blockers include tyrosine kinase gene amplification and point mutations in the ATP binding domain.

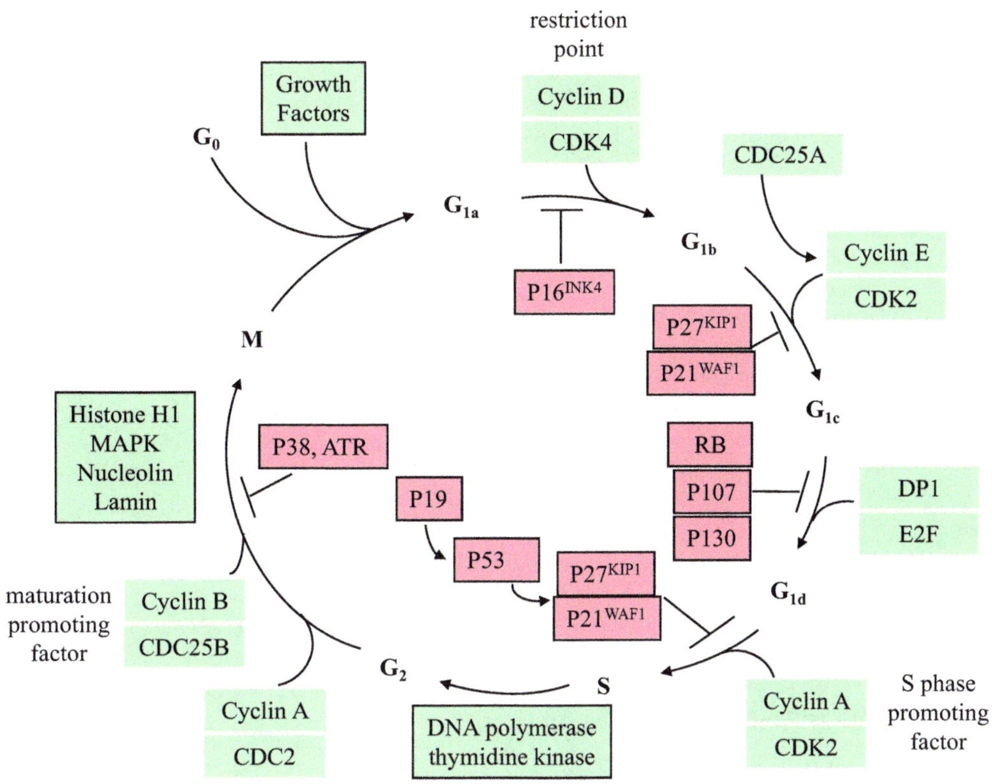

Fig. 4.2 Regulators of the cell cycle. The consecutive phases of the cell cycle are indicated between the *arrows* of the *circle*. Positive regulators mediate cell cycle progression and are shown on the outside in *green boxes*. Negative regulators activate cell cycle checkpoints or apoptosis and are shown in *red boxes* within the *circle*. The target points for action by the regulators are depicted. Three major checkpoints and their controlling complexes are named *unboxed*

4.1.1 EGFR Family Inhibitors

Cohen's discovery of Epidermal Growth Factor (EGF) in 1962 pioneered major progress in cell growth and differentiation research. In the early 1990s, the first clinical trials of anti-EGFR agents validated the drug target.

The EGFR (Epidermal Growth Factor Receptor, Human Epithelial Receptor, HER) family consists of receptor tyrosine kinases. Their excessive activity is common in solid tumors. It leads to a constitutive transduction of growth signals and correlates with decreased survival and a poor prognosis. ERBB1 (EGFR, HER1), ERBB2 (HER2/NEU), or ERBB3 may be over-expressed in lung, head and neck, breast, colon, and prostate cancers. ERBB2 is over-expressed in many adenocarcinomata, particularly in breast cancers. ERBB1 or ERBB2 may have gain-of-function mutations in lung cancer and glioblastoma multiforme.

The disruption of a transforming growth signal, caused by over-expressed ERBB gene products, can enforce remission. It may be accomplished with several strategies.

- Neutralization of the ligands before they can associate with their cognate receptors prevents them from initiating growth signals.
- Inhibition of the over-expressed receptors via blocking or disruption of their enzymatic activity can abrogate their excessive function.
- Inhibition of signaling by cytoplasmic second messengers, in particular serine-threonine kinases, can be therapeutic.

If there is a gain-of-function mutation, the affected receptor becomes independent of its ligand. Inhibitors acting upstream of the defect are ineffective. Inhibitors of the mutated receptors or their downstream targets may be therapeutic.

In addition to the growth promoting effects, ERBB1 protects malignant tumor cells from the cytotoxic effects of

Table 4.1 Molecular targets specific for cancer cells

1) Antigens encoded by *oncogenic viruses*. Epstein-Barr virus and Burkitt's lymphoma
2) *Mutations* of cancer-related genes. Expression of altered proteins
3) *Translocation* of proto-oncogenes. Frequent in leukemias. Unique domain at the junction
4) *Alternative transcripts*, including those from cryptic start sites, alternative reading frames, and pseudo-genes
5) *Post-translational modifications* of proteins differ between transformed and non-transformed cells, may open previously cryptic domains
6) Some *genes are silent* in normal tissue, *selectively expressed* on cells of a given differentiation. Oncofetal proteins
7) Malignancies of T- and B-lymphocytes express unique antigenic determinants in their T-cell antigen receptor or surface immunoglobulin. The *idiotype* of a given malignant clone provides a tumor specific marker

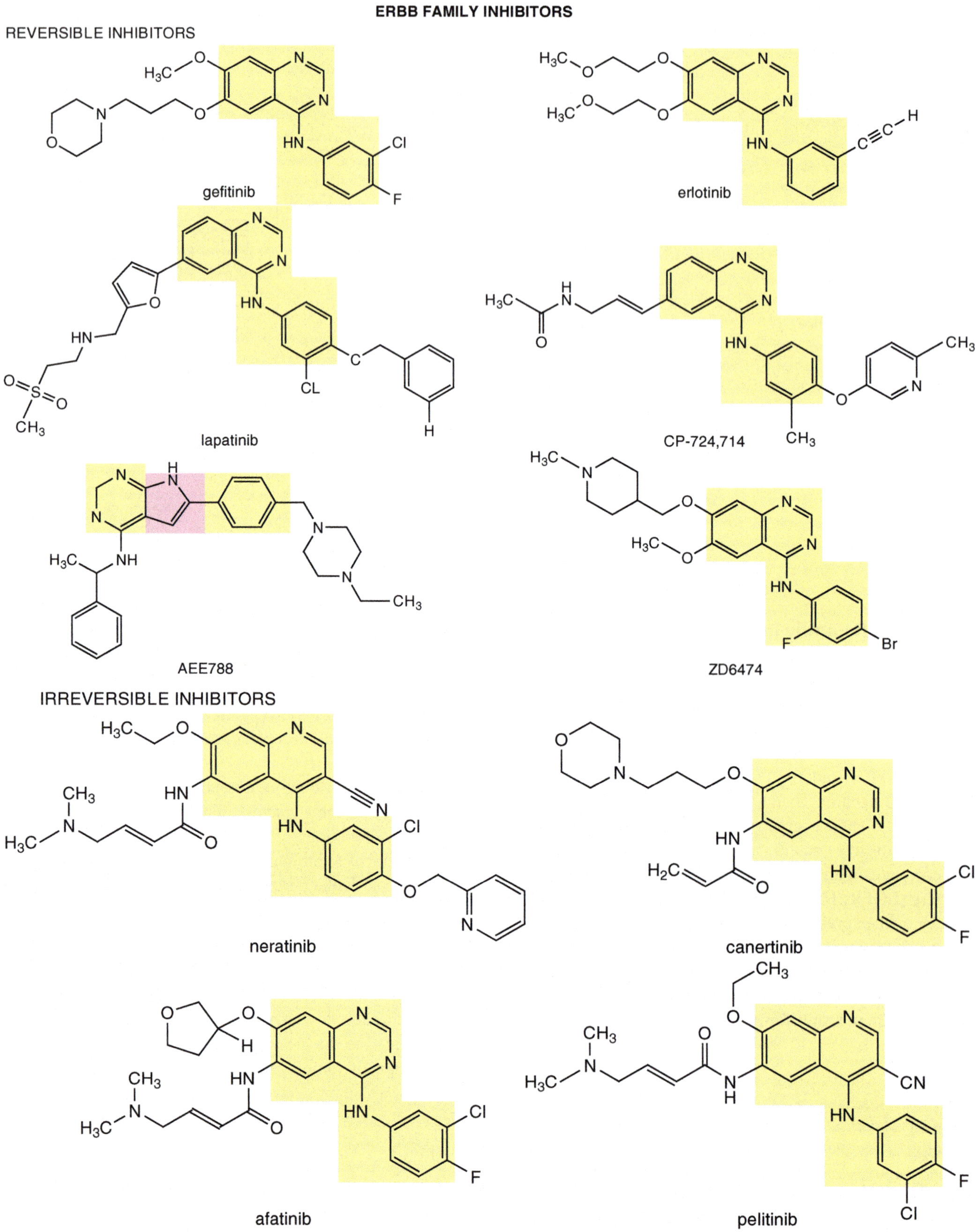

Fig. 4.3 Structures of ERBB family inhibitors. The 4-anilinoquinazoline core structure shared among all agents is highlighted in *yellow*, with one alteration in the core structure of AEE788 being marked in *pink*

Table 4.2 Treatment of EGFR mutations

Mutation	Cancers	Drug
EGFR mutation L858R (activation loop, kinase domain)	10% of lung cancers	Gefitinib (high affinity for mutated activation loop)
Various EGFR mutations	Non-small cell lung cancer, pancreatic cancer	Erlotinib (reversible binding to catalytic domain)
ErbB1 deletion of exons 2–7 (leads to the truncated EGFRvIII, aka 801EGFR)	Glioblastoma	Neratinib (irreversible binding to ATP pocket)
ErbB2 mutation A775insYVMA	Non-small cell lung cancer	Neratinib
ErbB2 mutation G776insV_G/C	Non-small cell lung cancer	Neratinib
ErbB1 gene amplification (leads to over-expression, homo- and hetero- oligomerization)	Breast cancer, lung cancer	Lapatinib (binds ErbB1 in locked conformation)
ErbB1 gene amplification (leads to over-expression, ligand-independent oligomerization)		Cetuximab
ErbB2 gene amplification (leads to over-expression, ligand-independent oligomerization)	Breast cancer	Trastuzumab (binds juxtamembrane, receptor internalization)
ErbB2 gene amplification (leads to over-expression, homo- and hetero-oligomerization)	Ovarian cancer	Pertuzumab (binds domain II, blocks dimerization)

conventional chemotherapy and radio-therapy, making these treatments less effective. Compared to those regimens, the specific inhibition of ERBB1 (Fig. 4.3) is characterized by higher efficacy and fewer adverse effects. One aspect to this modality is the relatively high specificity of small molecule kinase inhibitors to select mutations (Table 4.2), which requires knowledge of the underlying molecular defect for the most suitable choice of drug therapy.

Adverse Effects Skin rashes are common adverse effects of EGFR family inhibitors.

Drug Resistance Reversible ERBB1 tyrosine kinase inhibitors are active in a subset of patients. However, most cancers develop resistance and progress within the course of 1 year. In nearly 50% of the cases, acquired resistance is caused by the secondary ERBB1 mutation T790M.

Reversible specific inhibitors Gefitinib (Sirotnak 2000) is an anilinoquinazoline that inhibits the catalytic activity of multiple tyrosine kinases, including ERBB1 (EGFR, Human Epidermal Growth Factor Receptor 1, HER1). In initial clinical trials, there were no biomarkers available to predict outcome. In non-small cell lung cancer patients, gefitinib had only a 10% response rate, but displayed dramatic effects in the responders. The individuals who benefited mostly belonged to an uncommon sub-population of lung cancer patients, comprising Japanese, females, and non-smokers. These individuals were affected by point mutations in the kinase domain of the EGF Receptor. Seven years after the start of clinical trials, a predictive biomarker was developed. The drug was approved by the U.S. FDA in 2003, with new labeling announced in 2005.

Gefitinib (*N*-(3-chloro-4-fluoro-phenyl)-7-methoxy-6-(3-morpholin-4-ylpropoxy)quinazolin-4-amine) (ZD1839) <Iressa> competes with the binding of ATP to the tyrosine kinase domain of ERBB1, thereby inhibiting receptor auto-phosphorylation and resulting in the suppression of downstream signal transduction (Figs. 4.4, 4.5). The kinase inhibition may result in a suppression of tumor growth. The agent is indicated for the treatment of locally advanced or metastatic non-small cell lung cancer in patients who have previously received chemotherapy, but it is effective only in about 10% of patients, depending on the nature of the cancer causing mutation. Gefitinib has durable anti-tumor activity in the treatment of cancers with mutations in the tyrosine kinase domain of ERBB1. In contrast, it has limited efficacy in cancers with other ERBB1 defects (such as lung cancers with deletions in the extracellular domain or glioblastomas with the distinct variant III (vIII) in-frame deletion of exons 2–7). The common dose is 250 mg/day.

Pharmacokinetics Gefitinib is absorbed slowly after oral administration, and has a bioavailability of 60%. Elimination is by metabolism, primarily through CYP3A4. The molecule has three sites of biotransformation,

- metabolism of the N-propoxymorpholino-group,
- demethylation of the methoxy-substituent on the quinazoline,
- oxidative defluorination of the halogenated phenyl group.

Five metabolites accrue in the blood of patients. The elimination half-life is about 48 h. Daily oral administration of gefitinib to cancer patients results in a 2-fold accumulation compared to single dose administration. Steady state blood concentrations are achieved within 10 days. The drug is excreted in the feces.

Adverse Effects Adverse drug reactions include acne or other skin reactions, diarrhea, nausea and vomiting, asthenia or anorexia, conjunctivitis, blepharitis, corneal erosion, or aberrant eyelash growth. Asymptomatic elevations of liver Transaminases may arise. Interstitial lung disease is an infrequent, but serious adverse effect. About 1/3 of cases with interstitial lung disease are fatal. In the event of acute onset or worsening of pulmonary symptoms (dyspnea, cough, fever), gefitinib therapy should be interrupted, followed by a prompt investigation of the symptoms.

Drug Resistance Resistance to ERBB1 tyrosine kinase inhibitors, such as gefitinib, can arise through T790M mutation or activation of downstream pathways via *K- ras* mutation or *met* amplification.

Drug Interactions Gefitinib is sparingly soluble at pH 1, but is essentially insoluble above pH 7, with a sharp drop in the pH range of 4–6. Therefore, co-administration of high doses of ranitidine or sodium bicarbonate (which maintain the gastric pH above pH 5.0) reduces the mean gefitinib area under the concentration-time curve by 45 %. Gefitinib has no inhibitory effect on CYP1A2, CYP2C9, and CYP3A4 activities up to concentrations of 5000 ng/mL. However, exposure to metoprolol, a substrate of CYP2D6, is increased by 30 % when given in combination with gefitinib. The mean area under the concentration-time curve of gefitinib is reduced by 85 % by rifampicin, an inducer of CYP3A4, and is increased by the concomitant administration of itraconazole, an inhibitor of CYP3A4.

Erlotinib (*N*-(3-ethynylphenyl)-6,7-bis(2-methoxyethoxy) quinazolin-4-amine) (OSI-77) <Tarceva> was developed by OSI Pharmaceuticals, Genentech, and Roche. It is the hydrochloride salt of a quinazoline derivative. Erlotinib is designed to bind to the intracellular catalytic domain of the tyrosine kinase ERBB1, competing with ATP, thereby reversibly inhibiting auto-phosphorylation and blocking the tumorigenic signal transduction events associated with uncontrolled ERBB1 activation. The orally bioavailable erlotinib has largely replaced gefitinib in the U.S. (except in patients where gefitinib has had a proven response). It is indicated to treat lung cancer and pancreatic cancer. The agent was the first ERBB1 inhibitor to display a survival benefit in lung cancer patients, it has durable activity in the treatment of non-small cell lung cancers with

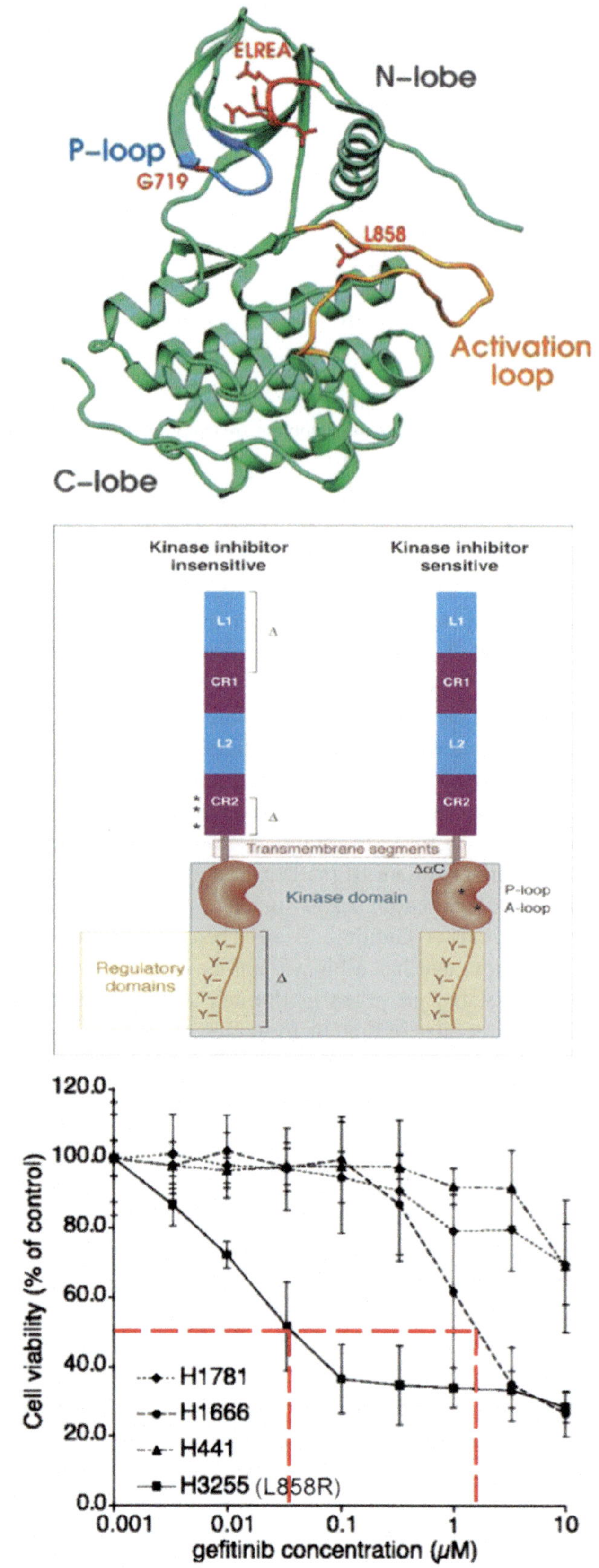

Fig. 4.4 Mode of action of gefitinib. (*Top panel*) Positions of missense mutations G719S and L858R and the Del-1 deletion in the 3-dimensional structure of the EGFR kinase domain. The *activation loop* is shown in *yellow*, the *P-loop* is in *blue*, and the *C-lobe* and *N-lobe* are as indicated. The residues targeted by mutation or deletion are highlighted in *red*. The Del-1 mutation targets the residues ELREA in codons 746–750. (*Middle panel*) EGFR mutations in tumors that are sensitive or insensitive to kinase inhibitors. Tumor mutations that are insensitive to kinase inhibitors, such as those in glioblastomata, include extensive deletions (Δ) or missense mutations (*) in the extracellular domain of EGFR, or deletions (Δ) of the regulatory intracellular domain (but not the kinase domain). In contrast, many non-small cell lung cancers carrying missense mutations (*) and deletions (Δ) in EGFR are sensitive to kinase inhibitors such as gefitinib. These mutations are in three distinct sites in the EGFR kinase domain: the P-loop, the activation loop (A-loop), and the αC helix. Tumor formation may require ligand binding to EGFR and receptor phosphorylation. The mutant EGFR allele also may be amplified (most notably with the ΔαC mutations). In kinase inhibitor-insensitive glioblastomata, tumors may be dependent or independent of ligand binding and the mutant EGFR locus is usually amplified. L1, L2: large (EGF binding) domain 1 and 2; CR 1, CR 2: cysteine-rich domain 1 and 2. Y, tyrosine residues in the regulatory domain that are available for phosphorylation. (*Bottom panel*) Cell survival after exposure to gefitinib at the indicated concentrations. Percentage of cell growth is shown relative to untreated controls. H3255 cells have the EGFR L858R mutation, whereas the three remaining cell lines have wild-type EGFR (WT). (Paez 2004; Minna 2004)

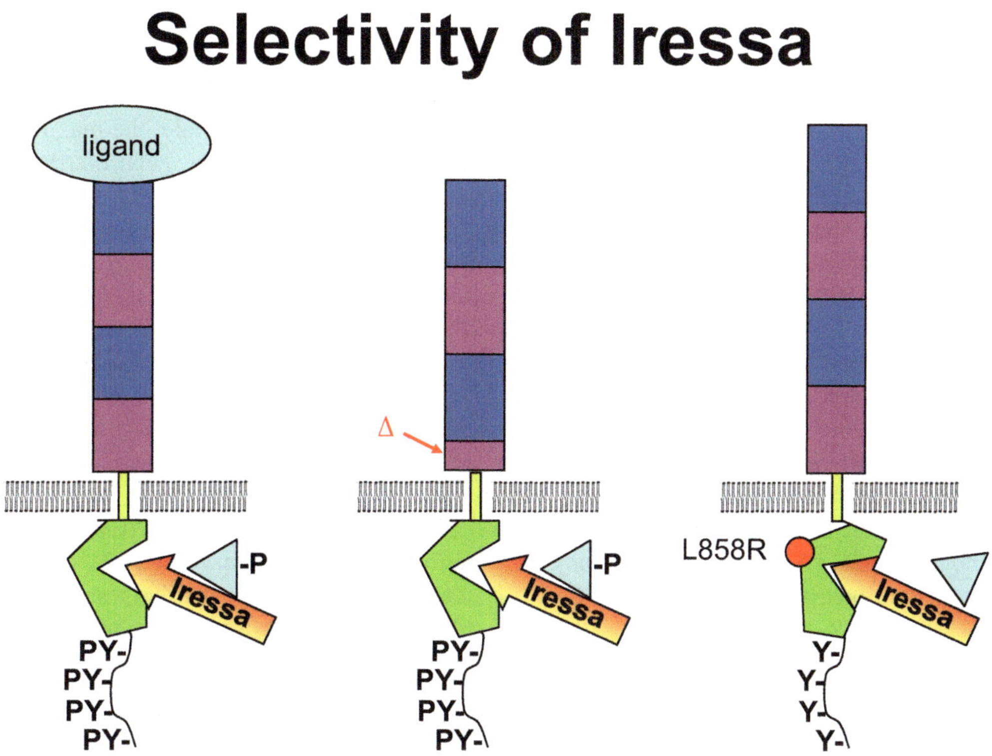

Fig. 4.5 Specificity of gefitinib to particular receptor mutations. Ligation of the EGF Receptor by its physiologic ligand leads to phosphorylation of the cytoplasmic tail and the transmission of a growth signal to the cell (*left*). Lung cancers may be caused by gain-of-function mutations of the EGF Receptor that lead to ligand-independent activation. Two such mutations include a deletion in the extracellular domain (*middle*), and a point mutation, L858R, in the catalytic domain (*right*). The anti-cancer drug gefitinib fits well into the altered conformation of the mutated catalytic domain (*right*) and blocks the phosphorylation of substrate. In contrast, the affinity of gefitinib to the unaltered catalytic domain (*left* and *center*) is low, thus allowing receptor kinase activity to persist

mutations in the tyrosine kinase domain of ERBB1. Erlotinib received U.S. FDA approval for the treatment of non-small cell lung cancer in 2004. European approval for treatment of non-small cell lung cancer in patients who have failed prior chemotherapy followed in 2005.

Adverse Effects Skin rashes occur in the majority of patients. They resemble acne and primarily involve the face and neck. In most cases, the rashes are self-limited and resolve. Other adverse effects comprise diarrhea, loss of appetite, fatigue, and ingrown hairs (such as eyelashes). Interstitial pneumonitis (characterized by cough and dyspnea) may become severe. Rare adverse effects may include serious gastrointestinal tract perforations, blistering and exfoliative skin conditions, or ocular disorders (such as corneal lesions).

Drug Resistance The T790M mutation of ERBB1 prevents erlotinib from binding to its drug target. The drug has limited efficacy in glioblastoma, where a distinct ERBB1 mutation, the variant III (vIII) in-frame deletion of exons 2–7, commonly arises. Drug resistance may occur through overexpression of MET.

Lapatinib ditosylate (GW572016) <Tykerb, Tyverb> is the salt of a synthetic, orally active quinazoline. The agent reversibly blocks the auto-phosphorylation of ERBB1, ERBB2 (HER2), and the kinases ERK-1, ERK-2, and PKB. It also suppresses the Cyclin D protein levels in tumor cells. Lapatinib is predominantly used with capecitabine in patients afflicted by advanced ERBB2-positive breast cancer with trastuzumab resistance. It is also approved with letrozole for the treatment of postmenopausal women with hormone receptor-positive metastatic breast cancer that over-expresses the ERBB2 receptor and for whom hormonal therapy is indicated. The drug is taken orally once a day.

Pharmacokinetics Absorption following oral administration of lapatinib is incomplete and variable. The systemic exposure is increased when administered with food. In the blood, more than 99 % of the drug is bound to Albumin and α-1 Acid Glycoprotein. Lapatinib is a substrate, and may act as an inhibitor, for the transporters ABCG2 and ABCB1, and the hepatic uptake transporter OATP1B1. The drug undergoes extensive metabolism, primarily by CYP3A4 and CYP3A5, with minor contributions from CYP2C19 and CYP2C8 to a variety of oxidized metabolites. The terminal phase half-life following a single dose is 14 h, which accumulates with repeated dosing to an effective half-life of 24 h. Elimination of lapatinib is predominantly through excretion in the feces, with renal excretion below 2 %.

Adverse Effects Cardiotoxicity is a potentially serious adverse effect. Lapatinib may cause liver damage and hepatitis, which can be severe or life-threatening. Liver damage may occur as soon as several days or as late as several months after the start of treatment.

Common adverse effects include nausea and vomiting, diarrhea, loss of appetite, heartburn, oral sores (lips, mouth, or throat), dysesthesias of hands and feet, pain (in arms, legs, or back), skin rashes, difficulty falling asleep or staying asleep.

CP-724,714 is an orally bioavailable quinazoline that selectively binds to the intracellular domain of ERBB2, reversibly inhibiting its tyrosine kinase activity and resulting in the suppression of tumor cell growth (Barbacci 2003). CP-724,714 suppresses ERBB2 auto-phosphorylation and selectively inhibits the growth of ERBB2 driven cells by inducing cell cycle arrest in G_1. The drug is under study for the treatment of metastatic breast cancer.

Reversible multi-kinase inhibitors AEE788 is an orally bioavailable, reversible multiple receptor tyrosine kinase inhibitor. It suppresses the phosphorylation of the tyrosine kinases of ERBB1 (EGFR), ERBB2 (HER2), and VEGFR2 (Vascular Endothelial Growth Factor Receptor 2), resulting in receptor inhibition, the inhibition of cellular proliferation, and the induction of tumor cell apoptosis and tumor associated endothelial cell apoptosis.

ZD6474 is an orally bioavailable inhibitor of EGFR and VEGFR2. It is in clinical trials for the treatments of non-small cell lung cancer and medullary thyroid carcinoma. The agent has shown efficacy in combination with cytotoxic chemotherapy.

Adverse Effects Adverse effects include diarrhea, hypertension, and skin rashes.

Irreversible inhibitors Neratinib (HKI-272) (Rabindran 2004) is an orally available, 6,7-disubstituted 4-anilinoquinoline-3-carbonitrile. It irreversibly binds to EGFR family kinases by targeting a cysteine residue in the ATP binding pocket, thereby reducing receptor auto-phosphorylation. Treatment with this agent results in an inhibition of downstream signal transduction events and cell cycle regulatory pathways, causing arrest at the G_1/S transition of the cell division cycle and ultimately decreasing cellular proliferation. Neratinib potently suppresses ERBB2 and is highly active against ERBB2 overexpressing breast cancer cells. It also inhibits ERBB1 and the proliferation of ERBB1 dependent cells. Anti-tumor activity is achieved at a daily oral dose of 10–40 mg/kg.

In approximately 2 % of primary non-small cell lung cancers, there are mutations in the *erbB2* gene, the most frequent one being A775insYVMA. While cells with this mutation are relatively resistant to erlotinib, they remain sensitive to neratinib (Minami 2007). The G776insV_G/C mutation in *erbB2*, present in a small percentage of non-small cell lung cancers, is also sensitive to neratinib (Shimamura 2006).

Adverse Effects When administered on a continuous, once-daily oral treatment schedule, the maximum tolerated dose of neratinib is 320 mg/day, with diarrhea as the most frequently occurring adverse effect.

Drug Resistance In glioblastoma, a characteristic EGFR mutation that commonly arises is the variant III (vIII) in-frame deletion of exons 2–7. EGFRvIII is also associated with 5 % of lung squamous cell carcinomata, but is not present in lung adenocarcinomata. Although this form of EGFR is resistant to multiple kinase inhibitors, treatment with neratinib may reduce the size of these EGFRvIII-driven tumors (Ji 2006). Neratinib is not a substrate for ABCG2.

Canertinib dihydrochloride (Cl-1033) is the salt of an orally bioavailable quinazoline, which binds to the intracellular domains of EGFR family tyrosine kinases. Along with the inhibition of tyrosine phosphorylation, small molecule kinase inhibitors enhance ubiquitylation, endocytosis, and subsequent intracellular destruction of ERBB molecules. Canertinib alkylates a cysteine specific to ERBB receptors and is particularly effective at inducing its degradation. Thus, it irreversibly inhibits ERBB associated signal transduction functions and results in tumor cell apoptosis and suppression of tumor cell proliferation. The kinase inhibition is selective for ERBB1, ERBB2, ERBB3, and ERBB4 without inhibiting the tyrosine kinase activity of receptors such as Platelet-Derived Growth Factor Receptor, Fibroblast Growth Factor Receptor, and Insulin Receptor, even at high concentrations. Canertinib effectively inhibits the growth of esophageal squamous cell carcinoma, which co-expresses ERBB1 and ERBB2, by mediating the inhibition of phosphorylation of both MAPK and AKT. It also acts as a radiosensitizing agent and displays synergistic activity with other chemotherapeutic agents.

Afatinib (BIBW 2992) <Gilotrif, Tomtovok, Tovok irreversibly inhibits ERBB1 and ERBB2. It is approved for the use in patients with metastatic non-small cell lung cancer, whose tumors have ERBB1 exon 19 deletions or exon 21 (L858R) substitution mutations. The drug is also in clinical trials for breast cancer, prostate cancer, and head and neck cancer. Afatinib is taken orally at least 1 h before or 2 h after a meal.

Adverse Effects Serious adverse effects that require permanent discontinuation of afatinib include life threatening skin lesions (bullous, blistering, or exfoliative), interstitial lung disease (may manifest as lung infiltration, pneumonitis, acute respiratory distress syndrome, or allergic alveolitis), severe drug-induced hepatic impairment, persistent ulcerative keratitis, left ventricular dysfunction.

Common adverse effects include diarrhea (may result in dehydration with or without renal impairment), reduced ap-

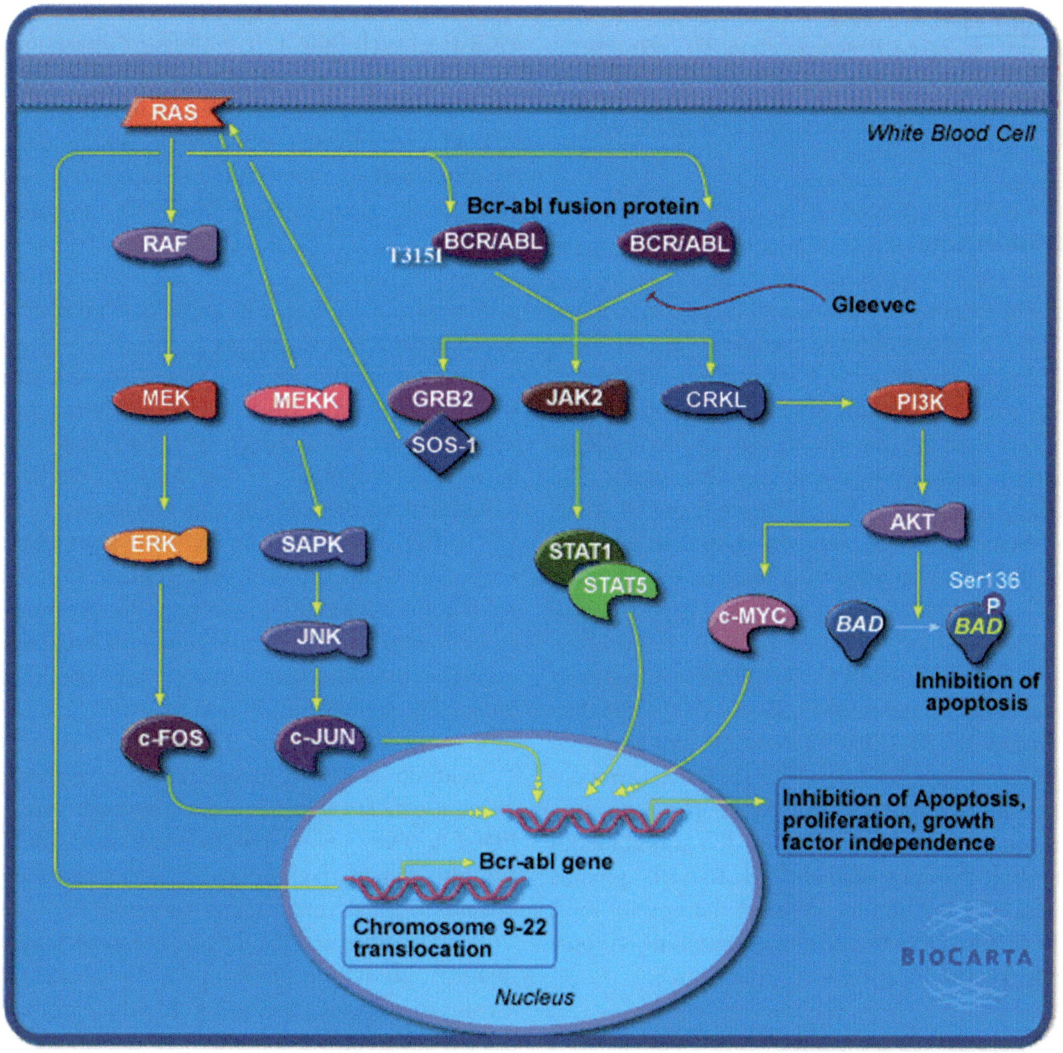

Fig. 4.6 BCR-ABL in cell proliferation. Chronic myelogenous leukemia (*CML*) is associated in most cases with a translocation between chromosomes 9 and 22 that occurs at the sites of *bcr* and the protein tyrosine kinase gene *abl*, creating the chimeric *BCR-ABL* protein. This leads to deregulation of the kinase activity of *ABL*, driving the uncontrolled cell growth in the disease. Blood cells containing the *BCR-ABL* fusion proliferate in the absence of growth factors they would normally require. In the cytoplasm, *BCR-ABL* is associated with a large signaling complex. Various of its cellular substrates may be involved in transformation, including PI-3 Kinase/PKB, the kinase JAK2, and STAT transcription factors. Specifically, STAT5 may contribute to the failure of apoptosis in *BCR-ABL* cells. The activation of *BCR-ABL* also represses apoptosis through the induction of *BAD*. *GRB-2* phosphorylation may play a regulatory role in tyrosine kinase signaling. Traditional cytotoxic anti-cancer drugs have serious adverse effects such as nausea, weight loss, hair loss and severe fatigue that result from their lack of specificity in killing cells. While such treatments kill all dividing cells, imatinib mesylate acts by a mechanism that is more specific to cancer cells. The drug was designed as a selective *BCR-ABL* inhibitor, and so produces less extensive adverse effects than other anti-cancer agents. (http://www.biocarta.com/pathfiles/h_gleevecpathway.asp)

petite, stomatitis, dermatitis, and paronychia. Afatinib may cause harm if administered during pregnancy.

Drug Interactions The concomitant treatment with ABCB1 inhibitors may cause increased systemic exposure to afatinib and require dose reduction. Concomitant ABCB1 inducers may require an afatinib dose increase.

Pelitinib (EKB-569) is a 3-cyanoquinoline that acts as an irreversible, covalent pan-ERBB tyrosine kinase inhibitor. It is under study for the treatment of colorectal cancer in combination with FOLFOX or FOLFIRI.

Adverse Effects The most common adverse effects are diarrhea and skin rashes.

Drug Resistance ABCG2 confers resistance to pelitinib.

Over-expression of EGFR family receptors is common in many solid tumors.

While reversible EGFR tyrosine kinase inhibitors are active in a subset of patients, most develop resistance within 1 year. In

nearly 50 % of the cases, acquired resistance is caused by the secondary ERBB1 mutation T790M.
In some cancers, the EGFR mutation variant III (vIII), an in-frame deletion of exons 2–7, commonly arises. Neratinib is effective against it.
Skin rashes are frequent adverse effects of EGFR inhibitors.

4.1.2 ABL Inhibitors

Physiologically, the tightly regulated activity of the tyrosine kinase ABL induces growth and resistance to apoptosis in hematopoietic cells. A common translocation[1] involving chromosomes 9 and 22 in chronic myeloid leukemia (CML) leads to the formation of the oncogenic, chimeric BCR-ABL, which transduces unregulated growth signals. The proto-oncogene product ABL signals through the PI 3-Kinase and JAK-STAT pathways, and it cross-talks to the RAS pathway (Fig. 4.6). The regulatory subunit of PI 3-Kinase binds directly to the SH3 domain of auto-phosphorylated, active ABL. Efficient transformation by ABL requires its protein tyrosine kinase activation and membrane association via NH_2-terminal myristoylation. BCR-ABL dependent JAK activation induces STAT5 to activate the expression of the anti-apoptotic protein BCL-x_L. The BCR-ABL oncoprotein also strongly associates with F-Actin. The formation of BCR-ABL oligomers is permissive for the simultaneous binding of multiple F-Actin filaments. BCR-ABL tyrosine kinase inhibitors (Fig. 4.7) are the first-line therapy for most patients with Philadelphia chromosome containing chronic myelogenous leukemia.

First generation BCR-ABL inhibitor Increasing insights into the molecular pathways associated with growth signals led to the development of small molecule inhibitors, including the salt imatinib mesylate <Gleevec, Glivec>(Druker 2000). Imatinib inhibits BCR-ABL, a fusion tyrosine kinase produced by chronic myelogenous leukemia cells, which harbor the Philadelphia chromosome. The drug suppresses ABL enzymatic activity by engaging with high specificity the ATP binding site of an inactive form of the kinase, thus preventing its auto-phosphorylation (Fig. 4.8). The interaction involves six hydrogen bond interactions at methionine 318, threonine 315, glutamine 286, asparagine 381, isoleucine 380, and histidine 361. This mechanism of action prevents ATP from reaching its binding site. Inhibition of the BCR-ABL kinase activity by imatinib induces cancer cell apoptosis. The agent was approved in 2001 in the U.S., Europe, and Japan for the treatment of chronic myelogenous leukemia.

Imatinib blocks auto-phosphorylation of the receptor tyrosine kinase CD117 (c-KIT, Stem Cell Factor Receptor, SCFR), as well as Stem Cell Factor stimulated downstream signaling events, such as the activation of ERK1, ERK2, and PKB (Heinrich 2000). It inhibits proliferation and induces apoptosis in cells that over-express the oncoprotein CD117. As CD117 is activated in gastrointestinal stromal tumor (GIST), imatinib was approved in 2002 by the U.S. FDA for the treatment of metastatic gastrointestinal stromal tumor, and as adjuvant treatment following the surgical resection of localized c-KIT positive-gastrointestinal stromal tumor. A fraction of melanomata harbor activating mutations or amplifications of *kit*. Some of the affected patients benefit from imatinib mesylate treatment.

Imatinib inhibits the receptor tyrosine kinase PDGFR (Platelet Derived Growth Factor Receptor). PDGF is a connective tissue cell mitogen with functions that include embryonal development, wound healing, and the control of interstitial fluid pressure in soft connective tissue. Paracrine PDGF signaling in the connective tissue tumor stroma plays a role in various types of solid tumors. It contributes to the regulation of interstitial fluid pressure. As most solid tumors have an increased interstitial fluid pressure, pharmacological reduction may be a way to increase the uptake of anti-cancer drugs. Through the inhibition of PDGFR, imatinib can significantly reduce the tumor interstitial fluid pressure.

Imatinib is under investigation as a treatment for additional cancers that have excessive activities of c-KIT or PDGFR. They include acute myelogenous leukemia, small cell lung cancer, ovarian cancer, testicular cancer, dermatofibrosarcoma protuberans, and glioma.

Pharmacokinetics At clinically relevant concentrations of imatinib, binding to plasma proteins is approximately 95 %, mostly to Albumin and α1-Acid Glycoprotein (AGP). The drug is metabolized by and is an inhibitor of the CYP3A4 enzyme system and caution needs to be exercised when substrates, inducers, or inhibitors of CYP3A4 are used concomitantly;. Additionally, imatinib mesylate is a substrate and inhibitor of CYP2D6 and the blood levels of CYP2D6 substrates can increase during imatinib mesylate therapy. CYPs 1A2, 2C9, and 2C19 are minor contributors to imatinib metabolism.

Adverse Effects While imatinib has been very successful in the treatment of chronic myelogenous leukemia and gastrointestinal stromal tumors, it is associated with uncommon, but severe cardiotoxicity[2]. The therapeutic effect on the kinase BCR-ABL is also linked to the cardiovascular adverse effects of the drug. Therefore, it is not possible to fully eliminate this toxicity. However, inhibition of the signaling intermediate JNK1 can ameliorate the imatinib effects on heart cells.

Drug Resistance Imatinib mesylate fails in approximately 20 % of patients within 5 years. Compromising factors in-

[1] The Philadelphia chromosome (Ph).

[2] Many receptor tyrosine kinase inhibitors may evoke cardiac dysfunction as potential adverse effects. They include lapatinib, imatinib, nilotinib, dasatinib, sorafenib, and sunitinib.

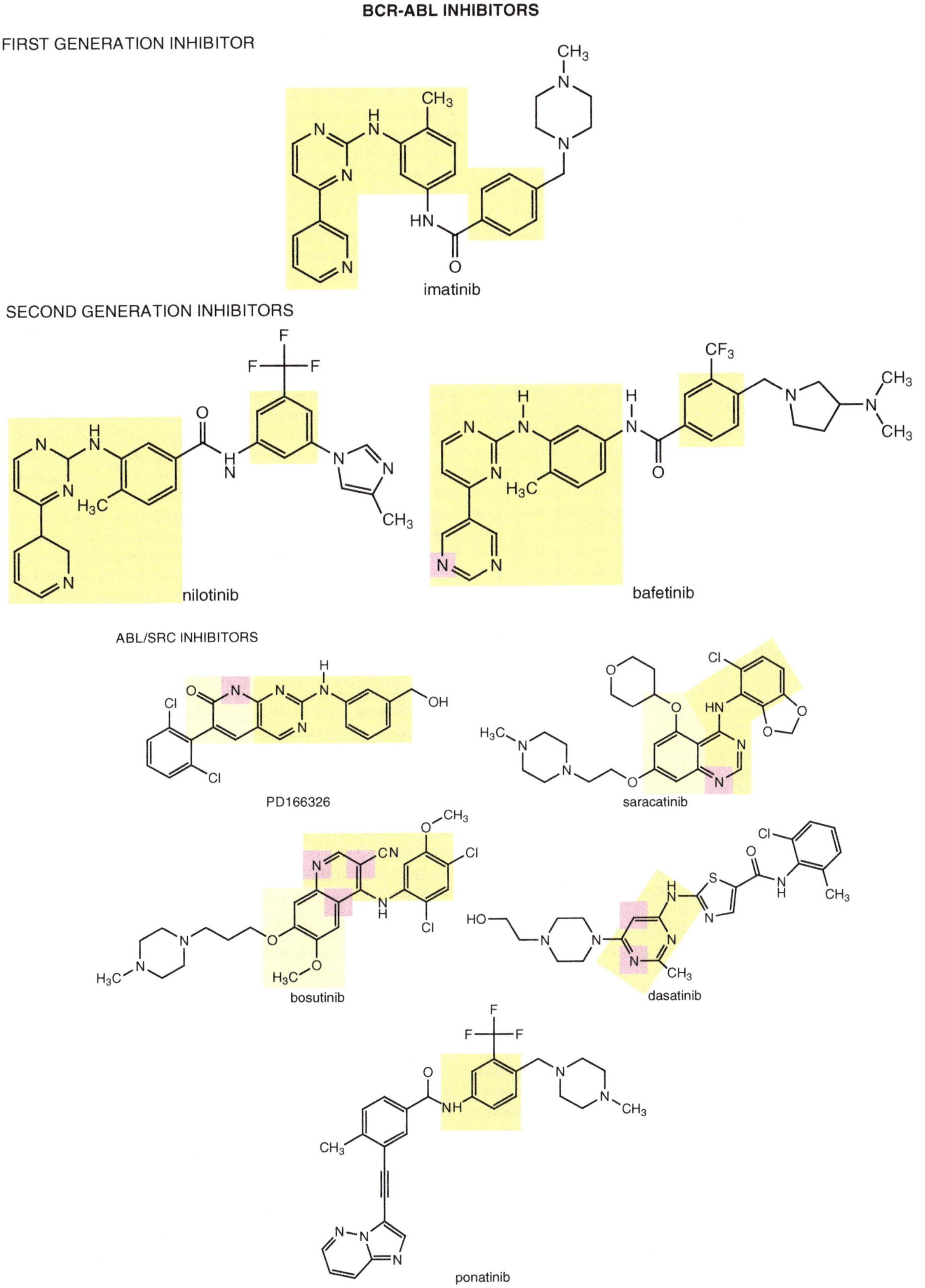

Fig. 4.7 Structures of BCR-ABL inhibitors. The subclasses comprise first and second generation BCR-ABL inhibitors, ABL/SRC inhibitors, and ABL/Aurora Kinase inhibitors. The core structure of the first generation inhibitor imatinib is common to the second generation inhibitors. Only in bafetinib a nitrogen is inserted (*pink*). The ABL/SRC inhibitors preserve some of the functional groups of the first and second generation inhibitors (*bright yellow*) and have subclass-specific elements in common (*light yellow*). Within the groups of ABL/SRC inhibitors and ABL/Aurora Kinase inhibitors, some core elements are common to several representatives

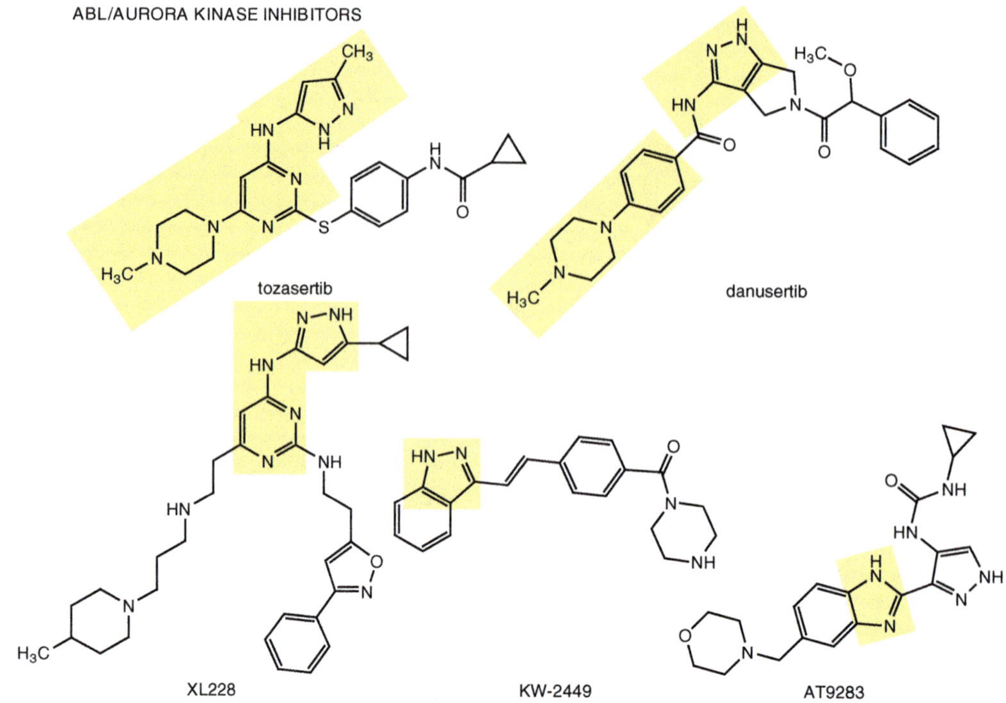

Fig. 4.7 (continued)

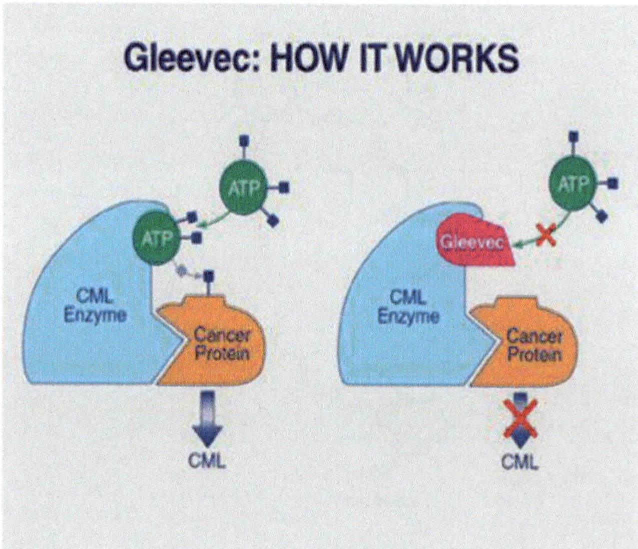

Fig. 4.8 Imatinib drug action. The drug targets the BCR-ABL protein in CML cells. (http://www.cancer.gov/PublishedContent/Images/images/documents/6ac3a026-8c6c-4a0f-97b0-df63d9f8ef92/poster_gleevec.gif) There are instances where we have been unable to trace or contact the copyright holder. If notified the publisher will be pleased to rectify any errors or omissions at the earliest opportunity

clude limited therapeutic activity and durability in advanced disease stages, persistence of minimal residual disease because of the limited effects of the drug on immature hematopoietic stem cells, and primary or acquired drug resistance (Gontarewicz 2008). In chronic myelogenous leukemia blast crisis, the initial rate of hematologic responses to imatinib is high. However, these responses are usually short-lived, most patients ultimately develop resistance and undergo disease progression. Mechanisms of resistance can be categorized into three main groups:

- BCR-ABL is reactivated and cell proliferation remains dependent on BCR-ABL signaling (amplification of the *bcr-abl* gene, mutations in the BCR-ABL kinase domain that prevent high affinity binding of imatinib). The emergence of transformed cell clones with resistance to imatinib and other small molecule inhibitors, mediated by mutations in BCR-ABL, has become a major challenge in the treatment of chronic myelogenous leukemia. Mutational frequencies increase as chronic myelogenous leukemia progresses from the chronic phase to the blast phase. More than 70 point mutations can be assigned to four major groups based on their location in the kinase domain, the ATP binding loop (40% of all mutations), the gatekeeper residue threonine 315 (25% of all mutations), the catalytic domain (25% of all mutations), or the activation loop (5% of all mutations). BCR-ABL contains the ATP binding P-loop and the activation loop, which stabilize the basal conformation. Mutations in these loops destabilize the protein structure, such that the kinase domain cannot assume the inactive conformation required for imatinib binding. Mutations in the P-loop region are the most common (Fig. 4.9). The mutation T315I is completely resistant to multiple BCR-ABL directed therapies. This substitution eliminates a critical oxygen molecule needed for

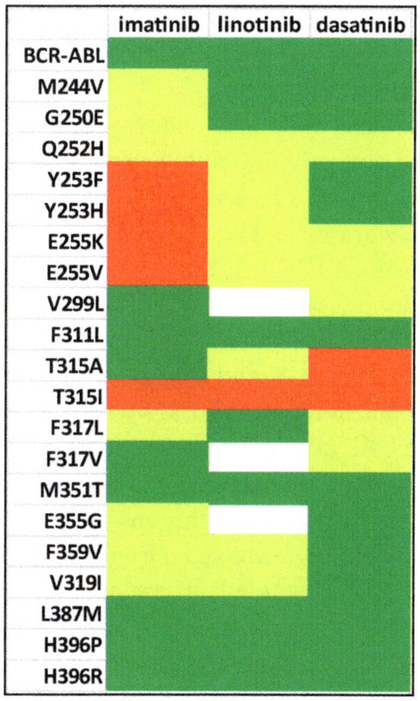

Fig. 4.9 Resistance to small molecule BCR-ABL inhibitors. The kinase inhibitors imatinib, nilotinib, and dasatinib are compared for their efficacy against BCR-ABL mutations (shown *top* to *bottom* in *N*-terminal to *C*-terminal order). The color coding indicates sensitivity (*green*), intermediate sensitivity (*yellow*), or resistance (*red*) according to IC_{50} values for cell proliferation (the IC_{50} value is the concentration of inhibitor resulting in a 50 % reduction in cell viability). Imatinib: sensitive (up to 1000 nM), intermediate (1001–3000 nM), insensitive (>3000 nM). Nilotinib: sensitive (up to 50 nM), intermediate (51–500 nM), insensitive (>500 nM). Dasatinib: sensitive (up to 3 nM), intermediate (4–60 nM), insensitive (>60 nM). The graph highlights the problematic nature of T315I. (Redrawn from (O'Hare 2007))

hydrogen bonding between imatinib and the ABL kinase. It also creates steric hindrance to the binding of most small molecule inhibitors. The development of an inhibitor for $BCR\text{-}ABL^{T315I}$ has been challenging, because most ATP competitive inhibitors directly interact with threonine 315 via hydrogen bonding and with the specificity imparting hydrophobic pocket, for which this residue serves as a gatekeeper. Several BCR-ABL mutations in the active site, such as Y235F/H or E255K/V, also confer imatinib mesylate resistance. Small molecule inhibitors of Aurora Kinase, including MK-0457 (VX-680), XL228, and AT9713, can effectively inhibit a mutant enzyme (Table 4.3).

- The BCR-ABL protein re mains inhibited by imatinib, but alternative or downstream signaling pathways become activated, often involving excessive activity of SRC kinases.
- The drug disposition is altered through increased efflux via up-regulated export transporters such as ABCB1, compromised influx by down-regulation of the organic cation transporter OCT1, or enhanced protein binding of imatinib to circulating α1-Acid Glycoprotein (AGP).

Approaches to overcome resistance include dose escalation, the use of alternative BCR-ABL inhibitors, combination chemotherapy (possibly comprising multiple BCR-ABL inhibitors), and inhibitors of downstream BCR-ABL targets (such as Farnesyl Transferase inhibitors).

In systemic mastocytosis, most cases have a point mutation in codon 17 of CD117, which results in a D816V amino acid substitution in the kinase-2 domain of CD117. This mutated CD117 is resistant to inhibition by imatinib (Frost 2002).

Second generation BCR-ABL inhibitors Nilotinib and bafetinib belong to the 2-phenylamino-pyrimidine based sub-class of inhibitors.

Although imatinib is an effective, frontline therapy for chronic phase chronic myelogenous leukemia, accelerated phase or blast crisis phase chronic myelogenous leukemia patients and Philadelphia chromosome positive acute lymphocytic leukemia, patients often relapse, resulting from the emergence of imatinib-resistant point mutations within the BCR-ABL tyrosine kinase domain.

Nilotinib monohydrate monohydrochloride (AMN107) <Tasigna> is an orally available phenylamino-pyrimidine, which was derived from the imatinib scaffold (Weisberg 2006). Nilotinib exhibits a similar binding mode as its model drug, however, its potency is increased by approximately 30-fold because of an improved topologic fit to the enzyme. Designed to overcome imatinib resistance, nilotinib binds to the ATP site in the inactive conformation of the ABL kinase domain, largely through lipophilic interactions. This agent inhibits (with decreasing potency) the auto-phosphorylation of DDR1, BCR-ABL, PDGFR, CSF-1R, and c-KIT. Nilotinib interrupts the downstream signaling targets of these tyrosine kinases, resulting in decreased cellular proliferation and the induction of apoptosis. The drug is indicated for the treatment of chronic phase and accelerated phase Philadelphia chromosome-positive (Ph^+) chronic myelogenous leukemia in adult patients—newly diagnosed or resistant of or intolerant to prior therapy that included imatinib.

Pharmacokinetics The recommended dose is 300–400 mg twice daily. As the bioavailability of nilotinib is variably increased with food, patients should avoid eating 2 h before and 1 h after taking a dose. Peak concentrations of nilotinib are reached 3 h after oral administration. The unaltered drug is the main circulating component in the blood. The main metabolic pathways are oxidation and hydroxylation, with none of the products contributing to the pharmacological activity. The apparent elimination half-life with daily dosing is approximately 17 h. Over 90 % of the drug is eliminated in the feces; the unmetabolized parent drug accounts for about 70 % of the eliminated agent. Dose reduction may be required in patients with hepatic impairment. Since nilotinib and its metabolites are not renally excreted, a decrease in total body clearance is not anticipated in patients with renal impairment.

Adverse Effects Nilotinib prolongs the QT interval, possibly leading to sudden deaths. The agent should not be used in patients with hypokalemia, hypomagnesemia, or long QT syndrome. As nilotinib causes myelosuppression, it may be given in combination with hematopoietic growth factors such as erythropoietin or G-CSF if indicated. The most common non-hematologic adverse drug reactions—occurring in over 10 % of patients—are rash, pruritus, headache, nausea, fatigue, and myalgia. Less common and of mild to moderate severity are upper abdominal pain, constipation or diarrhea, dry skin, alopecia, muscle spasms, arthralgia, peripheral edema, and asthenia. They are manageable and generally do not require dose reduction. Pleural and pericardial effusions may arise in 1 %, gastrointestinal hemorrhage in 0.5 % of patients. Because nilotinib can increase serum Lipase it requires caution in patients with a history of pancreatitis. If Lipase elevations are accompanied by abdominal symptoms, it necessitates dose interruption and diagnostics to exclude pancreatitis. The drug is Pregnancy Category D.

Nilotinib is a competitive inhibitor of UGT1A1 and can thus increase bilirubin levels. The largest increases in bilirubin arise in (TA)7/(TA)7 genotype (UGT1A1*28) patients relative to the (TA)6/(TA)6 and (TA)6/(TA)7 genotypes.

Drug Resistance In acute phase or blast crisis of chronic myelogenous leukemia, 30–60 % of patients are refractory to nilotinib. Resistance is associated with a limited spectrum of BCR-ABL kinase mutations that mostly affect the P-loop and T315I. As the drug is not a substrate for the efflux transporter ABCB1, its over-expression does not lead to resistance. Nilotinib influx is also independent of the uptake transporter OCT1.

Drug Interactions Nilotinib undergoes metabolism by CYP3A4, and concomitant administration of strong inhibitors or inducers of CYP3A4 can increase or decrease the nilotinib concentrations. The agent also acts as a competitive inhibitor of CYP3A4, CYP2C8, CYP2C9, CYP2D6. It may potentially increase the concentrations of drugs that are eliminated by these enzymes. Conversely, nilotinib can induce CYP2B6, CYP2C8, and CYP2C9, and may potentially decrease the concentrations of drugs which are eliminated by these enzymes. As nilotinib inhibits ABCB1, its administration with drugs that are substrates of this export transporter likely causes increased concentrations of the substrate drugs, and caution should be exercised. Drugs that prolong the QT interval need to be avoided in conjunction with nilotinib treatment. Due to decreased nilotinib solubility at increasing pH, drugs that suppress gastric acid secretion to elevate the gastric pH (such as proton pump inhibitors) may decrease the solubility of nilotinib and reduce its bioavailability.

The orally available, dual BCR-ABL/LYN inhibitor bafetinib (*N*-[3-([5,5′-Bipyrimidin]-2-ylamino)-4-methylphenyl]-4-[[(3S)-3-(dimethylamino)-1-pyrrolidinyl]methyl]-3-(trifluoromethyl)benzamide) (INNO-406, NS-187) was developed at Kyoto University Hospital in collaboration with Nippon Shinyaku. Its activity profile may overcome imatinib resistance. In addition to the BCR-ABL inhibitory properties, Bafetinib acts as a specific inhibitor of LYN kinase. Up-regulation of

Table 4.3 Specificities of ABl inhibitors

BCR-ABL inhibition										
	BCR-ABL	BCR-ABL^{T315I}	BCR-ABL^{T315N}	BCR-ABL^{V229L}	BCR-$ABL^{Y235F/H}$	BCR-$ABL^{E255K/V}$	BCR-ABL^{Q252H}	BCR-ABL^{M351T}	BCR-ABL^{F359V}	BCR-ABL^{H396P}
First generation										
Imatinib	S	R	R	S	R	R	S	S	S	
Second generation										
Nilotinib	S	R								
Bafetinib	S									
ABL/SRC inhibitors										
PD166326	S									
Saracatinib	S									
Bosutinib	S	R	R							
Dasatinib	S	R	S	R	S	S	S	S	S	S
Ponatinib	S	S								
ABL/Aurora Kinase inhibitors										
Tozasertib	S	S	S	S			S	S	S	S
Danusertib	S	S				S		S		
XL228	S	S								
KW-2449	S	S								
AT9283	S									

S sensitive, *R* resistant

Table 4.3 (continued)

	Off-target inhibition																
	SRC	SRC^{Y530F}	LYN	Auroa A	Aurora B	KIT	KIT^{D816V}	PDGFR	IGF-1R	FGFR	DDR1	DDR2	CSF-1R	JAK2	FLT3	EPHA2	GFR
First generation																	
Imatinib				R	R	S	R	S							R		
Second generation																	
Nilotinib						S		S			S		S				
Bafetinib			S														
ABL/SRC inhibitors																	
PD166326	S																
Saracatinib	S	S	S														
Bosutinib	S					R	R	R									
Dasatinib	S			R	R	S		S				S			R	S	S
Ponatinib	S																
ABL/Aurora Kinase inhibitors																	
Tozasertib				S	S										S		
Danusertib				S	S												
XL228	S			S	R				S	S							
KW-2449				S	S										S		
AT9283				S	S									S	S		

S sensitive, *R* resistant

LYN kinase activity is a common cause of imatinib resistance, and LYN activation is associated with a variety of solid tumors, including prostate cancer. Bafetinib has been granted orphan drug status by the U.S. FDA for the treatment of Philadelphia chromosome-positive chronic myelogenous leukemia.

ABL/SRC inhibitors SRC family protein tyrosine kinases interact with a variety of cell surface receptors and participate in intracellular signal transduction pathways to support growth. Tumorigenic forms can arise through altered regulation or expression of SRC. Over-expression of specific SRC kinases may be active in chronic myelogenous leukemia, and may contribute to the resistance by tumor cells to specific BCR-ABL inhibitors, such as imatinib. Therefore, dual ABL/SRC kinase inhibitors have the potential to suppress chronic myelogenous leukemia cells more effectively than ABL specific inhibitors.

PD166326 is a pyridopyrimidine type inhibitor of receptor tyrosine kinases that inhibits ABL induced or BCR-ABL induced cell growth with half maximal inhibitory concentrations in the low milimolar to sub-milimolar concentration range (Wolff 2005). PD166326 also potently inhibits SRC. Orally administered PD166326 is well tolerated.

Drug Resistance PD166326 can reduce the growth of some imatinib resistant forms of chronic myelogenous leukemia, such as $BCR\text{-}ABL^{H396P}$ and $BCR\text{-}ABL^{M351T}$.

Saracatinib (AZD0530) is a 5-, 7-substituted anilinoquinazoline that inhibits SRC and ABL by blocking the ATP binding site. Saracatinib sensitively inhibits SRC^{Y530F} as well as the SRC tyrosine kinase family members c-YES, FYN, LYN, BLK, FGR, and LCK. The orally available small molecule exerts anti-tumor and anti-invasive activities, as it has inhibitory effects on proliferation and survival, cell motility and invasion. In metastatic cancer, saracatinib inhibits SRC kinase-mediated osteoclast bone resorption.

Bosutinib (SKI-606) <Bosulif> is a synthetic 7-alkoxy-3-quinolinecarbonitrile and a dual kinase inhibitor that targets both ABL and SRC kinases, with minimal activity against PDGFR and c-KIT. It also inhibits select serine/threonine kinases. Bosutinib suppresses the auto-phosphorylation of ABL and SRC kinases, resulting in the inhibition of cell growth and the induction of apoptosis. Because of the dual mechanism of action, this agent may have activity in imatinib resistant chronic myelogenous leukemia, other myeloid malignancies, and solid tumors.

Adverse Effects Bosutinib causes nausea, vomiting and diarrhea, which diminish over time. Myelosuppression affecting platelets, white and red blood cells arises in 1–10% of patients. Fluid retention, particularly in the lungs, is possible. The symptoms of adverse events tend to be less severe than with other tyrosine kinase inhibitors.

Drug Resistance The T315 mutation is completely resistant to bosutinib. The drug is not an efficient substrate for multi-drug resistance export transporters.

Dasatinib hydrochloride (BMS-354825) <Sprycel> is a thiazolylaminopyrimidine dual BCR/ABL and SRC family kinase inhibitor that suppresses the growth promoting activities of these enzymes. In contrast to most other tyrosine kinase inhibitors, dasatinib binds to the active conformation of its target enzymes. At nanomolar concentrations, the drug inhibits BCR-ABL, SRC family (SRC, LCK, YES, FYN), c-KIT, EPHA2, PDGFRβ, and GFR. Mutations in the gene *discoidin domain receptor 2* (*ddr2*) are present in 4% of lung squamous cell carcinomata. These kinase mutations are associated with sensitivity to dasatinib. The drug has more than 300-fold increased potency to inhibit BCR-ABL compared with imatinib. Because it binds to ABL with less stringent conformational requirements than imatinib it exhibits increased potency but reduced selectivity. Likely because of its less stringent binding characteristics, dasatinib overcomes the resistance to imatinib of chronic myelogenous leukemia cells that harbor BCR-ABL kinase domain point mutations. In the U.S., dasatinib is approved for use in

- patients with chronic myelogenous leukemia who no longer benefit from imatinib treatment
- patients with Philadelphia chromosome-positive acute lymphoblastic leukemia (Ph^+ ALL) who no longer benefit from, or cannot tolerate prior treatment.

Dasatinib is given at 100–140 mg orally once per day. Dose escalation is permissible in patients who do not achieve a hematologic or cytogenetic response at the recommended starting dosage.

Pharmacokinetics Dasatinib is best absorbed from the stomach due to the presence of gastric acid. Therefore, medicines that reduce stomach acid or increase gastric pH should be avoided within 2 h before or after dasatinib administration. Following oral administration, maximum blood concentrations of dasatinib are reached after 0.5–6 h. The agent exhibits dose-proportional increases in blood concentration and linear elimination characteristics over the range of 15–240 mg/day. Binding of dasatinib and its major active metabolite to plasma proteins is in excess of 90%, however, the drug is abundantly distributed in the extravascular space. Dasatinib is extensively biotransformed, primarily by CYP3A4, the primary enzyme responsible for the formation of the active metabolite. Flavin-Containing Monooxygenase 3 (FMO-3) and Uridine Diphosphate-Glucuronosyltransferase (UGT) are also involved in the formation of dasatinib metabolites. However, dose adjustment is not necessary in patients with hepatic impairment. The overall mean terminal half-life is 3–5 h. 85% of dasatinib is eliminated in the feces.

Adverse Effects Dasatinib has a toxicity profile that includes nausea and vomiting, diarrhea, headache, musculoskeletal pain, and rash. Myelosuppression may require dose reduction or discontinuation of dasatinib treatment. Bleeding due to thrombocytopenia or platelet dysfunction can be serious. Severe brain hemorrhages may be fatal. Fluid retention can manifest in pleural effusions, pericardial effusions, ascites, superficial localized edema, or generalized edema and can lead to congestive heart failure. Dasatinib has the potential to prolong cardiac ventricular repolarization (the QT interval). The agent may increase the risk for developing pulmonary arterial hypertension, which may occur anytime after initiation, including after more than 1 year of treatment. The drug is Pregnancy Category D.

Drug Resistance In acute phase or blast crisis of chronic myelogenous leukemia, 20–40% of patients are refractory to dasatinib. Drug resistance to dasatinib occurs in patients with the BCR-ABL mutation T315I. The dasatinib resistant mutation V299L may develop under treatment. The resulting $BCR\text{-}ABL^{V299L}$ regains sensitivity for imatinib, and the mutated leucine enhances the affinity to the Aurora Kinase inhibitor tozasertib.

Since dasatinib is an inhibitor of ABL and SRC family kinases, it can overcome imatinib resistance due to SRC activation. Dasatinib is also not a substrate of multi-drug resistance efflux pumps.

Drug Interactions Similar to other tyrosine kinase inhibitors, dasatinib has extensive drug-drug interactions with agents metabolized by the enzyme CYP3A4. Drugs that inhibit CYP3A4 increase the blood levels of dasatinib (including ketoconazole, itraconazole, ritonavir, atazanavir sulfate, indinavir, nelfinavir, saquinavir, telithromycin, erythromycin, and clarithromycin). Grapefruit juice may also increase the blood concentrations of dasatinib and should be avoided. The use of concomitant strong CYP3A4 inducers (including dexamethasone, phenytoin, carbamazepine, rifampin, and phenobarbital) may decrease dasatinib concentrations. St. John's Wort may decrease dasatinib plasma concentrations unpredictably and should be avoided. Conversely, dasatinib may alter the blood levels of cyclosporine, alfentanil, fentanyl, pimozide, sirolimus, tacrolimus, and ergotamine. Antacids or proton pump inhibitors may reduce the absorption of dasatinib from the stomach.

Ponatinib (AP24534) <Iclusig> is an orally active BCR-ABL kinase inhibitor that is effective against the T315I mutation. The imidazo[1,2b]pyridazine core rests in the adenine pocket of the enzyme, the methylphenyl group occupies a hydrophobic pocket behind I315, the ethynyl linkage forms van der Waals interactions with the amino acid, and the trifluoromethyl group binds to a pocket of the inactive conformation kinase. Ponatinib was derived from the lead compound AP23464, which does not inhibit $BCR\text{-}ABL^{T315I}$.

Adverse Effects The most common adverse effects are diarrhea or constipation, abdominal pain, skin rashes, hypertension, fatigue, headache, dry skin, arthralgia, nausea, and pyrexia. Hematologic adverse reactions include thrombocytopenia, anemia, neutropenia, and leukopenia. Discontinuation may be required in cases of arterial thrombosis or hepatic toxicity. Ponatinib is Pregnancy Category D.

Drug Interactions The administration with strong CYP3A inhibitors may require dose reduction. Ponatinib inhibits ABCB1. It may affect the systemic exposure to drugs that are substrates for this export transporter. Drugs that elevate the gastric pH may reduce the bioavailability of ponatinib.

ABL/Aurora Kinase inhibitors The dual ABL/Aurora Kinase inhibitors are active against the mutant form BCR-ABL^{T315I}, which is associated with drug resistance against other BCR-ABL inhibitors. Therefore, they may serve as rescue treatments.

The pan-Aurora Kinase inhibitor tozasertib lactate (VX-680, MK-0457) is a synthetic small molecule drug that inhibits wild-type ABL, BCR-ABL^{Y253F}, and BCR-ABL^{T315I} at half-maximal concentrations below 50 nM. It anchors at the hinge region engaging asparagine-381 but does not reach as deep into the kinase domain as imatinib, which allows tozasertib to avoid the steric constraints imposed by the T315I mutations. Under dasatinib treatment, the resistant mutation BCR-ABL^{V299L} may develop. It remains sensitive to tozasertib because the mutated leucine enhances the drug affinity. The agent also induces apoptosis in tumor cells, in which Aurora Kinases are over-expressed.

Adverse Effects The main toxicities consist of myelosuppression, alopecia, and mucositis. QTc elongation in the electrocardiogram is a possible complication.

The pyrrolo-pyrazole danusertib (PHA-739358) is an ATP competitive pan-Aurora Kinase (Aurora Kinase A, B, and C) inhibitor that also has activity against BCR-ABL^{T315I}. Danusertib binds to the active conformation of BCR-ABL^{T315I} in a mode that accommodates the substitution of isoleucine for threonine, thus avoiding steric hindrance. Exposure of imatinib-resistant $CD34^{+}$, BCR-ABL^{T315I} carrying cells to danusertib decreases the phosphorylation of Histone H3 on serine-10 (reflective of Aurora Kinase inhibition) and CRKL (a downstream target of BCR-ABL). A regimen under study is the administration of 250–330 mg/m^2/day as a weekly 6-h infusion for 3 consecutive weeks, every 4 weeks.

Adverse Effects Adverse events comprise high grade neutropenia and infusion related reactions.

XL228 is an Aurora Kinase A inhibitor that also suppresses wild-type ABL and BCR-ABL^{T315I} at low nanomolar concentrations. It further acts as a kinase inhibitor of IGF1R, FGFR, and SRC. In sensitive cells, XL228 inhibits the phosphorylation of STAT5, a downstream target of BCR-ABL.

KW-2449 is a multi-kinase inhibitor of ABL, BCR-ABL^{T315I}, Aurora Kinase, and FLT3. As an ABL inhibitor, the drug may be of benefit in imatinib resistant leukemia. KW-2449 is also growth inhibitory for leukemia cells with FLT3 gain-of-function mutations, resulting in G_1 arrest, and apoptosis. In FLT3 wild-type leukemia cells, it induces G_2/M arrest and apoptosis. The orally available KW-2449 is under investigation to treat leukemia patients.

The pan-Aurora, ABL, FLT3, and JAK2 kinase inhibitor AT9283 (1-cyclopropyl-3[5-morpholin-4yl methyl-1*H*-benzomidazol-2-yl]-urea) induces a reduction in the phosphorylation of Histone H3, CRKL, and STAT5 (downstream targets of ABL, FLT3, and JAK2 signaling). AT9283 is in clinical trials and has activity in patients with refractory acute or chronic myelogenous leukemia (AML or CML).

Adverse Effects The maximum tolerated dose of AT9283, given as a 72-h intravenous infusion, is 100 mg/m^2/day. Dose limiting toxicities include myelosuppression and alopecia, tumor lysis syndrome may occur. Elevated Transaminases, non-cardiac Creatine Kinase, and Lactate Dehydrogenase rises can be reflective of muscle or liver damage.

A translocation involving chromosomes 9 and 22 generates the constitutively active fusion kinase BCR-ABL and causes chronic myelogenous leukemia (CML).
BCR-ABL inhibitors are drugs of choice for the disease.
While initially successful, small molecule kinase inhibitors of BCR-ABL loose effectiveness—often because of mutations in the drug target.
Second generation BCR-ABL inhibitors, ABL/SRC inhibitors or BCR-ABL^{T315I} inhibitors (also inhibit Aurora Kinase) are second line of defense.
In contrast to most tyrosine kinase inhibitors, dasatinib binds to the active conformation of the target enzyme.
BCR-ABL inhibitors are soluble at low pH and are absorbed in the stomach.
Many BCR-ABL inhibitors exert cardiotoxicity and cause fluid retention.

4.1.3 RAS Pathway Inhibitors

Signals transduced by various proto-oncogenic growth factors proceed through the small GTPase RAS. RAS functions as a cell membrane-associated switch that relays signals from ligand stimulated receptors to cytoplasmic cascades. These receptors include G-Protein coupled seven transmembrane spanning receptors, tyrosine kinase receptors, and cytokine receptors that cause the stimulation of associated non-receptor tyrosine kinases. The signal transduction may be initiated via the cascade Growth Factor Receptor→GRB→SOS→RAS and proceed through the canonical RAS→RAF→MEK→ERK signaling pathway (Fig. 4.10).

Kinases of the RAS family and some of their downstream targets are frequently up-regulated in neoplasms (Weber 2007). K-RAS mutations have the highest incidence in adenocarcinomata of the pancreas (90%), colon (50%), and lung (30%). N-RAS is predominantly mutated in myeloid

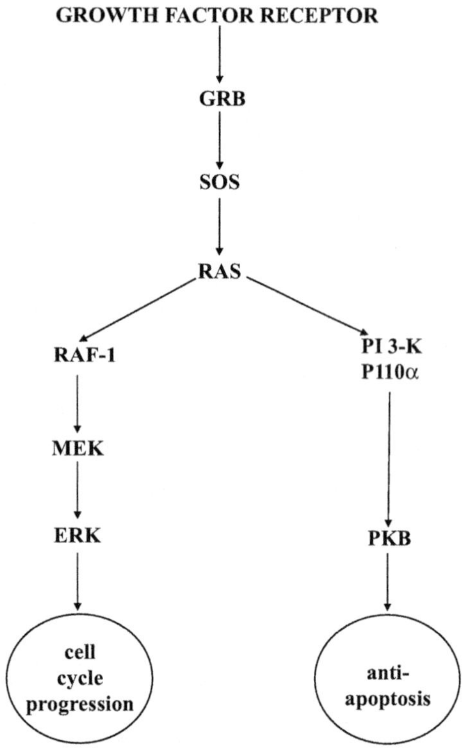

Fig. 4.10 RAS signaling pathways. RAS may mediate signals transduced by growth factor receptors. The latter may proceed through the cascade SHC→GRB-2→SOS. RAS induces cell growth through two principal downstream targets, namely the *ERK* (MAPK) pathway and the *PI3-K* pathway

leukemia (30 %) (Bos 1989). Inhibition of RAS signaling has the potential to cure those cancers by overcoming the excessive, RAS dependent cell growth (Table 4.4).

RAF inhibitors RAF is a serine/threonine kinase that is involved in the RAS dependent transduction of mitogenic signals from the cell membrane to the nucleus. There are three active *raf* genes (*A-raf*, *B-raf-1*, and *C-raf-1*), 2 of which have related pseudo-genes (*B-raf-2* and *C-raf-2*). *c-raf-1* RNA is present in many tissues, while *A-raf* and *B-raf-1* expression is restricted. *A-raf* and *c-raf* encode cytoplasmic serine/threonine protein kinases of 68 and 74 kD, which contain three conserved regions (CR). CR1 and CR2 are in the NH_2-terminal half with CR1 comprising the presumed ligand binding site, and CR3 represents the COOH-terminal kinase domain. RAF acts as a MAP Kinase Kinase Kinase and counteracts apoptosis by suppressing the activation of MST-2. RAF inhibitors may inhibit the excessive growth of some cancers. 40–60 % of melanomata carry a B-RAF mutation, in roughly 90 % of cases the specific mutation V600E.

RAF inhibitors suppress ERK signaling in mutant B-RAF cells but enhance ERK signaling in cells harboring wild-type B-RAF. RAF inhibitors bind to one member of the C-RAF/B-RAF hetero-dimer or C-RAF/C-RAF homo-dimer. While inhibiting one protomer, this allows transactivation of the other, drug-free binding partner.

Drug Resistance The development of drug resistance is a major limitation for the efficacy of small molecule B-RAF inhibitors. Mechanisms that mediate drug resistance include:

- expression of mutant N-RAS activates the signaling of MEK-1 and MEK-2 in some resistant tumors,
- an increase in RAS activation or RAF dimerization may be sufficient to cause drug resistance,
- over-expression of PDGF-β (Platelet Derived Growth Factor β) enables tumor cell survival,
- over-expression of MAP3K8 leads to resistance by activating MEK-1 and MEK-2 signaling.

Sorafenib tosylate (4-[4-[[4-chloro-3-(trifluoromethyl) phenyl]carbamoylamino] phenoxy]-*N*-methyl-pyridine-2-carboxamide) <Nexavar> is a synthetic compound that inhibits wild-type and mutant forms of the kinase RAF (Fig. 4.11[3]). The kinases KIT, FLT3, and RET are also targets. Sorafenib inhibits the VEGFR2/PDGFRβ signaling cascade, thereby blocking tumor angiogenesis. The drug is active orally and it is available as tablets. It is taken without food, 1 h before or 2 h after a meal, typically twice daily. Sorafenib was approved by the U.S. FDA in 2005, it received E.U. marketing authorization in 2006 to treat unresectable hepatocellular carcinoma and advanced renal cell carcinoma. The administration of sorafenib prolongs progression-free survival in patients with advanced clear cell renal carcinoma, in whom previous therapy has failed (Escudier 2007). Further, the agent is in testing for the treatment of soft tissue sarcoma.

Pharmacokinetics Following oral administration, sorafenib reaches peak blood levels after 3 h. With continuous exposure, steady state concentrations are achieved within 7 days, with a peak-to-trough concentration ratio below 2. The agent undergoes oxidative metabolism by hepatic CYP3A4, as well as glucuronidation by UGT1A9. Of eight sorafenib metabolites, five accumulate in the blood. The pyridine *N*-oxide is the main circulating product, comprising 10–15 % at steady state. The mean elimination half-life of sorafenib is 24–48 h. Neither renal impairment nor hepatic impairment substantially affects the pharmacokinetics.

Adverse Effects Common adverse effects of sorafenib include fatigue, weight loss, diarrhea, arthralgia or myalgia, alopecia, mucositis or stomatitis, hand-foot skin reactions, and skin rash or desquamation (in rare serious cases Stevens-Johnson syndrome and toxic epidermal necrolysis). Hypertension, congestive heart failure, and cardiac ischemia are rare serious adverse events. QT prolongation is rare, but increases the risk

[3] The structure of the representative XL281 has not been disclosed.

Table 4.4 RAS pathway inhibitors

	RAF	B-RAFV600E	PDGFR	VEGFR2	KIT	FLT3	RET	FGFR	MEK	ERK1	ERK2	CDKs	PKB	GSK3β	PKC
RAF inhibitors															
Sorafenib	S		S	S	S	S	S								
CHIR-265	S	S	S	S			S								
CHIR-258	S		S	S				S							
Vemurafenib	R	S													
PLX4032 and PLX4720	R	S	R												
Dabrafenib	R	S													
XL281	B and C, not A														
MEK/ERK inhibitors															
PD0325901									S						
Trametinib										S	S				
PKC inhibitors															
7-hydroxystaurosporine												S	S		S
Midostaurin			S	S		S									S
Enzastaurin				R									S	S	S
Safingol															S

S sensitive, *R* resistant, *CDKs* Cyclin Dependent Kinases

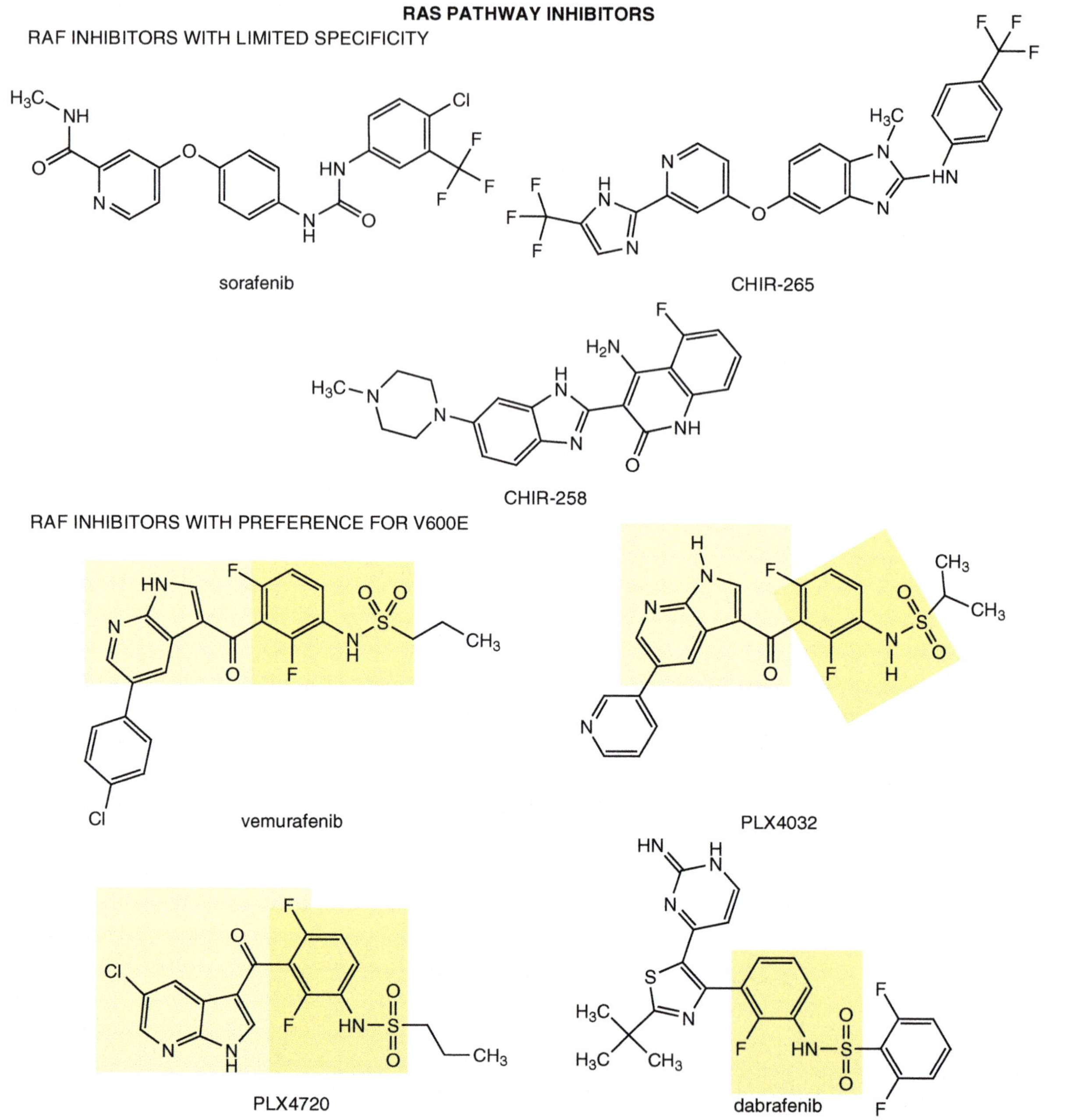

Fig. 4.11 Structures of RAS pathway inhibitors. Three sub-classes of RAF inhibitors comprise inhibitors with limited specificity, inhibitors with a preference for the mutant V600E, and (not shown) selective B-RAF/C-RAF inhibitors. The highlighted core structure (*bright yellow*) is common to all RAF^{V600E} inhibitors. The partially overlapping motif of joined 5- and 6-rings, a (C=O based) bridge, and a 6-ring (*light yellow*) bears similarity to the joined 6- rings, a (N-H based) bridge, and a 6-ring in the ERBB family inhibitors (see Fig. 4.3). MEK inhibitors suppress the RAS pathway downstream of RAF. Among the PKC inhibitors, the three staurosporin derivatives have an identical core structure, which is shared with indolocarbazoles (see Fig. 2.33 and 4.13). Their differences are highlighted in *pink*

for ventricular arrhythmias. An elevated risk of bleeding may arise following sorafenib administration. Gastrointestinal perforation is an uncommon adverse reaction in less than 1 % of patients. The drug is Pregnancy Category D.

Drug Interactions Concomitant use of strong CYP3A4 inducers (such as, carbamazepine, dexamethasone, phenobarbital, phenytoin, rifampin, rifabutin, St. John's Wort) is to be avoided, because they can decrease the systemic exposure to sorafenib. Neomycin can reduce the sorafenib bioavailability by as much as 50 %. Sorafenib inhibits glucuronidation catalyzed by UGT1A1 and UGT1A9 and transport mediated by ABCB1. It could increase the systemic exposure of simultaneously administered drugs that are substrates for these molecules.

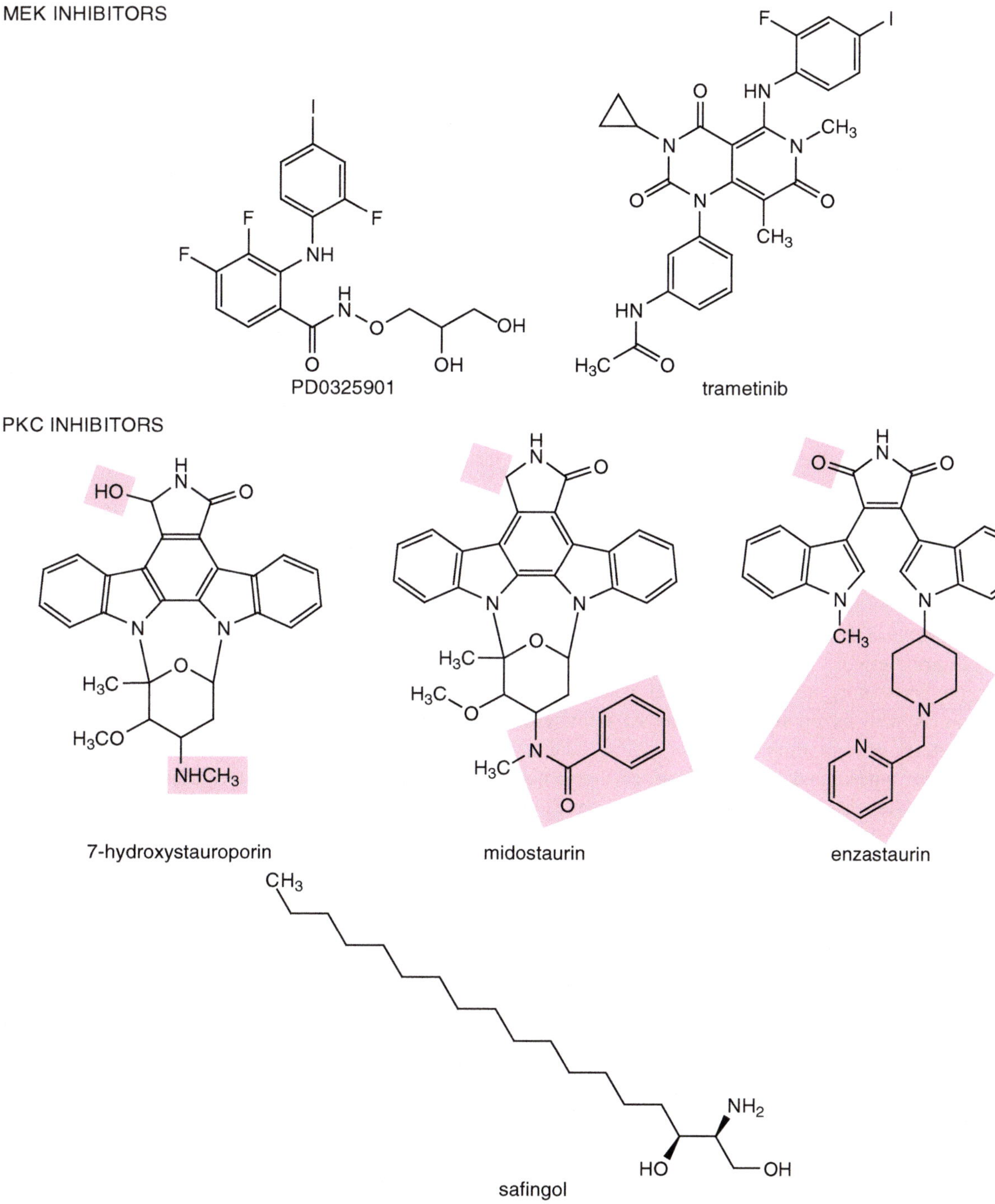

Fig. 4.11 (continued)

CHIR-265 (RAF265) is an orally active small molecule that binds to and inhibits RAF family kinases (C-RAF, B-RAF, B-RAF^{V600E}) and abrogates downstream ERK signaling. It also inhibits RET activity. This drug action results in a suppression of tumor cell proliferation and tumor cell death. In addition, CHIR-265 inhibits VEGFR-2, thereby disrupting tumor angiogenesis. Combination with the PI 3-K/mTOR (Phosphoinositol 3-Kinase/mammalian Target of Rapamycin) inhibitor BEZ235 achieves a synergistic effect leading to decreased cell proliferation. CHIR-265 is in clinical trials for the treatment of locally advanced or metastatic melanoma. The maximum tolerated oral dose is 48 mg daily, an intermittent schedule at higher dose may be possible.

- The related compound CHIR-258 is a small molecule with inhibiting properties against the kinases B-RAF, PDGFR-β, VEGFR-2, and FGFR. It is in clinical trials for the treatment of melanoma.

Adverse Effects Dose limiting toxicities within the first 28-day cycle include pulmonary embolism, visual disturbances, hyperlipasemia, diarrhea, and ataxia. Grade III and IV thrombocytopenia may also become dose limiting.

Vemurafenib (PLX4032) <Zelbroraf> blocks mutated B-RAF. It engages the ATP-binding domain of mutant B-RAF monomer and, under the condition that RAS is not constitutively activated, can block MEK and ERK signaling. The drug received U.S. FDA approval in 2011 for the treatment of unresectable or metastatic melanoma with the B-RAF^{V600E} mutation. It is not suitable for use in patients with wild-type B-RAF melanoma. The recommended dose is 960 mg twice daily without a meal.

Pharmacokinetics The vemurafenib concentration-time profile is adequately described by a one-compartment disposition model with first order absorption and first order elimination. At steady state, the drug exhibits linear pharmacokinetics within the 240–960 mg dose range. In the blood, over 99 % of vemurafenib is bound to Albumin and α1 Acid Glycoprotein. Over 95 % of a dose is excreted in the feces, only 1 % in the urine. The elimination half-life is 55 h.

Adverse Effects Serious hypersensitivity reactions, including anaphylaxis, may arise upon initial vemurafenib administration as well as upon re-initiation of treatment. Skin manifestations are common, including palmar-plantar erythrodysesthesia syndrome, keratosis pilaris, erythema nodosum, and rarely Stevens-Johnson syndrome. Patients have an increased risk for developing B-RAF-negative squamous cell skin cancers or basal cell carcinomata that are readily treatable. General adverse effects comprise arthritis, dizziness, folliculitis, vasculitis, uveitis, and mild photosensitivity. QT prolongation resulting in atrial or ventricular fibrillations may occur. The drug is Pregnancy Category D.

Drug Interactions Vemurafenib is a moderate CYP1A2 inhibitor, a weak CYP2D6 inhibitor, and a CYP3A4 inducer. Its concomitant use with agents with narrow therapeutic windows that are metabolized by CYP1A2, CYP2D6, or CYP3A4 is not recommended as vemurafenib may alter their concentrations. Co-administration of vemurafenib results in an increase in S-warfarin blood levels.

PLX4032 (RG7204, RO5185426) and PLX4720 are selective RAF inhibitors with a more than 10-fold higher selectivity for B-RAF^{V600E} than for wild-type B-RAF. Mutant B-RAF inhibition may lead to programmed cell death in the cancer cells. The orally bioavailable agents are in clinical trials for metastatic melanoma.

Adverse Effects Dose limiting toxicities include rash, fatigue, and joint pains. Serious adverse events can occur in some patients after long-term treatment, including the possibility of drug related cutaneous squamous cell carcinoma.

Drug Resistance Mechanisms of drug resistance, which is encountered in 40 % of patients after 2–18 months, include the over-expression of PDGFR-β, which creates an alternate survival pathway, and reactivation of the normal B-RAF survival pathway via N-RAS.

The orally bioavailable drug dabrafenib mesylate (GSK2118436) <Tafinlar> is a reversible, selective, ATP competitive B-RAF inhibitor with more than 100-fold selectivity for mutant B-RAF over wild type B-RAF. It is approved to treat patients with metastatic or unresectable melanoma whose tumors express the B-RAF^{V600E} gene mutation. There is a risk of paradoxical activation of MAP Kinase signaling and increased cell proliferation in B-RAF wild-type cells, which are exposed to B-RAF inhibitors. Dabrafenib has efficacy in shrinking brain metastases. The recommended dose is 150 mg orally taken twice daily, approximately 12 h apart, at least 1 h before or at least 2 h after a meal.

Pharmacokinetics Dabrafenib is primarily metabolized by CYP2C8 and CYP3A4. As it contains a sulfonamide moiety, dabrafenib confers a potential risk of hemolytic anemia in patients with Glucose-6-Phosphate Dehydrogenase (G6PD) deficiency.

Adverse Effects Cutaneous squamous carcinoma arises in 10 % of the patients. Hyperkeratosis, alopecia, palmar-plantar erythrodysesthesia syndrome, rash, headache, pyrexia, arthralgia or myalgia, back pain, constipation, or upper respiratory tract infections may occur. Serious febrile drug reactions[4] afflict fewer than 5 % of patients treated with dabrafenib. Hyperglycemia requiring an increase in the dose of, or initiation of insulin or oral hypoglycemic agent therapy is possible under treatment. The drug is Pregnancy Category D.

Drug Interactions Strong inhibitors or inducers of CYP3A4 or CYP2C8 may affect the concentrations of dabrafenib. Drugs that alter the pH of the upper gastrointestinal tract (such as proton pump inhibitors, H_2-receptor antagonists, or antacids) may alter the solubility of dabrafenib and reduce its bioavailability. Because dabrafenib induces CYP3A4 and CYP2C9 it decreased the systemic exposures of the CYP3A4 substrate midazolam, the CYP2C9 substrate S-warfarin, and the CYP3A4/CYP1A2 substrate R-warfarin.

XL281 (BMS-908662) is a highly selective inhibitor of B-RAF and C-RAF, but not A-RAF. The agent is orally bioavailable. The maximum tolerated dose is 150 mg/day.

Pharmacokinetics The time to peak blood concentration is 2 h. The half-life is 5–20 h. Steady-state levels after continuous administration are reached by day 8.

[4] Serious febrile drug reactions are defined as serious cases of fever or fever of any severity accompanied by hypotension, rigors or chills, dehydration, or renal failure in the absence of other identifiable causes (such as infections).

Adverse Effects Grade 3 adverse events include fatigue, vomiting, diarrhea, nausea, and arthralgia. Dose limiting toxicities occurring at 225 mg/day are grade 4 nausea, grade 3 fatigue, grade 3 diarrhea, and grade 3 vomiting.

MEK/ERK inhibitors MEK (MAP Kinase Kinase, MAPKK) is phosphorylated and activated by RAF in a growth factor signaling pathway that is frequently overactive in cancer cells.

PD0325901 (*N*-[(2R)-2,3-dihydroxypropoxy]-3,4-difluoro-2-[(2-fluoro-4-iodophenyl)amino]-benzamide) is a synthetic derivative of the selective, non-competitive MEK inhibitor CI-1040. PD0325901 has improved oral bioavailability and induces a longer duration of target suppression. The agent selectively binds to and inhibits MEK, thereby preventing the phosphorylation and activation of the downstream kinases ERK -1 and -2, which may result in the inhibition of tumor cell proliferation.

Trametinib (GSK-1120212) <Mekinist> is a reversible MEK-1/MEK-2 inhibitor approved for the treatment of patients with unresectable or metastatic melanoma harboring the B-RAF^{V600E} or B-RAF^{V600K} mutations. It is not indicated for the treatment of patients who have received prior B-RAF inhibitor therapy. The drug is also under study to treat leukemia, lymphoma, and pancreatic cancer. The recommended dose is 2 mg per day, 1–2 h before a meal, until disease progression or unacceptable toxicity is encountered.

Pharmacokinetics More than 95 % of the drug in circulation is protein-bound. Metabolism occurs via deacetylation with or without mono-oxygenation or glucuronidation.

Adverse Effects Rash, diarrhea, and lymphedema are common adverse effects. Discontinuation is required if retinal pigment epithelial detachments, retinal vein occlusion, or an intolerable rash occur. Interstitial lung disease or pneumonitis require permanent discontinuation. An asymptomatic decrease of the left ventricular ejection fraction of the heart is possible it may be a sign of cardiomyopathy. The drug is Pregnancy Category D.

PKC inhibitors Protein Kinase C (PKC) may activate RAS via the nucleotide exchangexe factor RAS-GRP. RAS-GRP activity also depends on the local availability of the signaling intermediate diacylglycerol. Abnormally high levels of RAS-GRP can lead to malignant transformation through excessive RAS pathway activity.

The indolocarbazole 7-hydroxystaurosporine (UCN-01) is a synthetic derivative of staurosporine that inhibits several kinases, including calcium dependent Protein Kinase C, the serine/threonine kinase PKB (AKT), and Cyclin-Dependent Kinases (CDKs). 7-hydroxystaurosporine promotes the accumulation of the negative cell cycle regulators P21 and P27, arresting tumor cells in the G_1/S phase of the cell cycle. The agent prevents nucleotide excision repair by inhibiting the G_2 checkpoint kinase CHK1, which results in apoptosis. Thus, it may enhance the effects of DNA damaging drugs. 7-hydroxystaurosporine is under study for treating melanoma and lymphoma.

Adverse Effects The maximum tolerated dose is 43 mg/m^2/day for 3 days. Dose limiting toxicities comprise nausea and vomiting, hypoxemia, and hyperglycemia.

Midostaurin ((9S,10R,11R,13R)-2,3,10,11,12,13-hexahydro-10-methoxy-9-methyl-11-(methylamino)-9,13-epoxy-1*H*,9*H*-diindolo[1,2,3-gh:3′,2′,1′-lm]pyrrolo[3,4-j][1,7]benzodiamzonine-1-one) (PKC412) is a synthetic indolocarbazole that acts as a non-specific inhibitor of Protein Kinase C family enzymes. Midostaurin inhibits oncogenic PKC signal transduction pathways involved in the regulation of the cell cycle in tumor cells. It also inhibits VEGF Receptors, Platelet-Derived Growth Factor Receptor, FLT3, and other receptor tyrosine kinases. Midostaurin thereby initiates tumor cell apoptosis. The agent is in clinical development.

Enzastaurin hydrochloride (3-(1-Methylindol-3-yl)-4-[1-[1-(pyridin-2-ylmethyl)piperidin-4-yl]indol-3-yl]pyrrole-2,5-dione) (LY317615) is the salt of a synthetic macrocyclic bisindolemaleimide. It acts as a potent inhibitor of PKCβ, PKCα, PKCγ and PKCε. Enzastaurin inserts into the ATP binding site and blocks catalytic activity. The drug also suppresses the phosphorylation of GSK3β and AKT. It may decrease tumor blood supply and so tumor burden. Enzastaurin has orphan drug status in Europe for the treatment of diffuse large B-cell lymphoma. In 2013 it failed a phase III clinical trial for lymphoma.

Safingol (L-threo-dihydrosphingosine, (2S,3S)-2-aminooctadecane-1,3-diol) <Kynacyte> is a saturated derivative of sphingosine. As an inhibitor of PKC, it competitively inhibits the regulatory, phorbol binding domain of PKC. This agent acts synergistically with other chemotherapeutic drugs, such as doxorubicin or cisplatin, and may potentiate chemotherapy-induced apoptosis.

Pharmacokinetics Despite its non-natural stereochemistry, safingol is metabolized preferentially by enzymes of the sphingolipid biosynthetic pathway. The cytotoxic potential of safingol is reduced via its metabolic conversion.

Excessive growth signals through constitutively active RAS pathways are common in some cancers.
RAF inhibitors may be first-line treatments of choice.
Some RAF inhibitors have low specificity, others bind preferentially to the RAF^{V600E} mutant in cancer cells.
Many RAF inhibitors exert cardiotoxicity, some increase the risk for cutaneous secondary malignancies.

Table 4.5 The phosphatidylinositol 3′OH kinase gene family. (Adapted from Wikipedia)

Group	Gene	Protein	Acronym	EC number
Class 2	PIK3C2A	PI3K, class 2, α polypeptide	PI3K-C2α	2.7.1.154
	PIK3C2B	PI3K, class 2, β polypeptide	PI3K-C2β	
	PIK3C2G	PI3K, class 2, γ polypeptide	PI3K-C2γ	
Class 3	PIK3C3	PI3K, class 3	VPS34	2.7.1.137
Class 1 catalytic	PIK3CA	PI3K, catalytic, α polypeptide	P110-α	2.7.1.153
	PIK3CB	PI3K, catalytic, β polypeptide	P110-β	
	PIK3CG	PI3K, catalytic, γ polypeptide	P110-γ	
	PIK3CD	PI3K, catalytic, δ polypeptide	P110-δ	
Class 1 regulatory	PIK3R1	PI3K, regulatory subunit 1 (α)	P85-α	(None)
	PIK3R2	PI3K, regulatory subunit 2 (β)	P85-β	
	PIK3R3	PI3K, regulatory subunit 3 (γ)	P55-γ	
	PIK3R4	PI3K, regulatory subunit 4	P150	
	PIK3R5	PI3K, regulatory subunit 5	P101	
	PIK3R6	PI3K, regulatory subunit 6	P87	

Inhibitors of various RAS pathway signaling molecules are in development.

4.1.4 Phosphoinositide 3-Kinase Pathway Inhibitors

PI3K inhibitors The Phosphoinositide 3′OH-Kinase (PI 3-Kinase, PI3K) family of gene products consists of three classes of lipid kinases that have a regulatory subunit (P85) and a catalytic subunit (P110), which combine to form an enzyme that phosphorylates the 3′ OH group of phosphatidylinositols (Table 4.5). The signaling pathway activated downstream of PI3K via PKB (AKT) and mTOR protects cells from apoptosis.

Whereas in healthy cells the Phosphoinositide 3′OH-Kinase pathway is tightly controlled, the inappropriate activation of PI3K is important in the pathogenesis of multiple cancers, in which activating somatic mutations may arise. Mutations in the catalytic subunit P110α (PIK3CA) are associated with approximately 30 % of epithelial cancers (Engelman 2009). Kinase domain and helical domain mutants comprise about 80 % of PI 3-Kinase dependent cancers. Kinase domain mutants, such as H1047R, have increased lipid kinase activity. Helical domain mutants, such as E545K or E542K, disrupt the inhibitory inter-molecular interaction between P85 and P110, thus excessively activating the kinase domain (Samuels 2004). Each type of mutant promotes uncontrolled cell expansion via anti-apoptosis. This renders the enzyme and its associated downstream signaling intermediates drug targets (Table 4.6).

Several agents that target the kinase domain of PI 3-Kinase (including BGT226, BKM120, XL765, XL147, GDC0941, GSK1059615) have entered early phase clinical trials. BEZ235, BGT226, PWT33597, and XL765 also possess mTOR inhibitory properties because the P110 kinase domain shares similar structural features with the serine/threonine kinase domain of mTOR.

PWT33597 mesylate[5] is a dual inhibitor of PI3Kα and mTOR with IC_{50} values around 20 nM. It is approximately 10-fold more selective for PI3Kα compared to PI3Kγand PI3Kδ. There is little or no cross-reactivity with either serine/threonine or tyrosine kinases. PWT33597 is in clinical trials for advanced solid tumors.

Pharmacokinetics PWT33597 is not extensively metabolized and shows little potential for interaction with Cytochrome P450 enzymes. There is high compound distribution into tumors. Also, administration of PWT33597 is associated with transient increases in Insulin blood levels, consistent with an effect on PI3K→PKB signaling.

Unlike other isoforms of PI3K, PI3Kδ is expressed primarily in hematopoietic lineage cells. The targeted inhibition of PI3Kδ is designed to suppress hematologic malignancies while preserving PI3K signaling in non-neoplastic cells. CAL101 (Fig. 4.12) is an oral small molecule inhibitor that targets the δ isoform of the 110 kD catalytic subunit of class IA PI3K. CAL-101 inhibits the production of the second messenger phosphatidylinositol-3,4,5-trisphosphate (PIP_3), thus preventing the activation of the PI3K signaling pathway and inhibiting tumor cell proliferation and survival. The agent is in clinical trials for certain forms of late-stage leukemias.

Semafore (SF1126) consists of the PI3K inhibitor LY294002 conjugated to an arginine-glycine-asparagine-serine (RGDS) peptide fragment. This peptide binds Integrin receptors in the tumor vasculature such that the LY294002 moiety inhibits PI3K dependent angiogenesis specifically in the tumor environment. SF1126 was granted orphan drug

[5] In veterinary use: VDC-597.

Table 4.6 PI3K pathway inhibitors

	PI3K	$PI3K^{H1047}R$	$PI3K^{E545K}$	$PI3^{KE542K}$	PKB	PKC	mTOR	FKBP12	Calcineurin
PI3K inhibitors									
PWT33597	PI3Kα						S		
CAL101	PI3Kδ								
Semafore	S								
NVP-BEZ235	S						S		
PX-866	S								
PKB inhibitors									
Miltefosine	S				S	S			
Perifosine	S	S	S		S				
MK-2206					S				
mTOR inhibitors									
Sirolimus							S	S	
Temsirolimus							S	S	S
Everolimus								S	
Ridaforolimus							S		

S sensitive, *R* resistant

status by the U.S. FDA in 2010 for the treatment of chronic B-cell lymphocytic leukemia.

The imidazoquinoline-derived dual PI3K and mTOR inhibitor NVP-BEZ235 is effective as a single agent and in combination with established cancer drugs. It is in clinical trials for advanced solid tumors. As gain-of-function mutations of RAS activate multiple pathways, including the PI3K pathway and the MEK→MAPK pathway, clinical trials combine NVP-BEZ235 with a MEK inhibitor.

PX-866 is a synthetic derivative from the fungal metabolite wortmannin (a product of Penicillium wortmannin). Compared to wortmannin, it has increased stability, reduced toxicity, and stronger drug activity. PX-866 is the only pan-isoform, irreversible PI3K inhibitor in clinical development (it forms a covalent bond with the PI3K molecule.). Due to its mechanism of action the agent results in sustained inhibition of the PI3K pathway. It is potent when delivered orally at 2–4 mg/kg.

Pharmacokinetics PX-866 is metabolized to produce an active metabolite, 17-OH, that is a more potent PI3K inhibitor than the parent drug and retains the same irreversible mechanism of action. PX-866 and the 17-OH metabolite inhibit all 4 PI3K family members and have the greatest potency for PI3Kα and β, the family members that are strongly linked to certain solid tumors.

PKB inhibitors The serine/threonine kinase PKB (AKT) is located at a critical signaling node downstream of Phosphatidylinositol 3′OH-Kinase. It is important in promoting cell survival and inhibiting apoptosis.

The PKB inhibitor miltefosine (hexadecylphosphocholine) <Impavido, Miltex> is an orally and topically active alkyl-phosphocholine compound that inhibits the anti-apoptotic MAPK (Mitogen-Activated Protein Kinase) pathway and modulates the balance between the MAPK and pro-apoptotic Stress-Activated Protein Kinase (SAPK/JNK) pathways, thereby inducing apoptosis. Synthetic phospholipids may exert anti-tumor activity through the inhibition of Protein Kinase C, an essential mediator in growth factor signal transduction, and m Miltefosine also targets cellular membranes, modulating cell membrane permeability, membrane lipid composition, and phospholipid metabolism. This results in cell differentiation and inhibition of cell growth. Acting further as an anti-protozoal immunomodulator, miltefosine stimulates T-lymphocytes, macrophages and the expression of IL-3 (Interleukin-3), GM-CSF (Granulocyte-Macrophage Colony Stimulating Factor), and IFN-γ (Interferon-γ).

Pharmacokinetics Administration can be oral or topical. Miltefosine is used as a 6% solution in an aqueous 3-alkyloxypropylene glycol mixture.

Adverse Effects With oral administration, hyperplastic gastrointestinal tract changes, nausea and vomiting, gonadal atrophy, hair loss, and ocular toxicity may arise. No systemic effects arise after dermal application, which may be indicated for breast cancer that is metastatic to the skin. The drug is teratogenic and should not be given to pregnant women.

Perifosine (octadecyl-(1,1-dimethyl-4-piperidylio) phosphate) (KRX-0401) is an alkylphospholipid that is structurally related to miltefosine. Perifosine inhibits PI3K and PKB. It is in clinical trials for colorectal cancer and multiple myeloma. It has orphan drug status for the treatment of multiple myeloma and neuroblastoma in the U.S., and for multiple myeloma in the E.U.

MK-2206 is a selective, allosteric inhibitor of PKB1, PKB2, and PKB3. The drug is activated by the pleckstrin homology domain and inhibits the auto-phosphorylation of both T308 and S473. This action results in an inhibi-

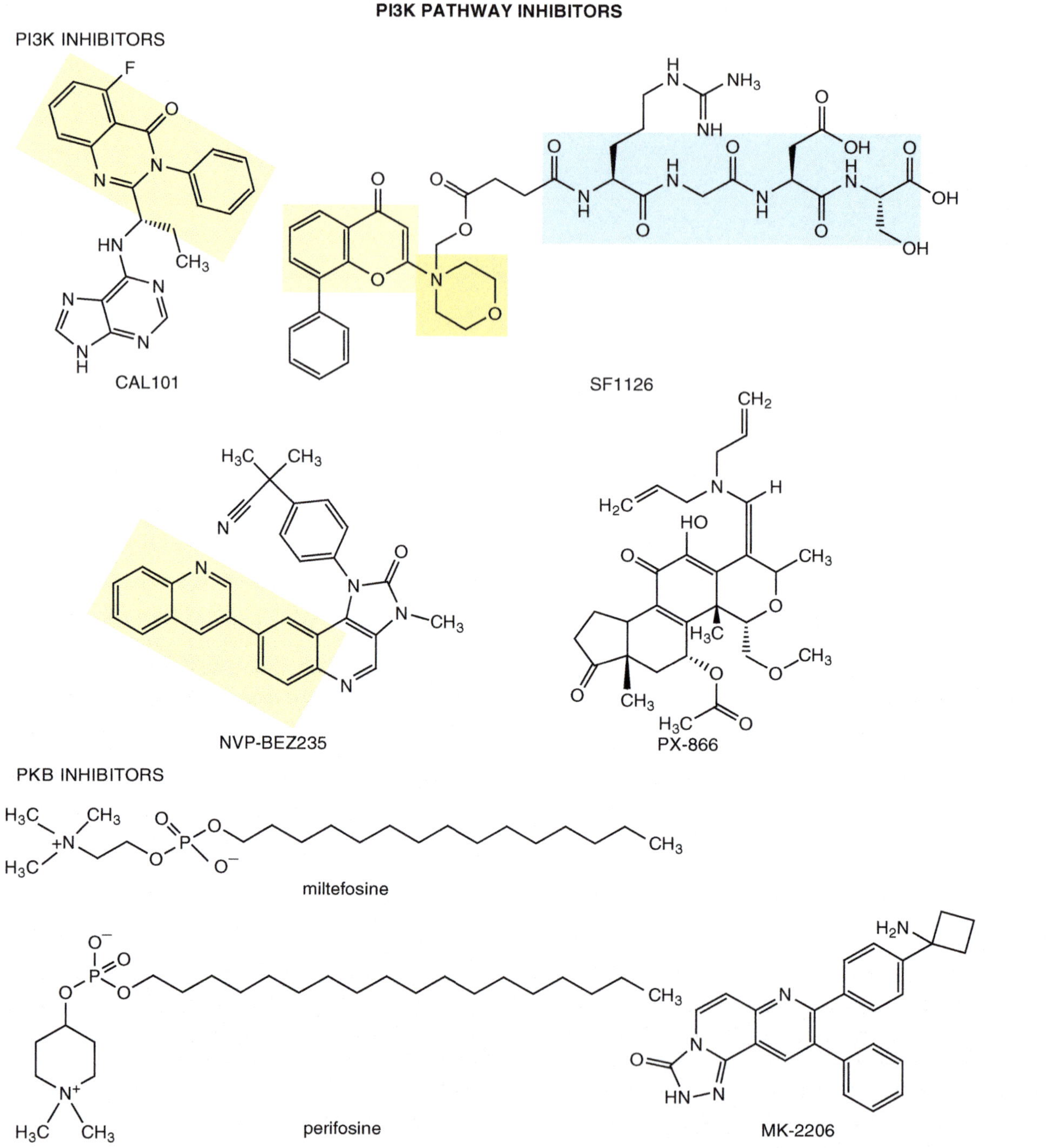

Fig. 4.12 Structures of PI3K pathway inhibitors. Subclasses include PI3K inhibitors, PKB inhibitors, and mTOR inhibitors. The loosely conserved core structure in a subset of PI3K inhibitors is highlighted in *light yellow*, the peptide bonds in the RGDS (arginine-glycine-asparagine-serine) of semaphore are shown on *blue* background. The mTOR inhibitors are derivatives of sirolimus. Structural differences among the representatives are highlighted in *pink*

tion of downstream signaling molecules, including TSC2, PRAS40 and Ribosomal S6 proteins. The orally bioavailable MK-2206 is in clinical trials for the treatment of ovarian cancer, primary peritoneal cancer, and fallopian tube cancer.

mTOR inhibitors mTOR (mammalian Target of Rapamycin, FRAP, FKBP-Rapamycin Associated Protein) is a serine/threonine kinase that controls cell growth and metabolism in response to nutrients, growth factors, and cellular energy levels. It plays a role in the PI3K→PKB→mTOR→RSK pathway that is up-regulated in several types of cancer. When the kinase activity of mTOR is activated, its downstream effects, entailing the synthesis of Cyclin D and HIF-1α, are increased. Cyclin D then stimulates cell cycle progression. HIF-1α (Hypoxia-Inducible Factor-1α) then stimulates VEGF (Vascular Endothelial Growth Factor), which results in angiogenesis.

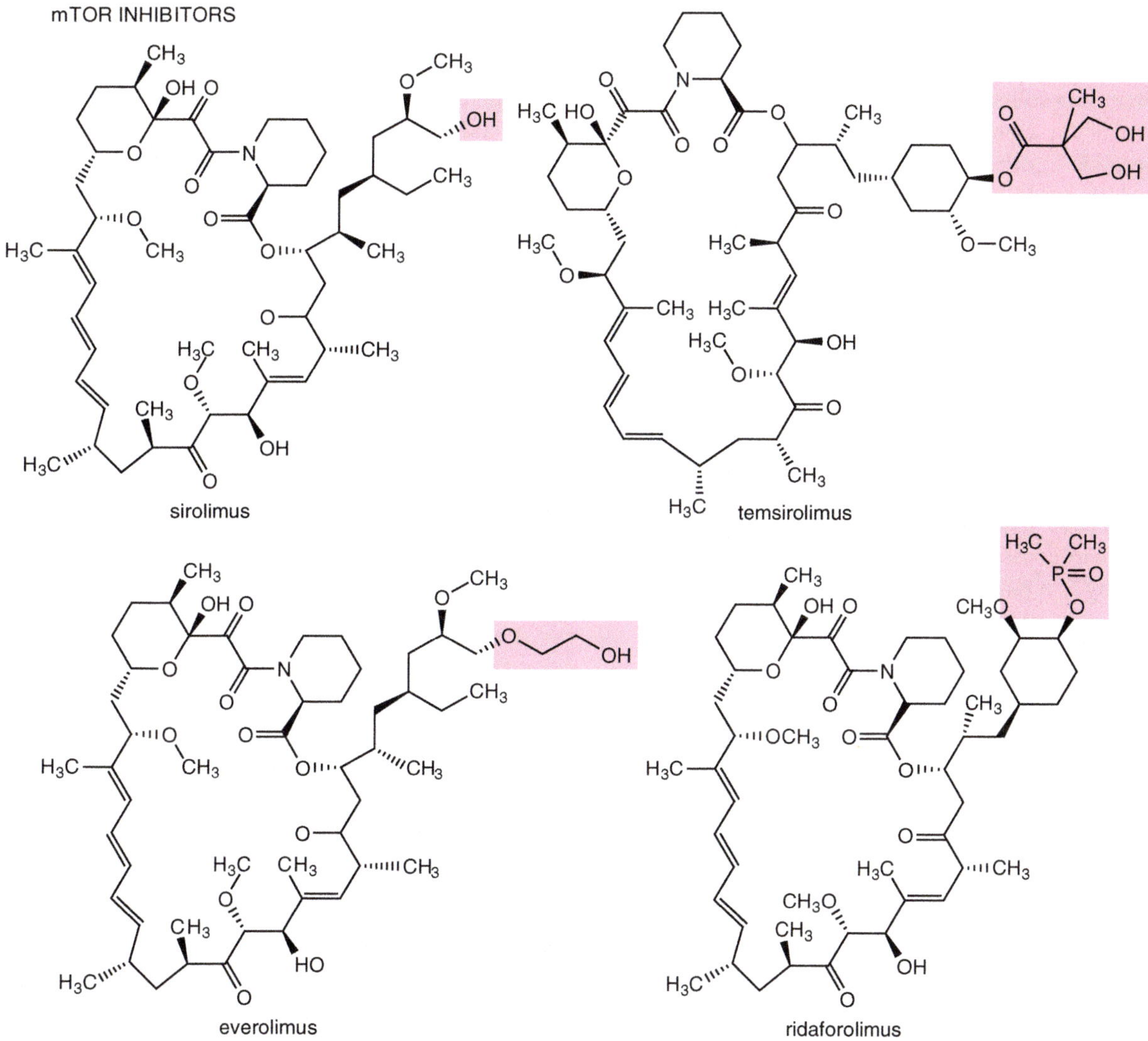

Fig. 4.12 (continued)

There are two mTOR multi-protein kinase complexes that may form. mTOR Complex-1 (mTORC1; comprised of mTOR, mLST8, AKT1S1, and RAPTOR) is the central component of a pathway that promotes growth in response to Insulin, energy levels, and amino acids. It activates protein synthesis, ribosome biogenesis, nutrient transport, and lipid synthesis, all resulting in cell growth. mTOR Complex-2 (mTORC2; consisting of mTOR, mLST8, PROTOR1, MAPKAP1, RICTOR) mediates Actin cytoskeletal organization via a mechanism involving PKB, SGK1, and PKC. Its dysregulation is implicated in tumor cell survival, motility, and invasiveness. The mTORC1 mediated consequences on cell cycle and cell size are distinct form the mTORC2 effects.

mTOR is particularly important in the biology of renal cell carcinoma, where HIF-1α plays a pathogenetic role. Mutation or loss of the tumor suppressor gene *vhl* (*von Hippel Lindau*) is common in this cancer and leads to a reduced degradation of HIF-1α. Activated mTOR further exacerbates the accumulation of the transcription factor HIF-1α by increasing its synthesis. There are familial cancer syndromes, in which mutations in negative regulators of the mTOR pathway give rise to transformation, including lymphangioleiomyomatosis and tuberous sclerosis complex (loss of TSC1 or TSC2), Peutz-Jeghers syndrome (loss of STK11), and Cowden syndrome (loss of PTEN).

- Derivatives of rapamycin (sirolimus, temsirolimus, everolimus, ridaforolimus) are allosteric mTOR inhibitors, and are sometimes referred to as rapalogs. Sirolimus inhibits only TORC1.
- ATP-competitive mTOR inhibitors are ATP analogs that inhibit mTOR kinase activity by competing with ATP for binding to the kinase domain in mTOR. The ATP analogs inhibit both mTORC1 and mTORC2. (Because of the similarity between the kinase domains of mTOR and the PI3Ks, mTOR inhibition by some of these compounds overlaps with PI3K inhibition. These drugs are discussed under PI3K inhibitors above.)

Sirolimus (rapamycin) was first discovered in the 1970s as a product of the bacterium Streptomyces hygroscopicus, present in a soil sample from Easter Island (Rapa Nui). The name of the compound was derived from that island. The macrolide sirolimus <Rapamune> binds the cytosolic immunophilin protein FKBP-12 (FK-Binding Protein 12). The bound molecules then engage the mTOR Complex-1 and inhibit it. Sirolimus strongly suppresses Interleukin-2 stimulated T-lymphocyte proliferation. It is mainly used as an immunosuppressant, but it possesses anti-proliferative properties. The agent suppresses the progression of dermal Kaposi sarcoma in patients with renal transplants. It also has modest clinical benefit in patients with tuberous sclerosis who have angiomyolipomata or sporadic lymphangioleiomyomatosis.

Adverse Effects Common adverse effects include stomach pain, headache, constipation, diarrhea, nausea, and joint pain. Lung toxicity is a potentially severe complication associated with sirolimus therapy. Allergic reactions may be serious.

Temsirolimus (CCI-779) <Torisel> is an ester analog of rapamycin that inhibits mTOR, causing decreased expression of genes necessary for cell cycle progression and resulting in consecutive cell cycle arrest in G_1. Temsirolimus is used to treat advanced renal cell carcinoma. It is also efficacious in the treatment of refractory mantle cell lymphoma. The intravenous dose is 25 mg over 30–60 min once weekly. The drug may also be administered orally. Temsirolimus received approval from the U.S. FDA and the European Medicines Agency (EMEA) in 2007.

Pharmacokinetics Cytochrome P450 3A4 is the primary enzyme responsible for the formation of five metabolites. Sirolimus, an active form of temsirolimus, is the principal metabolite following intravenous injection, while the other metabolites account for less than 10% of the drug in the blood. Elimination is primarily via the feces (80%) and less in the urine (5%).

Adverse Effects Premedication with an anti-histamine, such as 25–50 mg diphenhydramine, 30 min before the start of each dose is appropriate. Despite pretreatment, serious allergic reactions (anaphylaxis, dyspnea, flushing, chest pain) can occur.

The most common adverse reactions are rash, asthenia, mucositis, nausea, edema, and anorexia. There is the possibility of abnormal wound healing, bowel perforation, or intracranial bleeding. The use of temsirolimus may result in immunosuppression. Serious interstitial lung disease can develop. Increased blood glucose levels may require the initiation of Insulin therapy, while elevated triglycerides or cholesterol may require lipid lowering agents. The drug is Pregnancy Category D.

Drug Interactions The concomitant use of strong CYP3A4 inhibitors (including anti-retroviral protease inhibitors, ketoconazole, clarithromycin, nefazodone, telithromycin, voriconazole) or inducers (including dexamethasone, phenytoin, carbamazepine, rifampin, rifabutin, rifampacin, phenobarbital) should be avoided. Grapefruit juice may also increase the blood concentrations of sirolimus, a major metabolite of temsirolimus, and should be avoided. If the co-administration of strong CYP3A modulators is unavoidable, dose reduction (with CYP3A inhibitors) or dose increase (with CYP3A inducers) of temsirolimus need to be considered.

Everolimus (RAD001) <Zortress, Certican, Afinitor> is the *O*-(2-hydroxyethyl) derivative of sirolimus in position 40. Everolimus binds to FKBP-12, resulting in an inhibitory complex formation with mTORC1 and thus inhibition of mTOR. The effect of everolimus is solely on the mTORC1 protein complex and not on the mTORC2 complex. The drug was initially approved for use in Europe and Australia. It can be administered orally for use in

- advanced kidney cancer,
- subependymal giant cell astrocytoma (associated with tuberous sclerosis in patients who are not eligible for surgical intervention),
- progressive or metastatic pancreatic neuroendocrine tumors that are not surgically removable.

Pharmacokinetics Peak blood concentrations are reached 1–2 h after oral administration. Food may reduce the systemic exposure to oral everolimus. The drug is a substrate of CYP3A4. While the parent compound is the main circulating component in the blood, six main metabolites of everolimus are also present. They include three monohydroxylated metabolites, two hydrolytic ring-opened products, and one phosphatidylcholine conjugate. Everolimus is a substrate of ABCB1. 80% of the administered dose is excreted in the feces, while 5% is excreted in the urine. The agent should not be given to patients with severe hepatic impairment.

Adverse Effects Non-infectious pneumonitis (manifest in hypoxia, pleural effusion, cough, or dyspnea) is a class effect of rapamycin derivatives, including everolimus. The most common adverse reactions comprise stomatitis (leading to oral ulceration), rash, edema, diarrhea, abdominal pain, nausea, fatigue, fever, and headache. Everolimus has immunosuppressive properties and may predispose patients to bacterial, fungal, viral, or protozoal infections, including infections with opportunistic pathogens. The drug is Pregnancy Category D.

The selective inhibition of mTORC1 can lead to a hyperactivation of the kinase PKB via inhibition on the mTORC1 negative feedback loop, while not inhibiting the mTORC2-positive feedback to PKB. Because this effect may result in hypercholesterolemia and hypertriglyceridemia, monitoring of blood lipid levels is recommended.

Drug Interactions The concomitant use of strong CYP3A4 inhibitors or inducers should be avoided as they affect the blood concentrations of everolimus.

Ridaforolimus (deforolimus) (AP23573, MK-8669) contains a substitution of the secondary alcohol moiety at C-43 with a phosphate group. The drug is designed for improved aqueous solubility and oral delivery. Ridaforolimus improves the progression-free survival in patients with soft tissue or bone sarcomata.

Cell signaling via PI3K, PKB (AKT), and mTOR protects cells from apoptosis.
The inappropriate activation of PI3K pathways is an important step in the pathogenesis of multiple cancers.
PI3K inhibitors with various levels of specificity are in development.
mTOR inhibitors cause cell cycle arrest in G_1.
Sirolimus derivatives are substrates for CYP3A4.
As the mTOR pathway is important for glucose metabolism mTOR inhibitors increase blood glucose.
Non-infectious pneumonitis is a class effect of sirolimus derivatives.
Allergic reactions to sirolimus derivatives may be serious.
mTOR inhibitors are immunosuppressant.

4.1.5 FLT3 Inhibitors

The members of the proto-oncogene family *flt* encode receptors with protein tyrosine kinase activity that is important for the control of cell proliferation and differentiation. Expression of the cell surface receptor FLT3 (FMS Like Tyrosine Kinase 3, STK1, FLK2, CD135) is primarily restricted to the most undifferentiated hematopoietic progenitor cells. FLT3 Ligand is a member of a small family of growth factors that stimulate the proliferation of hematopoietic cells at select stages of their development and differentiation.

FLT3 is present on 80% of myeloid leukemia blast cells. Internal tandem duplication (FLT3 ITD[6]) is a common genetic defect in acute myelogenous leukemia (AML). Nearly 1/3 of AML patients have a gain-of-function mutation in the gene *flt3*, which is linked to an increased risk for relapse and reduced prospects for survival. For these cells, an excessive sensitivity to FLT3 dependent growth signals underlies their transformation.

FLT3 inhibitors may provide successful treatments for these cancers. These drugs fall into the categories of indolinones, and indolocarbazoles, FLT3/Aurora Kinase inhibitors, and others (Fig. 4.13). They all have cross-reactivities with multiple kinases and receptors. Members of the indolinone subgroup of inhibitors also block VEGFR2 (FLK1, KDR) and therefore have anti-angiogenic properties. Indolocarbazoles also inhibit Topoisomerase 1 and PKC. The FLT3/Aurora Kinase inhibitors also inhibit KIT (CD117) and ABL. They may be effective against tumors that over-express these molecules (Table 4.7).

[6] The duplicated stretch of DNA contains 18–108 nucleotides; it is always in frame and located in the juxtamembrane region of this class III tyrosine kinase receptor.

Drug Resistance In acquired resistance to FLT3 inhibitors, point mutations in the FLT3 molecule are rarely the cause. Much more common is anti-apoptosis through the up-regulation of MCL-1 (induced by FLT3 ITD627E, a non-juxtamembrane internal tandem duplication integrated into the first kinase domain), BCL-2 family proteins (may be overcome by adding the BH3 mimetic ABT-737), Survivin, or STAT signaling pathways. The resistance profiles of the FLT3 kinase inhibitors PKC412, SU5614, and sorafenib are non-overlapping, which suggests that combinations of FLT3 inhibitors may be therapeutically beneficial.

Indolinones Semaxanib (semoxind) (SU5416) is an intravenous indolinone that targets FLT3, KIT (CD117), PDGFR, and VEGFR (FLK-1, KDR). Twice weekly infusions of SU5146 administered on a 4-week cycle can reduce marrow blasts in AML or myeloproliferative disorders. In clinical trial, the agent displayed limited efficacy and substantial toxicity.

Sunitinib (SU11248) <Sutent> is an oral indolinone that acts as a more potent target inhibitor than semaxanib. The drug has higher success rates in patients with FLT3 mutations than in patients with wild-type FLT3. However, the duration of clinical responses is short, ranging 4–16 weeks. Sunitinib also inhibits c-KIT. The drug is used for the treatment of acute myelogenous leukemia, advanced renal cell carcinoma and gastrointestinal stromal tumors. Low dose treatment of 50 mg may be effective in combination chemotherapy with cytotoxic drugs.

Adverse Effects Target inhibition is achieved at dose levels of 75 mg at the expense of poor tolerability. Adverse effects include hand-foot syndrome, mucositis or stomatitis, and skin discoloration. Systemic adverse effects comprise fatigue, diarrhea, nausea, anorexia, and hypertension.

Indolocarbazoles Midostaurine (PKC412) is a semi-synthetic derivative of the alkaloid staurosporine, which is produced by Streptomyces staurosporeus. It is a multi-target protein kinase inhibitor that also inhibits FLT3. The drug is used for the treatment of acute myeloid leukemia. In 2004, orphan designation was granted by the European Commission to midostaurin for the treatment of AML.

Lestaurtinib (CEP-701, KT-5555, SPM-924) is an orally bioavailable indolocarbazole derivative. It inhibits the autophosphorylation of FLT3, resulting in a suppression of FLT3 activity and induction of apoptosis in tumor cells that over-express this kinase. The drug also acts as an inhibitor of RET, JAK2, TRK-A, TRK-B and TRK-C. Lestaurtinib is used to treat myeloproliferative disorders and AML in sequence with induction chemotherapy. The drug is administered in an oral dose of 80 mg twice daily for 16 weeks, beginning 2 days after the end of chemotherapy.

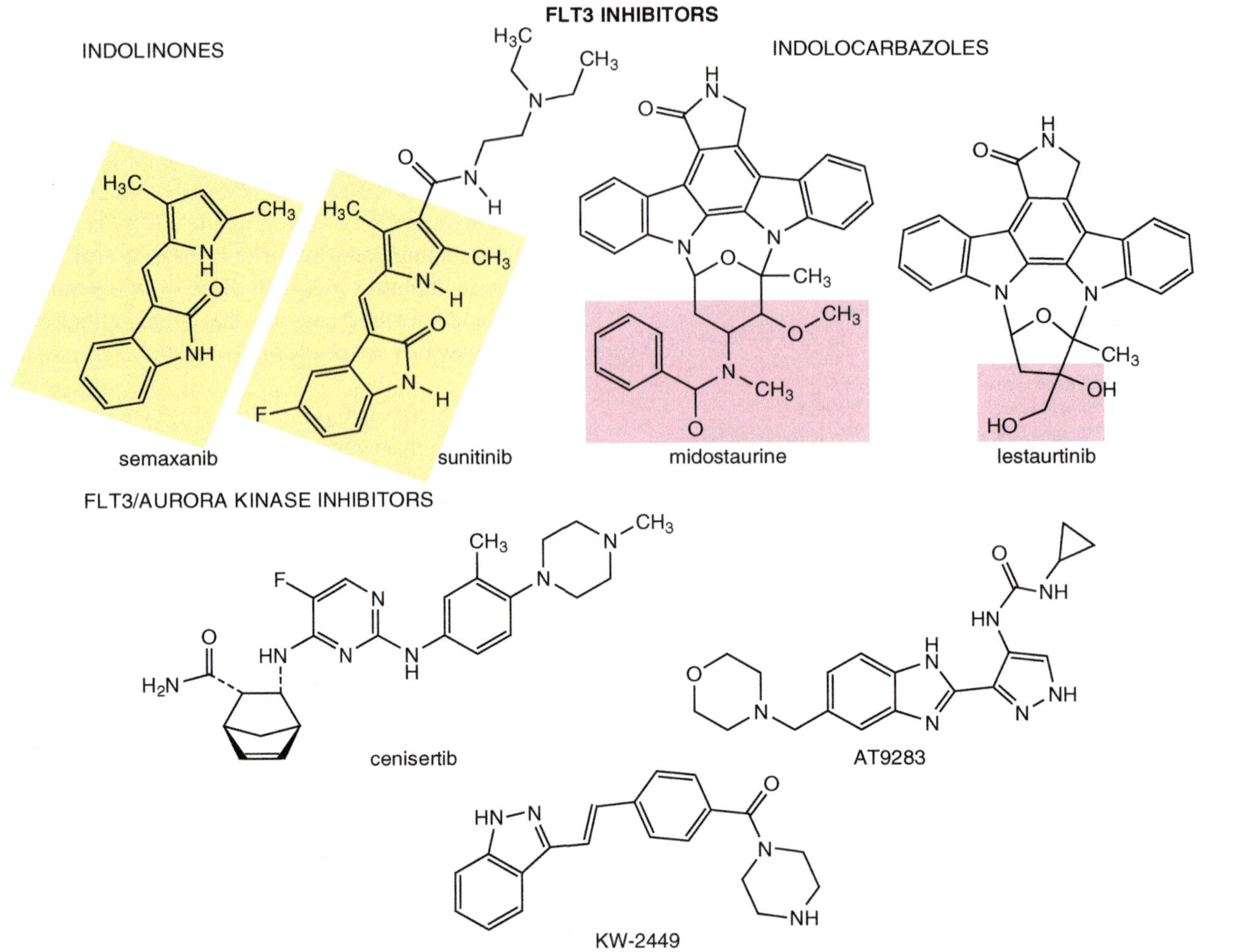

Fig. 4.13 Structures of FLT3 inhibitors. Sub-classes include indolinones (the indolinone-containing core moiety is highlighted in *yellow*), indolocarbazoles (the structural differences are shown on *pink* background), FLT3/Aurora Kinase inhibitors, and other inhibitors

Adverse Effects Most toxicities affect the gastrointestinal tract.

FLT3/Aurora Kinase inhibitors Some FLT3 inhibitors also inhibit Aurora Kinase. Cenisertib (AS703569, R-763) is an oral multi-kinase inhibitor that suppresses FLT3, Aurora A, Aurora B, and ABL kinases. The compound is in clinical trials for primary acute myelogenous leukemia (AML), secondary AML, chronic myelogenous leukemia (CML), myelodysplastic syndrome, and myeloproliferative disease.

Adverse Effects Common toxicities include neutropenia, thrombocytopenia, infection, mucositis and diarrhea.

The FLT3, pan-Aurora, ABL, and JAK2 kinase inhibitor AT9283 induces a reduction in the phosphorylation of Histone H3, CRKL, and STAT5 (a downstream target of ABL, FLT3 and JAK2 signaling). AT9283 is in clinical trials and has activity in patients with refractory acute and chronic myelogenous leukemias.

Adverse Effects The maximum tolerated dose of AT9283 as a 72-h intravenous infusion is 100 mg/m^2/day. Dose limiting toxicities include myelosuppression and alopecia, as well as tumor lysis syndrome. Elevated Transaminases, non-cardiac Creatine Kinase, and Lactate Dehydrogenase may occur.

KW-2449 is an orally available multi-kinase inhibitor of Aurora Kinases A and B, FLT3, ABL, and BCR-ABL^{T315I}. KW-2449 is growth inhibitory for leukemia cells with FLT3 gain-of-function mutations, resulting in G_1 arrest, and apoptosis. In FLT3 wild-type leukemia cells, it induces G_2/M arrest and apoptosis. KW-2449 is under investigation to treat leukemia patients.

Others Cabozantinib (XL184) <Cometriq> is an orally bioavailable, small molecule kinase inhibitor that strongly binds to and inhibits several receptor tyrosine kinases. This agent inhibits FLT3, KIT, TIE2 (TEK), MET (HGF Receptor), and VEGFR2. Cabozantinib was approved by the U.S. FDA in

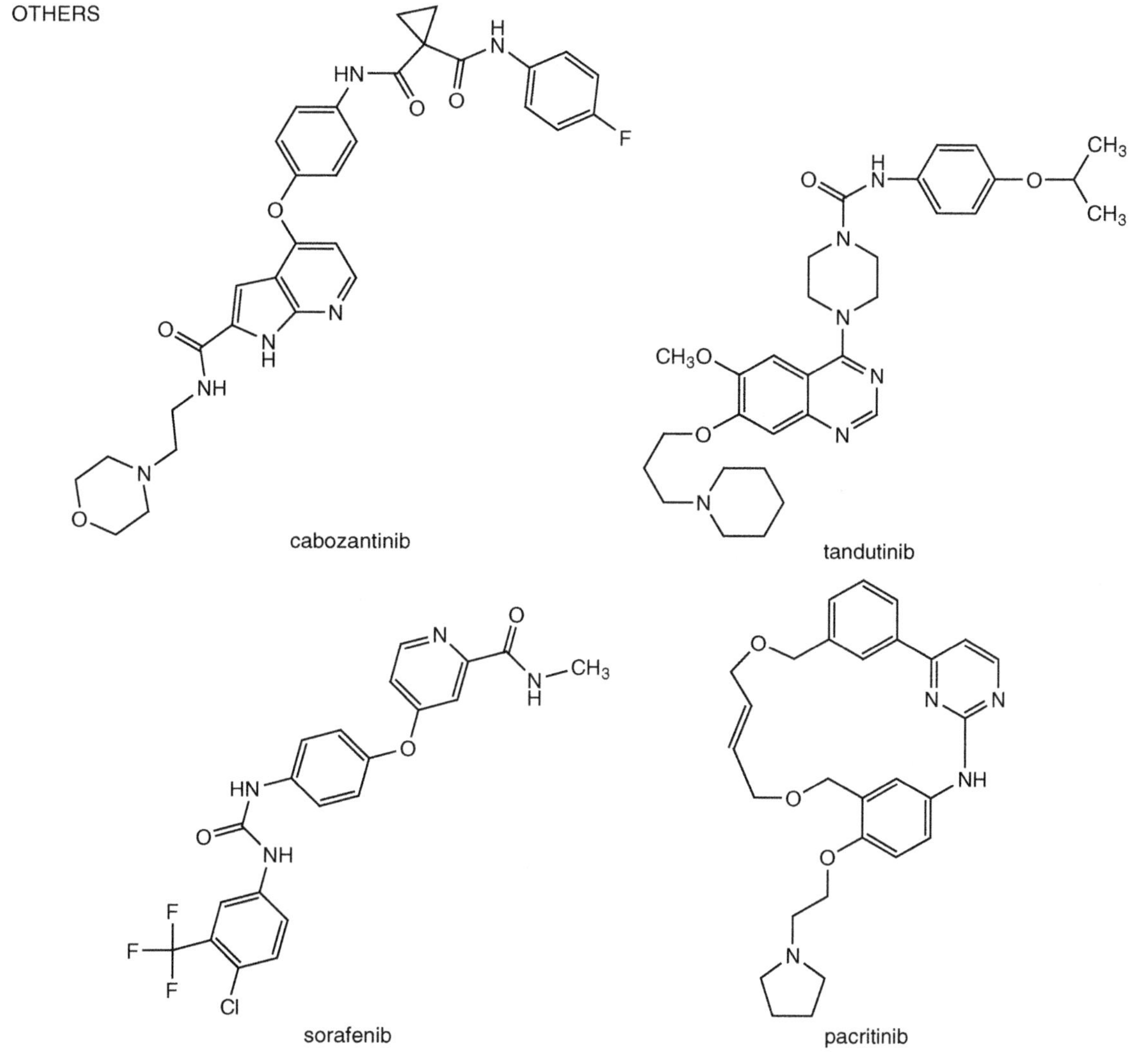

Fig. 4.13 (continued)

2012 for the treatment of medullary thyroid cancer. There is single agent activity in castration resistant prostate cancer, lung cancer, and ovarian cancer. The drug is in clinical trials for melanoma, brain, breast, non-small cell lung, hepatocellular, and kidney cancers.

Pharmacokinetics Cabozantinib has a long half-life of 60–120 h.

Adverse Effects Grade 3 dose limiting toxicities are palmar-plantar erythema, transaminitis, and mucositis. Permanent discontinuation of cabozantinib is required in cases of development of visceral perforation or fistula formation, severe hemorrhage, serious arterial thromboembolic event (such as myocardial or cerebral infarction), nephrotic syndrome, malignant hypertension or hypertensive crisis, persistent uncontrolled hypertension despite optimized medical management, osteonecrosis of the jaw, or reversible posterior leukoencephalopathy syndrome.

Tandutinib (*N*-(4-isopropoxyphenyl)-4-(6-methoxy-7-(3-(piperidin-1-yl) propoxy)quinazolin-4-yl)piperazine-1-carboxamide) (MLN518, CT53518) is a piperazinyl quinazoline that inhibits the auto-phosphorylation of receptor tyrosine kinases, thereby suppressing cellular proliferation and inducing apoptosis. Tandutinib acts as an ATP-competitive and reversible inhibitor of type III receptor tyrosine kinases, including FLT3 (and its cancer causing mutant W51 that results in a duplication of the amino acids 596–602, REYEYDL), PDGFRβ, and c-KIT, which are equally inhibited. The agent is much less active against CSF-1R. Tandutinib has no appreciable activity against EGFR, FGFR, or KDR. Non-receptor tyrosine kinases, serine-threonine kinases and MAP Kinases are not inhibited. The agent is under investigation in the treatment of glioblastoma and advanced androgen independent prostate cancer. Because of the correlation between FLT3 internal tandem duplication mutations and

Table 4.7 FLT3 inhibitors

	FLT3	FLT3(mut.)	KIT	KIT^{D816V}	PDGFR	VEGFR2	TIE2	RAF	RET	MET	PKC	Topoiso-merase 1	ABL	BCR-ABL^{T315I}	JAK2	TRK	Aurora Kinase A	Aurora Kinase B
Indolinones																		
Semaxanib	S		S		S	S												
Sunitinib	(S)	S	S	S		S												
Indolocarbazoles																		
Midostaurine	S		S								S	S						
Lestaurtinib	S								S		S	S			S	S		
FLT3/Aurora Kinase inhibitors																		
Cenisertib	S												S				S	S
AT9283	S												S		S		S	S
KW-2449	S												S	S			S	S
Others																		
Cabozantinib	S		S			S	S			S								
Tandutinib	S		S		S													
Sorafenib	S		S					S	S									
Pacritinib	S														S			

S sensitive, *R* resistant, (*mut.*) mutated

poor prognosis in acute myelogenous leukemia (AML), tandutinib may be beneficial against this form of leukemia.

Pharmacokinetics The major driver of tandutinib disposition are transporters, mainly ABCB1 (P-Glycoprotein) and ABCG2 (BCRP), with metabolism playing an insignificant role in its clearance.

Adverse Effects The principal dose limiting toxicity of tandutinib is reversible generalized muscular weakness or fatigue, occurring at doses of 525–700 mg (DeAngelo 2006).

Sorafenib tosylate (4-[4-[[4-chloro-3-(trifluoromethyl) phenyl]carbamoylamino] phenoxy]-*N*-methyl-pyridine-2-carboxamide) <Nexavar>is a synthetic, orally active compound that inhibits wild-type and mutant forms of the kinases FLT3, KIT, RAF, and RET (see Sect. 4.1.3). The drug also inhibits the VEGFR2/PDGFRβ signaling cascade, thereby blocking tumor angiogenesis.

Pacritinib (SB-1518) is a pyrimidine-based, ATP-competitive macrocyclic compound that inhibits FLT3 and JAK2. It also inhibits the JAK2 mutant V617F. As a consequence, the drug has anti-proliferative effects on myeloid and lymphoid cells driven by FLT3 or mutant or wild-type JAK2. Moreover, pacritinib is active against primary erythroid progenitor cells in myeloproliferative disease. The agent is in clinical studies in patients with myelofibrosis or lymphoma. Pacritinib has favorable pharmacokinetic properties after oral dosing and is well tolerated.

Acute myelogenous leukemia patients with gain-of-function mutations in flt3 have increased risk for relapse and reduced prospects for survival.
FLT3 inhibitors can treat these forms of AML.
FLT3 inhibitors have limited specificity. The indolinones also block VEGFR2. Indolocarbazoles also inhibit Topoisomerase 1 and PKC. Others also inhibit KIT.

4.1.6 Cell Cycle Kinase Inhibitors

The cell cycle describes the time period between two consecutive cell divisions and consists of four strictly regulated phases, referred to as gap 1 (G_1) for cell growth, DNA synthesis (S) for duplication of the genetic material, gap 2 (G_2) for preparation for cell division (G_1, S, and G_2 are collectively named interphase), and mitosis (M) for the execution of cell division. The cell cycle is driven by Cyclins and Cyclin-Dependent Kinases.

- The levels of Cyclins fluctuate with the phases of the cell cycle, due to changes in synthesis and degradation. Furthermore, their sub-cellular localization into the nucleus or the cytoplasm is important in cell cycle control. Cyclins serve as the regulatory subunits of cell cycle kinases. A Cyclin can assemble with an appropriate catalytic CDK subunit.
- Cyclin-Dependent Kinases (CDKs) are serine/threonine kinases. The regulation of their activities constitutes a rate limiting step in cell cycle progression, so that activation and inhibition of these kinases pace the progression through the cell cycle. While the expression levels of Cyclin-Dependent Kinases remain fairly constant, their activities are highly regulated.

DNA synthesis phase (S phase) occurs when the protein RB is phosphorylated by active CDK4 or CDK6, which releases the transcription factor E2F1 from RB and allows the free E2F1 to bind and activate E2F responsive genes necessary for progression to S phase. A majority of neoplasias have abnormalities in some component of the RB pathway.

During mitosis, Cyclin A is degraded. Cyclin B1, which is in the cytoplasm during S and G_2, translocates to the nucleus. The maturation promoting factor (MPF), consisting of Cyclin B and CDK1, initiates mitosis through the breakdown of the nuclear envelope, chromatin condensation, spindle formation, and fragmentation of the Golgi complex and endoplasmatic reticulum. The activation of M phase Cyclin-Dependent Kinases promotes the formation of the Ubiquitin Ligase complex called anaphase promoting complex (cyclosome, APC/C), which induces the loss of sister chromatid cohesion. The anaphase promoting complex is inactivated by the accumulation of G_1 Cyclin-Dependent Kinases at the end of M phase.

In prophase, the first mitotic stage, the Aurora Kinases phosphorylate Histone proteins (thereby promoting chromosome condensation) and interact with a number of chromosomal passenger proteins, including Inner Centrosome Proteins (INCEPs) and Survivin. Microtubules of the cytoskeleton, responsible for cell shape, motility, and attachment to other cells during interphase, dis-assemble. The building blocks of these microtubules are used to grow the mitotic spindle from the region of the centrioles.

Polo-Like Kinases, comprising PLK1, PLK2 (SNK), and PLK3 (FNK, PRK), are serine/threonine kinases that are required at several points during mitosis, including for the activation of the anaphase promoting complex, centrosome maturation, and mitotic exit. Polo-Like Kinases are localized to the kinetochore of chromosomes. The multi-protein complex Cohesin (SMC1, SMC3, SCC1/MCD1) creates physical links between sister chromatids. The phosphorylation of Cohesin by Polo-Like Kinases enhances its propensity to be cleaved by Separin (Separase), which then leads to chromatid separation (Fig. 4.14). The inhibition of Separin is released by the degradation of Securin (PDS1). APC/C acts as a Ubiquitin Protein Ligase, triggering the degradation of the anaphase inhibiting protein Securin.

Cell cycle kinase inhibition targets an essential step in tumor cell proliferation. However, the drug targets in this case are so far downstream in signal transduction that transformed and untransformed cells are affected alike. There-

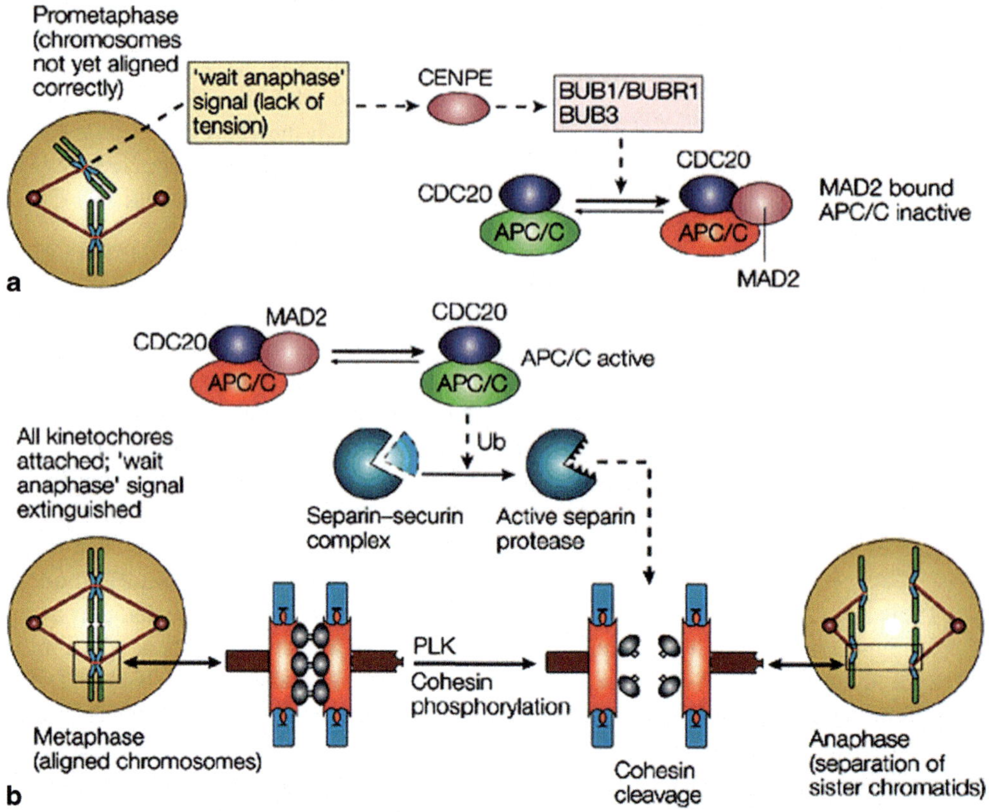

Fig. 4.14 Sister chromatid separation. **a** In prometaphase, cells contain condensed chromosomes that actively establish bipolar attachments to the mitotic spindle. Unattached chromosomes generate a signal that delays progress to anaphase until all sister chromatids are attached to the spindle apparatus. This signal is transduced by a relay of spindle checkpoint proteins that include CENPE and the MAD/BUB proteins. This ultimately results in inhibition of the anaphase promoting complex/cyclosome (APC/C), which is associated with the mitotic co-factor CDC20. **b** Following attachment of the last kinetochore to the mitotic spindle, the "wait anaphase" signal is extinguished. This allows APC/C and CDC20 to become active, resulting in the Ubiquitin dependent degradation of Securin and liberation of active Separin. This protease catalyses the cleavage of Cohesin complexes that bridge the aligned sister chromatids. The newly separated sister chromatids can then migrate to the poles along the spindle axis during anaphase. *PLK* Polo Like Kinases, *Ub* Ubiquitin. (Jallepalli 2001 with permission)

fore, adverse effects on rapidly proliferating, healthy tissues (hematopoietic system, gastrointestinal lining, hair roots) are likely. Further, while inhibition of an oncogenic pathway immediately downstream of a gain-of-function mutation is efficacious, the inhibition far downstream will capture only a fraction of the transforming activity as signaling pathways are branched, not linear.

A potential benefit of treatment with cell cycle kinase inhibitors may be the enhancement of concomitant cytotoxic therapy. The efficacy of cytotoxic agents is limited when cell cycle arrest and DNA repair reverse the drug induced damage. In the absence of cell cycle arrest, DNA repair cannot take place. Hence, the likelihood of cancer cell death is increased when cell cycle kinase inhibitors are used in conjunction with cytotoxic agents.

CDK inhibitors First generation ATP-site small molecule inhibitors (flavopiridol, bryostatin, seliciclib, 7-hydroxystaurosporin, BMS387032, E7070) and the second generation ATP-site small molecule inhibitors (PD-0332991, AT7519, SNS-032, P276-00, ZK304709, R-547, AG-24322, JNJ-7706621, GPC-286199, Bay80-3000) are in clinical trials. In general, second generation CDK inhibitors are more specific to individual Cyclin-Dependent Kinases (CDKs) (Table 4.8) and have improved pharmacokinetic and pharmacodynamic profiles compared to first generation inhibitors (Fig. 4.15).

Flavopiridol (HMR-1275, L86-8275) <Alvocidib> is derived from rohitukine, an alkaloid produced by an Indian medicinal plant that has been used in indigenous medicines. The drug acts as a pan-CDK inhibitor. It suppresses the activities of CKDs -1, -2, and -4 through competition with ATP. Flavopiridol blocks cell cycle progression at the G_1/S and G_2/M boundaries. This leads to apoptosis, which is correlated with the down-modulation of Cyclin D_1, up-regulation of P21, and induction of Caspase 3/7 activities. Flavopiridol has efficacy in hematologic malignancies, renal, colorectal, prostate, and gastric cancers.

Pharmacokinetics Because of the pharmacokinetic properties of flavopiridol, administration starts with a loading dose followed by continuous intravenous infusion.

Adverse Effects Main adverse effects are secretory diarrhea and a pro-inflammatory syndrome associated with hypotension.

In 1973, Lionel Rebhun observed that the puromycin analog 6-dimethylaminopurine prevents cell division without blocking protein synthesis. The compound was later found to inhibit the CDK1/Cyclin B complex. Consecutive screens identified 2,6,9-trisubstituted purines to represent a class of CDK inhibitors.

Seliciclib (R-roscovitine) (CYC202) is a 2,6,9-substituted purine analog that acts as a CDK inhibitor by competing with ATP. It has activity against CDK2/Cyclin E, CDK7/Cyclin H, and CDK9/Cyclin T, and also inhibits CDK1/Cyclin B and CDK5. The drug induces programmed cell death in various cell types independently of functional P53. Cell death is a consequence of the inhibition of CDK7/CDK9 dependent transcription (Fig. 4.16). Seliciclib reduces the level of the anti-apoptotic protein XIAP by down-regulating *xiap* mRNA expression. It also decreases the tyrosine phosphorylation and consequent activation of STAT5a, an upstream regulator of XIAP. Further, seliciclib down-regulates Survivin, which contributes to the activation of Caspase cascades (Kim 2004). Seliciclib is in clinical trials for B-cell malignancies, lung cancer, and breast cancer. Exposure to the drug overcomes glioma resistance to TRAIL mediated apoptosis. It can be given orally or by injection.

Pharmacokinetics After injection, seliciclib undergoes rapid passage into the blood, distribution into tissues, and metabolism. In accordance with a 2-compartment open model, the drug is subject to biphasic elimination with a 5-min and a 30-min half-life. It undergoes a rapid loss of the isopropyl group, several oxidations, and conjugation of a glucose residue. The carboxylated derivative is the main metabolite formed.

Palbociclib (PD-0332991) is an orally available, pyridopyrimidine derived CDK inhibitor that is selective for CDK4/Cyclin D_1 and CDK6. It may thus block RB protein phosphorylation and cause a down-regulation of genes under the transcriptional control of E2F. This prevents RB expressing tumor cells from entering the S phase of the cell cycle, leading to arrest in G_1. The drug results in a suppression of DNA reduplication, and consecutively in decreased tumor cell proliferation. The presence of a functional RB protein is a prerequisite for palbociclib efficacy.

In healthy cells, CDK4 and CDK6 are under the negative control of P16. However, in glioblastoma, P16 is often deleted. Thus, CDK4 and CDK6 are promising drug targets. Palbociclib can pass through the blood-brain barrier and is under study for the treatment of glioblastoma.

AT7519 is an orally available, multi-targeted inhibitor of CDKs -1, -2, -4, -5, and -9. In addition to its direct effects on the cell cycle (via CDKs 1–5), AT7519 also suppresses RNA Polymerase II dependent transcription (via inhibition of CDK9). The agent is under study for non-small cell lung cancer and pancreatic cancer. It is also under development for relapsed or refractory chronic lymphocytic leukemia (CLL), where the target is CDK9. As the survival of these transformed cells is very dependent on the cellular levels of certain anti-apoptotic proteins, which require RNA Polymerase II activity for their generation, AT7519 induces rapid cell death in leukemia cells.

Pharmacokinetics Over a wide dose range, AT7519 encounters multi-phasic elimination with a long terminal half-life of 8–12 h. There is only modest interpatient variation.

Adverse Effects The maximum tolerated dose is 30 mg/m^2 with the dose limiting toxicity being QTc prolongation. Adverse events are cyclical neutropenia[7], mucositis, and fatigue.

PNU-151807 (see Sect. 2.2.2.) is a synthetic minor groove binding antibiotic. Unlike other drugs in its class, PNU-151807 also abolishes the kinase activities of the CDK2/Cyclin A, CDK2/Cyclin E, and CDC2/Cyclin B complexes. PNU-151807 induces apoptosis via the activation of Caspases. While it may further induce the activation of P53, a disruption of P53 function does not substantially affect the cytotoxic activity of the drug. This property may make it useful for treating tumors with inactivating *p53* mutations.

Drug Resistance Mismatch DNA repair deficiency is associated with resistance to certain anti-cancer drugs. It may occur as a consequence of loss of MLH1 expression. By contrast, loss of mismatch repair does not mediate resistance to PNU-151807.

7-hydroxystaurosporine (UCN-01) is a synthetic derivative of staurosporine that arrests tumor cells in the G_1/S phase of the cell cycle by inhibiting Cyclin-Dependent Kinases (CDKs). This arrest leads to apoptosis. It promotes the accumulation of the cell cycle inhibiting proteins P21 and P27. The agent inhibits many kinases, including the G_2 checkpoint kinase CHK1, calcium dependent Protein Kinase C, and the serine/threonine kinase PKB (AKT). 7-hydroxystaurosporine is under study for treating melanoma and lymphoma.

CHK inhibitors In the presence of DNA damage or incomplete DNA reduplication, cells activate cell cycle checkpoints that temporarily halt the cell division cycle to permit DNA repair or the completion of DNA reduplication to take place. In the presence of extensive damage or absence of a timely repair, these checkpoint signaling pathways can also

[7] Cyclical neutropenia (cyclic neutropenia) is a form of the condition that tends to occur every 3 weeks and lasts 3–6 days at a time due to changing rates of cell production by the bone marrow.

trigger apoptosis. The physiologic functions of Checkpoint Kinases (CHKs) involve the initiation of cell cycle arrest and the up-regulation of gene transcription involved with DNA excision repair and deoxy-nucleotide synthesis.

Healthy tissues have a functioning G_1 checkpoint signaling pathway, allowing for DNA repair and cell survival. A large fraction of tumors are deficient in the G_1 DNA damage checkpoint, resulting in a dependence on the G_2 checkpoint for survival during cell reduplication. Specifically, high rates of *p53* loss-of-function mutations in cancer cells result in reliance on the S and G_2 checkpoints to repair DNA damage and promote cell survival. The S and G_2 checkpoints are regulated by the serine/threonine kinase CHK1, which is activated in response to DNA damage. Thus, inhibition of CHK1 signaling impairs DNA repair and increases tumor cell death (Fig. 4.17). G_2 checkpoint abrogation may be a relatively cancer cell specific therapy.

Checkpoint kinase inhibitors are in clinical development as combination therapies with DNA damaging cytotoxic agents. By preventing checkpoint activation, these drugs enhance the cell killing effects of the cytotoxic compounds. Potentiation of the effects of DNA damage is driven primarily through CHK1 inhibition rather than CHK2 inhibition. CHK2 inhibition may lead to the enhanced effect of sensitizing cancer cells that lack P53 while protecting normal cells. CHK inhibitors cause an increase in the levels of phospho-Histone 2A.X (p-H2A.X), which reflects double-stranded DNA damage. Tumor types that are particularly sensitive to CHK1 inhibition include triple negative breast cancer, where CHK1 is up-regulated, and colorectal cancer, where CHK1 levels are elevated in the tumor mucosa over healthy mucosa.

The oncogenic protein MYC induces DNA damage and results in genetic instability. This defect alone would lead to cell cycle arrest or apoptosis in early tumorigenesis, never allowing a clinically detectable cancer to form. For full transformation, loss of P53 or of DNA repair molecules is required. Further, ATR and CHK1 suppress a Caspase dependent apoptotic response following DNA reduplication stress induced by MYC. CHK1 inhibitors can effectively treat those cells in single agent regimens.

XL844 (EXEL-9844) is an orally available synthetic small molecule inhibitor of the checkpoint kinases CHK1

Table 4.8 Specificities of cell cyle kinase inhibitors

	CDK1	CDK2	CDK3	CDK4	CDK5	CDK6	CDK7	CDK9	CHK1	CHK2	Aurora Kinase A	Aurora Kinase B	PLK	ABL
CDK inhibitors														
Flavopiridol	S	S		S										
Seliciclib	S	S			S		S	S						
Palbociclib				S		S								
AT7519	S	S		S	S			S						
7-hydroxystaurosporine	S	S	S	S										
CHK inhibitors														
XL844									S	S				
AZD7762									S	S				
PF-00477736									S					
VRX0466617										S				
4,4′-diacetyl-diphenylurea-bis(guanylhydrazone)										S				
Aurora Kinase inhibitors														
Cenisertib											S	S		S
Tozasertib											S	S		S
Danusertib											S	S		
KW-2449											S	S		S
AT9283											S	S		S
MLN 8237											S			
XL228											S			S
Hesperadin												S		
AZD1152												S		
ZM447439												S		
PLK inhibitors														
BI2536													S	

S sensitive, *R* resistant, (*mut.*) mutated

Table 4.8 (continued)

	BCR-ABL^{Y253F}BCR-ABLY253F	BCR-ABL^{V299L}BCR-ABLV299L	BCR-ABL^{T315I}BCR-ABLT315I	FLT3	FLT3 (mut.)	FGFR	IGF-1R	PDGFR	RET	TRK-A	LYN	SRC	JAK2
CDK inhibitors													
Flavopiridol													
Seliciclib													
Palbociclib													
AT7519													
7-hydroxystaurospo-rine													
CHK inhibitors													
XL844				S				S					
AZD7762													
PF-00477736													
VRX0466617													
4,4′-diacetyl-diphenylurea-bis(guanylhydrazone)													
Aurora Kinase inhibitors													
Cenisertib				S									
Tozasertib	S	S	S										
Danusertib			S						S	S			
KW-2449			S	S	S								
AT9283				S									S
MLN 8237													
XL228			S			S	S				S	S	
Hesperadin													
AZD1152													
ZM447439													
PLK inhibitors													
BI2536													

S sensitive, *R* resistant, (*mut.*) mutated

and CHK2. XL844 also inhibits FLT-3, PDGFR, VEGFR2 and VEGFR3. The agent inhibits cell cycle arrest and DNA repair, which ultimately leads to tumor cell apoptosis. XL844 increases cancer cell radio-sensitivity through the promotion of mitotic catastrophe.

Checkpoint Kinase inhibitors have the potential to enhance the efficacy of both conventional chemotherapy and radio-therapy, and increase patient response rates. AZD7762 inhibits CHK1 and CHK2 via competition with ATP, and abrogates the DNA damage induced S and G_2 checkpoints. In combination with DNA damaging agents, the agent dose dependently potentiates the remission of cancers, in which the inhibition of Checkpoint Kinases results in an abrogation of DNA damage induced cell cycle arrest. AZD7762 enhances the efficacies of gemcitabine and topotecan.

The small molecule, ATP-competitive kinase inhibitor PF-00477736 has high selectivity for CHK1 over CHK2. PF-00477736 abrogates the S and G_2/M checkpoints and prevents the cell cycle arrest that is required for subsequent repair in DNA damaged tumor cells. The checkpoint abrogation results in sensitization to apoptosis. PF-00477736 displays chemopotentiation when given with DNA damaging agents. It is in clinical trials in combination with gemcitabine.

The selective CHK2 inhibitor VRX0466617 reduces the phosphorylation of the serines 19 and 33–35 on its target protein, but not of threonine 68 which is phosphorylated by ATM. VRX0466617 blocks the activation of CHK2 and downstream degradation of MDM4 in response to ionizing radiation, and may thus act as a radio-sensitizer. The agent is in preclinical development.

The inhibition of CHK2 sensitizes P53 deficient cells and may protect normal tissue after exposure to DNA damaging agents. 4,4′-Diacetyldiphenylurea-bis(guanylhydrazone) (NSC 109555) is a reversible, ATP-competitive CHK2 inhibitor that is under development.

Polo Like Kinase inhibitors PLK1 is a serine/threonine protein kinase that regulates cell division. It is important for the proliferation of tumor cells. Several Polo Like Kinase

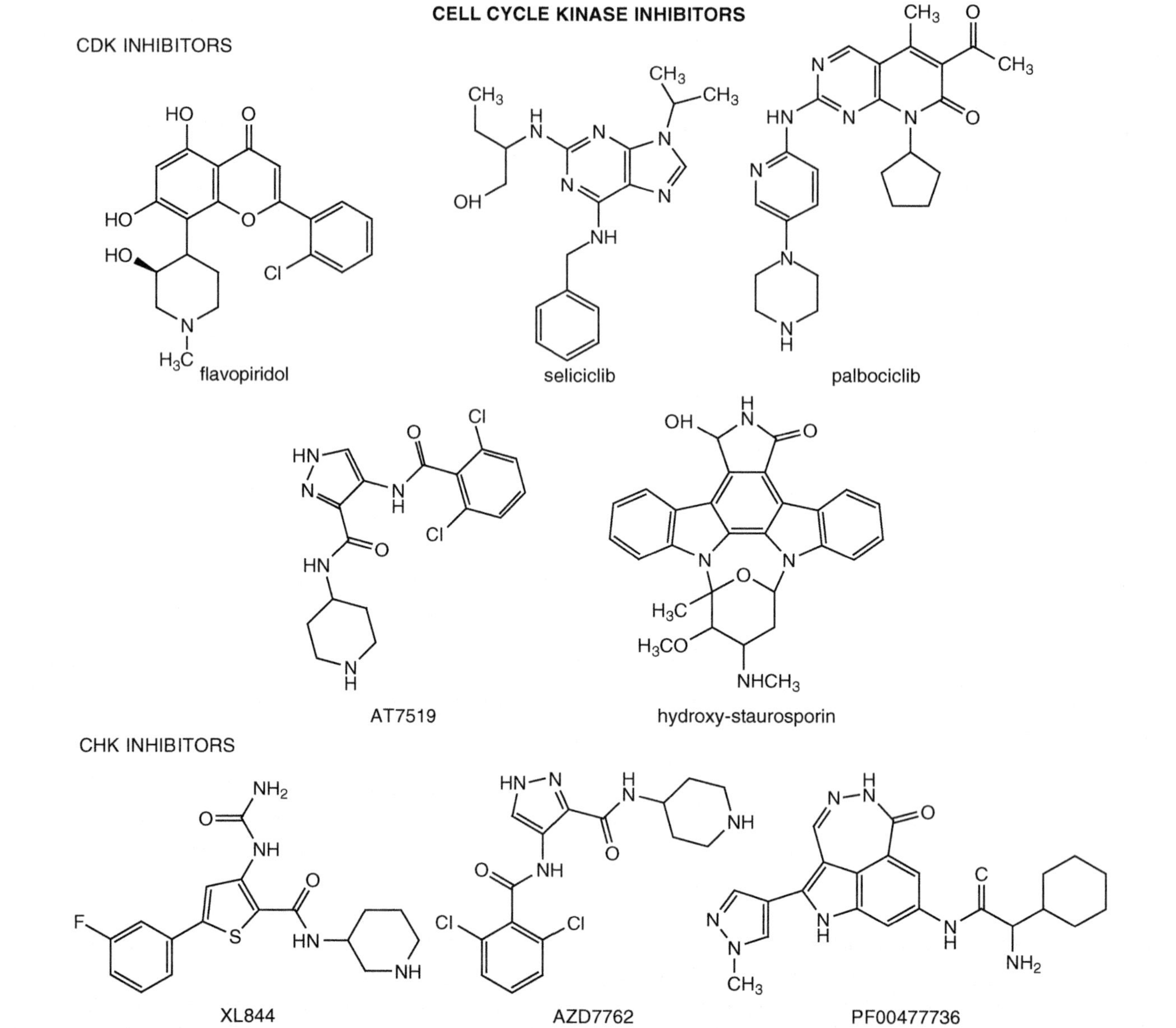

Fig. 4.15 Structures of cell cycle kinase inhibitors. Sub-classes include Cyclin Dependent Kinase (*CDK*) inhibitors, Checkpoint Kinase (*CHK*) inhibitors, and Polo-Like Kinase (*PLK*) inhibitors. The structural similarities among the representatives of a class are limited

small molecule inhibitors are in early clinical trials (BI2536, BI6727, GSK461364, ON 019190.Na, HMN-214) or in pre-clinical development (ZK-thiazolidinone, NMS-1, CYC-800, DAP-81, LC-445).

BI2536 is an anti-mitotic compound with anti-proliferative effects. BI2536 inhibits cell division by acting as a small molecule inhibitor of Polo Like Kinase 1 (PLK1). The inhibition of PLK1 by the drug results in mitotic arrest, disruption of cytokinesis and apoptosis in tumor cell populations. BI2536 induces the regression of large tumors with well tolerated intravenous dose regimens.

Aurora Kinase inhibitors Aurora kinases regulate cell cycle transit from G_2 through cytokinesis. They belong to a family of serine/threonine kinases that is essential for mitotic progression, spindle formation, centrosome maturation, chromosomal segregation, and cytokinesis. Aurora A is enriched at centrosomes, whereas Aurora B and its binding partners INCENP and Survivin act as chromosomal passenger proteins. Aurora Kinases are over-expressed or amplified in various types of cancer. Such up-regulation may result in drug resistance, as it disrupts the spindle checkpoint that is activated by paclitaxel or nocodazole treatment, thus inducing the cells to become unresoponsive to these drugs.

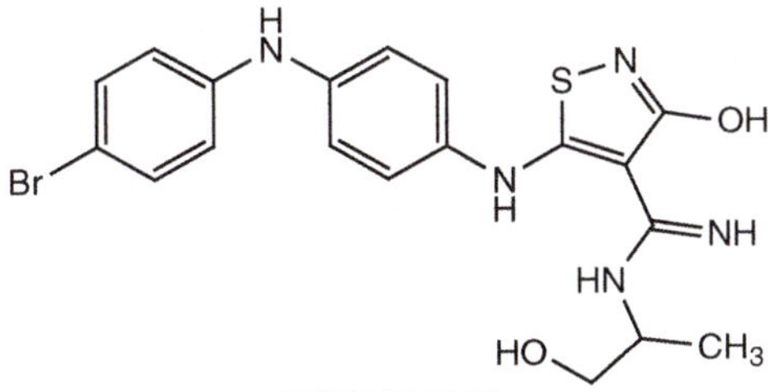

VRX0466617

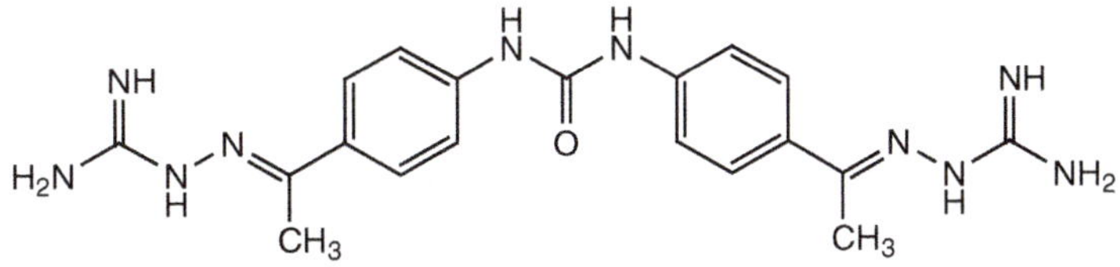

4,4'-diacetyldiphenylurea-bis(guanylhydrazone)

POLO LIKE KINASE INHIBIOTRS

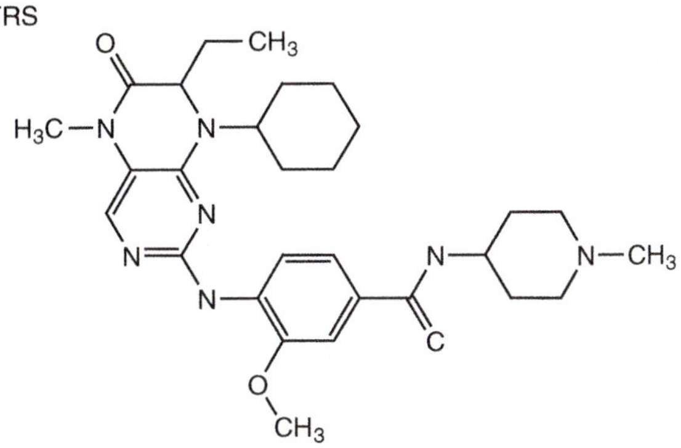

BI2536

Fig. 4.15 (continued)

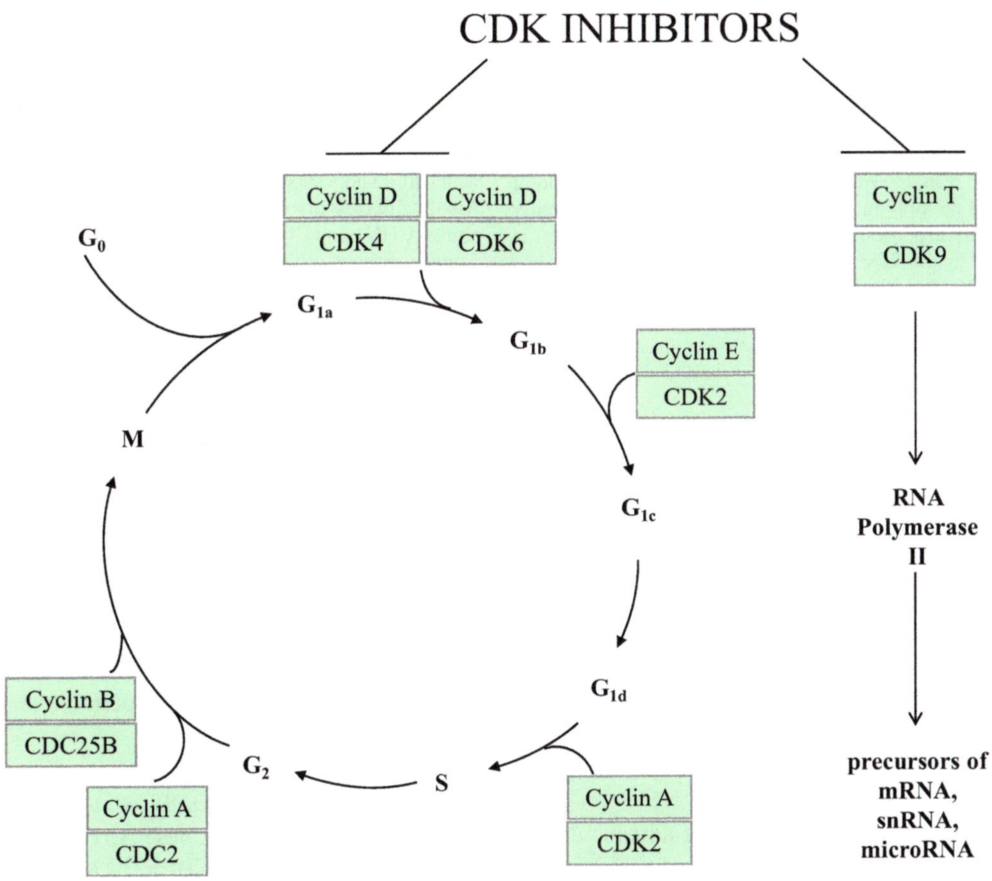

Fig. 4.16 Inhibition of CDK actions. CDK inhibitory drugs suppress the actions of Cyclins and Cyclin Dependent Kinases (*CDKs*), which entail furthering the progression of the cell division cycle (CDKs -2, -4, -6) at all phases and activating RNA Polymerase II (CDK9) to induce mRNA synthesis (and some small nuclear RNA and microRNA synthesis)

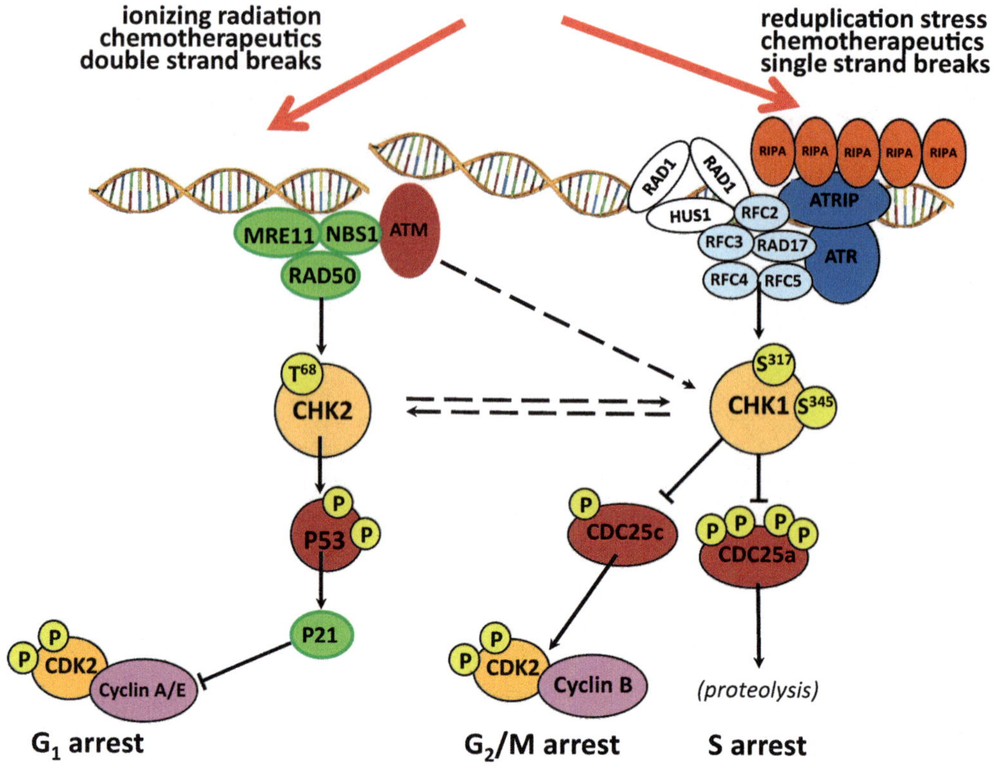

Fig. 4.17 DNA damage checkpoints. *CHK1* and *CHK2* are serine/threonine kinases that are activated in response to DNA damage by the kinases *ATM* and *ATR*. The checkpoint kinases are transducers of the DNA damage signal and both phosphorylate a number of substrates involved in the DNA damage response. *CHK1* and *CHK2* share a number of overlapping substrates, although it is clear that they have distinct roles in directing the response of the cell to DNA damage. Checkpoint kinases are involved not only in cell cycle regulation but also in other aspects of the cellular response to DNA damage. The G_1 checkpoint is modulated primarily by the ATM-CHK2-P53 pathway, as expression of *ATR*, *CHK1*, and *CDC25A* is limited until the cell passes this restriction point. At this point, levels of *ATR*, CHK1, and *CDC25A* all increase. If DNA damage is detected, *CHK1*/*CHK2* are activated, CDC25A is phosphorylated, and thus destabilized, resulting in a P53 independent S arrest. In S phase, the same cascade can result in an intra-S arrest in response to stalled replication forks. The G_2/M checkpoint prevents entry into mitosis with unrepaired DNA lesions. Initiation of this checkpoint is mediated by the ATM/ATR/CHK1/CHK2 cascades as shown, which ultimately suppresses the pro-mitotic activity of Cyclin B/CDC2. Along with their pivotal roles in the modulation of the cell cycle checkpoints, CHK1 and CHK2 are also involved in other aspects of the DNA damage response, including DNA repair, induction of apoptosis, and chromatin remodeling. (Redrawn from (Ashwell 2008))

Inhibition of Aurora Kinases does not arrest the cell cycle but leads to failure of cytokinesis, resulting in polyploidy and ultimately in cell death. Pan-Aurora Kinase inhibitors comprise tozasertib, AT9283, SNS-314, and PHA-739358. Inhibitors selective for Aurora Kinase A are MLN8054 and MLN8237. Aurora Kinase B inhibitors are hesperadin and AZD1152 (Fig. 4.18).

Some Aurora Kinase inhibitors also inhibit ABL, JAK2, or FLT3. Several of these compounds have promising applications in acute myelogenous leukemia with mutated FLT3, and as second line of defense in chronic myelogenous leukemia with imatinib resistant BCR-ABL.

Adverse Effects Among the most frequent adverse events caused by Aurora Kinase inhibitors are myelosuppression, febrile neutropenia, and gastrointestinal effects (nausea, diarrhea, mucositis).

Cenisertib (AS703569, R-763) is an oral multi-kinase inhibitor that suppresses Aurora A, Aurora B, FLT3 and ABL kinases. The compound is in clinical trials for primary or secondary acute myelogenous leukemia, chronic myelogenous leukemia, myelodysplastic syndrome, and myeloproliferative diseases.

Adverse Effects Common toxicities include neutropenia, thrombocytopenia, infection, mucositis, and diarrhea. Gastrointestinal bleeding can arise. Potential late effects from Aurora Kinase C inhibition on spermatogenesis and fertility are yet unknown.

Danusertib (PHA-739358) is a pyrrolo-pyrazole pan-Aurora Kinase (Aurora Kinase A, B, and C) inhibitor. The drug also inhibits BCR-ABL^{T315I}, RET, TRK-A, and (at a 4-fold higher half-maximal inhibitory concentration) FGFR-1. A regimen under study in the clinic is the administration of

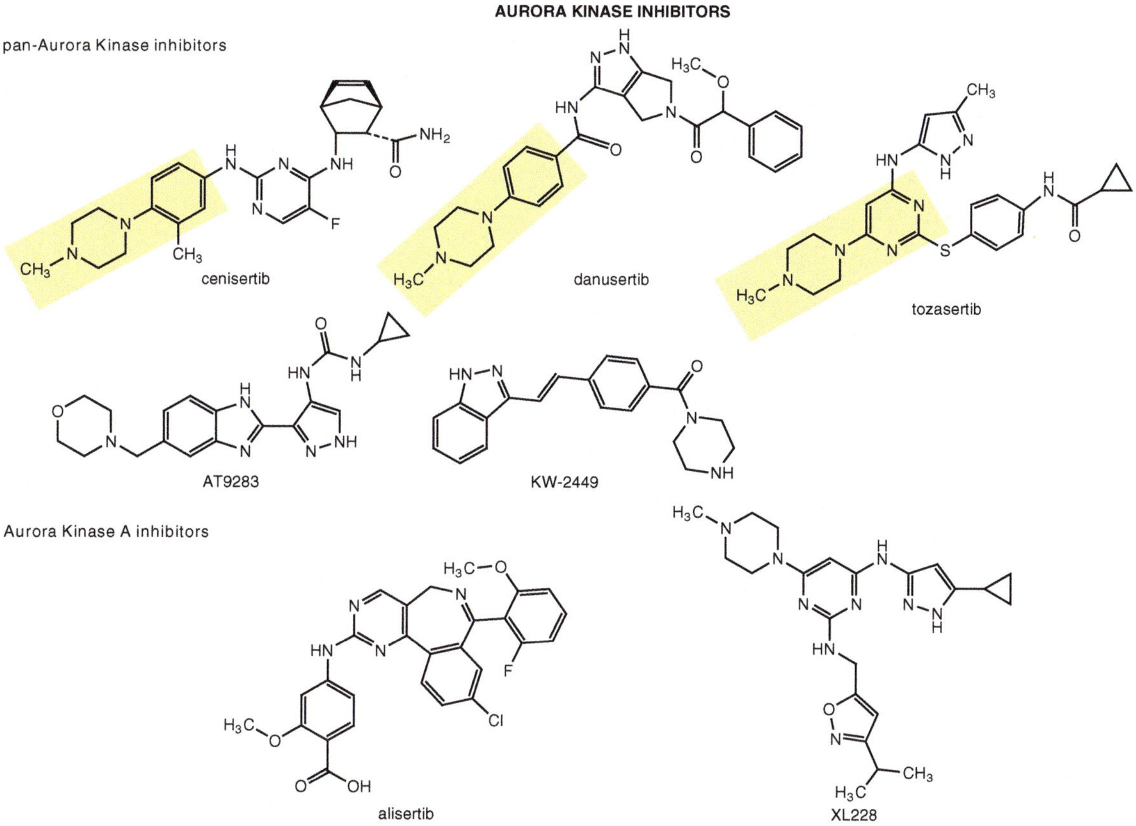

Fig. 4.18 Structures of Aurora Kinase inhibitors. Sub-classes include pan-Aurora Kinase inhibitors, Aurora Kinase A inhibitors, and Aurora Kinase B inhibitors. Common structural characteristics among the pan-Aurora Kinase inhibitors are highlighted in yellow. The Aurora Kinase B inhibitors AZD1152 and ZM447439 are related, and their differences are shown on *pink* background

250–330 mg/m^2/day as a weekly 6-h infusion for 3 consecutive weeks, every 4 weeks.

Adverse Effects Adverse events comprise high grade neutropenia and infusion related reactions.

The pan-Aurora Kinase inhibitor tozasertib (L-001281814, VX-680, MK-0457) is a synthetic small molecule drug that binds to and inhibits Aurora Kinases, thereby inducing apoptosis in tumor cells, in which Aurora Kinases are overexpressed. Tozasertib also inhibits wild-type BCR-ABL, BCR-ABL^{Y253F}, BCR-ABL^{V299L}, and BCR-ABL^{T315I}.

Adverse Effects The main toxicities consist of myelosuppression, alopecia, and mucositis. Long QT syndrome (QTc prolongation)[8] is a possible complication. Therefore, tosazertib (MK-0457) has been replaced in clinical trials by MK-5108 (VX-689).

[8] The QT interval describes the time between the start of the Q wave and the end of the T wave in the electrical cycle of the heart beat. It represents the electrical depolarization and repolarization of the ventricles. In long QT syndrome, delayed repolarization of the heart following a beat increases the risk of ventricular tachyarrhythmias. Such episodes may lead to fainting and sudden death.

The pan-Aurora, ABL, FLT3, and JAK2 kinase inhibitor AT9283 induces a reduction in the phosphorylation of Histone H3, CRKL, and STAT5 (a downstream target of ABL, FLT3 and JAK2 signaling). AT9283 is in clinical trials and has activity in patients with refractory acute or chronic myelogenous leukemia.

Adverse Effects The maximum tolerated dose of AT9283 as a 72-h intravenous infusion is 100 mg/m^2/day. Dose limiting toxicities include myelosuppression and alopecia. Tumor lysis syndrome may occur. Transaminases, non-cardiac Creatine Kinase, and Lactate Dehydrogenase may be elevated.

KW-2449 is a multi-kinase inhibitor of Aurora Kinases A and B, FLT3, ABL, and BCR-ABL^{T315I}. It is under investigation to treat leukemia patients. KW-2449 is growth inhibitory for leukemia cells with FLT3 gain-of-function mutations, resulting in G_1 arrest, and apoptosis. In FLT3 wild-type leukemia cells, it induces G_2/M arrest and apoptosis. As an ABL inhibitor, KW-2449 may be of benefit in imatinib resistant leukemia. KW-2449 is orally available.

Aurora Kinase A is required for cells to divide. In epithelial ovarian cancer, its frequent over-expression or up-reg-

Aurora Kinase B inhibitors

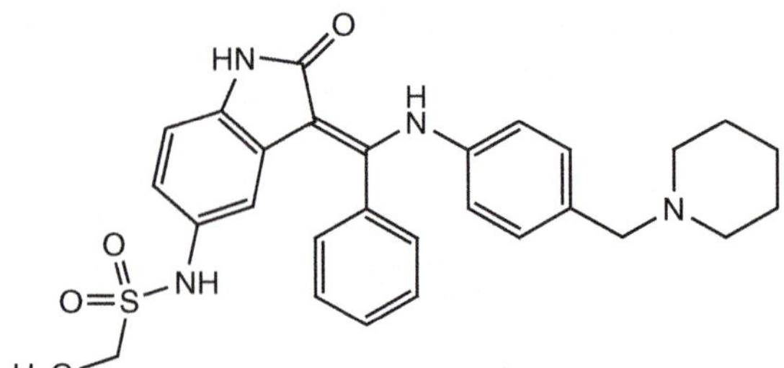

hesperadin

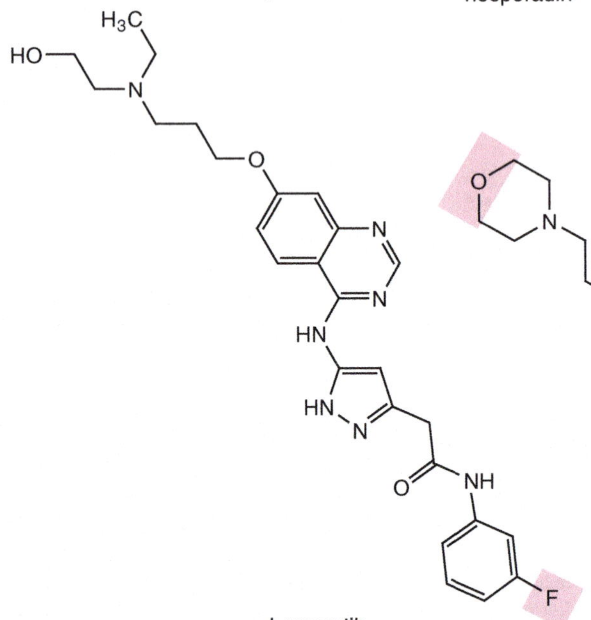

barasertib

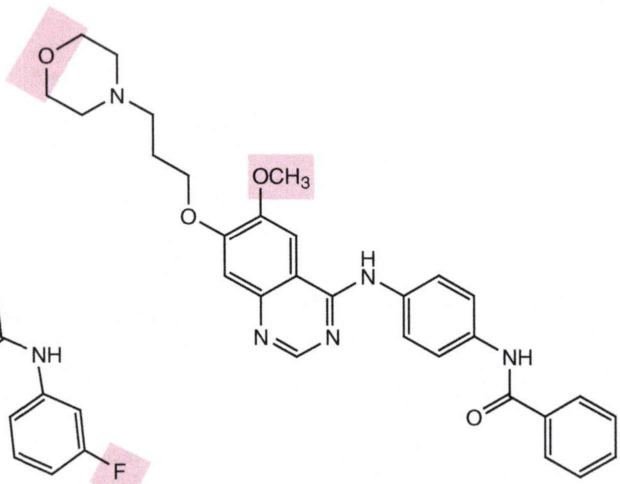

ZM447439

Fig. 4.18 (continued)

ulation is oncogenic. Alisertib (MLN8237) inhibits Aurora Kinase A. It was designed as a second line of defense in platinum resistant or refractory ovarian cancer.

Adverse Effects The predecessor lead compound MLN8042 was discontinued due to the induction of somnolence and lack of objective tumor responses in clinical trials. It has been replaced by the second generation agent alisertib (MLN8237).

XL228 is an Aurora Kinase A inhibitor that also suppresses wild-type ABL and BCR-ABL^{T315I} at low nanomolar concentrations. XL228 also inhibits the kinases FGFR, IGF-1R, LYN and SRC. It is in clinical trials.

Pharmacokinetics XL228 exhibits a long terminal half-life after administration through a 1-h infusion.

Adverse Effects Neutropenia may manifest as a dose limiting toxicity.

The indolinone hesperadin (Hauf 2003) is an inhibitor of Aurora Kinase B. Exposed cells enter anaphase in the presence of numerous mono-oriented chromosomes, many of which may have both sister kinetochores attached to 1 spindle pole. This effect prevents chromosome alignment and segregation, induces polyploidy, and overrides the spindle assembly checkpoint. In cancer cells treated with monastrol or taxol, hesperadin may induce mitotic exit.

High Aurora Kinase B activity may be associated with hepatocellular carcinoma, breast cancer, and some forms of leukemia. The dihydrogen phosphate prodrug barasertib (AZD1152-hydroxyquinazoline pyrazol anilide, AZD1152-HQPA) is under investigation. It is rapidly converted in the blood. The active drug AZD1152 is a selective inhibitor of Aurora Kinase B that suppresses downstream Histone phosphorylation and induces apoptosis in a dose dependent manner. A therapeutic dose is 1200 mg, administered as a continuous 7-day intravenous infusion every 21 days.

Adverse Effects Neutropenia and febrile neutropenia are the most common adverse events.

The quinazoline derivative ZM447439 (*N*-[4-[[6-Methoxy-7-[3-(4-morpholinyl)propoxy]-4-quinazolinyl]amino]phenyl] benzamide) is an ATP competitive Aurora Kinase inhibitor. It has higher affinity for Aurora Kinase B than for the forms A or C. Cells exposed to ZM447439 progress through interphase, enter mitosis and assemble bipolar spindles, but fail to properly align and segregate their chromosomes.

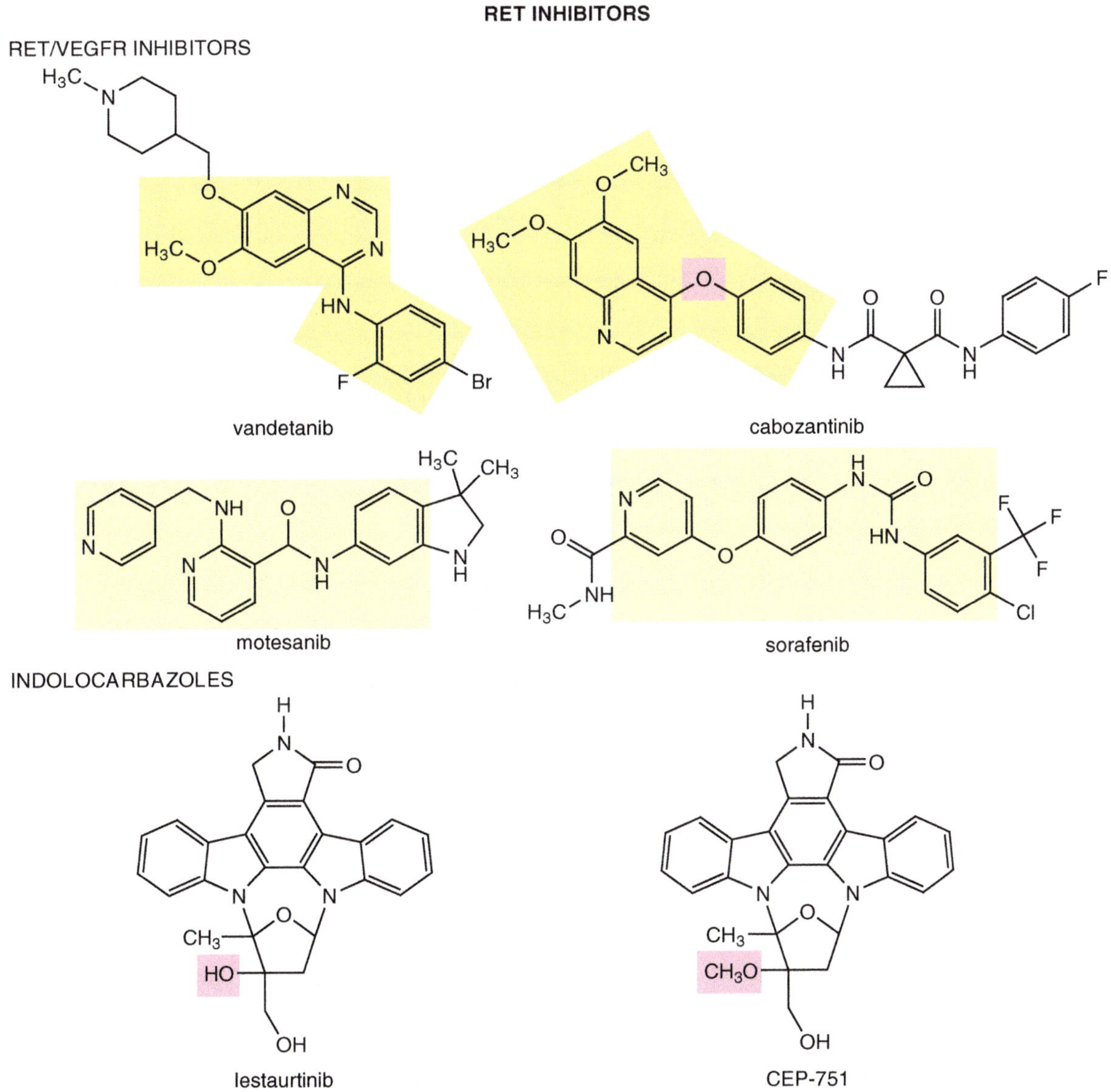

Fig. 4.19 Structures of RET inhibitors. Sub-classes include RET/VEGEF inhibitors and indolocarbazoles. The 4-anilinoquinazoline domain is highlighted in *yellow* in vandetanib and (with the modification of the bridging oxygen in *pink*) in cabozantinib. *Light yellow* shading shows a loosely conserved structure of 3 6-rings connected by bridges between motesanib and sorafenib. The difference in one chemical group between the indolocarbazoles is shown on *pink* background

The drug targets for cell cycle kinase inhibitors are far downstream signaling molecules.
A potential benefit of treatment with cell cycle kinase inhibitors may be the enhancement of concomitant cytotoxic therapy.
Adverse effects on rapidly proliferating normal tissues and incomplete inhibition of oncogenic pathways are likely.

CDK inhibitors are in clinical trials.

Many tumors are deficient in the G_1 DNA damage checkpoint pathway, which results in reliance on the S and G_2 checkpoints. These checkpoints are regulated by the serine/threonine kinase CHK1.
By preventing checkpoint activation, CHK inhibitors enhance the cell killing effects of cytotoxic therapy or radio-therapy.

Adverse events caused by Aurora Kinase inhibitors are myelosuppression, febrile neutropenia, and gastrointestinal effects.

4.1.7 Others

RET The proto-oncogene *ret* encodes a transmembrane receptor of the tyrosine kinase family. Activation of RET prompts its tyrosine phosphorylation. The ensuing signal transduction engages GRB2, SHC, and Phosphatidylinositol 3-Kinase. Oncogenic RET also activates RAS, RAF, MEKK1, and I-κB Kinase β. This leads to the phosphorylation and degradation of I-κB and results in the activation of NF-κB, which may promote cell expansion through its anti-apoptotic effects.

Gain-of-function mutations or translocations in the RET proto-oncogene are causative for medullary thyroid carci-

Table 4.9 Inhibitors of RET

	RET	VEGFR2	PDGFR	c-KIT	c-MET	EGFR	FLT3	RAF	RAF (mut.)	JAK	TRK
RET inhibitors											
Vandetanib	S	S				S					
Cabozantanib	S	S			S						
Motesanib	S	S	S	S							
Sorafenib	S	S	S	S			S	S	S		
Lestaurtinib	S						S			S	S
CEP-751	S										S

S sensitive, R resistant, *Raf (mut.)* mutant RAF

noma. Therefore, several therapies directed at this tyrosine kinase are in early phase clinical trials for thyroid cancer (Fig. 4.19; Table 4.9).

Vandetanib (*N*-(4-bromo-2-fluorophenyl)-6-methoxy-7-[(1-methylpiperidin-4-yl)methoxy]quinazolin-4-amine) (AZD6474, ZD6474) <Caprelsa, Zactima> targets RET, VEGFR2, and EGFR. It is an orally bioavailable 4-anilino-quinazoline[9] that is taken once per day. The drug has a half-life of more than 120 h.

Adverse Effects Vandetanib is well tolerated at doses of up to 300 mg/d. The main adverse effects are nausea, diarrhea, rash, and hypertension. Asymptomatic QTc prolongation of the heart beat may arise.

Cabozantinib (XL184) <Cometriq> is an oral multi-targeted inhibitor of RET, VEGFR2, and c-MET. It also binds to and inhibits FLT3, KIT, and TIE2 (TEK). Cabozantinib was approved by the U.S. FDA in 2012 for the treatment of medullary thyroid cancer. There is single agent activity in castration resistant prostate cancer, lung cancer, and ovarian cancer.

Motesanib (AMG706) is a multi-targeted tyrosine kinase inhibitor that suppresses RET, VEGFR, c-KIT, and PDGFR activity. It is in clinical trials for locally advanced and metastatic medullary thyroid cancer, and has resulted in partial responses.

Sorafenib tosylate <Nexavar> is a synthetic compound that inhibits RET. The kinases KIT, FLT3, and wild-type as well as mutant forms of the kinase RAF are also sorafenib targets. The drug inhibits the VEGFR2/PDGFRβ signaling cascade, thereby suppressing tumor angiogenesis.

Sorafenib is active orally and it is available as tablets. The drug is taken without food, 1 h before or 2 h after a meal, typically twice daily.

Indolocarbazoles with two bonds between the glycoside and the indolocarbazole heterocycle may act as inhibitors of Protein Kinases. Lestaurtinib (CEP-701) is an orally bioavailable indolocarbazole derivative that inhibits RET at nanomolar concentrations. The drug also acts as an inhibitor of FLT3, JAK2, TRK-A, TRK-B, and TRK-C.

Adverse Effects Most toxicities affect the gastrointestinal tract.

CEP-751 (KT-6587) is an indolocarbazole derivative that preferentially inhibits auto-phosphorylation and signaling of TRK family receptors. CEP-751 also inhibits constitutively active RET. It is effective at nanomolar concentrations.

MET The receptor tyrosine kinase MET (c-MET, Hepatocyte Growth Factor Receptor, HGFR) is amplified in some gastric cancers. It is mutationally activated in some head and neck cancers, is activated or over-expressed in glioblastomata, breast carcinomata, and non-small cell lung cancers. Single allele germline missense mutations in the *c-met* gene are oncogenic in hereditary papillary renal cell carcinoma type I and sporadic papillary renal cell carcinoma (trisomy 7 with non-random duplication of mutant *c-met*).

Most small molecule inhibitors of the MET intracellular kinase domain target the ATP binding site (crizotinib, MK2461, JNJ38877605, foretinib, BMS777607, cabozantinib, SGX523, MP470). They associate with the kinase hinge region by mimicking the purine in ATP (for this purpose, BMS777607 and crizotinib have a 2-amino-pyridine group, AMG-458 has a quinoline group, and MK2461 has a tricyclic aromatic group). MET inhibitors can be divided into two classes. Class I drugs (crizotinib, PF04217903, MK-2461, SU-11274) bind adjacent to the hinge region with a U-shaped conformation, whereas class II drugs (foretinib, cabozantinib, AM7) bind in an extended conformation that spans the area from to the C-helix of c-MET. Few small molecule drugs are allosteric c-MET inhibitors (ARQ197) (Fig. 4.20; Table 4.10).

The aminopyridine crizotinib (PF2341066) <Xalkori> is an orally bioavailable ATP-site small molecule inhibitor of c-MET, ALK (Anaplastic Lymphoma Kinase), and ROS1. The crizotinib derivative PF04217903 has a *N*-hydroxyethyl pyrazole group tethered to *C*-7 of the triazolopyrazine and

[9] Anti-cancer kinase inhibitors in the 4-anilinoquinazoline class include most ERBB inhibitors.

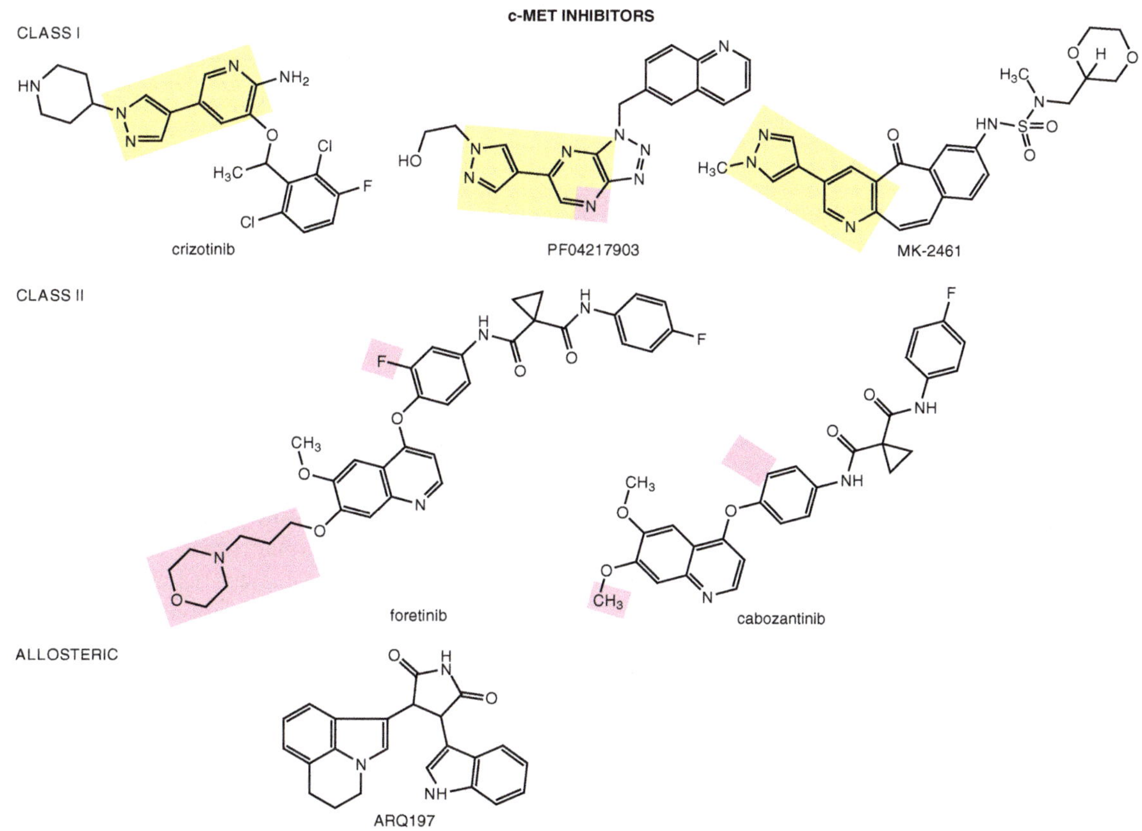

Fig. 4.20 Structures of MET inhibitors. Inhibitors of c-MET are categorized as class I inhibitors, class II inhibitors, and allosteric inhibitors. Class I inhibitors contain heterocyclic 5-and 6-rings connected by a bridge. The structural differences between the class II inhibitors are shown in *pink*

Table 4.10 Inhibitors of MET

	c-MET	VEGFR2	PDGFR	RON	KIT	TIE2	KDR	FLT-1	FLT-4	ALK	ROS1	RET
c-MET inhibitors												
Crizotinib	S									S	S	
MK-2461	S											
Foretinib	S	S	S	S	S	S	S	S	S			
Cabozantinib	S	S										S
ARQ197	S											

S sensitive, *R* resistant

possesses high selectivity for c-MET. The agent is under study for lung cancer and myofibroblastic tumors.

Adverse Effects At the maximum tolerated dose of 250 mg twice a day, the drug causes fatigue.

MK-2461 is an ATP-competitive multi-targeted inhibitor. The pyridine nitrogen in the molecule is necessary for inhibitory activity, and planarity of the molecule is essential for maximum potency. While the drug has low potency as an inhibitor of c-MET auto-phosphorylation at the kinase activation loop, MK-2461 binds preferentially to activated, phosphorylated c-MET. It inhibits the phosphorylation of c-MET substrates and its downstream signaling to the PI 3-K→PKB and RAS→ERK pathways. MK-2461 also displays inhibitory activities against Fibroblast Growth Factor Receptor (FGFR) and Platelet Derived Growth Factor Receptor. A well tolerated oral regimen of MK-2461 administered at 100 mg/kg twice daily effectively suppresses c-MET signaling and tumor growth.

Drug Resistance Mutations of c-MET are not likely to cause drug resistance to MK-2461.

Class II MET inhibitors are usually not as selective as class I inhibitors. The first ATP-site specific c-MET inhibitor to enter clinical trials was the orally bioavailable foretinib (XL880, GSK1363089), a class II ATP competitive antagonist. Foretinib also inhibits VEGFR2, PDGFR, RON, KIT, TIE2, KDR, FLT-1, and FLT-4.

Table 4.11 Inhibitors of PDGFR

	PDGFR	KIT	FLT3	BCR-ABL	VEGFR2	SRC	RAF	RET	CSF-1R	GFR	EPHA2	DDR1	DDR2	PKC	Topoiso-merase 1	FGFR
PDGFR inhibitors																
Imatinib	S	S	R	S												
Nilotinib	S	S		S					S			S				
Dasatinib	S	S	R	S		S				S	S		S			
Semaxanib	S	S	S		S											
Sorafenib	S	S	S				S	S								
Tandutinib	S	S	S													
Midostaurin	S	S	S											S	S	
Sorafenib	S	S	S		S		S	S								
CHIR-258	S				S		S									S

S sensitive, *R* resistant

Adverse Effects Foretinib is well tolerated with adverse events mostly limited to grade 1 or 2 hypertension, nausea, anorexia, fatigue, and asymptomatic liver function abnormalities.

Cabozantinib (XL184) <Cometriq> is an orally bioavailable, small molecule kinase inhibitor that strongly binds to and inhibits several receptor tyrosine kinases. Specifically, cabozantinib has a strong affinity for MET, which may result in the inhibition of tumor growth and possible tumor regression. The drug is also an inhibitor of RET and VEGFR2.

ARQ197 is a non-ATP-site competitive, selective small molecule inhibitor of the c-MET intracellular domain, which prevents auto-phosphorylation. ARQ197 selectively targets the inactive form of the kinase between the N- and C- lobes and occupies the ATP binding site. After prolonged treatment (12 weeks or longer), it may induce stable disease in otherwise refractory solid tumor patients, implicating potential anti-invasive activity. The agent is orally bioavailable.

PDGFR The cytokine Platelet Derived Growth Factor (PDGF) acts as a connective tissue cell mitogen with functions that include embryonal development, wound healing, and the control of interstitial fluid pressure in soft connective tissue. Paracrine PDGF signaling in the connective tissue stroma plays a role in various types of solid tumors. Further, gain-of-function mutations in *platelet-derived growth factor receptor* (*pdgfr*) or *c-kit* are the drivers in the pathogenesis of gastrointestinal stromal tumor (GIST). These properties render PDGF and its cognate receptor (PDGFR) potential drug targets.

Multi-kinase inhibitors that suppress PDGFR also inhibit ABL (imatinib, nilotinib, dasatinib; see Sect. 4.1.2.), FLT3 (semaxanib, sorafenib, tandutinib, midostaurin; see Sect. 4.1.5.), or RAF (sorafenib, CHIR-258) (Table 4.11).

Imatinib inhibits the receptor tyrosine kinase PDGFR. The agent also suppresses proliferation and induces apoptosis in cells that over-express the oncoproteins c-KIT or ABL. Imatinib is under investigation as a treatment for cancers that have excessive activity of PDGFR.

PDGF contributes to the regulation of interstitial fluid pressure. As most solid tumors have an increased interstitial fluid pressure, pharmacological reduction may be a way to increase the uptake of anti-cancer drugs. Through the inhibition of PDGFR, imatinib can substantially reduce tumor interstitial fluid pressure. In combination therapy, it may thus improve the pharmacokinetics of other agents.

Nilotinib monohydrate monohydrochloride (AMN107) <Tasigna> is an orally available phenylamino-pyrimidine, which was derived from the imatinib scaffold (Weisberg 2006). This agent inhibits the auto-phosphorylation of PDGFR, DDR1, BCR-ABL, CSF-1R, and c-KIT. Nilotinib interrupts the phosphorylation of these tyrosine kinases and their downstream signaling targets, resulting in decreased cellular proliferation or in the induction of apoptosis.

Dasatinib hydrochloride (BMS-354825) <Sprycel> inhibits PDGFRβ, BCR-ABL, SRC family kinases (SRC, LCK, YES, FYN), c-KIT, EPHA2, and GFR at nanomolar concentrations. In contrast to most tyrosine kinase inhibitors, dasatinib binds to the active conformation of the target enzyme. The agent is given at 100–140 mg orally once per day.

Semaxanib (SU5416) is an intravenous indolinone that targets PDGFR, FLT3, KIT, and VEGFR. Twice weekly infusions of semaxanib administered on a 4-week cycle can reduce marrow blasts in AML or myeloproliferative disorders. In clinical trials, the agent displayed substantial toxicity.

Midostaurine (PKC412) is a semi-synthetic derivative of the alkaloid staurosporine, which is produced by Streptomyces staurosporeus. It is a multi-target protein kinase inhibitor that inhibits PDGFR and FLT3. In 2004, orphan designation was granted to midostaurin for the treatment of acute myeloid leukemia (AML) by the European Commission.

Sorafenib tosylate <Nexavar> is a synthetic compound

Table 4.12 Inhibitors of KIT

	KIT	PDGFR	FLT3	BCR-ABL	VEGFR2	SRC	RAF	RET	CSF-1R	GFR	EPHA2	DDR1	DDR2	MET	TIE2
c-KIT inhibitors															
Imatinib	S	S	R	S											
Nilotinib	S	S		S					S			S			
Dasatinib	S	S	R	S		S				S	S		S		
Bosutinib	(S)	(S)		S		S									
Semaxanib	S	S	S		S										
Sorafenib	S		S				S	S							
Cabozantinib	S		S		S									S	S
Tandutinib	S	S	S												

S sensitive, *R* resistant

that inhibits the VEGFR2/PDGFRβ signaling cascade, thereby blocking tumor angiogenesis. The kinases RAF, KIT, FLT3, mutant and wild-type RAF, and RET are also drug targets. Sorafenib is active orally. It is taken without food, 1 h before or 2 h after a meal, typically twice daily.

Tandutinib (MLN518, CT53518) is a piperazinyl quinazoline that inhibits the auto-phosphorylation of receptor tyrosine kinases, thereby inhibiting cellular proliferation and inducing apoptosis. Tandutinib acts as a small molecule ATP competitive and reversible inhibitor of the type III receptor tyrosine kinases[10], including PDGFRβ, FLT3 (and its cancer causing mutant W51), and c-KIT, which are all equally suppressed. Non-receptor tyrosine kinases, serine-threonine kinases and MAP Kinases are not inhibited. The agent is under investigation in the treatment of glioblastoma and advanced androgen independent prostate cancer.

CHIR-265 is an orally active small molecule that binds to and inhibits PDGFR-β and RAF family kinases. The drug action results in a suppression of tumor cell proliferation and tumor cell death. In addition, CHIR-265 inhibits VEGFR-2, thereby disrupting tumor angiogenesis. This agent is in clinical trials for the treatment of locally advanced or metastatic melanoma.

The related compound CHIR-258 is a small molecule with inhibiting properties against the kinases B-RAF, PDGFR-β, VEGFR-2, and FGFR. It also is in clinical trials for the treatment of melanoma.

c-KIT c-KIT (Stem Cell Factor, SCF, CD117) is a cell surface receptor tyrosine kinase that is stimulated by the cognate ligand HGF (Hepatocyte Growth Factor, Scatter Factor, SCF). Gain-of-function mutations in *c-kit* are the drivers in the pathogenesis of a large fraction of gastrointestinal stromal tumors (GISTs). Multi-kinase inhibitors that suppress c-KIT (Table 4.12) also target ABL (imatinib, nilotinib, dasatinib, bosutinib; see Sect. 4.1.2.) or FLT3 (semaxanib, sorafenib, cabozantinib, tandutinib; see Sect. 4.1.5.).

Imatinib mesylate inhibits proliferation and induces apoptosis in cells that over-express the oncoproteins c-KIT, or ABL, or PDGF Receptor. The drug blocks c-KIT auto-phosphorylation, as well as downstream signaling events, such as the activation of ERK1, ERK2, and PKB (Heinrich 2000). In 2002, imatinib was approved by the U.S. FDA for the treatment of metastatic gastrointestinal stromal tumor. Other indications include adjuvant imatinib following surgical resection of localized c-KIT-positive gastrointestinal stromal tumor. A fraction of melanomas harbor activating mutations or amplifications of *kit*. Some of the affected patients benefit from imatinib mesylate treatment. The agent is under investigation for additional cancers that have excessive activities of c-KIT, including acute myelogenous leukemia, small cell lung cancer, ovarian cancer, testicular cancer, dermatofibrosarcoma protuberans, and glioma.

Drug Resistance Imatinib eventually fails in approximately 50 % of patients, who are then given salvage therapy with sunitinib malate. Sunitinib achieves a good response from cancers with exon nine mutants and wild-type KIT. However, patients with exon 11 mutations, in whom imatinib mesylate has failed, do not respond well to sunitinib because of secondary mutations within the activation loop of the kinase domain that cause resistance.

Nilotinib monohydrate monohydrochloride (AMN107) <Tasigna> is an orally available phenylamino-pyrimidine, which was derived from the imatinib scaffold (Weisberg 2006). This agent inhibits the auto-phosphorylation of DDR1, BCR-ABL, PDGFR, CSF-1R, and c-KIT. Nilotinib interrupts the phosphorylation of these tyrosine kinases and their downstream signaling targets, resulting in decreased cellular proliferation and the induction of apoptosis.

Dasatinib hydrochloride (BMS-354825) <Sprycel> inhibits c-KIT, BCR-ABL, SRC family kinases (SRC, LCK, YES, FYN), EPHA2, PDGFRβ, and GFR at nanomolar con-

[10] Close to 20 types of receptor tyrosine kinases have been identified. Type III comprises the PDGFR family of receptors. It also includes c-KIT, FMS, and FLT3.

centrations. In contrast to most other tyrosine kinase inhibitors, dasatinib binds to the active conformation of the target enzyme. The drug is given at 100–140 mg orally once per day.

Bosutinib (SKI-606) is a synthetic 7-alkoxy-3-quinolinecarbonitrile. While it targets ABL and SRC kinases, it has some activity against c-KIT and PDGFR. Bosutinib suppresses cell growth and apoptosis.

Semaxanib (SU5416) is an intravenous indolinone that targets PDGFR, FLT3, KIT, and VEGFR. Twice weekly infusions of SU5146 administered on a 4-week cycle can reduce marrow blasts in acute myelogenous leukemia (AML) or myeloproliferative disorders. In clinical trial, the agent displayed substantial toxicity.

The kinases KIT, FLT3, and RET, as well as wild-type and mutant forms of the kinase RAF are targets for sorafenib tosylate <Nexavar>. The drug also inhibits the VEGFR2/PDGFRβ signaling cascade, thereby blocking tumor angiogenesis. Sorafenib is active orally. It is taken without food, 1 h before or 2 h after a meal, typically twice daily.

Cabozantinib (XL184) <Cometriq> is an orally bioavailable, small molecule inhibitor that strongly binds to and suppresses several receptor tyrosine kinases. This agent inhibits KIT, FLT3, TIE2 (TEK), MET (HGF Receptor), and VEGFR2. There is single agent activity in medullary thyroid cancer, castration resistant prostate cancer, lung cancer, and ovarian cancer.

Tandutinib (MLN518, CT53518) is a piperazinyl quinazoline that inhibits the auto-phosphorylation of receptor tyrosine kinases, thereby suppressing cellular proliferation and inducing apoptosis. Tandutinib acts as a small molecule, ATP-competitive, reversible inhibitor of the type III receptor tyrosine kinases, including c-KIT, FLT3 (and its cancer causing mutant W51), and PDGFRβ, which are equally inhibited. The agent is much less active against CSF-1R. It is under investigation in the treatment of glioblastoma and advanced androgen independent prostate cancer. Because of the correlation between FLT3 internal tandem duplication mutations[11] and poor prognosis in acute myelogenous leukemia (AML), tandutinib may be beneficial against this form of leukemia.

[11] In FLT3 internal tandem duplication mutations, partial sequences in the juxtamembrane domain through the first tyrosine kinase domain are tandemly duplicated, generating a longer protein product. These mutations result in ligand independent dimerization and tyrosine autophosphorylation, as well as activation of downstream signaling pathways. The constitutive kinase activation confers factor-independent growth.

JAK/STAT Janus Kinases (JAKs) are universally required for signal transduction from cytokine receptors. Because receptors of this family do not have intrinsic kinase activity JAKs serve as the receptor associated tyrosine kinases. Cytokine receptor ligation and dimerization recruits two molecules of JAK, (Janus Kinase), which then bind to two molecules of STAT (Signal Transducer and Activator of Transcription), in turn leading to JAK/STAT dimerization and transmission of a growth signal. Similarly, the ligation of receptor tyrosine kinases, such as the EGF Receptor, can recruit JAK and SRC, which phosphorylate and activate two molecules of STAT, inducing their dimerization. JAK2 is the most commonly mutated gene in BCR-ABL negative myeloproliferative disorders.

Atiprimod (*N*, *N*-diethyl-8,8-dipropyl-2-azaspiro(4.5) decane-2-propanamine) (SK&F106615) (Fig. 4.21) was initially developed as a potential treatment for rheumatoid arthritis. The drug is an orally bioavailable small molecule belonging to the azaspirane class of cationic amphiphilic agents. Atiprimod inhibits the phosphorylation of STAT3, thus down-regulating the anti-apoptotic proteins BCL-2, BCL-X_L, and MCL-1. This induces cell cycle arrest and leads to apoptosis. The agent lowers the blood levels of IL-6, VEGF, TNF-α, and IL-1. Atiprimod is under evaluation for the treatments of multiple myeloma, metastastic carcinoid cancer, and hepatocellular carcinoma. It has activity against mantle cell lymphoma.

Lestaurtinib (CEP-701) is an orally bioavailable indolocarbazole derivative that inhibits JAK2 as well as RET, FLT3, TRK-A, TRK-B, and TRK-C.

Adverse Effects Most toxicities affect the gastrointestinal tract.

Pacritinib (SB-1518) is a pyrimidine based macrocycle that acts as an ATP competitive small molecule JAK2 kinase inhibitor. It also inhibits the mutant $JAK2^{V617F}$. The drug blocks JAK2 tyrosine phosphorylation on Y221, and dose dependently suppresses JAK2/STAT5 signaling. Pacritinib also suppresses FMS-Like Tyrosine Kinase-3 (FLT3). As a consequence, it has potent anti-proliferative effects on myeloid and lymphoid cells driven by mutant or wild-type JAK2 or FLT3. JAK1, JAK3, and TYK2 are not effectively inhibited. Pacritinib is active against megakaryoblastic leukemia and primary erythroid progenitor cells in myeloproliferative disease. The agent is in clinical studies in patients with myelofibrosis and lymphoma.

JNK The Stress-Activated Protein Kinase (SAPK) pathway is activated in response to noxious influences, including radiation, heat shock, reactive oxygen metabolites, and growth factor deprivation. c-JUN N-Terminal Kinases (JNK)

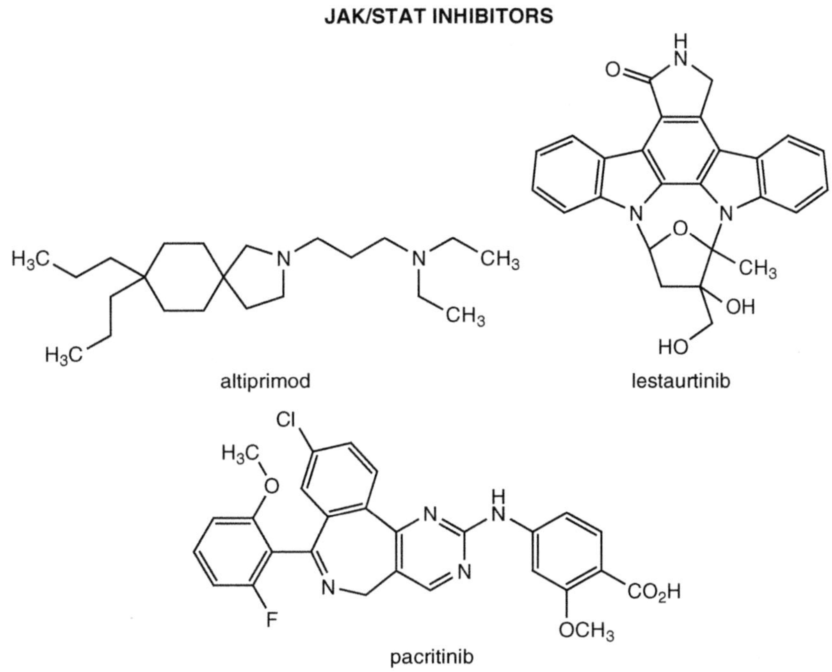

Fig. 4.21 Structures of JAK/STAT inhibitors

constitute a family of stress activated protein kinases derived from the genes, *jnk1*, *jnk2*, and *jnk3*. JNK-1 is required for the survival of the transformed cells in the absence of stromal support.

Robust over-expression of the JNK substrates and transcription factors JUN and JUN-B arises in Hodgkin lymphoma and anaplastic large cell lymphoma (ALCL), but not in other lymphoma types. This is associated with the proliferation of Hodgkin cells and suppression of apoptosis in ALCL cells. Furthermore, the oncogenic BCR-ABL fusion protein activates the JNK signaling pathway in hematopoietic cells. JNK therefore has promise as a drug target (Fig. 4.22).

1,9-pyrazoloanthrone (SP600125) is an anthrapyrazolone first generation, reversible, ATP competitive inhibitor with high selectivity for JNK over other kinases. The agent dose dependently inhibits the phosphorylation of JUN. Its half-maximal inhibitory dose for JNK1 and JNK2 is half that for JNK3. The compound is poorly water soluble, but cell permeable.

CC-401 (3-(3-(2-(piperidin-1-yl)ethoxy)phenyl)-5-(1*H*-1,2,4-triazol-3-yl)-1*H*-indazole hydrochloride) is a second generation, ATP competitive anthrapyrazolone JNK inhibitor. Similar to 1,9-pyrazoloanthrone, CC-401 competitively binds the ATP site of JNK. This leads to an inhibition of phosphorylation of the c-JUN NH_2-terminal activation domain, resulting in decreased transcriptional activity of c-JUN, and consequently decreased cellular proliferation.

ALK About 5 % of patients with non-small cell lung carcinoma have a chromosomal rearrangement that generates a fusion protein between EML4 and ALK (Anaplastic Lymphoma Kinase), which results in constitutive ALK kinase activity that contributes to carcinogenesis. Patients with this gene fusion are typically non-smokers, who do not have mutations in the *egfr* or *K-ras* genes. ALK gain-of-function mutations also may be important in driving the malignant phenotype in about 15 % of neuroblastomata.

Crizotinib ((R)-3-[1-(2,6-Dichloro-3-fluorophenyl) ethoxy]-5-[1-(piperidin-4-yl)-1H-pyrazol-4-yl]pyridin-2-amine) (PF2341066) <Xalkori> (see Fig. 4.22) is an orally bioavailable, ATP site competitive small molecule inhibitor of ALK. Crizotinib also inhibits the tyrosine kinases MET, which is involved in the oncogenesis of a number of other forms of cancer, and ROS1, which also may act as a proto-oncogene. The drug is approved in the U.S. for the treatment of non-small cell lung carcinoma. It is also undergoing clinical trials in anaplastic large cell lymphoma, neuroblastoma, myofibroblastic tumors, and other advanced solid tumors.

Pharmacokinetics Following oral single dose administration, crizotinib reaches a peak blood concentration in 4–6 h. With twice daily administration, steady state is reached within 15 days. Although the drug can be administered with or without food, a high-fat meal reduces crizotinib absorption by about 15 %. There is extensive distribution from the blood into tissues. Over a wide drug concentration the binding to

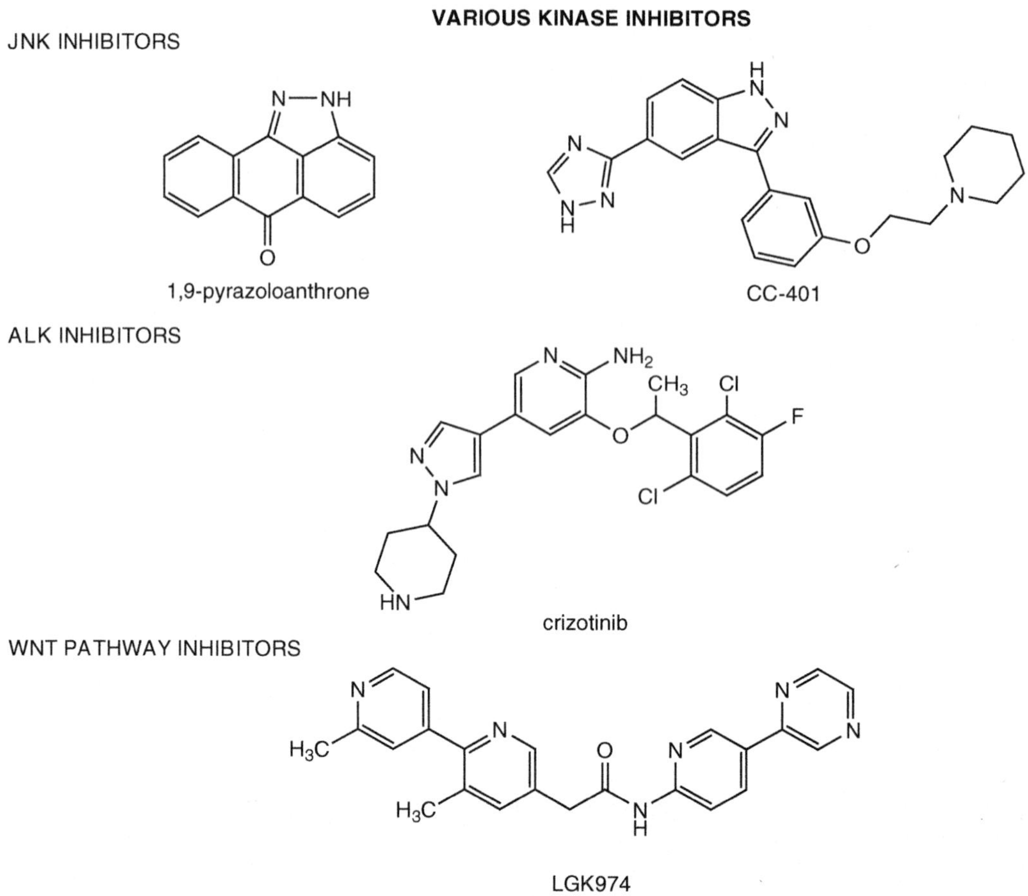

Fig. 4.22 Structures of various signal transduction kinase inhibitors

plasma proteins is 90 %. Following a single dose of crizotinib, the mean apparent terminal half-life is 40 h. 65 and 20 % of the administered are excreted in the feces and urine, respectively. About half of the fecal elimination is constituted by the unchanged drug, whereas the urine excretes mostly metabolites.

Crizotinib is predominantly metabolized by CYP3A4 and CYP3A5. The primary metabolic pathways are oxidation of the piperidine ring to crizotinib lactam and *O*-dealkylation, with subsequent conjugation of *O*-dealkylated metabolites. After multiple dosing, crizotinib acts as a time-dependent inhibitor of CYP3A.

Adverse Effects At the maximum tolerated dose of 250 mg twice a day, the drug causes increased fatigue. Other adverse events may include vision disorder (65 %), nausea or vomiting (50 %), diarrhea (50 %), constipation (40 %), esophageal discomfort (20 %), abdominal pain (15 %), or stomatitis (10 %). Severe pneumonitis and QTc prolongation are potentially dangerous complications. Drug induced hepatotoxicity with fatal outcome has occurred in fewer than 1 % of patients.

Drug Resistance Crizotinib is a substrate for the export transporter ABCB1 (P-Glycoprotein, MDR).

Drug Interactions Co-administration with strong CYP3A inhibitors (HIV protease inhibitors, triazole antifungals, macrolide antibiotics, ketoconazole, nefazodone) increases the crizotinib blood concentrations. Grapefruit or grapefruit juice should be avoided as they may slow the disposition of crizotinib. Co-administration of crizotinib with strong CYP3A inducers (carbamazepine, phenobarbital, phenytoin, rifabutin, rifampin, St. John's Wort) decreases its blood concentrations. As crizotinib itself inhibits CYP3A, dose reduction may be needed for co-administered drugs that are predominantly metabolized by CYP3A.

WNT The success of WNT pathway inhibitors is limited by the narrow therapeutic window afforded by the requirement for WNT signaling in healthy tissue homeostasis. The selective, orally bioavailable Porcupine inhibitor LGK974 (see Fig. 4.22) was the first small molecule WNT signal suppressor in clinical trials (Fig. 4.23). It limits the growth of WNT pathway driven tumors by reducing the expression of WNT target genes, such as *axin2*. LGK974 is efficacious at well tolerated doses against cancers that have NOTCH1 and mutations in RNF43. Head and neck cancer cells with loss-of-function mutations in the NOTCH signaling pathway have a high response rate to LGK974. All LGK974 sensitive pancreatic cancer cells carry inactivating mutations of RNF43.

Excessive activities of diverse kinases can be transforming, causing the development of various cancers.
Drug targets include RET, MET, PDGFR, KIT, JAK, JNK, ALK, WNT.
Drugs that inhibit these kinases have limited specificities.

4.2 Inhibitors of Oncogene Functions

4.2.1 Farnesyl Transferase Inhibitors

Prenylation (the attachment of a farnesyl group or a geranylgeranyl group) provides a mechanism for the membrane localization of proteins that lack a transmembrane domain. RAS proteins participate in numerous signaling pathways related to proliferation and cytoskeletal organization (see Sect. 4.1.3.). One function of RAS is to facilitate the localization of its cytosolic effectors to the plasma membrane, to which it is anchored via a COOH-terminal farnesyl group[12]. To support this function, a key step in the post-translational processing of RAS is its farnesylation by the enzyme Farnesyl Protein Transferase (Farnesyl Transferase). Some RAS proteins (H-RAS1, N-RAS, and K-RAS2) are further lipidated by palmitoylation at 1–2 cysteines near the farnesylated COOH-terminus.

Farnesyl Transferase is not specific for RAS. Other proteins are also subject to farnesylation. The centromeric proteins CENP-E and CENP-F depend on farnesylation for their association with the microtubules, which is important for mitosis. All farnesylated proteins end in a CAAX sequence (C = cysteine, A = aliphatic amino acid, X = methionine, glutamine, serine, or threonine).

Because constitutively activated forms of RAS contribute to a wide range of cancers, Farnesyl Transferase inhibitors were designed to block RAS signal transduction (Reuter 2000). However, they can prevent the farnesylation of various targets (Fig. 4.24) and exert their effects in part through inhibiting the functions of proteins other than RAS. Tumor cells that are sensitive to this class of drugs accumulate in G_2/M, except for cells with activated H-RAS, which accumulate in G_1. Based on the mechanism of action, there are three groups of Farnesyl Transferase inhibitors,

- compounds that act competitively with farnesylpyrophosphate,
- peptidomimetic and non-peptidomimetic compounds that compete with CAAX,
- bisubstrate analogs that combine features of both.

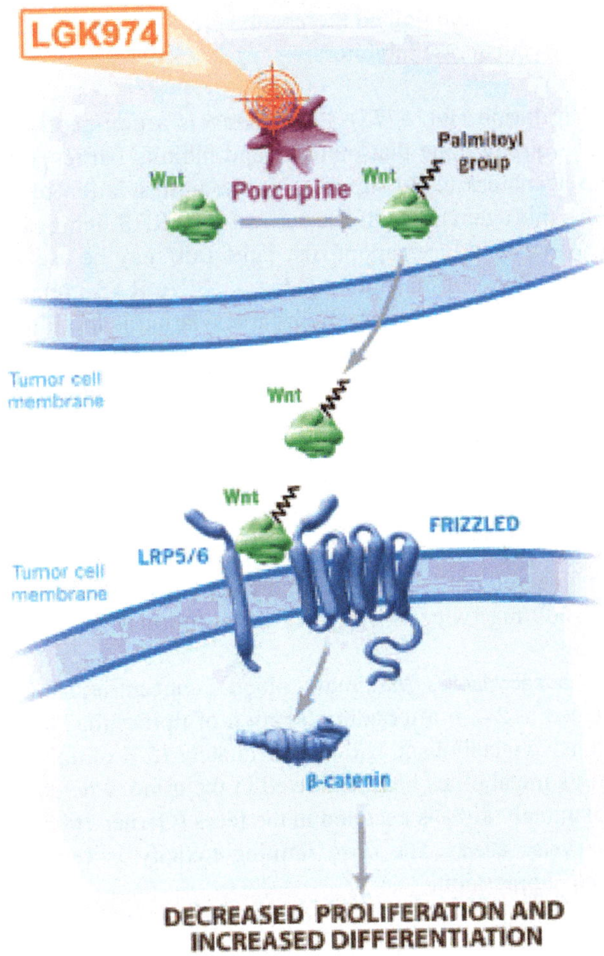

Fig. 4.23 Small molecule inhibitor of Porcupine. The WNT pathway regulates cellular morphology, differentiation, apoptosis, proliferation, and stem cell self-renewal. Dysregulation of this pathway plays a critical role in the development of melanoma, breast cancer, and squamous cell carcinoma. The canonical WNT signaling pathway is initiated by an interaction between WNT ligands and the co-receptors Frizzled LRP5/6. Activation of this pathway prevents the proteosomal degradation of β-Catenin, which translocates into the nucleus and activates the TCF/LEF family of transcription factors to activate specific WNT-target genes. This mechanism results in cell proliferation. WNT ligands require post-translational palmitoylation in order to be secreted and to be functionally active. The key enzyme regulating this process is the membrane-bound O-Acyl Transferase Porcupine, which is required and specific for palmitoylation of WNT ligands. LGK974 is a selective Porcupine inhibitor under development for the treatment of cancers that are driven by the WNT pathway in a WNT ligand-dependent manner ((http://www.novartisoncology.com/research-innovation/pipeline.jsp) with permission, ©2014 Novartis AG)

Adverse Effects The Farnesyl Transferase inhibitor group of drugs has mild toxicities, including neutropenia, thrombocytopenia, diarrhea, rash, neuropathy, and Transaminase elevations.

Drug Resistance Under conditions of inhibited Farnesyl Transferase, the related enzyme Geranyl-Geranyl Transferase 1 can catalyze the activation of RAS (Appels 2005). This

[12] farnesyl is a 15-carbon acyclic sesquiterpene alcohol.

may underlie the limited therapeutic effectiveness of the Farensyl Transferase inhibitors.

Tipifarnib (R115777) <Zarnestra> is a non-peptidomimetic quinolinone that binds to and inhibits Farnesyl Protein Transferase. By suppressing the farnesylation of proteins, this agent prevents the activation of RAS, inhibits cell growth and induces apoptosis. Tipifarnib may be useful in the treatment of multiple myeloma, where RAS mutations are common. Although protein farnesylation is inhibited in all patients exposed to the drug, the targeting of Farnesyl Transferase does not correlate with disease stabilization. Tipifarnib may also target a survival pathway, reflected in reduced levels of phosphorylated PKB and STAT3 in bone marrow from patients, in whom these tumor survival pathways are constitutively active. The reduced phosphorylation correlates with disease stabilization. The compound can be given orally. Dosing regimens frequently administer 300–600 mg twice daily for 21 days, followed by 1 week of rest.

Pharmacokinetics Maximal blood concentrations are reached at 2–4 h after administration of tipifarnib. There is extensive metabolism, with approximately 15% of tipifarnib and its metabolites being excreted in the urine, whereas approximately 80% is excreted in the feces (Garner 2002).

Adverse effects The dose limiting toxicity is reversible myelosuppression.

Lonafarnib (SCH66336) <Sarasar> is a synthetic tricyclic derivative of carboxamide that binds to and inhibits Farnesyl Transferase. The centromeric proteins CENP-E and CENP-F are substrates for Farnesyl Transferase, but not for Geranyl-Geranyl Transferase 1. Their prenylation is completely inhibited by lonafarnib. While this does not affect their localization to the kinetochores, it alters the association between CENP-E and the microtubules, resulting in the alteration of microtubule-centromere interactions during mitosis and leading to the accumulation of cells prior to metaphase (Ashar 2000). Lonafarnib is administered at 200 mg orally twice daily on a continuous regimen. The compound has oral bioavailability and metabolic stability, with maximal plasma concentrations being reached at 6–8 h.

Adverse Effects The main toxicity is diarrhea, but nausea, vomiting, and fatigue also frequently arise.

BMS-214662 is a non-sedating benzodiazepine derivative that belongs to the class of non-peptidomimetic Farnesyl Transferase inhibitors. The drug inhibits H-RAS and K-RAS. Its action is highly selective for Farnesyl Transferase over Geranyl-Geranyl Transferase.

Adverse Effects Because the oral formulation exhibits dose dependent gastrointestinal toxicity, intravenous administration is preferred. The maximum tolerated dose is around 200 mg/m^2, with dose limiting toxicities consisting of nausea, vomiting, and diarrhea. Besides, creatinine elevation, renal failure and acute pancreatitis can become dose limiting (Ryan 2004; Agus 2005).

Other Farnesyl Transferase inhibitors in development include L-778123, L744832, and FTI-277.

Farnesyl Transferase inhibitors suppress the prenylation of proteins, thus preventing their membrane association. This blocks signal transduction.
Multiple proteins may be affected.
The mechanism is not specific for cancer cells.

4.2.2 Inhibitors of Protein Turnover

Inhibitors of protein synthesis Inhibition of tumor cell proliferation by L-Asparaginase was described by Kidd, who observed that the growth of leukemia cells in culture was supported by horse serum or rabbit serum, but not by guinea pig serum. Guinea pig serum turned out to contain an enzyme that degrades asparagine in the medium, thus eliminating a required exogenous nutrient for the growth of leukemia cells.

L-asparagine is a non-essential amino acid that can be synthesized by most human cells, except for those of certain lymphoid malignancies, which lack or have very low levels of the Synthetase enzyme required for L-asparagine formation. L-Asparaginase (Colaspase) <Elspar> is an enzyme produced by various bacteria, such as Escherichia coli. It deaminates L-asparagine to aspartate and ammonia. The depletion of exogenous L-asparagine supplies and inhibition of protein synthesis results in tumor cell blockage of proliferation, especially in the G_1 phase of the cell cycle. L-Asparaginase also induces apoptosis in tumor cells. The drug is used in combination chemotherapy of childhood acute lymphocytic leukemia (ALL), particularly in patients who are refractory to first-line treatments. It has also been used to treat malignant mesothelioma.

- Pegaspargase <Oncaspar> is a complex of polyethylene glycol conjugated with L-Asparaginase. PEGylation decreases the antigenicity of the enzyme.

Drug Resistance Increased L-Asparagine Synthetase activity within tumor cells causes resistance to L-Asparaginase treatment (Kurtzberg 2003).

Ranpirnase is a natural homolog of Ribonuclease A isolated from the eggs of the frog Rana pipiens. Ranpirnase primarily degrades cellular transfer RNA (tRNA) with a substrate specificity for uridine-guanidine base pair sequences, resulting in the inhibition of protein synthesis and cytotoxicity. This agent also activates Caspase-9 in the mitochondria,

Treatment of Pancreatic Carcinoma

1. **Chemotherapy**

The high rate of relapse of pancreatic adenocarcinoma after surgery (85%) makes the combination of adjuvant postoperative therapy an important strategy. Postoperative adjuvant chemo-radiation with fluorouracil was the standard of care for more than 25 years (Kalser 1985; Abbruzzese 2008). However, the benefit of the radiation component was called into doubt by the EPAC-1 (European Study Group for Pancreatic Cancer-1) clinical trial. The treatment of pancreatic cancer depends on the stage. Fluorouracil, gemcitabine (approved by the U.S. FDA in 1996), and erlotinib (or other ERBB targeting drugs) are the chemotherapeutic agents of choice.

Fluorouracil-based regimens 5-fluorouracil is suitable for patients who cannot tolerate gemcitabine. Although pancreatic cancer is highly resistant to chemotherapy, response rates of approximately 25% can be achieved with 5-fluorouracil as a single agent or in combinations with other drugs. However, these treatments provide temporary relief with only small effects on overall survival.

Adjuvant postoperative therapy with fluorouracil and leucovorin (20 mg/m^2 folinic acid intravenous bolus, followed by 425 mg/m^2 fluorouracil intravenous bolus for 1–5 days every 28 days over 6 months) results in a survival benefit. Continuous infusion of 5-fluorouracil is associated with higher survival than bolus injection.

FAM (5-fluorouracil, doxorubicin <Adriamycin>, mitomycin C), FAM-S (5-fluorouracil, doxorubicin, mitomycin C with streptozocin), and the Mallinson regimen (sequential 5-fluorouracil, cyclophosphamide, methotrexate, vincristine, and mitomycin C) have response rates of 20–40% and median survival times up to 10 months. However, no survival advantages has been documented over single-agent 5-fluorouracil, and the toxicities are substantial.

First-line treatment for metastatic pancreatic adenocarcinoma with FOLFIRINOX (folinic acid (leucovorin), 5-fluorouracil, irinotecan, oxaliplatin) is superior to monotherapy with gemcitabine. The combination is associated with an improved response rate and increased progression free survival.

Adverse Effects Common adverse effects include vomiting, fatigue, diarrhea, neuropathy, myelosuppression, and febrile neutropenia. Because of the substantial adverse events, this regimen is limited to patients with very good performance status.

Gemcitabine-based treatments Adjuvant gemcitabine may have a slightly higher survival benefit compared to fluorouracil/leucovorin. Gemcitabine (1 g/m2 intravenous infusion once per week for 3 of every 4 weeks) also has a lower incidence of stomatitis and diarrhea. Monotherapy with this drug is common. While numerous gemcitabine based combination chemotherapy protocols (comprising 2–4 drug combinations) have been tested, none has yet evolved as superior.

Adverse Effects The use of gemcitabine is associated with an increased risk of myelosuppression and resulting hematologic toxicity (O'Reilly 2010).

The combination of gemcitabine with 5-fluorouracil is well tolerated, despite some additional toxicity over single-agent gemcitabine (grade 3/4 leukopenia and diarrhea are more frequent). However, it is not documented whether this combination has any advantage over single-agent gemcitabine.

GemCap is a combination chemotherapy treatment for pancreatic cancer that uses gemcitabine <Gemzar> and capecitabine <Xeloda>. Gemcitabine is given as an infusion over about 30 min on days 1 and 8. Capecitabine is taken in tablet form for 14 days, usually as a combination of 500 and 150 mg tablets. A rest period of 1 week completes the cycle. A usual regimen covers 4–8 cycles of treatment over a period of 3–4 months.

Gemcitabine/cisplatin combinations have modest additional benefits compared with outcomes for gemcitabine as a single agent. This therapy is tolerated without major compromises in the quality of life. Response rates and a longer median survival may favor the gemcitabine/cisplatin doublet over monotherapy.

Several Topoisomerase I inhibitors, including irinotecan, exatecan, and the oral drug rubitecan (9-nitrocamptothecin, 9NC), are undergoing clinical development in an effort to identify novel, improved gemcitabine based combinations.

ERBB-targeting treatments EGFR is overexpressed in a large fraction of pancreatic tumors. Resulting from a phase III randomized controlled trial, that demonstrated improved survival rates, improved tumor responses, and improved progression-free survival rates, the U.S. FDA has licensed the use of erlotinib <Tarceva> in combination with gemcitabine as a palliative agent for pancreatic cancer. The survival improvement with the combination is on the order of less than four weeks, causing the incremental value of adding erlotinib to gemcitabine treatment to be questioned. Erlotinib has now secured approval for the treatment of advanced pancreatic cancer in combination with gemcitabine in chemotherapy-naïve patients in both the U.S. and Europe.

As an alternative to erlotinib, the antibody cetuximab <Erbitux> (loading dose of 400 mg/m2 then 250 mg/m2 weekly) has been evaluated in conjunction with gemcitabine. The combination leads to disease stabilization in about 50% of patients and an increase in overall survival.

Adverse Effects The main adverse effects are dermatological, including acneiform rash (40%) and folliculitis (15%).

Approximately 20% of pancreatic tumors overexpress ERBB2 (HER-2/neu). Trastuzumab (loading dose of 4 mg/kg for the first week and then 2 mg/kg weekly) in combination with gemcitabine (1000 mg/m2 weekly) has a survival benefit in patients with metastatic, ERBB2-positive pancreatic cancer.

Adverse Effects Grade 3 hematologic toxicities and cardiotoxicity may occur.

Other drugs Blocking RAS signaling is highly promising for therapy since ras mutations arise in approximately 90% of pancreatic cancers. RAS inhibition may be achieved by small molecule kinase inhibitors or by blocking the posttranslational farnesylation of K-RAS. SCH66336, R1115777, and BMS 214662 are Farnesyl Transferase inhibitors in clinical development. They are available for oral and intravenous administration. Mostly, they are under study in combination with gemcitabine.

Leukocytes actively infiltrate the stroma of pancreatic ductal adenocarcinoma and orchestrate an immune response that is—in its result—immunosuppressive and leads to fibrosis. Activation of the TNF receptor CD40 is a key regulator in reversing this immunosuppression. Tumor regression requires macrophages, but not T-lymphocytes.

The fully human agonistic anti-CD40 antibody CP-870,893 may facilitate tumor regression in surgically incurable patients (Beatty 2011). The most common adverse effect is mild to moderate cytokine release syndrome (characterized by chills, fever, and rigors), which can be managed by supportive care.

TNFerade for the treatment of pancreatic cancer has orphan drug designation from the U.S. FDA. TNFerade is an adenovector, which contains the gene for tumor necrosis factor-α (tnf-α), an immune system protein with potent anti-cancer effects, for the direct injection into tumors. After administration, TNFerade stimulates the production of TNF-α in the tumor. The agent did not prove efficacious in clinical trials.

Endocrine cancer targets Z-360 is a selective, orally available, 1,5-benzodiazepine derivative that acts as a Gastrin/Cholecystokinin-2 Receptor antagonist. By binding to the receptor, Z-360 prevents its activation by Gastrin, a peptide hormone frequently associated with the proliferation of gastrointestinal and pancreatic tumor cells.

Streptozotocin is approved by the U.S. FDA for treating metastatic cancer of the pancreatic islet cells. The agent is generally limited to patients whose cancer cannot be resected surgically. Streptozotocin can reduce the tumor burden and ameliorate symptoms, such as hypoglycemia due to excessive Insulin secretion by insulinomata.

2. **Pain management**

The typical pain of locally advanced pancreatic cancer is a dull, fairly constant pain of visceral origin localized to the region of the middle and upper back. It results from tumor invasion of the celiac and mesenteric plexi (neuropathic and inflammatory type of pain). Some patients complain of vague, intermittent epigastric pain. The etiology of this discomfort may be secondary to pancreatic duct obstruction and resultant pancreatic insufficiency (obstructive and inflammatory types). In the early stages of the disease, only 10% of patients have severe pain.

Comprehensive pain management consists of a combination of anti-tumor therapy, analgesic drug therapy, anesthetic blocks, and behavioral approaches.

- Initially, pain associated with unresectable pancreatic cancer can be controlled with non-steroidal anti-inflammatory drugs (NSAIDs) or oral or transdermal narcotic analgesics. Upon disease progression, opioids alone may not be sufficient.
- The next major modality for pain control is an anesthetic block of the celiac plexus, using injection of a solution of 50–100% alcohol or a phenol solution. This offers pain control for a duration of 3–4 months in 80–90% of patients. Celiac block can be performed percutaneously (under radiologic guidance) or intraoperatively.
- While external beam radiation therapy with or without chemotherapy may be used to palliate pain asso-

ciated with pancreatic cancer, pain control may take several weeks to be achieved with radiation.

- Chemotherapy also can achieve pain control in pancreatic cancer patients, as is the case with the use of gemcitabine. Over 20 % of patients treated with gemcitabine experience a clinical benefit with regard to improved pain or fatigue (el-Kamar 2003).

3. **Obstruction**

About 70 % of pancreatic cancers are located in the head of the pancreas, and obstructive jaundice is often the first symptom leading to diagnosis. Biliary decompression can be accomplished by surgical bypass (including cholecystojejunostomy, choledochojejunostomy, or hepaticojejunostomy) or endobiliary stenting. Endoscopic stent placement has a higher success rate and lower 30-day mortality rate than percutaneous stenting and represents the procedure of choice. The choice of surgery versus stenting should be made in the context of the patient's overall treatment plan. For obstructive pain, pancreatic duct stenting or pancreatic enzyme replacement may be effective.

Gastric outlet obstruction is a late complication of advanced pancreatic cancer affecting approximately 10–20 % of patients who survive more than 15 months. However, fewer than 3 % of these patients require surgical bypass. 60 % of patients with advanced pancreatic cancer have no evidence of gastric or duodenal invasion but have abnormal gastric motility with delayed emptying. Also, nausea and vomiting may develop secondary to tumor infiltration of the nerve plexi of the stomach and duodenum. After gastric outlet and small bowel obstructions have been ruled out, empiric prokinetic drugs, such as metoclopramide, can be used to manage these symptoms (el-Kamar 2003).

4. **Cachexia**

Cachexia in the advanced pancreatic cancer patient results not only from loss of appetite and malnutrition but also from hyper-catabolism of lean tissue and anorexia/cachexia syndrome. The condition is reflected in weakness, fatigue, and poor quality of life. Weight loss also contributes to depression and is predictive of poor outcome and greater morbidity.

- The management of pancreatic exocrine insufficiency is especially important for managing cachexia. Pancreatic exocrine insufficiency is common but usually moderate in patients with pancreatic cancer. Approximately 65 % of patients have some degree of fat malabsorption and 50 % have some degree of protein malabsorption. These may contribute to weight loss, epigastric discomfort, and malabsorption symptoms such as excessive flatus, bloating, diarrhea, and steatorrhea. Pancreatic enzyme replacement improves malabsorption, bloating, and diarrhea and helps prevent further weight loss. Pancreatic enzyme therapy may sometimes be associated with gastrointestinal adverse effects such as nausea, vomiting, cramps, constipation, or diarrhea that can be ameliorated by adjusting doses or brands. Empiric Pancreolipase replacement should be considered for most patients.
- The initial management usually entails (preferably oral) supportive nutrition, comprising caloric supplementation and hydration.
- Anorexia is well treated with appetite stimulants, such as progestational drugs and corticosteroids. These agents are potent anti-emetics, act rapidly, and increase the non-fluid body weight in advanced cancer patients with anorexia. The most used agents are megesterol acetate, medroxyprogesterone acetate, and dexamethasone. Dexamethasone can be administered at doses ranging 3–8 mg/day and megesterol acetate doses range 400–800 mg/day. They are comparable in efficacy and produce an improvement in appetite with subsequent weight gain in approximately 15 % of patients. Dexamethasone has a short-lived duration of action (4 weeks) and a substantial adverse effect profile, including myopathy, mood changes, and hyperglycemia.
- A class of drugs in use is orexigenic (appetite stimulant) agents, such as the prokinetic medication metoclopramide and the cannabinoid dronabinol. Dronabinol at doses of 2.5–7.5 mg/day improves chemotherapy-induced nausea and vomiting in 65 % of cancer patients.
- An agent that may reverse cancer-associated cachexia is eicosapentaenoic acid (EPA, contained in fish oil pills) at doses of 1–6 g/day, which may result in weight stabilization after 3–4 weeks. Eicosapentaenoic acid works by suppressing the effect of the glycoprotein Proteolysis-Inducing Factor (PIF).
- Thalidomide at 100–200 mg/day at bedtime, provides some weight stabilization but no weight gain. It may shorten the half-life of *tnf-α* mRNA. Because of mixed results in clinical trials, thalidomide is not widely used.
- Ibuprofen has a role in abrogating the catabolic process and may lead to modest increases in weight. The combination of ibuprofen with megestrol acetate can reverse weight loss and improve the quality of life (el-Kamar 2003).

Treatment of Lung Cancer

Small cell lung cancer is treated primarily with chemotherapy, as surgery has no demonstrable influence on survival. Primary chemotherapy is also given in metastatic non-small cell lung cancer. The combination regimen depends on the tumor type.

- For non-small cell lung cancer, cisplatin or carboplatin, in combination with gemcitabine, paclitaxel, docetaxel, etoposide, or vinorelbine are used.
- For small cell lung cancer, cisplatin and etoposide are most commonly used. Combinations with carboplatin, gemcitabine, paclitaxel, vinorelbine, topotecan, and irinotecan are also applicable.

Adjuvant chemotherapy refers to the use of chemotherapy after surgery to improve outcome. In stage 2 or 3 disease (afflicted lymph nodes), adjuvant chemotherapy may improve survival by up to 15 %. Standard practice is to offer platinum based chemotherapy, such as cisplatin and vinorelbine.

Small cell lung cancer Chemotherapy has been used in patients with small cell lung cancer (SCLC) for more than 25 years.

- Lung cancers may be treated with CAP, a combination chemotherapy of cyclophosphamide, doxorubicin <Adriamycin>, and cisplatin (platinum alkylating agents).
- CAV is named after cyclophosphamide, doxorubicin <Adriamycin>, and vincristine. The chemotherapy drugs are then given separately, often starting with doxorubicin, followed by vincristine, and then cyclophosphamide. The cycle is completed with a rest period of 3 weeks. A course of the treatment comprises 4–6 cycles that are given over a period of 3–4 months.
- The COPE regimen includes cyclophosphamide, vincristine <Oncovin>, cisplatin (platinum alkylating agents), and etoposide.
- The PE (cisplatin, etoposide) regimen was developed in the early 1980s. For many years, it was a standard chemotherapy program most extensively used in clinical practice. Various modalities exist, in which cisplatin and etoposide are administered.

Non-small cell lung cancer Non-small cell lung cancer is more common than small cell lung cancer, accounting for around 80 % of all lung cancers. It is an aggressive disease, for which the overall 5 years survival rates are below 10 %. Cytotoxic chemotherapy is the standard of care for patients with unresectable stage 3 and stage 4 cancer and a good performance status. For the treatment of locally advanced or metastatic non-small cell lung cancer, platinum-based and taxane-based chemotherapies are the first line of treatment. Doublet chemotherapy including cisplatin or carboplatin with another drug (vinorelbine, paclitaxel, docetaxel, or gemcitabine) is recommended.

- Chemotherapy is initially conducted with docetaxel, paclitaxel, vinorelbine, gemcitabine, or pemetrexed.
- Second to third line therapy for non-small cell lung cancer includes small molecule tyrosine kinase inhibitors, such as gefitinib and erlotinib. In initial clinical trials, erlotinib was used as monotherapy in patients with chemo-refractory non-small cell lung cancer. 50 % of these achieved disease stabilization and 40 % survived for at least 12 months.
- The addition of bevacizumab to doublet chemotherapy improves the 1-year survival in selected patients with advanced non-small cell lung cancer. The drug is used in combination with carboplatin and paclitaxel as first-line treatment of patients with unresectable, locally advanced, recurrent or metastatic non-squamous non-small cell lung cancer.

GemCarbo chemotherapy (consisting of gemcitabine and carboplatin) is used to treat non-small cell lung cancer. It is usually given as a day patient treatment, involving a blood test the day before infusion of the drugs. The regimen is administered as a 21 day cycle. On the first day of treatment, the patient is given both agents. On day 8, there is an infusion of gemcitabine only. There then follows a rest period of 2 weeks which completes one cycle of chemotherapy. The next cycle of treatment is given after a rest period, which will be 3 weeks after the first injection. Usually 4–6 cycles of treatment are given over a period of 3–4 months and this makes up a course of treatment. This regimen may prevent the further spread of the cancer or in some cases may reduce the size of the tumor between 20–80 % depending upon the individual.

Inhibiting ERBB1 (EGFR) signaling is an effective strategy for treating non-small cell lung cancer patients. The first generation tyrosine kinase inhibitors, gefitinib and erlotinib, have temporary success. Second generation agents that aim to further improve patient outcomes are in preclinical and clinical trials. They include EKB-569, HKI-272, CI-1033, and ZD6474 (Sequist 2007).

Drug Resistance About half of all patients develop the ERBB1 mutation T790M, for which existing inhibitors do not work well. Over-expression of MET by the cancer cells may also cause resistance to small molecule ERBB1 inhibitors.

Adenocarcinoma 10–15 % of lung cancers involve patients who never smoked. In 70 % of the cases, these tumors are adenocarcinomata. These lung cancers constitute a distinct disease from lung cancers in smokers. Two mutations commonly occur.

- Many non-smoker type lung cancers have mutations in ERBB1 (EGFR). An activating mutation in exons 19 and 21 may be causative. Many patients initially respond to tyrosine kinase inhibitors, such as erlotinib, but resistance eventually develops. In relapsed patients, an activating mutation in exon 20 often arises. It may be selected for by treatment with tyrosine kinase inhibitors. The exon 20 mutation changes the structure of the tyrosine kinase inhibitor binding site, thus rendering the drugs ineffective. Amplification of *c-met* can be another mechanism to cause resistance to tyrosine kinase inhibitors by activating a rescue growth and survival pathway.
- A tumor driver in non-smoker type lung cancer can be mutated K-RAS. Until targeted therapies are developed, only conventional chemotherapy can be offered to those patients.

Mesothelioma Pemetrexed <Alimta> is a multi-target agent that inhibits several folate dependent enzymes. It is used in combination with cisplatin for the treatment of pleural mesothelioma. The average survival and time to cancer progression can be further improved by giving a vitamin supplementation of B12 and folic acid.

The chemotherapy regimen MVP includes mitomycin, vinblastine, and cisplatin. The drugs are given as consecutive injections or infusions over 8–12 h. Because the treatment contains a platinum drug, the ample consumption of fluids is recommended to protect kidney function. The cycle is completed by a rest period of 3 weeks.

resulting in tumor cell apoptosis. The agent is under study for the treatment of pleural and peritoneal mesothelioma.

KRN5500 (Fig. 4.25) is a semi-synthetic derivative of the nucleosidic antibiotic spicamycin, which was originally isolated from the bacterium Streptomyces alanosinicus. KRN5500 inhibits protein synthesis by interfering with endoplasmic reticulum and Golgi apparatus functions. This agent also induces cell differentiation and Caspase dependent apoptosis. It is under investigation for B-cell chronic lymphocytic leukemia

Homoharringtonine (omacetaxine mepesuccinate, cephalotaxine 4-methyl (2R)-2-hydroxy-2-(4-hydroxy-4-methylpentyl)butanedioate) <Synribo> is a cytotoxic plant alkaloid isolated from the evergreen trees Cephalotaxus fortuneii and Cephalotaxus hainanensis. The molecule binds to the ribosome. It suppresses the elongation phase of translation by preventing substrate binding to the acceptor site on the 60S ribosomal subunit and blocking aminoacyl-tRNA binding[13] and peptide bond formation.

Homoharringtonine induces differentiation or apoptosis in some cancer cell types. It has been used in China to treat adults with chronic or accelerated phase chronic myeloid leukemia (CML) who are no longer responding to, or who could not tolerate, at least two tyrosine kinase inhibitors. Homoharringtonine is also active in patients carrying the BCR-ABL^{T315I} mutation. The recommended starting schedule for induction is 1.25 mg/m^2 administered subcutaneously twice daily for 14 consecutive days over a 28-day cycle. Cycles should be repeated until the patient achieves a hematologic response. The recommended maintenance schedule is 1.25 mg/m^2 administered subcutaneously twice daily for 7 consecutive days over a 28-day cycle. Treatment should continue as long as the patient is clinically benefiting from the therapy.

Adverse Effects In chronic and accelerated phase patients, the most common adverse reactions (over 20 % of patients) include thrombocytopenia, anemia, neutropenia, diarrhea, nausea, fatigue, asthenia, injection site reaction, pyrexia, infection, and lymphopenia. The drug is Pregnancy Category D.

Didemnins are cyclic depsipeptides, originally isolated in 1978 from a tunicate of the genus Trididemnum collected in the Caribbean Sea. A didemnin was the first marine peptide that entered clinical trials in U.S. for the treatment of cancer. Didemnins inhibit protein synthesis and arrest cells in G_1.

[13] The interaction of homoharringtonine with the ribosomal A site prevents the correct positioning of amino acid side chains of incoming aminoacyl-tRNAs.

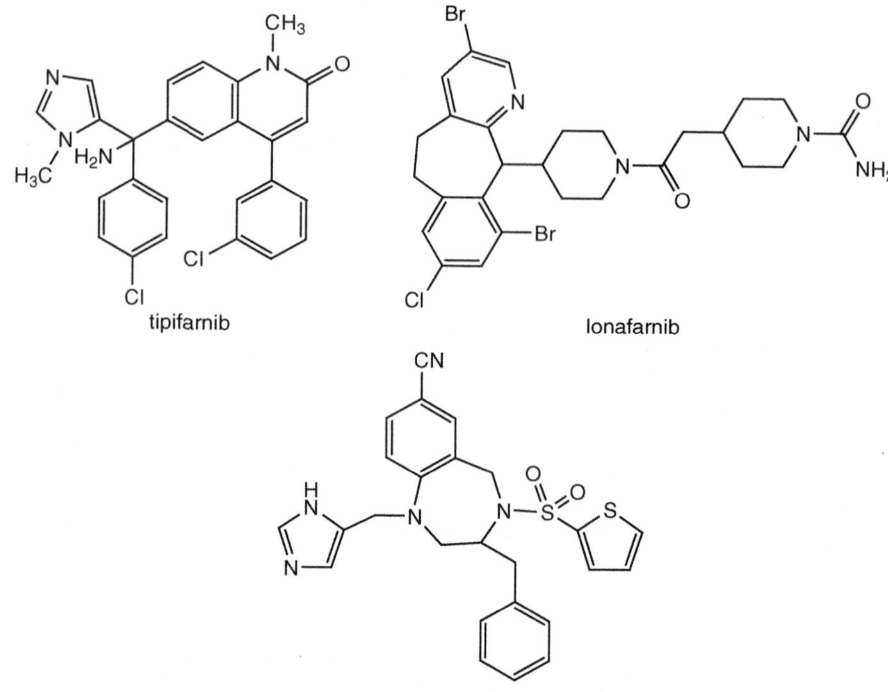

Fig. 4.24 Structures of Farnesyl Transferase inhibitors

They display GTP dependent binding to the translation elongation factor EF1α. They also bind to Palmitoyl Thioesterase (the enzyme removes palmitate from H-RAS and from the $G\alpha_s$ subunits of hetero-trimeric GTP binding proteins). Didemnins are under study against renal adenocarcinoma, advanced epithelial ovarian cancer, and metastatic breast cancer.

- Dihydrodidemnin B (aplidine) is produced by the ascidian Aplidium albicans. It is in clinical trials. In 2003, aplidine was granted orphan drug status by the European Medicines Agency for treating acute lymphoblastic leukemia.

Adverse Effects Didemnins are immunosuppressive. Didemnin B exhibits a high incidence of anaphylactic reactions, which have led to the termination of its clinical development.

Proteasome inhibitors The proteasome is a multi-catalytic protease complex that degrades most endogenous proteins, including those that are misfolded or damaged, to ensure normal cellular function. The attachment of Ubiquitin moieties to a protein typically marks it for transport to the proteasome. The Ubiquitin-proteasome degradation pathway plays essential roles in multiple cellular processes, including cell cycle progression and proliferation. Cancer cells are more sensitive than untransformed cells to proteasome inhibition. Healthy cells often are able to recover from intermittent inhibition of proteasome function, but many types of cancer cells undergo apoptosis when their proteasomes are inhibited longer. The drug names of proteasome inhibitors end on -zomib.

Bortezomib (PS-341, MLN341, LDP-341) <Velcade> is a first-in-class reversible proteasome inhibitor. It exerts its effects in part through its ability to block the activation of the transcription factor NF-κB by preventing the proteasomal degradation of the inhibitor I-κB. Upon activation, NF-κB sends a message for cells to increase the expression of various adhesion molecules, which allow myeloma cells to attach to cells in the bone marrow. This interaction stimulates the bone marrow cells to produce growth and survival factors, such as IL-6 and VEGF. Therefore, by blocking NF-κB, bortezomib blocks myeloma cell growth, inhibits the interactions between myeloma and bone marrow cells, and suppresses angiogenesis.

In 2005, bortezomib was approved by the U.S. FDA. In the same year, the European Commission also approved it for use in mono-therapy for myeloma patients who have received at least one prior therapy and who have already undergone or are unsuitable for stem cell transplantation. The recommended dose of bortezomib for treating multiple myeloma or mantle cell lymphoma is 1.3 mg/m^2 administered as an intravenous injection twice weekly for 2 weeks (days 1, 4, 8, and 11), followed by a 10-day rest period (days 12–21) to complete the cycle. For extended therapy of more than eight cycles, bortezomib may be administered on this standard schedule or on a maintenance schedule of once weekly injections for 4 weeks (days 1, 8, 15, and 22) followed by a 13-day rest period (days 23–35). At least 70–72 h should elapse between consecutive doses.

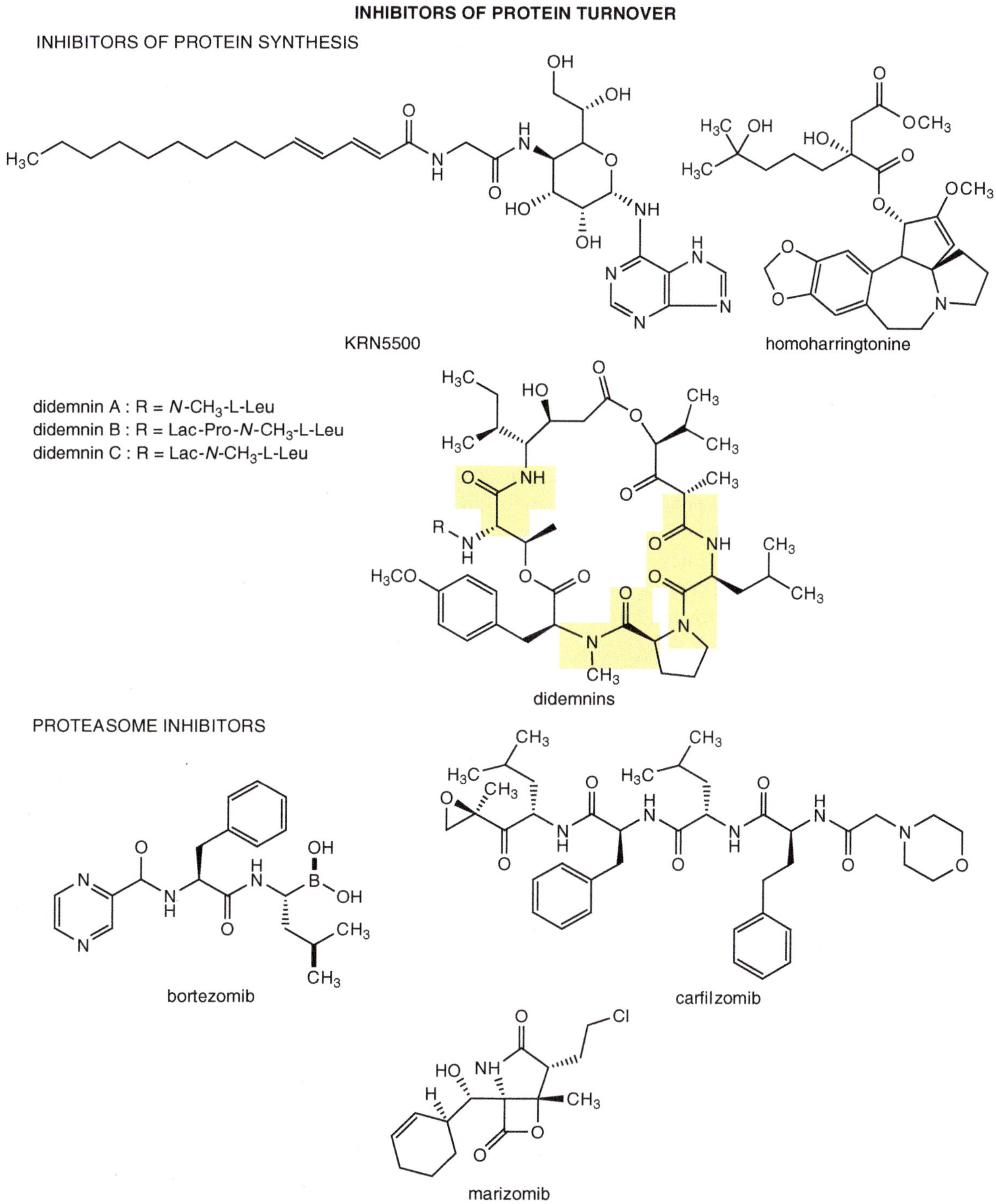

Fig. 4.25 Structures of inhibitors of protein turnover. The peptide bonds in didemnins are highlighted in *yellow*

Pharmacokinetics Bortezomib undergoes hepatic metabolism primarily via the Cytochromes P450 CYP3A4, CYP2C19, and CYP1A2. Its pharmacokinetics is not affected by renal impairment, however, dialysis may reduce the bortezomib blood concentrations.

Adverse Effects Common adverse effects comprise asthenic conditions (fatigue, malaise, weakness) in about 60 %, digestive irregularity (60 % diarrhea, 40 % constipation), nausea (55 %) and vomiting (35 %), peripheral neuropathy (35 %), fever (35 %), thrombocytopenia (35 %), psychiatric disorders (35 %), and decreased appetite or weight loss in 35 % of cases. Patients who experience neuropathic pain or peripheral neuropathy (abnormal or decreased sensation, burning, or tingling) should have their dose and schedule adjusted. Bortezomib is contraindicated in patients with hypersensitivity to bortezomib, boron, or mannitol.

Carfilzomib <Kyprolis> is derived from epoxomicin, a natural product that was found in the laboratory of Craig Crews at Yale University to inhibit the proteasome. The drug is approved for the treatment of patients with multiple myeloma, who have already received at least two other treatments including bortezomib and an immunomodulatory agent (lenalidomide or thalidomide), and whose disease has progressed on or within 60 days of their last therapy. Carfilzomib for injection has efficacy as single agent therapy, however, improvement in survival has not been proven.

Adverse Effects Anemia and thrombocytopenia are the most common adverse effects. Carfilzomib can cause heart problems or worsen pre-existing heart conditions, and death due to cardiac arrest may occur. Shortness of breath arises in 35 % of patients. There is a risk for pulmonary hypertension. Potential infusion reactions include fever, chills, joint or muscle pain, facial flushing or swelling, nausea, weakness, low blood pressure, fainting, and chest tightness. These symptoms can occur immediately following infusion or up to 24 h after administration.

The β-lactone-γ-lactam proteasome inhibitor marizomib ((-)-salinosporamide A) (NPI-0052) was discovered from the marine-obligate actinomycete Salinispora tropica. The agent is distinct from bortezomib in its chemical structure and mechanism of action. It covalently modifies the active site threonine residues of the 20S proteasome. Inhibition of Ubiquitin-proteasome mediated proteolysis leads to an accumulation of poly-ubiquitinated proteins, which may result in the disruption of cellular processes, the induction of apoptosis, and the inhibition of tumor growth. Marizomib can be given orally. It is in clinical trials.

Several natural compounds, including the microbial metabolite lactacystin, green tea polyphenols, and traditional medicinal triterpenes, are potent proteasome inhibitors. This suggests the potential use of natural proteasome inhibitors as chemopreventive and chemotherapeutic agents, but also as tumor sensitizers to conventional radio-therapy and chemotherapy.

HSP90 inhibitors Chaperones, such as HSP90 (90 kD Heat Shock Protein) are critical to maintaining the normal protein folding environment. The HSP90 protein family consists of four members (HSP90α, HSP90β, GRP94, TRAP1). HSP90 comprises three conserved domains, the N-terminal lobe that contains an adenine nucleotide binding pocket (responsible for the ATPase activity), the highly charged middle region (modulates the ATPase activity), and the C-terminal lobe (contains an additional ATP binding pocket). HSP90 mediated protein folding requires energy that depends on the hydrolysis of ATP by the N-terminal ATP binding pocket. This nucleotide binding domain is unique compared to other ATP binding proteins because the nucleotide is bound in a bent conformation[14] as opposed to the extended conformation utilized by most proteins. Activation of HSP90 results in its association with a series of co-chaperones, which form a complex that interacts with client proteins. The increased expression of chaperones enhances cell survival in tissues damaged by a variety of stressors. Such conditions are common within tumors, and there is increased expression of chaperone proteins in several types of solid tumors. Several HSP90 client proteins play important roles in the regulation of the cell cycle and cell survival.

Specific inhibitors of HSP90 have entered clinical trials for metastatic cancer. Inhibition of the HSP90 ATPase activity with high affinity natural product inhibitors results in proteasome mediated degradation of the client proteins (including oncogenic signaling proteins that are over-expressed by tumor cells) and subsequent interruption of their signaling function. Cancers that are not driven by HSP90 client proteins are not sensitive to HSP90 inhibitors.

HSP90 inhibitors may be useful in combination with DNA damaging agents, because of their ability to abrogate S and G_2/M cell cycle checkpoint controls by promoting the degradation of the client kinases CHK1 and WEE1. The effect is independent of the P53 status in the tumor, which is advantageous as about 50 % of cancers are defective in P53 function.

Inhibition of the molecular chaperone HSP90 promotes the transcription of both Major Histocompatibility (MHC) class I encoding genes (*mica* and *micb*) in myeloma cells. MICA and MICB are ligands for a receptor on natural killer cells, which is important for tumor cell recognition and lysis by the immune system. Consequently, HSP90 inhibitors increase myeloma cell stimulation of natural killer cell degranulation, possibly enhancing host immune surveillance.

Ansamycins were discovered in 1959 in the actinomycete Amycolatopsis mediterranei. The ansamycin (ansa macrolide) class of antibiotics is structurally characterized by a medium sized to large macrolide or macrolactam handle fused to a mono- or bicyclic aromatic core. Representatives of this class differ mainly in the aromatic moiety, which can be a naphthalene ring (in rifamycin, naphthomycins), a naphthoquinone ring (in hygrocins), a benzene or benzoquinone ring system (in geldanamycin, ansamitocin). Ansamycins (Fig. 4.26) bind to the N-terminal domain and inhibit the cytosolic chaperone functions of HSP90 via blocking the essential ATPase activity.

[14] This binding conformation is shared by only four proteins, DNA Gyrase, HSP90, Histidine Kinase, and MUT-L.

- Geldanamycin (geldenamycin) was first described in 1970. It is a naturally occurring benzoquinone ansamycin. Geldanamycin preferentially induces the degradation of proteins that are mutated in tumor cells such as v-SRC, BCR-ABL, and P53 over their normal cellular counterparts.
- Tanespimycin (17-allylamino,17-demethoxygeldanamycin, 17-AAG) (NSC 330507) is a benzoquinone derived from geldanamycin. In 1999, it was the first HSP90 inhibitor to enter clinical trials. The drug has possible clinical activity in metastatic melanoma, prostate cancer, and multiple myeloma with manageable toxicity. In clinical trials, it has shown signs of effectiveness against ERBB2-positive breast cancers[15]. However, tanespimycin has unfavorable physiochemical properties, including poor water solubility, making its formulation for clinical delivery difficult.
- Alvespimycin hydrochloride (17-DMAG) (KOS-1022) is a tansepimycin derivative with improved water solubility that may be given intravenously or orally.
- Retaspimycin hydrochloride (IPI-504) is the hydroquinone hydrochloride salt of alvespimycin. It is administered intravenously.
- 17-Aminogeldanamycin (17-AG) (IPI-493) is the major metabolite of tanespimycin (17-AAG) and retaspimycin (17-DMAG). It can be administered as an orally available HSP90 inhibitor.
- The rifamycins are a group of ansamycins, in which the aromatic moiety is a naphthalene ring. They are synthesized either naturally by the bacterium Amycolatopsis mediterranei or synthetically. Beside acting as HSP90 inhibitors, rifamycins may inhibit RNA tumor viruses via inhibition of their DNA Polymerase.
- Maytansinoid anti-tumor agents are members of the ansamycin group. They are 19-membered macrocyclic lactams that target the microtubules (see Sect. 3.1.6.) and thus inhibit cell proliferation.

Adverse Effects Hepatotoxicity (due to the presence of a reactive quinone moiety) limits the use of geldanamycin and its derivatives.

Drug Resistance The co-chaperone of HSP90, Prostaglandin E Synthase 3 (PTGES3, P23), modulates the rate of the HSP90 cycle by affecting the conformational dynamics of the chaperone. Over-expression of PTGES3 protects cells from geldanamycin. NQO1 (NAD(P)H/Quinone Oxidoreductase 1) reduces the quinone moiety of geldanamycin to its dihydroquinone form, which enhances the HSP90 binding properties. A loss of the enzyme NQO1 leads to tanespimycin resistance. The cytotoxic activity of ansamycin antibiotics is compromised by over-expression of BCL-2 in the tumor cells. Ansamycin antibiotics are ABCB1 substrates, and are inactive against cells that express high levels of the export transporter.

HSP90 client proteins play important roles in the regulation of the cell cycle. A pocket region in the N-terminal domain of HSP90 serves as an ATP/ADP-binding site. The macrocyclic antifungal radicicol (monorden) is a natural product that binds to this site. Like ansamycins, radicicol inhibits the binding of the accessory protein P23. It interferes with the assembly of the mature Progesterone Receptor complex and depletes cells of ERBB2, RAF1, and mutant P53. Radicicol does not diminish cellular HSP90, but rather increases synthesis and steady-state levels of this protein, similar to a stress response. Through an ATPase domain common to HSP90, radicicol also binds to and inhibits DNA Topoisomerase 2 and GRP94.

Novobiocin (albamycin, cathomycin), first reported in 1955 under the name streptonivicin (Hoeksema 1955), is an aminocoumarin antibiotic that is produced by the actinomycetes Streptomyces niveus and Streptomyces spheroides, members of the order Actinobacteria. The HSP90 inhibitor engages a C-terminal motif[16]. Whereas small molecule inhibitors of the canonical N-terminal nucleotide binding site (ansamycins, radicicol) have half-maximal inhibitory concentration values in the low nanomolar range, novobiocin exhibits half-maximal inhibition at 700 μM, which is substantially less potent. The agent also inhibits Topoisomerase 2[17], increases the cytotoxicity of several alkylating agents by the formation of lethal DNA-DNA inter-strand cross-links, perhaps by decreasing the repair of drug mono-adducts.

Representatives of the Pu class (purine based molecules) of HSP90 inhibitors specifically bind to the HSP90 N-terminal regulatory pocket. They include Pu24FCl (8-(2-chloro-3,4,5-trimethoxybenzyl)-2-fluoro-9-(pent-4-ynyl)-9Hpurin-6-amine), Pu-H58 (8-(6-bromobenzo[d][1,3]dioxol-5-ylthio)-9-(pent-4-ynyl)-9H-purin-6-amine), and Pu-H71 (8-(6-iodobenzo[d][1,3]dioxol-5-ylthio)-9-(3-(isopropylamino)propyl)-9H-purin-6-amine).

---

15 ERBB2 (HER2/NEU) is a HSP90 client protein.

16 Other coumarin antibiotics, such as clorobiocin and coumermycin A1, also target the HSP90 C-terminal domain. However, the poor affinity of these compounds for HSP90 in conjunction with their high affinity for Topoisomerase 2 has precluded their further development as clinically useful HSP90 inhibitors.

17 Due to similarities to the ATP binding sites between HSP90 and DNA Gyrase (an enzyme present in prokaryotes and some eukaryotes), novobiocin is also a DNA Gyrase inhibitor.

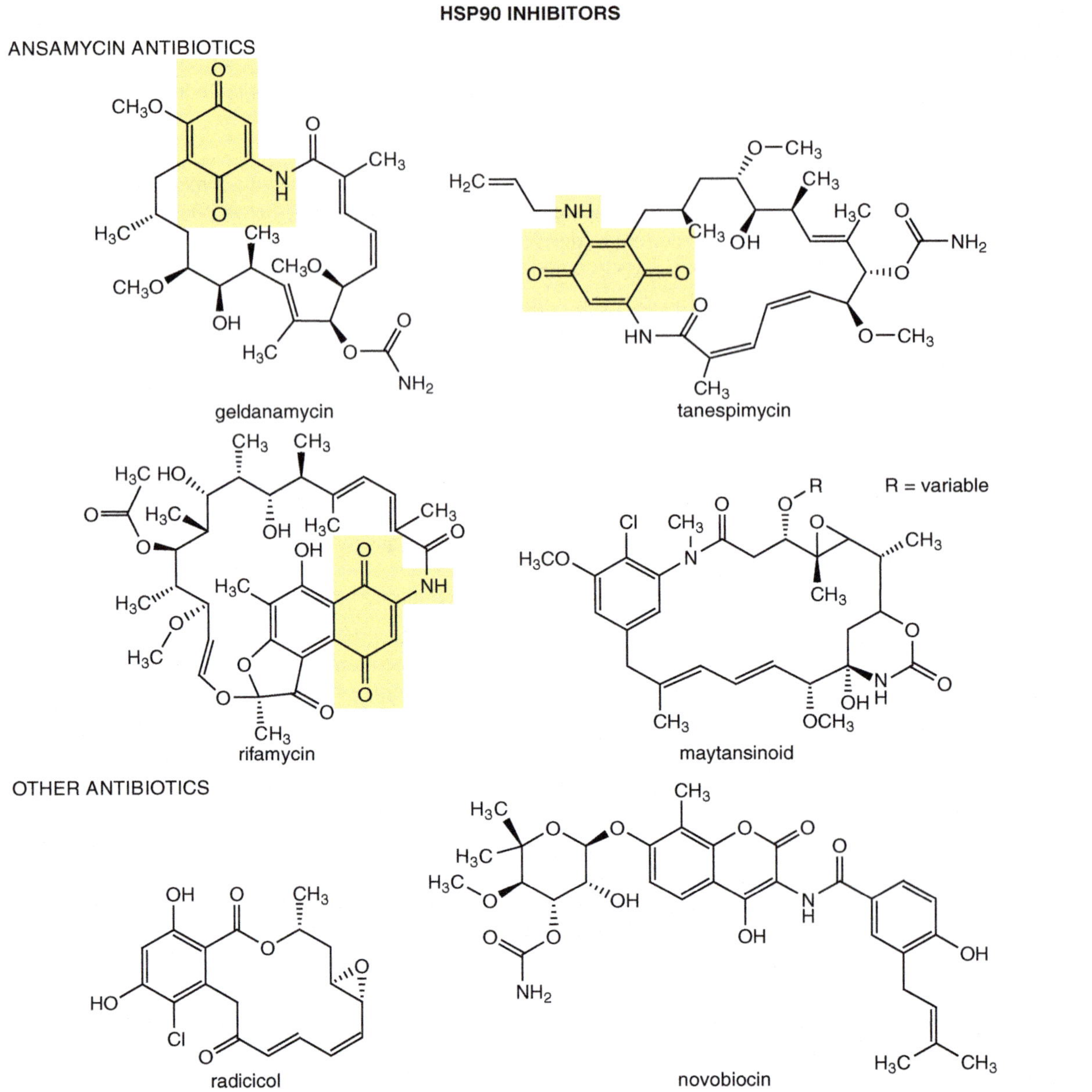

Fig. 4.26 Structures of HSP90 inhibitors. Sub-classes include ansamycin antibiotics, other antibiotics, PU class inhibitors, various inhibitors, and peptidomimetic inhibitors. The amioquinone domain in ansamycins is highlighted in *yellow* (not present in the ansamycin analog mytansinoid), as is the purine domain in the PU class inhibitors

- Pu-H71 exerts durable anti-cancer effects in triple negative breast cancers. It causes the down-regulation of various HSP90 client proteins, including components of the RAS-RAF-MAPK pathway, the PKB pathway, cell cycle regulators, and anti-apoptotic factors. Due to the critical role of HSP90 in the disease, small cell lung cancer is particularly susceptible to HSP90 inhibitors, including Pu-H71, Pu24FCi and Pu-H58.
- BIIB021 (CNF2024) is an orally active 2-amino-6-halopurine HSP90 inhibitor (Kasibhatla 2007) that depletes NF-κB. It may sensitize tumors to radio-therapy or immune surveillance. The cytotoxic activity of BIIB021 is also not influenced by loss of NQO1 or BCL-2 over-expression.

Pharmacokinetics The Pu class of compounds exhibits favorable pharmacological features, including negligible micro-environmental inactivation.

Drug Resistance Pu inhibitors are not subject to ABCB1 mediated export.

Treatment with AUY922 (5-(2,4-dihydroxy-5-isopropylphenyl)-N-ethyl-4-[4-(morpholinomethyl)phenyl]isoxazole-3-carboxamide) results in the binding of HSP90 to client proteins and setting them up as targets for degradation by the proteasome. AUY922 causes P23 dissociation from HSP90 and can then recruit HSP70 to the HSP90 complex. The agent reduces the expression of VEGFR-1, -2, -3, PDGFR-α,

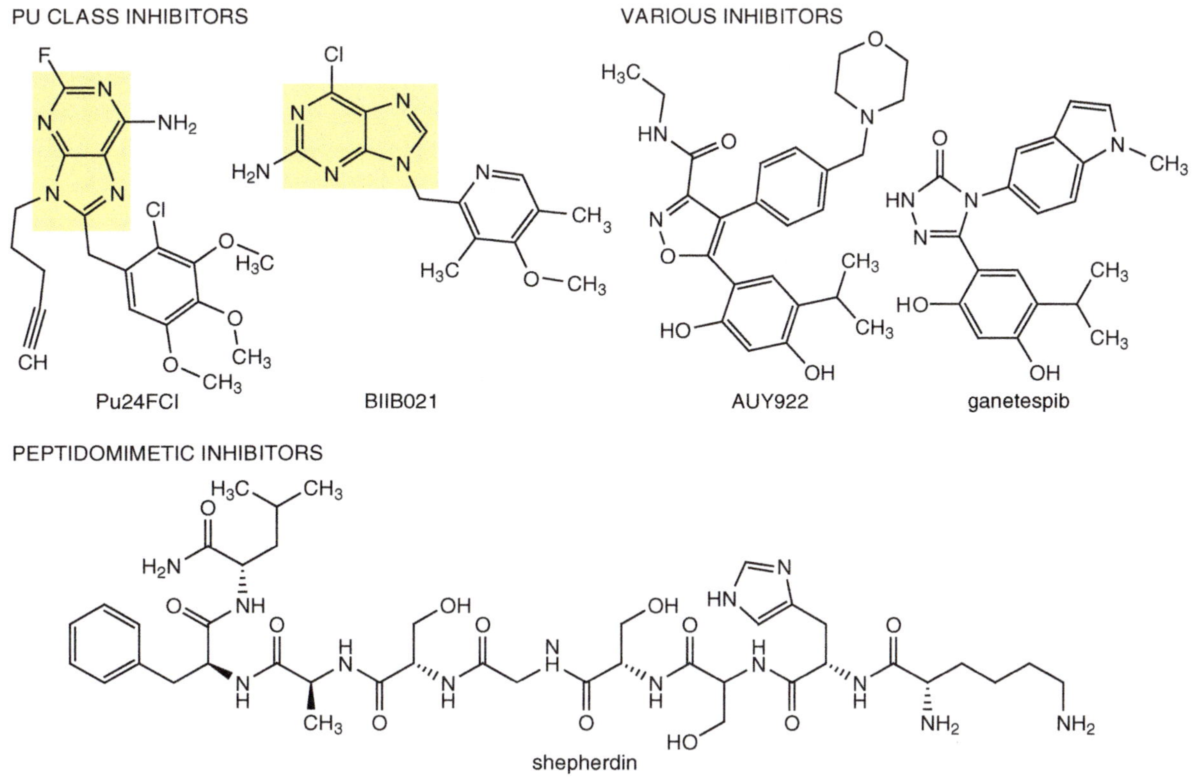

Fig. 4.26 (continued)

and PKB (AKT). AUY922 does not influence the expression of HSP90, but like other HSP90 inhibitors it leads to a compensatory increase in expression of HSP70. The agent is administered intravenously.

Ganetespib (STA-9090) is an intravenous HSP90 inhibitor that also inhibits multiple kinases with comparable potency. The drug suppresses c-KIT and EGFR, which as client proteins depend on functional HSP90 for maintenance. In chronic myelogenous leukemia (CML) caused by the chimeric oncoprotein BCR-ABL, the secondary mutation BCR-ABL^{T315I} is cross-resistant to several tyrosine kinase inhibitors, however, the transformed cells remain sensitive to HSP90 inhibition. Compensatory elevation of HSP72 levels occurs. Treatment with ganetespib has shown objective responses in clinical trials.

Adverse Effects The most common adverse event is diarrhea, which is manageable with standard supportive care. There is no evidence of the serious bone marrow toxicities and neuropathy that are associated with conventional chemotherapy, or of the severe liver and common ocular toxicities associated with other HSP90 inhibitors.

Shepherdin (L-lysyl-L-histidyl-L-seryl-L-serylglycyl-L-cysteinyl-L-alanyl-L-phenylalanyl-L-leucine) is a peptidomimetic drug. It was modeled on the binding interface between the molecular chaperone HSP90 and the anti-apoptotic and mitotic regulator Survivin. The agent makes extensive contacts with the ATP pocket of HSP90, destabilizes its client proteins (specifically Survivin), and induces death of tumor cells by apoptotic and non-apoptotic mechanisms. The fusion of its N-terminus to either helix III of the Antennapedia homeodomain protein or the human immunodeficiency virus TAT sequence has generated membrane permeant forms of Shepherdin. They accumulate in the mitochondria, bind to HSP90 and TRAP1, and rapidly trigger Cyclophilin D mediated mitochondrial pore transition and cell death, independently of P53 and BCl-2 expression levels.

Protein synthesis inhibitors do not target cancer specific mechanisms, but they reduce the levels of proteins that are over-abundant in cancers.
Protein turnover can be targeted with inhibitors of protein synthesis, proteasome inhibitors, or HSP90 inhibitors.
The proteasome is a clinically relevant target for the treatment of hematologic malignancies.
Only cancers that are driven by HSP90 client proteins are sensitive to HSP90 inhibitors.
The exposure to HSP inhibitors may lead to a compensatory up-regulation of HSP proteins.

4.2.3 Others

The Notch, Hedgehog, and WNT pathways may facilitate the expansion of the stem-like cancer initiating cells. This sub-population is often responsible for the aggressiveness of a tumor. It also tends to be highly treatment resistant against conventional chemotherapy. Somatostatin is an endocrine suppressor. It may exert growth inhibitory effects on some tumors.

Notch signaling The Notch signaling pathway importantly contributes to cell fate determination, cell survival, and cell proliferation. However, the outcome of Notch signaling is highly context dependent. The engagement by one of the Notch ligands, Delta Like-1 (DLL-1), Delta Like-3 (DLL-3), Delta Like-4 (DLL-4), Serrate/Jagged-1 (JAG-1), or Serrate/Jagged-2 (JAG-2), presented on adjacent cells, initiates a proteolytic cascade that leads to its cleavage and release of the Notch intracellular domain, which then translocates to the nucleus and functions as a transcriptional activator. This setting causes the gene expression of *hes-1* and may lead to the regulation of programmed cell death (Fig. 4.27).

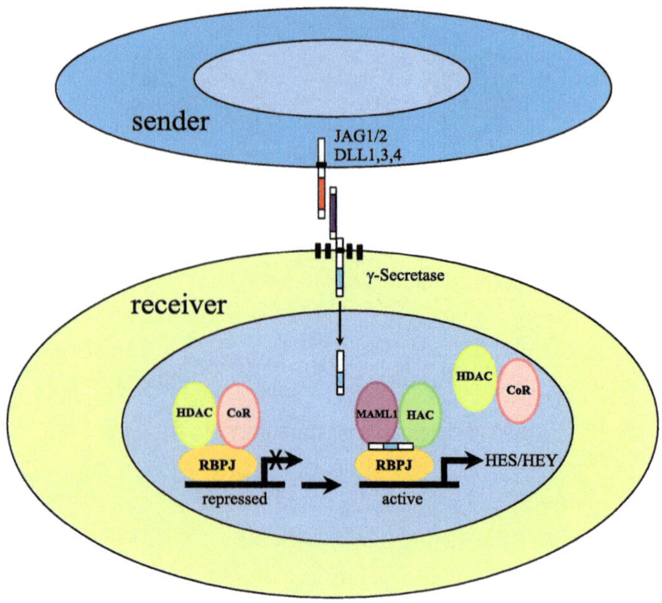

Fig. 4.27 Core components of the canonical Notch signaling pathway. Ligands of the Jagged (*JAG1* and *JAG2*) and Delta-Like (*DLL1*, *DLL3*, *DLL4*) families (*upper* cell, shown in *green*) interact with Notch family receptors (NOTCH1 through to NOTCH4) on an adjacent cell (*lower* cell, shown in *yellow*). The Notch receptor exists at the cell surface as a proteolytically cleaved hetero-dimer consisting of a large ectodomain and a membrane-tethered intracellular domain. The receptor-ligand interaction induces two additional proteolytic cleavages that free the Notch Intracellular Domain (*NICD*) from the cell membrane. The NICD translocates to the nucleus (*blue*), where it forms a complex with the *RBPJ* protein, displacing a Histone Deacetylase (*HDAc*) co-repressor (*CoR*) complex from the *RBPJ* protein. Components of an activation complex, such as *MAML1* and Histone Acetyl Transferases (*HAc*), are recruited to the NICD-RBPJ complex, leading to the transcriptional activation of Notch target genes. (Redrawn from Gridley 2007)

Ligand binding leads the release of NICD (Notch Intracellular Domain) from the endothelial cell plasma membrane by γ-Secretase dependent proteolytic cleavage of Notch. NICD translocates to the nucleus, where it binds to the transcription repressor CSL thus activating the transcription of target genes. Inhibitors of γ-Secretase can suppress Notch signaling.

MK0752 (Fig. 4.28) is a synthetic small molecule that inhibits the Notch signaling pathway by inhibiting γ-Secretase[18]. The agent may cause growth arrest and apoptosis in tumor cells, in which the Notch signaling pathway is over-activated. The drug can be administered orally.

Adverse Effects Dose limiting toxicities include grade 3 diarrhea or constipation, nausea, and abdominal cramping. Grade 2–3 fatigue may require dose reduction.

RO4929097 is a selective inhibitor of γ-Secretase. The drug suppresses Notch signaling. While it does not block tumor cell proliferation or induce apoptosis, it produces a less transformed, slower growing phenotype. The agent is in clinical studies for advanced cancer.

Hedgehog pathway Signaling by the Hedgehog family of secreted glycoproteins contributes to the determination of embryonic cell fate, the maintenance of somatic cell fate, the specification of organ size, and the patterning of skin, lung, brain, bone, and blood. Hedgehog (HH) signaling promotes the expression of G_1/S Cyclins, including Cyclins D and E, and results in the growth of cells. It also opposes epithelial cell cycle arrest through $P21^{CIP1/WAF1}$ (Fig. 4.29).

Vismodegib <Erivedge> inhibits the Hedgehog signaling pathway. The agent acts as a cyclopamine-competitive antagonist of the receptor SMO (Smoothened) which is part of the hedgehog signaling pathway. SMO inhibition causes the transcription factors GLI1 and GLI2 to remain inactive, which prevents the expression of oncogenes within the Hedgehog pathway. In 2012, vismodegib gained U.S. FDA approval. The drug is indicated for patients with basal cell carcinoma, which has spread, relapsed after surgery, or cannot be treated with surgery or radiation. Vismodegib is also undergoing clinical trials for basal cell naevus syndrome (Grolin syndrome), metastatic colorectal cancer, small cell lung cancer, advanced stomach cancer, pancreatic cancer, medulloblastoma and chondrosarcoma.

Adverse Effects Vismodegib has a high rate of adverse effects, including dysgeusia (loss of taste), gastrointestinal disorders (nausea and vomiting, diarrhea or constipation), hair loss, muscle cramps, and fatigue, which lead to frequent of non-compliance.

[18] The γ-Secretase complex is composed of four proteins, Presenilin, Nicastrin, APH-1, and PEN-2.

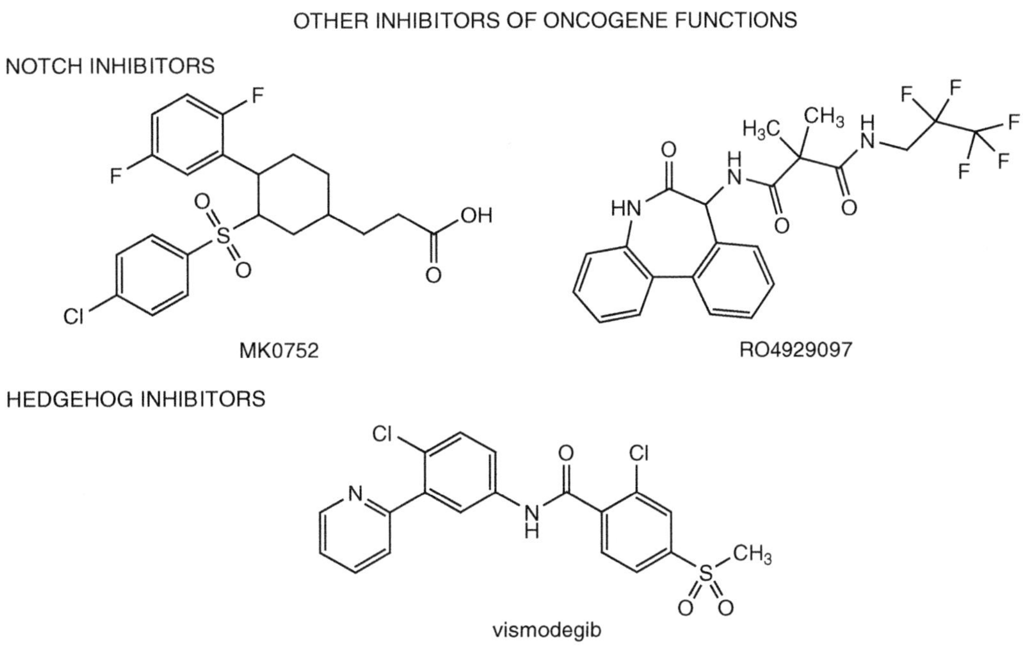

Fig. 4.28 Structures of various inhibitors of oncogene function

Somatostatin Somatostatin is an endogenous cyclic tetradecapeptide that inhibits the release of growth hormone and all gastrointestinal hormones. Somatostatin Receptors are expressed by some neuroendocrine and non-neuroendocrine tumor cells.

The mode of action of Somatostatin analogs is the suppression of hormone production, particularly Growth Hormone and serotonin. It helps to control the diarrhea and skin flushing associated with carcinoid syndrome[19]. Reducing these hormones also has anti-proliferative effects on some tumors, involving the hyper-phosphorylation of RB with resulting G_1 cell cycle arrest in addition to Somatostatin Receptor mediated apoptosis. Somatostatin analogs may enhance the therapeutic effects of hormonal intervention in patients with breast cancer, prostate cancer, or pancreatic cancer. However, only a small number of patients treated with Somatostatin analog therapy experience partial tumor regression.

Pharmacokinetics The clinical utility of native Somatostatin has been limited by its short half-life of 1–3 min. This has led to the development of Somatostatin analogs that are long-acting and more potent than native Somatostatin-14. The typical duration of treatment with Somatostatin analogs is approximately 12 months because of the development of tachyphylaxis (less frequent with long-acting formulations than short-acting formulations) or disease progression.

Octreotide pamoate (SMS 201–995) <Sandostatin> is a synthetic, long-acting octapeptide analog of Somatostatin. It binds to Somatostatin Receptors, thereby initiating apoptosis. Other possible anti-neoplastic activities of this agent include the suppression of the tumor growth promoting effects of IGF-1 (Insulin Like Growth Factor 1). The main indication is carcinoid syndrome. The drug is administered up to three times per day subcutaneously. The half-life is 40–60 min after intravenous administration and close to 2 h when given subcutaneously.

Adverse Effects The main adverse effects are loss of appetite, nausea, fatigue, bloating and stomach pain, diarrhea or steatorrhea, and soreness at the injection site. Over the course of months, gallstones may develop.

Drug Interactions Drugs that prolong the QT interval of the electrocardiogram or that slow down the heart (β–blockers, digoxin), certain blood pressure medicines (calcium channel blockers), and anti-arrhythmic drugs can cause dangerously slow heartbeats. Agents that lower the blood potassium or magnesium levels (such as diuretics) can worsen this effect. As somatostatin analogs affect the blood sugar levels, diabetic patients may need to reduce their medication or Insulin. Octreotide may lower the levels of cyclosporine and thus require an increase in cyclosporine dose.

Lanreotide <Somatuline LA> is a long acting (slow release) drug which is given as an intramuscular injection every 2 or 4 weeks. The effects of lanreotide on symptom relief are comparable to those of octreotide, with 75–80 % of carcinoid syndrome patients having decreased diarrhea

[19] Carcinoid syndrome may be caused by over-abundant endogenous secretion of serotonin and kallikrein. It manifests in flushing and diarrhea, as well as possibly heart failure and bronchoconstriction.

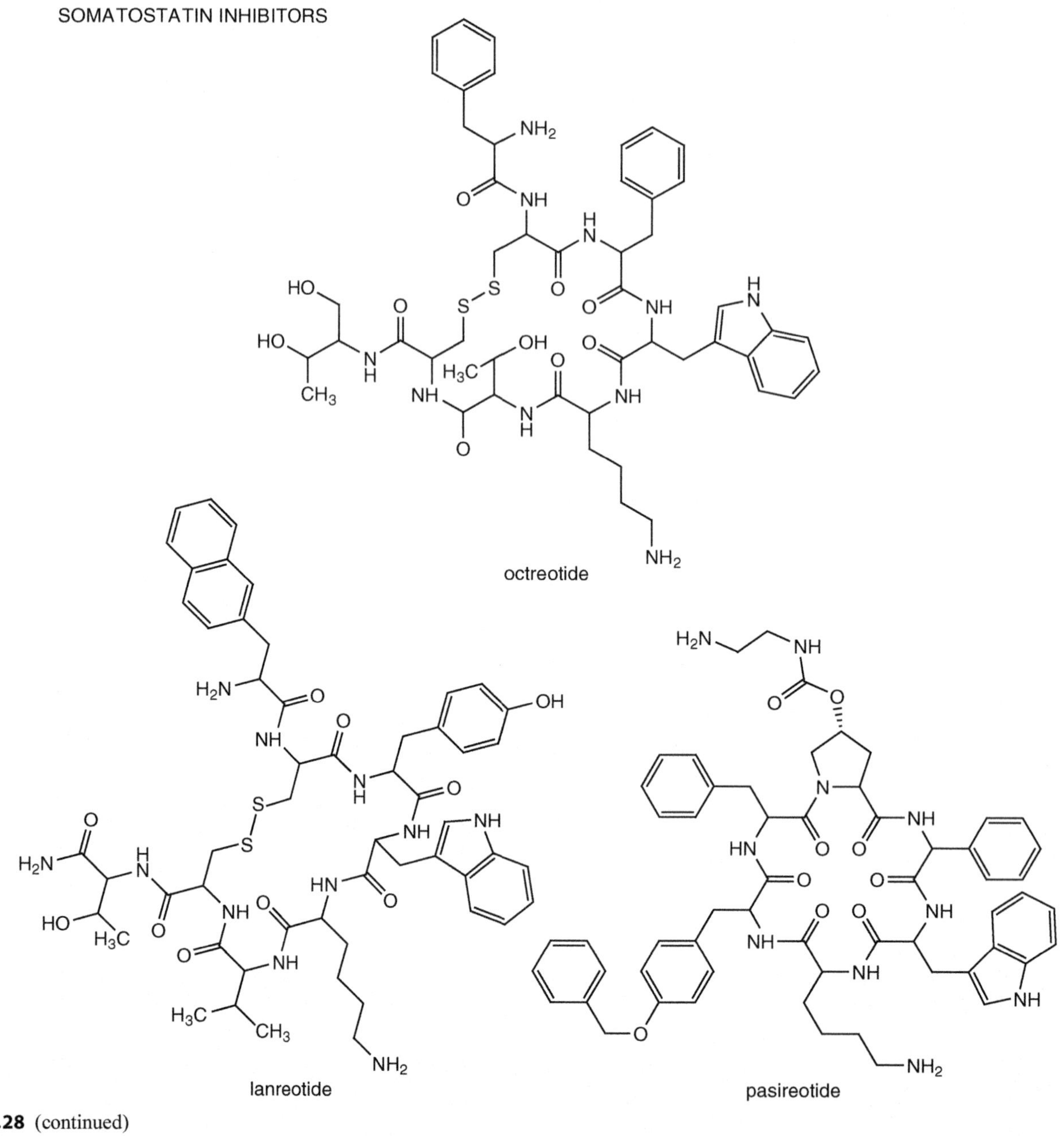

Fig. 4.28 (continued)

and flushing. However, there is little improvement in tumor responses over octreotide.

Pasireotide <Signifor> is injected subcutaneously 1–2 times per day. It is used to treat Cushing disease, a common syndrome associated with pituitary tumors. The drug is also under study to treat carcinoid tumors.

Vapreotide (octastatin) (RC-160) is an octapeptide analog of Somatostatin. It is under study for various palliative applications.

Adverse Effects Abscess formation at the infusion site, erythema, and discomfort have occurred in clinical studies.

Ligand and receptors that contribute to cell fate decisions may also facilitate the expansion of cancer stem cells. These pathways are suitable drug targets in cancer therapy.

4.3 Antibodies

The investigation of antibodies began in 1890, when Emil von Behring and Shibasaburo Kitasato described antibody activity against diphtheria and tetanus toxins. They put forward the theory of humoral immunity, proposing that a mediator in serum could react with a foreign antigen. In the 1920s, Michael Heidelberger and Oswald Avery observed that an-

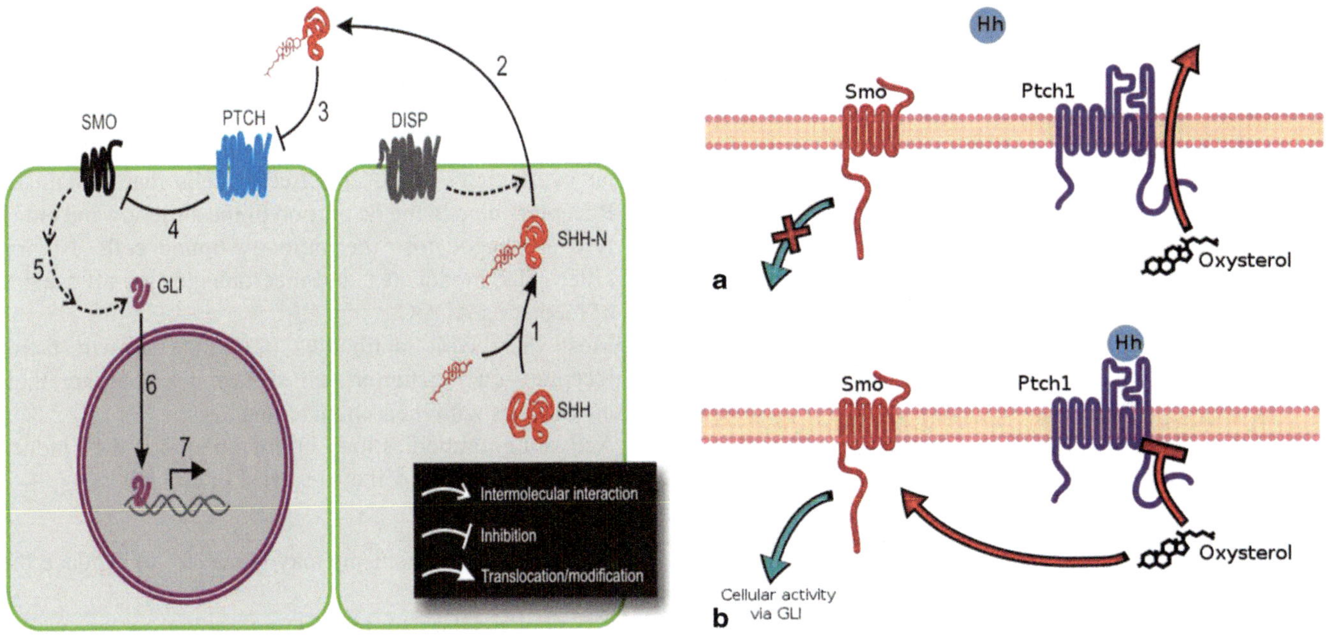

Fig. 4.29 The Hedghog signaling pathway. (*Left panel*) Overview of Sonic Hedgehog signaling. (*Right panel*) Pathway of Smoothened (*Smo*) regulation via Hedgehog (*Hh*) and Patched (*Ptch1*) When the protein Hedgehog is absent (*A*), the transmembrane Patched (*Ptch1*) removes oxysterols, thus preventing them from interacting with the transmembrane protein Smoothened (*Smo*). When Hedgehog is bound to Patched (*B*), *Ptch1* no longer removes oxysterols, allowing them to accumulate and activate *Smo*. (http://en.wikipedia.org/wiki/Hedgehog_signaling_pathway)

tibodies are proteins that can precipitate antigens. In 1948, Astrid Fagreaus discovered that plasma cells (differentiated B-lymphocytes) were responsible for generating antibodies. Consecutively in the 1950s and 1960s, many efforts to devise "magic bullets" for targeted cancer therapy were undertaken[20], but stalled due to technical limitations. In 1975, Köhler and Milstein develoepd hybridoma technology for the essentially unlimited generation of monoclonal antibodies. These agents quickly became valuable diagnostic tools (Yelton 1981). The specificity of binding also made antibodies attractive as potential therapeutics and reignited thoughts in the cancer research community about the potential of therapeutic antibodies being used to treat cancer, as illustrated by the 1984 publication of the book "Magic Bullets" (Fjermedal 1984). The development of antibodies as therapeutic agents, however, was hampered by the immune response of patients, which readily inactivated murine antibodies. A fast development of human anti-mouse antibody (HAMA) responses in the treated patients accounted for an accelerating clearance rate, resulting in ineffectiveness of the treatment after about 3 weeks[21]. HAMA responses could also be associated with symptoms that can range from mild (fever, chills, nausea, rash) to severe, life threatening anaphylaxis with cardiopulmonary collapse. Technical advances in antibody humanization were therefore required to gain safety and efficacy. To this end, the first chimeric antibodies were generated in the late 1980s (Liu 1987; Riechmann 1988), later followed by CDR grafting (Fig. 4.30). In 1997, the first therapeutic anticancer antibody, rituximab, was approved by the U.S. FDA for the treatment of B-cell non-Hodgkin lymphoma[22]. Since then, monoclonal antibody based therapies have become a major strategy in cancer treatment. The humanization of antibodies has allowed them to function as drug molecules. They are generally very well tolerated and lead to clinical results. However, none of them are able to cure cancer as single agents.

The fundamental structure of all antibodies is identical and consists of two heavy chains and two light chains joined by disulfide bonds. The constant region (Fc fragment) determines the effector function of the antibody. The Fab portion is composed of heavy (V_H) and light chains (V_L), which are

[20] The metaphoric term "magic bullets" to describe ideal therapeutic agents goes back to Paul Ehrlich, who reasoned that the selective targeting of a disease causing agent would provide a therapeutic with high efficacy and low toxicity.

[21] The immunologic memory generated in the HAMA response renders ensuing treatments with xenogeneic antibodies of the same species ineffective for the life of the patient.

[22] The first monoclonal antibody to be approved as a drug was muromonab (anti-CD3), which received U.S. FDA approval in 1986 as an immunosuppressant to reduce the acute rejection of organ transplants.

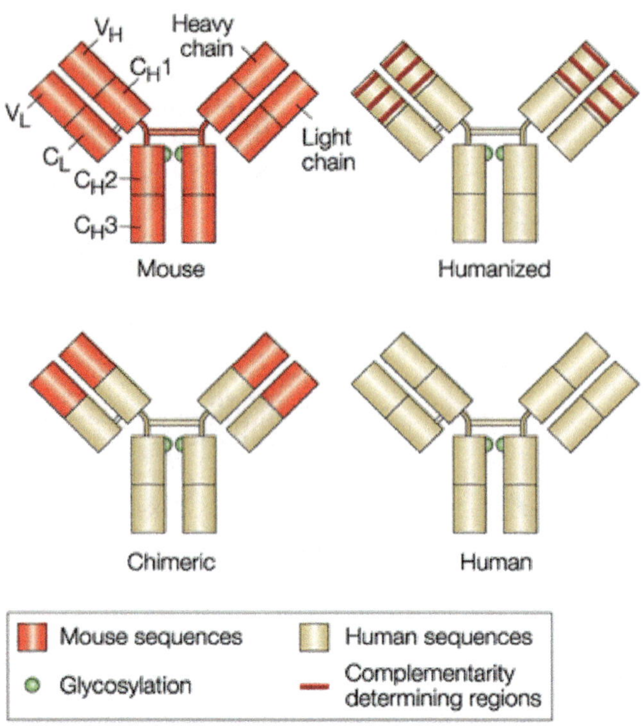

Fig. 4.30 Antibody humanization. Murine antibodies: Derived by hybridoma technology following immunization of mice or, less commonly, rats. Chimeric antibodies: Obtained by joining the antigen-binding variable domains of a mouse monoclonal antibody (*mAb*) to human constant domains: mouse *VL* to human *CL* and mouse *VH* to human *CH1–CH2–CH3* for *light* and *heavy* chains, respectively. Humanized antibodies: In the simplest case, these are created by grafting the antigen-binding loops, known as complementarity-determining regions (*CDRs*), from a mouse mAb into a human IgG. The generation of high-affinity humanized antibodies generally requires the transfer of one or more additional residues from the so-called framework regions (*FRs*) of the mouse parent mAb. Several variants of the humanization technology have been developed. Human antibodies: These have high affinity for their respective antigens and are routinely obtained from very large, single-chain variable fragments (*scFvs*) or Fab phage display libraries. Moreover, the difficulty in obtaining antibodies to self-antigens that are highly conserved between mouse and humans using hybridoma technology is readily overcome using phage display technology. High-affinity human antibodies have also been obtained from transgenic mice that contain some, or preferably many, human immunoglobulin genes and genetically disrupted endogenous immunoglobulin loci. Immunization elicits the production of human antibodies recoverable using standard hybridoma technology. A human anti-epidermal growth factor (*EGF*) receptor mAb obtained using transgenic mice eradicates large, established tumours in some preclinical xenograft models10, auguring well for ongoing oncology trials. (Carter 2001 with permission)

responsible for binding to antigens. Within the Fab fragment, the variable region of antibodies differs greatly and is composed of three complementarity determining regions (CDRs) on each arm. Most of the therapeutic antibodies used in oncology are of the IgG_1 sub-class, which is most effective at engaging Fcγ receptors on natural killer cells, macrophages, and neutrophils.

Antibodies can suppress tumor growth in various ways.

- Antibodies may induce anti-tumor immune responses by complement dependent cytotoxicity (CDC). It results when the Fc portion of the antibody activates the complement system leading to tumor cell lysis.
- Antibodies can stimulate antibody dependent cellular cytotoxicity (ADCC). Effector cells that contain Fc Receptors bind to the Fc portion of the antibody and either lyse or phagocytose the antibody bound cells. Natural killer cells, monocytes, and macrophages are all capable of mediating ADCC.
- Most therapeutic antibodies neutralize growth factor receptors on the tumor cell surface by blocking their interactions with their cognate ligands.
- Activating antibodies may be therapeutic if they induce signals that lead to cell cycle arrest or apoptosis.

Several of these mechanisms may synergize to produce the therapeutic effect.

The nomenclature of monoclonal antibodies assigns generic (non-proprietary) names to therapeutic monoclonal antibodies. The World Health Organization's International Nonproprietary Names defines this scheme. In general, suffixes are used to identify classes of medicines; all monoclonal antibody pharmaceuticals end with the suffix -mab. It is preceded by an infix that denotes the animal origin of the antibodies. The infix preceding the source of the antibodies refers their targets. Most of these consist of a consonant, vowel, then another consonant. For ease of pronunciation, the final consonant is dropped if the following infix begins with a consonant. The prefix carries no special meaning and should be unique for each antibody. A second word may be added if there is another substance attached or linked to the antibody (Table 4.13).

Pharmacokinetics Antibodies are protein drugs of about 150 kD molecular mass. They cannot be given orally and are administered by injection. The half-life of antibody drugs is comparatively long. This is in part due to the minor role played by drug-metabolizing enzymes in the liver. Antibodies are internalized in cells of the monocyte-phagocyte system (MPS, reticuloendothelial system, RES), either directly or by phagocytosis after binding to their target cells. This is followed by catabolism via proteolysis. Antibody half-life and degradation are also regulated by binding to the neonatal receptor FcRn, mostly on cells of the monocyte-phagocyte system. This binding initially protects from clearance. After dissociation, the IgG is taken up into endosomes and degraded.

Adverse Effects To avoid anaphylactic reactions, most antibodies require pre-medication with anti-histamines and acetaminophen (e.g. 25–50 mg diphenhydramine, 650 mg acetaminophen orally). Recommended infusion rates are usually lower for the initial dose, with incremental increases as tolerated by individual patients. Chills during the infu-

Table 4.13 Stems for monoclonal antibody nomenclature. (Adapted from Wikipedia)

Prefix	Target substem			Source substem		Stem
	Old	New	Meaning		Meaning	
Variable	*-anibi-*	–	Angiogenesis (inhibitor)	*-a-*	Rat	*-mab*
	-ba(c)-	*-b(a)-*	Bacterium	*-e-*	Hamster	
	-ci(r)-	*-c(i)-*	Circulatory system	*-i-*	Primate	
	-fung-	*-f(u)-*	Fungus	*-o-*	Mouse	
	-ki(n)-	*-k(i)-*	Interleukin	*-u-*	Human	
	-les-	–	Inflammatory lesions	*-xi-*	Chimeric (human/foreign)	
	-li(m)-	*-l(i)-*	Immune system	*-zu-*	Humanized	
	-mul-	–	Musculoskeletal system	*-xizu-*	Chimeric/humanized hybrid rat/mouse hybrid (including *trifunctional antibody*)	
	-ne(u)(r)-	*-n(e)-*	Nervous system	*-axo-*		
	-os-	*-s(o)-*	Bone			
	-toxa-	*-tox(a)-*	Toxin			
	-co(l)-		Colonic tumor			
	-go(t)-		Testicular tumor			
	-go(v)-		Ovarian tumor			
	-ma(r)-	*-t(u)-*	Mammary tumor			
	-me(l)-		melanoma			
	-pr(o)-		prostate tumor			
	-tu(m)-		miscellaneous tumor			
	-vi(r)-	*-v(i)-*	virus			

sion may require medication (e.g. 25 mg intravenous meperidine). For patients experiencing symptoms of serious infusion related reactions, the administration needs be interrupted and prompt treatment with corticosteroids and other supportive measures needs to be initiated. Pulmonary toxicity may occur as part of the infusion related reaction or as a distinct entity. Additionally, the toxicities of monoclonal antibodies are determined by the selectivity of their target antigens.

Antibodies may suppress cancer by inducing complement mediated cytotoxicity, antibody dependent cytotoxicity, inhibition of oncogenic signaling, or activation of cell cycle arrest or apoptosis.
Administration is by infusion.
As foreign proteins, antibodies may induce anaphylactic infusion reactions. The risk is highest at the first infusion and can be reduced by pre-treatment.

4.3.1 EGFR Family Targets

The growth factor EGF (Epidermal Growth Factor) is a 53 amino acid polypeptide, constrained by 3 internal disulfide bonds. It stimulates many epithelial and mesenchymal cells. EGF binds to a transmembrane receptor, which then becomes internalized and activated as a tyrosine kinase. The EGF Receptor was first cloned as a surface molecule related to a viral oncogene in 1984. The four related genes *erbB1* (*egfr*), *erbB2* (*her-2/neu*), *erbB3* (*her-3*), and *erbB4* (*her-4*) encode the family of EGF Receptor tyrosine kinases. They are composed of a cysteine rich extracellular domain, a single transmembrane domain, and an intracellular catalytic domain. ERBB2 (HER-2/NEU, $P185^{HER2}$) transduces signals through Phospholipase C, phosphatidylinositol 1,4,5-trisphosphate, and diacylglycerol. Ensuing effects are the cellular influx of calcium ions from the exterior and the up-regulation of the anti-apoptotic proteins BCL-X_L and BCL-2. ERBB2 is over-expressed by various adenocarcinomata including breast adenocarcinoma.

anti-ERBB2 HER-2/NEU (ERBB2) is a member of the EGF Receptor family that is amplified in about 30 % of breast cancers. Trastuzumab (anti-HER-2/NEU monoclonal antibody) <Herceptin> is a recombinant humanized monoclonal antibody directed to the extracellular domain IV of ERBB2. The drug was jointly developed by Axel Ullrich at Genentech and Dennis Slamon at the Jonsson Cancer Center at UCLA by humanizing a mouse monoclonal antibody (antibody 4D5, previously defined in 1990). Trastuzumab received U.S. FDA approval in 1998. Since 2006, the antibody has been made available through a public benefits scheme for Australian women with early stage breast cancer. As a molecularly targeted treatment, trastuzumab benefits patients whose cancer cells over-express ERBB2. Routine ERBB2 status analysis is performed on tissue biopsies by immunohistochemistry to stratify patients. Multiple mechanisms may contribute to the therapeutic effects of this antibody:

- After binding to its cognate receptor on the tumor cell surface, trastuzumab induces antibody dependent cell mediated cytotoxicity against tumor cells that over-express ERBB2.
- Cells treated with trastuzumab undergo arrest during the G_1 phase of the cell cycle. Trastuzumab induces a down-regulation of ERBB2, leading to the disruption of receptor dimerization and signaling through the downstream PI-3 Kinase cascade.
- A contribution to the unregulated growth of breast cancer cells may be the proteolytic cleavage of ERBB2 that releases the extracellular domain and results in constitutive activation of the tyrosine kinase domain with consecutive unrestricted cell cycle progression. Trastuzumab inhibits ERBB2 ectodomain cleavage by blocking the protease site on domain IV.

Based on sensitization theory, the co-administration of trastuzumab and ERBB ICD (a peptide fragment of the C-terminal and the intracellular domain of ERBB2) may result in the potentiation of an ERBB specific cytotoxic T-lymphocyte response in breast cancer patients via MHC class I antigen presentation.

- Ado-trastuzumab emtansine (T-DM1) <Kadcyla> is an antibody-drug conjugate consisting of trastuzumab linked to the cytotoxic agent mertansine (DM1). The linker is designed not to be cleaved by lysosomal proteases. The drug is administered by injection for intravenous use, as a single agent. It is indicated for the treatment of patients with ERBB2-positive, metastatic breast cancer, who previously received trastuzumab and a taxane, separately or in combination.

Pharmacokinetics Although trastuzumab treatment is the standard of care for ERBB2-positive breast cancer, it shows only a 15 % response rate as a mono-therapy and a 50 % response rate in combination with paclitaxel. The antibody is administered either once a week or once every 3 weeks intravenously over 30–90 min.

Adverse Effects ERBB2 is an important developmental growth factor receptor, which is vital to normal cardiac development and myocardial trabeculation. One of the substantial complications associated with trastuzumab is cardiac dysfunction in about 5 % of cases. Approximately 10 % of patients are unable to tolerate this drug because of pre-existing heart problems. The risk of cardiomyopathy is increased when trastuzumab is combined with anthracycline chemotherapy, which itself has cardiac toxicity (myocardial ERBB2 may be unregulated early in response to anthracycline injury, rendering the myocardium particularly vulnerable to trastuzumab exposure).

Drug Resistance A problem of therapy with trastuzumab is the rapid development of resistance in virtually all patients. It is based on

- truncation of the receptor that leads to reduced antibody binding but retains active signaling,
- activation of downstream signaling via PTEN inactivation or increased Protein Kinase B activity, or
- compensation due to alternative signaling; one potential underlying mechanism is the lack of $P27^{KIP1}$ translocation into the nucleus, which enables CDK2 to sustain cell proliferation.

Pertuzumab (2C4) <Perjeta> is a humanized monoclonal IgG_1 antibody designed to target ERBB2 at the extracellular domain II. It blocks the formation of ERBB2 hetero-dimers with other members of the ERBB family and thus reduces signaling through the multiple pathways associated with ERBB2 activation (Agus 2005). Because it inhibits ERBB2/ERBB3 hetero-dimer formation, pertuzumab may be useful in suppressing ERBB3 over-expressing tumors, some of which include ovarian, breast, prostate, colon, and lung cancers. The agent is given in combination with trastuzumab (which binds a different domain of the receptor) and docetaxel. It received U.S. FDA approval in 2012.

Adverse Effects Common adverse effects in combination therapy (with trastuzumab and docetaxel) comprise diarrhea, alopecia, neutropenia, nausea, fatigue, and rash. Grade 3–4 adverse reactions may include neutropenia, leukopenia, anemia, diarrhea, or peripheral neuropathy. Other adverse reactions to pertuzumab can include left ventricular dysfunction, infusion reactions, and hypersensitivity. The antibody may be associated with embryo-fetal toxicity and birth defects.

anti-ERBB1 Cetuximab <Erbitux> is a chimeric monoclonal antibody, composed of the Fv regions of a murine anti-EGFR antibody (m225) with human IgG_1 heavy and κlight chain constant regions and has an approximate molecular weight of 152 kD. It is specific for ERBB1 (Epidermal Growth Factor Receptor, EGFR, HER1), a receptor tyrosine kinase that triggers cell division. Cetuximab inhibits EGF Receptor dependent signal transduction and leads to the inhibition of tumor growth by cancers that over-express EGF Receptors. The agent can mediate antibody dependent cellular cytotoxicity (ADCC) against certain tumor types. Cetuximab was approved by the U.S. FDA in 2004 for the second-line treatment of metastatic colorectal cancer with over-expression of ERBB1. Treatment with cetuximab is given intravenously,

- in combination with irinotecan <Camptosar> for patients whose tumor growth has progressed after receiving chemotherapy with irinotecan
- as a single agent for patients who are unable to tolerate chemotherapy with irinotecan.

Cetuximab, in combination with radiation therapy, is indicated for the treatment of locally or regionally advanced squamous cell carcinoma of the head and neck. It may also be indicated as mono-therapy for the treatment of patients with recurrent or metastatic squamous cell carcinoma of the head and neck, for whom prior platinum based therapy has failed.

Pharmacokinetics Cetuximab is formulated in a preservative-free salt solution for injection. The half-life is approximately 110 h. In patients with colorectal cancer, female patients have a 25 % lower intrinsic clearance of cetuximab than male patients. However, the gender difference in clearance does not necessitate any alteration of dosing because of comparable safety profiles.

Adverse Effects Severe allergic reactions, with symptoms including difficulty breathing, rash, itching, low blood pressure, and loss of consciousness occur in about 3 % of patients treated. On rare occasions, these reactions can result in death. Severe cases require that treatment with cetuximab be stopped immediately and not started again. Additional adverse effects include serious lung disease (1 %), fever (5 %), infection, kidney failure, and pulmonary embolism. Heart attacks or sudden death occur in 2 % of patients with head and neck cancer treated with radiation therapy and cetuximab.

Panitumumab (ABX-EGF) <Vectibix> is a fully human monoclonal IgG_2 antibody that engages the ligand-binding region of ERBB1 (EGFR, HER1) on transformed and untransformed cells. Panitumumab[23] may inhibit autocrine EGF stimulation of tumor cells that express the EGF Receptor, thereby suppressing tumor cell proliferation. The agent received U.S. FDA approval in 2006 for the treatment of ERBB1 expressing metastatic colorectal cancer with disease progression despite prior treatment.

Pharmacokinetics Following a single dose 1-h infusion of panitumumab, the area under the concentration-time curve increases in a greater than dose proportional manner, and clearance of panitumumab decreases as the dose is increased. Following the recommended dose regimen (6 mg/kg once every 2 weeks as a 1-h infusion), panitumumab concentrations reach steady state levels by the thrid infusion. The elimination half-life is approximately 7.5 days.

Adverse Effects Dermatologic toxicities (acneiform dermatitis, pruritus, erythema, rash, exfoliation, paronychia, dry skin, skin fissures) occur in 90 % of patients and reach grade 3 or higher in 10 % of patients. Pulmonary fibrosis or pulmonary embolism may become serious. Other common adverse events comprise hypomagnesemia, paronychia, fatigue, abdominal pain, nausea, vomiting, and diarrhea (possibly resulting in dehydration). Ocular toxicities (conjunctivitis, ocular hyperemia, increased lacrimation, eyelid irritation) affect 15 % of patients. Severe infusion reactions arise in approximately 1 %. The drug is Pregnancy Category C.

Panitumumab is not indicated for use in combination with chemotherapy. In clinical studies, the addition of panitumumab to the combination of bevacizumab and chemotherapy resulted in decreased overall survival and increased incidence of grade 3–5 adverse reactions.

Drug Resistance There is no treatment benefit in patients whose tumors have K-RAS mutations in codon 12 or 13.

Nimotuzumab <BIOMAb EGFR, TheraCIM, Theraloc, CIMAher> is a humanized monoclonal antibody that binds to and inhibits ERBB1, resulting in growth inhibition of tumor cells that over-express this receptor. In addition, this antibody may act synergistically with radiation therapy. Nimotuzumab is in testing for the treatment of non-small cell lung cancers, refractory colorectal tumors, squamous cell carcinomata of the head and neck, recurrent or refractory high grade malignant gliomata, and for intrinsic diffuse pontine glioma (an inoperable, treatment-resistant malignant brain cancer in children). Nimotuzumab is approved in India, China, Argentina, Columbia, and Cuba.

Adverse Effects Most adverse reactions are mild to moderate and are considered infusion reactions, including chills, fever, nausea and vomiting, dizziness and hypotension, dryness of the mouth, asthenia, flushing.

Hypomagnesemia and debilitating skin rashes, which may be caused by other anti-ERBB1 antibodies, do not arise in patients treated with nimotuzumab.

Zalutumumab <HuMax-EGFr> is a fully human IgG_1 that binds to the ERBB1 extracellular domain III. This locks the receptor in an inactive conformation. The antibody is designed for the treatment of squamous cell carcinoma of the head and neck, as over 90 % of head and neck cancers over-express ERBB1.

Matuzumab (EMD 72000) is a humanized monoclonal antibody that binds ERBB1 with high affinity. It competitively blocks the binding of endogenous ligands and suppresses receptor mediated downstream signaling. This results in an impairment of tumor cell proliferation. Due to a lack of efficacy of the antibody in clinical trials its further development is on hold.

Ligand binding to the ERBB1 and ERBB3 receptors leads to their activation, dimerization, and downstream cell signaling. When these receptors are dysregulated in cancer, overactive signaling may lead to tumor cell survival and proliferation. The monoclonal anti-ERBB1/ERBB3 antibody MEHD7945A is a human IgG_1 with dual binding specificity. It inhibits ligand binding to both receptors. Each antigen-binding arm of the dual-action antibody engages a unique

[23] The agent was produced by immunization of transgenic mice (xenomice) that are able to generate human immunoglobulin heavy and light chains. A specific clone of B-lymphocytes secreting an antibody to ERBB1 was selected and immortalized.

epitope target. Simultaneously binding two receptors may inhibit the activity of multiple cancer signaling pathways. MEHD7945A is designed to block downstream signaling by inhibiting ligand binding and thus preventing the activation of all major ERBB pathways.

ERBB1 inhibition is efficacious in cancer therapy, but initially sensitive tumors often develop resistance, in some cases through compensatory ERBB3 signaling. In cancer cells resistant to the ERBB1 inhibitors cetuximab and erlotinib, MEHD7945A (but not single-target EGFR inhibitors) can suppress tumor growth and cell cycle progression due to ERBB1/ERBB3 signaling pathway modulation. MEHD7945A is more effective than a combination of cetuximab and anti-ERBB3. The agent may also limit the cross-resistance to radiation by cells resistant to EGFR inhibitors via modulating cell cycle progression and repair processes that control apoptotic cell death.

anti-ERBB3 MM-121 is a human monoclonal antibody that targets ERBB3 (HER3). It was the first selective ERBB3 antagonist to have entered clinical development. MM-121 prevents the phosphorylation of ERBB3 and its downstream targets.

Antibody inhibition of ERBB is suitable in cancers where the ligand or receptor is over-expressed.
Among the adverse effects are skin rashes and heart problems because of the important roles for ERBB molecules in these organs.

4.3.2 Lymphocytic Surface Targets

anti-CD20 In some forms of non-Hodgkin lymphoma, B-lymphocytes expressing the surface molecule CD20 expand excessively. Rituximab <Rituxan, Mabthera> is a recombinant chimeric murine/human antibody that selectively targets CD20. Following binding, this agent triggers a host cytotoxic immune response against CD20 bearing cells. Rituximab is indicated

- for the treatment of patients with relapsed or refractory, low grade or follicular, CD20-positive, B-cell non-Hodgkin lymphoma
- for the first-line treatment of diffuse large B-cell, CD20-positive, non-Hodgkin lymphoma in combination with CHOP (cyclophosphamide, doxorubicin, vincristine, prednisone) or other anthracycline-based chemotherapy regimens
- for the first-line treatment of follicular, CD20-positive, B-cell non-Hodgkin lymphoma in combination with CVP (cyclophosphamide, vincristine, prednisolone) chemotherapy
- for the treatment of low grade, CD20-positive, B-cell non-Hodgkin lymphoma in patients with stable disease or who achieve a partial or complete response following first-line treatment with CVP chemotherapy.

Rituximab is administered intravenously. Approved by the U.S. FDA in 1997, rituximab was the first therapeutic antibody marketed for treating cancer in the U.S. In 1998, rituximab was approved in the European Union (the antibody is sold by Genentech, one of the first biotechnology companies, founded in 1976).

Adverse Effects Serious adverse effects associated with the use of rituximab include

- potentially fatal allergic and infusion reactions: Deaths within 24 h of rituximab infusion follow an infusion reaction complex, which includes hypoxia, pulmonary infiltrates, acute respiratory distress syndrome, myocardial infarction, ventricular fibrillation, or cardiogenic shock. Approximately 80 % of fatal infusion reactions occur in association with the first infusion. Prior to the rituximab infusion, patients should receive diphenhydramine and acetaminophen as premedications. Discontinuation of infusion is required in patients who develop severe infusion reactions
- tumor lysis syndrome: Acute renal failure requiring dialysis with instances of fatal outcome may arise following treatment with rituximab
- mucocutaneous reactions: Rituximab may cause skin reactions, in rare cases with fatal outcome. Toxic epidermal necrolysis is a severe manifestation
- progressive multifocal leukoencephalopathy: Patients treated with rituximab may experience JC virus activation[24], resulting in progressive multifocal leukoencephalopathy and death
- in some patients treated with rituximab, reactivation of the hepatitis B virus (HBV) may occur. Carriers of hepatitis B should be closely monitored during therapy.

Drug Resistance Patient populations likely to respond to rituximab have the drug target, CD20, expressed on the transformed cells. In addition, specific polymorphisms can predict the response rate. Antibody dependent cytotoxicity is associated with the FcγRIIIA (CD16) genotype, determined by a SNP at residue 158 (either phenylalanine, F, or a valine, V). Patients with the 158VV genotype show higher affinity for human IgG_1 and better clinical responses to rituximab than 158F carriers. Similarly, FcγRIIA (CD32) residue 131

[24] The JC virus is a polyomavirus that resides in latent form in up to 80 % of healthy adults. It usually remains latent, typically only causing disease in immunocompromised patients.

affects the rituximab response rate, which is higher in histidine/histidine carriers (131HH) than in arginine carriers (131R). C1q is a complement neutralizing molecule that functions in the clearance of apoptotic bodies. Polymorphisms in C1q also affect the response rate to rituximab.

Ofatumumab (HuMax-CD20) <Arzerra> is a human IgG_1 antibody directed to CD20. It binds in proximity to the membrane to the small and large loops of CD20, which may allow for effective complement deposition and subsequent B-cell killing. Ofatumumab is indicated for chronic lymphocytic leukemia that is refractory to fludarabine and alemtuzumab. It is also under study for follicular non-Hodgkin lymphoma, diffuse large B-cell lymphoma, and refractory chronic lymphocytic leukemia.

Ofatumumab is administered in 12 doses, with dose 1 of 300 mg, followed 1 week later by 2000 mg weekly for 7 doses (doses 2–8), followed 4 weeks later by 2000 mg every 4 weeks for 4 doses (doses 9–12).

Pharmacokinetics Ofatumumab is subject to dose dependent clearance. The antibody is eliminated through a target independent route and a B-lymphocyte mediated route. Due to the depletion of B-cells, the clearance decreases substantially after subsequent infusions compared to the first infusion. Renal impairment does not have a clinically important effect on ofatumumab pharmacokinetics.

Adverse Effects Serious adverse reactions may include infusion reactions (the risk can be reduced by premedication with acetaminophen, an anti-histamine, and a corticosteroid), cytopenias (prolonged severe neutropenia and thrombocytopenia), progressive multifocal leukoencephalopathy, Hepatitis B reactivation (possibly fulminant and fatal), and intestinal obstruction. The most common adverse reactions are neutropenia, anemia, fatigue, pyrexia, rash, diarrhea, nausea, cough, dyspnea, pneumonia, bronchitis, and upper respiratory tract infections. The drug is Pregnancy Category C.

Tositumomab <Bexxar> is a murine IgG_2 monoclonal antibody directed to the cell membrane antigen CD20 on the surface of B-lymphocytes. Upon receptor binding, the antibody induces apoptosis, and it may stimulate anti-tumor cell mediated or antibody dependent cytotoxicity. Tositumomab is administered as a radio-immunotherapeutic, conjugated to ^{131}iodine (see Sect. 13.2.). It is a drug for the treatment of follicular lymphoma.

Adverse Effects The most serious adverse reactions are prolonged cytopenias, the sequelae of cytopenias which included infections (sepsis) and hemorrhage in thrombocytopenic patients, allergic reactions (bronchospasm and angioedema), secondary leukemia, and myelodysplasia.

Drug Interactions Drugs or supplements that interfere with blood clotting (vitamin E, non-steroidal anti-inflammatory drugs, warfarin, ticlopidine, clopidogrel) can raise the risk of bleeding during treatment with tositumomab.

Ibritumomab tiuxetan <Zevalin> is a monoclonal antibody radio-immunotherapy treatment for some forms of B-cell non-Hodgkin lymphoma. The drug combines a mouse monoclonal $IgG_1\kappa$ that recognizes CD20 with the chelator tiuxetan, to which a radioactive isotope (either ^{90}yttrium or ^{111}indium) is added (see Sect. 13.2.). Tiuxetan is a modified version of diethylene triamine pentaacetic acid (DTPA), the carbon backbone of which contains an isothiocyanatobenzyl and a methyl group.

Others Epratuzumab (AMG 412) <LymphoCide> is a recombinant, humanized monoclonal antibody (LL2) directed to CD22, a cell surface glycoprotein present on mature B-lymphocytes and on many types of malignant B-cells. After binding to CD22, the predominant anti-tumor activity of epratuzumab may be mediated through antibody dependent cellular cytotoxicity, but not by complement dependent cytotoxicity. The drug may be radio-conjugated (see Sect. 13.2.). It is under study for follicular lymphoma and acute lymphoblastic leukemia (ALL).

Pharmacokinetics The half-life of the drug increases over repeated infusions and may reach 25 days.

Adverse Effects Epratuzumab is well tolerated when infused over 30 min. Headache, nausea, dizziness, and upper respiratory tract infections are the most common adverse events.

CD33 is a cell surface receptor, the expression of which is restricted to cells of the myelomonocytic lineage, mostly to progenitor cells. CD33 is a member of the SIGLEC (Sialic Acid Binding Immunoglobulin-Like Lectin) family of receptors, which contains cytoplasmic immune receptor based tyrosine signaling motifs typical of inhibitory receptors of the immune system. Engagement of the receptor by specific antibodies results in a dose dependent induction of apoptotic cell death. Because of its almost universal presence on over 90% of acute myeloid leukemia (AML) blast cells and lack of expression in most non-hematopoietic tissues, antibodies to CD33 have been developed to treat patients with acute myeloid leukemia.

Lintuzumab (HuM195, SGN-33) <Zamyl> is a humanized recombinant monoclonal IgG_1 antibody directed to CD33. Lintuzumab stimulates antibody dependent cell mediated cytotoxicity against tumor cells that express the antigen. This results in a decrease in tumor burden. The U.S. FDA and the European EMA had granted lintuzumab orphan drug status for the treatment of acute myeloid leukemia and myelodysplastic syndromes. However, while this agent was safe in clinical studies, its efficacy is low and it was pulled from further development.

Brentuximab vendotin (SGN-35, cAC10-vcMMAE) <Adcetris> consists of the chimeric monoclonal antibody brentuximab, which targets CD30, connected via a protease cleavable linker to 3–5 units of the anti-mitotic (microtubule disrupting) agent monomethyl auristatin E (MMAE). Approved by the U.S. FDA in 2011, the agent is used for Hodgkin lymphoma and anaplastic large cell lymphoma. The antibody is a second line of defense after failure of autologous stem cell transplant or of two prior multi-agent chemotherapy regimens. The recommended dose is 1.8 mg/kg administered as an intravenous infusion over 30 min every 3 weeks, continued over a maximum of 16 cycles, or until disease progression or unacceptable toxicity occurs.

Pharmacokinetics Brentuximab vendotin exposure is increased in patients with hepatic impairment or severe renal impairment.

Adverse Effects Adverse effects include peripheral neuropathy, neutropenia, upper respiratory tract infection, fatigue, nausea, and diarrhea. Brentuximab vendotin is associated with progressive multifocal leukoencephalopathy due to JC virus reactivation. The drug is Pregnancy Category D.

CD2 (Sheep Red Blood Cell Receptor) is a specific receptor on T-lymphocytes and natural killer cells. It is expressed by most peripheral T-cell lymphomata, cutaneous T-cell tumors, and T-cell prolymphocytic leukemia. Further, CD2 is also expressed by the malignant cells of large granular lymphocytic leukemia, extranodal T/NK cell lymphoma, nasal type and blastic or aggressive NK cell leukemia.

Siplizumab (MEDI-507) is a monoclonal IgG_1 κ antibody that binds to CD2 and causes the depletion of T-lymphocytes. Receptor engagement by the antibody triggers a host immune response that results in cell lysis, selective suppression of the immune system, and control of activated T-cell growth.

Pharmacokinetics Siplizumab pharmacokinetics follows a 1-compartment model with linear FcRn mediated[25] and non-linear target mediated clearance.

Adverse Effects The antibody is safe and well tolerated in patients with $CD2^+$ T-cell lymphomata and leukemias. The most common adverse effects comprise lymphopenia, chills, headaches, pyrexia, and infusion reactions.

CD52 is a differentiation antigen typically expressed at high levels on thymocytes, lymphocytes, monocytes, and macrophages. The molecule is also present on the epithelial cells lining the male reproductive tract; it is shed into seminal plasma and acquired by spermatozoa. CD52 is expressed at variable levels on the majority of lymphoid malignancies.

Alemtuzumab <Campath, Campath-1H, MabCampath> is a humanized IgG_1 to CD52 that can activate complement and antibody dependent cell mediated cytotoxicity. It is used as a second-line therapy to treat B-cell chronic lymphocytic leukemia. The agent was approved by the U.S. FDA in 2001. Alemtuzumab is administered by dose escalation over 3–7 days. Once the recommended dose is achieved, the treatment is given 3 times a week for 4–12 weeks.

Adverse Effects Adverse effects comprise infusion related events. They include syncope, pulmonary infiltrates, adult respiratory distress syndrome (ARDS), respiratory arrest, cardiac arrhythmias, myocardial infarction, and cardiac arrest. A complication of therapy with alemtuzumab is that it increases the risk for opportunistic infections, in particular the reactivation of cytomegalovirus (CMV). Active vaccinations should be avoided during treatment with the antibody.

Alemtuzumab is contraindicated for patients with active systemic infections, underlying immunodeficiency, or known type I hypersensitivity or anaphylactic reactions to Campath or to any of its components.

Lymphocytic surface molecules are highly accessible targets for lymphoma and leukemia treatment.
Antibodies that recognize lymphocytic surface receptors may cause the depletion of white blood cells.

4.3.3 Various Targets

Antibodies to HGF and MET Hepatocyte Growth Factor (HGF, Scatter Factor, SF) and its receptor MET are involved in the initiation, progression, and metastasis of lung cancer, colorectal cancer, renal cancer, and glioma. Blockage of the HGF-MET interaction with an anti-HGF monoclonal antibody has therapeutic potential through abrogation of the excessive growth signal. As there is interdependence between the HGF/MET pathway and the ERBB1 (EGFR) pathway in colorectal and lung cancers, anti-HGF antibody may be beneficial if used in combination with blockers of EGFR. Similarly, combination with SHH blockers in medulloblastoma may enhance therapeutic efficacy. However, targeting the HGF/MET pathway may not be effective if downstream signaling is activated by a K-RAS mutation.

DN-30 is a monoclonal anti-MET antibody that recognizes the extracellular portion of the receptor. It induces the proteolytic cleavage of the MET extracellular region (receptor shedding), thus decreasing the number of cell surface receptors and generating a decoy effect for HGF binding. DN30 also induces cleavage of the intracellular domain, which is successively degraded by the proteasome. However, DN-30 binding to MET also results in a partial activation of the kinase due to antibody-mediated receptor homo-dimer-

[25] The neonatal Fc receptor (FcRn) plays a critical role in regulating IgG homeostasis.

ization. To dissociate shedding activity from agonistic activity, the use of a DN-30 Fab fragment has been suggested. The antibody inhibits tumor growth and prevents metastasis.

OA-5D5 is a one-armed monovalent anti-MET Fab antibody fragment that prevents HGF binding. OA-5D5, composed of murine variable domains for the heavy and light chains with human IgG_1 constant domains, is produced as a recombinant protein in Escherichia coli. The agent is in clinical development. It has an intracerebral tumor suppressive effect when given topically.

Rilotumumab (AMG102) is a fully humanized monoclonal antibody (IgG_2) that binds to and neutralizes HGF, preventing its binding to the receptor c-MET. The inhibition of c-MET mediated signal transduction may result in the induction of apoptosis. Rilotumumab is in clinical trials for the treatment of glioblastoma, renal cell carcinoma, and metastatic colorectal cancer.

The antibody L2G7 is a neutralizing anti-HGF antibody that may have efficacy against lung cancer. It crosses the blood-brain barrier, potentially causing intracranial tumor regression.

Antibodies to IGF-1R Insulin, Insulin Like Growth Factors -1 and -2, and Relaxin stimulate DNA synthesis and cell growth. Insulin Like Growth Factors are expressed in two types, IGF-1 (Somatomedin C) and IGF-2 (Somatomedin A, Multiplication-Stimulating Factor, MSF). They are bound to carrier proteins and are maintained at relatively steady blood levels. While IGF-2 is a primary growth factor required for early development, IGF-1 expression mostly occurs in later life. The biological actions of the Insulin Like Growth Factors are predominantly exerted through the type 1 Insulin Like Growth Factor Receptor (IGF-1R), which binds IGF-1 and IGF-2 with high affinity. Activation of the hetero-tetrameric tyrosine kinase receptor IGF-1R occurs following IGF-1 binding to the receptor σ ubunit ⟨, and leads to auto-phosphorylation of the subunit β IGF-1R is linked to the RAS→RAF→MAPK and PI 3-K→PKB signal transduction cascades, which are involved in mitogenesis and cell survival. The IGF-1 Receptor displays potent mitogenic, anti-apoptotic, and transforming activities, which may be a prerequisite for oncogenesis. IGF-1R is expressed on many tumor cells, where it may contribute to proliferation and progression.

Several anti-IGF-1R antibodies have not succeeded in clinical trials.

Figitumumab (CP-751,871) is a human monoclonal antibody directed to IGF-1R. Figitumumab selectively binds to IGF-1R, thus preventing IGF-1 from engaging the receptor and inducing receptor auto-phosphorylation. Inhibition of IGF-1R auto-phosphorylation can result in a reduction of the anti-apoptotic effect of IGF and cause an inhibition of tumor growth. The antibody is under investigation for the treatment of adrenocortical carcinoma and non-small cell lung cancer. Responses may be achieved with combination therapy of figitumumab plus paclitaxel and carboplatin.

Adverse Effects The most common adverse events are hyperglycemia, fatigue, neutropenia, and neuropathy.

Ganitumab (AMG479) blocks IGF-1R and consecutively inhibits the PI3K→AKT signaling pathway downstream of the receptor. It is under study in pancreatic cancer.

The monoclonal antibody cixutumumab (IMC-A12) is a fully human IgG_1 monoclonal antibody directed to IGF-1R. It prevents the binding of the natural ligand IGF-1 and the subsequent activation of PI 3-K→PKB signaling pathway. The effects may result in the induction of cancer cell apoptosis and may decrease cancer cell proliferation. cixutumumab has not progressed to phase III clinical trials.

R1507 is a human monoclonal antibody that blocks the action of IGF-1R. Its development was abandoned.

Others Apolizumab <Remitogen> is a humanized monoclonal antibody directed to 1D10, a polymorphic determinant on the HLA-DR β chain that is expressed on normal and neoplastic B-lymphocytes. Apolizumab induces complement mediated cytotoxicity, antibody dependent cell mediated cytotoxicity, and apoptosis of 1D10 expressing B-lymphocytes. It is under investigation for treating low grade or follicular B-cell non-Hodgkin lymphomata and chronic lymphocytic leukemia (CLL).

The ganglioside GD2 is over-expressed in malignant melanoma, neuroblastoma, osteosarcoma, and small cell carcinoma of the lung. 14G2A is a murine monoclonal antibody directed to GD2. Binding of this antibody to its cognate antigen induces antibody dependent cell mediated cytotoxicity and complement dependent cytotoxicity against GD2 expressing tumor cells.

Pharmacokinetics The peak serum levels and elimination are dose dependent. The decay from the plasma is biphasic with the longer half-life plateauing at doses of 250 mg/m^2. There likely exists a saturable mechanism for antibody elimination.

The human/mouse chimeric antibody ch14.18 recognizes GD2. It triggers tumor cell lysis via antibody dependent cellular cytotoxicity and complement dependent cytotoxicity. In clinical trials against melanoma, neuroblastoma, and osteosarcoma ch14.18 has displayed an acceptable safety profile.

The effects may be enhanced by administering the antibody in combination with systemic cytokines (GM-CSF or IL-2).

For most patients with advanced ovarian cancer, the front-line treatments, surgery and chemotherapy, do not suffice to control the high recurrence rate. CA125 is a Mucin-like glycoprotein that is expressed on the surface of more than 95 % of all non-mucinous stage III/IV epithelial ovarian cancers, which serves as a clinical marker.

Oregovomab (MAb B43.13) <OvaRex> is a murine monoclonal antibody (B43.13) that attaches to the tumor associated carbohydrate antigen CA125. Vaccination with this antibody may stimulate a host cytotoxic immune response against tumor cells that express CA125. Patients who mount a T-cell response to CA125 show significantly improved survival compared to patients who do not.

MUC-1 is a heavily glycosylated transmembrane glycoprotein that is over-expressed in many carcinomata. MUC-1 consists of 3 domains, a large extracellular motif, a transmembrane motif, and a cytoplasmic tail. The molecule mediates signal transduction events that stimulate the motility, invasion, and metastasis of cancer cells. In cancer patients, humoral and cellular responses to MUC-1 may arise, implicating MUC-1 as a potential target for immunotherapy.

A murine monoclonal antibody to Human Milk Fat Globule 1 (muHMFG1) recognizes an epitope localized in the extracellular MUC-1 domain. A humanized variant of muHMFG1, AS1402, is in clinical trials. It could represent a potential treatment agent for patients with ovarian cancer, possibly as a radiotherapeutic after labeling with ^{90}yttrium.

Phosphatidylserine is a highly immunosuppressive molecule that is usually located inside cells. It becomes exposed on the outer membrane of cells that line tumor blood vessels, creating a specific target for treatment.

Treatment of B-cell Lymphocytic Leukemia

1. **B-cell acute lymphocytic leukemia**

The standard treatment of acute lymphocytic leukemia (ALL) is generally divided into three phases,

- induction chemotherapy for the rapid restoration of bone marrow function
- central nervous system prophylaxis or treatment
- post-remission therapies to eliminate minimal residual disease.

Acute lymphoblastic leukemia in pediatric patients and young adolescents is highly responsive to conventional chemotherapy. In older patients, clinical remission is more difficult to obtain and early relapse is more common. Corticosteroid therapy, in combination with other anti-leukemic drugs or in cyclic combinations including methotrexate, has produced rapid and effective responses. When used for induction, methotrexate in doses of 3.3 mg/m^2 in combination with 60 mg/m^2 of prednisone, given daily, produces remissions in 50 % of patients treated, usually within a period of 4–6 weeks. When remission is achieved and supportive care has produced general clinical improvement, maintenance therapy is considered essential. Methotrexate is administered two times weekly either by mouth or intramuscularly in total weekly doses of 30 mg/m^2. It can also be given in doses of 2.5 mg/kg intravenously every 14 days. Alternatively, the usual daily maintenance dose of 6-mercaptopurine is 1.5–2.5 mg/kg/day as a single dose. It may also be combined with methotrexate. If or when relapse does occur, the re-induction of remission can usually be obtained by repeating the initial induction regimen.

Daunorubicin hydrochloride <Cerubidine> for infusion is indicated in combination chemotherapy for remission induction in acute lymphocytic leukemia in children and adults.

- A representative regimen in pediatric patients comprises daunorubicin 25 mg/m^2 (1 mg/kg in children less than 2 years of age) by infusion on day 1 every week, vincristine 1.5 mg/m^2 intravenously on day 1 every week, oral prednisone 40 mg/m^2 daily. If after 4 weeks remission is incomplete one or two additional courses may be given.
- In adult patients the dose schedule may combine daunorubicin 45 mg/m^2/day by infusion on days 1, 2, and 3 with intravenous vincristine 2 mg on days 1, 8, and 15 and oral prednisone 40 mg/m^2/day on days 1 through 22, then tapered between days 22 to 29, and intravenous L-Asparaginase 500 IU/kg/day for 10 days on days 22–32.

Cyclophosphamide <Cytoxan, Neosar> shows activity against acute leukemias. It may be combined with other agents (in CALGB 8811 with daunorubicin, vincristine, prednisone, and Pegaspargase). However, cyclophosphamide treatment may induce secondary leukemais.

Hyper-CVAD chemotherapy consists of two courses of drug combinations administered in an alternating fashion. The acronym stands for hyper-fractionated CVAD (cyclophosphamide, vincristine, doxorubicin <Adriamycin>, and dexamethasone). Compared to conventional protocols, it is given in smaller doses and more frequently, to minimize the adverse effects. The protocol was originally developed to treat leukemia in young patients with good overall health, due to its intensity, but has since been used more widely.

- Course A comprises intravenous cyclophosphamide <Cytoxan> (at 300 mg/m^2 every 12 h over 3 h on days 1, 2, and 3), vincristine <Oncovin>(at 2 mg on days 4 and 11), doxorubicin <Rubex>(50 mg/m^2 on day 4), dexamethasone <Decadron> (40 mg/day on days 1–4 and 11–14; it may be given orally), intrathecal cytarabine <Cytosar> (70 mg on day 7), methotrexate (12 mg on day 2), and infusion of mesna <Uromitexan> (to reduce the incidence of hemorrhagic cystitis associated with cyclophosphamide).
- Course B entails intravenous methotrexate (1000 mg/m^2 over 24 h on day 1), cytarabine (3000 mg/m^2 over 2 h every 12 h on days 2 and 3), leucovorin (25 mg/m^2, six doses over 6 h each, 24 h after starting methotrexate), oral sodium bicarbonate (600 mg starting a day before methotrexate, continued over 4 days).

The dosages are individualized, based on body weight, body surface area, and the overall health of the patient. Each course is given up to four times, over up to eight cycles that are 2–3 weeks apart. While the aim is to administer the largest number of cycles in the shortest time period possible, adjustments may be required based on patient recovery.

Post-remission therapy for adult acute lymphocytic leukemia includes intensive short-term chemotherapy followed allogeneic bone marrow transplant. The transplant of matched, unrelated bone marrow results in a lower incidence of leukemic relapse, when compared to syngeneic or autologous bone marrow transplant. This may be caused by an immunologic graft-versus-leukemia effect. Yet, the improvement in disease-free survival is partially offset by the treatment-induced morbidity and mortality from graft-versus-host disease, veno-occlusive disease of the liver, and interstitial pneumonitis. Therefore, allogeneic bone marrow transplantation is reserved for patients in second remission or beyond. As an alternative, hematopoietic stem cell transplant may be considered.

2. **B-cell chronic lymphocytic leukemia**
Chronic lymphocytic leukemia (CLL) is the most common type of leukemia in North America and Europe. It mainly affects the elderly, and has a highly variable course, with survival ranging from months to decades. Most patients with chronic lymphocytic leukemia are identified through blood tests performed for unrelated reasons rather than because of symptoms of the disease. Approximately 1/3 of patients never require treatment. Standard management of most patients has therefore traditionally involved a period of observation to assess disease progression. For those patients with chronic lymphocytic leukemia who are treated, therapy is generally palliative. Need-to-treat criteria include hematopoietic insufficiency, B-symptoms[26], rapidly progressive disease, or risk of complications from bulky lymphadenopathy. Regimens based on DNA alkylating agents, such as chlorambucil and cyclophosphamide, have been used for more than 30 years. In the 1980s, purine analogs (such as fludarabine) achieved more complete remissions than alkylator-based regimens. Since then, considerable efforts have focused on developing combination therapy protocols that are built on fludarabine. In a third phase of development, combination protocols have included targeted monoclonal antibodies. Throughout, the identification of agents with activity against resistant or treatment-refractory chronic lymphocytic leukemia has remained a high priority (Keating 2008).

Drug Resistance Expression of the efflux transporter ABCC1 (MRP1) occurs on the transformed cells in chronic lymphocytic leukemia. It may contribute to anti-cancer drug resistance.

Conventional chemotherapy With the possible exception of stem cell transplants, there is no curative treatment currently available but standard chemotherapy regimens can prolong survival. Induction chemotherapy may be started with an alkylating agent. Continuous or intermittent treatment with chlorambucil or cyclophosphamide reduces total lymphocyte mass and may prevent bone marrow failure until the disease becomes refractory. Chlorambucil can be given as first-line, single-agent treatment. Cyclophosphamide is often part of the COP (cyclophosphamide, vincristine <Oncovin>, prednisolone) or CHOP (cyclophosphamide, hydroxy-daunorubicin, vincristine <Oncovin>, prednisolone) regimens.

Fludarabine phosphate, a purine analog, is a mainstay in the treatment of patients with chronic lymphocytic leukemia. It was developed by John Montgomery. In

[26] B-symptoms refer to fever (greater than 38°C), night sweats, and weight loss (more than 10% of normal body weight over 6 months or less). Their presence or absence has prognostic significance for leukemias or lymphomata.

1989, the drug was found to be very effective in patients resistant to alkylating agents, and it was able to achieve complete remissions, leading to its approval for refractory chronic lymphocytic leukemia (Keating 1989). Combinations of purines and alkylators have been demonstrated to be superior to single agents, and combinations of rituximab with fludarabine or fludarabine and cyclophosphamide have led to a dramatic improvement in complete responses and progression-free survival.

Flavopiridol (alvocidib) (HMR 1275, L86-8275), a flavonoid derived from an indigenous plant from India, specifically inhibits Cyclin Dependent Kinases (CDKs 1, 2, 4, 7, and 9) with resulting blocks in cell cycle progression at the G_1/S and G_2/M boundaries. It generates responses in about one half of patients with advanced chronic lymphocytic leukemia. The drug effects are limited by binding to plasma proteins, leaving an ineffective level of free drug in circulation. This needs to be accounted for with a suitable dosing schedule.

Antibody therapy The monoclonal antibody alemtuzumab <Campath> binds to the cell surface molecule CD52. It was initially approved against chronic lymphocytic leukemia for the treatment of fludarabine-refractory patients, where there was no other available option. Alemtuzumab has demonstrated a higher response rate and longer progression-free survival than chlorambucil. It is now approved by the U.S. FDA as a single agent for first-line therapy.

Rituximab <Rituxan>, the first therapeutic antibody approved for cancer treatment, is a chimeric anti-CD20 antibody with efficacy against chronic lymphocytic leukemia, both as a single agent and in combination with traditional chemotherapies. In relapsed chronic lymphocytic leukemia, higher doses or more dose-intensive strategies can yield positive results.

There are a variety of combination regimens of rituximab with chemotherapy. FCR combines fludarabine, cyclophosphamide, and rituximab every 28 days in conjunction with infectious disease prophylaxis.

- Cycle 1 entails on day 1 intravenous rituximab 375 mg/m^2 at 50 mg/h (adjusted every 30 min by 50 mg/h until the goal of 400 mg/h is reached), on days 1–3 intravenous cyclophosphamide at 250 mg/m^2 over 10–30 min plus fludarabine at 25 mg/m^2 over 20–30 min.
- Cycles 2–6 comprise intravenous rituximab 500 mg/m^2 at 50 mg/h (adjusted every 30 min by 50 mg/h until the goal of 400 mg/h is reached), on days 1–3 intravenous cyclophosphamide at 250 mg/m^2 over 10–30 min plus fludarabine 25 mg/m^2 over 20–30 min.

Treatment of hairy cell leukemia Hairy cell leukemia is treated with the purine analog deoxycoformycin (pentostatin) <Nipent>, Interferon-α, and cladribine (2-chlorodeoxyadenosine, 2-CDA) <Leukostatin, Litak, Movectro>.

- Interferon-α improves the blood counts in about 80% of patients treated, however, only 10% of patients enter complete remission and relapse if the treatment is discontinued.
- Deoxycoformycin is indicated for patients who are refractory to Interferon-α treatment. Although it is an inhibitor of the enzyme ADA, deoxycoformycin has proved to be exceptionally active in hairy cell leukemia, a B-cell neoplasm with low intracellular concentrations of ADA.
- Cladribine is an adenosine analog. Because the agent is resistant to Adenosine Deaminase (ADA), an enzyme that inactivates some anti-neoplastic agents, it is selectively toxic to lymphocytes and monocytes, which exhibit little Deoxynucleotide Deaminase activity. Cladribine is mostly used for the treatment of hairy cell leukemia. The drug is administered by injection or infusion. The recommended dose and schedule for active hairy cell leukemia is as a single course given by continuous infusion for 7 consecutive days at 0.09 mg/kg/day.

35–40% of patients on standard therapy relapse. Second line therapy may be implemented with LMB-2, an immunotoxin that targets CD25.

Bavituximab <Peregrine> is a monoclonal antibody to phosphatidylserine. It binds to various aminophospholipids in a manner that is dependent on its interaction with the plasma protein β_2-Glycoprotein I. Bavituximab induces the immune cell mediated destruction of cells with exposed phosphatidylserine and may reactivate the immune response to cancer by blocking phosphatidylserine induced immunosuppression. Binding of bavituximab to the phosphatidylserines in the cell membrane helps mobilize the immune system to attack tumor associated blood vessels. Additionally, as chemotherapy increases the exposure of phosphatidylserine on tumor blood vessels, bavituximab combined with conventional chemotherapy, specifically carboplatin and paclitaxel, may hold potential for synergistic therapeutic effects. The antibody is in clinical trials to treat cancers of the lungs, liver, breast, and pancreas.

Farletuzumab is a humanized monoclonal antibody with high affinity for Folate Receptor α. This receptor, while almost absent from normal tissue, is over-expressed in most ovarian cancers. Farletuzumab mediates antibody dependent cellular cytotoxicity and complement dependent cytotoxicity. The antibody has shown clinical efficacy in early phase trials as single agent and combination therapy with minimal drug specific toxicity. It displays a safe toxicology profile.

4.3.4 Antibody Mimetics

Antibody mimetics are organic compounds that, like antibodies, can specifically bind antigens, but are structurally not related to antibodies. They are usually synthetic peptides or proteins with a molecular mass of about 3–20 kD. Nucleic acids and small molecules may sometimes act as antibody mimetics as well.

References

Abbruzzese JL (2008) Adjuvant therapy for surgically resected pancreatic adenocarcinoma. J Am Med Assoc 299:1066–1067

Agus DB, Gordon MS, Taylor C, Natale RB, Karlan B, Mendelson DS, Press MF, Allison DE, Sliwkowski MX, Lieberman G, Kelsey SM, Fyfe G (2005) Phase I clinical study of pertuzumab, a novel HER dimerization inhibitor, in patients with advanced cancer. J Clin Oncol 23:2534–2543

Appels N, Beijnen JH, Schellens JHM (2005) Development of farnesyl transferase inhibitors: a review. Oncologist 10:565–578

Ashar HR, James L, Gray K, Carr D, Black S, Armstrong L, Bishop WR, Kirschmeier P (2000) Farnesyl transferase inhibitors block the farnesylation of CENP-E and CENP-F and alter the association of CENP-E with the microtubules. J Biol Chem 275:30451–30457

Ashwell S, Zabludoff S (2008) DNA damage detection and repair pathways-recent advances with inhibitors of checkpoint kinases in cancer therapy. Clin Cancer Res 14:4032–4037

Barbacci EG, Pustilnik LR, Rossi AM, Emerson E, Miller PE, Boscoe BP, Cox ED, Iwata KK, Jani JP, Provoncha K, Kath JC, Liu Z, Moyer JD (2003) The biological and biochemical effects of CP-654577, a selective erbB2 kinase inhibitor, on human breast cancer cells. Cancer Res 63:4450–4459

Beatty GL, Chiorean EG, Fishman MP, Saboury B, Teitelbaum UR, Sun W, Huhn RD, Song W, Li D, Sharp LL, Torigian DA, O'Dwyer PJ, Vonderheide RH (2011) CD40 agonists alter tumor stroma and show efficacy against pancreatic carcinoma in mice and humans. Science 331:1612–1616

Bos JL (1989) ras oncogenes in human cancer: a review. Cancer Res 49:4682–4689

Carter P (2001) Improving the efficacy of antibody-based cancer therapies. Nat Rev Cancer 1:118–129

DeAngelo DJ, Stone RM, Heaney ML, Nimer SD, Paquette RL, Klisovic RB, Caligiuri MA, Cooper MR, Lecerf JM, Karol MD, Sheng S, Holford N, Curtin PT, Druker BJ, Heinrich MC (2006) Phase 1 clinical results with tandutinib (MLN518), a novel FLT3 antagonist, in patients with acute myelogenous leukemia or high-risk myelodysplastic syndrome: safety, pharmacokinetics, and pharmacodynamics. Blood 108:3674–3681

Druker BJ, Lydon NB (2000) Lessons learned from the development of an abl tyrosine kinase inhibitor for chronic myelogenous leukemia. J Clin Investig 105:3–7

el-Kamar FG, Grossbard ML, Kozuch PS (2003) Metastatic pancreatic cancer: emerging strategies in chemotherapy and palliative care. Oncologist 8:18–34

Engelman JA (2009) Targeting PI3K signalling in cancer: opportunities, challenges and limitations. Nat Rev Cancer 9:550–562

Escudier B, Eisen T, Stadler WM, Szczylik C, Oudard S, Siebels M, Negrier S, Chevreau C, Solska E, Desai AA, Rolland F, Demkow T, Hutson TE, Gore M, Freeman S, Schwartz B, Shan M, Simantov R, Bukowski RM, TARGET Study Group (2007) Sorafenib in advanced clear-cell renal-cell carcinoma. N Engl J Med 356:125–134

Fjermedal G (1984) Magic bullets. Macmillan, New York

Frost MJ, Ferrao PT, Hughes TP, Ashman LK (2002) Juxtamembrane mutant V560GKit is more sensitive to Imatinib (STI571) compared with wild-type c-kit whereas the kinase domain mutant D816VKit is resistant. Mol Cancer Ther 1:1115–1124

Garner RC, Goris I, Laenen AA, Vanhoutte E, Meuldermans W, Gregory S, Garner JV, Leong D, Whattam M, Calam A, Snel CA (2002) Evaluation of accelerator mass spectrometry in a human mass balance and pharmacokinetic study-experience with 14C-labeled (R)-6-[amino(4-chlorophenyl) (1-methyl-1H-imidazol-5-yl)methyl]-4-(3-chlorophenyl)-1-methyl-2(1H)-quino-linone (R115777), a farnesyl. Drug Metab Dispos 30:823–830

Gontarewicz A, Balabanov S, Keller G, Colombo R, Graziano A, Pesenti E, Benten D, Bokemeyer C, Fiedler W, Moll J, Brümmendorf TH (2008) Simultaneous targeting of aurora kinases and Bcr-Abl kinase by the small molecule inhibitor PHA-739358 is effective against imatinib-resistant BCR-ABL mutations including T315I. Blood 111:4355–4364

Gridley T (2007) Notch signaling in vascular development and physiology. Development 134:2709–2718

Hauf S, Cole RW, LaTerra S, Zimmer C, Schnapp G, Walter R, Heckel A, van Meel J, Rieder CL, Peters JM (2003) The small molecule Hesperadin reveals a role for Aurora B in correcting kinetochore-microtubule attachment and in maintaining the spindle assembly checkpoint. J Cell Biol 28:281–294

Heinrich MC, Griffith DJ, Druker BJ, Wait CL, Ott KA, Zigler AJ (2000) Inhibition of c-kit receptor tyrosine kinase activity by STI 571, a selective tyrosine kinase inhibitor. Blood 96:925–932

Hoeksema H, Johnson JL, Hinman JW (1955) Structural studies on streptonivicin, a new antibiotic. J Am Chem Soc 77:6710–6711

Jallepalli PV, Lengauer C (2001) Chromosome segregation and cancer: cutting through the mystery. Nat Rev Cancer 1:109–117

Ji H, Zhao X, Yuza Y, Shimamura T, Li D, Protopopov A, Jung BL, McNamara K, Xia H, Glatt KA, Thomas RK, Sasaki H, Horner JW, Eck M, Mitchell A, Sun Y, Al-Hashem R, Bronson RT, Rabindran SK, Discafani CM, Maher E, Shapiro GI, Meyerson M, Wong KK (2006) Epidermal growth factor receptor variant III mutations in lung tumorigenesis and sensitivity to tyrosine kinase inhibitors. Proc Natl Acad Sci USA 103:7817–7822

Kalser MH, Elenberg SS (1985) Pancreatic cancer. Adjuvant combined radiation and chemotherapy following curative resection. Arch Surg 120:899–903

Kasibhatla SR, Hong K, Biamonte MA, Busch DJ, Karjian PL, Sensintaffar JL, Kamal A, Lough RE, Brekken J, Lundgren K, Grecko R, Timony GA, Ran Y, Mansfield R, Fritz LC, Ulm E, Burrows FJ, Boehm MF (2007) Rationally designed high-affinity 2-amino-6-halopurine heat shock protein 90 inhibitors that exhibit potent antitumor activity. J Med Chem 14:2767–2778

Keating MJ, Kantarjian H, Talpaz M, Redman J, Koller C, Barlogie B, Velasquez W, Plunkett W, Freireich EJ, McCredie KB (1989) Fludarabine: a new agent with major activity against chronic lymphocytic leukemia. Blood 74:19–25

Keating MJ, Bach C, Yasothan U, Kirkpatrick P (2008) Bendamustine. Nat Rev Drug Discov 7:473–474

Kim EH, Kim SU, Shin DY, Choi KS (2004) Roscovitine sensitizes glioma cells to TRAIL-mediated apoptosis by downregulation of survivin and XIAP. Oncogene 23:446–456

Kurtzberg J, Yousem D, Beauchamp N Jr (2003) Asparaginase. In: Pollock RE, Weichselbaum RR, Kufe DW (eds) Cancer medicine. DC Becker, Hamilton, pp 823–830

Liu AY, Robinson RR, Hellström KE, Murray ED Jr, Chang CP, Hellström I (1987) Chimeric mouse-human IgG1 antibody that can mediate lysis of cancer cells. Proc Natl Acad Sci USA 84:3439–3443

McMillan R, Matsui W (2012) Molecular pathways: the Hedgehog signaling pathway in cancer. Clin Cancer Res 18:4883–4888

Minami Y, Shimamura T, Shah K, LaFramboise T, Glatt KA, Liniker E, Borgman CL, Haringsma HJ, Feng W, Weir BA, Lowell AM, Lee JC, Wolf J, Shapiro GI, Wong KK, Meyerson M, Thomas RK (2007) The major lung cancer-derived mutants of ERBB2 are oncogenic and are associated with sensitivity to the irreversible EGFR/ERBB2 inhibitor HKI-272. Oncogene 26:5023–5027

Minna JD, Gazdar AF, Sprang SR, Herz J (2004) A bull's eye for targeted lung cancer therapy. Science 304:1458–1461

O'Hare T, Eide CA, Deininger MW (2007) Bcr-Abl kinase domain mutations, drug resistance, and the road to a cure for chronic myeloid leukemia. Blood 110:2242–2249

O'Reilly EM (2010) Refinement of adjuvant therapy for pancreatic cancer. J Am Med Assoc 304:1124–1125

Paez JG, Jänne PA, Lee JC, Tracy S, Greulich H, Gabriel S, Herman P, Kaye FJ, Lindeman N, Boggon TJ, Naoki K, Sasaki H, Fujii Y, Eck MJ, Sellers WR, Johnson BE, Meyerson M (2004) EGFR mutations in lung cancer: correlation with clinical response to gefitinib therapy. Science 304:1497–1500

Rabindran SK, Discafani CM, Rosfjord EC, Baxter M, Floyd MB, Golas J, Hallett WA, Johnson BD, Nilakantan R, Overbeek E, Reich MF, Shen R, Shi X, Tsou HR, Wang YF, Wissner A (2004) Antitumor activity of HKI-272, an orally active, irreversible inhibitor of the HER-2 tyrosine kinase. Cancer Res 64:3958–3965

Reuter WM, Morgan MA, Bergmann L (2000) Targeting the Ras signaling pathway: a rational, mechanism-based treatment for hematologic malignancies?. Blood 96:1655–1669

Riechmann L, Clark M, Waldmann H, Winter G (1988) Reshaping human antibodies for therapy. Nature 332:323–327

Ryan DP, Eder JP Jr, Puchlaski T, Seiden MV, Lynch TJ, Fuchs CS, Amrein PC, Sonnichsen D, Supko JG, Clark JW (2004) Phase I clinical trial of the farnesyltransferase inhibitor BMS-214662 given as a 1-hour intravenous infusion in patients with advanced solid tumors. Clin Cancer Res 10:2222–2230

Samuels Y, Wang Z, Bardelli A, Silliman N, Ptak J, Szabo S, Yan H, Gazdar A, Powell SM, Riggins GJ, Willson JK, Markowitz S, Kinzler KW, Vogelstein B, Velculescu VE (2004) High frequency of mutations of the PIK3CA gene in human cancers. Science 304:554

Sequist LV (2007) Second-generation epidermal growth factor receptor tyrosine kinase inhibitors in non-small cell lung cancer. Oncologist 12:325–330

Shimamura T, Ji H, Minami Y, Thomas RK, Lowell AM, Shah K, Greulich H, Glatt KA, Meyerson M, Shapiro GI, Wong KK (2006) Non-small-cell lung cancer and Ba/F3 transformed cells harboring the ERBB2 G776insV_G/C mutation are sensitive to the dual-specific epidermal growth factor receptor and ERBB2 inhibitor HKI-272. Cancer Res 66:6487–6491

Sirotnak FM, Zakowski MF, Miller VA, Scher HI, Kris MG (2000) Efficacy of cytotoxic agents against human tumor xenografts is markedly enhanced by coadministration of ZD1839 (Iressa), an inhibitor of EGFR tyrosine kinase. Clin Cancer Res 6:4885–4892

Weber GF (2007) Molecular mechanisms of cancer. Springer, Dordrecht

Weisberg E, Manley P, Mestan J, Cowan-Jacob S, Ray A, Griffin JD (2006) AMN107 (nilotinib): a novel and selective inhibitor of BCR-ABL. Br J Cancer 94:1765–1769

Wolff NC, Veach DR, Tong WP, Bornmann WG, Clarkson B, Ilaria RL Jr (2005) PD166326, a novel tyrosine kinase inhibitor, has greater antileukemic activity than imatinib mesylate in a murine model of chronic myeloid leukemia. Blood 105:3995–4003

Yelton DE, Scharff MD (1981) Monoclonal antibodies: a powerful new tool in biology and medicine. Annu Rev Biochem 50:657–680

Anti-Metastasis Therapy

5

Cancers that metastasize release their cells early in carcinogenesis. The aberrant expression or splicing of metastasis genes in cancer makes their products quite cancer specific. Further, these molecules are not known to be mutated in cancer or to be altered under genomic instability. Because metastasis molecules tend to be shared among large subsets of invasive cancers, anti-metastasis agents may be efficacious against a broad spectrum of malignant tumors. There are 2 complementary anti-metastasis strategies, the prevention of cancer cell dissemination and the suppression of already existing metastases. Drug molecules in the former category will not be successful when given at a late disease stage, but may be life saving if administered immediately after diagnosis. About 5 % of cancer diagnoses are based on the discovery of metastases before the identification of the primary tumor. The most suitable treatment of these metastases is dictated by their location rather than their origin.

Although the presence of metastases generally implies a poor prognosis, some metastatic cancers can be forced into remission with conventional therapy. The treatment of metastatic cancers is compromised by multiple morbidities associated with systemic disease, and frequently by acquired drug resistance if the metastatic cancer represents a recurrence.

5.1 Integrin Inhibitors

Integrins are hetero-dimeric transmembrane receptors composed of non-covalently bound α and β chains that serve as receptors to the extracellular matrix. As direct mechano-receptors for adhesion, Integrins play a major role in the migration of healthy and neoplastic cells. Adhesion is also linked to cell survival, and the loss of Integrin mediated adhesion to the extracellular matrix can lead to cell death. Integrins play a role in blood vessel formation by facilitating the adhesion of stimulated endothelial cells to the extracellular matrix. This triggers the secretion of extracellular matrix degrading proteases, and propagates signaling events that promote the survival and differentiation of cells in the newly formed vasculature.

A subset of Integrins recognizes a common motif in their ligands, the RGD sequence (arginine-glycine-aspartate, Arg-Gly-Asp). Based on this motif, many peptidic and non-peptidic heterocyclic mimetics have been identified that can block the interaction between certain Integrins and their ligands (Tucker 2006). Integrin inhibitors in clinical development (Fig. 5.1) have distinct mechanisms of action,

- the peptide cilengitide and the antibodies etaracizumab and CNTO-95 target the α_v Integrin subunit, in particular in the Integrin $\alpha_v\beta_3$, that may also be affected by ATN-161
- the peptide ATN-161 and the antibody volociximab target the Integrin $\alpha_5\beta_1$
- the small molecule E7820 directly alters the expression of the Integrin $\alpha_2\beta_1$ at the RNA level
- additional small molecule, peptidomimetic Integrin blocking agents are in development.

5.1.1 Peptide Inhibitors

Cilengitide (EMD121974) is a head-to-tail cyclic peptide containing the RGD triad, wedged into a small constrained sequence that is flanked by D-phenylalanine and *N*-methylated valine residues. The molecule is based on the sequence cyclo[-RGDf(*N*Me)V-], where cyclization is accomplished by a peptide bond. Cilengitide binds to and inhibits the activities of the Integrins $\alpha_{5v}\beta_3$ and $\alpha_v\beta_5$, thereby suppressing endothelial cell-cell interactions, endothelial cell-matrix interactions, and angiogenesis. The drug has been under study for the treatment of prostate cancer, melanoma, myeloid leukemia, and brain tumors. The European EMA has granted cilengitide orphan drug status.

ATN-161 (ac-PHSCN-NH_2) is a capped, 5-amino-acid peptide. ATN-161 was derived from the sequence PHSRN in the synergy region of the Integrin ligand Fibronectin. The motif acts in synergy with the RGD containing binding site to strengthen the Integrin $\alpha_5\beta_1$-Fibronectin interaction. ATN-161 competes with this interaction. The drug action may result in an anti-angiogenesis effect. ATN-161 is under study for advanced renal cancer.

G. F. Weber, *Molecular Therapies of Cancer*, DOI 10.1007/978-3-319-13278-5_5,

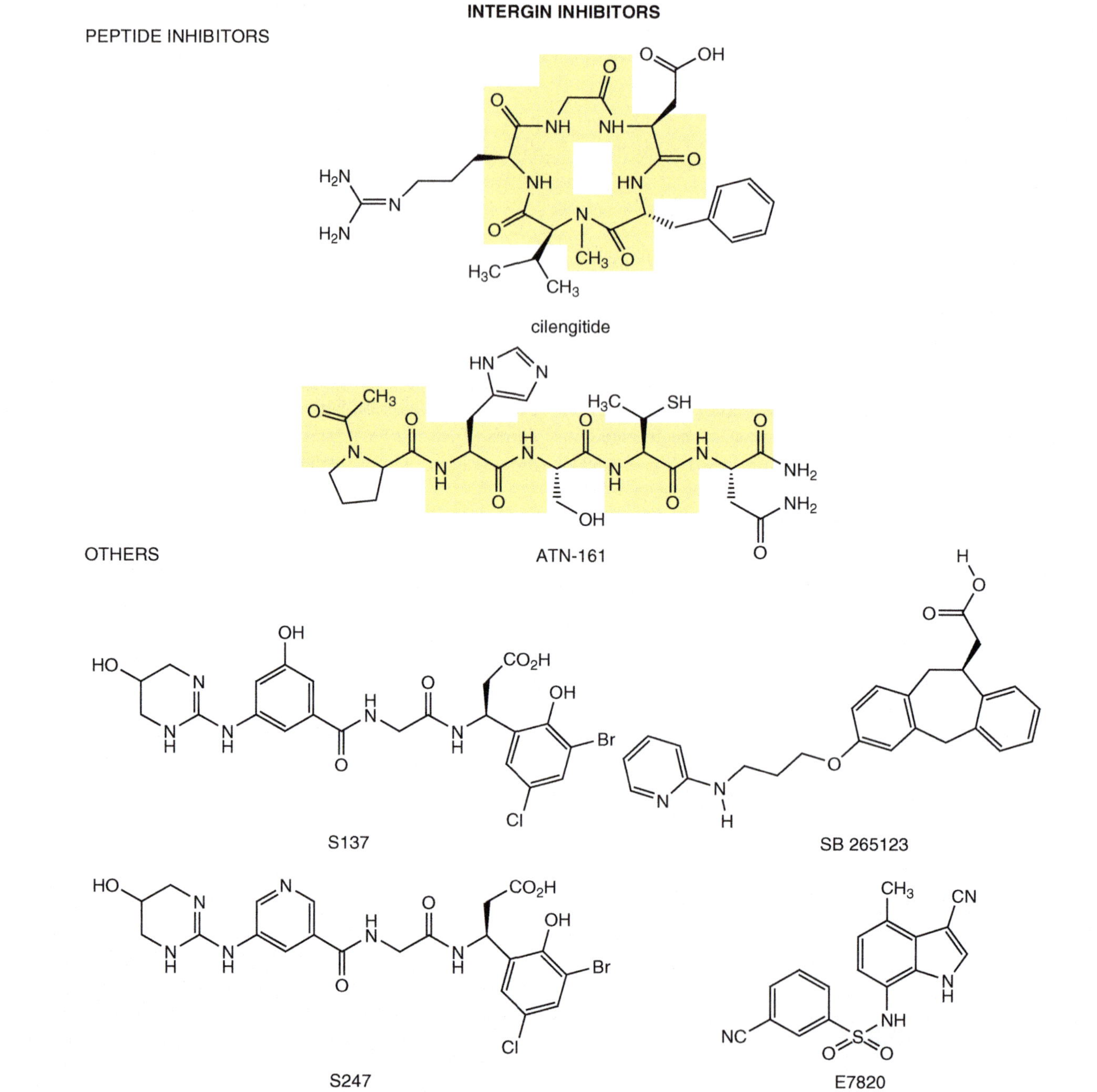

Fig. 5.1 Structures of Integrin inhibitors. In the peptide drugs, the backbones are highlighted in *yellow*

5.1.2 Antibodies

Integrin $\alpha_v\beta_3$ is a cell adhesion and signaling receptor that is expressed on the surface of tumor vessel endothelial cells, some tumor cells, and osteoclasts. It is important in angiogenesis, tumor invasion, and bone metastasis.

LM609 is a mouse anti-human monoclonal antibody that binds to Integrin $\alpha_v\beta_3$ Its primary mechanism of action is the suppression of FGF-2 and TNF-α signaling, which inhibits angiogenesis. Because the Integrin $\alpha_v\beta_3$ is barely expressed on preexisting resting vessels, there is little impact on them. MEDI-522 and MEDI-523 are humanized derivatives of the antibody LM609, with MEDI-522 having higher affinity for Integrin $\alpha_v\beta_3$ than MEDI-523. Antibody dependent cellular cytotoxicity contributes to their anti-tumor activity. In 1997, the IgG_1 etaracizumab (MEDI-522) <Abegrin, Vitaxin[1]>

[1] Although the name Vitaxin has been used in the literature for a humanized LM609 derivative, Vitaxin is the trademark for a supplement made from the branch tips and the needles of the Pacific yew tree. It is

was the first Integrin antagonist to enter clinical trials for cancer. It blocks the binding of ligands, such as Vitronectin or Osteopontin, resulting in the inhibition of metastasis and angiogenesis. Etaracizumab has been under study for the treatment of leiomyosarcoma and metastatic melanoma. It is also under investigation for the treatment of prostate cancer, ovarian cancer, and Kaposi sarcoma.

The monoclonal antibody intetumumab (CNTO-95) is an anti-pan-α_v antibody that was generated in mice transgenic for part of the human immunoglobulin repertoire. This antibody recognizes the Integrins $\alpha_v\beta_1$, $\alpha_v\beta_3$, $\alpha_v\beta_5$, and $\alpha_v\beta_6$. It competitively binds to and blocks these receptors, resulting in an inhibition of Integrin dependent tumor expansion and angiogenesis. Besides the use as a single agent, intetumumab is also under investigation for combination with fractionated radiation. With a good tolerance of up to 10 mg/kg/week, intetumumab displays tumor penetration and achieves a reduction of BCL-2 expression, thus facilitating tumor cell death. The antibody can achieve responses in angiosarcoma and ovarian carcinosarcoma.

Volociximab (Eos200-4, M200) is a chimeric monoclonal antibody that binds to and inhibits the activity of Integrin $\alpha_5\beta_1$, thereby inhibiting endothelial cell-cell interactions, endothelial cell-matrix interactions, and angiogenesis. This induces apoptosis in proliferating endothelial cells. The antibody is under investigation, alone or in combination with chemotherapy, for the treatment of metastatic kidney cancer.

Abciximab (c7E3 Fab) <ReoPro> is a mouse/human chimera derived from a mouse anti-Integrin $\alpha_{IIb}\beta_3$ (GPIIb–IIIa) monoclonal antibody. This antibody retains the variable region of the underlying mouse antibody, ligated to the constant domain of human IgG. It inhibits platelet aggregation by targeting Integrin $\alpha_{IIb}\beta_3$, and it also binds to Integrin $\alpha_v\beta_3$ with comparable affinity. As Integrin $\alpha_v\beta_3$ is important in mediating cancer angiogenesis and metastasis, abciximab may inhibit Integrin $\alpha_v\beta_3$ mediated endothelial and cancer cell adhesion, as well as migration and invasion[2].

Pharmacokinetics Abciximab is eliminated from the blood with 2 half-lives of 10 and 30 min. Platelet aggregation is prolonged and returns to normal about 95–120 h after discontinuation of the drug.

Adverse Effects Many of the adverse effects are due to the anti-platelet effects, including an increased risk of bleeding (often gastrointestinal hemorrhage) and thrombocytopenia.

5.1.3 Others

The Integrin $\alpha_v\beta_3/\alpha_v\beta_3$ antagonists S137 and S247 are low molecular weight peptidomimetics of the RGD motif. They have a broad potency against the family of α_v containing Integrins, with substantially less potency against $\alpha_v\beta_1$ and $\alpha_{IIb}\beta_3$. The agents are in preclinical development.

SB265123 is an orally active RGD peptidomimetic Integrin $\alpha_V\beta_3$ antagonist. SB 265123 engages $\alpha_V\beta_3$ and the closely related integrin $\alpha_V\beta_5$ with high affinity, but binds only weakly to the related, RGD-engaging Integrins $\alpha_{IIb}\beta_3$ and $\alpha_5\beta_1$.

Various Integrin blockers are under investigation. GLPG 0187 inhibits multiple Integrins that bind RGD. The low molecular weight, imidazole-containing, non-peptide Integrin $\alpha_v\beta_3$ antagonist SM256 is in preclinical development. SD983 is a small molecule Integrin antagonist. It is in preclinical development as a potential angiogenesis inhibitor. SC68448 and DE19548709-A are Integrin inhibitors in development.

Disintegrins are components in viper snake venoms, which entail a family of low molecular mass RGD proteins. Two sub-classes comprise the monomeric and dimeric Disintegrins. Some Disintegrins have entered clinical trials.

E7820 is an aromatic sulfonamide derivative. It acts as a modulator of the expression of *integrin α_2* subunits in endothelial cells. This may result in anti-metastatic or anti-angiogenic activity. E7820 is orally bioavailable.

Adverse Effects The compound has a good safety profile up to 100 mg/day.

5.2 CD44 Inhibitors

In the absence of candidate small molecule drugs, 3 general strategies exist for therapeutic interference with receptor ligation. They include the use of neutralizing antibodies, the interference with peptide antagonists, and the decoy activity of soluble receptors.

- Due to their high affinity binding, antibodies are often employed to block receptor/ligand interactions. The malignant phenotype of various cancers is caused by a splice variant of CD44 that contains variant exon 6. Metastasis formation by such cancers may be blocked by intravenous injection of an anti-variant CD44 antibody. This treatment strategy is only effective when given before lymph node colonization. Previously developed anti-CD44v6 did not induce complement mediated cytotoxicity or antibody dependent cellular cytotoxicity. This may be a consequence of the drug action: A lack of T-lymphocyte activation may

derived from healing traditions of the Indian tribes in the Northwest of the United States and in Canada, and is unrelated to Integrin inhibitors.

[2] While abciximab is efficacious in preventing coronary restenosis after angioplasty, its use for the treatment of cancers is still under investigation.

be due to blocking of CD44v on activated T-cells with possible immunosuppressive consequences (Seiter 1993).
- Attempts have been made to utilize peptide antagonists of receptors in cancer therapy. Because they often model the binding domain of physiological ligands, such peptide antagonists may have substantial specificity. However, the concentrations needed for effective blocking are often high, and parenteral application is mandatory to avoid destruction of the peptides in the stomach.
- Soluble receptors can be used to sequester growth factors from their specific membrane-bound receptors. CD44 can be shed from the cell surface by ectodomain cleavage (Kawano et al. 2000) and exert distinct effects as a soluble molecule (Bazil and Horejsi 1992). The soluble receptor may act as a scavenger by engaging the physiological ligands thus preventing them from binding to the receptor on the cell surface (Alpaugh et al. 2000). This implies potential therapeutic use for engineered soluble CD44 molecules in cancer (Peterson et al. 2000). Because shedding occurs through proteolytic cleavage of the extracellular portion of CD44 by chymotrypsin-like activity (Lee et al. 2000), it is conceivable that therapeutic application of a protease that sheds CD44 from the membrane would also inhibit dissemination by two mechanisms, removal of a surface receptor that is important for invasion and scavenging of the physiological ligands by the released extracellular receptor domain.

5.3 MMP Inhibitors

Matrix Metalloproteinases (MMPs) are enzymes critical for a variety of physiological and patho-physiological processes. In cancer, they support dissemination by degrading the tumor surrounding stroma, including components of the extracellular matrix such as Collagen, Elastin, Laminin, Fibronectin, and the protein cores of proteoglycans. In osteolytic cancer lesion formation, Matrix Metalloproteinases are produced directly by the tumor cells and by osteoclasts after induction by tumor cells. Osteoclast mediated osteolysis is dependent on Matrix Metalloproteinases, not in the initial phase of bone mineral resorption but for unmineralized matrix degradation.

As Matrix Metalloproteinases play a pivotal role in the process of malignant dissemination, their pharmacological inhibition could markedly suppress tumors invasiveness. Therefore, they are promising targets for anti-metastasis therapy. All Matrix Metalloproteinases share a common active site motif, in which 3 histidine residues bind to a zinc ion. Conceptually, these biomolecules are inhibitable through the design of small organic chelators that bind the metal in the active center to inactivate a metalloenzyme.

Matrix Metalloproteinase inhibitors (Figs. 5.2 and 5.3) have been tested in clinical trials in several solid malignancies. Most of these studies did not show any survival benefit. In some cases, the initiation of therapy may have commenced at too late a stage in carcinogenesis, where the cancer had already spread. Also, the pleiotropic effects of several Matrix Metalloproteinases allow them to play protective roles in specific settings.

5.3.1 Hydroxamates

Peptidomimetic Matrix Metalloproteinase inhibitors are pseudo-peptidic derivatives that mimic the structure of the MMP-sensitive site in Collagen. These inhibitors bind at the active site of Matrix Metalloproteinases in a stereospecific manner and chelate the zinc atom on the enzyme activation site. In this group of agents, hydroxamates covalently bind and inactivate the zinc atom in the active center of the enzymes. Members of this class of drugs have names that typically end on -mastat.

Problems with the peptidic Matrix Metalloproteinase inhibitors include poor oral bioavailability (except for marimastat) and a relative lack of specificity for individual Matrix Metalloproteinases. Further, the hydroxamate group is metabolically labile.

Adverse Effects Dose limiting muscular and skeletal pain (musculoskeletal syndrome), occurring after several weeks of treatment in a substantial number of patients, is a class effect.

First generation hydroxamates Marimastat (BB-2516, TA 2516) is an orally active synthetic hydroxamate that covalently binds to the zinc^{II} ion in the active site of Matrix Metalloproteinases, thereby inhibiting the enzymatic action. This agent acts as a broad spectrum inhibitor, suppressing the activities of MMP-1, -2, -3, -7, and -9. It may also inhibit TACE (Tumor Necrosis Factor-α Converting Enzyme), an enzyme involved in TNF-α production that may play a role in some malignancies. Marimastat is orally administered. The drug has shown positive effects against prostate cancer in clinical trials, but several other trials have failed to demonstrate efficacy.

Pharmacokinetics The pharmacokinetics of marimastat is linear, with dose-proportional increases in blood concentrations. Their peaks are reached within 1.5–3 h after oral administration. The elimination half-life range is 8–10 h. Continuous administration of oral doses of 50–200 mg twice a day over a week does not result in blood accumulation.

Adverse Effects Single oral doses of up to 800 mg are well tolerated. Adverse effects include frozen shoulder syndrome[3] and frozen hand syndrome. Prolonged treatment with broad

[3] In frozen shoulder syndrome (adhesive capsulitis), the articular shoulder capsule swells and stiffens, restricting its mobility.

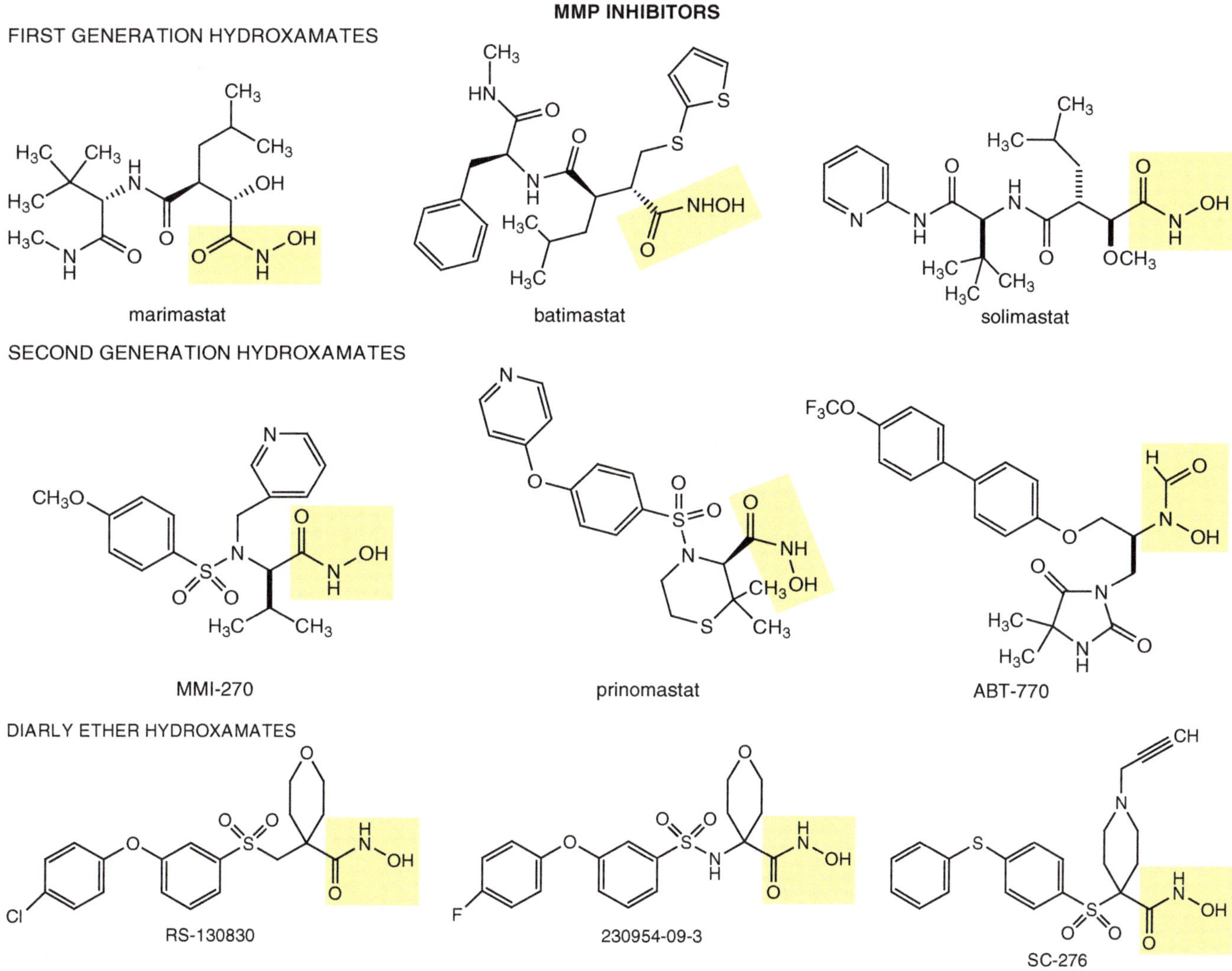

Fig. 5.2 Structures of hydroxamate Matrix Metalloproteinase inhibitors. Sub-classes comprise first generation, second generation, and diaryl ether hydroxamate Matrix Metalloproteinase inhibitors. The common hydroxamate moiety in all representatives is highlighted in *yellow*

spectrum Matrix Metalloproteinase inhibitors causes musculoskeletal pain and inflammation, thus limiting the cumulative dosages administrated.

Batimastat ((2R,3S)-*N*4-Hydroxy-*N*1-[(1S)-2-(methylamino)-2-oxo-1-(phenylmethyl)ethyl]-2-(2-methylpropyl)-3-[(2-thienylthio) methyl]butanediamide) (BB-94) is a synthetic hydroxamate, broad spectrum Matrix Metalloproteinase inhibitor that covalently binds to the zinc in the active site of the enzymes. Batimastat is relatively non-specific with activity against MMP-1, -2, -3, -7, and -9. It is cannot be given orally.

Solimastat is a broad spectrum Matrix Metalloproteinase and TACE (ADAM) inhibitor. Although it has diminished toxicity compared to the structurally related marimastat, its toxicity caused the prematurely termination of clinical studies.

Second generation hydroxamates The hypothesis that MMP-1 sparing structures would avoid the adverse effects of causing musculo-skeletal pain, second generation compounds were directed away from the shallow binding pocket of MMP-1 (Collagenase), and toward the deep binding pockets of the Gelatinases (MMP-2 and MMP-9). This goal may be accomplished by 2 phenyl rings that are connected directly or via an oxygen atom (as is the case in ABT-770 and PD-166793).

MMI-270 is a water soluble, low molecular mass, broad spectrum inhibitor of Matrix Metalloproteinases. It contains the basic structural features that confer Matrix Metalloproteinase inhibition, including a substituted aryl and an acyl hydrogen bond acceptor that is separated by 2 atoms from the hydroxamate group. There is an amino acid side-chain type substituent on the carbon α to the hydroxamate. The *N*-arylsulfonyl-α-amino acid hydroxamate of MMI-270 mim-

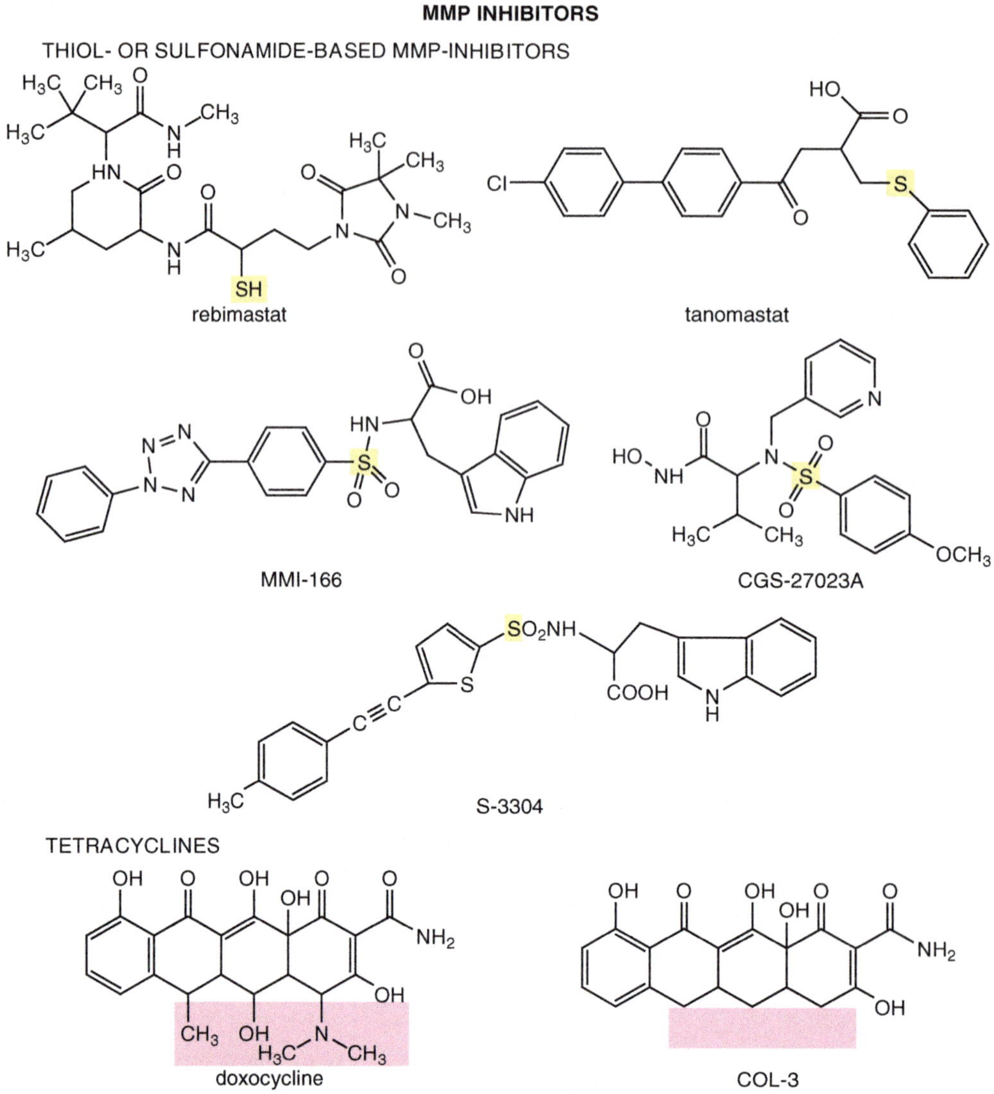

Fig. 5.3 Structures of non-hydroxamate Matrix Metalloproteinase inhibitors. Within the group of thiol- or sulfonamide-based inhibitors, the sulfur is highlighted in *yellow*. Within the group of pyrimidine 2,4,6-triones, the core group is highlighted in *yellow*. The difference between the tetracyclines is shaded in *pink*

ics the marimistat succinate motif (butanedioate motif; substituted as half hydroxamate and half amide). The agent is orally available. The prototype drug MMI-270 is limited by metabolic lability and risk for musculo-skeletal syndrome.

Prinomastat ((3S)-*N*-hydroxy-2,2-dimethyl-4-{{4-(4-piridinyloxy)phenyl}sulfonyl}-3-thiomorpholinecarboxamide) (Ag 3340) is an inhibitor of the Matrix Metalloproteinases MMP-2 (Gelatinase A), MMP-9 (Gelatinase B), MMP-13, and MMP-14, with some MMP-1 selectivity. It has a *N*-arylsulfonyl-α-amino acid hydroxamate motif, with the cyclization of the side-chain back to the nitrogen. While prinomastat inhibition of Metalloproteinases may counteract metastasis, its inhibition of the MT1-MMP catalyzed proteolysis of Vitronectin can promote metastasis. As a lipophilic agent, prinomastat crosses the blood-brain barrier. The drug has not shown efficacy in clinical trials.

Adverse Effects Prinomastat causes moderate but reversible arthralgia, myalgia, and muscolo-skeletel syndrome at high doses, beginning 2 months after therapy initiation.

ABT-770 is an orally available retro-hydroxamate that is optimized for suppressing MMP-2 and -9 activity over MMP-1 activity.

Fig. 5.3 (continued)

PYRIMIDINE-2,4,6-TRIONES

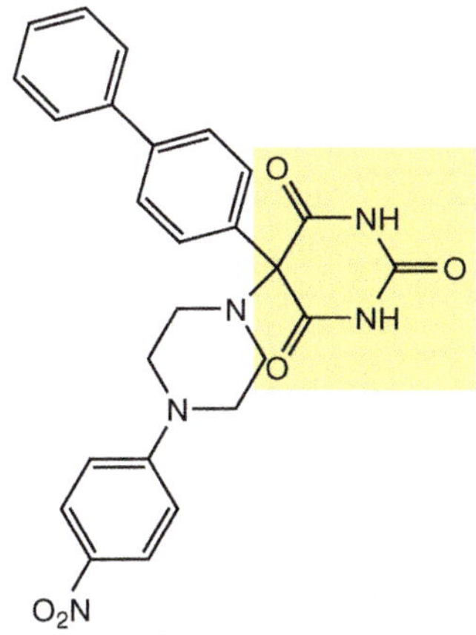

Ro 28-2653

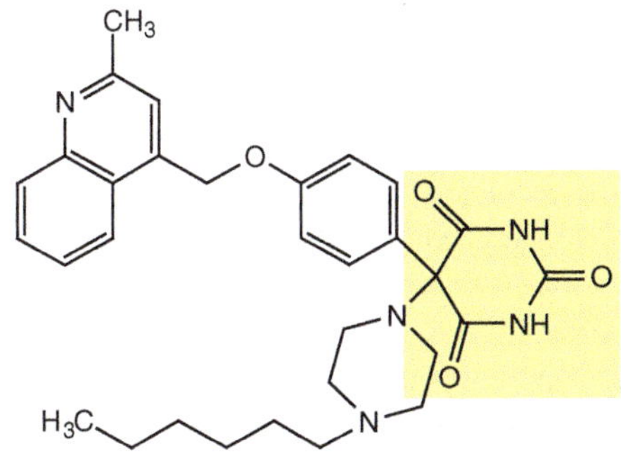

556052-30-3

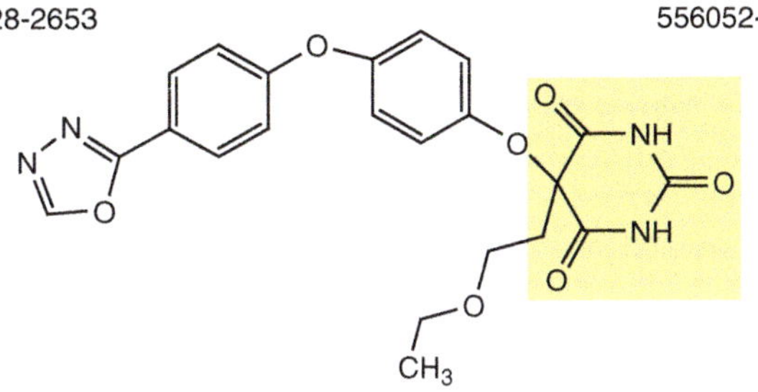

420121-84-2

OTHERS

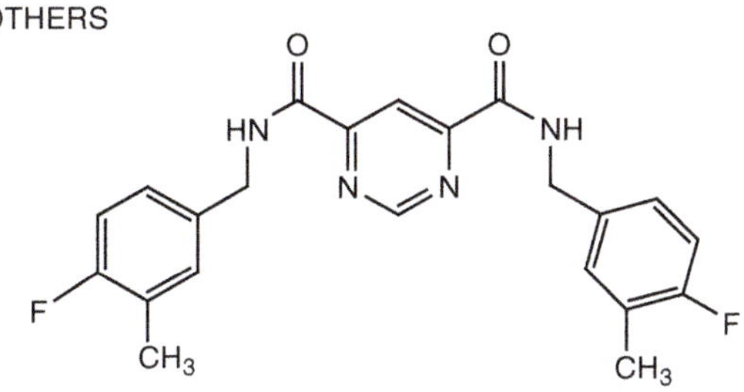

544678-85-5

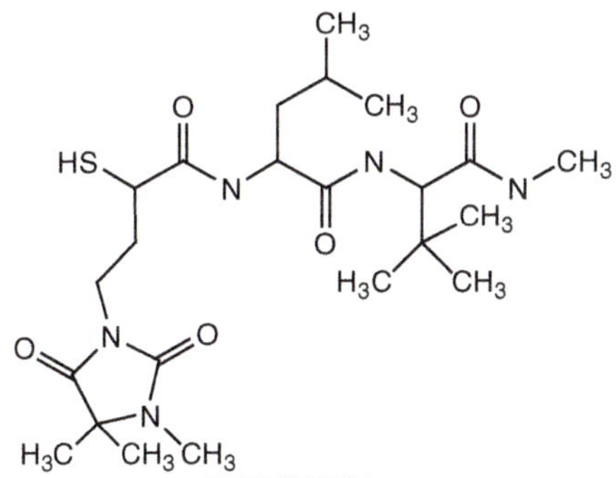

BMS-275291

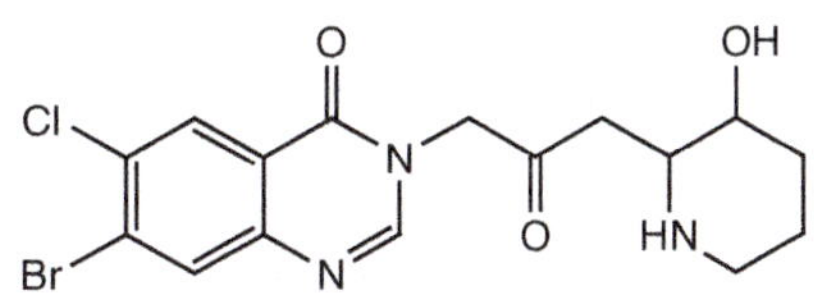

halofuginone

Adverse Effects ABT-770 is readily metabolized to an amine metabolite that can cause phospholipidosis[4].

Diaryl ether hydroxamates A recurring limitation to the efficacy of second generation hydroxamates is inactivating drug metabolism, including the loss of the zinc-binding hydroxamate group by its reduction to an amide, its hydrolysis to a carboxylate, and its conjugation as a glucuronide. The ensuing generation of hydroxamate structures focused on the suppression of metabolism, the minimization of MMP-1 inhibitory activity, and the control of subtype selectivity (especially toward the Gelatinases MMP-2 and MMP-9, the Collagenase MMP-13, and TACE). Diaryl ether hydroxamates contain a linked diaryl that is specific for Matrix Metalloproteinases with a long and narrow pocket. Their structures achieve MMP-1 sparing selectivity. While these Matrix Metalloproteinase inhibitors possess the requisite subtype potency and improved pharmacokinetic

[4] Phospholipidosis is a lysosomal storage disorder characterized by the excess accumulation of phospholipids in tissues. It may be induced by certain drugs.

properties for anti-cancer activity, their utility for the treatment of cancer remains to be confirmed.

The first compound of the class of diaryl ether hydroxamates, RS-130830 (4-[4-(4-Chloro-phenoxy)-benzenesulfonylmethyl]-tetrahydro-pyran-4-carboxylic acid hydroxyamide), entered into clinical evaluation as an MMP-13 specific inhibitor. Its annulated tetrahydropyran, located in α position to the hydroxamate, introduces a steric block that suppresses metabolism while achieving the desired Matrix Metalloproteinase selectivity. The agent is orally active.

The phenoxyphenyl α-sulfonylpiperidine hydroxamate 230954–09-3 is an orally available compound that has high metabolic stability. 239796–97-5 is an effective MMP-9 and MMP-13 inhibitor, which has a good TACE sparing and an excellent MMP-1 sparing profile.

Adverse Effects Despite its MMP-1 sparing properties, the drug induces musculo-skeletal syndrome.

The thiophenoxyphenyl structure of SC-276 inhibits MMP-2 and MMP-13 at sub-nanomolar concentrations. It displays greatly improved MMP-1 sparing over earlier compounds. SC-276 is orally active as an anti-angiogenic and as an anti-cancer drug.

New generation hydroxamates The transition to structures with narrower MMP or ADAMS selectivity characterizes the new generation inhibitors. In many cases this objective is accomplished by combining the biaryl S1' space with new cyclic and acyclic substituted hydroxamates.

- Both enantiomers of a β-trifluoromethyl sulfone, 851371-13-6 and 851371-11-4, are potent MMP-3 inhibitors with good selectivity for MMP-9.
- The *N*-isopropoxy substituted compound 849773-63-3 is MMP-1 sparing (MT1-MMP, 15-fold selective and MMP-2, 1500-fold selective against MMP-1).
- ONO-4817, an orally available and water soluble broad spectrum MMP inhibitor, is MMP-1 and MMP-7 sparing, and has efficacy against some cancer activities.
- The 4-butynoxyphenylsulfonamides 287405-83-8 and TMI-1 are dual MMP-TACE inhibitors.

5.3.2 Thiol- or Sulfonamide- Based MMP Inhibitors

Rebimastat (*N*-((2S)-2-Mercapto-1-oxo-4-(3,4,4-trimethyl-2, 5-dioxo-1-imidazolidinyl)butyl)-L-leucyl-*N*,3-dimethyl-L-valinamide) (BMS-275291, D2163) is a sulfhydryl based Matrix Metalloproteinase inhibitor. The structural scaffold for its thiol is a deep-pocket, Collagen non-peptide mimetic. This agent rather selectively inhibits the Matrix Metalloproteinases MMP-2 and MMP-9, but also has activity against MMP-1, -8, and -14, thereby preventing extracellular matrix degradation, inhibiting angiogenesis, and protecting from tumor invasion and metastasis. The agent is orally bioavailable. It does not inhibit the Metalloproteinases that release TNF-α, L-Selectin, IL-1-RII, and IL-6-R cytokines.

Adverse Effects Rebim astat does not cleave the extracellular domain of the TNF Receptor, a mechanism that may be responsible for some of the musculoskeletal effects of other non-peptidic Matrix Metalloproteinase inhibitors.

The α-[(phenylthio)methyl]carboxylate tanomastat (BAY12-9566) contains a thioether zinc binding group. It has a biphenyl deep-pocket segment, and constitutes a better inhibitor of MMP-2, MMP-3, and MMP-9 than it is of MMP-1 or MMP-13. The agent is associated with good tolerance, but may be ineffective if given late in disease.

Pharmacokinetics The oral bioavailability of tanomastat is 70–95 %. The drug reaches peak blood concentrations at 0.5–2 h after dosing. The pharmacokinetics is linear at doses of up to 100 mg/day. Enterohepatic recirculation may occur. Repeated administration of the drug results in increa sed clearance, and thus a reduction in drug exposure.

Adverse Effects The agent has low toxicity. Administration results in only mild anemia (thrombocytopenia), hepatotoxicity, and renal toxicity.

MMI-166 *N*α-[4-(2-phenyl-2H-tetrazole-5-yl) phenyl sulfonyl]-D-tryptophan) has a *N*-arylsulfonyl-α-aminocarboxylate zinc binding group. Key features of the structure are 2 phenyl rings connected by a tetrazole ring and a triaryl substitution. MMI-166 is a selective inhibitor of MMP-2, -9 and -14 that spares MMP-1, -3 and -7.

CGS-27023A (MMI270) is a broad-spectrum Matrix Metalloproteinase inhibitor. The agent does not suppress the proliferation of cancer cells, but it does reduce their invasion. CGS-27023A can be administered orally. The combination of CGS-27023A with conventional cytotoxic agents results in additive or synergistic effects. CGS-27023A is in clinical trials. Doses range 150–600 mg.

Adverse Effects The major toxic effects are encountered at doses exceeding 300 mg twice a day. They consist of cutaneous and musculoskeletal toxicity.

The tryptophan derivative N^{α}-[2-[5-[4-methylphenyl] ethynyl]thienyl]sulfonyl]-d-tryptophan (S-3304) is an orally active agent that inhibits Matrix Metalloproteinases, thereby inducing extracellular matrix degradation and inhibiting angiogenesis, tumor invasion, and metastasis.

Adverse Effects When administered orally in doses up to 800 mg twice daily for 10–17 days, S-3304 is devoid of musculoskeletal symptoms, and the most common adverse events are headache and somnolence.

5.3.3 Tetracyclines

Tetracyclines act as broad-spectrum Matrix Metalloproteinase inhibitors by suppressing not only their activities but also their synthesis. Tetracyclins inhibit the Collagenases (MMP-1, -3, and -13) and the Gelatinases (MMP-2 and -9). Because these drugs are highly osteotropic, they may be suited for treating bone metastases. Their concentrations needed to achieve the desired effects in bone are such that the blood concentrations stay below toxic levels.

Adverse Effects Gastrointestinal toxicity is the principal dose-related adverse effect of tetracycline antibiotics.

Doxycycline non-selectively inhibits Matrix Metalloproteinases by binding to the active zinc site and secondarily to the inactive calcium ion site, causing conformational changes that lead to the loss of enzymatic activity. Doxycycline suppresses the activities of MMP-8 and MMP-9 and the activation of pro- MMP-2. It inhibits the expression of MMP-9 mRNA, but not MMP-2 mRNA.

Adverse Effects Oral doses of 400 mg, administered twice a day, result in dose limiting toxicity that consists of fatigue, confusion, nausea, and vomiting.

6-deoxy-6-demethyl-4-dedimethylamino-tetracycline (COL-3, CMT-3) <Metastat> is a chemically modified tetracycline that competitively inhibits Matrix Metalloproteinases, with specificity for MMP-2 and MMP-9. This agent also causes mitochondrial depolarization in tumor cells and induces both cellular apoptosis and tissue necrosis.

Adverse Effects The maximum tolerated dose is 50 mg/m^2/day. The most common adverse events are dose related photosensitivity and rash. Drug-induced lupus may result in rare cases.

5.3.4 Pyrimidine-2,4,6-triones

Because the pyrimidine-trione template is an efficient zinc chelating moiety (Grams et al. 2001), pyrimidine-2,4,6-triones (barbiturates) are under development as a sub-type specific class of Matrix Metalloproteinase inhibitors. The structural basis for the inhibition involves pyrimidine-trione chelation of the active site zinc. These compounds bind to the Matrix Metalloproteinases in a manner that saturates nearly all possible interactions of the pyrimidine core moiety to the protein. Pyrimidine-triones have oral availability.

Ro 28-2653 (5-biphenyl-4-yl-5-[4-(-nitro-phenyl)-piperazin-1-yl]-pyrimidine-2,4,6-trione) is a Matrix Metalloproteinase inhibitor with high affinity for MMP-2, MMP-9, and MMP-14 (Membrane Type 1-MMP). It also inhibits MT-3-MMP and MMP-8, while sparing MMP-1 activity. Ro 28-2653 does not inhibit the zinc endoprotease Meprin, which is sensitive to hydroxamate based Matrix Metalloproteinase inhibitors. It only moderately up-regulates MMP-2 and MT1-MMP, and (unlike batimastat) does not up-regulate MMP-9 angiogenic activity. Ro 28-2653 reduces tumor vascularization and inhibits the tumor promoting effects of fibroblasts. The drug is orally bioavailable, but has poor water solubility. It is in clinical trials for non-small cell lung cancer.

Adverse Effects Ro 28-2653 was designed to avoid the adverse neuromuscular effects of earlier generation MMP inhibitors.

Compound 556052-30-3 is TACE selective over Matrix Metalloproteinases (with inhibitory doses in the nanomolar and micromolar range, respectively) as it incorporates the 4-[(2-methylquinolin-4-yl)methoxy]phenyl side-chain.

Selectivity for MMP-13 over MMP-14 (MT-1 MMP) is achievable within the pyrimidine-trione zinc binding group. Substitution of a 1,3,4-oxadiazol-2-yl hetero-aryl at C-4 of the diphenylether segment gives the pyrimidinetrione 420121-84-2. This compound has a 200-fold lower inhibitory dose for MMP-13 than for MMP-14.

Pharmacokinetics The compound is orally available. It has a half-life of 4 h, low clearance, and low volume of distribution.

5.3.5 Others

The MMP-13 selective pyrimidine-4,6-dicarboxamide inhibitor 544678-85-5 has high MMP-13 selectivity over MMP-1, -2, -3, -7, -8, -9, -10, -12, -14, and -16. The MMP-13 complex with this drug has extensive hydrogen bonding interactions involving the tyrosine 244-to-leucine 255 loop in the active site, but without direct contact to the catalytic zinc. The 2 distal 3-methyl-4-fluorophenyl segments of the inhibitor occupy opposing faces of the leucine 218 side-chain. The 3-methyl-4-fluoro substituents are sufficiently proximal to the zinc to displace the water ensemble around the metal.

AG3340, BAY 12–9566, and BMS-275291 were designed to be relatively selective inhibitors of MMP-2.

AG3340 is a non-peptidic Collagen mimicking Matrix Metalloproteinase inhibitor. The drug inhibits MMP -2, -9, -3, and -13. It may have anti-tumor activity against a broad spectrum of cancers. The compound is in clinical trials.

Halofuginone hydrobromide is a quinazolinone alkaloid anticoccidial. It inhibits *matrix metalloproteinase-2* (*mmp-2*) gene expression and type I Collagen synthesis, which results in the suppression of tumor progression, tumor stromal cell development, and angiogenesis. These effects may be due to an effect of halofuginone on the activity of the *mmp-2* promoter.

Neovastat (AE941) is a drug made from a concentrated extract of shark cartilage. Rather than being a specific mono-molecular compound, AE-941 is a defined standardized liquid extract comprising the smaller than 500 kD fraction. Cartilage lacks blood vessels and can prevent their growth. Neovastat interferes with several steps of angiogenesis through its ability to inhibit Matrix Metalloproteinases, to induce endothelial apoptosis, and to suppress signaling pathways mediated by VEGF. It is in clinical trials for multiple myeloma, non-small cell lung cancer and renal cell cancer.

An experimental approach to the inhibition of Matrix Metalloproteinase expression is via the use of specific antisense oligonucleotides. Because MMP-7 is implicated in the progression of colon cancer, there is potential benefit for the use of an antisense phosphorothioate oligodeoxyribonucleotide to MMP-7.

In cancer, Matrix Metalloproteinases support dissemination by degrading the tumor surrounding stroma.

Metalloproteinase inhibitors may act as anti-metastasis drugs. Metalloproteinase inhibitors often have names that end on -mastat.
Muscular and skeletal pain (musculoskeletal syndrome) is a dose limiting class effect, especially for drugs that inhibit MMP-1 or TACE.

5.4 Chemokine Receptor Inhibitors

Chemokines are a super-family of small cytokines that induce directional cell migration. According to the number and spacing of conserved cysteine residues in the sequence of these 8–10 kD proteins, there are four major groups, consisting of CC containing Chemokines and their corresponding receptors CCR1 through CCR10, CXC containing Chemokines with receptors CXCR1 through CXCR5, a CXXXC Chemokine with receptor CXXXCR1, and a XC Chemokine with receptor XCR1. Chemokine receptors are specific 7 transmembrane spanning, G-Protein coupled cell surface receptors. Upon ligand binding, the hetero-trimeric G-Proteins dissociate into α and βγ subunits, which activate target enzymes. Mostly, they are functionally linked to Phospholipases and to members of the RHO family. Chemokines and their receptors are critically important in tissue specific leukocyte homing. When expressed on cancer cells, Chemokine Receptors mediate metastatic dissemination.

CXCR1 and CXCR2 are receptors for Interleukin-8 (IL-8, Neutrophil Chemotactic Factor) and closely related glutamate-leucine-arginine (ELR) containing CXC chemokines. At nanomolar concentrations, the compounds SB225002 (*N*-(2-bromophenyl)-*N*'-(2-hydroxy-4-nitrophenyl)-urea) and SB265610 are antagonists of CXCR2 that have relatively weak activity on CXCR1 (150-fold less). These agents cause the inhibition of intracellular calcium mobilization mediated by IL-8 or CXCL1 (GROα) (Fig. 5.4).

Reparixin (repertaxin) was originally designed to target CXCR1 and CXCR2 on the surface of neutrophils to prevent their migration to sites of inflammation. Although the compound is no longer in development for preventing graft dysfunction, reparixin is safe and is under study for the treatment of cancer.

Pharmacokinetics Reparixin is metabolized to ibuprofen and suppresses the blood levels of thromboxane B2.

J113863 (1,4-cis-1-(1-Cycloocten-1-ylmethyl)-4-[[(2,7-dichloro-9*H*-xanthen-9-yl)carbonyl]amino]-1-ethylpiperidinium iodide) is an antagonist of CCR1 and CCR3.

- UCB35625 is the trans-isomer of J113863 and is also under study as a drug candidate.

SB328437 ((S)-Methyl-2-naphthoylamino-3-(4-nitrophenyl)propionate) is a selective CCR3 antagonist. It inhibits the effects of Eotaxin, Eotaxin-2, and MCP-4.

CXCR4 regulates the proliferation and migration of neural precursor cells. It is also expressed at high levels in brain tumors of neuronal and astrocytic lineage. Systemic administration of the CXCR4 antagonist AMD3100 (JM3100) may inhibit the progression of glioblastoma and medulloblastoma. AMD3100 lacks oral bioavailability.

Adverse Effects Development of AMD3100 was halted because of adverse cardiac effects that were likely caused by antagonism of CXCR4 mediated receptor activity on atrial smooth muscle.

The hexapeptide antileukinate (ac-RRWWCR-NH_2) is an inhibitor of CXC Chemokine binding to their cognate cell membrane receptors. Antileukinate can inhibit the progression of melanoma cells and certain adenocarcinoma cells.

Neutralizing antibodies to Chemokines or Chemokine Receptors may interfere with cancer dissemination. Anti-CXCR4 antibodies can inhibit the spread of breast cancer cells to the lymph nodes. The proliferation of various adenocarcinomata is inhibited by anti-CXCL1 antibodies.

Chemokines mediate directed cell migration and may contribute to organ specific metastasis through cognate receptors on tumor cells.
Chemokine receptor blockers may have anti-metastatic effects.

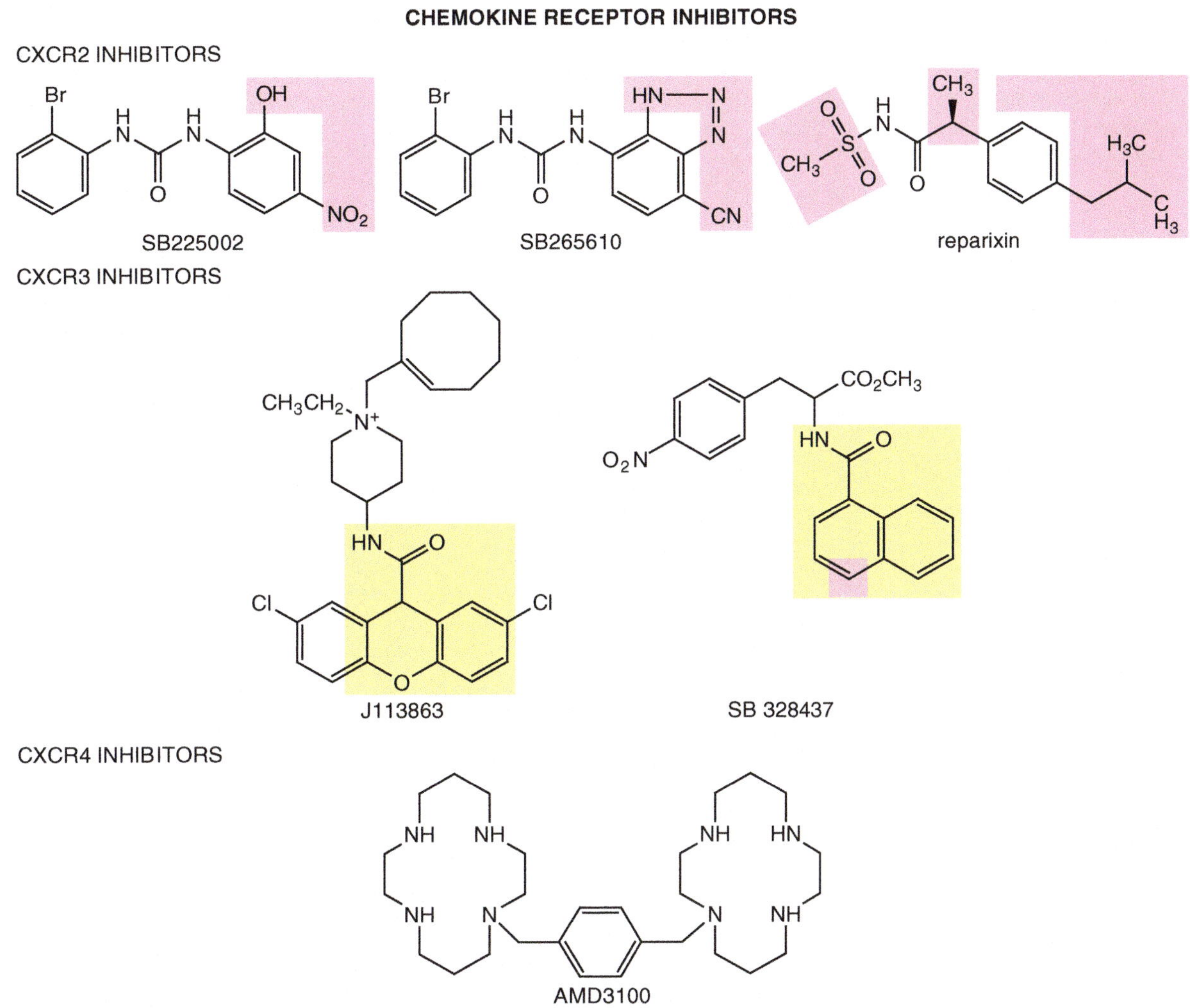

Fig. 5.4 Structures of Chemokine Receptor inhibitors. 3 Chemokine Receptors serve as confirmed drug targets, CXCR2, CXCR3, and CXCR4. The structural differences among the CXCR2 inhibitors are highlighted in *pink*. The shared motif of CXCR3 inhibitors is shown in *yellow*, with a difference in 1 oxygen (*pink*)

5.5 TGF-β Inhibitors

Transforming Growth Factor β (TGF-β) is implicated in the progression of late stage tumors through pro-metastatic activity and immune suppression[5]. The cytokine has a role in the conversion of early stage epithelial tumors to invasive tumors by promoting epithelial-to-mesenchymal transition (EMT)[6]. In breast cancer, TGF-β may synergize with ERBB2 to promote progression.

Ligands of the TGF-β family (TGF-β1, -β2 or -β3) exert their effects through type I and the type II serine/threonine kinases, which form a heteromeric signaling complex upon ligation. Type I receptors are referred to as Activin Receptor-Like Kinases (ALKs), while the type II receptors are named for the ligands they bind. Signaling procedes via SMAD2/SMAD3 phosphorylation. The inhibition of the TGF-β signaling pathway with selective agents is intended to abrogate tumor-stroma interactions, thus preventing invasion and metastasis.

The TGF-β_2 specific 18-mer phosphorothioate antisense oligonucleotide AP12009, which contains neither G-4 tracts nor CpG motifs, decreases TGF-β_2 secretion from various types of cancer cells. AP12009 was developed for the intravenous treatment of pancreatic carcinoma and malignant melanoma. It is under study for the treatment of malignant glioma, where it is directly infused into the tumor.

[5] TGF-β up-regulates the production of regulatory T-cells and down-regulates the responsiveness of cytotoxic T-lymphocytes, leading to compromised immune capability.

[6] In epithelial-mesenchymal transition (EMT), epithelial cells lose their cell polarity and cell-cell adhesion, and gain migratory and invasive properties that are typical of mesenchymal stem cells.

Fig. 5.5 Structures of TGFβ inhibitors. The loosely conserved motif of 6-ring, 5-ring, 6-ring is shaded in *light yellow*. (note the differing positions of the nitrogen hetero-atoms)

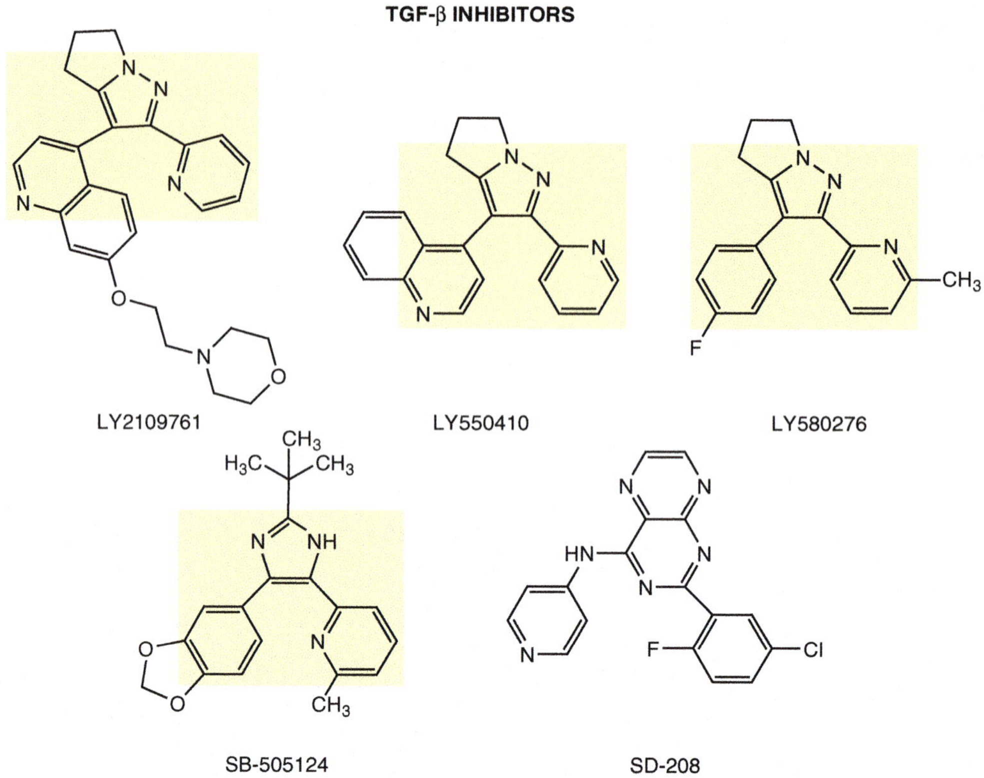

- The related antisense oligonucleotide AP11014 targets TGF-β_1.

Adverse Effects The application of AP12009 as continuous intracerebral infusion results in reversible lymphocytic leptomeningo-encephalitis, which reflects an immunological reaction to AP12009.

Fresolimumab (GC1008) is a pan-neutralizing IgG$_4$ human antibody directed against all 3 isoforms of TGF-β. Metastatic melanoma and renal cell carcinoma are under investigation as possible targets for anti-TGF-β therapy.

Lerdelimumab (CAT-152) <Trabio> is a recombinant human IgG$_4$ anti-TGF-β_2 monoclonal antibody derived from phage display. It neutralizes TGF-β2 and TGF-β3 at low nanomolar concentrations, while showing no binding to TGF-β1.

The human IgG$_4$ metelimumab (CAT-192) targets TGF-β_1. Its use in cancer treatment has not been determined.

The signaling of TGF-β through the receptor kinase TGF-βRI (ALK5) has opened the possibility to design small molecule kinase inhibitors as suppressors of TGF-β signaling. Molecules in this class (Fig. 5.5) have common features. The small molecule ATP-competitive compounds LY550410, LY580276 and SB-505124 each contain a different set of heteroaryl rings appended from a central heterocyclic scaffold. Generally, the most essential functionality of TGF-βRI inhibitors consists of a warhead group that contains an adequate hydrogen bond acceptor (4-fluorophenyl in LY580276, quinoline in LY550410) and forms a specific hydrogen bond to the ATP binding site backbone (N-H of histidine 283). LY550410 and LY580276 bind to the conformationally active T204D mutant of the TGF-βRI kinase domain.

The dihydropyrrolopyrazole LY2109761 is a small molecule inhibitor of the receptor serine/threonine kinases TGF-βRI and II. Treatment with LY2109761 completely prevents TGF-β induced SMAD2 phosphorylation. It has only a small effect on ERK-1 or -2 phosphorylation and no effect at all on the JNK pathway.

SB-505124 is an imidazole based structure derived from a series of P38 MAP Kinase inhibitors. It also inhibits ALK4 (which results in modulation of the Activin dependent activation of SMAD2 and SMAD3) and ALK7, but not ALK2. The drug suppresses the TGF-β stimulated activation of MAP Kinase pathways.

SD-208 (2-(5-Chloro-2-fluorophenyl)-4-[(4-pyridyl) amino]pteridine) is an orally active, ATP competitive TGF-β Receptor I kinase inhibitor that displays high selectivity over TGF-βRII and other common kinases. The drug blocks the TGF-β induction of SMAD3 phosphorylation, SMAD3/4 specific transcription, expression of the TGF-β target genes *pthrp*, *il-11*, *ctgf*, and *runx2*. SD-208 exhibits anti-inflammatory and anti-tumor activity, reduces the development and progression of melanoma bone metastases, and suppresses the invasiveness of glioma cells.

> *TGF β inhibitors may act through suppression of TGF β secretion (antisense drug), receptor blockage (neutralizing antibodies), or suppression of receptor kinase activity (small molecule kinase inhibitors).*

5.6 Bone Targeting Agents

Cancer in bones can cause pain, fractures, hypercalcemia, and nerve/spinal cord compression. The pathophysiology of bone metastases includes increased bone turnover, imbalance and uncoupling of the processes of resorption and remodeling. Osteoclastic metastases are characterized by an erosion of bone due to excess osteoclast activity, while osteoblastic metastases have bone deposits due to excess osteoblast activity. Historically, the management of symptomatic bone disease has depended on analgesics, radio-therapy, endocrine therapy, and chemotherapy. Despite these treatments, progressive skeletal destruction has frequently led to ongoing symptoms and deterioration of the quality of life.

5.6.1 Bisphosphonates

Bisphosphonates (diphosphonates) are synthetic analogs of pyrophosphate, which have 2 phosphonate (PO_3) groups (Fig. 5.6). They were developed in the nineteenth century for the non-medical use to soften water in irrigation systems used in orange groves. These compounds were first studied in the 1960s for the use in disorders of bone metabolism. An indication is the treatment of hypercalcemia in patients with malignancies and bone metastasis. Bisphosphonates act primarily by reducing the activity of osteoclasts. When cancer has spread to the bones, the inclusion of bisphosphonate drugs in the anti-cancer treatment can reduce pain, fractures and other bone problems. In multiple myeloma, they improve the quality of life by reducing the number of and time to skeletal events. In advanced breast cancer and clinically evident bone metastases, these drugs reduce the risk of developing a skeletal event by about 15%. However, treatment with bisphosphonates may not affect survival in women with advanced breast cancer (Pavlakis et al. 2005).

Adverse Effects Adverse effects of bisphosphonates include mild gut reactions, transient fever, and hypocalcemia. The intensity of these symptoms may vary among individual representatives of this drug class. Oral bisphosphonates can cause serious esophagitis in some users, however, they do not increase the risk for esophageal or gastric cancer. Infusion of bisphosphonates causes a substantial increase in the number of γδ T-lymphocytes over a month, leading to an influenza-like acute phase reaction. Atypical, low energy or low trauma fractures of the femoral shaft may occur in bisphosphonate treated patients. They can be

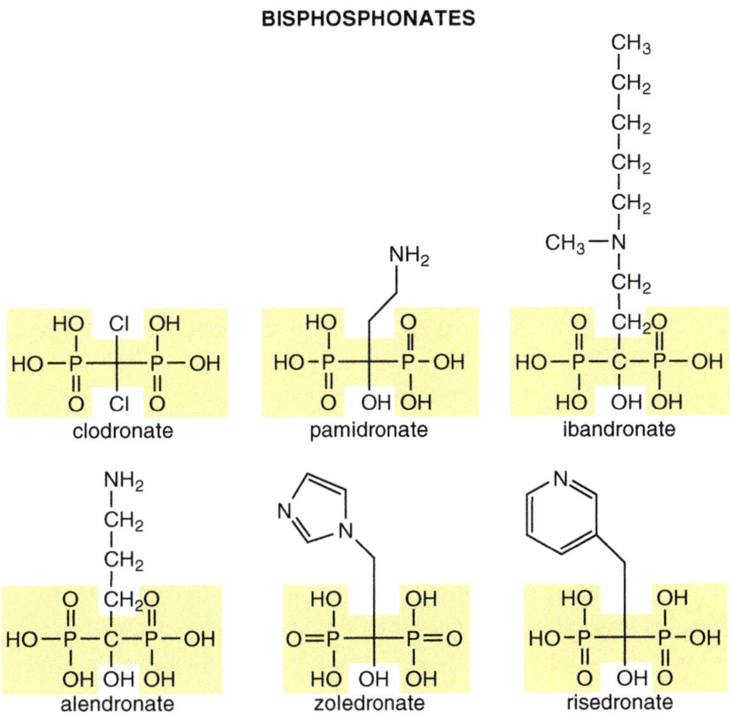

Fig. 5.6 A structures of bisphosphonates. The common bisphosphonate moiety is highlighted in *yellow*

located anywhere in the femoral shaft from just below the lesser trochanter to above the supracondylar flare.

Since 2003, bisphosphonate associated osteo-necrosis has become an increasing problem associated with long term intravenous bisphosphonates. The pathogenesis of bone necrosis of the jaws may be associated with defects in vascularization. The pharmacological activity of bisphosphonates is exerted through the inhibition of osteoclastic function, which leads a reduction of bone vascularization. The most common predisposing factors for the development of bisphosphonate associated osteonecrosis of the jaw may be the type and total dose of bisphosphonate, a history of dental surgery (such as tooth extraction), dental trauma or dental infection—with half of all reported cases (60 %) occurring after dentoalveolar surgery (such as tooth extraction) to treat infections (Woo et al. 2006). The vast majority of patients with osteonecrosis have received the amino-bisphosphonates pamidronate or zoledronate with a median duration of drug use of 20–40 months. The cumulative hazard appears to increase with time and is higher for zolendronate than pamidronate. It is recommended that patients obtain baseline dental review prior to bisphosphonate treatment to identify and treat oral infections that could lead to the subsequent need for dental surgery and to maintain regular dental review.

Clodronate disodium ((dichloro-phosphono-methyl)phosphonic acid) <Bonefos, Loron, Clodron> is the salt of a nitrogen-free bisphosphonate analog of naturally occurring pyrophosphate. Clodronate binds to calcium. It inhibits osteoclastic bone resorption as well as hydroxyapatite crystal formation and dissolution, resulting in a reduction of bone turnover. The drug also acts as a competitive inhibitor of Adenine Nucleotide Transferase (ANT, one of the components of the mitochondrial permeability transition pore), leading to the reduction of mitochondrial oxygen consumption, dissipation of the mitochondrial membrane potential and apoptosis. Clodronate may control malignancy associated hypercalcemia, inhibit osteolytic bone metastasis, and decrease pain. 1600 mg oral clodronate, taken daily in addition to chemotherapy or hormone therapy, is effective in reducing the incidence and rate of skeletal events, and delaying skeletal events in women with advanced breast cancer and clinically evident bone metastases. It may also reduce bone pain in women with clinically evident bone metastases and may decrease the rate of skeletal events but not the incidence of skeletal events in women with advanced breast cancer without clinically evident bone metastases. In women with early breast cancer, adjuvant oral clodronate does not significantly reduce the risk of developing skeletal or visceral metastases (Pavlakis et al. 2005).

Adverse Effects Mild gastrointestinal toxicity is the most frequent adverse effect of oral clodronate. Gastrointestinal events are more frequent with oral administration, while acute phase reactions are more frequent after i.v. administration. Nausea can arise.

Pamidronate disodium (APD) <Aredia> is the salt of a synthetic bisphosphonate. The drug may adsorb to calcium phosphate crystals in bone, blocking their dissolution by inhibiting osteoclast mediated bone resorption. It does not inhibit bone mineralization and formation. Intravenous pamidronate (90 mg every 3–4 weeks) delays the time to a skeletal event, reduces the rate of skeletal events, and significantly reduces the risk for developing a skeletal event.

Adverse Effects Fever and asymptomatic hypocalcemia are the most common adverse effects in women receiving intravenous pamidronate. Nausea and vomiting may be a cause for withdrawal from therapy. Phlebitis or renal impairment may occur. Oral administration is hampered by toxicity.

Ibandronate sodium <Boniva, Bondronat, Bonviva> is the sodium salt of ibandronic acid, a synthetic nitrogen-containing bisphosphonate. Ibandronate inhibits Farnesyl Pyrophosphate Synthase, resulting in a reduction in Geranylgeranyl GTPase signaling proteins and apoptosis of osteoclasts. This agent increases bone mineral density, decreases bone remodeling, inhibits osteoclast mediated bone resorption, and reduces bone pain related to metastases or corticosteroids. It reduces the risk for vertebral, but not non-vertebral fracture. Intravenous or oral ibandronate treatment leads to improved global quality of life in women with breast cancer. Intravenous administration (6 mg every 3–4 weeks) delays the time to a skeletal event. Oral administration 50 mg daily), in addition to chemotherapy or hormone therapy, is effective in reducing bone pain and improving global quality of life. It also may delay the time to skeletal events and may diminish the likelihood of developing a new skeletal event.

Adverse Effects An influenza-like syndrome and arthralgia may occur after intravenous application. At high oral doses, gastrointestinal toxicity (dyspepsia, nausea, esphagitis) and hypocalcemia can be caused.

Alendronate sodium <Fosamax> is the salt of a second generation bisphosphonate and a synthetic analog of pyrophosphate. The drug has anti-resorption activity. It binds to and inhibits the activity of Farnesyl Pyrophosphate Synthase (Farensyl Diphosphate Synthase, Geranyl Transtransferase). Inhibition of this enzyme prevents the formation of isoprenoid lipids[7] that are donor substrates of farnesylation and geranylgeranylation during the post-translational modification of small GTPase signaling proteins, which is important in osteoclast activity. As a result, bone resorption and turnover

[7] The isoprenoid lipids (terpenoids) comprise farnesyl pyrophosphate (FPP) and geranyl-geranyl pyrophosphate (GGPP).

are suppressed. Alendronate can reduce the risk for vertebrate and non-vertebrate fractures in patients.

Pharmacokinetics The systemic bioavailability after oral dosing is below 1 %. Intake together with meals and beverages other than water further reduces the bioavailability. The drug rapidly partitions, with approximately 50 % binding to the exposed bone surface and the remainder being excreted unchanged by the kidneys. Due to the strong negative charge on the 2 phosphonate moieties, the exposure to tissues other than bone is very low. After absorption in the bone, alendronate has an estimated terminal half-life of 10 years.

Adverse Effects Ulcerations of the esophagus, skin rashes, and osteo-necrosis of the jaw are potential adverse effects. Aledronate use constitutes a risk factor for atrial fibrillation in women. Rare instances of auditory hallucinations and visual disturbances may be associated with the drug.

The third generation bisphosphonate Zoledronate <Zometa, Zomera, Aclasta, Reclast> is a synthetic imidazole bisphosphonate analog of pyrophosphate. The bone resorption inhibiting activity contributes to the analgesic properties for painful osteoblastic lesions.

- Zoledronate binds to hydroxyapatite crystals in the bone matrix, slowing their dissolution, and inhibiting the formation and aggregation of these crystals.
- Zolendronate inhibits Farnesyl Pyrophosphate Synthase, thereby preventing protein prenylation within the mevalonate pathway. This leads to the loss of downstream metabolites essential for osteoclast function and induces apoptosis, ultimately resulting in cell death. The inhibitory effects on osteoclast mediated bone resorption result in decreased bone turnover and stabilization of the bone matrix.

The drug is indicated for the treatment of multiple myeloma and of bone metastases from solid tumors (in conjunction with standard anti-neoplastic therapy). It is given intravenously at 4 mg every 3–4 weeks. Zolendronate can treat hyper-calcemia of malignancy, defined as Albumin-corrected calcium (Ca_{ac}) of ≥ 12 mg/dL[8].

Pharmacokinetics Zoledronate is approximately 20 % bound to plasma proteins. The drug does not inhibit microsomal CYP450 enzymes, and is not metabolized. It is excreted into the urine as the intact drug.

Adverse Effects Bone pain flare, fever, nausea, vomiting, constipation, diarrhea, and myalgias are the most common adverse effects. Although renal impairment occurs only in a fraction of patients, dose related and infusion time related renal toxicity is the main problem with intravenous zolendronate. The agent constitutes a risk factor for atrial fibrillation in women. Rarely, allergic reactions can arise with intravenous zoledronic acid, including angioedema and bronchoconstriction. The drug is Pregnancy Category D.

Drug Interactions Aminoglycosides and loop diuretics may have an additive effect to lower blood calcium level for prolonged periods and need to be applied with caution. Caution is also indicated when zolendronate is used with other potentially nephrotoxic drugs.

Risedronate sodium <Actonel> is a salt of a synthetic pyridinyl bisphosphonate. Risedronate binds to hydroxyapatite crystals in the bone and inhibits osteoclast dependent bone resorption. The drug is indicated for the treatment of Paget disease of the bone in men and women.

Pharmacokinetics Due to limited oral bioavailability (less than 1 % of the drug is absorbed within 1 h), risedronate should be taken at least 30 min before the first food or drink of the day other than water. Plasma protein binding of the drug is about 25 %. Risedronate is not metabolized and does not induce or inhibit microsomal drug metabolizing enzymes. It is excreted in the urine, and is not recommended for use in patients with severe renal impairment.

Adverse Effects Gastrointestinal irritation, musculo-skeletal pain, and osteo-necrosis of the jaw are potential adverse effects. Adequate intake of calcium and vitamin D is important in all patients, especially in patients with Paget disease, in whom bone turnover is substantially elevated. The drug is Pregnancy Category C.

Drug Interactions Co-administration of calcium, antacids, or oral medications containing divalent cations interferes with the absorption of risedronate.

Bisphosphonates suppress bone metastasis via binding to hydroxyapatite crystals and inhibiting osteoclast activity.
Oral bioavailability is low, bisphosphonates are not metabolized and are excreted in the urine.
Adverse class effects of bisphosphonates include gastrointestinal reactions, transient fever, hypocalcemia, musculo-skeletal pain, and osteo-necrosis of the jaw.
Oral bisphosphonates can cause serious esophagitis in some users.

5.6.2 Antibodies

Bone remodeling is the process that removes old material from the bone and adds new bone. It is driven most notably by osteoblasts, which produce new bone, and osteoclasts, which break down bone. The cytokine RANKL (Receptor Activator of Nuclear Factor-κB Ligand, TNFSF11, Osteoprotegerin Ligand, Osteoclast Differentiation Factor) is

---

[8] The formula is: Ca_{ac} [mg/dL] = Ca_{total} · [mg/dL] + 0.8. · (4.0 [g/dL] − Albumin [g/dL]).

a protein of the Tumor Necrosis Factor family that is expressed by osteoblastic cells and plays an important role in osteoclastic differentiation and activation.

Denosumab (AMG162) <Xgeva, Prolia> is a fully human monoclonal IgG_2 antibody with anti-osteoclast activity. Denosumab specifically binds to RANKL and blocks its interaction with the receptor RANK on osteoclast cell surfaces. This blockage results in an inhibition of osteoclast activity, a decrease in bone resorption, and a potential increase in bone mineral density. Denusomab is indicated as a treatment to increase bone mass

- in men at high risk for fracture receiving androgen deprivation therapy for non-metastatic prostate cancer
- in women at high risk for fracture receiving adjuvant aromatase inhibitor therapy for breast cancer.

The drug is administered by subcutaneous injection.

Pharmacokinetics The antibody is metabolized by proteolysis. No dose adjustment is necessary in patients with renal impairment.

Adverse Effects The most common adverse effects include potentially serious infections of the urinary and respiratory tract. There may be increased rates of eczema, infections of the skin, and rashes (concomitant treatment with immunosuppressants increases this risk). Osteonecrosis of the jaw is generally associated with tooth extraction or local infection followed by delayed healing. Back pain, pain in the extremities, musculoskeletal pain, hypercholesterolemia, cataract, constipation, rashes, pancreatitis, and endocarditis are possible. Hypocalcemia is a contraindication for denusomab treatment, and pre-existing hypocalcemia must be corrected prior to treatment. The drug is Pregnancy Category C.

As a poly-hormone with diverse biological roles, Parathyroid Hormone-Related Protein (PTHrP) is expressed by healthy tissues, acting in local micro-environments. It is commonly over-expressed by breast and prostate cancers, acting systemically by promoting bone resorption, inhibiting calcium excretion from the kidney, and inducing hypercalcemia. Thus, it has a possible role in the formation of bone metastases.

Monoclonal antibody CAL is a humanized monoclonal antibody directed against PTHrP. By blocking the effects of PTHrP on calcium metabolism, monoclonal antibody CAL may inhibit cancer related hypercalcemia and bone colonization.

5.6.3 Others

Cathepsin K is a lysosomal cysteine protease that is expressed by osteoclasts during the process of bone resorption. It acts as the major Collagenase responsible for the degradation of the organic bone matrix during the remodeling process. Because excessive bone remodeling is a key element in the pathogenesis of skeletal disorders, cathepsin K is a potential target for therapeutic intervention.

Cathepsin inhibitors are in clinical trials. Odanacatib (MK-0822, MK-822) is an orally administered Cathepsin K inhibitor. Weekly doses of odanacatib increase bone mineral density.

Systemic treatment of bone metastases can be attempted with radio-pharmaceuticals (see Sect. 13.2.). These types of drugs may be used to deliver radiation to many bones at once. However, they are limited by the cancer non-specific action of radiation.

5.7 Others

To metastasize, tumor cells take advantage of proteases to invade and remodel surrounding tissues. The 3-amidinophenylalanine based synthetic small molecule WX-UK1 (*Nα*-(2,-4,6-triisopropylphenylsulfonyl)-3-amidino-(L)-phenylalanine-4-ethoxycarbonylpiperazide) is an intravenously applied inhibitor of uPA (Urokinase-Type Plasminogen Activator) and other serine proteases. WX-UK1 inhibits tumor invasion and thus blocks the metastatic process. The compound was designed for the treatment of patients with breast, gastric, ovarian, colon, and pancreatic cancers. In clinical trials, it has been well tolerated.

- Upamostat (mesupron) (WX-671) is an orally bioavailable prodrug that is metabolized to the active WX-UK1.

Proteoglycans are complex glycoconjugates that regulate critical biological pathways. Bikunin, with a single glycosaminoglycan chain the simplest proteoglycan, is a Kunitz-type protease inhibitor. Bikunin, down-regulates the expression of *upa* and its receptor *upar* at the mRNA and protein levels in various types of tumor cells. Daily oral administration of bikunin is under study in clinical trials against ovarian carcinoma.

Prostacyclin (PGI_2), which may be synthesized by endothelial cells, is an eicosanoid with anti-inflammatory and anti-metastatic properties. Iloprost is a prostacyclin analog with potential chemopreventive activity against cancer cell dissemination. Iloprost binds to the Prostacyclin Receptor in various target cells, thereby causing vasodilation, inhibition of platelet aggregation, and decreased tumor cell adhesion to endothelium.

β-Adrenergic Receptors are G-Protein Coupled Receptors that activate Adenylate Cyclase to elevate intracellular 3',5'-cyclic adenosine monophosphate (cAMP) and activate Protein Kinase A. β-Adrenergic Receptor signaling is involved in the pathogenesis of various cancer metastases.

Inhibiting β_2-adrenergic signaling can reduce cancer progression and mortality. The commonly prescribed class of β-Adrenergic Receptor antagonist drugs (β-blockers) may favorably impact the progression of breast cancer, prostate cancer, or melanoma because there is a potential role for targeting this pathway. Non-selective blockers, such as propranolol and nadolol, are under consideration in future use.

References

Alpaugh ML, Lee MC, Nguyen M, Deato M, Dishakjian L, Barsky SH (2000) Myoepithelial-specific CD44 shedding contributes to the anti-invasive and antiangiogenic phenotype of myoepithelial cells. Exp Cell Res 25:150–158

Bazil V, Horejsi V (1992) Shedding of the CD44 adhesion molecule from leukocytes induced by anti-CD44 monoclonal antibody simulating the effect of a natural receptor ligand. J Immunol 149:747–753

Grams F, Brandstetter H, D'Alò S, Geppert D, Krell HW, Leinert H, Livi V, Menta E, Oliva A, Zimmermann G, Gram F, Brandstetter H, D'Alò S, Geppert D, Krell HW, Leinert H, Livi V, Menta E, Oliva A, Zimmermann G (2001) Pyrimidine-2,4,6-triones: a new effective and selective class of matrix metalloproteinase inhibitors. Biol Chem 382:1277–1285

Kawano Y, Okamoto I, Murakami D, Itoh H, Yoshida M, Ueda S, Saya H (2000) Ras oncoprotein induces CD44 cleavage through phosphoinositide 3-OH kinase and the rho family of small G proteins. J Biol Chem 275:29628–29635

Lee MC, Alpaugh ML, Nguyen M, Deato M, Dishakjian L, Barsky SH (2000) Myoepithelial-specific CD44 shedding is mediated by a putative chymotrypsin-like sheddase. Biochem Biophys Res Commun 279:116–123

Pavlakis N, Schmidt RL, Stockler MR (2005) Bisphosphonates for breast cancer (Review). The Cochrane Collaboration. Wiley. doi:10.1002/14651858.CD003474.pub2

Peterson RM, Yu Q, Stamenkovic I, Toole BP (2000) Perturbation of hyaluronan interactions by soluble CD44 inhibits growth of murine mammary carcinoma cells in ascites. Am J Pathol 256:2159–2167

Seiter S, Arch R, Reber S, Komitowski D, Hofmann M, Ponta H, Herrlich P, Matzku S, Zoeller M (1993) Prevention of tumor metastasis formation by anti-variant CD44. J Exp Med 177:443–455

Tucker G (2006) Integrins: molecular targets in cancer therapy. Curr Oncol Rep 8:96–103

Woo SB, Hellstein JW, Kalmar JR (2006) Systematic review: bisphosphonates and osteonecrosis of the jaws. Ann Intern Med 144:753–761

6 Induction of Senescence

Sencescence is an essential mechanism to protect from excessive tissue proliferation. After about 50 population doublings, somatic cells enter irreversible cell cycle arrest. During cell division, the ends of chromosomes (telomeres) cannot be fully reduplicated and, in the absence of a mechanism for maintaining telomere length, erode 50–100 bases per cell division. The telomere shortening with every cell division reflects the history of population doublings. In addition, chromosome shortening may be caused by single strand breaks derived from oxidative stress (accumulation of reactive oxygen metabolites). Senescence is overcome in cancer cells.

6.1 Telomerase Inhibitors

The ends of the chromosomes have specialized, non-coding DNA sequences that together with their associated proteins constitute the telomeres. The telomere sequences contain variable numbers of the nucleotide repeats TTAGGG. These have developed to protect the chromosome ends from being recognized by the harboring cell as sites of DNA breakage. Because telomeres protect the gene encoding regions of the chromosomes they are essential for maintaining the stability of the genome.

Maintenance of the telomeres depends on the enzyme complex Telomerase, which is activated in more than 80% of cancer cells, but is absent from most healthy cells[1]. Therefore, targeting Telomerase in drug treatment has the potential to be very cancer-specific. The immediate outcome of Telomerase inhibition is to halt telomere extension, leading to progressive chromosome shortening, until eventually the critically short length is reached that leads to senescence. For cells with telomeres of an average length of 5 kb, about 50 rounds of reduplication need to occur before the onset of senescence and subsequent apoptosis, if the telomeres must be completely eroded before an effect is achieved. This implies an extensive lag time before the positive effects of a Telomerase inhibitor can occur. Hence, anti-Telomerase drugs may be of benefit predominantly in tumor cells that have short telomeres, and as a second-line therapy after tumor debulking (Neidle and Parkinson 2002). The principal approaches that are being pursued for the inhibition of Telomerase action involve

- targeting the RNA domain template, often with an antisense approach
- inhibiting the catalytic site of Reverse Transcriptase activity
- interacting with the telomeric DNA template.

6.1.1 Non-Nucleoside Telomerase Inhibitors

For non-nucleoside Telomerase inhibitors, the emphasis is on G-quadruplex interacting ligands, which generally have planar aromatic chromophores.

BIBR1532 is a non-nucleoside Telomerase inhibitor with a nanomolar effective concentration. This compound produces progressive telomere shortening from 4 to 1.5 kb over a period of 140 population doublings, a loss of 30 base pairs per round of reduplication, resulting in the appearance of a senescent phenotype in treated cells.

The distamycin derivative MEN 10716 is a minor groove DNA binding antibiotic (see Sect. 2.2.2.). After prolonged exposure, the drug also acts as a Telomerase inhibitor.

6.1.2 Antisense Telomerase Inhibitors

The Telomerase template antagonist GRN163L is a synthetic, lipid conjugated 13-mer oligonucleotide *N3'P5'*-thiophosphoramidate. Being complementary to the template region of *telomerase* RNA, GRN163L acts as a competitive inhibitor that binds and blocks the active site of the enzyme Telomerase. The inhibition of Telomerase expression by GRN163L results in telomere shortening, which leads to cell

[1] Germ line cells and stem cells typically have active Telomerase.

G. F. Weber, *Molecular Therapies of Cancer*, DOI 10.1007/978-3-319-13278-5_6,

cycle arrest or apoptosis. GRN163L has anti-tumor activity predominantly targets tumor stem cells.

6.1.3 G-quadruplex Ligands

Almost all of several 100 DNA quadruplex ligands that have been discovered so far share the common structural feature of an extended planar aromatic chromophore. Anthraquinone compounds inhibit the activity of Telomerase (Sun et al. 1997). These compounds can have selectivity for specific types of DNA structure and they can interact with quadruplex DNA.

BR-ACO-19 (9-[4-(*N*, *N*-dimethylamino)phenylamino]-3,6-bis(3-pyrrolodino-propionamido)acridine) is a 3,6,9-trisubstituted acridine compound that causes hTERT (Telomerase Reverse Transcriptase, the catalytic subunit of the enzyme Telomerase) to be bound to Ubiquitin and targeted for proteasomal degradation. It induces the single stranded G-rich overhang at telomere 3' ends to fold into 4-stranded quadruplex complexes. Formation of a quadruplex DNA structure is incompatible with Telomerase attachment to the 3' end. Therefore, potent quadruplex binding ligands produce telomere shortening and senescence in cancer cells. BR-ACO-19 is highly water soluble but poorly penetrates through cell membranes, which is its main pharmacokinetic limitation.

Screening of the metabolites of the micro-organism Streptomyces anulatus identified the 8-ring cyclic molecule telomestatin (Shin-ya et al. 2001) as a Telomerase inhibitor. Telomestatin inhibits Telomerase by binding to G-quadruplex forming sequences. It also inhibits POT1 binding to the telomeric overhang. These functions inhibit reduplication and induce the senescence of cancer cells. Telomestatin suppresses the proliferation of Telomerase positive cells at non-cytotoxic concentrations.

The telomere associated proteins TRF1, TRF2, and POT1 are important regulators of Telomerase activity that might represent potential targets against cancer. However, these telomere associated proteins have limited tumor cell specificity.

References

Neidle S, Parkinson G (2002) Telomere maintenance as a target for anticancer drug discovery. Nat Rev Drug Discov 1:383–393

Shin-ya K, Wierzba K, Matsuo K, Ohtani T, Yamada Y, Furihata K, Hayakawa Y, Seto H (2001) Telomestatin, a novel telomerase inhibitor from Streptomyces anulatus. J Am Chem Soc 123:1262–1263

Sun D, Thompson B, Cathers BE, Salazar M, Kerwin SM, Trent JO, Jenkins TC, Neidle S, Hurley LH (1997) Inhibition of human telomerase by a G-quadruplex-interactive compound. J Med Chem 40:2113–2116

7 Combination Chemotherapy

The often adverse effects of conventional chemotherapy were diminished when it was realized that these agents could be effectively used in combination (Frei et al. 1958, 1965). This approach conceptually followed the strategy of antibiotic therapy for tuberculosis, which used combinations of drugs with different mechanisms of action. The rationales for combination chemotherapy are

- to use drugs that work by distinct mechanisms of action, thereby decreasing the likelihood that resistant cancer cells will develop.
- to reduce the incidence of severe adverse effects when drugs with different properties are combined.

Frei, Freireich, and Holland simultaneously administered 6-mercaptopurine <Purinethol>, vincristine <Oncovin>, methotrexate, and prednisone (together referred to as the POMP regimen) and induced long term remissions in children with acute lymphoblastic leukemia (ALL).

The realization of this concept was extended to lymphomata in 1963 by Vincent T. DeVita and George Canellos at the U.S. National Cancer Institute, who later demonstrated that the MOPP regimen consisting of nitrogen mustard, vincristine <Oncovin>, procarbazine and prednisone could cure patients with Hodgkin and non-Hodgkin lymphoma. Currently, nearly all successful cancer chemotherapy regimens use the strategy of administering multiple drugs simultaneously.

A desirable combination regimen may consist of agents with distinct mechanisms of action, that are not subject to cross-resistance, and have adverse event profiles that do not overlap. Synergistic or additive effects should reach beyond the single agent activities. It is not advisable to combine, simultaneously or sequentially, cancer chemotherapeutic modalities that have the same mechanism of action.

Induction regimen refers to a chemotherapy that is used for the initial treatment of a disease. Maintenance regimen refers to a protocol given after the cancer growth has been arrested by prior chemotherapy treatments.

7.1 Treatment of Hematologic Malignancies

7.1.1 Vincristine and Prednisone Based Regimens

POMP (Table 7.1) is comprised of 6-mercaptopurine <Purinethol>, vincristine sulfate <Oncovin>, methotrexate, and prednisone. It is used for the treatment of ALL, where it achieves about 90 % remissions. POMP may also be used in adult AML for remission induction and maintenance. It achieves a response rate of 50 % and a complete remission rate of 40 %. For responding patients, the median survival time is increased by several months. Age and previous therapy are major factors influencing responsiveness.

Adverse Effects Adverse effects include myelosuppression, liver function abnormalities, minor gastrointestinal intolerance, and paresthesias.

The combination chemotherapy regimen MOMP (nitrogen mustard, vincristine <Oncovin>, methotrexate, and prednisone) was the first to achieve substantial remission rates in advanced Hodgkin disease. It was later replaced with the MOPP regimen, comprising mechlorethamine, vincristine <Oncovin>, procarbazine, and prednisone, which can lead to remission in almost 70 % of patients with advanced stage Hodgkin lymphoma. Unlike the stepwise increase in remission duration achieved in childhood acute leukemia, about 60 % of patients with advanced Hodgkin disease who attained a complete remission in the original MOPP study never relapsed with follow-up into the 40th year (DeVita and Chu 2008).

Adverse Effects The toxicity of MOPP is substantial. Frequent adverse effects include bone marrow suppression, nerve damage caused by vincristine, and allergic reactions to procarbazine. Long term effects include infertility. MOPP chemotherapy used to treat Hodgkin lymphoma inhibits close to 90 % of sperm function in men. There is a 15-fold increased risk of developing treatment related myelodysplasia or acute leukemia. These secondary hematologic malig-

G. F. Weber, Molecular *Therapies of Cancer,* DOI 10.1007/978-3-319-13278-5_7,

Table 7.1 Vincristine and prednisone based combination chemotherapy

	Vincristine	Prednisone	Procarba-zine	Cyclophos-phamide	Chloram-bucil	Nitrogen mustard	Mitoxan-trone	Mechlor-ethamine	Metho-trexate	6-Mercap-topurine	Cytarabine	Bleomycin	Etoposide	Doxorubi-cin
POMP	+	+							+	+				
MOMP	+	+				+			+					
MOPP	+	+	+					+						
MVPP	+ (vinblastine)	+	+					+						
ChlVPP	+	+	+		+									
COPP	+	+	+	+										
BEACOPP	+	+	+	+								+	+	+
VAPEC-B	+	+		+								+	+	+
PMit-CEBO	+	+		+			+					+	+	
CHOP	+	+		+										+
COAP	+	+		+							+			

nancies peak at 5–9 years after treatment for Hodgkin lymphoma and are associated with a very poor prognosis.

The long-term adverse effects of sterility (especially in males) and myelodysplasia are most likely due to alkylating agent toxicity and are not likely to be ameliorated by the common MOPP variants, such as MVPP (mechlorethamine, vinblastine, procarbazine, prednisone), ChlVPP, and COPP.

ChlVPP (chlorambucil, vinblastine, procarbazine, prednisolone) was devised by the substitution of chlorambucil for nitrogen mustard and vinblastine for vincristine to improve the tolerability of the MOPP regimen. Vinblastine is administered as an infusion on day 1, the other drugs are given as tablets or capsules over a 2-week course. This is followed by a rest period of 2 weeks. Usually 4–6 cycles are given over a period of 4–6 months. Hodgkin lymphoma may be treated with ChlVPP.

Adverse Effects ChlVPP has relieved many of the MOPP toxicities, but not myelosuppression with ensuing risks for infections (leucopenia), bleeding (thrombocytopenia), and fatigue (anemia). Other adverse effects include hair loss, sore mouth, taste changes, stomach ulcers, weight gain, peripheral neuropathy, and fluid retention.

COPP comprises cyclophosphamide (650 mg/m^2 intravenously on days 1 and 8), vincristine <Oncovin> (1.4 mg/m^2 intravenously on days 1 and 8), procarbazine (100 mg/m^2 orally on days 1–14), and prednisone (40 mg/m^2 orally on days 1–14). The cycle is repeated every 28 days. COPP is used for the treatment of advanced T-cell and B-cell lymphomata.

- BEACOPP comprises bleomycin (10 mg/m^2 intravenously on day 8), etoposide (100 mg/m^2 intravenously on days 1–3), adriamycin (25 mg/m^2 intravenously on day 1), cyclophosphamide (650 mg/m^2 intravenously on day 1), vincristine <Oncovin> (1.4 mg/m^2 intravenously on day 8), procarbazine (100 mg/m^2 orally on days 1–7), and prednisone (40 mg/m^2 orally on days 1–14). It is a chemotherapy regimen for the treatment of advanced Hodgkin lymphoma. Patients typically receive the drugs in cycles of 21 days, which include a rest phase on days 15–21. A more intensive variant of the regimen has cycles of 14 days. Usually a therapy consists of 6–8 cycles.

Adverse Effects BEACOPP may induce secondary neoplasias, such as leukemias. Because of myelosuppression, BEACOPP requires G-CSF support.

VAPEC-B is a combination chemotherapy protocol containing vincristine, doxorubicin <Adriamycin>, prednisolone, etoposide, cyclophosphamide, and bleomycin. Vincristine, doxorubicin, and cyclophosphamide are administered by infusion, etoposide and prednisolone are taken as tablets. On day 1, doxorubicin and cyclophosphamide are given. On day 8, vincristine and bleomycin follow. On day 15, there is doxorubicin and the start of a 4-day course of etoposide capsules. The cycle is completed with vincristine on day 22. Usually, a course of treatment comprises 3 cycles of 4 weeks over a period of 12 weeks. The regimen is used for the treatment of Hodgkin lymphoma and non-Hodgkin lymphoma.

Drug Interactions Reversible decreases in steady state digoxin blood concentrations and renal glycoside excretion can arise in patients receiving β-acetyldigoxin while being treated with chemotherapy regimens that contain cyclophosphamide, vincristine, and prednisone. Therefore, monitoring of plasma digoxin levels may be indicated in heart patients. The utilization of digitoxin for such patients may be considered as an alternative.

A chemotherapy treatment for non-Hodgkin lymphoma is called PMitCEBO. It comprises the steroid prednisolone, plus the chemotherapy drugs mitoxantrone, cyclophosphamide, etoposide, bleomycin, and vincristine <Oncovin>. On day 1, the chemotherapy drugs are given by infusion. On day 7, additional infusions of vincristine and bleomycin are included. At the end of the cycle, there is a 6 day rest period. Each cycle takes 2 weeks. Usually, 4–8 cycles are given over a period of 2–4 months. The steroid is taken every day for 4 weeks, and then every other day for the next 4 weeks.

CHOP is named after the drugs cyclophosphamide, hydroxydaunorubicin (doxorubicin), vincristine <Oncovin> and prednisolone (or prednisone). Typically, courses are administered at an interval of 2 weeks (CHOP-14) or 3 weeks (CHOP-21).

- With the advent of molecularly targeted drugs, monoclonal antibodies have been added to conventional combination chemotherapy. R-CHOP is named after the monoclonal antibody rituximab and the drugs of CHOP. The regimen may be used if the lymphoma is of B-lymphocyte origin.

Adverse Effects Alopecia is common. Allopurinol is typically co-administered prophylactically to prevent hyperuricemia that results from tumor lysis syndrome. Chemotherapy induced nausea and vomiting may require anti-emetics. Hemorrhagic cystitis may be prevented with the administration of mesna. Neutropenia generally develops in the second week and may be controlled with pegfilgrastim. Antibiotic prophylaxis with ciprofloxacin can be beneficial. If fever develops in the neutropenic period, urgent medical assessment for neutropenic sepsis is required.

COAP contains cyclophosphamide, vincristine <Oncovorin>, cytarabine <Ara-C>, and prednisolone. This regimen achieves 50 % remissions in the treatment of AML. The complete remission rate for acute leukemias with the COAP regimen is similar to that obtained with cytarabine plus cyclophosphamide, but the median duration of remission is increased. COAP has activity in childhood ALL. However, effectiveness in markedly diminished in patients with prior bone marrow relapse.

Adverse Effects Vincristine and prednisone have low myelosuppressive toxicity and can be combined without modifying the dose of cytarabine or cyclophosphamide.

One important modification of high dose combination chemotherapy is the combination with autologous bone marrow transplantation as a means that allows the administration of otherwise lethal doses of anti-cancer drugs. Bone marrow is first harvested from the patient, the chemotherapy is administered, and the harvested marrow is returned a few days later. This approach, initially considered to be of benefit to a large fraction of patients, has not lived up to expectations. The curative benefits of high doses of chemotherapy afforded by autologous bone marrow rescue have mainly been limited to the subgroup of Hodgkin disease patients, for whom prior conventional combination chemotherapy has failed.

7.1.2 Doxorubicin Based Regimens

Doxorubicin containing regimens, such as ABVD (doxorubicin <Adriamycin>, bleomycin, vinblastine, dacarbazine) and ABDIC (doxorubicin <Adriamycin>, bleomycin, dacarbazine <DTIC>, lomustine, CCNU, prednisone), have been treatments for Hodgkin disease (Table 7.2).

ABVD (doxorubicin <Adriamycin>, bleomycin, vinblastine, dacarbazine) is a chemotherapy regimen used in the first-line treatment of Hodgkin lymphoma (Bonadonna et al. 1975). It was developed to overcome some of the adverse effects of the MOPP regimen. Because ABVD has higher efficacy and lower toxicity than MOPP (Santoro et al. 1987; Canellos et al. 1992) it has replaced MOPP in the first-line therapy of Hodgkin lymphoma.

A cycle of ABVD chemotherapy is given over 4 weeks, with 2 doses (on day 1 and day 15) per cycle. The treatment is usually administered in the outpatient setting. Typical dosages for 1 cycle of 28 days include doxorubicin 25 mg/m^2 intravenously, bleomycin 10 mg/m^2 intravenously, vinblastine 6 mg/m^2 intravenously, and dacarbazine 375 mg/m^2 intravenously. The total number of cycles given depends on the disease stage and on how well an individual patient tolerates the chemotherapy. Doses may be delayed because of adverse effects.

Adverse Effects ABVD has a unique toxicity profile. Acute adverse effects comprise transient alopecia, nausea and vomiting, low blood counts (neutropenia, thrombocytopenia) in about 50 % of patients, allergic reactions to bleomycin, and neuropathy (numbness in the tips of fingers and toes). Delayed adverse effects include cardiomyopathy from doxorubicin, and secondary malignancies in up to 30 % of patients within 25 years after treatment. Pulmonary fibrosis (especially in conjunction with radiation therapy to the chest) is unique to ABVD. Myelodysplasia and infertility have a low likelihood to occur.

Patients often receive a combination of 5-HT$_3$ receptor antagonists, corticosteroids, and benzodiazepines before chemotherapy to prevent nausea. Blood growth factors, such as G-CSF and Erythropoietin may be given with ABVD to prevent neutropenia and anemia related to the chemotherapy.

ABVD has been incorporated into alternating MOPP/ABVD schemes and into hybrids that attempt to offer all active agents together, such as MOPP/ABV. In some cases, they have achieved high and durable complete remissions. MOPP/ABVD × 12 months and MOPP-2/ABVD-2 have been compared with MOPP alone, resulting in apparent superiority for the alternating regimens.

The single dose activity of etoposide in Hodgkin disease prompted its inclusion in second-line programs, such as EVA (etoposide, vincristine or vinblastine, doxorubicin <Adriamycin>). Such second-line treatments achieve responses around 60 %.

Derived from EVA, the Stanford V regimen is a chemotherapy that is intended as a first-line treatment for Hodgkin lymphoma. Stanford V was developed in 1988, with the objective to maintain a high remission rate while reducing the incidence of acute and long term toxicity, pulmonary damage, and sterility that may arise in alternative treatment

Table 7.2 Doxorubicin based combination chemotherapy

	Doxorubicin	Vinblastine	Vincristine	Corticosteroid	Cyclophosphamide	Mechlorethamine	Lomustine	CCNU	Dacarbazine	Bleomycin	Etoposide
ABVD	+	+							+	+	
ABDIC	+			+ (prednisone)			+	+	+	+	
EVA	+	+									+
Stanford V	+	+	+	+ (prednisone)		+				+	+
C-VAMP	+		+	+ (methylprednisone)	+						
VAD	+		+	+ (dexamethasone)							

regimens (such as ABVD). Stanford V consists of 7 drugs: etoposide, vinblastine, vincristine, doxorubicin, mechlorethamine, bleomycin, and prednisone. It may be combined with radiation therapy. The chemotherapy part of Stanford V treatment lasts from 8 to 12 weeks, depending on the stage of the disease. In many cases, this is followed by radiation therapy for 2–6 weeks to the affected areas of the body.

C-VAMP is used to treat multiple myeloma. The regimen is named after its constituents, cyclophosphamide, vincristine, doxorubicin <Adriamycin>, and methylprednisolone. Cyclophosphamide is given as either an infusion or an injection. Methylprednisolone can be given as an infusion or as tablets. Following cyclophosphamide, vincristine and doxorubicin are administered together through a portable pump over 4 days. The cycle is completed with additional cyclophosphamide on days 8 and 15, followed by a week of rest (to complete 3 weeks). Usually, 4–6 cycles over a period of 3–5 months complete the treatment.

A simpler form of chemotherapy treatment for myeloma is VAD. On day 1, vincristine and doxorubicin are given together through a portable pump continuously for 4 days. Dexamethasone is then given as tablets on days 1–4, 9–12, and 17–20. A rest period ensues for the next 8 days to complete a 4 week cycle. Usually, 4–6 cycles are administered over a period of 4–6 months.

7.1.3 Others

A treatment for non-Hodgkin lymphomata is ICE, which includes ifosfamide, carboplatin, and etoposide (Table 7.3). This regimen is commonly used to treat primary progressive and poor risk recurrent lymphomata. Cycles are administered every 21 days in the outpatient setting, and may consist of ifosfamide 5000 mg/m^2 intravenously (fractionated into 3 equal doses over 3 days), carboplatin (mg dose = 5-fold area under the concentration-time curve) intravenously on day 1, and etoposide 100 mg/m^2 intravenously daily for 3 days.

- In R-ICE, this regimen is combined with rituximab, an anti-B-lymphocyte antibody.

Adverse Effects Common adverse effects include nausea, vomiting, myelosuppression, and hair loss. Ifosfamide can irritate the bladder lining and cause bleeding (hemorrhagic cystitis). To ameliorate this, mesna <Uromitexan> is given as a separate infusion simultaneously with the ifosfamide.

DHAP is a combination chemotherapy regimen for the treatment of recurring high grade non-Hodgkin B-cell lymphoma. DHAP is comprised of the steroid dexamethasone (orally on days 1 and 4), cytarabine <Ara-C> (2 doses on day 2 by infusion over 2–3 h; HA = high dose Ara-C), and cisplatin (infusion over 24 h on day 1). Patients undergo 2–6 cycles of treatment, with 3 weeks per cycle.

- R-DHAP also includes the monoclonal antibody rituximab.

Adverse Effects Neutropenia, anemia, and thrombocytopenia are common. So are fatigue, nausea, diarrhea, and mouth ulcers. Dexamethasone may cause changes in blood sugar levels. Long term adverse effects may include loss of fertility, secondary cancers, and heart disease.

To protect the patient from kidney damage, this treatment may be combined with the infusion of mannitol as a diuretic. Steroid eye drops should be used for 1 week after treatment because cytarabine can cause sore eyes (conjunctivitis).

The ESHAP regimen entails the chemotherapy drugs etoposide, methylprednisolone, cytarabine <Ara-C>, and cisplatin. It is a 5-day inpatient regimen. On days 1–4, infusions are administered of etoposide for 1 h, methylprednisolone for 15–30 min, cytarabine for 2 h, and cisplatin continuing for the entire 4 days. On day 5, the cisplatin infusion is complete, and a final dose of methylprednisolone and cytarabine is given. With the following rest period, a cycle lasts 21 days. Depending on the disease status, 1–6 cycles may be required. ESHAP is used to treat Hodgkin and non-Hodgkin lymphomata, or it may be given before a stem cell transplant.

- R-ESHAP also includes the monoclonal antibody rituximab.

Adverse Effects Common adverse effects (afflicting more than 10% of patients) include bone marrow depression, fatigue, nausea, hair loss, tinnitus, loss of taste or metallic taste, conjunctivitis, and amenorrhea. Occasional adverse effects comprise numbness in hands and feet, skin rashes, mouth sores, mood changes, and indigestion. Allergic reactions to the infusions can occur.

Table 7.3 Various combination chemotherapies for hematologic malignancies

	Dexamethasone	Platinum drug	Thioguanine	Cytarabine	Etoposide	Methylprednisolone	Asparaginase	Daunorubicin	Ifosfamide	Cyclophosphamide	BCNU
ICE		+ (carboplatin)			+				+		
DHAP	+	+ (cisplatin)		+							
ESHAP				+	+	+					
CART			+	+			+	+			
CBV					+					+	+

CART contains cytarabine (100 mg/m^2, days 1–5), Asparaginase (30,000 IU/m^2, days 1, 4, 7, 10, 13), daunorubicin <Rubidomycin> (40 mg/m^2, day 1), and thioguanine (100 mg/m^2, days 1–5). It is indicated for acute lymphoblastic leukemia (ALL). This combination exploits synergies among the anti-leukemic drugs.

Adverse Effects Patients with adult acute non-lymphocytic leukemia may develop peripheral motor and sensory neuropathies after consolidation with high dose cytarabine, daunorubicin, and Asparaginase. These patients should be observed accordingly because dose schedule alterations may be needed to avoid irreversible neurologic disorders.

The anti-lymphoma regimen CBV comprises cyclophosphamide <Cytoxan>, BCNU, and etoposide <VP-16>. CBV is a treatment of choice for patients who have relapsed or who have refractory disease that is unresponsive to standard chemotherapy. As one course of the regimen suffices to severely damage the bone marrow, the patient must receive an allogeneic or autologous transplant of stem cells.

Successful treatment of pediatric ALL and AML involves intensive, multi-cyclic therapy with several drugs that have various mechanisms of action and dosing regimens. It includes DNA and RNA alkylation (cyclophosphamide), anti-folates (methotrexate), anti-purines and anti-pyrimidines (6-mercaptopurine, 6-thioguanine), incorporation into DNA or RNA (cytarabine), microtubule inhibition (vincristine), membrane stabilization (prednisone), and inhibition of Topoisomerase 1 (topotecan) and 2 (anthracycline) (Bonate et al. 2006).

- Induction: vincristine, prednisone, L-Asparaginase, possibly including anthracyclines, depending on whether the patient is at high or low risk.
- Consolidation: 5 weeks of prednisone, cyclophosphamide, 6-mercaptopurine, vincristine, cytarabine, and methotrexate, plus radio-therapy.
- Interim maintenance: 8 weeks of mercaptopurine and methotrexate.
- Delayed intensification: re-induction with 4 weeks of dexamethasone, vincristine, doxorubicin, Asparaginase; or re-consolidation with 3 weeks of vincristine, cyclophosphamide, 6-thioguanine, cytarabine, methotrexate.
- Maintenance: 12 weeks of vincristine, prednisone, mercaptopurine, and methotrexate for standard risk ALL patients.

In general, approximately 25 % (ALL) to 50 % (AML) of leukemic pediatric patients will experience disease recurrence. Once a pediatric patient relapses, the primary therapeutic alternatives include further chemotherapy, bone marrow transplant, or hematopoietic stem cell transplant, with the timing of patient relapse being an important prognostic indicator and determinant of the type of treatment to be considered. Treatment outcomes for patients who relapse in their 2nd or 3rd remission are characterized by substantially decreased long term probability for a complete cure.

Treatment of Hodgkin Lymphoma

Hodgkin lymphoma was one of the first cancers, in which chemotherapy treatments were investigated with some success. It was originally treated with nitrogen mustard, the first conventional anti-cancer chemotherapeutic. In 1963, Scott recommended the use of chlorambucil as maintenance chemotherapy following nitrogen mustard treatment for Hodgkin lymphoma. In the same year, the first combination chemotherapy (MOMP, consists of cyclophosphamide, vincristine Oncovin, methotrexate, and prednisone) was developed. By 1970, the survival curves for MOPP-treated patients confirmed that advanced Hodgkin lymphoma is curable with combination chemotherapy. In 1972, Frei reported a remission success of 56 % in previously untreated patients with Hodgkin lymphoma using dacarbazine DTIC, DTIC-Dome, which has now become part of the ABVD regimen of combination chemotherapy, a standard treatment for Hodgkin lymphoma.

Adverse Effects Since studies in 1972, it has been known that secondary cancers can arise following therapy for Hodgkin disease (Arsenau et al. 1972).

Mechlorethamine hydrochloride (nitrogen mustard, chlormethine hydrochloride, mustine) Mustargen exhibits lympholytic properties. It is a useful chemotherapy drug in treating Hodgkin disease. The MOPP regimen, comprising mechlorethamine, vincristine Oncovin, procarbazine, and prednisone, can lead to remission in almost 70 % of patients with advanced stage Hodgkin lymphoma. However, its toxicity is substantial.

Adverse Effects Frequent adverse effects include bone marrow suppression, nerve damage caused by vincristine, and allergic reactions to procarbazine. Long term effects include infertility and a 15-fold increased risk of developing treatment-related myelodysplasia or acute leukemia. These secondary hematologic malignancies peak at 5–10 years after treatment for Hodgkin lymphoma and are associated with a dismally poor prognosis. MOPP chemotherapy used to treat Hodgkin lymphoma inhibits virtually 90 % of sperm function in men.

For the treatment of Hodgkin disease, bleomycin is useful in drug combinations. ABVD (adriamycin, bleomycin, vinblastine, dacarbazine) is a chemotherapy regimen used in the first line treatment of Hodgkin lymphoma (Bonadonna et al. 1975). It was developed to overcome some of the adverse effects of the MOPP regimen. Because ABVD has higher efficacy and lower toxicity than MOPP (Santoro et al. 1987; Canellos et al. 1992) it has replaced the older combination in the first line therapy of Hodgkin lymphoma.

A cycle of ABVD chemotherapy is administered in the outpatient setting. Typical dosages for 1 cycle of 28 days of ABVD include intravenous doxorubicin 25 mg/m^2, bleomycin 10 mg/m^2, vinblastine 6 mg/m^2, and dacarbazine 375 mg/m^2, with 2 doses (on day 1 and day 15) per cycle. The total number of cycles given depends on the disease stage and how well the patient tolerates the chemotherapy. Doses may be delayed because of neutropenia, thrombocytopenia, or other adverse effects.

Adverse Effects Acute adverse effects comprise transient alopecia, nausea and vomiting, low blood counts in about 50 % of patients, allergic reactions to bleomycin, and neuropathy (numbness) in the tips of fingers and toes. Delayed effects include infertility in rare cases, pulmonary toxicity especially in conjunction with radiation therapy to the chest, cardiomyopathy from doxorubicin, and secondary malignancies in up to 30 % of patients at 25 years after treatment.

In 1986, the MOPP/ABV hybrid chemotherapy was developed and published by Canadian researchers. Intended to improve the efficacy of each, MOPP and ABV, it improves relapse-free and overall survival. However, MOPP/ABV is associated with a greater incidence of acute toxicity, myelodysplasia, and leukemia.

VAPEC-B is a combination chemotherapy protocol containing vincristine, doxorubicin Adriamycin, prednisolone, etoposide, cyclophosphamide, and bleomycin. Vincristine, doxorubicin, and cyclophosphamide are given by infusion, etoposide and prednisolone are taken as tablets. The regimen is used for the treatment of Hodgkin lymphoma and non-Hodgkin lymphoma. On day 1, doxorubicin and cyclophosphamide are administered. On day 8, vincristine and bleomycin follow. On day 15, there is doxorubicin and the start of a 4-day course of etoposide capsules. The cycle is completed with vincristine on day 22. Usually, a course of treatment comprises 3 cycles of 4 weeks over a period of 12 weeks.

A chemotherapy regimen that is widely used in Hodgkin lymphoma is the Stanford V regimen, which consists of intravenous mechlorethamine (sometimes replaced by cyclophosphamide) every 4 weeks, doxorubicin every odd week, vinblastine every odd week, vincristine every even week, bleomycin every even week, etoposide 2 days in a row in weeks 3, 7, 11, and oral prednisone every other day. The chemotherapy part of Stanford V treatment can last 8–12 weeks, depending on the stage of the disease. In many cases, this is followed by radiation therapy for 2–6 weeks to the affected areas of the body. The regimen is a rigorously administered form of chemotherapy, with treatments roughly twice as fast as those of other Hodgkin lymphoma treatments.

Numerous attempts to improve on Hodgkin lymphoma therapy have yielded various combination chemotherapy protocols.

- In 1987, EBVP (epirubicin, bleomycin, vinblastine, prednisone) was introduced by Zittoun (Hoerni et al. 1991) and tested in the EORTC H7 trial.
- In 1992, the German Hodgkin's Study Group designed the BEACOPP regimen that used similar drugs as in the COPP/ABVD regimen, excluding velban and dacarbazine and adding etoposide, in an attempt to increase efficacy. Hodgkin lymphoma may be treated with ChlVPP. It entails chlorambucil, vinblastine, procarbazine, and prednisolone. Vinblastine is administered as an infusion on day 1, the other drugs are given as tablets or capsules over a 2-week course. This is followed by a rest period of 2 weeks. Usually 4–6 cycles are given over a period of 4–6 months.

NHPHL is the only form of Hodgkin lymphoma that is CD20 positive. For this subtype, rituximab may be a treatment choice (in conjunction with ABDV or for the treatment of a relapse after ABVD has failed).

7.2 Treatment of Solid Tumors

7.2.1 Cyclophosphamide Based Regimens

Lung cancer may be treated with COPE. It includes cyclophosphamide, vincristine <Oncovin>, cisplatin (platinum alkylating agents), and etoposide. The regimen has been studied in combination with radiation therapy (Table 7.4).

A combination chemotherapy for breast cancer may be CMF, which combines cyclophosphamide, methotrexate, and 5-fluorouracil. Cyclophosphamide is given by infusion,

Table 7.4 Cyclophosphamide based regimens

	Cyclophos-phamide	Doxorubicin	Fluorouracil	Methotrexate	Cisplatin	Vincristine	Etoposide	Epirubicin	Docetaxel	Prednisone
COPE	+				+	+	+			
CMFVP	+		+	+		+				+
CMF	+		+	+						
E-CMF	+		+	+				+		
FEC	+		+					+		
CAF	+	+	+							
CAP	+	+			+					
CAV	+	+				+				
AC	+	+								
TAC	+	+							+	

followed by an injection of methotrexate, and an injection of 5-fluorouracil. There are multiple different schedules in use, which are usually all administered 4–6 times over a period of 3–6 months. This constitutes a course of treatment. Adjuvant therapy with CMF conveys survival benefit to breast cancer patients. In postmenopausal patients there is poorer tolerance to the chemotherapy, leading to a decrease in the delivered CMF doses within the classical schedule and consecutively lower benefit.

- The regimen E-CMF (Epi-CMF) adds epirubicin to this mix. An epirubicin dose of 100 mg/m^2 is considered more effective than 50 mg/m^2.
- CMFVP (Cooper regimen), entailing cyclophosphamide, methotrexate, 5-fluorouracil, vincristine, and prednisone, was initially devised in 1979 for enhanced efficacy over CMF (see below). The increase in the number of agents from 3 in CMF to 5 in CMFVP brings increased benefit only to patients with a greater burden of disease. CMFVP achieves 70 % disease free survival in breast cancer patients with multiple metastatic axillary nodes.
- In the related regimen FEC, 5-fluorouracil, epirubicin, and cyclophosphamide are administered.

CAF includes cyclophosphamide, doxorubicin <Adriamycin>, and 5-fluorouracil. It is used for the treatment of breast cancer. A cycle comprises

- on day 1 an injection of doxorubicin alongside a drip of saline, cyclophosphamide by infusion or as an injection alongside a drip of saline, then an injection of 5-fluorouracil. This is followed by a rest period of 3 weeks (schedule A)
- injections of 5-fluorouracil and doxorubicin on day 1, 14 days of treatment with cyclophosphamide tablets, after 7 days doxorubicin and 5-fluorouracil are administered again. From days 15 through 28, there is a rest period to complete the cycle (schedule B).

Lung cancers and endometrial cancers may be treated with CAP. It is a combination chemotherapy of cyclophosphamide, doxorubicin <Adriamycin>, and cisplatin (platinum alkylating agents). On day 1, cyclophosphamide 400–600 mg/m^2, doxorubicin 40–45 mg/m^2, and cisplatin 50–60 mg/m^2 are administered intravenously. This cycle is repeated every 28 days.

CAV is named after cyclophosphamide, doxorubicin <Adriamycin>, and vincristine. The chemotherapy drugs are given separately, often starting with doxorubicin followed by vincristine and then cyclophosphamide. The cycle is completed with a rest period of 3 weeks. A course of the treatment comprises 4–6 cycles, which are given over a period of 3–4 months. After its introduction, the CAV regimen was the standard of care for the treatment of small cell lung cancer. It is used for palliation and is not considered to have curative potential.

- Several variations of this regimen have been applied. They include CAVE (addition of etopiside), CEV (doxorubicin is replaced by etopiside), and PACE (vincristine is replaced by cisplatin).

AC is a breast cancer chemotherapy regimen that combines doxorubicin <Adriamycin> and cyclophosphamide <Cytoxan>. The drugs are given separately by infusion in an outpatient setting. The order is first a steroid and anti-emetic medication to limit adverse effects, then doxorubicin (sucking on ice cubes during infusion may reduce the risk of mouth sores by causing vasoconstriction), then cyclophosphamide. A course of treatment comprises 4–6 cycles of 3 weeks, usually over a period of 3–4 months.

Adverse Effects In patients who had prior radio-therapy, the treated areas may sometimes become red and sore during chemotherapy ("radiation recall reaction"). The effects are reversible upon completion of chemotherapy.

TAC treatment for breast cancer involves docetaxel <Taxotere>, doxorubicin <Adriamycin>, and cyclophosphamide. On the first day of treatment, all 3 drugs are administered by infusion or injections. After this, there is a rest period

Table 7.5 Epirubicin based regimens

	Epirubicin	Capecitabine	Cisplatin	Fluorouracil	Oxaliplatin
ECF	+		+	+	
ECX	+	+	+		
EEX	+	+			+
ELF	+			+ (+ leukovorin)	

with no chemotherapy for the next 3 weeks. This completes a cycle of treatment. Usually, 4–6 cycles are given over 3–4 months to complete a course of treatment.

7.2.2 Epirubicin Based Treatments

Combination chemotherapy treatments based on epirubicin (Table 7.5) are in use for the treatment of stomach cancer or esophageal cancer. This treatment may also be applied to treat cancers of the breast, ovary, and less common malignancies.

ECF comprises epirubicin, cisplatin, and 5-fluorouracil. It is used for gastric and esophageal cancers. The treatment is preceded by an anti-emetic drug (tablet or injection). The chemotherapy agents are then given separately, epirubicin as an injection along with an infusion of saline (less commonly as an infusion), cisplatin as an infusion (with abundant fluid to ameliorate kidney toxicity), then 5-fluorouracil through a portable pump. A cycle completes after 3 weeks. There may be up to 8 cycles of ECF chemotherapy over a 24-week period. Sometimes, 4 cycles of ECF chemotherapy can be given before surgery followed by 4 cycles after surgery.

The treatment regimen ECX combines epirubicin with cisplatin and capecitabine <Xeloda>. The treatment is preceded by an anti-emetic drug (tablet or injection). On day 1, epirubicin is administered along with an infusion of saline. Consecutively, cisplatin is given as an infusion. Starting on the evening of day 1, capecitabine is then taken for 21 days in the form of tablets twice a day within 1/2 h of finishing a meal. A course of treatment lasts 21 days. There may be up to 8 cycles over 24 weeks.

EEX (EOX) is a combination of epirubicin, oxaliplatin <Eloxatin>, and capecitabine <Xeloda>. The regimen is preceded by anti-emetic tablets or injection. Then epirubicin is given as an injection along with an infusion of saline, followed by an infusion of oxaliplatin. Starting on the evening of day 1, capecitabine is then taken for 21 days in the form of tablets twice a day within 1/2 h of finishing a meal. A course of treatment lasts 21 days. There may be up to 8 cycles over 24 weeks.

ELF is named after etoposide, leucovorin, and 5-fluorouracil. Etoposide and 5-fluorouracil are the active anti-cancer agents, while leucovorin ameliorates the adverse effects of 5-fluorouracil. The treatment starts with anti-emetic medication as tablets or via injection. On days 1–3, the chemotherapy drugs are then given separately, etoposide as an infusion over 30–60 min, leucovorin as a slow injection or an infusion over 15 min, 5-fluorouracil as an infusion, over about 60 min. This is followed by a rest period with no chemotherapy for 25 days to complete a 28-day cycle of treatment. Usually, 6 cycles of treatment are given over 6 months to make up a course of treatment.

7.2.3 Platinum Based Chemotherapy

In the 1970s, the use of cisplatin in combination chemotherapy (Table 7.6) dramatically increased the cure rate of testicular cancer to around 80%. In 1973, Einhorn recognized that cisplatin had activity in testis cancer and was a suitable drug for combining with the best agents of the time that were known to act synergistically, vinblastine and bleomycin. The predominant adverse effects of cisplatin were nausea, vomiting, and kidney toxicity, whereas vinblastine had bone marrow toxicity and bleomycin had lung toxicity. The diverse mechanisms of adverse effects allowed these drugs to be used in conjunction without cumulative damage. With this combination, the cure rate went from 10–80%. Vinblastine was replaced by etoposide in the 1980s due to its fewer adverse effects and is slightly higher efficacy.

In platinum based combination therapy, a common approach is the combination of one or more non-platinum anti-cancer drugs with a platinum compound. Cisplatin, carboplatin, and oxaliplatin have been evaluated in combination with etoposide, mitomycin C, vinblastine, paclitaxel, docetaxel, vinorelbine, gemcitabine, cyclophosphamide, doxorubicin, epirubicin, methotrexate, lonidamine, and 5-fluorouracil. When combined with 5-fluorouracil, cisplatin improves response rates in head and neck cancer, oxaliplatin with 5-fluorouracil significantly improves survival in colon cancer. Rational combination therapies take advantage of known platinum processing pathways (Wang and Lippard 2005).

- Cisplatin affords survival benefit in germ cell cancers and in patients with metastatic breast cancer when used

Table 7.6 Platinum based regimens

	Cisplatin	Ifosfamide	Bleomycin	Etoposide	Mitomycin	Vinblastine	Paclitaxel
BEP	+		+	+			
MIC	+	+			+		
VIP	+	+				+	
TIP	+	+					+

with the Topoisomerase 2 inhibitor etoposide, which suppresses cell cycle progression before mitosis.

- Nucleosome structure and DNA accessibility can be altered by several multi-protein remodeling complexes or by the covalent post-translational modification of Histones. Pre-treatment with the HDAC inhibitors trichostatin A (TSA) or suberoylamilide hydroxamic acid (SAHA) enhances the cancer cell-killing efficiency of cisplatin, reflecting that relaxation of the chromatin structure by Histone acetylation increases the cytotoxicity of the drug. Similarly, the combination of arginine butyrate and cisplatin results in a concentration responsive increase in cisplatin-DNA adduct formation, and a resulting enhancement of the cytotoxicity of cisplatin. A compromised chromatin configuration may affect cisplatin adduct formation and modulate the drug effect.
- Carboplatin combined with paclitaxel, a microtubule disassembly inhibitor, has been increasingly applied in ovarian cancer, non-small cell lung cancer, and head and neck cancer.
- The use of pharmacological means to inhibit DNA repair by using trastuzumab or DNA Polymerase inhibitors is a potential approach to overcome acquired cisplatin resistance.

For germ cell tumors with favorable prognosis, standard therapy comprises 3 cycles of cisplatin, etoposide plus bleomycin (BEP × 3). Cisplatin and etoposide are given over 5 days. The approach achieves approximately 90 % response rates. About 75 % of intermediate risk and 45 % of poor risk patients display a durable complete response with BEP × 4.

- Potentially curative options in the salvage setting include ifosfamide plus cisplatin containing standard dose therapy, and high dose carboplatin plus stem cell rescue (Kondagunta and Motzer 2006).
- Sometimes, 4 cycles of etoposide plus cisplatin (EP) is used to treat testicular cancers with favorable prognosis.

MIC uses the chemotherapy drugs mitomycin, ifosfamide, and cisplatin. These agents are given separately as consecutive infusions on day 1. Mitomycin is usually administered as an infusion (sometimes as a slow injection into an infusion of saline), then ifosfamide is infused, followed by cisplatin. Cisplatin treatment is administered with large amounts of fluid to protect from kidney damage. After a rest period of 3 weeks, the same drugs are given again to begin the next cycle of treatment. Usually 4–6 cycles of treatment are administered over a period of 3–5 months. This makes up a course of treatment.

VIP comprises vinblastine, ifosfamide, and a platinum agent (cisplatin). The regimen is used in testicular cancer and germ cell tumors[1].

If a germinal cancer recurs, salvage therapy is required. It is very important that salvage therapy is not given unless a relapse is documented by a biopsy or clearly rising and elevated levels of biomarkers. Most salvage chemotherapy for testicular cancer is VeIP (vinblastine, mesna, ifosfamide, cisplatin), which results in 30–50 % of patients being cured on the condition that the patient is not cisplatin refractory. During this type of therapy, it is general routine to add G-CSF <Neupogen>.

TIP chemotherapy combines paclitaxel <Taxol>, ifosfamide, and a platinum agent (cisplatin). It is used for testicular cancer and germ cell tumors in salvage therapy. Treatment is preceded by the administration of anti-emetic drugs, usually by injection, and steroid tablets to prevent anaphylactic reactions to paclitaxel. Cisplatin is combined with plenty of fluid to maintain normal kidney function, ifosfamide is combined with mesna. On day 1, the chemotherapy drugs are then given separately as infusions, paclitaxel over 3 h, cisplatin over 4 h, and ifosfamide over 2 h. On days 2–5, cisplatin and ifosfamide are given. This is followed by a rest period with no chemotherapy for the ensuing 16 days to complete a 21-day cycle. A course of treatment usually comprises 4 cycles of TIP over a period of 3–4 months.

7.2.4 Others

A common regimen involves fluorouracil and folinic acid (leucovorin) (Table 7.7). These 2 drugs are often used together in various ways. In the Mayo scheme for bowel cancer, folinic acid is given by injection, then 5-fluorouracil is administered by infusion. This is repeated daily, for 5 days of treatment. The cycle is completed by a rest period of 3 weeks. The treatment is usually given for 6 cycles over a period of 6 months to complete a course of treatment.

The LV5FU2 regimen administers biweekly fluorouracil plus leucovorin in 48-h infusions. Typical doses are 200 mg/m^2 leucovorin infusion, 400 mg/m^2 5-fluorouracil bolus, and 600 mg/m^2 5-fluorouracil infusion. LV5FU2 may be combined with other agents as in irinotecan/LV5FU2 or oxaliplatin/LV5FU2. For colon cancer, IFL was often used, which comprised a weekly bolus of irinotecan, 5-fluorouracil, and leucovorin. It is no longer recommended.

Oxaliplatin displays synergy with fluorouracil, with little toxicity overlap. Commonly used first-line chemotherapy

[1] Note with caution that the acronym VIP is also used to denote etoposide <VP-16>, ifosfamide, and cisplatin.

Table 7.7 Other combination chemotherapy regimens

	Oxaliplatin	Irinotecan	Capecitabine	Fluorouracil	Mitomycin	Mitoxantrone	Methotrexate	Procarbazine	Lomustine	Vincristine	Dacarbazine	Doxorubicin	Ifosfamide
Mayo				+ (+ leukovorin)									
LV5FU2				+ (+ leukovorin)									
FOLFOX	+			+ (+ leukovorin)									
FOLFIRI		+		+ (+ leukovorin)									
XELOX	+		+										
XELIRI		+	+										
IROX	+	+											
MMM					+	+	+						
PVC								+	+	+			
MAID											+	+	+ (+ mesna)

regimens for colorectal cancer involve the combination of infusional 5-fluorouracil, leucovorin, and oxaliplatin (FOLFOX), possibly in combination with bevacizumab, or infusional 5-fluorouracil, leucovorin, and irinotecan (FOLFIRI), possibly with bevacizumab. Maximum reduction in tumor size is usually seen within 3 months.

FOLFOX regimens differ in agent dosing and administration schedule and include FOLFOX 4, FOLFOX 6, modified FOLFOX 6, and FOLFOX 7. A FOLFOX regimen may cover 12 cycles every 2 weeks. On day 1, it starts with an infusion of 85 mg/m^2 oxaliplatin and 200 mg/m^2 leucovorin, both given over 2 h in separate bags using a Y-line. This is followed by a 400 mg/m^2 bolus of 5-fluorouracil over 2–4 min, and then 600 mg/m^2 5-fluorouracil by continuous infusion over 22 h. On day 2, leucovorin is infused at 200 mg/m^2 over 2 h, followed by a 400 mg/m^2 bolus of fluorouracil, and then 600 mg/m^2 5-fluorouracil infusion over 22 h.

Adverse Effects Adverse effects include severe fatigue, bouts of insomnia after each chemotherapy cycle, and myelosuppression. Longer periods of chemotherapy can lead to non-alcoholic steatohepatitis. 5-fluorouracil can cause heart problems such as myocardial infarction, arrhythmias, angina, and heart failure. Patients with a history of heart disease are likely at higher risk.

Oxaliplatin can cause early onset or chronic neuropathies. Early onset neuropathy starts within a few hours to 2 days and usually lasts for 14 days. Exposure to cold temperatures and cold objects can cause or worsen the symptoms. Chronic neuropathy usually starts after several treatments and can last for weeks or months. A less common oxaliplatin related neuropathy is pharyngolaryngeal dysesthesia (tightness or discomfort in the throat, which can make it feel difficult to breathe or swallow).

Capecitabine is an orally administered fluoropyrimidine carbamate, which was developed as a prodrug of 5-fluorouracil with the goal to improve its tolerability and intra-tumoral drug concentrations. Capecitabine has high efficacy as a first-line treatment for metastatic colorectal cancer, making it a candidate to replace 5-fluorouracil plus leucovorin in combination therapy with oxaliplatin. The XELOX regimen (oxaliplatin plus capecitabine) was designed to improve on FOLFOX protocols (infused oxaliplatin with fluorouracil and leucovorin). XELOX is an effective first-line treatment for metastatic colorectal cancer. Response rates, median time to disease progression, and overall survival are similar to those observed with fluorouracil/leucovorin/oxaliplatin combinations. XELOX is administered in 3-week treatment cycles. On day 1, oxaliplatin is given intravenously at 130 mg/m^2 followed by oral capecitabine 1000 mg/m^2 twice daily (from day 1, evening through day 15, morning).

Whereas the XELOX regimens include oxaliplatin at 130 mg/m^2 on day 1 every 3 weeks, CAPOX regimens (capecitabine <Xeloda> and oxaliplatin <Eloxatin>) split the oxaliplatin dose to 70 mg/m^2 on days 1 and 8.

The replacement of 5-fluorouracil and leucovorin in FOLFIRI with capecitabine results in XELIRI regimen. It entails intravenous irinotecan at 250 mg/m^2 on day 1 plus oral capecitabine at 1000 mg/m^2 twice daily on days 1–15, every 3 weeks.

Adverse Effects In XELOX (unlike FOLFOX) myelosuppression is uncommon (7 % incidence of grade 3 or 4 neutropenia). Most adverse events are mild to moderate, the most common one being acute sensory neuropathy (85 %).

In metastatic colorectal cancer, irinotecan and oxaliplatin act synergistically, their dose limiting toxicities are largely non-overlapping (diarrhea and myelosuppression for irinotecan and peripheral sensory neuropathy for oxaliplatin). IROX for colorectal cancer combines irinotecan with oxaliplatin, without 5-fluorouracil. Irinotecan is given at 150 mg/m^2, and oxaliplatin at 85 mg/m^2 on day 1 over 90 min. This is repeated every 2 weeks.

Adverse Effects IROX has a higher incidence of adverse effects than FOLFOX. Major hematologic toxicities include grade 1–2 anemia (90 %), neutropenia (35 %, grade 3–4 neutropenia 10 %), and thrombocytopenia (30 %). The most frequent non-hematologic toxicity is grade 3 diarrhea (15 %).

The MMM chemotherapy regimen for breast cancer comprises mitomycin, methotrexate, and mitozantrone. These drugs are administered separately as consecutive infusions, which are followed by a 3 week rest period. In the next part, only methotrexate and mitoxantrone are given, followed by a 3 week rest period to complete the first cycle of 6 weeks (42 days). Usually 3–4 cycles are administered over a period of 3–6 months to complete a course of treatment.

PCV, including procarbazine, lomustine <CCNU>, and vincristine, is used to treat brain tumors. This involves an injection of vincristine and intake of lomustine capsules on day 1, plus initiation of a 10 day treatment with procarbazine capsules. Then, there is a rest period of 32 days to complete a cycle. The treatment is repeated over a total of 2–3 cycles.

The MAID regimen as one of the standard treatments for disseminated soft tissue sarcoma entails mesna, dacarbazine <Adriamycin>, ifosfamide, and doxorubicin. The chemotherapy is given in the in-patient setting. The schedule may be mesna 120 mg/m^2 prior to ifosfamide on day 1 and 1.2 mg/m^2 infusion over 8 h starting immediately after the ifosfamide on days 1–3, doxorubicin 15 mg/m^2 on days 1–3, ifosfamide 1.2 gm/m^2 on days 1–3, and dacarbazine 200 mg/m^2 on days 1–3.

- AIM is a variation of MAID that lacks dacarbazine. It combines 20–25 mg/m^2 doxorubicin on days 1–3 plus 2000–3000 mg/m^2 ifosfamide (plus 225 mg/m^2 intravenous mesna over 1 h before ifosfamide and at 4 and 8 h after ifosfamide) on days 1–3, which is repeated every 21–28 days. It is a standard treatment for disseminated soft tissue sarcomata.

Adverse Effects This regimen is associated with substantial toxicity, including a risk of death from neutropenic sepsis.

Drug combinations may be inferior to mono-therapies. Combining monoclonal antibodies and small molecule ki-

Treatment of Colorectal Cancer

Chemotherapy is used to slow tumor growth, shrink tumor size, or reduce the likelihood of metastasis developing from colorectal cancer. Chemotherapy is often applied after surgery (adjuvant), before surgery (neo-adjuvant), or as the primary therapy if surgery is not indicated (palliative).

1. Adjuvant Chemotherapy

Fluorouracil and folinic acid (leucovorin) are often used together in various ways. In the Mayo scheme for bowel cancer, folinic acid is injected, then 5-fluorouracil is infused. This is repeated daily, for 5 days of treatment. The cycle is completed by a rest period of 3 weeks. The treatment is usually administered for 6 cycles over a period of 6 months to complete a course of adjuvant treatment.

Another regimen covers 500 mg/m^2 leucovorin intravenously plus bolus 500 mg/m^2 5-fluorouracil intravenously on day 1, repeated weekly for 6 weeks. This is followed by 2 weeks of rest. The 8-week cycles are repeated 4 times.

FOLFOX comprises leucovorin (folinic acid), 5-fluorouracil, and oxaliplatin. On day 1, 85 mg/m^2 oxaliplatin plus 200 mg/m^2 leucovorin are given intravenously, followed by 400 mg/m^2 5-fluorouracil (5-FU) as an intravenous bolus, then 600 mg/m^2 5-fluorouracil as a 22-h continuous intravenous infusion. On day 2, 200 mg/m^2 leucovorin is administered as an intravenous infusion over 120 min, followed by 400 mg/m^2 5-fluorouracil intravenous bolus, then 600 mg/m^2 5-fluorouracil intravenously as a 22-h continuous infusion. Each cycle is repeated every 14 days.

FLOX also contains 5-fluorouracil, leucovorin, and oxaliplatin. For 6 weeks, once a week (on days 1, 8, 15, 22, 29, and 36) 500 mg/m^2 5-fluorouracil and 500 mg/m^2 leucovorin are given intravenously. 85 mg/m^2 oxaliplatin is administered intravenously on days 1, 15, and 29. 2 weeks of rest complete a 8-week cycle, of which 3 rounds are given.

XELOX (CapeOX) is a combination of capecitabine <Xeloda> and oxaliplatin. It entails 130 mg/m^2 oxaliplatin intravenously on day 1 plus 1000 mg/m^2 capecitabine orally twice daily for 14 days in a 21-day cycle for 8 cycles.

The levels of prostaglandins are elevated in colon cancers and their precursor lesions (adenomatous polyps). They may be generated by 2 forms of Cyclooxygenases, COX-1 and COX-2. As COX-1 is constitutively expressed, COX-2 is likely responsible for the increased prostaglandin production in transformed lesions. COX-2 inhibitors may be beneficial in the prophylaxis and treatment of colon cancer. They are approved by the U.S. FDA for the prevention of polyps.

2. Therapy for Advanced or Metastatic Colon Cancer

There are various regimens for the chemotherapy of metastatic disease.

- FOLFOX, involves the combination of leucovorin (LV, folinic acid), infusional 5-fluorouracil (5-FU), and oxaliplatin Elotaxin. In FOLFOX, patients receive infusions of leukovorin and oxaliplatin, followed by an injection or infusion of 5-fluorouracil, every 2 weeks. Maximum reduction in tumor size usually occurs within 3 months. Longer periods of chemotherapy can lead to non-alcoholic steatohepatitis. There are variations of the FOLFOX regimen (such as FOLFOX-4, FOLFOX-6, mFOLFOX-6)

- A standard FOLFIRI regimen includes a 90 min infusion of 180 mg/m^2 irinotecan plus 400 mg/m^2 leukovorin concurrently with a bolus of 400 mg/m^2 5-fluorouracil, then a 2400 mg/m^2 5-fluorouracil infusion over 46 h. The cycle is repeated every 2 weeks. IFL uses the same drugs as FOLFIRI. It consists of concurrent treatment with irinotecan, leucovorin (folinic acid), and fluorouracil, however, the fluorouracil component is given as a bolus injection rather than as an infusion.
- FOLFOXIRI (leucovorin, 5-fluorouracil, oxaliplatin, irinotecan) comprises on day 1 165 mg/m^2 irinotecan plus 85 mg/m^2 oxaliplatin plus 200 mg/m^2 leucovorin intravenously; on days 1 and 2, 5-fluorouracil 1600 mg/m^2/day continuous infusion intravenously over 48 h (the total dose of 5-fluorouracil equals 3200 mg/m^2).
- For fluorouracil intolerant individuals, the IROX regimen is an appropriate alternative. IROX for colorectal cancer combines irinotecan with oxaliplatin (without 5-fluorouracil). It comprises 85 mg/m^2 oxaliplatin intravenously plus 200 mg/m^2 irinotecan intravenously; repeat cycle every 21 days.
- CapeOX (XELOX) (oxaliplatin plus capecitabine) gives on day 1, 130 mg/m^2 oxaliplatin intravenously plus 850–1000 mg/m^2 capecitabine orally twice daily for 14 days in 16 21-day cycles.
- In the XELIRI regimen, a 22 day cycle includes 1000 mg/m^2 capecitabine <Xeloda> twice daily on days 1 and 14, 100 mg/m^2 irinotecan twice daily on days 1 and 8.

In a comparison of combination chemotherapy regimens, FOLFOX is associated with a median time to progression of 9 months, response rate of 45 %, and median survival time of 20 months. This is superior to all endpoints achieved with IFL (median time to progression 7 months, response rate 30 %, median survival time 15 months) and to 2 endpoints of IROX (median time to progression 6 months, response rate 35 %, median survival time 17 months). The FOLFOX regimen is associated with more sensory neuropathy and neutropenia, but otherwise has a more favorable adverse event profile (Goldberg et al. 2004).

Targeted therapy includes bevacizumab <Avastin>, cetuximab <Erbitux>, and panitumumab <Vectibix>.

As a single agent, bevacizumab has minimal activity. However, the addition of bevacizumab (5–10 mg/kg every 2 weeks) to conventional chemotherapy regimens may result in a significant improvement of survival. The agent is approved in combination with 5-fluorouracil based chemotherapy as a first-line and second-line treatment of metastatic colorectal cancer.

Cetuximab is a monoclonal antibody that specifically blocks ERBB2 (EGF Receptor). Although the antibody has efficacy when given alone, the response rates are higher when it is combined with chemotherapy. Cetuximab may be administered in combination with FOLFOX or FOLFIRI.

Panitumumab is a humanized antibody designed to be different from cetuximab. It binds specifically to ERBB2 and completely blocks ligand binding. The antibody is only used for tumors with wild-type K-RAS, at a dose of 6 mg/kg intravenously every 14 days. Panitumomab has fewer infusion related adverse effects than cetuximab.

Bevacizumab plus conventional chemotherapy containing regimens may be administered in diverse combinations.

- Bevacizumab 5 mg/kg intravenously every 14 days plus 5-fluorouracil 500 mg/m^2 intravenously every 7 days for 6 weeks plus leucovorin 500 mg/m^2 intravenously every 8 weeks.
- Bevacizumab plus FOLFOX: On day 1, bevacizumab 10 mg/kg plus oxaliplatin 85 mg/m^2 plus leucovorin 200 mg/m^2 intravenously, then 5-fluorouracil 400 mg/m^2 intravenous bolus, followed by 5-fluorouracil 600 mg/m^2 intravenously as a 22-h continuous infusion. On day 2, leucovorin 200 mg/m^2 intravenous infusion over 120 min, followed by 5-fluorouracil 400 mg/m^2 intravenous bolus, then followed by 5-fluorouracil 600 mg/m^2 intravenously as a 22-h continuous infusion. The cycles are repeated every 14 days.
- Bevacizumab plus FOLFIRI-B: On day 1, bevacizumab 5 mg/kg plus irinotecan 180 mg/m^2 intravenously. On days 1 and 2, 200 mg/m^2 intravenous leucovorin followed by a 400 mg/m^2 intravenous bolus of 5-fluorouracil, then followed by 5-fluorouracil 600 mg/m^2 intravenously as a 22-h continuous infusion. The cycles are repeated every 14 days.
- CAPIRI-B (capecitabine, irinotecan, bevacizumab): On day 1, intravenous irinotecan 250 mg/m^2 plus

bevacizumab 7.5 mg/kg. On days 1–14, 2000 mg/ m^2 oral capecitabine. The cycles are repeated every 3 weeks.

Fewer than 10% of patients with *K-ras* codon 12 or 13 mutated tumors respond to anti-ERBB2 therapy with cetuximab. The G13D mutation in K-RAS does benefit from treatment with this antibody, displaying increased progression-free survival and overall survival. Cetuximab may be combined with irinotecan.

- On day 1, cetuximab 400 mg/m^2 intravenously, then 250 mg/m^2 intravenously every 7 days.
- On day 1, cetuximab 500 mg/m^2 intravenously every 14 days plus
  - irinotecan 300–350 mg/m^2 intravenously every 21 days or
  - irinotecan 180 mg/m^2 intravenously every 14 days or
  - irinotecan 125 mg/m^2 intravenously on days 1 and 8; repeat cycle every 21 days.

While systemic chemotherapy can cause a regression in size of liver metastases, the long-term survival without local therapy is poor. Surgical resection of hepatic metastases continues to be the first line treatment.

If liver metastases are present or to prevent recurrence after the resection of liver metastases, hepatic artery infusion is a therapeutic option. It is the infusion of chemotherapy drugs into the hepatic artery via a surgically implanted pump. Fluorodeoxyuridine (FUDR) has been the therapy of choice for this approach, because it has a high rate of extraction in the liver.

Transcatheter arterial chemoembolization (TACE) is used for the palliative treatment of liver metastases. It is based on the concept of tumor embolization plus local drug release. The administered drug eluting beads (microspheres) are biocompatible, non- resorbent, and loaded with a chemotherapy agent (such as irinotecan).

3. Anal Cancer

Principles of adjuvant therapy for anal cancer comprise regimens that include both concurrent chemotherapy and radiotherapy, administration of radio-chemotherapy either pre- or post-operatively, preference for 6 months of peri-operative therapy.

Anal cancer is typically a squamous cell carcinoma that arises near the squamocolumnar junction at the anus. Anal canal carcinoma is mostly a local-regional cancer with metastatic potential (mostly to liver and lungs) in only 15% of patients. The 5-year survival rates decrease precipitously in tumors larger than 5 cm in diameter at the time of diagnosis. Similarly, the presence of node infiltration results in a reduction of the cure rate. The cancer is highly sensitive to chemoradiation, resulting in full remission in 60% of cases. Radiation therapy plus fluorouracil and mitomycin is superior to radiotherapy alone, and it is superior to radiation plus fluorouracil. By comparison, cisplatin based chemo-radiation therapy results in substantially increased colostomy rates (Ajani et al. 2008).

- Cancers of the anal margin (distal to the dentate line until the junction between the perineal skin and the hair-bearing skin of the buttocks) are treated like skin cancers with either excision or chemo-radiotherapy depending on the tumor size and differentiation. T1 tumors of the anal margin that are well differentiated are primarily locally excised. Larger tumor size or node positive cancers of the anal margin are all treated with chemo-radiation in the form of mitomycin/5-fluorouracil and radiation.
- Squamous cell cancers constitute 80% of anal canal cancers (from anorectal ring above to dentate line below). Combination chemo-radiotherapy is used for stages I-III. Patients with T1–2, N0 are treated with mitomycin (10 mg/m^2 on day 1) plus 5- fluorouracil (750 mg/m^2 continuous infusion days 1–5) every 4 weeks with radiotherapy. Patients with larger tumor size or lymph node positivity are treated with mitomycin plus 5-fluorouracil and radiotherapy at higher doses. Chemotherapy in the form of cisplatin plus 5-fluorouracil (FUP) is used for systemic salvage of metastatic (stage IV) disease.

Local recurrences or persistent disease after treatment may be controlled by using abdomino-perineal resection or inguinal node dissection for local salvage after radiation and local radiation for local salvage after surgery. In some cases, chemo-radiation salvage with 5-fluorouracil plus cisplatin plus a radiation boost can be used to treat residual disease and avoid a permanent colostomy.

Anal adenocarcinomata, which are not common, behave like rectal cancers and have higher incidence of recurrence and metastasis. They are treated with the same protocols as rectal cancer.

Post-operative adjuvant therapy for patients who do not receive preoperative therapy FOLFOX (oxaliplatin <Eloxatin>, leucovorin, 5-fluorouracil <5-FU>), comprising on day 1 oxaliplatin 85 mg/m^2 plus leucovorin 200 mg/m^2 intravenously, then 5-fluorouracil 400 mg/m^2 intravenous bolus, followed by 5-fluorouracil 600 mg/m^2 as a 22-h continuous infusion. On day 2, leucovorin 200 mg/m^2 infusion over 120 min, followed by 5-fluorouracil 400 mg/m^2 intravenous bolus, then followed by 5-fluorouracil 600 mg/m^2 as a 22-h continuous infusion. Each cycle is repeated every 14 days.

CapeOX (XELOX) (oxaliplatin, capecitabine) entails on day 1 intravenous oxaliplatin 130 mg/m^2 plus capecitabine 1000 mg/m^2 orally twice daily for 14 days in a 21 day cycle for 8 cycles. Capecitabine <Xeloda> monotherapy can be given at 1250 mg/m^2 orally twice daily for days 1–14 every 3 weeks, over 24 weeks.

Concurrent chemotherapy plus radiotherapy External beam radiotherapy may be combined with 5-fluorouracil plus leucovorin. All patients receive an initial 2 cycles of intravenous bolus 5-fluorouracil-based chemotherapy, followed by pelvic radiation therapy plus chemotherapy, then 2 more cycles of chemotherapy. It entails on days 1–5 and days 29–33 intravenous 5-fluorouracil 425 mg/m^2/day and leucovorin 20 mg/m^2/day for 4 cycles. During radiotherapy, 5-fluorouracil 400 mg/m^2/day intravenously and leucovorin 20 mg/m^2/day are given for 4 days during weeks 1 and 5. After radiotherapy, 5-fluorouracil 380 mg/m^2/day intravenously and leucovorin 20 mg/m^2/day intravenously for 5 consecutive days for 2 cycles for 4 cycles are administered.

Advanced or metastatic rectal cancer is treated like advanced or metastatic colon cancer.

nase inhibitors in the treatment of ERBB1-positive cancers is ineffective. Similarly, the combination of ERBB1 antagonism with cytotoxic chemotherapy has failed to show clinical benefit. By contrast, ERBB2 antagonists are very effective in combination with conventional chemotherapy.

7.3 Emerging Combination Chemotherapies

Three decades of molecular biology research (around 1970–2000) have become vested in the development of targeted drugs (described in Chap. 4). The promise of these new agents has not yet been fully realized, as they often cause only temporary remission followed by relapse, resulting in very modest gains in overall survival. Some cancers rapidly develop resistance because of their genetic instability and the selective pressure exerted by the treatment. An initially successful drug becomes ineffective due to mutations in the tumor. In other cancers, multiple signaling pathways (often linked to receptor tyrosine kinases) are co-activated, so that redundant inputs drive oncogenic signaling. In those cases, the efficacy of therapies targeting single receptor tyrosine kinases is limited.

To overcome the acquired resistance of cancer cells to tyrosine kinase inhibitors (caused by mutations in the drug target, such as T790M in EGFR or T315I in BCR-ABL), second and third generation tyrosine kinase inhibitors have been developed. As single agents, however, they are also subject to losing efficacy.

To increase the success rates, past efforts have combined the new-generation molecular drugs with conventional chemotherapy (see examples in Chaps. 7.1 and 7.2). This has maintained the toxicity of those regimens and yielded only moderate gains. In development are combination chemotherapy strategies constituted of multiple molecularly targeted agents. After periods of non-specific anti-proliferative or cytotoxic mono-therapy (around 1945 through 1965), conventional combination chemotherapy (1965 through the late 1990s), and molecularly targeted single agents (since 1997), combination therapy with multiple molecularly targeted drugs will constitute the fourth major phase in the history of anti-cancer drug treatment. Its successful realization will require the analysis of the molecular defects of the primary and metastatic growths to identify the drivers of pathogenesis, and to characterize suitable drug targets through which these drivers can be silenced.

Targeted therapies that inhibit receptor tyrosine kinases and the downstream Phosphatidylinositol 3-Kinase signaling pathway have anti-cancer activity, but their efficacy in solid tumors, including glioblastoma multiforme, has been modest. These cancers display multiple concomitantly activated receptor tyrosine kinases. Hence, combinations of tyrosine kinase inhibitors, but not single agents, decrease signaling, cell survival, and anchorage-independent growth. Response may be achieved even in glioma cells deficient in PTEN, a frequently inactivated inhibitor of Phosphatidylinositol 3-Kinase. Thus, effective glioblastoma multiforme therapy may require combined regimens targeting multiple receptor tyrosine kinases (Stommel et al. 2007).

Within months of starting therapy, breast cancer resistance typically occurs to the antibody trastuzumab and the tyrosine kinase inhibitor lapatinib, either as single agents or in combination with chemotherapy in the metastatic setting. Trastuzumab resistance can be caused by signaling from other ERBB receptors, signaling from receptor tyrosine kinases outside of the ERBB family, increased Phosphatidylinositol 3-Kinase signaling, or the presence of truncated forms of ERBB2. Lapatinib resistance may be due to increased Phos-

Cancer (current):

Targets:	Agents:
DNA damage	redox-cycling antibiotics
DNA damage	anti-metabolites
DNA damage	alkylating agents
mitosis inhibitors	vinca alcaloids

conventional chemotherapy (e.g. COPP, MOPP) combines several DNA damaging agents to limit the impact of their adverse effects

Cancer (vision):

Targets:	Agents:
Tumor growth	small molecule kinase inhibitors, neutralizing antibodies
Immortalization	telomerase inhibitors
Metastasis	blockers of homing receptors protease inhibitors
Host interactions	angiogenesis inhibitors tumor vaccines/ immuno-therapy

Combination chemotherapy targets the major characteristics of cancer to maximize efficacy

Fig. 7.1 Combination drug treatment. Current combination chemotherapy for cancer combines agents that uniformly exert DNA damage to suppress cell division, thus predominantly reducing the adverse effects of high dose monotherapy (*top*). Increasing insights into the molecular mechanisms of malignant transformation have defined multiple candidate drug targets. This should lead to combination chemotherapy protocols that target the major characteristics of cancer cells to maximize efficacy (*bottom*). (Weber 2008)

phatidylinositol 3-Kinase signaling as well as derepression or activation of compensatory survival pathways (Garrett and Arteaga 2011). Elevated expression of ERBB3 induces resistance to therapeutic agents, including trastuzumab, in ERBB2 over-expressing breast cancer. ERBB3 can form a hetero-trimeric complex with ERBB2 and IGF-1 Receptor, thus activating a growth signal. The addition of an anti-ERBB3 antibody to the regimen may overcome resistance and induce apoptosis in the transformed cells (Huang et al. 2013). A neutralizing antibody to ERBB3 that inhibits ligand-induced and ligand-independent ERBB3 dimerization, may be combined with trastuzumab and an ATP competitive inhibitor of Phosphatidylinositol 3-Kinase to treat breast or gastric cancers that over-express ERBB2. The combination inhibits tumor growth and improves survival. Dual blockade of the ERBB2 signaling network with an ERBB3 antibody that inhibits ERBB2/ERBB3 dimers in combination with a specific inhibitor of Phosphatidylinositol 3-Kinase in the absence of a direct ERBB2 antagonist may be an effective treatment approach (Garrett et al. 2013).

The mortality of cancer patients is largely caused by tumor invasiveness, leading to local or metastatic tissue destruction. Conventional anti-cancer drugs mostly exert their effects through the inhibition of cell cycle progression, leaving two major intrinsic characteristics of transformed cells, invasiveness and extension of lifespan, under-treated. Because receptors and cytokine ligands that mediate metastasis formation are sparsely expressed in the adult healthy organism and are more readily reached by pharmaceuticals than intracellular drug targets they may represent a particularly suitable focus for therapeutic intervention. Conventional combination chemotherapy predominantly reduces the adverse effects of agents that by-and-large have the same drug target: rapidly dividing cells. The benefit of the combination is the enhanced tolerability of the treatment. Emerging concepts of combination chemotherapy, using molecularly targeted drugs, will be directed at several components of transformation. The inclusion of anti-metastatic agents in new generation cancer chemotherapy is expected to improve treatment success (Fig. 7.1).

References

Ajani JA, Winter KA, Gunderson LL, Pedersen J, Benson AB III, Thomas CR Jr, Mayer RJ, Haddock MG, Rich TA, Willett C (2008) Fluorouracil, mitomycin, and radiotherapy vs fluorouracil, cisplatin, and radiotherapy for carcinoma of the anal canal. JAMA 299:1914–1921

Arseneau JC, Sponzo RW, Levin DL, Schnipper LE, Bonner H, Young RC, Canellos GP, Johnson RE, DeVita VT (1972) Nonlymphomatous malignant tumors complicating Hodgkin's disease. Possible association with intensive therapy. N Engl J Med 287:1119–1122

Bonadonna G, Zucali R, Monfardini S, De Lena M, Uslenghi C (1975) Combination chemotherapy of Hodgkin's disease with adriamycin, bleomycin, vinblastine, and imidazole carboxamide versus MOPP. Cancer 36:252–259

Bonate PL, Arthaud L, Cantrell WR Jr, Stephenson K, Secrist JA III, Weitman S (2006) Discovery and development of clofarabine: a nucleoside analogue for treating cancer. Nat Rev Drug Discov 5:855–863

Canellos G, Anderson J, Propert K, Nissen N, Cooper M, Henderson E, Green M, Gottlieb A, Peterson B (1992) Chemotherapy of advanced Hodgkin's disease with MOPP, ABVD, or MOPP alternating with ABVD. N Engl J Med 327:1478–1484

DeVita VT Jr, Chu E (2008) A history of cancer chemotherapy. Cancer Res 68:8643–8653.

Frei E 3rd, Holland JF, Schneiderman MA, Pinkel D, Selkirk G, Freireich EJ, Silver RT, Gold GL, Regelson W (1958) A comparative study of two regimens of combination chemotherapy in acute leukemia. Blood 13:1126–1148

Frei E 3rd, Karon M, Levin RH, Freireich EJ, Taylor RJ, Hananian J, Selawry O, Holland JF, Hoogstraten B, Wolman IJ, Abir E, Sawitsky A, Lee S, Mills SD, Burgert EO Jr, Spurr CL, Patterson RB, Ebaugh FG, James GW 3rd, Moon JH (1965) The effectiveness of combinations of antileukemic agents in inducing and maintaining remission in children with acute leukemia. Blood 26:642–656

Garrett JT, Arteaga CL (2011) Resistance to ERBB2 directed antibodies and tyrosine kinase inhibitors: mechanisms and clinical implications. Cancer Biol Ther 11:793–800

Garrett JT, Sutton CR, Kurupi R, Bialucha CU, Ettenberg SA, Collins SD, Sheng Q, Wallweber J, Defazio-Eli L, Arteaga CL (2013) Combination of antibody that inhibits ligand-independent HER3 dimerization and a p110α inhibitor potently blocks PI3K signaling and growth of HER2+ breast cancers. Cancer Res 73:6013–6023

Goldberg RM, Sargent DJ, Morton RF, Fuchs CS, Ramanathan RK, Williamson SK, Findlay BP, Pitot HC, Alberts SR (2004) A randomized controlled trial of fluorouracil plus leucovorin, irinotecan, and oxaliplatin combinations in patients with previously untreated metastatic colorectal cancer. J Clin Oncol 22:23–30

Hoerni B, Orgerie MB, Eghbali H, Blanc CM, David B, Rojouan J, Zittoun R (1991) Novel combination of epirubicin, bleomycin, vinblastine and prednisone (EBVP II) before radical radiotherapy in localized stages (I–IIIA) of Hodgkin's disease. Early results in 100 consecutive patients. Pierre-et-Marie-Curie Group. J Cancer Res Clin Oncol 117:377–380

Huang J, Wang S, Lyu H, Cai B, Yang X, Wang J, Liu B (2013) The anti-erbB3 antibody MM-121/SAR256212 in combination with trastuzumab exerts potent antitumor activity against trastuzumab-resistant breast cancer cells. Mol Cancer 12:134

Kondagunta GV, Motzer RJ (2006) Chemotherapy for advanced germ cell tumors. J Clin Oncol 24:5493–5502

Santoro A, Bonadonna G, Valagussa P, Zucali R, Viviani S, Villani F, Pagnoni A, Bonfante V, Musumeci R, Crippa F (1987) Long-term results of combined chemotherapy-radiotherapy approach in Hodgkin's disease: superiority of ABVD plus radiotherapy versus MOPP plus radiotherapy. J Clin Oncol 5:27–37

Stommel JM, Kimmelman AC, Ying H, Nabioullin R, Ponugoti AH, Wiedemeyer R, Stegh AH, Bradner JE, Ligon KL, Brennan C, Chin L, DePinho RA (2007) Coactivation of receptor tyrosine kinases affects the response of tumor cells to targeted therapies. Science 318:287–290

Wang D, Lippard SL (2005) Cellular processing of platinum anticancer drugs. Nat Rev Drug Discov 4:307–320

Weber GF (2008) Molecular mechanisms of metastasis. Cancer Lett 270:181–190

Part III
Emerging and Alternative Treatment Modalities

8 Gene Therapy

The roots of gene therapy go back to the 1960s (Table 8.1). One basic concept that emerged was the replacement of a defective gene with exogenous DNA representing the intact sequence. The notion that gene expression can be modified through the use of exogenous nucleic acids largely derives from studies that in 1977 first used single stranded DNA to inhibit the translation of a complementary RNA in a cell free system (Paterson et al. 1977). In the following year (Stephenson and Zamecnik 1978; Zamecnik and Stephenson 1978), it was shown that a 13-mer DNA oligodeoxynucleotide, which was antisense to the Rous sarcoma virus, could inhibit viral reduplication in culture. In the 1980s, gene therapy was conceptualized (Anderson 1984). In 1980, Martin Cline attempted to correct an inherited metabolic defect in children by transfecting and re-infusing bone marrow cells. The study had not received prior permission and was unsuccessful. Cline lost his university chair at the University of California, Los Angeles and much of his NIH (National Institute of Health) funding. The molecular biology and clinical medicine communities working on gene therapy came together effectively for the first time at the Banbury Conference Center, Cold Spring Harbor Laboratories in 1983. The first approved gene therapy in the United States was undertaken in 1990 to correct an inherited enzyme deficiency. In that same year, gene therapy was tested on melanoma patients (the first successful gene therapy of metastatic melanoma was reported only in 2006, using killer T-cells genetically re-targeted to attack the cancer cells). In 1992, Claudio Bordignon at the Vita-Salute San Raffaele University at Milan, Italy performed the first procedure of gene therapy using hematopoietic stem cells as vectors to deliver genes that were intended to correct hereditary diseases. In 2003, a University of California, Los Angeles research team inserted genes into the brain using liposomes coated in polyethylene glycol.

Gene therapy requires specific functional nucleotide sequences in cloned form and efficient methods for their transfer. Genes may be delivered in multiple ways, including in vivo (the gene is delivered to a targeted site within the patient) or ex vivo (cells are collected, the gene is transduced, cells are re-infused). There are nucleotide based (mostly DNA based, in vivo) and cell based (ex vivo) treatment regimens. DNA based gene therapy uses vectors to deliver modified genes to their target cells. Cell based gene therapy techniques remove cells from the patient, alter their genetic makeup, and then reintroduce them to the body.

8.1 Gene Silencing

Agents for gene silencing are comprised of nucleic acids or nucleic acid analogs capable of Watson-Crick base pairing. The target sequence is either DNA or RNA. Most compounds target and bind to the mRNA of specific genes, resulting in post-transcriptional gene silencing. However, native DNA does not easily penetrate through cell membranes. Inside cells, it is subject to relatively rapid degradation, primarily through the action of 3' Exonucleases, but also through Endonuclease attack. Modifications of the nucleic acids destined for clinical use facilitate delivery, confer increased resistance to Nucleases, provide distinct affinities for DNA or RNA, and increase the specificity for a given target.

8.1.1 Antisense

The antisense principle was originally described in experiments that blocked the reduplication of Rous Sarcoma Virus in infected chicken fibroblasts (Stephenson and Zamecnik 1978; Zamecnik and Stephenson 1978). In the mid-1980s, the existence of naturally occurring antisense RNAs and their roles in regulating gene expression was shown (Simons and Kleckner 1983; Mizuno et al. 1984). These observations lent credibility to the notion that antisense was more than just a laboratory phenomenon, and supported the hypothesis that reverse complementary antisense nucleic acids could be used in patients to manipulate gene expression. On this basis, the development of technologies that use nucleic acids to manipulate gene expression was stimulated.

Antisense oligodeoxynucleotides are short stretches of 12–30 bases, DNA or RNA, that down-regulate gene

G. F. Weber, *Molecular Therapies of Cancer*, DOI 10.1007/978-3-319-13278-5_8,

Table 8.1 Time line of DNA technology

1869	Miescher identifies weakly acidic substance in the nuclei of white blood cells (later known as deoxyribonucleic acid, DNA)
1909	The term gene is used by Johanssen to explain the hereditary basis of traits
1944	Avery, McLeod, McCarthy show that DNA constitutes the genetic material
1953	Watson and Crick deduce the double helical structure of DNA (from X-ray diffraction data generated by Rosalind Franklin)
1961	Brenner and Crick establish that codons (3 nucleotide bases) specify individual amino acids
1966	The genetic code is cracked by Nierenberg and Matthaei
1960s	Evidence for uptake and expression of exogenous DNA by mammalian cells
1973	Cohen and Boyer clone genes inserted into plasmids
1973	Development of calcium phosphate cell transformation
1977	Sanger and Gilbert independently devise methods for sequencing DNA
1981	Stable in vitro correction of gene deficiency
1982	Development of retroviral vectors
1982	Palmiter and Brinster generate the first transgenic mouse
1983	PCR is invented by Mullis
1985	Hood invents an automated DNA sequencer
1987–1989	Evans, Smithies, and Capecchi create knockout mice
1989	First approved human clinical gene therapy study
1990	The Human Genome Project (HUGO) is launched
1998	Competition to HUGO by a private enterprise (Venter)
2000	Draft sequence of the human genome

expression. These oligodeoxynucleotides can be designed to complement a region of a particular gene or messenger RNA and serve as potential inhibitors of transcription or translation through sequence specific hybridization. The ability of an antisense molecule to form a stable hybrid is a function of its binding affinity and sequence specificity. Binding affinity is determined by the number of hydrogen bonds that are formed between the drug and its target. Tertiary structure and mRNA associated proteins also influence the ability of an antisense molecule to hybridize with its target. Sequence specificity reduces adverse effects. Additional factors that affect the pharmacological properties of antisense compounds are

- secondary and tertiary structure of the targeted mRNA,
- generic sequence motifs (such as G-4 tracts, composed of 4 consecutive guanosines), which inhibit cell proliferation non-specifically,
- CpG motifs, which can non-specifically activate certain parts of the immune system,
- sequence dependent cellular uptake.

Safety, specificity, efficacy and cellular uptake of oligodeoxynucleotides strongly depend on an appropriate selection of the target sequence.

Virtually all of the available antisense technologies rely on some type of nucleotide sequence recognition for targeting specificity, but differ as to where and how they perturb the flow of genetic information. Strategies for targeting genes focus primarily on homologous recombination or triple-helix-forming oligonucleotides. While homologous recombination involves vector technology, triple-helix-forming oligonucleotides bind in the major groove of duplex DNA in a sequence specific manner (Opalinska and Gewirtz 2002). Gene targeting with these molecules is constrained by the fact that triple-helix forming oligonucleotides require runs of purines on one strand and pyrimidines on the other (10–30 nucleotides in length) for stable hybridization. The triple-helix forming oligonucleotides can be composed of either poly-purine or poly-pyrimidine tracts, but hybridization always occurs on the purine strand of the duplex through the formation of Hoogsteen bonds. The frequency of repairs accomplished with triple-helix forming oligonucleotides, in most cases, has been far too low to be of clinical use at the present time.

The major challenge to antisense therapeutic strategies is the stability of the agents. Phosphorothioate antisense oligonucleotides (isoelectronic congeners of phosphodiester oligodeoxynucleotides that contain internucleoside linkages, in which one of the non-bridging oxygen atoms has been replaced by a sulfur atom) have enhanced Nuclease resistance with a half-life in the blood of approximately 9–10 h compared to less than 1 h for unmodified antisense oligonucleotides. DNA-RNA duplexes are short lived in cells because they are strong inducers of RNAse H activity that hydrolyses the RNA in the duplex. Antisense oligonucleotide analogs with 2' modifications to the ribose increase DNA-RNA stability. There have been 3 generations of nucleic acid analogs capable of binding RNA or DNA.

- The first generation analogs add a sulfur to the non-bridging oxygen atom of the phosphodiester bond, conferring additional stability through Nuclease resistance. The addition of a charged group enhances water solubility.

- Second generation analogs add alkyl modifications at the 2' position of the ribose, which avoids stimulating RNAse H activity when bound to RNA.
- Third generation analogs add substantial modifications to the sugar or to the phosphate backbone, conferring resistance to DNAses.

Adverse Effects The efficacy and toxicity profiles of antisense oligonucleotides may be highly dependent on the schedule of administration. Adverse effects induced by antisense oligodeoxynucleotides can result not only from the suppression of the targeted gene, but also from effects of the chemical backbone. In the case of phosphorothioates, this problem is addressed by infusion continuously and slowly at low doses. In clinical trials, phosphorothioates have been well tolerated.

Pro-apoptosis The anti-apoptotic protein BCL-2 is an important regulator of programmed cell death. Its over-abundance is implicated in the pathogenesis of some lymphomata. Specifically, BCL-2 is highly over-expressed in CLL cells and plays a role in pathogenesis of the disease, preventing lymphocyte apoptosis and being strongly correlated with poor clinical outcome. Up-regulation of BCL-2 in certain types of cancer is also linked to tumor drug resistance. The proliferation of lymphoma cells with a t(14;18) translocation can be inhibited by antisense RNA targeted at the start codon region of *bcl-2* messenger RNA. A potential limitation to this approach is a poor correlation of substantial suppression of BCL-2 protein expression with clinical responses.

The phosphorothioate antisense oligonucleotide oblimersen (G3139) <Genasense, Augmerosen>was developed by Genta to target BCL-2. It is complementary to the first 6 codons of *bcl-2* mRNA. Targeted to the initiation site, oblimersen inhibits *bcl-2* translation, resulting in a decreased expression of the BCL-2 protein. It is under study as a possible treatment for several types of cancer, including chronic lymphocytic leukemia, B-cell lymphoma, and breast cancer.

This agent may enhance the efficacy of standard cytotoxic chemotherapy. Oblimersen down-regulates *bcl-2* mRNA within 48 h and protein levels within 96 h. This down-regulation is associated with sensitization of myeloma cells to the cytotoxic activity of dexamethasone and doxorubicin.

Oligonucleotide SPC2996 constitutes a synthetic phosphorothioate antisense 16-mer oligonucleotide, of which 4 DNA nucleotides are replaced with locked nucleic acid nucleotides[1]. The incorporation of locked nucleic acids into the molecule may offer increased target sequence affinity, specificity, and higher biostability. SPC2996 is the first drug in the class of locked nucleic acid based (LNA based) RNA antagonists. It differs in only 3 nucleotides from the oblimersen sequence. The drug is efficiently incorporated into various tumor cell types. It binds to and inactivates *bcl-2* mRNA, thereby inhibiting the expression of the BCL-2 protein. While the oligonucleotide alone does not consistently display strong anti-tumor responses, it may have benefit in potentially enhancing the efficacy of standard cytotoxic chemotherapy.

Adverse Effects SPC2996 has immunostimulatory effects in chronic lymphocytic leukemia (CLL) patients.

XIAP (X-Linked Inhibitor of Apoptosis Protein) is a pivotal inhibitor of apoptosis that is over-expressed in many tumors. It may render tumor cells resistant to apoptosis by interfering with both the intrinsic and extrinsic death program pathways. XIAP is an inhibitor of the initiator Caspase-9 and the effector Caspases -3 and -7. In acute myeloid leukemia (AML), XIAP may be over-expressed, contribute to chemo- and radio-resistance, and lead to poor clinical outcome.

AEG35156 (GEM 640) is a second generation synthetic antisense oligonucleotide. The drug is a 19-mer, fully phosphorothioated oligonucleotide, in which the 11 core DNA bases are flanked by 4 2'-*O*-methyl-modified RNA residues at the 3' and 5' ends. The sequence of this mixed backbone oligonucleotide was designed for specificity and cellular potency in the absence of CpG residues (to avoid CpG mediated immunostimulation). AEG35156 selectively blocks the cellular expression of XIAP. This agent reduces the total levels of XIAP in tumor cells, working synergistically with cytotoxic drugs to overcome tumor cell resistance to apoptosis. AEG35156 is administered at a maximum dose of 350 mg/m^2.

Survivin (BIRC5) is a member of the IAP (Inhibitor of Apoptosis) family. It plays a key role in cell division, as well as in inhibiting programmed cell death. Survivin is up-regulated in a variety of cancers, while being absent from most normal adult cells. Its expression in cancers is associated with an aggressive phenotype, decreased patient survival, and increased resistance to chemotherapy.

EZN-3042 hybridizes to *survivin* mRNA, thereby blocking the translation of the Survivin protein. This inhibits Survivin induced anti-apoptotic activity and promotes tumor cell apoptosis in cancers that over-express the target molecule.

[1] Locked nucleic acids (LNAs) are high-affinity RNA analogs, in which the ribose ring is locked in a favorable conformation for Watson-Crick binding. They contain a methylene bridge linking the 2' oxygen and 4' carbon of the ribose sugar ring, thereby increasing their stability and decreasing their degradation. Locking also results in high stability after hybridization with a complementary DNA or RNA strand. Locked nucleic acid oligonucleotides typically consist of a mixture of locked and conventional bases. This allows optimization of their sensitivity and specificity.

EZN-3042 is based on locked nucleic acids. EZN-3042 may chemosensitize as it potentiates the anti-tumor activity of paclitaxel.

Anti-growth signal Protein Kinase C (PKC) comprises a family of biochemically and functionally distinct cytoplasmic Serine/Threonine Kinases. These proteins have a crucial role in transducing the signals that regulate cell proliferation and differentiation. PKC is over-expressed in various cancers.

Aprinocarsen (d(P-thio)GTT CTC GCT GGT GAG TTT CA-3' deoxyribonucleic acid) (ISIS-3521, LY900003) is a 20-mer antisense phosphorothioate oligonucleotide that hybridizes to the 3' untranslated region of the *pkcα* (*protein kinase C-α*) mRNA and degrades it through RNase H mediated cleavage, thereby inhibiting PKC-α expression and growth of PKC-α dependent tumor cells.

Pharmacokinetics With continuous infusion, steady state blood concentrations of aprinocarsen are reached within 4 h.

Adverse Effects Adverse effects may entail fever, hemorrhage, nausea, chills, myalgias, headache, and fatigue. Transient grade 4 neutropenia may be a serious event. These changes correlate with dose and are transient, with recovery to baseline by day 7. Drug induced coagulation and complement changes result in a maximum tolerated dose of 25 mg/kg.

RAS is a component of several interconnected receptor signaling pathways. The protein is constitutively active, and promotes proliferation and malignant transformation in multiple cancers. RAF is a serine/threonine kinase that functions as an effector immediately downstream of RAS signal transduction via the ERK pathway **(see Fig. 4.10)**. Constitutive activation of this pathway directly contributes to malignant transformation in various tumors.

ISIS-5132 (CGP 69846A) is a synthetic 20-base antisense phosphorothioate oligodeoxynucleotide that hybridizes to the 3' untranslated region of *c-raf* mRNA. ISIS-5132 specifically suppresses RAF-1 expression. In clinical trials, while no major tumor responses were achieved, some patients had stabilization of their disease.

Pharmacokinetics Half-lives in tissues generally are 15–60 h, compared to blood half-lives of 30–45 min. Rapid clearance of the oligonucleotide from the blood is predominantly the result of distribution to tissue and Exonuclease mediated base deletion. Urinary excretion is a minor pathway for the elimination of oligonucleotide over the 24-h period immediately following intravenous administration, however, the amount of oligonucleotide excreted in the urine increases as a function of dose.

Adverse Effects The maximum tolerated dose is 25 mg/kg/week, limited by acute hemolytic anemia, acute renal failure, and anasarca (extreme generalized edema). Dose dependent complement activation can occur.

The proto-oncogene *c-myb* encodes a protein that is a regulator of cell cycle progression and maturation, primarily in hematopoietic cells. In experimental treatment, antisense targeting of *c-myb* is used to purge $CD34^+$ cells from marrow autografts that are administered to patients with allograft-ineligible chronic myelogenous leukemia (CML). Post-purging, *c-myb* mRNA levels decline substantially in about 50 % of the patients, and in some patients complete remission is achieved (Luger et al. 2002).

The proto-oncogene *c-myc* contributes to progression and is associated with prognosis in melanoma. Over-expression of c-MYC may also contribute to chemoresistance to cisplatin and other drugs.

AVI-4126 is a *c-myc* antisense phosphorodiamidate morpholino oligomer[2]. The drug is in clinical trials. Intravenous administration allows its accumulation in tumor tissues.

Members of the *erbb* gene family are over-expressed in many cancers. They play roles in the regulation of cell proliferation and carcinogenesis. *egfr* antisense DNA represents the antisense orientation to a sequence of DNA in *epidermal growth factor receptor* (*egfr*), an *erbb* gene family member. *egfr* antisense DNA suppresses the expression of ERBB1 (EGFR) by tumor cells, thereby inhibiting tumor cell proliferation and decreasing tumor growth. This agent also may reduce the invasiveness of certain breast cancer cells by blocking the downstream activation of metastasis genes. Further, *egfr* antisense molecules are under study as sensitizers for chemo-radio-therapy.

A 39-base pair *egfr* antisense sequence in clinical trials (5'-CCG GCC GTC CCG GAG GGT CGC ATC GCT GCT CCC CGA AGA-3') spans the translation start site. It is administered in a modified pNGVL vector and expressed under the U6 promoter (Lai et al. 2009).

Others High grade gliomata, pancreatic cancers, and malignant melanomata typically over-express the cytokine TGF-β_2, which suppresses the immune system and prevents immune surveillance.

The *tgf-β_2* specific phosphorothioate antisense oligonucleotide trabedersen (AP-12009) is under study for the treatment of malignant glioma. It is directly infused into the tumor.

[2] Phosphorodiamidate morpholino oligomers are neutrally charged antisense agents, wherein the deoxyribose moiety of DNA is replaced with a 6-membered morpholine ring and the charged phosphodiester internucleoside linkage is replaced with phosphorodiamidate linkages. These agents are steric blockers that inhibit gene expression by preventing components of the splicing or translational machinery from binding. The neutral character avoids the binding to other cellular and extra-cellular proteins that can occur with charged oligonucleotide chemistries.

GTI-2040 is a 20-mer phosphorothioate oligonucleotide that is complementary to a mRNA coding region of the R2 small subunit component of Ribonucleotide Reductase. GTI-2040 is in clinical evaluations for the treatment of solid tumors and acute myelogenous leukemia as a single agent or in combination therapy.

Hypoxia Inducible Factors (HIFs) are transcription factors that respond to decreased availability of oxygen in the cellular environment. HIF-1 is a hetero-dimer composed of an α and a β subunit. Whereas HIF-1β is constitutively expressed, HIF-1α is inducible by hypoxia. As a master regulator of oxygen homeostasis, HIF-1 activates the transcription of genes that are involved in angiogenesis, cell survival, and glucose metabolism. EZN2968, a locked nucleic acid based *hif-1α* inhibitor, is under investigation in clinical trials against a variety of cancers.

8.1.2 Ribozymes

RNA can have catalytic activity. Ribozymes cleave or ligate their target RNA in the absence of accessory proteins. They are important for RNA splicing. Ribozymes rely on secondary and tertiary structure to orient the substrate in the catalytic core. Their catalytic motifs are surrounded by flanking sequences that are responsible for guiding the ribozymes to their mRNA targets and giving stability to their structures. There are various classes of ribozymes. The hammerhead ribozymes and the hairpin ribozyme have been extensively studied owing to their small size and rapid kinetics, which make them candidates for the use as drugs. Ribozymes can be expressed from a vector that offers the advantage of continued production of these molecules intracellularly.

RPI 4610 <Angiozyme> is a chemically stabilized (nuclease resistant) ribozyme that targets *vascular endothelial growth factor receptor 1* (*flt-1*) (Fig. 8.1). It is under investigation in combination with carboplatin and paclitaxel in patients with advanced solid tumors (Kobayashi et al. 2005). RPI 4610, given intravenously or subcutaneously, is largely non-toxic at doses up to 300 mg/m^2.

Adverse Effects Adverse effects include nausea and vomiting, anorexia, neuropathy, myalgias, arthalgias, and fatigue. Injection site reactions and generalized skin rashes can arise. Hematologic toxicity includes neutropenia and thrombocytopenia.

Clinical trials are underway with Herzyme, a ribozyme that targets *her2* mRNA. The agent is intended for the treatment of breast and ovarian cancers, as well as a broad spectrum of solid tumors. Herzyme is well tolerated, but efficacy is not yet established.

8.1.3 RNA Interference

A developing approach for targeting messenger RNA is RNA interference (RNAi, co-suppression, post-transcriptional gene silencing). Two types of small RNA molecules, microRNA (miRNA) and small interfering RNA (siRNA), are central to the process. These small RNAs can bind to other specific mRNA molecules and either increase or decrease their activity. Small nuclear RNA (snRNA) is a variant form

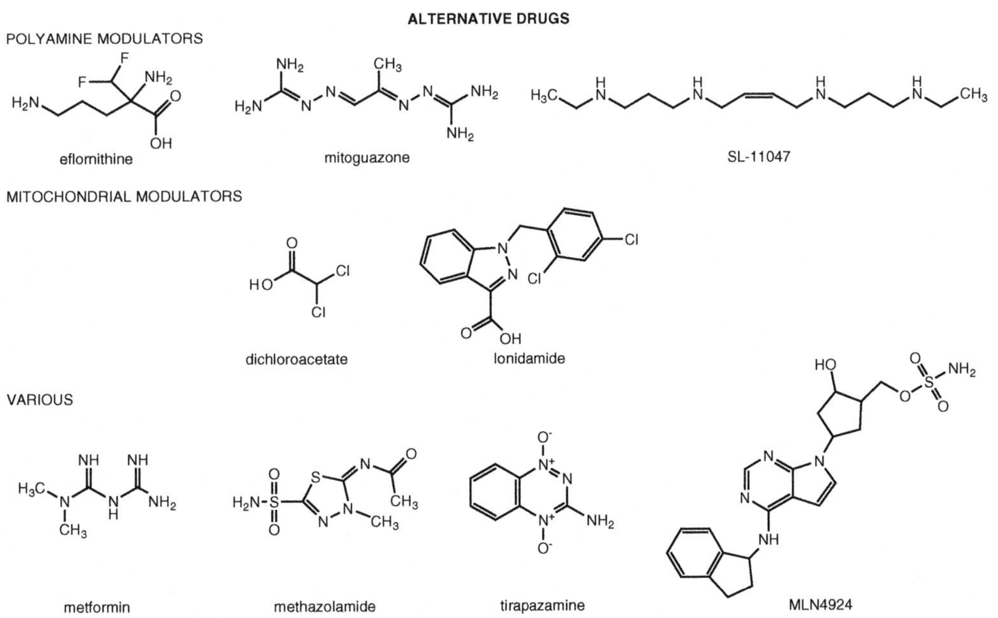

Fig. 8.1 Structure of angiozyme. *Uppercase letters* indicate ribonucleotides, *lowercase letters* designate 2'-*O*-methyl ribonucleotides. The *subscript s* denotes a phosphorothioate linkage. *B* inverted 2'-deoxy abasic, u_4 2'-*C*-allyl uridine. (Redrawn from Sandberg et al. 2000)

comprised of 90–300 nucleotides. It has regulatory roles in RNA processing.

The RNA interference pathway is initiated by the enzyme Dicer, which cleaves long double stranded RNA molecules into short fragments of around 20 nucleotides, which are unwound into 2, a passenger strand and a guide strand. Whereas the passenger strand is degraded, the guide strand is incorporated into the RNA induced silencing complex (RISC). When the guide strand base pairs with a complementary sequence of a messenger RNA molecule and induces cleavage by the enzyme Argonaute (the catalytic component of the RISC complex), post-transcriptional gene silencing results.

Silencing of oncogenes may be accomplished with antisense, ribozyme, or RNA interference constructs.
Due to the size and charge characteristics of the drug compounds, their delivery is a major limitation.

8.2 Suicide Genes

Ganciclovir (9-(1,3-dihydroxy-2-propoxymethyl)guanine, GCV) <Cytovene> is a synthetic guanine derivative with anti-viral activity. Herpes simplex virus Thymidine Kinase is different from mammalian Thymidine Kinase; it is able to metabolize the non-toxic prodrug, ganciclovir, into a monophosphate derivative, then into a triphosphate. The active metabolite ganciclovir-5-triphosphate (ganciclovir-TP) may inhibit viral DNA synthesis by competitive inhibition of viral DNA Polymerases and incorporation into viral DNA, resulting in the eventual termination of viral DNA elongation. The host cells do not activate the prodrug and are not killed.

Suicide gene therapy with herpes simplex virus *thymidine kinase* plus ganciclovir is a prodrug activation therapy (Plautz et al. 1991). In this mode, the transduced herpes simplex virus *thymidine kinase* gene is expressed in tumor cells and activates the prodrug ganciclovir. Activated ganciclovir consecutively inhibits DNA Polymerase and kills proliferating cells. It is not necessary to transduce all cancer cells with the suicide gene. The modality also kills non-transduced tumor cells through a bystander effect, possibly by passage of the activated ganciclovir through cell-cell contacts (gap junctions) or by immunostimulation through the lysed tumor cells.

Ganciclovir has higher cytotoxic efficacy than the other herpes simplex virus Thymidine Kinase substrates acyclovir and 1-β-D-arabinofuranosylthymine (araT). Liposomal encapsulation of ganciclovir may further enhance its efficacy.

Adverse Effects Adverse effects include nausea, confusion, seizure, headache, cerebral edema, and meningitis.

An advanced form of the suicide gene strategy is a combination of prodrug activation therapy and gene based immunotherapy. The herpes simplex virus *thymidine kinase* gene and a cytokine gene are introduced into the tumor cells of a patient. The tumor cells that produce the cytokine attract immune response cells, while the cells that express the herpes simplex virus Thymidine Kinase phosphorylate ganciclovir. Activated ganciclovir kills the tumor cells, and the immune response cells eliminate them.

Genetic variants of HSV-1 have been engineered for use in suicide gene therapy with various agents (see Sect. 8.3.1.)

8.3 Oncolytic Viruses

Oncolytic viruses preferentially infect and lyse cancer cells. This may allow their therapeutic use for the destruction of tumor cells or for delivering anti-cancer agents to the tumor site. However, blood-borne viruses can be inactivated by antibodies and cleared from the blood stream by Kupffer cells. Avoidance of the immune system is one of the major challenges in oncolytic virus therapy. The virus should also be able to tolerate storage and production at high titers. A double stranded DNA genome is advantageous because it has greater stability during storage, which reduces the risk of hazardous mutations.

8.3.1 Engineered Oncolytic Viruses

In 2005, the first oncolytic virus to be approved by a regulatory agency (China's State Food and Drug Administration, SFDA) was the genetically modified adenovirus H101 (recombinant human adenvirus type 5, for injection) <Oncorine>. H101 is engineered to remove a viral defense mechanism from adenovirus that interacts with P53 to allow virus reduplication. As P53 is very commonly inactivated in cancer cells H101 can selectively multiply in these cells.

Upon infection of cells by adenovirus, the early proteins E1A and E1B are expressed and support viral reduplication. The infected cells respond by activating P53 expression, which curbs virus production by mediating cell cycle arrest, apoptosis, and DNA damage repair. E1B can degrade P53, favoring virus reduplication. H101 is reconstructed from the wild-type adenovirus type 5 by deletion of the genes for E1B and E3. Due to the deletion of E1B, H101 cannot reduplicate in untransformed cells, but P53 deficient cells are susceptible. The partial deletion of E3, which encodes the adenovirus death protein, enhances the safety profile of the administered treatment. While the virus does not specifically infect cancer cells, it kills cancer cells preferentially. When combined with chemotherapy, H101 increases the treatment response rate. Injection into the tumor is the preferred route of administration, but may be replaced by intravenous infusion for metastatic disease. The drug is used for the treatment of head and neck cancer.

Adverse Effects Fever commonly results and should not be suppressed for the full effect of the viral therapy.

ONYX-015 is an adenovirus with deleted E1B that is able to selectively reduplicate in and lyse P53 deficient cells. After tumor cell lysis, released viruses infect neighboring cancer cells, tripping a chain of ONYX-015 mediated tumor cell cytotoxicity.

G207 is a genetically engineered mutant strain of herpes simplex virus 1 (HSV-1). It has defects in the genes encoding for both Ribonucleotide Reductase and the neurovirulence factor ICP34.5 (γ34.5)[3]. G207 can be used as a cancer cytotoxic agent and as a gene transfer vector. While the virus is reduplication competent, it is engineered to selectively multiply within cancer cells.

HSV1716 <Seprehvir> is a first generation oncolytic virus developed to selectively destroy cancer cells. Based on herpes simplex virus-1 (HSV-1), the HSV1716 strain contains a deletion of the neurovirulence gene ICP34.5, the absence of which suppresses reduplication in untransformed cells (compared to HSV-1, it also reduces the reduplication in transformed cells, but to a lesser extent). Due to the lack of ICP34.5, the HSV-1716 variant is unable to overcome the Protein Kinase R mediated defenses of healthy cells, but these defenses are much weaker in tumor cells.

- The variant HSV1716NTR is generated by the insertion of the gene for Nitroredcutase into the HSV1716 genome to initiate a gene-directed enzyme prodrug therapy[4]. It is used in conjunction with the prodrug 5-(1-aziridinyl)-2,4-dinitrobenzamide (CB1954) to force a reduction in tumor volume.
- A variant of HSV1716 expresses the Noradrenaline Transporter. Based on gene expression from the virus, the Noradrenaline Transporter becomes abundant on the cancer cells and specifically imports a co-treatment containing radioactive iodine across the cell membrane.

GL-ONC1 (GLV-1h68) is a genetically stable, attenuated vaccinia virus. Upon administration, GL-ONC1 preferentially enters tumor cells due to the permeable nature of the tumor vasculature. Once inside a cell, the virus reduplicates, resulting in tumor cell lysis and the release of mature viral particles into the tumor micro-environment. These viral particles may then infect and destroy neighboring tumor cells. The virus encodes the light-emitting fusion protein Renilla Luciferase-Aequorea Green Fluorescent Protein (RUC-GFP), which allows for both detection and monitoring of virally infected tumor cells with luciferase mediated bioluminescence imaging and fluorescence imaging techniques. GL-ONC1 is in clinical trials for treating solid tumors.

8.3.2 Immunostimulatory Oncolytic Viruses

OncoVEX GM-CSF is an oncolytic virus based on herpes simplex virus. In contrast to other oncolytic viruses, the efficacy of OncoVEX GM-CSF (Granulocyte-Macrophage Colony-Stimulating Factor) is not compromised by host immunity. By contrast, this virus stimulates a systemic anti-tumor immune response, enhanced through the release of GM-CSF into the micro-environment of the dying tumor cells. It is in clinical trials for melanoma and head and neck cancer. Mono-therapy has resulted in a 30 % response rate following local injection into accessible tumors.

CGTG-102 (Ad5/3-D24-GMCSF) is a recombinant, oncolytic serotype 5/3 capsid modified adenovirus that encodes the immune-stimulatory cytokine GM-CSF. The replacement of the Ad5 capsid protein knob with a knob domain from serotype 3 causes higher transduction in cancer cells as compared to normal cells. CGTG-102 is designed to reduplicate only in cells with defects in the P16/RB/E2F pathway, which are common in solid tumors. Upon administration, the oncolytic adenovirus selectively infects and reduplicates in tumor cells, which may result in tumor cell lysis. Synergistically, the produced GM-CSF enhances antigen presentation, promotes natural killer cell mediated killing, and causes a cytotoxic T-lymphocyte response against the infected tumor cells. CGTG-102 (Ad5/3-D24-GMCSF) is in clinical trials.

Adverse Effects The most common adverse reactions are pain (mostly tumor pain or pain in the injected tumor), fever, fatigue, nausea, and anemia.

JX-594 is a vaccinia poxvirus engineered to contain a disruption of the viral *thymidine kinase* gene and to produce GM-CSF. JX-594 is intended to selectively reduplicate in tumor cells that have an activated EGFR→RAS pathway, but not in untransformed tissue. Delivered either directly into tumors or infused intravenously, it induces tumor shrinkage via

- the lysis of cancer cells through viral reduplication
- the reduction of the blood supply to tumors through vascular targeting and destruction

[3] ICP34.5 enables HSV-1 to reduplicate in neurons of the brain and spinal cord by conditioning post-mitotic cells for viral reduplication.

[4] Directed enzyme prodrug therapies use enzymes that are artificially introduced into the body to convert prodrugs to their active forms in the desired location within the body. Such strategies aim at reducing the systemic toxicity of a drug by achieving high levels of the active form only at the desired site. Due to the lack of specificity y many anti-cancer chemotherapy agents, directed enzyme prodrug therapies have been studied particularly for their use in cancer treatment. Specific strategies include antibody-directed, gene-directed, virus-directed, polymer-directed, and clostridia-directed enzyme prodrug therapies.

- the stimulation of the immune response against cancer cells.

The virus is in clinical trials for the treatment of hepatocellular carcinoma.

Vaccinia-PSA-TRICOM vaccine is a formulation consisting of a mixture of recombinant vaccinia virus that encodes Prostate Specific Antigen (PSA) and recombinant vaccinia virus that encodes the 3 immuno-co-stimulatory transgenes B7.1, ICAM-1, and LFA-3 (TRICOM). This vaccine may enhance antigen presentation over preparations that lack co-stimulation, resulting in the augmentation of a cytotoxic T-lymphocyte immune response against tumor cells that express PSA.

Poxviruses may serve as immunomodulatory cancer therapeutics. Recombinant fowlpox-TRICOM vaccine is a cancer vaccine comprised of a recombinant fowlpox virus vector encoding TRICOM (B7.1, ICAM-1, LFA-3). These 3 co-stimulatory molecule transgenes may enhance antigen presentation and activate cytotoxic T-lymphocytes. Fowlpox virus is reduplication incompetent in mammalian cells.

8.3.3 Wild-Type Oncolytic Viruses

Vesicular stomatitis virus (VSV) is a rhabdovirus that consists of 5 genes encoded by a negative-sense, single stranded RNA genome. The virus has low pathogenicity, due in large part to its sensitivity to Interferons. These molecules activate genetic anti-viral defense programs that protect cells from infection and prevent the spread of the virus. Defects in Interferon response pathways render cancer cells highly sensitive to infection with VSV. Attenuation of the virus by engineering a deletion of the matrix protein MET-51 ablates virtually all infection of untransformed tissues, while reduplication in tumor cells is unaffected.

Pharmacokinetics Because VSV undergoes a rapid cytolytic reduplication cycle, infection leads to death of the transformed cells and roughly a 1000-fold amplification of virus within 24 h. Systemically administered VSV can reach a tumor site, where it reduplicates and induces disease regression.

Poliovirus has a plus-strand RNA genome, the translation of which depends on a tissue specific internal ribosomal entry site (IRES) within the 5' untranslated region of the viral genome, which is active in cells of neuronal origin and allows the translation of the viral genome without a 5' cap. The replacement of the poliovirus IRES with a rhinovirus IRES alters tissue specificity. The resulting PV1(RIPO) virus is able to selectively destroy malignant glioma cells, while leaving healthy neuronal cells unaffected.

Reovirus (respiratory enteric orphan virus) generally infects mammalian respiratory and bowel systems. The majority of humans have been exposed to reovirus by adulthood, without having experienced symptoms. Yet, the virus reproduces well in cancer cells and lyses them. Wild-Type Reovirus, Serotype 3 Dearing <Reolysin> is a formulation of reovirus that is in clinical trials for the treatment of head and neck cancer and colorectal cancer.

NTX-010 (seneca valley virus-001) is a naturally occurring picorna virus. It was originally discovered as a contaminant in cell cultures. NTX-010 is not transmissible among humans and is non-pathogenic to healthy cells, but it displays selectivity for cancers with neuroendocrine features, including small cell lung cancer. As preexisting antibodies are rare in patients NTX-010 can be systemically administered. Neutralizing antibodies are generated within 7–25 days post-treatment. Under investigation is a single dose of 1×10^7 vp/kg.

Coxsackievirus A21 (CVA21) <Cavatak> is a naturally occurring virus that contains a single positive-stranded RNA genome. The virus binds to and enters through the cognate receptor ICAM-1, which is present in abundance on the surface of many cancer cells. Its ensuing exponential reduplication causes the cells to lyse, which also triggers an antitumor immune response. Coxsackievirus A21 is in clinical trials for head and neck cancer and malignant melanoma. Infection remains unsymptomatic or induces mild upper respiratory symptoms.

The oncolytic effect of the newcastle disease virus (NDV) was documented in the 1950s. In 1999, promising results were reported using an attenuated strain, code-named MTH-68, in cancer patients by the researchers who had isolated it in 1968. The virus preferentially targets and fuses with certain types of tumor cells, leaving untransformed cells largely unaffected. It reduplicates within the cytoplasm of the infected cells independently of their cell cycle state. The virus triggers apoptosis via the intrinsic pathway through a loss of mitochondrial membrane potential and release of Cytochrome *c*. At a later stage, the extrinsic pathway is also activated by TRAIL mediated apoptosis. Newcastle disease virus also has aggregating properties that cause syncytia formations of tumor cell, which results in necrosis and amplifies immune system based cell killing. One of the main limitations to the use of newcastle disease virus in treatment is the patient immune response against the virus, which may limit efficacy. Variants have been engineered to circumvent or focus the immune response on the cancer.

- The variant NDV-HUJ has promise in the treatment of glioblastoma multiforme.

- A hyper-fusogenic variant, NDV/F3aa(L289A), has refined abilities of fusing with somatic cells. There is a substantial accumulation of NK-cells and neutrophils following the infusion of NDV/F3aa(L289A).
- The engineered Hitcher B1 NDV/F3aa strain expresses a highly fusogenic F-Protein in combination with immune-stimulatory molecules (Interferon-γ, Interleukin-2, or Tumor Necrosis Factor α). NDV/F3aa IL-2 induces an increase in $CD4^+$ and $CD8^+$ T-lymphocytes, as well as cytotoxic activity within the tumor.
- NDV/F3aa can be modified to express NS1, an influenza virus protein with capability to modulate the innate immune response by suppressing the induction of Interferons.

Oncolytic viruses preferentially infect and lyse cancer cells. Avoidance of neutralization by the immune system is one of the major challenges in oncolytic virus therapy.
Virus forms may be engineered, immunostimulatory, or wild-type.

8.4 Gene Delivery

The development of efficient gene transfer methods has allowed principal proof that phenotype correction with gene therapy is technically feasible. Suitable vehicles include diverse viruses and non-viral delivery systems. The promoters under which genes are expressed may be inducible or constitutive, lineage specific or general. The genes to deliver to cancer cells are predominantly undamaged versions of tumor suppressor genes, although other strategies are also possible.

8.4.1 Viral Gene Delivery Systems

The transduction with non-pathogenic, reduplication defective viral vectors may cause a latent-like infection. Viral genomes can persist in cancer cells for long terms.

By 1981, much of the life cycle and transduction capabilities of retroviruses had become well understood through the work by Mizutani, Temin, and Baltimore. New techniques allowed augmenting these viruses with potentially therapeutic genes. Commercial viral transfection systems contain a number of modifications to limit viral reduplication (and thus increase safety), specify tropism, and generate sites for gene insertions.

- Some adenovirus-5 vectors have deletions of the genes for the structural glycoproteins E1 and E3. While E3 is non-essential and its deletion mainly enables larger sequence insertions, E1 is required and its removal renders the virus incapable of reduplication. It must therefore be supplied either by a packaging cell line or a helper plasmid.
- Some lentiviral and adeno-associated virus based systems have transferred structural and enzymatic genes from the viral vector to helper plasmids. Lentiviral vectors sometimes contain deletions of the 3' long terminal repeat (LTR) enhancer that has no effect on packaging but ensures inactivation following genome insertion.
- Gene sequences may be altered in helper plasmids to prevent homologous recombination and subsequent regeneration of functional virus.
- If viral tropism is unsuitable for therapeutic purposes, it can be altered using different surface glycoproteins to direct virions toward specific targets. The lentiviral coat envelope gene can be replaced with the G Glycoprotein from vesicular stomatitis virus.

Adverse Effects Gene therapy is associated with a unique set of adverse effects. Viral vectors may be oncogenic[5].

Adenoviral Vectors Adenoviruses are large, double stranded DNA viruses that have genomes of 36 kB. As icosahedral, non-enveloped viruses with broad tropism, adenoviruses can infect both dividing and quiescent cells. They do not integrate into the genome, rendering them limited to transient epichromosomal expression. Adenoviruses use both cellular and viral gene products to produce the proteins necessary for building new virion particles.

The tumor suppressor protein P53 is defective in about 50 % of cancers. Recombinant adenovirus-p53 (SCH-58500) is a genetically engineered adenovirus that contains the human *p53* gene. Recombinant adenovirus-p53 delivers this gene into tumor cells in order to initiate P53 expression and consecutively P53 dependent cell cycle arrest and apoptosis.

Contusugene ladenovec (INGN-201) <Advexin> is a reduplication deficient non-integrating, serotype 5 adenoviral vector that carries *p53* under the control of the CMV promoter. Its intended use is for recurrent or refractory head and neck cancer and for Li-Fraumeni syndrome.

rAd-p53 <Gendicine> is an infectious, reduplication-incompetent, recombinant adenoviral particle, composed of the adenoviral vector (serotype 5) and the human wild-type *p53* tumor suppressor gene. It is intended to replenish a functional tumor suppressor P53 in cancer cells with loss of function of this protein. Gendicine does not reduplicate in the infected cells and is incapable of multi-cycle infection and

[5] Since 1999, gene therapy of X-SCID has restored the immune systems of children with the disorder. In 2002, two patients developed T-cell leukemia in a French trial of X-SCID, a 3rd child followed. The leukemias were caused after a retrovirus carrying a gene called γc (common γ chain) inserted into the oncogene *lmo2* in bone marrow cells in infants less than 3 months old. Retroviruses tend to insert into active genes, perhaps because the condensed DNA containing chromatin opens up in these regions.

spreading to the neighboring cells. The infected adenoviral DNA does not integrate into the human host cell genome. In 2003, the agent became the first gene therapy product in clinical use when it was approved by China's State Food and Drug Administration. rAd-p53 is used for treating head and neck cancer. In combination with chemo- and radio-therapy, Gendicine has improved treatment efficacy more than 3-fold.

Adverse Effects The most prominent adverse effect is limited fever in nearly 80 % of patients, occurring usually 2–4 h after administration and lasting for approximately 2–6 h. The fever tends to diminish spontaneously and without medical intervention. Generally, fever occurs at the beginning of the treatment, and then decreases gradually in severity and incidence. Rare events include chills, pain at the injection site, fatigue, nausea, and diarrhea. The treatment is not known to cause allergic reactions.

Adeno-associated viral vectors Adeno-associated virus (AAV) is a non-pathogenic virus of the family parvoviridae with a single stranded DNA genome of 4.7 kb. It was discovered fortuitously by researchers working with adenovirus. Like adenovirus, adeno-associated virus can infect non-dividing cells, but it has the characteristic of integration competence, specifically into the long arm of chromosome 19. Adeno-associated virus vectors typically contain inverted terminal repeats necessary for genomic integration and coercion of the host cells into synthezising the complementary DNA strand. As a naturally reduplication-deficient virus, adeno-associated virus requires co- or super-infection with a helper virus, such as adenovirus or herpes simplex virus. Alternatively, the missing but required viral genes (E1, E2A, E4, and VA) can be supplied by co-transfection. Adeno-associated virus vectors have been evaluated for clinical use. An obstacle to their application is a low transgene expression efficiency, mainly due to a limited second strand synthesis and transgene expression, which may be enhanceable by γ-ray irradiation.

Herpes simplex virus based vectors Herpes simplex virus (HSV) is a highly infectious double stranded DNA virus with a 152 kb genome. The pathogen responsible for the common cold sore is transmitted by direct contact. Attachment of the virus to cells occurs through binding to glycosaminoglycan moieties of cell surface proteoglycans. Herpes simplex virus reduplicates in epithelial cells of the skin or mucosa at the site of contact. Progeny particles are taken up by the terminals of sensory neurons that innervate the infected epithelium. The uptake of the virus via interactions of specific envelope glycoproteins with their cognate receptors on host cells is followed by retrograde transport of the virion to the nucleus where the viral DNA is injected through a nuclear pore. Viral genes may be expressed resulting in lytic infection, or the viral lytic cycle genes may be silenced resulting in persistence of the viral DNA in the transcriptionally quiescent state of latency. Latent infection with wild-type virus results in life-long episomal viral persistence in peripheral sensory neuronal nuclei of the host.

Because herpes simplex virus is highly infectious, vectors based on its genome are efficient vehicles for the delivery of exogenous genetic material to cells. As the virus is naturally neurotropic, many applications for gene therapy have been directed toward the nervous system. Viral reduplication is readily disrupted by null mutations in immediate early genes thus allowing the virus to be used as a non-pathogenic vector. HSV DNA consists of two unique sequences, each of which is surrounded by a pair of inverted repeat sequences. These genes can be replaced with large or multiple transgenes. The latency active promoter complex can be exploited in vector design to achieve long term stable transgene expression. The virus may be turned into a vector by

- deleting non-essential genes so it becomes conditionally reduplicating
- deleting essential genes to obtain a reduplication defective virus
- generating amplicons in which the transgenes (plus viral packaging signal) are administered as plasmids separate from the viral genome (sans packaging signal).

Deletion of essential immediate early genes (IE genes) prevents herpes simplex virus reduplication and thus eliminates the component of cytopathogenicity that is attributable to viral reduplication. Quintuple mutants that lack ICP0, ICP4, ICP22, ICP27 and ICP47 are non-toxic to cells and the genomes are able to persist for long periods of time. However, their amplification and transgene expression are poor. For many applications, where immune evasion is desirable, triple mutants lacking ICP42, ICP222, and ICP272 show minimal cytotoxicity, are efficient vehicles for transgene delivery, and can grow efficiently in cells that complement the absence of ICP4 and ICP27.

Lentivirus vectors The use of gene delivery vectors based on retroviruses was introduced in the early 1980s (Mann et al. 1983). Lentivirus is a member of the retroviridae family with a genome of 9.2 kb. It displays a tropism for helper T-lymphocytes, macrophages, monocytes, intestinal epithelia, and brain. A single stranded RNA virus, lentivirus can transduce quiescent cells and provide stable expression of transgenes through integration into the host DNA. It uses viral Reverse Transcriptase to create DNA copies of its RNA genome, and the cellular machinery to create the second strand. The resulting double stranded molecule can integrate anywhere within the genome using a virally encoded Integrase.

Once inserted into a lentiviral vector, a fragment is flanked by the 5' and 3' long-terminal repeats (LTRs) and the Ψ packaging signal necessary for incorporation into an infective, but reduplication incompetent virion. Helper plasmids are often used to supply the missing viral activities needed to build the virus particles (such as the *gag*, *pol*, and *rev* genes).

Lentiviral vectors have emerged as potential tools for immunotherapy. They are capable of transducing dendritic cells with tumor antigens. This may induce strong antigen specific T-lymphocyte responses. One advantage of retroviral vectors is their low intrinsic immunogenicity due to the removal of most genes that encode viral proteins, thus enabling the repeated use of these vectors for immunization with tumor associated antigens. Limitations associated with retroviral vectors include the instability of the viral particle and low viral titers.

8.4.2 Non-Viral Gene Delivery Systems

Methods of non-viral gene delivery use physical and chemical approaches. The physical methods include needle injection, electroporation, gene gun, ultrasound, and hydrodynamic delivery to permeate the cell membrane and facilitate intracellular gene transfer. The chemical methods use carrier compounds to deliver the transgene into cells. Although progress has been made in the applications of non-viral gene delivery systems, they are generally much less efficient than viral vectors. A particular problem for the application of most non-viral systems is their poor efficiency at transducing non-proliferating cells. This may be attributable to the integrity of the nuclear membrane, which provides a physical barrier to entry. The mode of delivery is often intravenous, by inhalation as aerosol, or by intra-tumoral injection.

The low in situ stability, low cellular uptake, and lack of tissue specificity limit the therapeutic applications of oligonucleotides. Beside chemical modifications, the use of lipid based delivery systems represents a strategy for improving the pharmacokinetic properties. Liposomal formulations enhance the blood and tissue levels of nucleotide drugs, leading to improvements in their anti-tumor effects. Sterically stabilized immunoliposomes, which have cell surface-directed antibodies grafted on their exteriors, can be efficient tools for the selective delivery of drugs and diagnostic agents to target cells. On tumors of neuroectodermal origin, GD2 may be a suitable target because it has high levels of expression on these tumors while being less common in non-malignant tissues.

Cationic liposomes Non-viral gene delivery was discovered in 1987, when the double-chain monovalent quaternary ammonium lipid *N*-[1-(2,3-dioleyloxy)propyl]-*N, N,N*-trimethylammonium chloride was found to effectively bind and deliver DNA to cells (Felgner et al. 1987). Cationic lipids are soluble in aqueous solution, forming micellar structures (liposomes). Upon mixing with cationic liposomes, plasmid DNA is condensed into quasi-stable lipoplexes with diameters of 100–200 nm. Complexing DNA with cationic carrier molecules neutralizes its electrostatic charge. Therefore, lipoplexes facilitate cellular uptake, protect the DNA from Nucleases, and trigger the release of the DNA from the intracellular vesicles before reaching the lysosomal compartments, where degradation would take place.

The transfection activities of the lipoplexes are determined by

- the chemical structure of the cationic lipid
- the charge ratio between the cationic lipid and the DNA
- the structure and proportion of the helper lipid in the complexes
- the size and structure of the assembled liposomes.

In general, multivalent lipids with long and unsaturated hydrocarbon chains tend to be more efficient than monovalent cationic lipids with the same hydrophobic chains.

The cationic lipid is always in slight excess over the DNA such that the lipoplexes have net positive charges. Cationic liposomes are often formulated with an uncharged phospholipid or cholesterol as helper lipids. Suitable compositions may differ by the number of charges in the hydrophilic head group and the specific structure of the hydrophobic moiety of the lipid. Spontaneous lipid mixing in endosomes becomes more profound when a non-bilayer-forming lipid, such as dioleoylphosphatidylethanolamine (DOPE), is used as the helper lipid, rather than a bilayer forming lipid, such as dioleoylphosphatidylcholine (DOPC). Inclusion of dioleoylphosphatidylethanolamine may increase membrane fluidity, facilitate lipid exchange and membrane fusion between the lipoplexes and the endosomal membrane, and promote endosomal rupture (purportedly by a mechanism involving transition from a bilayer phase to an inverted micellar structure).

Pharmacokinetics Many cationic lipids do not maintain their integrity in the presence of blood plasma, and only a few are active in this environment. Changes in size, surface charge, and lipid composition occur when lipoplexes are exposed to the negatively charged, often amphipathic proteins and polysaccharides in blood, mucus, epithelial lining fluid, or tissue matrix. Whereas the helper lipid dioleoylphosphatidylethanolamine makes the formulation more efficient for airway gene delivery, it has a compromising effect on intravenous delivery because its formulations tend to disintegrate in the presence of blood components. Cholesterol is a better helper lipid for systemic gene delivery, as it stabilizes the lipoplex structure in blood.

Gene transfer by systemic administration of lipoplexes mainly transfects endothelial cells in the pulmonary vasculature. Although lipoplexes often show high levels of transgene expression following direct administration or injection into target tissues, their non-specific membrane activity usually precludes cell selective targeting. Lipoplexes have been investigated for gene delivery to the lungs by intravenous and airway administration. Inhibitory factors for lipoplex gene delivery include a negatively charged and viscous mucus layer that often traps and neutralizes the surface charges of the lipoplexes. Well differentiated upper airway epithelial cells are less active in taking up lipoplexes than are those in the lower airways.

The hydrophobic or positively charged surface of lipoplexes frequently leads to non-specific interactions with plasma proteins and other extracellular proteins, which may result in inactivation. To limit this effect, protein resistant lipoplexes have been developed. Many proteoglycans in cell membranes or extracellular matrix are sulphated, and therefore are negatively charged, allowing them to interact with positively charged lipoplexes. Gene expression is abolished or markedly inhibited by heavily sulphated of these proteins, including those that contain heparin sulphate and chondroitin B. These proteins can compete with DNA contained within the lipoplex, causing it to dissociate away from cationic carrier molecules. Most of the glycosaminoglycans may adhere to the complexes and are involved in the process of internalization.

Adverse Effects Toxicity related to gene transfer by lipoplexes may be due to inflammatory reactions, including influenza-like symptoms with fever and airway inflammation. Systemically administered cationic lipids can cause acute pulmonary hypotension, induction of inflammatory cytokines, tissue infiltration of neutrophils in lungs, decrease in white cell counts, and in some cases tissue injury in liver and spleen.

A factor related to the severity of adverse effects is complement activation and adsorption of plasma proteins onto their surface, which act as opsonins to trigger the uptake of opsonized particles by macrophages and other immune cells. The incorporation of polyethylene glycol (PEG) conjugates into the lipoplexes as a cover may reduce the non-specific interaction of lipoplexes with blood components. Once at the target cells, polyethylene glycol lipids fall off, revealing highly active lipoplexes. The polyethylene glycol lipid shield for lipoplexes can be made detachable using an acid sensitive linker, so that the polyethylene glycol moiety is removed when lipoplexes are inside the endocytic compartment.

Cationic polymers Synthetic and naturally occurring cationic polymers, linear or branched, constitute a category of DNA carriers that has been extensively tested for gene delivery. Poly-L-lysine was one of the first cationic polymers used in gene transfer in vivo. Others include polyethylenimine, polyallylamine, cationic dextran, chitosan, cationic proteins, polyamidoamine and polypropylamine dendrimers, and cationic peptides. Although most cationic polymers condense DNA into small particles and facilitate cellular uptake via endocytosis through charge-based interactions with anionic sites on cell surfaces, they differ widely in their transfection efficiency and toxicity.

The group of Jean Paul Behr first introduced polyethylenimine as a synthetic polymeric gene transfer agent. The densely charged polyethylenimine is one of the most active known polymers for this purpose.

- Depending on its process of synthesis, polyethylenimine may be either linear or branched.
- Polyethylenimine oligomers are generated by treatment with bifunctional cross-linking reagents.
- Polyethylenimine derivatives with lipid conjugation form aggregated micelles that are biologically active.
- Conjugation of the lytic peptide Melittin to polyethylenimine results in an increase in transfection efficiency.
- Surface modification with polyethylene glycol can drastically reduce the surface charge of polyethylenimine and the tendency to form large aggregates in the presence of blood plasma.

For gene transfer, the DNA/polyethylenimine ratio, the molecular weight and configuration of polyethylenimine, and the ionic strength of the solvent for preparation are all important factors that determine the physical properties and transfection activity of the DNA/polyethylenimine complexes (polyplexes). Linear complexes dissociate more efficiently inside cells and lead to higher and faster gene expression in target cells than branched complexes. Linear complexes also enter the nucleus more readily than branched ones. The intravenous injection of polyplexes of linear polyethylenimine is as efficient as the intravenous injection of lipoplexes in transfecting pulmonary endothelial cells.

Adverse Effects Polyethylenimine is non-biodegradable, which underlies some of its adverse effects. Linear polyethylenimine is less toxic to cells than its branched variants, low molecular weight compounds are less toxic than high molecular weight polymers. Polyethylenimine of 2 kD or smaller is relatively non-toxic but not active in transfection. While low dose, well dispersed polyplexes administered by aerosolization are relatively non-toxic, large doses are injurious to the respiratory tract.

A successful class of cationic polymers is comprised of aminoesters. The intrinsic ester bonds limit stability, thus reducing overall toxicity. Branched polyaminoesters are chemically more stable than those with linear configurations when the polymer contains primary amine groups. Cationic polymers with disulfide bond linkages assembled from low-molecular-weight polyamines have good transfection efficiency and relatively low toxicity.

Cationic peptides may serve as carriers for gene delivery. Short cationic peptides may act as membrane penetrating molecules bringing into cells a variety of substances. This mechanism may be employed to enhance the efficiency of polyplex mediated gene delivery. An arginine-rich peptide derived from the small basic protein Protamine is able to transfect cells, whereas the whole protein has minimal activity. Synthetic peptides that contain an arginine-rich dimer derived from the HIV TAT protein are active in transfection.

Lipid/polymer hybrid systems Lipid/polymer hybrid systems contain DNA pre-condensed with poly-cations, then coated with either cationic liposomes, anionic liposomes, or amphiphilic polymers, with or without helper lipids. Linear poly-L-lysine, protamine, Histone, or synthetic polypeptides may serve as the DNA condensation components. When anionic liposomes, rich in dioleoylphosphatidylethanolamine, are added to DNA/poly-cation complexes, an extensive reorganization of the lipid membranes takes place, resulting in lipid polymer/DNA complexes with anionic lipid coatings. Advantages of the hybrid system include the protection of the DNA to be transferred and efficient DNA transfection. The structure of polyplexes makes receptor mediated targeting possible without interference from non-specific charge-based interaction.

Polyelectrolyte complexes formed by self-assembly of DNA with cationic polymers (typically poly-L-lysine or polyethyleneimine) are referred to as polyplexes. Such polyplexes are usually nano-particulate with diameters below 100 nm. Complexes based on polyethyleneimine often exhibit high transfection activity, possibly due to endosomal buffering capacity. Consequently, increased osmolarity of the endosome might cause rupture of the endosomal membrane and release of entrapped DNA complexes.

Adverse Effects The cytotoxicity of the polyplexes is reduced compared to liposomes or polymers.

Targeted delivery is one of the major limitations to gene therapy. Gene therapy may be delivered by viral or non-viral vehicles.

8.5 Other Strategies

Decoy molecules Short, double stranded DNA decoy molecules can disrupt gene expression at the level of transcription. These oligodeoxynucleotides are designed to compete for transcription factor complexes, with the ultimate goal of attracting them away from the promoter that they would ordinarily activate (Sharma et al. 1996). Due to limited gene accessibility in the nucleosome structure, the clinical application of these methods has encountered technical challenges.

One approach uses oligoribonucleotides. Similar to the strategy of the DNA decoys, the RNA decoys are designed to provide alternate, competing binding sites for proteins that act as translational activators or mRNA stabilizing elements. By attracting away the desired protein, the decoy can prevent translation or induce instability, resulting in the destruction of the mRNA (Beelman and Parker 1995).

Aptamers Aptamers (developed in 1990 independently by Szostak and Gold) may be based on nucleotides or amino acids as building blocks. DNA or RNA aptamers consist of short strands of oligonucleotides. Peptide aptamers consist of a short variable peptide domain, attached at both ends to a protein scaffold. Aptamers are usually created by selecting them from a large random sequence pool to bind to a specific target molecule. They are under study as potential macromolecular drugs.

References

Anderson WF (1984) Prospects for human gene therapy. Science 226:401–409

Beelman CA, Parker R (1995) Degradation of mRNA in eukaryotes. Cell 81:179–183

Felgner PL, Gadek TR, Holm M, Roman R, Chan HW, Wenz M, Northrop JP, Ringold GM, Danielsen M (1987) Lipofection: a highly efficient, lipid-mediated DNA-transfection procedure. Proc Natl Acad Sci U S A 84:7413–7417

Kobayashi H, Eckhardt SG, Lockridge JA, Rothenberg ML, Sandler AB, O'Bryant CL, Cooper W, Holden SN, Aitchison RD, Usman N, Wolin M, Basche ML (2005) Safety and pharmacokinetic study of RPI.4610 (ANGIOZYME), an anti-VEGFR-1 ribozyme, in combination with carboplatin and paclitaxel in patients with advanced solid tumors. Cancer Chemother Pharmacol 56:329–336

Lai SY, Koppikar P, Thomas SM, Childs EE, Egloff AM, Seethala RR, Branstetter BF, Gooding WE, Muthukrishnan A, Mountz JM, Lui VW, Shin DM, Agarwala SS, Johnson R, Couture LA, Myers EN, Johnson JT, Mills G, Argiris A, Grandis JR (2009) Intratumoral epidermal growth factor receptor antisense DNA therapy in head and neck cancer: first human application and potential antitumor mechanisms. J Clin Oncol 27:1235–1242

Luger SM, O'Brien SG, Ratajczak J, Ratajczak MZ, Mick R, Stadtmauer EA, Nowell PC, Goldman JM, Gewirtz AM (2002) Oligodeoxynucleotide-mediated inhibition of c-myb gene expression in autografted bone marrow: a pilot study. Blood 99:1150–1158

Mann R, Mulligan RC, Baltimore D (1983) Construction of a retrovirus packaging mutant and its use to produce helper-free defective retrovirus. Cell 33:153–159

Mizuno T, Chou MY, Inouye M (1984) A unique mechanism regulating gene expression: translational inhibition by a complementary RNA transcript (micRNA). Proc Natl Acad Sci U S A 81:1966–1970

Opalinska JB, Gewirtz AM (2002) Nucleic-acid therapeutics: basic principles and recent applications. Nat Rev Drug Discov 1:503–514

Paterson BM, Roberts BE, Kuff EL (1977) Structural gene identification and mapping by DNA-mRNA hybrid-arrested cell-free translation. Proc Natl Acad Sci U S A 74:4370–4374

Plautz G, Nabel EG, Nabel GJ (1991) Selective elimination of recombinant genes in vivo with a suicide retroviral vector. Nat Biol 3:709–715

Sandberg JA, Parker VP, Blanchard KS, Sweedler D, Powell JA, Kachensky A, Bellon L, Usman N, Rossing T, Borden E, Blatt LM (2000) Pharmacokinetics and tolerability of an antiangiogenic ribozyme (ANGIOZYME) in healthy volunteers. J Clin Pharmacol 40:1462–1469

Sharma HW, Perez JR, Higgins-Sochaski K, Hsiao R, Narayanan R (1996) Transcription factor decoy approach to decipher the role of NF-kB in oncogenesis. Anticancer Res 16:61–69

Simons RW, Kleckner N (1983) Translational control of IS10 transposition. Cell 34:683–691

Stephenson ML, Zamecnik PC (1978) Inhibition of Rous sarcoma viral RNA translation by a specific oligodeoxyribonucleotide. Proc Natl Acad Sci U S A 75:285–288

Zamecnik PC, Stephenson ML (1978) Inhibition of Rous sarcoma virus replication and cell transformation by a specific oligodeoxynucleotide. Proc Natl Acad Sci U S A 75:280–284

9 Drugs with Diverse Modes of Action

Complementary and alternative medicines[1] are treatments that are not used in the practice of conventional medicine. Complementary medicines are used in combination with treatments administered by standard medical practice. Alternative medicines, on the other hand, are treatments used in place of accepted practice. The branch of medicine referred to as integrative care involves treatment plans that utilize both conventional medicine and less proven complementary methods.

Biologics Biologics are emerging drug categories that are distinct from small molecule drugs primarily in their origin. Biologics typically are long-chain proteins, heavily glycosylated proteins, or proteins with considerable folding2. They are in contrast to simple short peptides, which in general can be completely humanized. The production of recombinant proteins is often efficient and inexpensive, in potentially limitless quantity. Among their benefits over purified native proteins is the reduction of exposure to animal or human diseases. Recombinant technologies allow the modification of a protein or the selection of a particular genetic variant to improve function or specificity, even the production of proteins that provide novel functions or activities (Table 9.1).

Proteins are large molecules with both hydrophilic and hydrophobic properties that can make entry into cells and compartments of the body difficult. Protein solubility, route of administration, distribution and stability can affect the application as a therapy. The half-life of a therapeutic protein can be drastically affected by Proteases, protein-modifying chemicals, or other clearance mechanisms. An important challenge is that the body may mount an immune response against the therapeutic protein, which can neutralize the protein or cause a harmful anaphylactic reaction in the patient. The risk for an immune reaction is lower for humanized proteins than for xenogeneic (non-human) proteins.

Biosimilars are biopharmaceutical products that are similar to the innovator product (original drug), but have the potential to exhibit different therapeutic effects. The biologic nature of these classes of agents limits their interchangeability (compared to chemically synthesized drugs), which has created regulatory issues for generic versions, called follow-on compounds. A requirement by the U.S. FDA is that the biosimilar is as similar to the reference products as may be achieved given the state of scientific knowledge and technology at the time.

- Follow-on protein products are manufactured using biotechnology or are derived from sources that are intended to be sufficiently similar to a product already approved
- Second generation protein products are biopharmaceuticals with structural differences designed to improve performance while maintaining the same mechanism of action as the original product.

In contrast to small molecule drugs, the actions of which are largely independent of the manufacturing process, the performance of biologics is inextricably linked to the mode of production. Therefore, the production technology is often patented and cannot be copied by generic manufacturers. Comparability testing requires analytical methods, bioassays, preclinical animal studies, and clinical studies. The development time and cost are much higher for follow-on biologics than for generic small molecule drugs.

Metabolic intervention Polyamines (organic compounds with more than 1 primary amino group) are involved in nucleosome oligomerization and DNA conformation, creating a chromatin environment that stimulates the neoplastic transformation of cells. In tumor cells, there is an increased dependence on polyamines compared to untransformed cells. The polyamine metabolic pathway is dysregulated, resulting in abnormal or sustained tumor growth. The polyamines

[1] Complementary and alternative medicine approaches are backed by limited evidence to support efficacy and safety.

[2] The first commercially available recombinant protein therapeutic was Insulin, approved by the U.S. FDA in 1982 for the treatment of diabetes mellitus.

G. F. Weber, *Molecular Therapies of Cancer*, DOI 10.1007/978-3-319-13278-5_9,

Table 9.1 Functional classification of protein therapeutics. Protein therapeutics can be organized by function and therapeutic application. (adapted from Leader et al. 2008)

Group I: Protein therapeutics with enzymatic or regulatory activity
Ia: Replacing a protein that is deficient or abnormal
Ib: Augmenting an existing pathway
Ic: Providing a novel function or activity
Endocrine and metabolic disorders with defined molecular etiologies dominate Group Ia. Group Ib is dominated by therapies that augment hematological and endocrine pathways and immune responses. Group Ic demonstrates the rational use of naturally occurring proteins to modify the pathophysiology of human diseases
Group II: Protein therapeutics with special targeting activity
IIa: Interfering with a molecule or organism
IIb: Delivering other compounds or proteins
Group IIa therapeutics use their special targeting activity to interfere with molecules by binding specifically to them and blocking their function, targeting them for destruction, or stimulating a signaling pathway. This group has grown as monoclonal antibody technology has matured. Group IIb therapeutics deliver other compounds or proteins to a specific site
Group III: Protein vaccines
IIIa: Protecting against a deleterious foreign agent
IIIb: Treating an autoimmune disease
IIIc: Treating cancer
Although this is currently a small class of therapies, there is potential for the production of recombinant vaccines that provide broad protection against infectious or cancers. Many of the U.S. FDA approved vaccines include synthetic, recombinant and purified protein components

spermine and spermidine are essential for the translation of thymidine kinase mRNA.

Eflornithine (α-difluoromethylornithine, DFMO) was initially developed for cancer treatment at Merrell Dow Research Institute in the late 1970s. Eflornithine (Fig. 9.1) is a difluoromethylated ornithine compound that irreversibly inhibits Ornithine Decarboxylase, an enzyme required for polyamine biosynthesis. Thereby the drug inhibits the formation and proliferation of tumor cells. It induces apoptosis in leiomyoma cells but has not proven efficacious in cancer treatment[3].

Mitoguazone (methylglyoxal, bis(guanylhydrazone), MGBG) is a guanylhydrazone that competitively inhibits S-Adenosyl-L-Methionine Decarboxylase, an enzyme involved in the synthesis of polyamines. This results in decreased proliferation, anti-mitochondrial effects, and P53 independent apoptosis. Mitoguazone may be effective in patients with leukemias or lymphomata, head and neck cancers, and esophageal cancer. One of several possible schedules administers 600 mg/m^2 by intravenous infusion on days 1 and 8, and then every 2 weeks.

Pharmacokinetics Mitoguazone is cleared from the plasma triexponentially with a harmonic mean terminal half-life of 175 h and a mean residence time of 190 h. Renal excretion of unchanged mitoguazone accounts for 15 % of the administered dose. The drug enters the cerebrospinal fluid with CSF/blood concentration ratios well below 10 %. The tissue levels of mitoguazone are highest in the liver followed by lymph node, spleen and the brain.

Adverse Effects The dose limiting toxicity is muscle weakness. Flushing during infusion, primarily on the face, is common. Other adverse effects are usually mild, consisting of mucositis, tingling in the face or extremities, tinnitus, nausea and vomiting, somnolescence and fatigue. At moderate doses, mitoguazone lacks substantial myelosuppression, which is favorable in combination regimens with conventional agents.

*N*1,*N*12-bis(ethyl)-cis-6,7-dehydrospermine (SL-11047, PG11047) is a second generation polyamine analog synthesized through the restriction of molecular conformations of parent polyamine compounds. It may displace endogenous polyamines from DNA binding sites, thereby interfering with cell cycle processes that depend on polyamine binding and function. This results in cell-cycle arrest or apoptosis, and interferes with gene activities involved in cell growth.

Adverse Effects This agent may exhibit decreased toxicity and enhanced efficacy profiles compared to first generation polyamine compounds.

As a result of metabolic and mitochondrial defects, tumor cells often preferentially use glycolysis to generate adenosine triphosphate (ATP), even in the presence of oxygen, a phenomenon known as aerobic glycolysis, or the Warburg effect.

Dichloroacetate (DCA) <Ceresine> is an inhibitor of mitochondrial Pyruvate Dehydrogenase Kinase, which inhibits Pyruvate Dehydrogenase, a gatekeeping enzyme for the entry of pyruvate into the mitochondrial tricarboxylic acid cycle. Dichloroacetate treatment may reactivate mitochondrial respiration in tumor cells, induce their selective killing, and suppress cancer growth (Bonnet et al. 2007).

[3] Eflornithine is in clinical use as a cream for the treatment of facial hirsutism and for injection against sleeping sickness.

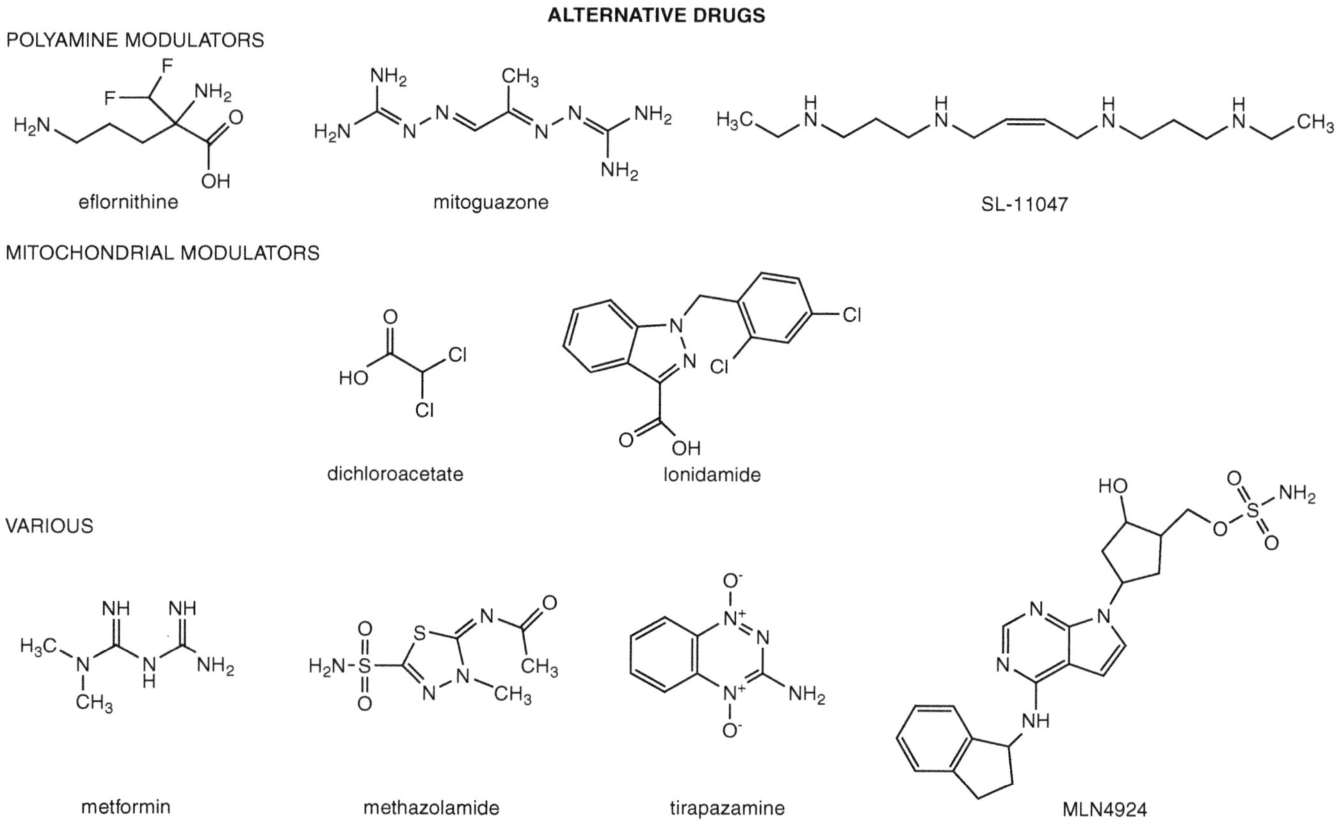

Fig. 9.1 Structures of alternative anti-cancer drugs

Dichloroacetate has been in use to reduce hyperglycemia in diabetes mellitus, because it affects pathways of the intermediary metabolism to stimulate peripheral glucose utilization and inhibit gluconeogenesis. It suppresses lipogenesis and cholesterolgenesis, thereby decreasing circulating lipid and lipoprotein levels in patients with acquired or hereditary disorders of lipoprotein metabolism. By stimulating the activity of Pyruvate Dehydrogenase, dichloroacetate facilitates the oxidation of lactate and decreases morbidity in acquired and congenital forms of lactic acidosis.

Pharmacokinetics Dichloroacetate is dehalogenated to monochloroacetate and glyoxylate, from which it can be further catabolized to glycolate, glycine, oxalate, and carbon dioxide.

Adverse Effects At sustained, higher doses (generally 25 mg/kg/day taken orally), there is an increased risk of reversible peripheral neuropathy, neurotoxicity, and gait disturbance. Dichloroacetate can cause a reversible peripheral neuropathy that may be related to thiamine deficiency and may be ameliorated or prevented with thiamine supplementation. The drug can also be carcinogenic at high doses.

Lonidamine, an indazole carboxylate, suppresses aerobic glycolysis in cancer cells but enhances it in untransformed cells, likely through the inhibition of mitochondrial Hexokinase. This causes a decrease in cellular ATP. The drug may also act as a putative ANT ligand that triggers apoptosis. Lonidamine is in clinical trials for the treatment of brain tumors.

Various In many cancers, the PI 3-kinase pathway is up-regulated, either by elevated levels of Insulin or IGF (Insulin-Like Growth Factor) or by loss-of-function mutations of the tumor suppressor gene pten. Obesity and diabetes are associated with increased cancer risk, which may be associated with high circulating levels of the growth factors Insulin and IGF. Type 2 diabetics who receive Insulin therapy or drugs that stimulate Insulin secretion have a higher incidence of cancer than those who receive metformin.

Diabetics treated with metformin have 25–40 % less cancer than those who receive Insulin as therapy or take sulfonylurea drugs that increase Insulin secretion from the pancreas (a phenomenon first identified in 2005 by the group of Andrew Morris). Metformin seems to work by lowering the blood Insulin and IGF levels. Metformin also activates the enzyme AMPK in the liver, which then reduces the synthesis and secretion of glucose, thereby lowering the blood glucose levels. Further, the drug stimulates the tumor suppressor gene *lkb1*.

As a hypoxia inducible transmembrane glycoprotein, Carbonic Anhydrase IX (CAIX) catalyzes the rapid interconversion of carbon dioxide and water into carbonic acid, protons, and bicarbonate ions, helping to maintain acidification of the tumor micro-environment and enhance resistance to cytotoxic therapy in some hypoxic tumors.

Methazolamide (*N*-[5-(aminosulfonyl)-3-methyl-1,3,4-thiadiazol-2(3*H*)-ylidene]-acetamide) is a sulfonamide derivate that inhibits tumor associated Carbonic Anhydrase IX, which may result in increased cell death in hypoxic tumors.

Adverse Effects Common adverse reactions, occurring most often early in therapy, include paresthesias, tinnitus, fatigue, malaise, loss of appetite, taste alteration, gastrointestinal disturbances (nausea, vomiting, diarrhea), polyuria, and occasional instances of drowsiness and confusion. Metabolic acidosis and electrolyte imbalance may arise. Transient myopia subsides upon diminution or discontinuance of the medication. Rare but dangerous adverse events can be caused by severe reactions to sulfonamides and include toxic epidermal necrolysis (Stevens-Johnson syndrome), fulminant hepatic necrosis, agranulocytosis, or aplastic anemia.

Drug Interactions Methazolamide should be used with caution in patients on steroid therapy because of the potential for developing hypokalemia. Under concomitant use of high dose aspirin, Carbonic Anhydrase inhibitors can lead to anorexia, tachypnea, lethargy, coma or death.

Tirapazamine (3-amino-1,2,4-benzotriazine-1,4 dioxide) (SR-4233) was prepared in a screening for new herbicides in 1972 and was introduced into clinical use in 1986. Cancer cells in hypoxic regions are resistant to killing by radiotherapy and many anti-cancer drugs. Tirapazamine is a benzotriazine di-*N*-oxide prodrug. The compound is selectively activated by multiple Reductases to form a free radical in hypoxic cells, thereby inducing single-strand and double-strand DNA breaks and base damage, which lead to cell death. This agent also sensitizes hypoxic cells to ionizing radiation and counteracts the repair of radiation induced DNA strand breaks via inhibition of Topoisomerase 2. Tirapazamine is under study for the treatment of head and neck cancer and gynecological cancers.

The name laetrile originally refered to the contraction of laevo-mandelonitrile glucoside, a cyanogenic glycoside, which occurs naturally in some plants. The meaning of laetrile has evolved to cover preparations, where amygdalin is the major constituent (laetrile and amygdalin are often used interchangeably, but are different agents). Cyanide and benzaldehyde are metabolites of both laetrile and amygdalin. Both metabolites may possess anti-neoplastic properties. Although laetrile has been used as an anti-cancer treatment, it has not been proven to be effective. It is not approved for use in the United States.

In 1996, aminoflavone (NSC 686288), a synthetic material that is related to flavonoids, which modulate various biological activities in plants, showed promising properties in screening. Aminoflavones are under investigation as anti-cancer agents.

AFP464 is a synthetic lysyl prodrug of the amino-substituted flavone derivate aminoflavone. Aminoflavone activates AhR (Aryl Hydrocarbon Receptor) signaling pathway, leading to an increase in CYP1A1 enzyme activity and, to a lesser extent, in CYP1B1 enzyme activity and gene expression. Subsequently, aminoflavone is metabolized by the CYP1A1 and CYP1B1 enzymes that it induces. Toxic metabolites covalently bind to DNA, thereby inhibiting cell proliferation and inducing apoptosis.

Pharmacokinetics AFP464 is rapidly converted to aminoflavone in the blood.

Adverse Effects Pulmonary toxicity may be dose limiting.

The Cullin-RING Ubiquitin Ligases are a sub-set of E3 enzymes that control the ubiquitination and subsequent degradation of proteins with key roles in cell cycle progression (P27, Cyclin E, c-MYC) and DNA damage (CDT1). NEDD8 Activating Enzyme (NAE) is the proximal regulator of the NEDDylation pathway. NAE activates NEDD8 (Neural Precursor Cell Expressed, Developmentally Down-regulated 8), an Ubiquitin like protein that modifies Cullin-RING Ubiquitin Ligases. Given the essential functions of its protein substrates in suppressing the malignant phenotype, the NEDD8 degradation pathway is a potential treatment target.

MLN4924 is a selective inhibitor of NAE, which may result in the suppression of tumor cell proliferation and survival. The induction of oxidative stress is a key event in MLN492 induced apoptosis. Elevated antioxidant defenses contribute to resistance to platinum based chemotherapy in ovarian cancer, and targeting NAE with MLN4924 augments the anti-cancer activity of cisplatin. MLN4924 and cisplatin synergize to induce DNA damage, oxidative stress, and increased BIK (BCL-2 Interacting Killer) expression.

Drug Resistance Mutations in the drug target, NEDD8, can lead to MLN4924 resistance.

Shark cartilage may have some positive effects. Some of its components, such as alkyl glycerols, inhibit certain types of cancer. A yet unidentified component acts as an angiogenesis inhibitor that is under investigation for the treatment of Kaposi Sarcoma or some solid tumors (prostate, uterus, colon).

References

Bonnet S, Archer SL, Allalunis-Turner J, Haromy A, Beaulieu C, Thompson R, Lee CT, Lopaschuk GD, Puttagunta L, Bonnet S, Harry G, Hashimoto K, Porter CJ, Andrade MA, Thebaud B, Michelakis ED (2007) A mitochondria-K+ channel axis is suppressed in cancer and its normalization promotes apoptosis and inhibits cancer growth. Cancer Cell 11:37–51

Leader B, Baca QJ, Golan DE (2008) Protein therapeutics: a summary and pharmacological classification. Nat Rev Drug Discov 7:21–39

Part IV

Molecular Targeting of Tumor-Host Interactions

10 Hormone Therapy

Over the decades, the roles of hormones in carcinogenesis have received increasing attention. The observation by Bernardino Ramazzini in 1713 of a virtual absence of cervical cancer and relatively high incidence of breast cancer in nuns was an important step toward identifying and understanding the importance in modifying cancer risk of hormonal factors, such as those associated with pregnancy. In 1878, Thomas Beatson discovered that the breasts of rabbits stopped producing milk after he removed the ovaries. He suggested to the Edinburgh Medico-Chirurgical Society in 1896: "This fact (…) pointed to one organ holding control over the secretion of another and separate organ". Beatson found that oophorectomy often resulted in the improvement of breast cancer patients and inferred the stimulating effect of a female ovarian hormone on breast cancer, before the hormone itself was discovered (Beatson 1896). Allen and Doisey identified this ovarian hormone they referred to as "estrus stimulating principle" (Allen and Doisy 1923), later called estrogen. The benefit of ablation of the adrenal gland (Dao/Huggins) or hypophysectomy (Pearson/Ray) for some women with breast cancer highlighted the importance of estrogens and Gonadotropins for mammary cancer growth. From the late 1950s to the 1970s Elwood Jensen demonstrated that such hormones do not undergo redox modifications to become activated. Instead, they bind to a receptor protein within their target cells (Jensen and Jacobson 1962). This hormone/receptor complex then travels to the cell nucleus, where it regulates gene expression. The first non-steroidal anti-estrogen, ethamoxytriphetol (MER25), was described by Lerner and co-workers in 1958 (Lerner et al. 1958) as an agent that had no other hormonal or anti-hormonal properties. The drug failed in clinical trials because the large doses required caused serious adverse central nervous system effects (hallucinations and psychotic episodes). Tamoxifen, discovered in 1962, is a non-steroidal anti-estrogen that serves a dual role as breast cancer preventive and therapeutic. It was approved for the treatment of advanced breast cancer by the U.S. FDA in 1977.

Awareness of the androgen dependence of prostate tissue can be traced back to the Scottish surgeon John Hunter, who observed in 1786 that castrated bulls had small prostates. In 1941, Charles Brenton Huggins (1901–1997), a urologist at the University of Chicago, together with his students Clarence V. Hodges and William Wallace Scott, published 3 papers that demonstrated the relationship between the endocrine system and the normal functioning of the prostate gland. In the 1940s, Huggins also reported a dramatic regression of metastatic prostate cancer following removal of the testes (Huggins and Hodges 1941). Later, drugs that blocked male hormones were found to be effective treatments for prostate cancer. Androgen ablation in prostate cancer patients with Gonadotropin Releasing Hormone agonists (GnRH-As) was first reported in 1982 (Tolis et al. 1982). In 1988, the Androgen Receptor was cloned (Chang et al. 1988), identifying an additional drug target.

The phenanthrene steroid hormone nucleus is not necessary for estrogenic activity. Synthetic phenolic and triphenolic compounds may exert strong activity. Iatrogenic causes for cancer predisposition were incriminated by a study published in 1971, which documented an association between clear cell adenocarcinoma of the vagina and in utero exposure to diethylstilbestrol (Herbst et al. 1971)[1]. In July 2002, the Women's Health Initiative study was stopped after an elevated number of breast cancers and heart problems occurred among women taking estrogen-progestin pills. In 2006, multiple clinical studies showed that breast cancer rates in the United States dropped in 2003, consecutive to a drastic reduction in the use of hormone replacement therapy. Some of the numbers came from the National Cancer Institute's surveillance database, which uses cancer registries around the country to project national incidence and death rates.

---

[1] Dodds and associates had characterized diethylstilbestrol as an extremely potent estrogen (Dodds et al. 1938). It had been prescribed for close to 30 years to prevent certain complications of pregnancy and as a treatment for advanced breast cancer in post-menopausal women.

G. F. Weber, *Molecular Therapies of Cancer*, DOI 10.1007/978-3-319-13278-5_10,

10.1 Anti-estrogens

About 1/3 of breast cancers retain the hormone dependency of the original breast tissue. The deprivation of this growth support by endocrine ablation (ovariectomy, adrenalectomy, hypophysectomy), blocking estrogen biosynthesis (Aromatase and Sulfatase inhibitors, progesterone derivatives), or blocking the estrogen action (selective estrogen receptor modulators) at its receptor level have emerged as therapeutic strategies. Candidate breast cancers for such treatments are Estrogen Receptor- or Progesterone Receptor-positive or receptor unknown.

10.1.1 Selective Estrogen Receptor Modulators

Selective Estrogen Receptor modulators (SERMs) suppress the effects of estrogen by blocking the Estrogen Receptors, relatively selectively in breast cells (Fig. 10.1). This disrupts the estrogenic growth signal. Cells in other tissues, such as bones, liver, and uterus, have Estrogen Receptors with slightly different structures and lower affinities to SERMs. Hence, these drugs, while blocking estrogenic actions on breast cells, may activate estrogen signaling in others. As a benefit, SERMs also can improve bone density, which reduces the risk of osteoporosis, and may lower cholesterol levels. These drugs are taken daily as pills.

Adverse Effects The most common adverse effects of selective Estrogen Receptor modulators are fatigue, hot flashes, night sweats, vaginal discharge, and mood swings. Hot flashes or night sweats from taking a SERM can be troubling, but are likely associated with a reduced risk of cancer recurrence.

SERMs may cause serious adverse effects, including blood clots, stroke, and endometrial cancer. The risk is increased in smokers and patients with a history of thromboses or heart attacks. Symptoms potentially associated with emboli are abnormal vaginal bleeding or discharge, pain or pressure in the pelvis, leg swelling or tenderness, chest pain, shortness of breath, weakness, tingling, or numbness in the face, arm, or leg, dizziness, sudden difficulty seeing, or sudden severe headache.

The triphenylethylene tamoxifen competitively inhibits the binding of estradiol to Estrogen Receptors, thereby preventing the receptors from engaging the cognate estrogen-response elements in the DNA[2] (Figs. 10.2 and 10.3). The result is a reduction in the cellular response to estrogen. In addition, tamoxifen up-regulates the production of Transforming Growth Factor β (TGF-β), a molecule that inhibits tumor cell growth, and down-regulates Insulin-Like Growth Factor 1 (IGF-1), a molecule that stimulates breast cancer cell growth.

- Tamoxifen citrate (ICI 46,474) <Nolvadex, Soltamox> is the salt of the non-steroidal selective Estrogen Receptor modulator.
- 4-Hydroxytamoxifen (afimoxifene) <TamoGel> is a tamoxifen metabolite with both estrogenic and anti-estrogenic effects. 4-hydroxytamoxifen has a higher affinity for the Estrogen Receptor than tamoxifen, and functions as an antagonist in breast cancer cells. It is under study for transdermal application.

Since its original FDA approval in 1977, tamoxifen has been considered the "gold standard" treatment for Estrogen Receptor-positive postmenopausal breast cancer patients. In 1998, tamoxifen was also approved for breast cancer prevention by the U.S. FDA. Tamoxifen is used for

- women and men diagnosed with hormone receptor-positive, early stage breast cancer after surgery (or possibly chemotherapy and radiation) to reduce the risk of recurrence
- women and men diagnosed with advanced stage or metastatic hormone receptor-positive disease
- women who are at higher-than-average risk for breast cancer to reduce the likelihood of its occurrence.

Some women may take tamoxifen for 5 years. Other women may take it for 2–3 years and then switch to an Aromatase inhibitor.

Pharmacokinetics Tamoxifen is a prodrug, converted to its active form, primarily through *N*-demethylation and hydroxylation. The main active enzyme is the Cytochrome P450 CYP2D6, which catalyzes the formation of both 4-OH-tamoxifen and 4-OH-*N*-demethyl-tamoxifen (endoxifen). This activity may be compromised by a low activity polymorphism in CYP2D6, which exists in about 10% of the population (for those patients, toremifene is a better drug choice). The Flavin Monooxygenases FMO1 and FMO3 convert tamoxifen into its *N*-oxide.

Adverse Effects Tamoxifen is associated with harmful, sometimes life threatening adverse effects attributable to its partial estrogen agonist properties. These include hot flashes, vaginal discharge, thromboembolism (deep vein thrombosis or pulmonary emboli), stroke, cataract, and secondary cancers. Tamoxifen is genotoxic and long-term use may cause endometrial carcinoma or hepatocellular carcinoma. 4-Hydroxytamoxifen may be further oxidized to an electrophilic quinone methide, which has the potential to alkylate

[2] The receptors, once bound to their natural ligands, shuttle into the nucleus and act as transcription factors.

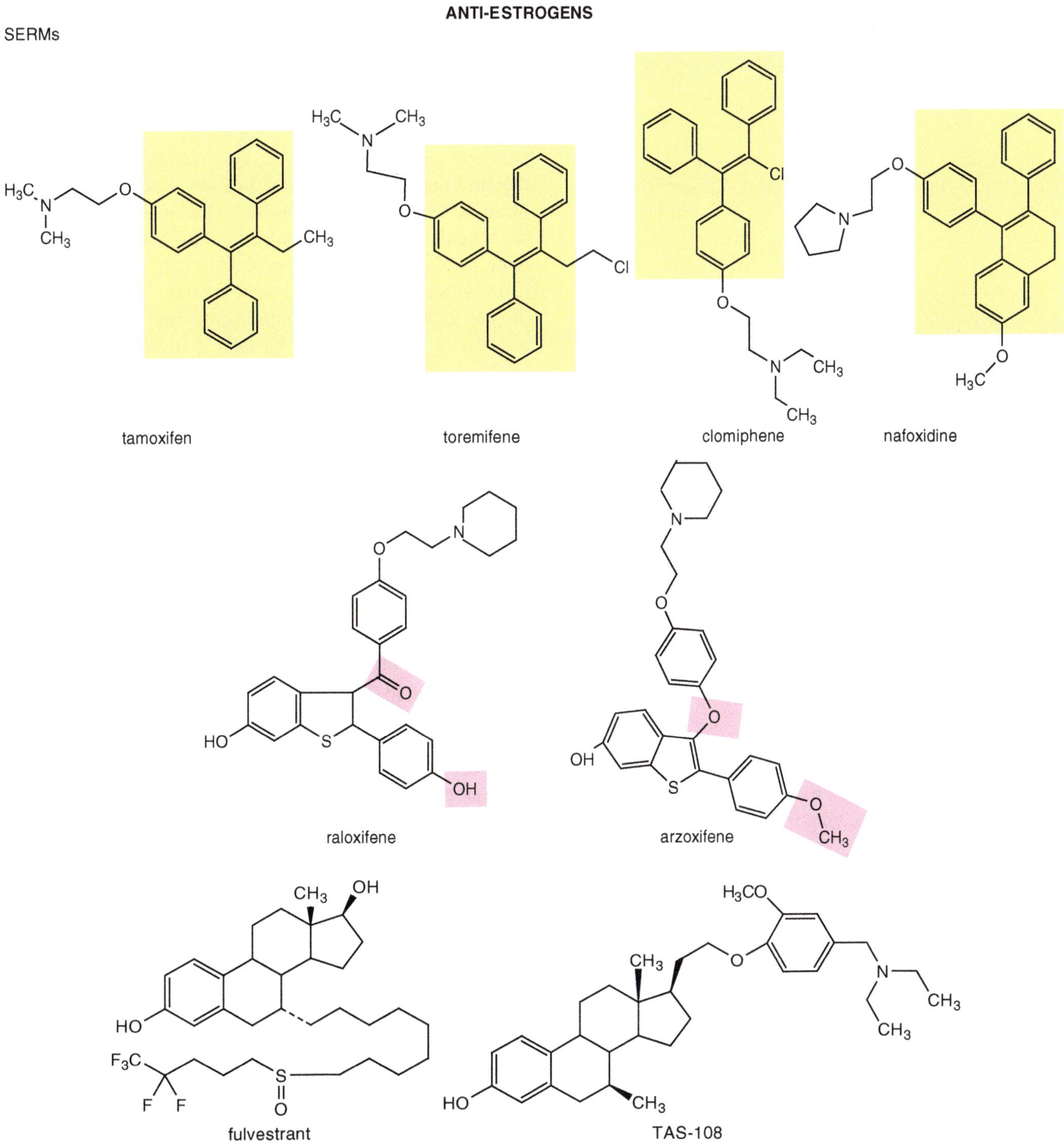

Fig. 10.1 Structures of anti-estrogen *SERMs*. The triphenylethylene moiety that is common to a subset of representatives in this class of drugs is highlighted in *yellow*. Differences between the benzothiophenes raloxifene and arzoxifene are shown on a *pink* background

DNA and may initiate carcinogenesis. Patients receiving tamoxifen tend to have an increase in spine and hip bone mineral density.

Drug Interactions There are medications that can block the activity of CYP2D6 to varying degrees, including some antidepressants of the serotonin specific reuptake inhibitor (SSRI) and serotonin norepinephrine reuptake inhibitor (SNRI) classes, quinidine <Cardioquin>, diphenhydramine <Benadryl>, and cimetidine <Tagamet>. Those agents reduce the effectiveness of tamoxifen.

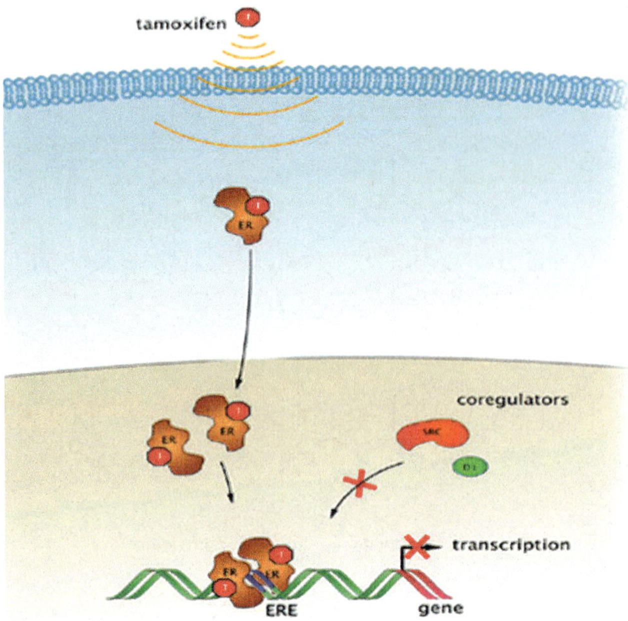

Fig. 10.2 Tamoxifen drug action. ERα-complex binds to its cognate ERE recognition site in the promoter of estrogen responsive genes. Transcription is mediated through the subsequent recruitment of a number of co-activators, an interaction stabilized by Cyclin D1. The binding of tamoxifen (*T*) to ER prevents the recruitment of the co-activator SRC-1 and impedes ER-mediated transcription. (Michalides et al. 2004)

Toremifene <Fareston> is a chlorinated non-steroidal triphenylethylene anti-estrogen. Chemically related to tamoxifen, toremifene acts as a selective Estrogen Receptor modulator that binds competitively to Estrogen Receptors, thereby interfering with estrogen activity. Toremifene also has intrinsic estrogenic properties, which are manifested according to tissue type. The agent is available in tablet form for oral administration at a dose of 60 mg per day. It is indicated for the treatment of metastatic breast cancer in postmenopausal women with Estrogen Receptor-positive or Estrogen Receptor-unknown tumors.

Pharmacokinetics In the blood, toremifene is mostly bound to protein. Its terminal half-life is about 6 days. The drug is extensively metabolized, principally by CYP3A4 to *N*-demethyltoremifene, which is also anti-estrogenic but with weak anti-tumor potency. At steady state, the blood concentrations of *N*-demethyltoremifene are 2–4 times higher than those of the parent drug. Toremifene is eliminated as metabolites predominantly in the feces, with about 10% excreted in the urine. The elimination is slow, in part because of enterohepatic circulation. Hepatic or renal insufficiency does not commonly have a strong effect on the pharmacokinetics of toremifene.

Adverse Effects Adverse drug reactions are mostly due to the anti-estrogenic hormonal actions of toremifene and typically occur at the beginning of the treatment. Common adverse effects include hot flashes (30%), sweating (15%), nausea (15%), vaginal discharge (15%), dizziness, edema, vomiting, and vaginal bleeding. Endometrial hyperplasia may occur, but it is not known whether the risk of endometrial cancer is increased by toremifene treatment. The DNA damaging properties of the drug are 150-fold lower than those of tamoxifen. The agent is pregnancy category D.

As with other anti-estrogens, hypercalcemia and tumor flare can arise in some breast cancer patients with bone metastases during the first weeks of treatment. Tumor flare is a syndrome of diffuse musculoskeletal pain and erythema with increased size of tumor lesions that later regress. It is often accompanied by hypercalcemia. Tumor flare does not imply

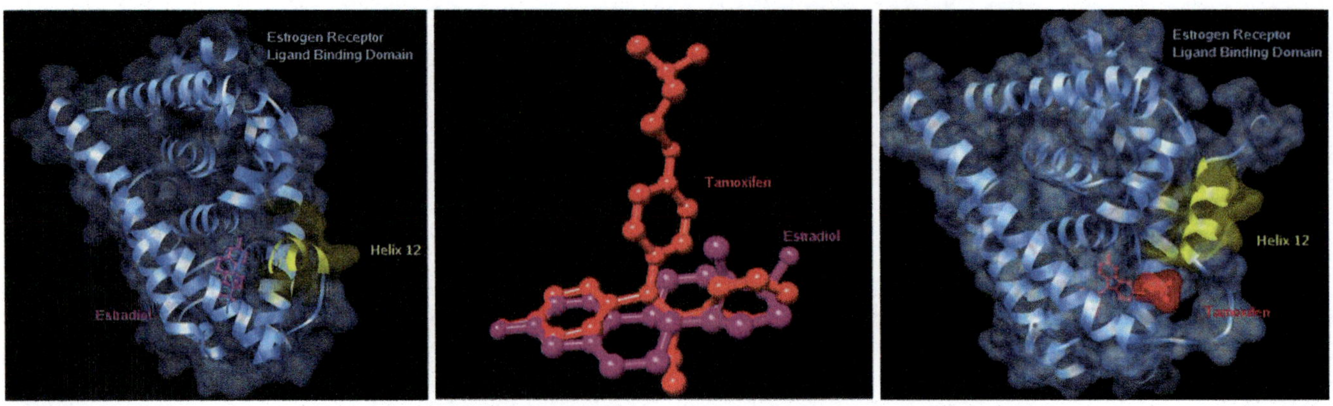

Fig. 10.3 Tamoxifen drug action. (*left*) Ligand binding domain of estrogen receptor alpha bound to estradiol, which is completely embedded in the binding pocket. Highlighted in *yellow* is helix 12, which caps the binding pocket. (Gangloff et al. PDB 1qku X RAY). (*middle*) Overlap of estradiol and drug tamoxifen, highlighting the fact that tamoxifen mimics the structure of extradiol, but has an extra tail that sticks out of the binding pocket in the ligand binding domain, preventing helix 12 from capping the pocket and therefore inactivating the receptor. (PDB 1qku, 3ert). (*right*) Ligand binding domain of estrogen receptor alpha bound to drug tamoxifen, which is sticking out of the binding pocket. Highlighted in *yellow* is the displaced helix 12. (Shaiu et al. PDB 3ert X RAY). [http://maptest.rutgers.edu/drupal/?q=node/273]

failure of treatment or represent tumor progression. If hypercalcemia occurs, appropriate measures need to be instituted and if it is severe, toremifene should be discontinued.

Drug Interactions Drugs that decrease renal calcium excretion, such as thiazide diuretics, may increase the risk of hypercalcemia in patients receiving toremifene. There are interactions between anti-estrogenic compounds of the triphenylethylene derivative class and coumarin-type anticoagulants, leading to an increased prothrombin time. When concomitant use of anticoagulants with toremifene is necessary, careful monitoring of the prothrombin time is required. Cytochrome P450 3A4 enzyme inducers, such as phenobarbital, phenytoin, and carbamazepine increase the rate of toremifene metabolism, lowering the steady state concentration in the blood. Conversely, the metabolism of toremifene may be inhibited by drugs that inhibit the CYP3A4-6 enzymes, such as ketoconazole and similar antimycotics, as well as erythromycin and similar macrolides.

The citrate salt of the triphenylethylene clomiphene <Clomid, Serophene, Milophene> has both estrogenic and anti-estrogenic activities that compete with estrogen for binding to Estrogen Receptor sites in target tissues. This agent causes the release of the pituitary Gonadotropins Follicle Stimulating Hormone (FSH) and Luteinizing Hormone (LH), leading to ovulation. While mostly used as non-steroidal ovulatory stimulant (for the treatment of ovulatory dysfunction or polycystic ovary syndrome), clomiphene may also have activity against breast cancer.

Nafoxidine (1-(2-(4-(3,4-dihydro-6-methoxy-2-phenyl-1-naphthyl)phenoxy)ethyl)pyrrolidine) (U 11100A) was synthesized by Daniel Lednicer at Upjohn. It is a triphenylethylene that is administered in the form of its hydrochloride. Nafoxidine binds to the cytoplasmic and nuclear forms of the Estrogen Receptor and acts as a partial antagonist. The agent also induces oxidative stress, Protein Kinase C, and calcium signaling. Further, it inhibits angiogenesis in some tissues by blocking the effects of Fibroblast Growth Factor (FGF) and Vascular Endothelial Growth Factor (VEGF). Nafoxidine is under study for the treatment of breast cancer. The response to nafoxidine is strongly correlated to the presence of Estrogen Receptors in the tumor and to the response to prior hormonal treatment.

Adverse Effects Adverse effects include dryness of skin, photosensitivity reactions, and (less commonly) partial hair loss. In a paradoxical reaction, nafoxidine may enhance angiogenesis in uterine tissue.

A benzothiophene selective Estrogen Receptor modulator, raloxifene <Evista> binds to the Estrogen Receptor as a mixed estrogen agonist/antagonist. It displays both an ERα selective partial agonist/antagonist effect and an ERβ selective pure antagonist effect. Due to these properties, this agent functions as an estrogen mimic in some tissues and processes (bones, lipid metabolism) and as an estrogen inhibitor in others (endometrium and breasts), with the potential for producing some of the beneficial estrogen effects without exerting its adverse effects. Indications are

- reduction in the risk of invasive breast cancer in postmenopausal women with osteoporosis
- reduction in the risk of invasive breast cancer in postmenopausal women at high risk of invasive breast cancer.

The recommended dosage is a 60 mg tablet daily, which may be administered any time of day without regard to meals.

Pharmacokinetics Raloxifene is not dependent on CYP2D6 for activation and may be a treatment alternative for patients with compromised CYP2D6 activity. In the blood, raloxifene is more than 95 % bound to plasma proteins.

Adverse Effects The most serious adverse reaction related to raloxifene is venous thrombembolism (deep venous thrombosis, pulmonary embolism, and retinal vein thrombosis) in about 1 % of patients. Superficial thrombophlebitis also arises with increased frequency. There is an increased risk for death from stroke. The drug is Pregnancy Category X.

Drug Interactions Raloxifene can be concomitantly administered with ampicillin, amoxicillin, antacids, corticosteroids, and digoxin. It should not be co-administered with other anion exchange resins, such as cholestyramine. The safety of the concomitant use of raloxifene with systemic estrogens has not been established and the combination is not recommended.

The hydrochloride salt of arzoxifene is a synthetic benzothiophene. Arzoxifene is a potent estrogen antagonist in mammary and uterine tissue, while acting as an estrogen agonist by maintaining bone density and low serum cholesterol. It exhibits reduced estrogenicity in the uterus compared with either tamoxifen or raloxifene. This agent may have beneficial effects on bone and on the cardiovascular system.

Pharmacokinetics In comparison to other selective Estrogen Receptor modulators, arzoxifene exhibits greater bioavailability and higher anti-estrogenic potency in the breast than raloxifene.

Adverse Effects Adverse effects include endometrial polyps, vulvular and vaginal inflammation (including mycotic infections), vaginal discharge, and urinary tract infections.

Fulvestrant <Faslodex> is a synthetic competitive Estrogen Receptor antagonist with no agonist activity. The bulky side chain of fulvestrant prevents Estrogen Receptor dimerization. This results in Estrogen Receptor degradation and a substantial decline in its expression levels. Because of this mechanism of action, fulvestrant is also referred to a selective Estrogen Receptor down-regulator (SERD)[3]. The drug reversibly inhibits the growth of tamoxifen resistant, estrogen sensitive breast cancer cells. It is indicated for drug treatment of hormone receptor-positive metastatic breast cancer in postmenopausal women with disease progression following anti-estrogen therapy. Fulvestrant is approved by the U.S. FDA for post-menopausal women with hormone receptor-positive metastatic breast cancer after other hormonal treatments (such as Aromatase inhibitors or selective Estrogen Receptor modulators) have stopped working. Sustained exposure via continuous administration is required for activity. The recommended dose is 500 mg administered intramuscularly on days 1, 15, 29 and once monthly thereafter.

Pharmacokinetics Following a single intramuscular injection of long-acting fulvestrant preparation, the time to maximum blood concentrations varies over 2–19 days, reflecting the prolonged release from the injection site. The time course fits a 2-compartment model. Fulvestrant is extensively metabolized, with substantial contributions by CYP3A4. Fulvestrant is mainly excreted in the feces. The major excretory products are fulvestrant and its 17-ketone or sulphone derivatives together with sulphate conjugates. In patients with hepatic impairment, the dose may need to be reduced to 250 mg per injection.

Adverse Effects The most frequent adverse reactions are injection site pain (10%), nausea (10%) and bone pain (10%), back pain may also arise. Because fulvestrand is administered intramuscularly, it should be used with caution in patients with bleeding diatheses, thrombocytopenia, or anticoagulant use. The drug is Pregnancy Category D.

TAS-108 (SR16234) is a synthetic, orally available, steroidal compound that binds to and inhibits ERα, which is mainly expressed in the mammary gland and uterus, and is up-regulated in estrogen dependent tumors. Blockage of ERα by TAS-108 prevents the binding and signaling by estrogen and may lead to an inhibition of estrogen dependent cancer cell proliferation. TAS-108 also is a partial agonist of ERβ, which is expressed in many tissues, including the central nervous system, urogenital tract, bone, and cardiovascular system. The agent thereby exerts a positive effect on these tissues. In addition, it activates the co-repressor SMRT (Silencing Mediator for Retinoid and Thyroid Hormone Receptor), which inhibits the transactivating activities of the Estrogen Receptors. This may contribute to the anti-tumor activity of TAS-108.

Pharmacokinetics The drug has linear pharmacokinetics. It is metabolized by 4 major pathways including conjugation of the 3-hydroxyl group, steroid ring hydroxylation, and *N*-oxidation resulting in *N*-oxide and *N*-deethylated forms. The deethylation is catalyzed mainly by CYP3A4 in the liver.

Adverse Effects Common toxicities include hot flashes, headache, nausea and vomiting.

[3] Estrogen Receptor down-regulators block and break down Estrogen Receptors. With fewer hormone receptors available, fewer cancer cells receive the growth signal.

CC-8490 (SPC8490) is a benzopyran that acts as a selective Estrogen Receptor modulator (SERM), inhibiting the proliferation of estrogen sensitive breast cancer cells. This agent also inhibits growth and induces apoptosis of glioblastoma cells via a mechanism independent of Estrogen Receptor related mechanisms. The drug is under investigation for breast and brain cancers.

Soy isoflavones or soy protein isolates are dietary supplements, isolated from soybeans, which contain phytoestrogens. These phytoestrogens mimic estrogen action, mediated through Estrogen Receptors, and modulate estrogen metabolism. As a result, soy extracts may reduce tumor cell proliferation and induce tumor cell apoptosis. They may also be able to regulate hormone balance and reduce the risks of breast cancer.

Anti-estrogens aim at neutralizing the responsible growth factor for transformed breast tissue.
Selective Estrogen Receptor modulators (SERMs) block Estrogen Receptors relatively selectively in breast cells.
SERMs may cause blood clots, stroke, and endometrial cancer.

10.1.2 Progesterone Derivatives

High doses of progesterone inhibit the release of Luteinizing Hormone (LH) and Follicle Stimulating Hormone (FSH) from the hypophysis. This suppresses the aromatization of androstendione to estrogen and increases the catabolism of androgens in the liver, thus reducing the levels of steroids that are growth promoting to certain cancers (Fig. 10.4).

Adverse Effects High gestagen therapy is limited by substantial adverse effects, comprising weight gain, sweating, constipation, and Cushing-like symptoms. In rare cases, disorientation and depression can become manifest. Long-term treatment with estrogens and progestins may increase the risk of heart attack, embolism, or stroke.

Medroxyprogesterone acetate (17α-hydroxy-6α-methylpro gesterone acetate, MPA) <Provera, Depo-Provera, Depo-Sub Q Provera 104>, discovered in 1956, is an orally available synthetic derivative of progesterone with anti-estrogenic effects. Medroxyprogesterone (Fig. 10.5). acts as an agonist of the Progesterone Receptor (PR), Androgen Receptor (AR), and Glucocorticosteroid Receptor (GR). It inhibits the hypothalamic-pituitary-adrenal and hypothalamic-pituitary-gonadal axes, resulting in a marked suppression in the levels of androgen, estrogen, cortisol, Gonadotropin, Adrenocorticotropic Hormone, and Sex Hormone Binding Globulin (SHBG). This agent may

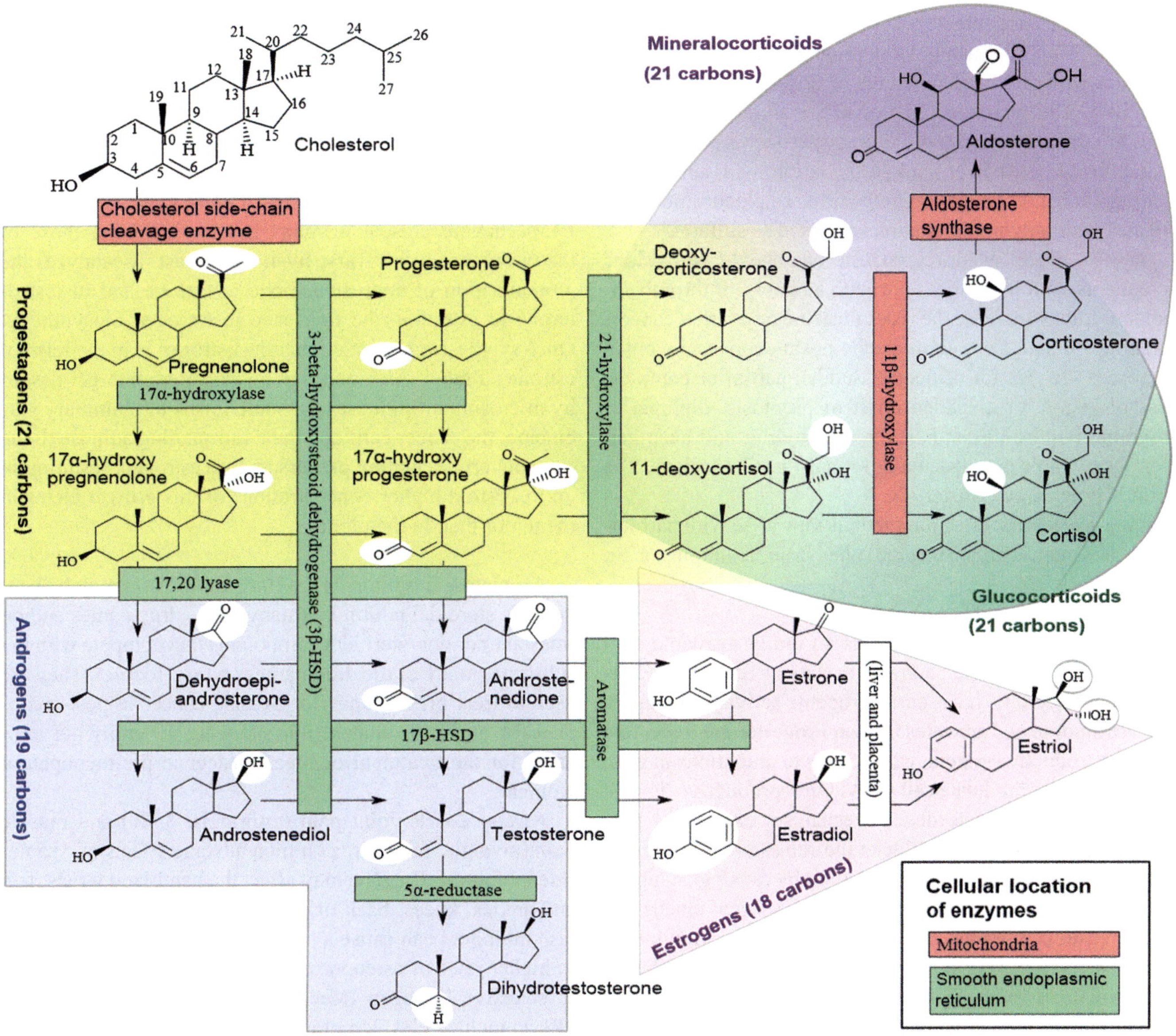

Fig. 10.4 Steroid biosynthesis. [http://en.wikipedia.org/wiki/File:Steroidogenesis.svg]

inhibit the growth stimulating effects of estrogen on estrogen sensitive tumor cells. It decreases the risk for endometrial hyperplasia, a condition that may lead to uterine cancer.

Pharmacokinetics The bioavailability of medroxyprogesterone is increased when taken with food. The drug is rapidly absorbed from the gastrointestinal tract, and maximum blood

Fig. 10.5 Structures of anti-estrogens. The difference between the progesterones is highlighted in *pink*

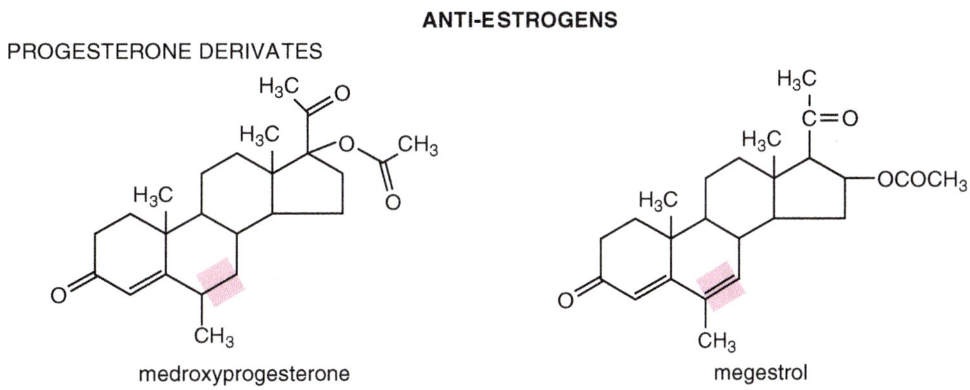

concentrations are achieved 2–4 h after oral administration. The drug is approximately 90 % protein bound, primarily to albumin while no binding occurs to Sex Hormone Binding Globulin. The pharmacokinetics may vary between single and multiple doses. Medroxyprogesterone is extensively metabolized in the liver via hydroxylation, with subsequent conjugation and elimination in the urine as glucuronide conjugates with only minor amounts excreted as sulfates.

Adverse Effects Medroxyprogesterone should be avoided in patients with liver disease or with a history of thrombembolism. It may increase the risk of uterine or ovarian cancers in some women. Long-term use by postmenopausal women increases the risk for dementia. Sudden partial or complete loss of vision, or a sudden onset of proptosis, diplopia or migraine require discontinuation of the drug and examination for possible papilledema or retinal vascular lesions. The drug is Pregnancy Category X.

Drug Interactions Drug interactions may arise with barbiturates, bosentan, carbamazepine, phenytoin, rifampin, or St. John's Wort.

Megestrol acetate <Megace> is an orally available synthetic derivative of the naturally occurring female sex hormone progesterone. It has anti-estrogenic activity. Megestrol acetate binds to and activates nuclear Progesterone Receptors in the reproductive system, which leads to alterations in gene expression that modulate cell growth in reproductive tissues. Engaging a negative feedback mechanism exerted by progesterone, megestrol also blocks the release of Luteinizing Hormone from the pituitary gland, thereby causing an inhibition of ovulation and an alteration in the cervical mucus and endometrium. Without Luteinizing Hormone stimulation, estrogen release from the ovaries is suppressed, and hence the growth of estrogen sensitive tumor cells is impeded. Megestrol acetate is used in the treatment of advanced breast cancer and advanced endometrial cancer. It may be indicated for endometriosis or endometrial hyperplasia.

Adverse Effects The most common adverse effects are weight gain, nausea, rash, impotency, insomnia, mood swings, sweating, breakthrough menstrual bleeding, high blood pressure, and flatulence. Blood clots in the legs and lungs may occur. Megestrol may worsen existing diabetes or lead to new onset diabetes. Allergic reactions are possible.

Drug Interactions Indinavir <Crixivan> reduces the blood concentrations of megestrol. An increase in the dose of the progesterone derivative should be considered.

Progesterone inhibits the release of Luteinizing Hormone (LH) and Follicle Stimulating Hormone (FSH) from the hypophysis, thus reducing the levels of steroids.
High gestagen therapy is limited by weight gain, sweating, constipation, and Cushing-like symptoms.
Long-term treatment with estrogens and progestins may increase the risk of heart attack, embolism, or stroke.

10.1.3 Aromatase and Sulfatase Inhibitors

In pre-menopausal women, estrogen is predominantly synthesized by the ovaries. Post-menopausally, adrenal Aromatase and adipose tissue are mainly responsible for the residual estrogen production from androgenic precursors. Aromatase (Estrogen Synthase, CYP19A1) is a Cytochrome P450 enzyme present in many tissues, including those of the pre-menopausal ovary, liver, and breast. It catalyzes the aromatization of androstenedione to estrone and of testosterone to estradiol, the final step in estrogen biosynthesis. Once synthesized, most circulating estrogen is in the form of estrone sulfate, which needs to be activated in target tissues by microsomal Sulfatases. In some forms of mammary carcinoma, the cancer cells and their surrounding adipose tissue can convert circulating precursors into estrogen, resulting in up to 20-fold higher concentrations of this growth factor in the tumor than in the blood.

Aromatase inhibitors (Fig. 10.6, Table 10.1) may be irreversible steroidal inhibitors (many of the drug names end on -mestane) or non-steroidal compounds that compete with the substrate (many of the drug names end on -rozole). They are used to treat breast cancer or ovarian cancer in post-menopausal women. Aromatase inhibitors are generally not indicated for the treatment of breast cancer in pre-menopausal women[4].

Adverse Effects Joint pain (arthralgia, 35 %) and muscle pain (myalgia, 15 %) are common adverse effects of Aromatase inhibitors. The pain may affect the hands and wrists, feet and ankles, knees, back or other parts of the body. Aromatase inhibitors can cause a loss of bone density, which leads to higher rates of osteoporosis and bone fractures compared to selective Estrogen Receptor modulators. Other adverse effects include elevated blood pressure and elevated cholesterol.

Steroidal Aromatase inhibitors The steroid exemestane (10,13-dimethyl-6-methylidene-7,8,9,10,11,12,13,14,15,16-decahydrocyclopenta[a]phenanthrene-3,17-dione) <Aromasin> is a third generation Aromatase inhibitor that is orally active. It forms a permanent bond with the Aromatase enzyme complex and is thus irreversible. Exemestane is used

[4] Pre-menopausally most of the circulating estrogen is produced by the ovaries (not by conversion of androgens to estrogen), and blocking Aromatase does not decrease this synthetic path of estrogen. When Aromatase inhibitors are used in pre-menopausal women, the limited decrease in estrogen activates the hypothalamus and pituitary axis to increase Gonadotropin secretion, which in turn stimulates the ovary to increase androgen production. This counteracts the effect of the Aromatase inhibitor.

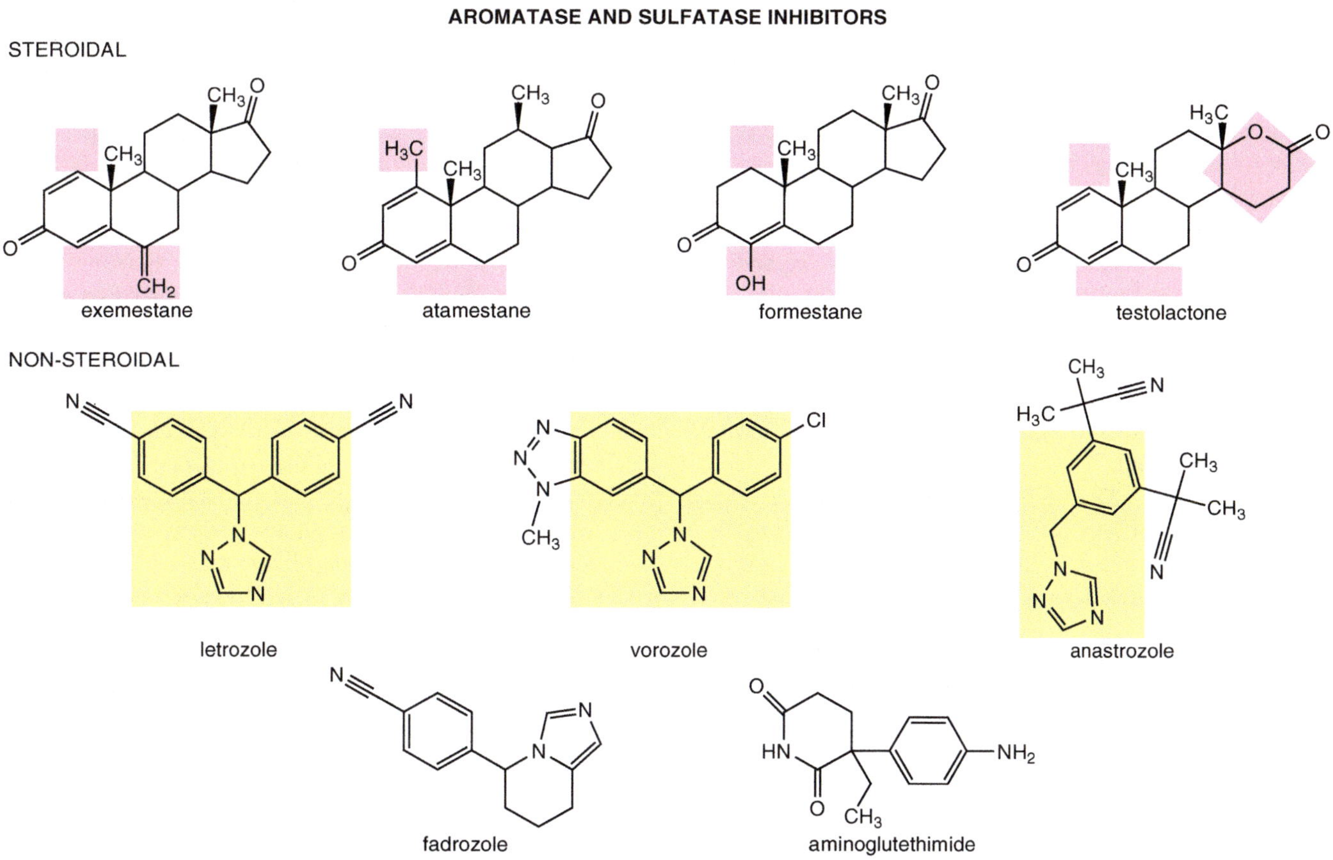

Fig. 10.6 Structures of Aromatese and Sulfatase inhibitors. The core structure for steroidal inhibitors is common. Differences in molecular structure are highlighted in *pink*. The common core of the non-steroidal inhibitors letrozole and vorozole (partially preserved in anastrozole) is shown on *yellow* background

in post-menopausal women for the treatment of advanced breast cancer that has become refractory to conventional hormone therapy.

Pharmacokinetics Consecutive to oral intake of 25 mg tablets, the plasma levels increase by 40 % when exemestane is taken after a fatty meal. The distribution is extensive. 90 % of the drug is bound to protein, primarily to Albumin and 1-Acid Glycoprotein. The half-life for elimination is 24 h. Exemestane is a substrate for CYP3A4. This enzyme oxidizes the methylene group, which is followed by a reduction of the 17-keto group and results in the formation of multiple inactive metabolites.

Adverse Effects Adverse reactions to exemestane include fatigue, pain, insomnia, depression, anxiety, hot flashes, nausea, edema, hypertension, chest pain, dizziness, headache, fever, hypoesthesia, and confusion. The drug is not recommended for use in pre-menopausal women. Hypersensitivity to exemestane or any component of the formulation is a contraindication for its use.

Drug interactions Exemestane should not be administered concurrently with estrogen containing drugs. Inducers of CYP3A4 may decrease the levels of exemestane. Such inducers include aminoglutethimide, carbamazepine, nafcillin, nevirapine, phenobarbital, phenytoin, and rifamycin. Dosage adjustments are required if administered simultaneously.

Table 10.1 Generations of Aromatase inhibitors

Aromatase inhibitors	
First generation	Aminoglutethimide
Second generation	Formestane, fadrozole
Third generation	Letrozole, anastrozole, vorozole, exemestane

Atamestane (1-methyl-1,4-androstadiene-3,17-dione) is a synthetic steroidal substance that binds competitively and irreversibly to the enzyme Aromatase and inhibits it, thereby blocking the conversion of cholesterol to pregnenolone and the peripheral aromatization of androgenic precursors into estrogens. Atamestane lacks other intrinsic hormonal or anti-hormonal activities and displays no inhibition of other Cytochrome P450 dependent enzymes involved in adrenal steroidogenesis. However, it inhibits the estrogen related negative feedback to the central nervous system. The extent and consequence of the induced counter-regulation of the pituitary-hypothalamic axis show major sex specific differences. Atamestane may be beneficial for the management of benign prostate hyperplasia.

The synthetic steroid formestane (4-hydroxyandrost-4-ene-3,17-dione, 4-OHA) (CGP 32349) <Lentaron> is a second generation, competitive and irreversible Aromatase inhibitor. It is administered at 500 mg intramuscularly every 14 days, to be reduced to 250 mg once efficacy is achieved. Formestane permanently deactivates Aromatase by forming an irreversible bond.

Pharmacokinetics Due to its poor oral bioavailability and the availability of orally active Aromatase inhibitors formestane is not widely used. Following formestane discontinuation, it takes several days for Aromatase to become active again.

Adverse Effects The adverse effects that accompany formestane use are common for this class of drugs. They include fatigue, mood swings, depression, joint pain, hot flashes, head aches, swelling of the arms and legs, and high blood pressure. Formestane also suppresses high density lipoprotein (HDL cholesterol) levels and may decrease bone density, thus increasing the susceptibility to osteoporosis or fractures.

Testolactone <Teslac> is a progesterone derivative that inhibits Aromatase by competing with its substrate, thereby preventing the formation of estrogen from adrenal androstenedione and reducing endogenous estrogen levels. Testolactone is structurally distinct from the androgen steroid nucleus in possessing a 6-membered lactone ring in place of the usual 5-membered carbocyclic D-ring. The drug is recommended as adjunctive therapy in the palliative treatment of advanced or disseminated breast cancer in post-menopausal women when hormonal therapy is indicated. It may also be used in pre-menopausal women with disseminated breast carcinoma, in whom ovarian function has been terminated. The drug is effective in approximately 15 % of patients. An oral dose of 250 mg should be continued for a minimum of 3 months before evaluating the response, unless there is active progression of the disease.

Pharmacokinetics Despite some structural similarity to testosterone, testolactone has no androgenic effect. The agent is well absorbed from the gastrointestinal tract. It is metabolized to several derivatives in the liver, all of which preserve the lactone D-ring. These metabolites, as well as a fraction of the unmetabolized drug, are excreted in the urine.

Adverse Effects Reactions include maculopapular erythema, increase in blood pressure, paresthesia, malaise, aches and edema of the extremities, glossitis, anorexia, nausea and vomiting. Alopecia alone and with associated nail growth disturbance is rare and normally subsides without interruption of treatment. Testolactone is contraindicated in the treatment of breast cancer in men and in patients with a history of hypersensitivity to the drug. The agent is Pregnancy Category C.

Drug Interactions When administered concurrently, testolactone may increase the effects of oral anticoagulants. Monitoring and anticoagulant dosage adjustments are necessary.

Non-steroidal Aromatase Inhibitors The third generation Aromatase inhibitor letrozole <Femara> is an orally active, non-steroidal inhibitor of estrogen synthesis. Letrozole selectively and reversibly inhibits Aromatase by competitively binding to the heme component. At a dose of 2.5 mg/day, the drug lacks estrogen agonist activity and produces complete suppression of estrogen synthesis in post-menopausal patients. Letrozole is indicated in post-menopausal women for

- first-line treatment of hormone receptor-positive or hormone receptor unknown, locally advanced, or metastatic breast cancer
- treatment of advanced breast cancer with disease progression following anti-estrogen therapy
- extended adjuvant treatment of early breast cancer after 5 years of adjuvant tamoxifen therapy (even when started within years after completion of standard therapy, letrozole can reduce the risk of breast cancer recurrence by half).

Pharmacokinetics Following oral administration, letrozole is rapidly absorbed. It has near complete systemic bioavailability and a large volume of distribution. Protein binding is moderate (60 %, mainly to Albumin). Maximum drug concentrations in the blood are achieved within 1 h after intake, and the terminal half life is approximately 2 days. The major route of elimination is via metabolism to an inactive carbinol metabolite (4,4'-methanol-bis-benzonitrile) by CYP3A4 and CYP2A6. Letrozole and its metabolites are then excreted mainly via the kidneys.

Adverse Effects Patients on letrozole therapy exhibit large inter-individual variability in their efficacy and toxicity profiles. In some patients, letrozole is ineffective, while in others a high incidence of arthralgia, myalgia, and cardiovascular events occurs. The typical response rate varies from 20–50 %[5].

Adverse reactions to letrozole may include hot flashes, headache, fatigue, nausea, musculoskeletal pain, arthralgia,

[5] In addition to environmental and physiological factors, such inter-patient variation is commonly associated with polymorphisms in genes that encode drug metabolizing enzymes, drug transporters, or drug targets.

dyspnea, and cough. Letrozole is better tolerated than tamoxifen and is associated with lower incidence of endometrial cancer, vaginal bleeding or discharge, and thromboembolic events.

Drug Interactions If taken together with other CYP2A6 substrates, such as dexmedetomidine or ifosfamide, letrozole may increase their blood levels.

The third generation Aromatase inhibitor vorozole (6-[(4-chlorophenyl)(1,2,4-triazol-1-yl)methyl]-1-methylbenzotriazole) (CGS 16949A, R83842) <Rivizor> is a triazole derivative, which binds competitively to the Cytochrome P450 moiety of Aromatase, thus causing reversible inhibition of the enzyme. The drug reduces the blood estradiol levels in post-menopausal women by about 90%. It was withdrawn from further development when it failed to induce a survival benefit (compared to standard therapy) in breast cancer patients.

Adverse Effects The tolerability of vorozole is better than that of aminoglutethimide. The most common adverse events are hot flashes, and nausea, which are generally mild.

Anastrozole <Arimidex> is a third generation, competitive and reversible Aromatase inhibitor. In estrogen dependent breast cancers, anastrozole may inhibit tumor growth. The dose is one 1 mg tablet once a day, taken with or without food. For patients with advanced breast cancer, anastrozole should be continued until tumor progression sets in. Indications are

- adjuvant treatment of post-menopausal women with hormone receptor-positive early breast cancer
- first-line treatment of post-menopausal women with hormone receptor-positive or hormone receptor-unknown locally advanced or metastatic breast cancer
- second-line treatment of advanced breast cancer in post-menopausal women with disease progression following tamoxifen therapy.

Patients with Estrogen Receptor-negative disease and patients who have not responded to preceding tamoxifen therapy rarely respond to anastrozole.

Pharmacokinetics Orally administered anastrozole is well absorbed into the systemic circulation. Food reduces the rate, but not the overall extent of absorption. Uptake is rapid and maximum blood concentrations occur within 2–5 h. The pharmacokinetics of anastrozole are linear over the dose range of 1–20 mg, and do not change with repeated dosing. Blood concentrations approach steady state levels at about 7 days of once daily dosing. 40% of the drug is bound to plasma proteins. The inhibition of Aromatase activity is primarily due to the action of the parent drug. Hepatic metabolism via *N*-dealkylation, hydroxylation, and glucuronidation accounts for approximately 85% of anastrozole elimination. The 3 metabolites in blood and urine are triazole, a glucuronide conjugate of hydroxy-anastrozole, and a glucuronide conjugate of anastrozole itself. 75% of anastrozole is excreted in the feces, renal elimination accounts for approximately 10% of the total clearance. The mean elimination half-life of anastrozole is 50 h. No dosage adjustment is necessary for patients with renal impairment or for elderly patients. No changes in dose are recommended for patients with mild-to-moderate hepatic impairment.

Adverse Effects Serious adverse reactions with anastrozole, occurring in fewer than 1 in 10,000 patients, are skin reactions (lesions, ulcers, blisters) allergic reactions (swelling of the face, lips, tongue, or throat), changes in liver function (inflammation, jaundice, liver pain). Common adverse reactions, occurring with an incidence over 10%, include hot flashes, rash, asthenia, depression, insomnia, headache, arthritis, arthralgia, bone pain, osteoporosis, hypertension, nausea and vomiting, peripheral edema, cough, dyspnea, pharyngitis, and lymphedema. Patients receiving anastrozole have a decrease in lumbar spine and hip bone mineral density. Women with pre-existing ischemic heart disease have an increased incidence of ischemic cardiovascular events. The drug is Pregancy Category X.

Drug Interactions Estrogen containing therapies should not be used with anastrozole as they may diminish its pharmacological action. The combination of anastrozole and tamoxifen does not have any efficacy benefit and should not be used. It is considered unlikely that co-administration of 1 mg anastrozole can affect other drugs as a result of inhibition of Cytochrome P450 1A2, 2C8/9, or 3A4. Anastrozole has no inhibitory effect on reactions catalyzed by cytochrome P450 2A6 or 2D6.

Aromatase over-expression is linked to the development of pre-neoplastic and neoplastic changes in breast tissue. Fadrozole hydrochloride (CGS 16949A) <Afema> is a second generation Aromatase inhibitor. The agent specifically and selectively inhibits Aromatase, blocking the aromatization of androstenedione into estrone and of testosterone into estradiol. The resulting reduction in estrogen levels may inhibit the growth of estrogen dependent cancers. Fadrozole has been introduced in Japan for the treatment of breast cancer.

Adverse Effects Toxicity is limited to mild to moderate hot flashes (30%), nausea and vomiting (15%), fatigue (10%), and loss of appetite (5%).

Aminoglutethimide (3-(4-aminophenyl)-3-ethyl-2,6-piperidinedione, AG-1) <Orimeten, Cytadren> is a first generation non-steroidal Aromatase inhibitor. It is also an inhibitor of other Cytochrome P450 dependent enzymes. The drug suppresses the enzymatic conversion of cholesterol to D5-pregnenolone, resulting in a decrease in the production of adrenal glucocorticoids, mineralocorticoids, estrogens, and androgens. A decrease in adrenal secretion of cortisol is followed by an increased secretion of pituitary Adrenocorticotropic Hormone (ACTH), which can overcome the blockade of adrenocortical steroid synthesis by aminoglutethimide. This compensatory increase in ACTH secretion may be suppressed by the simultaneous administration of hydrocortisone. Aminoglutethimide is clinically used in the treatment of metastatic breast cancer.

Pharmacokinetics Aminoglutethimide is rapidly and completely absorbed from the gastrointestinal tract. Its main metabolite is acetylaminoglutethimide. The excretion is predominantly renal.

Adverse Effects Adverse effects can be caused through the inhibition of the Desmolase complex[6] by aminoglutethimide. This prevents the conversion of cholesterol to pregnenolone. In extreme cases, the agent can trigger adrenal insufficiency and an Addison crisis. The drug is contraindicated in patients with serious forms of hypersensitivity to glutethimide or aminoglutethimide. The most frequent and reversible adverse effects are drowsiness (30%), morbilliform skin rash (15%), nausea (10%), anorexia (10%), and dizziness (5%). The dizziness is possibly caused by lowered vascular resistance or orthostasis. These reactions often disappear spontaneously with continued therapy. The drug is Pregnancy Category D.

Drug Interactions Aminoglutethimide accelerates the metabolism of dexamethasone. Therefore, if glucocorticoid replacement is needed, hydrocortisone should be prescribed. Aminoglutethimide diminishes the effects of coumarin and warfarin.

Aromatase catalyzes the aromatization of androstenedione to estrone and testosterone to estradiol, the final step in estrogen biosynthesis.
Aromatase inhibitors may be non-steroidal compounds or irreversible steroidal inhibitors that compete with the substrate.
Aromatase inhibitors are used to treat breast cancer or ovarian cancer in post-menopausal women, they are not indicated for the treatment of breast cancer in pre-menopausal women.
Arthralgia and myalgia are common adverse effects of Aromatase inhibitors.

10.1.4 Others

Among the key processes by which the body eliminates toxic chemicals as well as hormones, such as estrogen, is the attachment of glucuronate to them in the liver, followed by excretion of the complex in the bile. When β-Glucuronidase (an enzyme present in certain bacteria that reside in the human gut) breaks this chemical bond, it prolongs the stay of the hormone or toxic chemical in the body. Elevated β-Glucuronidase activity is implicated in an increased risk for hormone dependent cancers, like breast, prostate, and colon cancers.

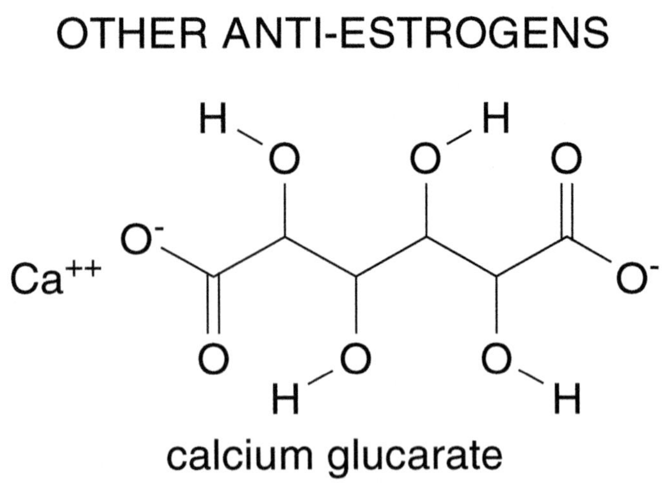

Fig. 10.7 Structure of calcium glucarate

The calcium salt form of glucaric acid (Fig. 10.7), a natural substance in many fruits and vegetables, may have anti-estrogenic properties. The active metabolite of calcium glucarate, D-glucaro-1,4-lactone, is an inhibitor of the enzyme β-Glucuronidase. Through this mechanism, supplementing calcium glucarate may suppress the developments of hormone dependent cancers.

10.2 Anti-androgens

Activation of the Androgen Receptor (AR) is critical for prostate cancer growth. Androgen ablation therapy is the first line of treatment. Anti-androgens (androgen antagonists), first discovered in the 1960s (starting with cyproterone acetate in 1962), prevent androgens from exerting their effects on responsive tissues, such as the prostate.

Drug Resistance Most prostate cancer patients relapse within 18–36 months of anti-androgen therapy and progress to an androgen independent state. However, castration resistant prostate cancers remain dependent on Androgen Receptor function for growth by evolving mechanisms to activate receptor signaling. Underlying alterations include the over-expression of the receptor, receptor mutations that allow activation by anti-androgens or other steroids (progesterone, hydrocortisone), ligand independent activation by growth factor signaling pathways, or changes in the levels of Androgen Receptor transcriptional cofactors.

[6] Desmolases catalyze the formation or destruction of carbon-carbon bonds within a molecule. These enzymes play roles in respiration and fermentation and are involved in steroidogenesis.

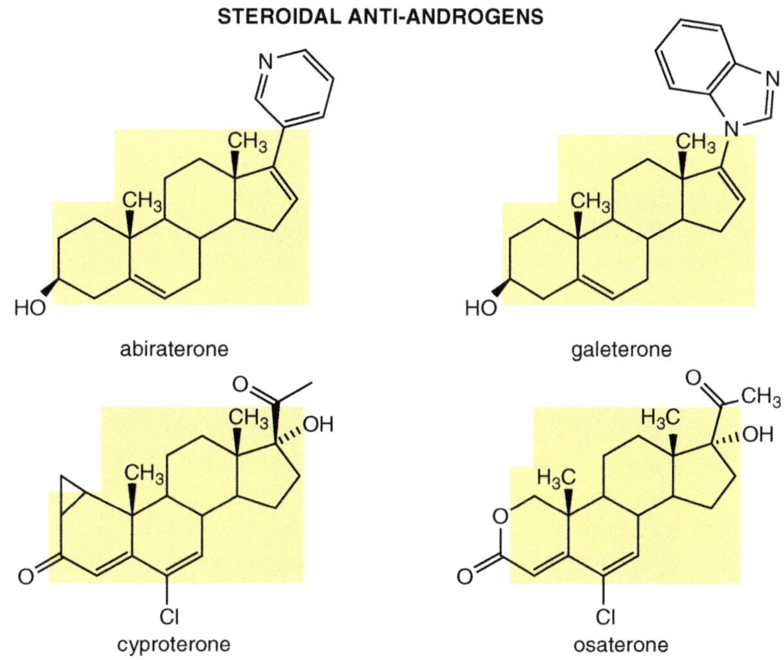

Fig. 10.8 Structures of steroidal anti-androgens. The common steroid core structure is highlighted in *yellow*

10.2.1 Steroidal Anti-androgens

Due to their lipophilicity, steroidal anti-androgens (Fig. 10.8) diffuse through the plasma membrane and prevent the binding of testosterone or dihydrotestosterone to the Androgen Receptor in the cytoplasm. The drug names of steroidal anti-androgens end on -terone.

A negative feedback loop controls androgen production at the hypothalamic-pituitary level, such that elevated testosterone blood levels suppress Gonadotropin secretion, which leads to an inhibition of further androgen production. Anti-androgens interrupt this negative feedback loop, which causes a counter-regulatory increase in androgen concentration and consequently diminished efficacy of the anti-androgen. Due to their progestational property (progesterone-like actions), the steroidal anti-androgens also exert anti-gonadotropic activity, which prevents the counter-regulation, and even decreases peripheral testosterone concentrations. However, in males, but not in females, the anti-androgenic activity partially neutralizes the anti-gonadotropic effect at the hypothalamic-pituitary level.

CYP17A1 (17 α-Hydroxylase, C17,20 Lyase) catalyzes the conversion of pregnenolone and progesterone to didehydroepiandrosterone (DHEA) and 4-androstenedione, which are precursors to testosterone. Abiraterone ((3β)-17-(pyridin-3-yl)androsta-5,16-dien-3-ol) <Zytiga> inhibits CYP17A1 in testicular, adrenal, or prostatic tumor tissues. The inhibition of CYP17A1 activity thus decreases the circulating levels of testosterone. Abiraterone was approved by the U.S. FDA in 2011.

Pharmacokinetics Abiraterone must be taken on an empty stomach (no food for at least 2 h before and 1 h after) because the exposure to the drug variably increases up to 10-fold when it is taken with meals. After oral administration, abiraterone acetate is converted into the active abiraterone by Esterases. The drug is highly protein bound (>99%), and is metabolized in the liver by CYP3A4 and SULT2A1 to inactive products. With a terminal half life of 12 h, close to 90% is excreted via the feces and about 5% in the urine.

Adverse Effects Abiraterone causes a mineralocorticosteroid excess that may lead to hypertension, hypokalemia, and fluid retention. The drug is to be used with caution in patients with a history of cardiovascular disease or with medical conditions that might be compromised by mineralocorticosteroid effects. Abiraterone is hepatotoxic (increases in liver enzymes can enforce dose modification or discontinuation). The most common adverse reactions (occurring in at least 5% of patients) include joint swelling, edema, muscle pain, hot flashes, diarrhea, urinary tract infection, cough, hypertension, arrhythmia, altered urinary frequency or nocturia, dyspepsia, and upper respiratory tract infection. The drug is Pregnancy Category X.

Drug Resistance Most prostate cancer patients on abiraterone eventually progress. One possible mechanism for Androgen Receptor reactivation is the expression of a truncated, constitutively active form of the receptor.

Drug Interactions Abiraterone is an inhibitor of the hepatic drug metabolizing enzyme CYP2D6. It should not be given together with CYP2D6 substrates that have a narrow therapeutic index. Additionally, abiraterone is a substrate of

CYP3A4. Strong inhibitors and inducers of CYP3A4 should be avoided or used with caution.

Cyproterone acetate <Androcur, Cyprostat> is a synthetic derivative of 17-hydroxyprogesterone that acts as a competitive inhibitor of the Androgen Receptor. Cyproterone binds to the receptor, thereby preventing androgen induced signal transduction in target tissues and inhibiting the growth of testosterone sensitive tumor cells. The drug has low specificity and can activate the receptors for glucocorticosteroids, mineralocorticosteroids and progesterone. Cyproterone acetate inhibits the steroidogenic enzyme 21-Hydroxylase and to a lesser extent 3β-Hydroxysteroid Dehydrogenase, both of which are needed to synthesize endogenous corticosteroids such as cortisol and aldosterone. It also exerts progestational agonist properties[7] at the level of the pituitary that reduce Luteinizing Hormone (LH) and Follicle Stimulating Hormone (FSH), resulting in reductions in testicular androgen secretion and blood testosterone levels. Due to the multiple effects of the drug, treatment with cyproterone acetate alone results in a partial suppression of testosterone.

Pharmacokinetics Steroidal anti-androgens are active when given orally. Peak blood levels for cyproterone acetate are achieved within 3–4 h after administration. The terminal half-life is about 38 h. A portion of the drug is metabolized by hydrolysis to cyproterone and acetic acid. However, in contrast to many other steroid esters hydrolysis is not extensive, and much of the pharmacological activity is exerted by the acetate form. Excretion is about 70 % in the feces, mainly in the form of glucuronidated metabolites, and about 30 % in the urine, predominantly as non-conjugated metabolites.

Adverse Effects The most serious adverse effect is liver toxicity, especially at high dose treatment. The drug may cause a suppression of adrenal function, the resulting low cortisol levels can impair carbohydrate metabolism, low aldosterone levels can lead to salt loss and hyperkalemia. The glucocorticosteroid activity of cyproterone acetate is associated with striae of the skin. Androgen deprivation can lead to depressive mood changes (although the adrenal suppression could have the opposite effect). As cyproterone acetate suppresses the production of estrogen, long term use may result in osteoporosis, gynecomastia, galactorrhea, and erectile dysfunction.

Drug Resistance The Androgen Receptor mutation T877A confers agonist properties to cyproterone acetate.

The steroid galeterone (3β-hydroxy-17-[1*H*-benzimidazole-1-yl]androsta-5,16-diene) (VN/124–1, TOK001) binds to and inhibits the Androgen Receptor with 10-fold increased affinity compared to bicalutamide (see Sect. 10.2.2). This blocks androgen signaling. Upon binding, galeterone also causes the degradation of the Androgen Receptor, thus desensitizing prostate cancer cells to the growth stimulatory androgen signal. In addition, galeterone inhibits CYP17. The agent is in development for the treatment of advanced prostate cancer.

The synthetic steroid osaterone acetate (17α-acetoxy-chloro-2-oxa-4,6-pregnadiene-3,20-dione) (TZP-4238) is a derivative of the less potent chlormadinone acetate, which was previously used in the clinical treatment of prostatic hypertrophy and prostate cancer. Osaterone acetate has anti-androgenic and gestagenic effects with virtually no estrogenic and androgenic activity. The agent possesses a similar pharmacological profile to other steroidal anti-androgens. It is in clinical development in Japan for prostate cancer and benign prostatic hyperplasia.

Pharmacokinetics The primary routes of osaterone acetate metabolism involve 11β-, 15β- and 21-hydroxylation, 17α-deacetylation, and dechlorination. Other metabolites arise from combinations of these pathways to form multiple oxidized metabolites.

10.2.2 Non-steroidal Anti-androgens

Non-steroidal anti-androgens (Fig. 10.9) were developed in the 1970s to circumvent the off-target effects of the steroidal agents. They were not believed to have major interaction with nuclear receptors other than the Androgen Receptor or to activate Androgen Receptor dependent genes in prostate cancer cells. The drug names end on -lutamide.

Adverse Effects Given as a mono-therapy to patients with non-castrate levels of testosterone, non-steroidal anti-androgens as a class are better tolerated than androgen lowering agents. They produce less impotence, hot flashes, anemia, and bone loss, but cause gynecomastia and breast tenderness.

Drug Resistance After long-term use of anti-androgens in combination with testosterone lowering treatment, a proportion of patients will respond to the selective discontinuation of the drug with tumor regression (the anti-androgen withdrawal syndrome), which implies that these anti-androgens can serve as agonists under some circumstances.

Flutamide (2-methyl-*N*-[4-nitro-3(trifluoromethyl)phenyl]propanamide) <Eulexin> is a toluidine derivative and first generation non-steroidal anti-androgen. Flutamide and its more potent active metabolite 2-hydroxyflutamide competitively block dihydrotestosterone binding to Androgen Receptors, forming inactive complexes, which cannot translocate into the cell nucleus. The formation of inactive

[7] The progestational effect of the drug is linked to the presence of the acetyl group at position C17 of the steroid. The free alcohol of cyproterone acetate, cyproterone, which lacks the acetyl group, is devoid of progestational properties.

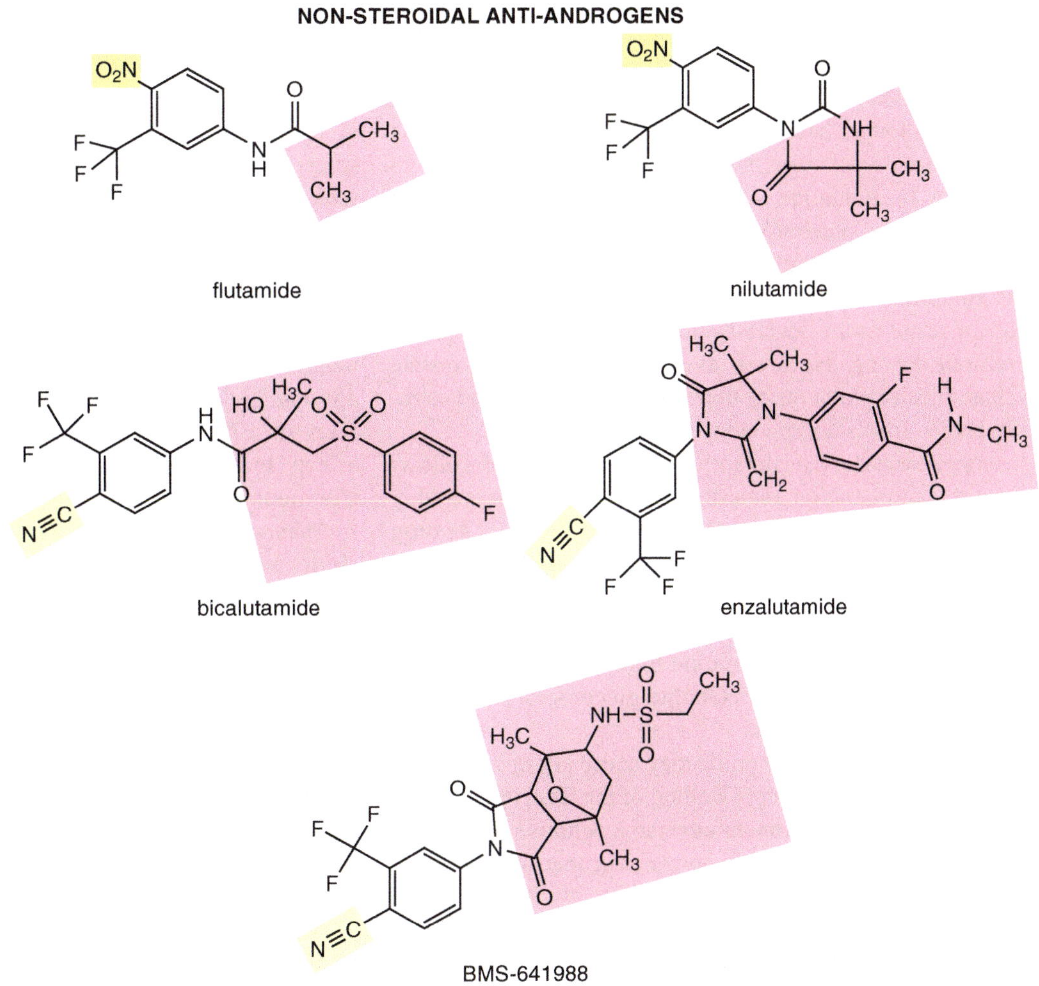

Fig. 10.9 Structures of non-steroidal anti-androgens. The core structure is common. Variations in the side chain are highlighted in *pink*. Two sub-classes have either a nitro group or a nitrile group attached to the 6-ring (bright or pale *yellow*)

receptors inhibits androgen dependent gene expression, resulting in tumor cell growth arrest or transient tumor regression. The drug is approved to block the exacerbation of disease that can occur following the rise in serum testosterone consecutive to the initial administration of Gonadotropin Releasing Hormone (GnRH, Luteinizing Hormone Releasing Hormone, LHRH) agonists.

Pharmacokinetics Flutamide is rapidly and completely absorbed, with food having no effect on its bioavailability. The drug is rapidly metabolized, resulting in at least 6 derivates. Following a 250 mg oral dose, the biologically active α-hydroxylated metabolite reaches maximum blood concentrations in about 2 h. Excretion is mainly in the urine, the major metabolite being 2-amino-5-nitro-4-(trifluoromethyl)phenol.

Adverse Effects Adverse effects include diarrhea, cystitis, alcohol intolerance, and interstitial lung disease. Allergic reactions to the drug are possible. Potentially dangerous hepatotoxicity can occur and may require the discontinuation of treatment.

Drug Resistance The Androgen Receptor mutation T877A confers agonist properties to flutamide.

Nilutamide <Anandron, Nilandron>is a synthetic, non-steroidal anti-androgenic agent. Nilutamide preferentially binds to Androgen Receptors and blocks Androgen Receptor activation by testosterone and other androgens. This drug may inhibit the androgen dependent growth of normal and neoplastic prostate cells. It has pharmacokinetic properties that permit once daily dosing. The drug was approved in 1996 in combination with orchiectomy because of improved disease free and overall survival.

Adverse Effects Adverse effects include diarrhea, alcohol intolerance, interstitial lung disease, and hepatotoxicity. Nilutamide has a unique ocular toxicity that affects the perception of color and the ability to adapt to light.

Drug Resistance The Androgen Receptor mutation T877A confers agonist properties to nilutamide.

The toluidide bicalutamide <Casodex> is a synthetic, non-steroidal anti-androgen. It was derived from flutamide by the addition of a bulky 4-fluorophenylsulfonyl moiety. The drug competitively binds to cytosolic Androgen Receptors in target tissues, thereby inhibiting the receptor engagement by androgens. Compared to flutamide and nilutamide, bicalutamide has a 2-fold increased affinity for the Androgen Receptor, a longer half-life, and substantially decreased toxicities. Based on a more favorable safety profile relative to flutamide, bicalutamide is indicated for use in combination therapy with a Gonadotropin Releasing Hormone analog for the treatment of advanced metastatic prostate carcinoma. In this combination, bicalutamide does not affect the suppression of testosterone levels by the Gonadotropin Releasing Hormone analog. However, as a single agent for prostate cancer, bicalutamide raises the blood testosterone and estradiol levels. It was approved in 1995.

Pharmacokinetics Bicalutamide is well absorbed following oral administration, regardless of food intake. It is highly protein bound (95 %) and has a half-life of 1 week. The drug undergoes stereospecific metabolism. The inactive S enantiomer is metabolized primarily by glucuronidation and is rapidly cleared. The active R enantiomer is predominantly oxidized to an inactive metabolite followed by glucuronidation. Both the parent and metabolite glucuronides are eliminated in the urine and feces.

Adverse Effects Bicalutamide may cause allergic reactions (hives, difficulty breathing, swelling of the face, lips, tongue, or throat). The most frequent adverse reaction is hot flashes (50 %). The hepatotoxicity is lower than that of other non-steroidal anti-androgens.

Drug Resistance Bicalutamide does not bind to most mutated forms of the Androgen Receptor. However, amplification of the Androgen Receptor or the mutations W741L or W741C can confer agonist properties to bicalutamide.

Drug Interactions Caution should be exercised when the drug is co-administered with CYP3A4 substrates. Bicalutamide can displace coumarin anti-coagulants from their binding sites. Monitoring and adjustment of the anticoagulant dose may be necessary.

The diarylthiohydantoin enzalutamide (MDV3100) <Xtandi> is an anti-androgen specifically engineered for activity in prostate cancers with over-expressed Androgen Receptor. When enzalutamide binds the Androgen Receptor, nuclear translocation is inefficient, a substantial fraction of the receptor remains in the cytosol, and DNA binding plus recruitment of co-activators are completely inhibited. The drug was approved by the U.S. FDA in 2012.

Drug Resistance Not all patients respond to enzalutamide treatment and resistance develops in many initial responders. One possible escape mechanism may be the emergence of drug-resistant Androgen Receptor mutants, while another could arise from alternate Androgen Receptor splice forms, which can result in constitutively active receptors that are truncated right before the ligand binding domain. Enzalutamide does not activate the Androgen Receptor mutants T877A or W741C.

BMS-641988 was identified in a structure assisted drug screen using nilutamide as the parent compound. Molecules with a hydantoin ring display high affinity for the Androgen Receptor; combinatorial chemistry produced derivatives that were screened for Androgen Receptor affinity and for the inhibition of transcriptional activation.

BMS-641988 binds the Androgen Receptor with approximately 20-fold increased affinity compared to bicalutamide and has higher therapeutic efficacy. The transcriptional effects of BMS-641988 treatment are more similar to the effects that occur with castration than with bicalutamide treatment. BMS-641988 is in clinical trials.

Pharmacokinetics BMS-641988 has good oral bioavailability and a half-life of 30 h. Metabolism of the drug occurs via CYP3A4 mediated oxidation of the C5 position, followed by elimination of the sulfonamide and rapid reduction by cytosolic Reductase.

Adverse Effects The therapeutic index for QT prolongation is relatively low. Although BMS-641988 is an antagonist of the $GABA_A$ receptor, it does not induce seizures.

Drug Resistance BMS-641988 has agonist activity toward the T877A mutant Androgen Receptor.

Activation of the Androgen Receptor is critical for prostate cancer growth.
Androgen ablation therapy is the first line of treatment.
There are steroidal and non-steroidal anti-androgens.
Most prostate cancer patients relapse within 18–36 months of anti-androgen therapy and progress to an androgen independent state.
Castration resistant prostate cancers remain dependent on Androgen Receptor function for growth by evolving mechanisms to activate receptor signaling.

10.2.3 Dihydrotestosterone Reductase Inhibitors

In castration resistant prostate cancer, the enzymes involved in androgen synthesis, CYP17, 3-β-Hydroxysteroid Dehydrogenase, 17-Ketoreductase, 5α-Reductase, are highly active. They contribute to cancer progression.

The development and enlargement of the prostate gland is dependent on 5α-dihydrotestosterone (DHT) (Fig. 10.10). The 5α-Reductase isoenzyme type 2 is primarily active in reproductive tissues (the prostate gland), while the type 1 isoenzyme is also active in skin and the liver. Type 2 5α-Reductase metabolizes testosterone to dihydrotestosterone, which then induces androgenic effects by binding to Androgen Receptors in the cells of these organs.

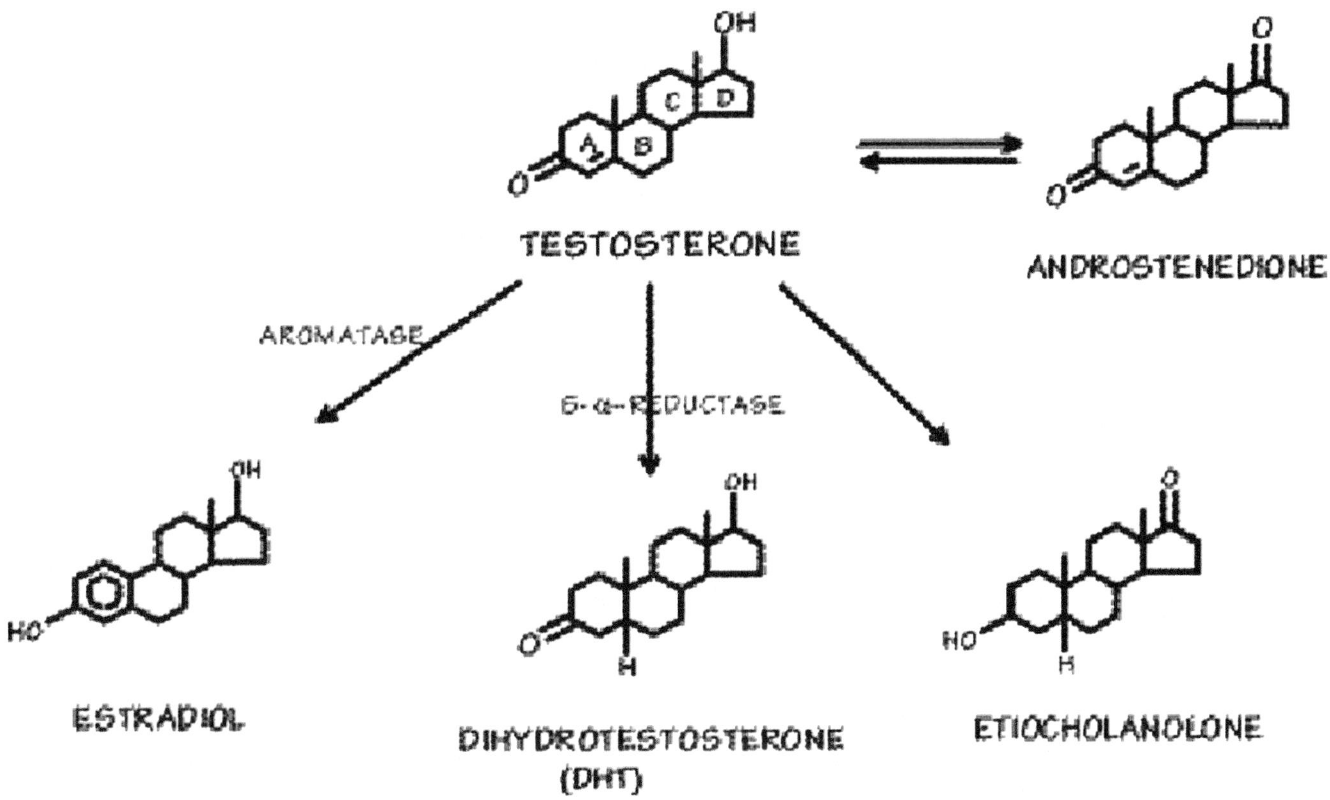

Fig. 10.10 Metabolism of testosterone. Testosterone is reduced by the enzyme 5α-Reductase to dihydrotestosterone. ([http://www.antiaging.com/andropause/andropause2.html] with permission)

Finasteride <Proscar> is a synthetic 4-azasteroid compound (Fig. 10.11) that competitively binds to and inhibits the type 2 Steroid 5α-Reductase in the prostate gland, liver, and skin. It thereby interferes with the enzymatic conversion of testosterone to 5-dihydrotestosterone, and reduces the dihydrotestosterone levels in the blood. This results in a diminished stimulation of Androgen Receptors in the nuclei of prostate cells and consecutively diminished prostate cell proliferation. Finasteride is indicated for the treatment of symptomatic benign prostatic hyperplasia and as adjuvant mono-therapy after radical prostatectomy in the treatment of prostatic cancer. A minimum of 6 months of treatment may be required to determine whether an individual responds to finasteride.

Pharmacokinetics The bioavailability of finasteride is not affected by food. A single 5 mg oral dose produces a rapid reduction in blood dihydrotestosterone levels that reaches a maximum effect after 8 h and is maintained throughout the 24-h dosing interval. Approximately 90 % of the circulating drug is bound to plasma proteins. Finasteride is extensively metabolized in the liver, primarily by Cytochrome P450 3A4. 2 major metabolites comprise the t-butyl side chain monohydroxylated and monocarboxylic acid derivatives, which possess no more than 20 % of the 5α-Reductase inhibitory activity of the parent drug. The mean elimination half-life is 6 h. 40 % of the dose is excreted in the urine in the form of metabolites, while close to 60 % is excreted in the feces.

Adverse Effects Allergic reactions (hives, difficulty breathing, swelling of the face, lips, tongue, or throat) may pose an emergency situation. Male breast cancer can arise in rare cases. Less serious adverse effects may include impotence, loss of libido, abnormal ejaculations, swelling of the hands or feet, swelling or tenderness in the breasts, dizziness. Caution is indicated in patients with hepatic dysfunction. Patients with a large residual urinary volume or severely diminished urinary flow need to be monitored for obstructive uropathy. These patients may not be candidates for finasteride therapy.

Dutasteride <Avodart> is a synthetic 4-azasteroid compound. Dutasteride competitively and specifically binds to the isoenzymes 1 and 2 of 5α-Reductase, forming stable enzyme complexes and inhibiting the conversion of testosterone to 5α-dihydrotestosterone. The reduction in dihydrotestosterone activity may mitigate or prevent the enlargement of the prostate gland. The drug is used for the treatment of benign prostate hypertrophy. It is not approved for the prevention of prostate cancer.

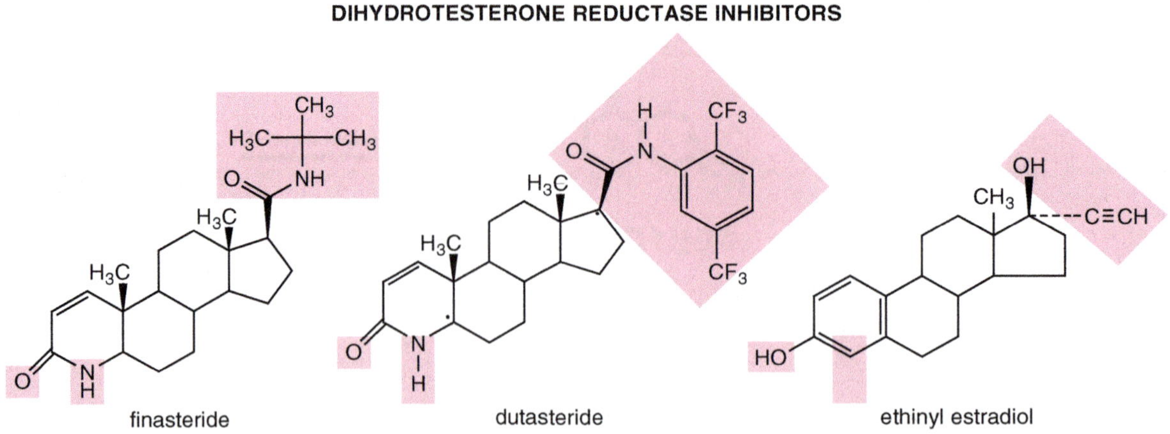

Fig. 10.11 Structures of Dihydrotestosterone Reductase inhibitors. The drugs have a common steroid core structure. Differences among the representatives of the class are highlighted in *pink*

Adverse Effects The most common adverse effects of dutasteride include impotence, a decrease in libido, ejaculation problems, enlarged or painful breasts.

Ethinyl estradiol (19-nor-17α-pregna-1,3,5(10)-trien-20-yne-3,17-diol) is a semi-synthetic estrogen that inhibits 5α-Reductase in epididymal tissue, which lowers testosterone levels and may delay the progression of prostate cancer. This agent also binds to the Estrogen Receptor complex and enters the nucleus, activating the transcription of genes involved in estrogenic cellular responses. In addition to its anti-neoplastic effects, ethinyl estradiol protects against osteoporosis. Short term therapy with this agent provides long term protection against breast cancer, mimicking the antitumor effects of pregnancy. The agent can be used in the treatment of prostate cancer.

The enlargement of the prostate gland is dependent on 5α-dihydrotestosterone (DHT), which is produced by 5α-Reductase type 2.
Dihydrotestosterone induces androgenic effects by binding to Androgen Receptors.
Dihydrotestosterone Reductase inhibition results in diminished stimulation of Androgen Receptors in the nuclei of prostate cells and consecutively diminished prostate cell proliferation.

10.2.4 Peptide Modulators

Gonadotropin Releasing Hormone (GnRH, Luteinizing Hormone Releasing Hormone, LHRH) modulators represent hormonal treatments for prostate cancer (Fig. 10.12). These agents are synthetic peptide derivatives of the natural decapeptide[8], which is produced by neurons in the hypothalamus. GnRH antagonists (drug names end on -relix) compete with Gonadotropin Releasing Hormone for binding to the GnRH Receptors in the pituitary gland. Thus, they block the release of the Gonadotropins Luteinizing Hormone (LH) and Follicle Stimulating Hormone (FSH) from the pituitary. The reduction in Luteinizing Hormone leads to a rapid and sustained suppression of testosterone release from the testes and subsequently reduces the growth of prostate cancer. Some GnRH peptide drugs may act as agonists (drug names end on -relin).

Adverse Effects GnRH agonists are associated with an increased risk of developing diabetes, myocardial infarction, sudden cardiac death, or stroke. Cases of spinal cord compression, which may contribute to weakness or paralysis with or without fatal complications, are possible under treatment with GnRH agonists.

GnRH antagonists do not cause a surge in testosterone or clinical flare.

The Gonadotropin Releasing Hormone antagonist abarelix(acetyl-D-β-naphthylalanyl-D-4-chlorophenylalanyl-D--3-pyridylalanyl-L-seryl-L-*N*-methyl-tyrosyl-D-asparagyl-L-leucyl-L-*N*(e)-isopropyl-lysyl-L-prolyl-D-alanyl-amide) <Plenaxis> is a synthetic decapeptide. It directly and competitively binds to and blocks the Gonadotropin Releasing Hormone Receptor in the anterior pituitary gland, thereby inhibiting the secretion and release of Luteinizing Hormone and Follicle Stimulating Hormone. In males, the inhibition of Luteinizing Hormone secretion prevents the release of testosterone. As a result, this may relieve symptoms associated with prostate hypertrophy or prostate cancer, since testosterone is required to sustain prostate growth. Abarelix is used for the palliative treatment of advanced symptomatic prostate cancer in patients in whom Gonadotropin Releasing

[8] The amino acid sequence of Gonadotropin Releasing-Hormone is pyroGlu-His-Trp-Ser-Tyr-Gly-Leu-Arg-Pro-Gly-NH_2. The starting amino acid pyroGlu (pyroglutamate) is a derivative of glutamic acid. The NH_2 at the carboxyl terminus indicates the protein terminates as a carboxamide.

PEPTIDE ANTI-ANDROGENS

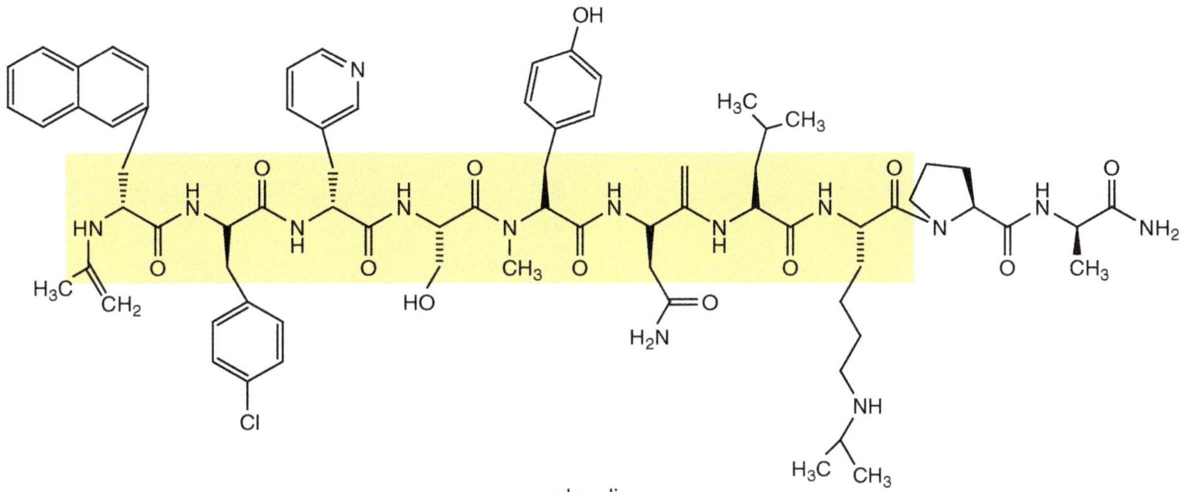

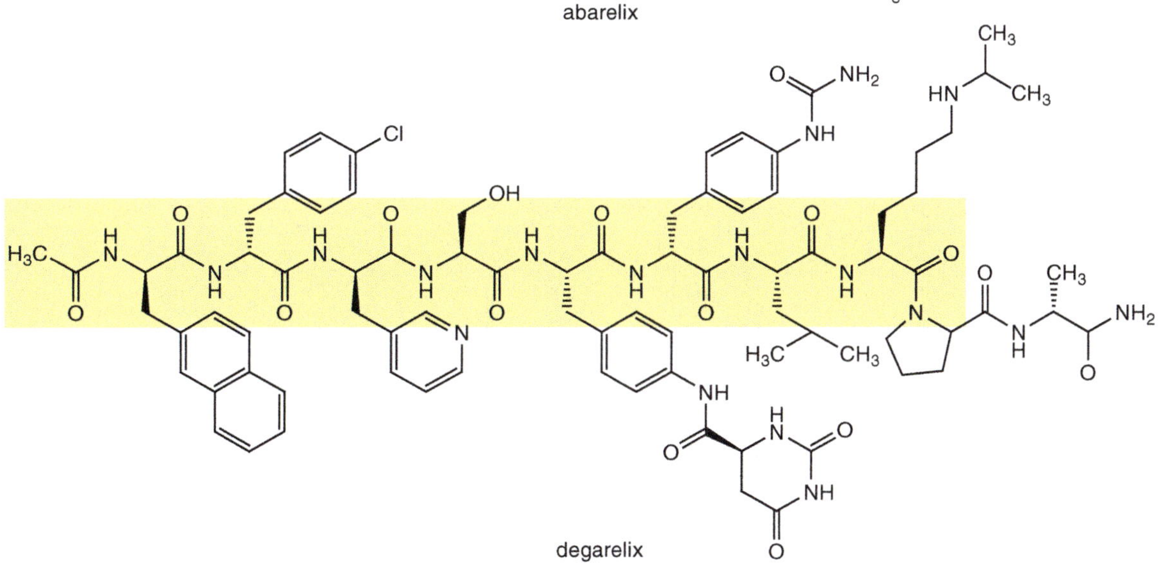

Fig. 10.12 Structures of peptide anti-androgens. The common peptide bond backbone is highlighted in *yellow*

Hormone agonist therapy is not appropriate and who do not undergo surgical castration, while having

- a risk of neurological compromise due to metastases
- or urinary outlet obstruction due to local encroachment or metastatic disease
- or severe bone pain from skeletal metastases persisting on narcotic analgesia.

A single dose contains 100 mg of free base peptide supplied in a carboxymethylcellulose complex that is administered intramuscularly in solution on days 1, 15, 29 and every 4 weeks thereafter.

Pharmacokinetics After intramuscular administration, the drug is absorbed slowly, reaching its peak blood concentration after 3 days. Over 95 % of the agent is bound to plasma proteins. Cytochrome P450 is not involved in the metabolism of abarelix. The major metabolites are formed via hydrolysis of the peptide bonds.

Adverse Effects Immediate onset systemic allergic reactions after administration, some resulting in hypotension and syncope, are an acute risk. The cumulative risk of such reactions increases with the duration of treatment. Adverse events associated with the drug may be caused by androgen deprivation, including hot flashes (80 %), sleep disturbance (45 %), pain (30 %), breast enlargement (30 %), and nipple tenderness (20 %). Other adverse effects can comprise back pain (15 %), peripheral edema (15 %), constipation (15 %), diarrhea (10 %), headache (10 %), fatigue (10 %), dizziness (10 %), nausea (10 %), upper respiratory tract infections (10 %), altered micturition frequency (10 %), urinary

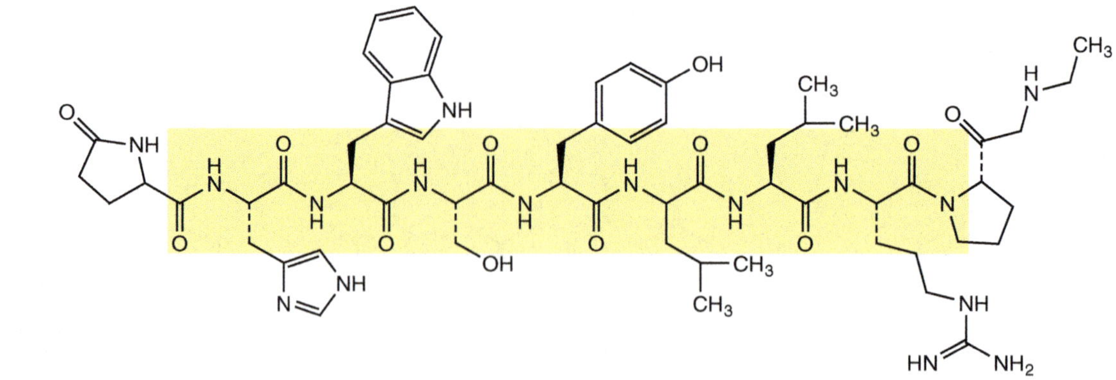

leuprorelin

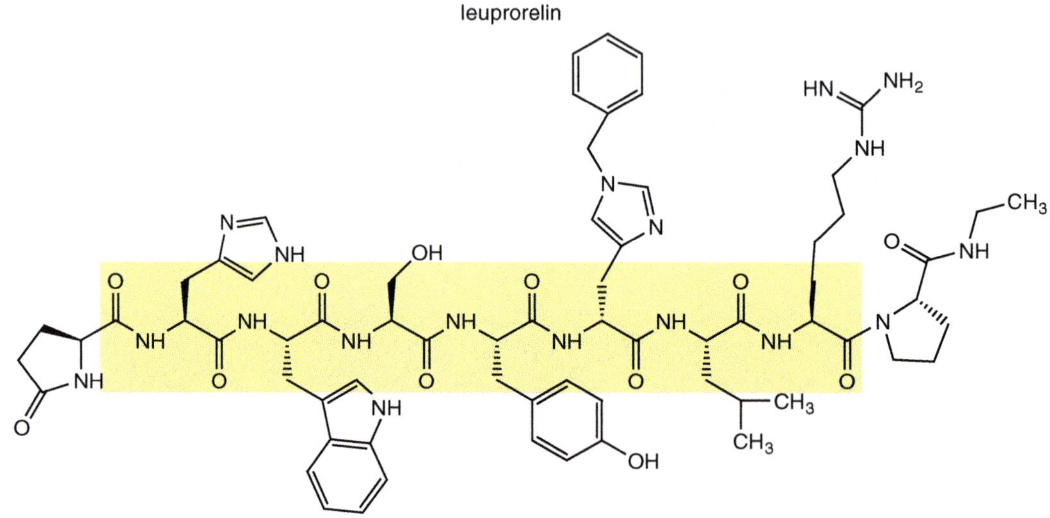

histrelin

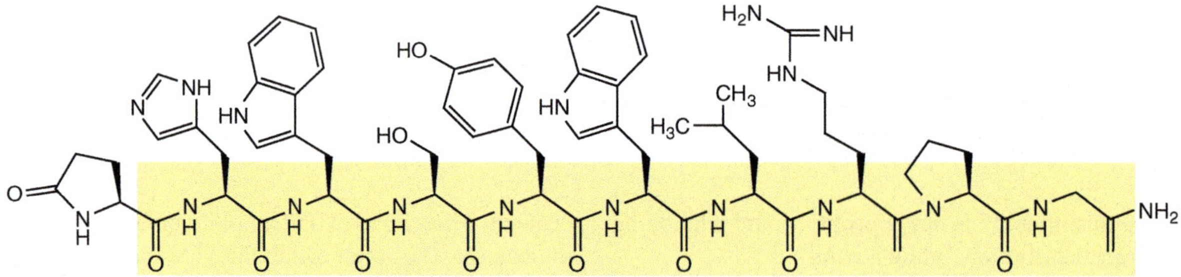

triptorelin

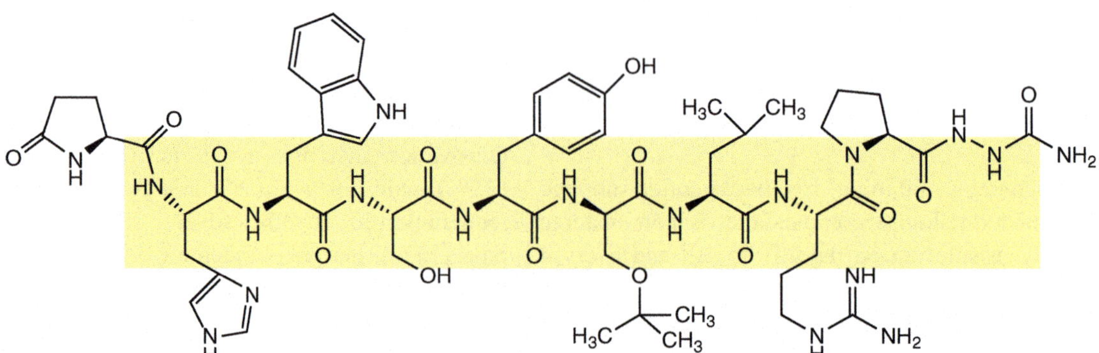

goserelin

Fig. 10.12 (continued)

tract infections (10 %), dysuria (10 %), and urinary retention (10 %). The agent is Pregnancy Category X.

Abarelix may prolong the QT interval of the heart beat. Therefore, careful consideration is in place when treating patients with baseline QTc values over 450 ms, and in patients who take Class IA or Class III anti-arrhythmic medications.

Drug Resistance The effectiveness of Abarelix decreases with continued dosing and is not established beyond 12 months. Therefore, treatment should be monitored according to total testosterone blood concentrations just prior to administration, on day 29, and every 8 weeks thereafter.

Degarelix (FE200486) <Firmagon> is a long acting synthetic peptide with Gonadotropin Releasing Hormone antagonistic properties. It targets and blocks Gonadotropin Releasing Hormone Receptors located on the surfaces of gonadotroph cells in the anterior pituitary, thereby reducing the secretion of Luteinizing Hormone by these cells and consecutively decreasing testosterone production by interstitial Leydig cells in the testes. The drug was approved in 2008 by the U.S. FDA and in 2009 by the European Commission. It is used for the treatment of patients with advanced hormone dependent prostate cancer.

Adverse Effects Adverse effects are commonly hormonal, including hot flashes and weight gain. Degarelix is also associated with mild or moderate injection site reactions such as pain, erythema or swelling.

Luprorelin (leuprolide acetate) <Lupron> is the acetate salt of a synthetic nonapeptide analog of Gonadotropin Releasing Hormone. Leuprolide binds to and activates Gonadotropin Releasing Hormone Receptors. Continuous, prolonged administration of leuprolide in males results in pituitary receptor desensitization and inhibition of pituitary secretion of Follicle Stimulating Hormone and Luteinizing Hormone, leading to a significant decline in testosterone production. In females, prolonged administration results in a decrease in estradiol production. Leuprolide may be used in the treatment of hormone responsive cancers such as prostate cancer or breast cancer, or of estrogen dependent conditions such as endometriosis or uterine fibroids. This agent reduces testosterone production to castration levels and may inhibit Androgen Receptor dependent tumor progression.

Adverse Effects Gonadotropin Releasing Hormone agonists may cause a surge in testosterone or clinical flare, usually manifested by an increase in bone pain. Rarely, a temporary worsening of existing hematuria and urinary tract obstruction can arise during the first week. Temporary weakness and paresthesia of the lower limbs is possible.

Histrelin acetate <Vantas> is a nonapeptide analog of Gonadotropin Releasing Hormone. Histrelin stimulates gonadotrope pituitary gland cells to release Luteinizing Hormone and Follicle Stimulating Hormone. Histrelin is used to treat hormone sensitive cancers of the prostate in men and uterine fibroids in women. It is available as a daily intramuscular injection or as a 12-month subcutaneous implant for the palliative treatment of advanced prostate cancer. The agent was approved by the U.S. FDA in 2005 and in the U.K. in 2010.

- <Vantas implant> is a sterile, non-biodegradable, diffusion controlled polymer reservoir containing histrelin acetate. It is designed to deliver approximately 50 micrograms histrelin acetate per day over 12 months.

Adverse Effects Gonadotropin Releasing Hormone analogs cause a transient increase in blood testosterone concentrations during the first week of treatment. Therefore, potential exacerbations of the disease during the first few weeks of treatment are of concern in patients with vertebral metastases or urinary obstruction or hematuria. If these conditions are aggravated, they may lead to neurological problems, including weakness or paresthesia of the lower limbs or worsening of urinary symptoms.

Acetate or pamoate salts of triptorelin <Decapeptyl, Diphereline, Gonapeptyl, Trelstar> act as analogs of Gonadotropin Releasing Hormone. By causing constant stimulation of the pituitary, triptorelin decreases the secretion of the Gonadotropins (Luteinizing Hormone and Follicle Stimulating Hormone). Like other Gonadotropin Releasing Hormone agonists, this drug may be used in the palliative treatment of advanced prostate cancer.

Pharmacokinetics Triptorelin has higher receptor affinity and is more active than native Gonadotropin Releasing Hormone in stimulating the release of Luteinizing Hormone from pituitary cells. Following the first administration, there is a transient surge in the circulating levels of Luteinizing Hormone, Follicle Stimulating Hormone, testosterone, and estradiol. After 2–4 weeks of continuous administration, a sustained decrease in Luteinizing Hormone and Follicle Stimulating Hormone secretion and marked reduction of testicular steroidogenesis arise. Consequently, functions that depend on these hormones become quiescent. These effects are usually reversible after cessation of the therapy.

Adverse Effects Common adverse effects include hot flashes, skeletal pain, peripheral edema, and impotence. Anaphylactic shock, hypersensitivity, and angioedema related to triptorelin administration are possible.

The decapeptide goserelin acetate <Zoladex> is an injectable Gonadotropin Releasing Hormone super-agonist. It is used to suppress the production of the sex hormones testosterone and estrogen, particularly in the treatment of breast and prostate cancer. The stimulation of non-pulsatile sex hormone secretion causes a disruption of the endogenous hormonal feedback systems, resulting in eventual down-regulation.

Pharmacokinetics Goserelin bioavailability is almost complete, reaching peak blood concentrations in about 2 h. The drug is poorly protein bound and has an elimination half-life of 2–4 h (which increases in patients with impaired renal function). Drug binding to the Gonadotropin Releasing Hormone Receptors in the pituitary gland leads to an initial increase in the incretion of Luteinizing Hormone (the initial flare may be treated by co-administration of bicalutamide). After a period of 14–21 days, Luteinizing Hormone is suppressed due to compensatory receptor down-regulation, and sex hormones are generally reduced.

Adverse Effects During the first few weeks of treatment, goserelin may cause a tumor flare effect, that manifests in a temporary increase in bone pain and worsening symptoms of prostate cancer. It is the result of an initial increase in Luteinizing Hormone production, before the receptors are desensitized and hormonal production is inhibited. This window can be counteracted by co-administration of anti-androgens during the first 2–3 weeks, particularly in patients with pre-existing bone symptoms.

Goserelin may cause bone pain, hot flashes, headache, upset stomach, weight gain, depression, swelling and tenderness of the breasts, decreased erections, and reduced libido. Memory loss can be severe and may not return to pre-treatment levels.

Synthetic peptide derivatives of Gonadotropin Releasing Hormone (GnRH) serve as agonists (-relin drugs) or antagonists (-relix drugs) for the hormonal treatment of prostate cancer.
Gonadotropin Releasing Hormone antagonists compete for binding to the Gonadotropin Releasing Hormone Receptors in the pituitary gland, thus blocking the release of Luteinizing Hormone and Follicle Stimulating Hormone, leading to a suppression of testosterone release from the testes.
Gonadotropin Releasing Hormone antagonists do not cause a surge in testosterone or clinical flare.
Gonadotropin Releasing Hormone agonists or super-agonists effect transient increases of Luteinizing Hormone, Follicle Stimulating Hormone, testosterone, and estradiol over the first weeks. Thereafter, a compensatory receptor down-regulation leads to suppressed Luteinizing Hormone levels.

10.2.5 Others

Estrogens may exert anti-androgenic effects. The masking of diethylstilbestrol by 2 phosphate groups has produced the transport form fosfestrol tetrasodium ([4-[4-(4-phosphonooxyphenyl)hex-3-en-3-yl] phenoxy]phosphonic acid, diethyldihydroxystilbene diphosphate) <Honvan>. From the prodrug[9], the active form is liberated selectively in prostate tissue. The drug is used for the treatment of metastatic prostate carcinoma.

Prednisone and hydrocortisone (see Sect. 10.3) lower serum testosterone and adrenal androgen levels, displaying modest efficacy in castration resistant prostate cancer. In addition, these agents reduce pain and raise the energy levels. Glucocorticosteroids are commonly administered adjunct to chemotherapy in castration resistant prostate cancer.

10.3 Corticosteroids

Steroids are lipid soluble. They diffuse freely through the cell membrane and into the cytoplasm of target cells. There, steroids bind to cognate nuclear receptors, which then dimerize and shuttle into the nucleus. Ligated, dimerized nuclear receptors form one functional DNA binding unit that can act as a transcription factor and induce the expression of target genes.

- Corticosteroid hormones can serve as anti-cancer agents because of their lymphotoxic effects. Their primary use is in the management of hematologic malignancies, especially Hodgkin and non-Hodgkin lymphomata, lymphocytic leukemias, and multiple myeloma.
- Corticosteroids have a potential role in the hormone therapy of prostate cancer as they can suppress the production of androgens by the adrenal glands.
- Corticosteroids have applications in the supportive care of cancer patients, such as reducing swelling and inflammation that cause cancer pain (predominantly used is dexamethasone).
- Corticosteroids can be used palliatively in the treatment of brain tumors. The reduction of swelling around the neoplasms may reduce headaches.
- Corticosteroids are commonly used together with ondansetron <Zofran> and aprepitant <Emend> to control and prevent nausea and vomiting caused by chemotherapy.

Pharmacokinetics In patients on corticosteroid therapy subjected to unusual stress, increased dosage of rapidly acting corticosteroids before, during, and after the stressful situation is indicated.

Adverse Effects Corticosteroids in chronic or high dose use can cause osteoporosis, cataract formation, high blood pressure, or the development of diabetes. They are generally well tolerated in the short term therapies that are commonly applied to cancer patient care.

To avoid withdrawal effects, the therapy with corticosteroids needs to be tapered, not stopped abruptly. Eliminating doses too quickly can result in

- adrenal crisis (a life threatening state caused by insufficient production of cortisol by the adrenal glands) or
- steroid withdrawal syndrome, which is the body's exaggerated response to removal of the drug (fever, muscle pain, joint pain) or
- rebound effect (exacerbation of prior disease symptoms).

[9] A prodrug (latent drug) is a chemically masked, inactive transport form that is converted by specific enzymes into the active form in its target cells or organs (Druckrey 1952).

Drug Interactions Corticosteroids are subject to multiple drug-drug interactions. Agents that can reduce the effectiveness of corticosteroids include anticonvulsants (such as carbamazepine, primidone, phenytoin), phenylbutazone (used to treat fever, pain, and inflammation), aminoglutethimide (administered in some tumor treatments), griseofulvin (used to treat skin infections), barbiturates (including phenobarbital), and mitotane (used to treat cancers that affect the adrenal cortex). Anti-diabetic agents or Insulin can increase blood glucose levels when taken with corticosteroids.

Taken together with corticosteroids, medicines containing potassium (used to treat high blood pressure) may interfere with the potassium levels in the blood. Diuretics may be less effective and may increase the loss of potassium. Amphotericin B by injection, used to treat fungal infections, can decrease the amount of potassium in the blood. The decreasing blood potassium levels can lead to an irregular heartbeat.

Dexamethasone <Dexamethasone Intensol, Decadron> is commonly used in the combination chemotherapy of some leukemias and lymphomata. The drug may reduce swelling (edema), especially for tumors in the brain, spinal cord, or bones. In patients with bone metastases, it may help lower the blood calcium levels.

Adverse Effects Dexamethasone, if given too rapidly intravenously, may cause temporary itching or burning in the vaginal or rectal area, which goes away after a few minutes. Adverse effects can include nausea, vomiting, stomach upset or ulcers (risk can be reduced by taking the pills with a full glass of fluid and a small snack), fluid retention that causes swelling of the hands and feet, increased appetite, heightened risk of infection, menstrual period changes, behavioral alterations (such as symptoms of paranoia or psychosis), muscle wasting (resulting in difficulty to climb stairs or rise from sitting to standing without assistance). Dexamethasone is contraindicated in patients with systemic fungal infections, and in patients with known hypersensitivity to the drug or its constituents.

Most therapeutic corticosteroids are synthetic derivatives of the physiologically most abundant glucocorticosteroid hydrocortisone (cortisol) <Cortef, Hydrocortone>. Hydrocortisone acts as a stress response hormone that regulates carbohydrate, fat, and protein metabolism by inhibiting cellular glucose uptake, elevating blood glucose, and increasing the levels gluconeogenic enzymes. Hydrocortisone also acts as immunosuppressive and anti-inflammatory through the inhibition of Phospholipase A_2 (PLA_2) and a resulting reduction in the release of arachidonic acid. Hydrocortisone is indicated for the palliative management of leukemias and lymphomata in adults and acute leukemias of childhood.

Adverse Effects Cushing disease is a malfunction of the adrenal glands resulting in an over-production of cortisol. The same symptoms may be induced by therapeutic hydrocortisone. They comprise increased appetite and weight gain (deposits of fat in chest, face, upper back), water and salt retention leading to swelling, edema, high blood pressure, diabetes, delayed wound healing, osteoporosis, cataracts, muscle weakness, thinning of the skin, acne, increased susceptibility to infection, stomach ulcers, mood swings, and depression. Glucocorticosteroids inhibit vitamin D mediated intestinal calcium uptake, retard the rate of wound healing, and interfere with the rate of growth.

The synthetic glucocorticosteroid prednisone <Deltasone, Prednisone Intensol> is used in combination chemotherapy for leukemias and lymphomata, where it is anti-proliferative. Prednisone may reduce the nausea and vomiting induced by other anti-cancer drugs. It may help lower blood calcium levels in people with primary or metastatic bone cancers. Prednisone is flexible in the route of administration (oral, intramuscular, or intravenous).

Pharmacokinetics Prednisone is a prodrug that is converted to the active form prednisolone by the liver.

Adverse Effects Adrenocortical insufficiency can arise after an interruption of daily steroids or with concurrent infection or stress. Caution is advised if prednisone is stopped or withdrawn or if the patient experiences unusual stress. Increased dosages of corticosteroids may be used before, during and after stressful situations.

Prednisolone <Delta-Cortef, Orapred, Pediapred, Prelone, Solone> is a corticosteroid drug with predominantly glucocorticosteroid and low mineralocorticosteroid activity. It is used as a treatment for a variety of cancers, including leukemia, lymphoma, and multiple myeloma. Prednisolone may be administered to treat nausea and vomiting associated with some chemotherapy drugs. It can also stimulate appetite in cancer patients with severe appetite problems. Prednisolone is taken orally with food or after meals. The generally recommended dosages are 10–100 mg daily in divided doses for adults, 2.5–10 mg twice a day for children up to 5 years, and 5–20 mg twice a day for children 6–12 years.

Adverse Effects Adverse effects include Cushing syndrome[10] with fluid retention of the face (dubbed "moon face"), acne, constipation, and mood swings. Other effects include insomnia, decreased or blurred vision, increased eye pressure, increased thirst, and confusion.

Methylprednisolone as the free form, acetate, or sodium acetate <Medrol, Depo-Medrol, Hybrisil> is used for the

[10] Cushing syndrome describes the symptoms associated with prolonged exposure to inappropriately high levels of the hormone cortisol.

palliative management of leukemias and lymphomata in adults, and acute leukemia of childhood. The drug has anti-inflammatory effects.

- A sodium succinate form of methylprednisolone <Solu-Medrol, A-Methapred> is used for injection.

Adverse Effects Adverse effects of methylprednisolone depend on the dose and duration of administration. Short courses are usually well tolerated with few, mild adverse effects. Long term, high doses may produce potentially serious side effects. Whenever possible, the lowest effective doses of methylprednisolone should be used for the shortest length of time to minimize adverse effects. Alternate day dosing also can help to reduce toxicity.

Drug Interactions Methylprednisolone may increase the clearance of chronic high dose salicylate <Aspirin>. This could lead to decreased salicylate blood levels or increase the risk of salicylate toxicity when methylprednisolone is withdrawn. Salicylate should be used cautiously in conjunction with corticosteroids in patients suffering from hypoprothrombinemia. Mutual inhibition of metabolism occurs with the concurrent use of cyclosporin and methylprednisolone, which may manifest in convulsions. Drugs that induce hepatic enzymes such as phenobarbital, phenytoin and rifampin may increase the clearance of corticosteroids and may require increases in methylprednisolone dose to achieve the desired response. Troleandomycin and ketoconazole affect Cytochrome P450 and may inhibit the metabolism of methylprednisolone, thus decreasing its clearance. Estrogens, including birth control pills, can increase the effects of corticosteroids by 50 %. Higher doses of diabetes medications may be required because corticosteroids increase blood glucose.

Mineralocorticosteroids maintain the blood volume. They control the excretion of electrolytes (sodium reabsorption in kidneys, colon, sweat glands), the retention of chloride and water (expansion of extracellular volume), and the excretion of potassium and hydrogen ions from kidneys. The mineralocorticoid analog spironolactone <Aldactone, Spirotone> has partial Androgen Receptor agonist activity. It induces a limited response and is not suitable as a first-line therapy of prostate cancer.

The primary use of corticosteroids is in the management of hematologic malignancies.
Corticosteroids have applications in the supportive care of cancer patients, such as reducing swelling, inflammation, nausea and vomiting.
Corticosteroids in chronic or high dose use can cause osteoporosis, cataract formation, high blood pressure, or the development of diabetes.
To avoid withdrawal effects, corticosteroid therapy needs to be tapered, not stopped abruptly.

Treatment of Prostatic Neoplasms

1. Prostate Carcinoma

The majority of prostate cancers are diagnosed as low risk, clinically localized disease. The treatment of these cancers is associated with substantial morbidity and needs to be weighed against the prognosis. Treatment choices include active surveillance, brachytherapy (internal radiotherapy, sealed source radiotherapy, endocurietherapy), intensity-modulated radiation therapy, and radical prostatectomy. In addition, chemotherapy options can be considered.

Androgen ablation Because prostate cancer typically originates from excessive androgen sensitivity, the first-line therapy is androgen ablation. Hormonal treatments for advanced, hormone dependent prostate cancer include

- the LHRH analogs (antagonists of Luteinizing Hormone Releasing Hormone) include goserelin <Zoladex>, triptorelin <Trelstar>, histrelin <Vantas>, leuprolide subcutaneous injection or intramuscular depot <Lupron>, leuprolide subcutaneous depot <Eligard>, leuprolide subcutaneous implant <Viadur>. When LHRH analogs are first given, the testosterone levels transiently increase before falling to very low levels. The flare results from the mechanism of action of this class of drugs. During this initial phase, patients with bone metastases may experience bone pain
- LHRH antagonists reduce the testosterone levels more quickly than LHRH analogs and do not cause tumor flare like the LHRH agonists do. Degarelix <Firmagon> is given as a monthly subcutaneous injection
- anti-androgens, such as flutamide <Eulexin>, bicalutamide <Casodex>, and nilutamide <Nilandron>, are taken daily as tablets. Enzalutamide <Xtandi> is a newer type of anti-androgen that suppresses the androgenic signal from the Androgen Receptor to the cell nucleus
- abiraterone acetate <Zytigia> is an inhibitor of androgen biosynthesis that works by blocking cytochrome P450 17A1 (CYPC17A1). It is indicated in combination with prednisone for the treatment of patients with metastatic castration resistant prostate cancer, who have received prior chemotherapy containing docetaxel
- the anti-fungal ketoconazole <Nizoral> blocks the production of androgens and thus rapidly lowers the testosterone levels. It is most often used upon diagnosis of advanced stage prostate cancer. It can also be tried if other forms of hormone therapy are

no longer effective. As ketoconazole can block the production of cortisol, it should be taken together with hydrocortisone to compensate for the low endogenous corticosteroid levels

- the female sex hormones, estrogens, have been largely replaced in prostate cancer therapy due to their adverse effects, including blood clots and gynecomastia (breast enlargement). These agents may be tried in cases where androgen deprivation is no longer working.

Adverse Effects Gynecomastia, hot flashes, and impotence are estrogenic effects that are commonly associated with androgen ablation. In addition, osteoporosis, anemia, loss of muscle mass, weight gain, and fatigue may arise.

Chemotherapy Chemotherapy for prostate cancer utilizes alkylating agents, anti-mitotic drugs, and corticosteroids.

Estramustine phosphate sodium <Emcyt> is the orally available monohydrate disodium salt of estramustine phosphate, a synthetic molecule that combines estradiol and nornitrogen mustard through a carbamate link. This agent exhibits anti-androgenic effects and is used for the palliative treatment of metastatic or progressive prostate cancer. It was designed with the intent that the estradiol portion of the molecule would facilitate uptake of the alkylating agent into hormone sensitive prostate cancer cells.

Adverse Effects There is an increased risk of thrombosis, including fatal myocardial infarction, in men receiving estrogens for prostatic cancer.

Docetaxel <Taxotere> is a standard treatment for hormone refractory (castration resistant) metastatic prostate cancer. The recommended dose is 75 mg/m^2 every 3 weeks as a 1 h intravenous infusion.

Mitoxantrone, a microtubule inhibitor, has not shown a survival benefit compared to docetaxel-based chemotherapy regimens in metastatic, castration-resistant prostate cancer. However, it is used in combination with prednisone.

Prednisone 5 mg orally twice daily is administered continuously. Improved pain control can be achieved in patients with hormone-resistant prostate cancer treated with mitoxantrone plus prednisone compared with those treated with prednisone alone.

Treatment of metastases Osteoblastic bone metastases are common in prostate cancer patients, in particular in hormone refractory cancer.

- Bisphosphonates act primarily by reducing the activity of osteoclasts. When cancer has spread to the bones, the inclusion of bisphosphonate drugs in the anti-cancer treatment can reduce pain, fractures and other bone problems. Zolendronate prevents skeletal-related events, including pathologic fractures and spinal cord compression.
- Denosumabmay prevent skeletal-related events in prostate cancer with bone metastases. The antibody neutralizes RANKL (RANK Ligand), a protein that acts as the primary signal for bone removal. As prostate cancer metastases are typically osteogenic, denusomab is approved as a prophylaxis to increase bone mass in non-metastatic prostate cancer.
- Endothelin-1 is integrally involved in the progression of prostate cancer. Tumor produced Endothelin-1 stimulates new bone formation in osteoblastic metastases via engagement of the Endothelin A Receptor. Zibotentan (ZD4054) is an orally available selective antagonist of the Endothelin A Receptor (the names of Endothelin Receptor antagonists end on -entan). It binds selectively to the Endothelin Receptor, thereby inhibiting Endothelin mediated mechanisms that promote tumor cell proliferation. Nebentan (YM598) is an orally active synthetic substituted phenylethenesulfonamide. As a selective Endothelin A Receptor antagonist, nebentan inhibits Endothelin mediated mechanisms involved in tumor cell growth and progression, angiogenesis, and metastasis.

Immunotherapy Sipuleucel-T, an active cellular immunotherapy, can increase overall survival in patients with hormone-refractory metastatic prostate cancer. The treatment consists of autologous peripheral blood mononuclear cells that have been exposed ex vivo to a recombinant fusion protein (PA2024) composed of Prostatic Acid Phosphatase fused to Granulocyte-Macrophage Colony-Stimulating Factor. These patient specific, activated cells are re-infused.

Chemoprevention Patients with a modest elevation of Prostate Specific Antigen (PSA) (below 4.0 ng/mL) have a risk of prostate cancer that is reduced by finasteride, however, many of these cases may represent clinically inconsequential tumors[11]. Therefore, the effectiveness of finasteride in preventing prostate cancer (including cancers with Gleason scores

[11] Lower cutoff levels for treatment increase the detection of insignificant disease, but the cure rates are comparatively high, whereas higher cutoff levels make the detection of significant cancer more likely, but cure is less likely.

below 7) with meaningful rates of significant disease suggests that cutoff values for PSA screening should be individualized. Men undergoing screening should be informed of the opportunity to reduce their risk of disease with finasteride (Lucia 2007).

Digoxin is a cardiac glycoside. Long term treatment with digoxin is associated with a 25% lower prostate cancer risk. The protection is increased with increasing length of treatment. The mechanism of action is unknown. While the observed association is clinically relevant, the use of digoxin for chemoprevention in non-cardiac patients is prohibitive due to its risks.

2. Benign Prostate Hyperplasia

Benign prostate hyperplasia (BPH) is a common benign growth in aging men and is the most frequent cause of urinary flow obstruction at the bladder neck. Benign prostate hyperplasia displays androgen dependency, stromal-epithelial interaction, and a role for estrogens. Treatments include surgical procedures, minimally invasive procedures, and pharmacotherapy. Commonly, the first line of therapy is the use of

- α blockers, which work through adrenergic pathways. The use of these agents may lead to orthostatic hypotension, or affect bone metabolism and result in an increased risk of hip fracture.
- 5α-Reductase inhibitors, which work through hormonal mechanisms. 5α-Reductase catalyzes the conversion of testosterone to dihydrotestosterone and has broad biological effects. Adverse effects of the use of 5α-Reductase inhibitors, such as the type II enzyme inhibitor finasteride <Proscar, Propecia, Fincar, Finpecia, Finax, Finast, Finara, Finalo, Prosteride, Gefina, Appecia, Finasterid IVAX, Finasterid Alternova>, may include erectile dysfunction, decreased ejaculate volume, breast pain, and gynecomastia (Jacobsen 2008).

Treatment of Breast Cancer

Surgery alone can cure most patients with in situ cancers, 70–80% of patients with stage I, and about half of all patients with stage II cancers. While adjuvant endocrine therapy reduces the rates of relapse and death in patients with hormone receptor-positive early breast tumors, adjuvant chemotherapy reduces the rates of relapse and death in all patients with early stage breast tumors. Neoadjuvant chemotherapy, followed by local therapy and further adjuvant systemic therapy, is appropriate for patients with locally advanced or inflammatory breast cancer.

Most chemotherapy regimens combine multiple agents simultaneously. The benefit of sequential combination chemotherapy (treatment with a second agent after disease progression following treatment with a first agent) is subject to debate. Sequential single-agent therapy may be considered the treatment of choice, except when patients have life-threatening symptoms (Bernard-Marty et al. 2004).

Pharmacogenetics in breast cancer Uncontrolled growth of breast cancer cells may be caused by excess activity of estrogen pathways, WNT pathways, or EGF Receptor family pathways. The genetic makeup of the disease determines the appropriate pharmacotherapy.

- Breast cancers with uncontrolled EGF Receptor pathways may over-express ERBB2 (HER-2/NEU). This affects about 30% of breast cancer patients. The antibody trastuzumab <Herceptin> binds to ERBB2 and blocks its activity. It is highly effective in the treatment of breast cancers that over-express ERBB2, but it is ineffective in the treatment of breast cancers based on other mechanisms. Viable alternatives for this group of tumors are lapatinib and pertuzumab.
- The initial treatment of metastatic breast cancer in women with hormone receptor-positive tumors should consist of hormonal therapy. Women with metastatic breast cancer who have hormone receptor-positive tumors and respond to an initial hormonal manipulation will usually respond to a second hormonal manipulation. Anti-estrogens are most effective against breast cancers with deregulated estrogen pathways. They include selective Estrogen Receptor modulators (SERMs), progesterone derivatives, and Aromatase and Sulfatase inhibitors.

Estrogen sensitive breast cancer Hormone receptors are also transcription factors, which upon ligand binding travel to the nucleus and activate gene expression that results in cell growth and proliferation. The hormone receptors clinically useful in breast cancer treatment include the Estrogen Receptor (ER) and the Progesterone Receptor (PR). The presence of the Progesterone Receptor protein is important for the functional effects of the Estrogen Receptor protein to occur. Patients with Estrogen Receptor-negative and Progesterone Receptor-negative tumors rarely respond to hormonal manipulation.

The Estrogen Receptor antagonist Fulvestrant <Faslodex> is used for hormone receptor-positive metastatic breast cancer in post-menopausal women with disease progression following anti-estrogen therapy. Devoid of agonist effects, the drug works by down-regulating the estrogen receptor. The agent is administered as monthly injection.

Selective Estrogen Receptor modulators (SERMs) are taken daily as tablets. They can be used to treat women before and after menopause. For pre-menopausal women diagnosed with hormone receptor-positive breast cancer, the selective Estrogen Receptor modulator and tamoxifen is the hormonal therapy treatment standard.

In 1971, tamoxifen was approved by the U.S. FDA for the treatment of late stage breast cancer. In 1980, it was shown that tamoxifen plus chemotherapy could improve survival rates. It is important to always determine the hormone receptor status of a breast cancer, because tamoxifen treatment for 5 years may be considered in some women with ductal carcinoma in situ (DCIS) to reduce the risk for recurrence.

Indications for the use of Aromatase inhibitors include:

- Anastrozole <Arimidex> is approved by the U.S. FDA for post-menopausal women with early-stage disease right after surgery.
- Exemestane <Aromasin> is approved by the U.S. FDA for women with early-stage disease who have completed 2–3 years of tamoxifen.
- Letrozole <Femara> is approved by the U.S. FDA for women with early-stage disease right after surgery and for women with early-stage disease who have completed 5 years of tamoxifen.
- All 3 Aromatase inhibitors are also approved for women with advanced (metastatic) disease.

For treating early-stage, hormone receptor-positive breast cancer in post-menopausal women, there is a choice between selective Estrogen Receptor modulators and Aromatase inhibitors.

- An Aromatase inhibitor is considered the best type of hormonal therapy to start with for post-menopausal women. When treating early-stage, hormone receptor-positive breast cancer, Aromatase inhibitors have more benefits and fewer serious adverse effects than tamoxifen.
- Switching to an Aromatase inhibitor after taking tamoxifen for 2–3 years (for a total of 5 years of hormonal therapy) offers more benefits than 5 years of tamoxifen. Taking an Aromatase inhibitor for 5 years after taking tamoxifen for 5 years continues to reduce the risk of cancer recurrence, compared to no treatment after tamoxifen.

Endocrine resistant breast cancer For de novo endocrine resistant (negative for Estrogen Receptor and Progesterone Receptor) metastatic breast cancer, chemotherapy is the most appropriate first-line treatment option. Increasingly patients receive the most active agents, anthracyclines and taxanes, in the adjuvant setting. This has increased the number of metastatic breast cancer patients, who may be resistant to these agents when they relapse with metastatic disease. Some patients may have acquired resistance to the most effective agents because of exposure to systemic adjuvant therapy at the non-metastatic stage.

Anthracyclines (doxorubicin <Adriamycin>, epirubicin <Ellence>) are the most active single agents in the treatment of breast cancer. The primary therapeutic target molecule of anthracyclines is Topoisomerase 2α, and efficacy is particularly high in cancers with over-expression of this protein. However, only 1/3 of patients with ERBB2-positive mammary carcinoma (and none with ERBB2-negative breast cancers) have co-amplified Topoisomerase 2α Therefore, only 8% of all breast cancers contain the makeup to respond to anthracyclines, however their responses are typically very strong. Nearly all patients on anthracyclines eventually progress, while some may experience unacceptable toxicity after an initial period of response.

- TAC treatment for breast cancer involves docetaxel <Taxotere>, doxorubicin <Adriamycin>, and cyclophosphamide <Cytoxan>. On the first day of treatment, all 3 drugs are given by infusion or injections. After this, there is a rest period with no chemotherapy for the next 3 weeks. This completes a cycle of treatment. Usually, 4–6 cycles of treatment are given over 3–4 months to complete a course of treatment.
- CAF includes cyclophosphamide, doxorubicin <Adriamycin>, and 5-fluorouracil. A cycle comprises an injection of doxorubicin alongside a drip of saline, cyclophosphamide by infusion or as an injection alongside a drip of saline, followed by an injection of 5-fluorouracil on day 1. This is followed by a rest period of 3 weeks (schedule A). Alternatively, injections of 5-fluorouracil and doxorubicin are given on day 1, and 14 days of treatment with cyclophosphamide tablets are initiated. After 7 days, doxorubicin and 5-fluorouracil are administered again. From days 15 through 28, there is a rest period to complete the cycle (schedule B).
- The CEF-120 regimen comprises oral cyclophosphamide 75 mg/m^2 on days 1–14, intravenous epirubicin 60 mg/m^2 on days 1 and 8, intravenous

5-fluorouracil 500 mg/m^2 on days 1 and 8, repeated every 28 days for 6 cycles.
- The FEC-100 regimen contains 5-fluorouracil 500 mg/m^2, epirubicin 100 mg/m^2, cyclophosphamide 500 mg/m^2, all drugs administered intravenously on day 1 and repeated every 21 days for 6 cycles.

Supportive treatment with dexrazoxane <Zinecard> is indicated for reducing the incidence and severity of the cardiomyopathy associated with doxorubicin administration in women with metastatic breast cancer who have received a cumulative doxorubicin dose of 300 mg/m^2 and who continue to receive doxorubicin therapy to maintain tumor control.

Drug Resistance Because the anthracyclines are among the more effective chemotherapeutic agents in metastatic breast cancer they are often used in first line treatment. In many patients, intrinsic or acquired drug resistance is a reason for treatment failure. In addition, the increasing use of anthracyclines for adjuvant treatment has led to a concomitant increase in the number of patients with resistant or refractory disease in the metastatic setting. An approved therapy for this population is capecitabine. Epothilones have low susceptibility to classic tumor drug resistance mechanisms. The epothilone ixabepilone has efficacy as a single agent and in combination with capecitabine in the treatment of metastatic breast cancer in patients with multi-drug resistant tumors. Ixabepilone may act synergistically with capecitabine, and this combination is indicated for patients with metastatic or locally advanced breast cancer after the failure of anthracycline. The toxicity profiles of ixabepilone and capecitabine do not overlap. Although the incidence of grade 3/4 toxicities (peripheral neuropathy, arthralgia, and neutropenia) is elevated, the combination regimen is generally well tolerated. Another drug for second-line treatment is vinorelbine.

The taxanes are among the more effective chemotherapeutic agents in estrogen sensitive and estrogen resistant metastatic breast cancer and are often used as first line therapeutics. Many patients have tumors that fail to respond to these agents, and nearly all will eventually progress, while some may experience unacceptable toxicity after an initial period of response.

Drug Resistance 30% of patients who take taxanes do not respond or become resistant. Resistance is associated with abnormally high expression of the micro-RNAs miR-221 and miR-222. These micro-RNAs down-regulate the levels of P27^{KIP1} in the cancer cells.

The microtubule stabilizer ixabepilone may act synergistically with capecitabine, and this combination is indicated for patients with metastatic or locally advanced breast cancer after the failure of taxane.

The MMM combination of mitomycin C, mitoxantrone, and methotrexate produced good response rates in advanced breast cancer (Hortobagyi 1993). However, this regimen has received only limited use because of its high toxicity.

Radiation and systemic chemotherapy have no role in the management of lobular carcinoma in situ (LCIS). The use of chemoprevention in pre-menopausal women with tamoxifen, or in postmenopausal women with tamoxifen or raloxifene can be considered as a risk reduction option.

HER-2 positive breast cancers The ERBB2 (HER-2/NEU) protein is physiologically expressed at low levels in the epithelial cells of healthy breast tissue. The receptor is a member of the Epidermal Growth Factor Receptor family. ERBB2 over-expression occurs in approximately 20–30% of breast cancers, and is associated with the transmission of growth signals that support aspects of cell division. ERBB2 is linked to increased tumor aggressiveness, increased rates of recurrence, and increased mortality. ERBB2 positive status predicts responsiveness to trastuzumab <Herceptin> therapy, which is a monoclonal antibody directed to the receptor ERBB2.

Adding trastuzumab to standard chemotherapy leads to an increase in the time to progression, a higher rate of objective responses, a longer median duration of response, and improved survival. The most important adverse event associated with the combination of anthracyclines and trastuzumab is cardiac dysfunction. Hence, this combination chemotherapy is no longer recommended. By contrast, the combination of taxanes with trastuzumab may have a synergistic effect. Trastuzumab combined with paclitaxel is U.S. FDA approved as a first line therapy for ERBB2 over-expressing metastatic breast cancer patients, who have not yet received chemotherapy.

Pertuzumab is a humanized monoclonal IgG1 antibody designed to target ERBB2 at the extracellular domain II. The agent is given in combination with trastuzumab (which binds a different domain of the receptor) and docetaxel.

The small molecule lapatinib acts as a reversible kinase inhibitor for ERBB1, ERBB2, ERK-1, ERK-2, and PKB. The drug is predominantly used with capecitabine in patients afflicted by advanced ERBB2-positive breast cancer with trastuzumab resistance. It is also approved with letrozole for the treatment of postmenopausal women with hormone receptor-positive metastatic breast cancer that over-expresses the ERBB2 receptor and for whom hormonal therapy is indicated.

Treatment of metastases Once metastases are present, breast cancer patients need to expect a compromised life expectancy. Some patients may have acquired resistance to the most effective agents because of prior exposure to systemic adjuvant therapy. A large fraction of relapsing metastatic breast cancer patients has received anthracyclines and taxanes as first line treatment and is resistant to these drugs. The cumulative risk of anthracycline cardiotoxicity is also a limiting factor (after adjuvant chemotherapy, patients typically have been exposed to 240–300 mg/m^2 of doxorubicin). Therefore, many standard combination chemotherapy approaches use 2 non-anthracycline cytotoxic agents.

Drug Resistance About 40 % of breast cancers express the efflux transporter ABCB1 (Pgp, MDR1). ABCB1 expression increases after therapy and is associated with a greater likelihood of treatment failure.

When breast cancer has spread to the bones, bisphosphonate drugs added to the anti-cancer treatment can reduce pain, fractures and other bone problems. In advanced breast cancer and clinically evident bone metastases, bisphosphonates reduce the risk of developing a skeletal event by about 15 %. However, treatment with bisphosphonates does not appear to affect survival in women with advanced breast cancer.

Treatment regimens approved by the U.S. FDA for metastatic breast cancer may include a targeted therapeutic with a conventional chemotherapy agent. Lapatinib is a dual kinase inhibitor that blocks signaling through ERBB2 and the ERBB1 (EGF Receptor). It is indicated in combination with capecitabine in advanced or metastatic ERBB2 over-expressing breast cancer, following treatment with other agents, including taxanes, anthracyclines, and trastuzumab.

Many standard combination chemotherapy approaches for metastatic breast cancer use 2 non-anthracycline cytotoxic agents, such as an alkylating agent, an anti-metabolite, or a vinca alkaloid. Ixabepilone, nano-particle albumin-bound paclitaxel (nab-paclitaxel), trastuzumab, lapatinib, and bevacizumab have all been approved by the U.S. FDA for use as part of combination regimens for defined sub-groups of patients with metastatic breast cancer. Paclitaxel may be administered as a monotherapy. Advanced breast cancer therapy favors weekly paclitaxel administration over administration every 3 weeks.

Treatment of adverse effects 20–30 % of breast cancer patients under chemotherapy are afflicted by memory and attention problems. The symptoms are sometimes referred to as chemo-brain (chemo-fog). However, the relative contributions to this condition by the chemotherapeutic agents, genetic factors, and the underlying disease are subject to discussion. Often, the symptoms improve after the completion of chemotherapy. Memory and adaptation training (MAAT) may aid in cognitive rehabilitation.

Relatively small metastases to the pleura can cause large effusions. Topical infusion of quinacrine <Atebrine> has been used in experimental protocols to provide symptomatic control[11]. Its interstitial injection stimulates the migration of leukocytes and local accumulation of various lymphokines, and the reaction is followed by cicatricial fibrosis.

Lymph edema is a frequent complication in breast cancer survivors, despite lymphatic-sparing procedures such as sentinel biopsy. Lymphedema causes swelling and discomfort leading to impaired arm function. No effective drug treatments are available.

Risk mitigation Daily intake of non-steroidal anti-inflammatory drugs may protect from breast cancer and aid in the treatment of women already diagnosed with breast cancer. Potential serious adverse effects may include gastrointestinal bleeding, gastrointestinal perforation, and heart disease (Agrawal and Fentiman 2008). According to a 2006 alert from European regulatory agencies, high doses of non-steroidal anti-inflammatory drugs are associated with a small increased risk of heart attacks or strokes when taken over a long period of time. So, the risk of the treatment needs to be weighed against the risk to develop cancer.

Prophylaxis with the selective estrogen receptor modulator (SERM) tamoxifen reduces the risk of hormone-sensitive breast cancers in women at high cancer risk. There is no benefit from tamoxifen in preventing hormone resistant breast cancers. Raloxifene is as effective as tamoxifen in reducing breast cancer risk in postmenopausal women. Both drugs reduce the risk of

[11] Quinacrine is in use as an anti-malaria drug.

developing invasive breast cancer by about 50 percent (Vogel 2009).

In 2002, a clinical trial of hormone replacement therapy for postmenopausal women was stopped early when it turned out that women who took hormones had an increased risk of developing breast cancer (Rossouw et al. 2002). Since then, the use of hormone replacement therapy has been limited.

References

Agrawal A, Fentiman IS (2008) NSAIDs and breast cancer: a possible prevention and treatment strategy. Int J Clin Pract 62:444–449

Allen E, Doisy EA (1923) An ovarian hormone: preliminary report on its localization, extraction and partial purification and action in test animals. J Am Med Assoc 81:819–821

Beatson GT (1896) On the treatment of inoperable cases of carcinoma of the mamma: suggestions for a new method of treatment with illustrative cases. Lancet 2:104–107

Bernard-Marty C, Cardoso F, Piccart MJ (2004) Facts and controversies in systemic treatment of metastatic breast cancer. Oncologist 9:617–632

Chang CS, Kokontis J, Liao ST (1988) Molecular cloning of human and rat complementary DNA encoding androgen receptors. Science 240:324–326

Dodds EC, Golberg L, Lawson W (1938) Oestrogenic activity of esters of diethylstilboestrol. Nature 142:211–212

Druckrey H (1952) Experimentelle Grundlagen der Chemotherapie des Krebses. Deutsche Medizinische Wochenschrift 77:1534–1537

Herbst AL, Ulfelder H, Poskanzer DC (1971) Adenocarcinoma of the vagina. Association of maternal stilbestrol therapy with tumor appearance in young women. N Engl J Med 284:878–881

Hortobagyi, GN. (1993) Mitomycin: its evolving role in the treatment of breast cancer. Oncology (Basel) 50(Suppl 1):1–8

Huggins C, Hodges CV (1941) Studies on prostatic cancer, I: the effect of estrogen and of androgen injection on serum phosphatases in metastatic carcinoma of the prostate. Cancer Res 1:293–297

Jacobsen SJ, Cheetham TC, Haque R, Shi JH, Loo RK (2008) Association between 5-a reductase inhibition and risk of hip fracture. J Am Med Assoc 300:1660–1664

Jensen EV, Jacobson HI (1962) Basic guides to the mechanism of estrogen action. Recent Prog Horm Res 18:387–414

Lerner LJ, Holthaus JF, Thompson CR (1958) A nonsteroidal estrogen antagonist 1-(p-2 diethylaminoethoxyphenyl)-1-phenyl-2-p-methoxyphenyl-ethanol. Endocrinology 63:295–318

Lucia MS, Epstein JI, Goodman PJ, Darke AK, Reuter VE, Civantos F, Tangen CM, Parnes HL, Lippman SM, La Rosa FG, Kattan MW, Crawford ED, Ford LG, Coltman CA Jr, Thompson IM (2007) Finasteride and high-grade prostate cancer in the prostate cancer prevention trial. J Nat Cancer Inst 99:1375–1383

Michalides R, Griekspoor A, Balkenende A, Verwoerd D, Janssen L, Jalink K, Floore A, Velds A, van't Veer L, Neefjes J. (2004) Tamoxifen resistance by a conformational arrest of the estrogen receptor α after PKA activation in breast cancer. Cancer Cell 5:597–605

Rossouw JE, Anderson GL, Prentice RL, LaCroix AZ, Kooperberg C, Stefanick ML, Jackson RD, Beresford SA, Howard BV, Johnson KC, Kotchen JM, Ockene J (2002) Writing Group for the Women's Health Initiative, Investigators. Risks and benefits of estrogen plus progestin in healthy postmenopausal women: principal results From the Women's Health Initiative randomized controlled trial. J Am Med Assoc 288:321–333

Tolis G, Ackman D, Stellos A, Mehta A, Labrie F, Fazekas ATA, Comaru-Schally AM, Schally AV (1982) Tumor growth inhibition in patients with prostatic carcinoma treated with luteinizing hormone-releasing hormone agonists. Proc Natl Acad Sci USA 79:1658–1662

Vogel VG (2009) The NSABP Study of tamoxifen and raloxifene (STAR) trial. Expert Rev Anticancer Ther 9:51–60

11 Immunotherapy

Cancers can interact with the immune system in various ways.

- Chronic inflammation can cause DNA damage and thus increase the susceptibility to transformation.
- Immune surveillance may protect from tumorigenesis by recognizing and eliminating transformed cells.
- Some cancers can induce immune deviation, which may aid the progression of the neoplastic disease.

In the seventeenth and eighteenth centuries, some believed that cancer was contagious. In fact, the first cancer hospital in France was forced to move from the city in 1779 because of the fear that cancer could spread throughout the population. Decades later, the potentially protective role of the immune system against transformed cells was recognized. In 1813, Vautier reported that tumors regressed in patients, who had suffered from gas gangrene, a condition that is caused by Clostridial infection. In 1909, Paul Ehrlich carried out immunizations in animals with tumor cells and suggested that cell transformations occur at high frequency in humans, but are kept under control by the immune system (Ehrlich 1909).

Attempts at immune-based cancer therapies have a long history. Busch in 1868 and Fehleisen in 1882 undertook efforts to inoculate erysipelas (the etiology of erysipelas is Streptococcus pyogenes) to treat cancer patients with inoperable tumors (Busch 1868; Fehleisen 1882). In the 1890s, the New York surgeon William B. Coley found a record of a young patient with round cell sarcoma on the neck, who had been listed as a hopeless patient when he developed a severe infection of erysipelas. He survived the infection and his tumor went into remission. Based on this case, Coley devised a killed vaccine of Streptococcus pyogenes with Serratia marcescens. After a few years of its use, he reported to have successfully treated some sarcoma patients with the application of his bacterial toxins (Coley's toxin) (Coley 1893; Coley 1896). After his death, his daughter Helen Coley Nauts reviewed his records, published several reviews of his work, and founded the Cancer Research Institute, which promotes immune therapies for cancer. In 1935, Connell used sterile filtrates from Clostridium histolyticum to treat advanced cancers and attributed the observed tumor regression to the production of proteolytic enzymes (Connell 1935). However, further research did not show significant therapeutic effects. This modality has received renewed attention with the possibility to genetically engineer Clostridium spores to improve the bacterial oncolytic capability (Wei et al. 2008). The first substantial success in bacterial cancer therapy was achieved in 1976, when Morales, Eidinger and Bruce reported the successful treatment of superficial bladder cancer with Bacillus Calmette-Guerin (BCG) (Morales et al. 2002). Based on this observation, Bacillus Calmette-Guerin has become a widely used treatment of choice for high risk, superficial bladder cancer (Shintani et al. 2007). The injection of the attenuated bacterium Bacillus Calmette-Guerin together with a lipopolysaccharide endotoxin from gram negative bacteria induces the secretion of the cytokine Tumor Necrosis Factor (TNF), in some cases causing tumor regression.

Contemporary immunotherapy is based on immunology research that has identified cell subsets and humoral factors. Antibodies have been recognized as therapeutic entities or as delivery vehicles for cytotoxic drugs. Some Immunotherapy strategies have focused on activating cells of the immune system to fight tumor associated antigens or whole tumor cells. Based on the importance of the cytotoxic components of the immune system for anti-cancer responses, many immunotherapies have focused on the potential to generate cancer specific cytotoxic T-lymphocytes with memory (in the form of vaccines), or increasing the numbers of T-lymphocytes that can attack the tumor (adoptive therapy).

11.1 Immunotoxins

The treatment of cancer should be as aggressive as possible to completely destroy the tumor, but this aggressiveness often causes severe adverse effects and is a reason why some therapeutics cannot be applied systemically. Targeting strategies can increase the specificity of the therapeutic interven-

G. F. Weber, *Molecular Therapies of Cancer,* DOI 10.1007/978-3-319-13278-5_11,

Table 11.1 Immunotoxins

Category	Drug Name	Trade Name	Antigen	Toxin
Antibody based				
	Gemtuzumab ozogamicin	Mylotarg	CD33	Ozogamicin
	Brentuximab vendotin	Adcetrics	CD30	Monomethyl auristatin E
	HuC242-DM4		CA242	Maytansine DM4
	MLN2704		PSMA	Maytansinoid DM1
	Ado-trastuzumab emtansine	Kadcyla	ERBB2	Maytansinoid DM1
	erb-38		ERBB2	PE38
	SS1(dsFv)-PE38		Mesothelin	PE38
	BL-22	CAT-3888	CD22	PE38
	HA-22	CAT-8015	CD22	PE38
	LMB-2		IL-2R CD25	PE38
	LMB-1		Lewis Y	PE38
	LMB-7		Lewis Y	PE38
	LMB-9		Lewis Y	PE38
Cytokine based				
	TGFa-PE38		TGF-α	PE38

tion and thus minimize adverse effects while maximizing the desired effects. A way to accumulate therapeutic agents at the tumor site is their conjugation to specific monoclonal antibodies that bind to cancer cells (Schrama et al. 2006). If a suitable antigen is targeted, the conjugate, which is generally inactive without further modification, is internalized via receptor mediated endocytosis and the parent drug is released from the lysosome into the cell to restore its cytotoxic activity. Drug loading is generally an important measure for the potential efficacy of antibody-drug conjugates. The cytotoxic potency of antibody-drug conjugates can be augmented by either increasing the number of molecules that can be delivered per cell or by taking advantage of highly cytotoxic compounds, such as calicheamicin, maytansine or its derivatives, or monomethyl auristatin E (Table 11.1).

There are various chemical reactions suitable for coupling cytotoxic agents to antibodies.

- Peptide linkers are stable in blood but can be readily degraded in intracellular compartments by specific enzymes. They are superior to hydrazone linkers (Doronina et al. 2003).
- Disulfide linkers are suitable for the conjugation of some drugs to antibodies. They have the benefit of providing relative tumor specificity because they are cleaved by disulfide exchange with an intracellular thiol such as glutathione which is present at much higher concentrations in tumor cells than in normal cells (Jaracz et al. 2005).

Drug Resistance Immunotoxins may be antigenic, in particular if the toxin is a xenoprotein. Whereas patients with hematologic malignancies tend to be immunocompromised and respond to treatment, patients with solid tumors have strong immune systems and may neutralize the toxin after only 1–2 cycles.

Gemtuzumab ozogamicin <Mylotarg> is a recombinant humanized anti-CD33 monoclonal IgG_4 antibody, attached to the cytotoxic antibiotic ozogamicin (N-acetyl-γ-calicheamicin)[1]. In this conjugate, the antibody binds to and is internalized by tumor cells expressing CD33, a sialic acid dependent glycoprotein commonly present on the surface of leukemic blasts. It thereby delivers the attached calicheamicin to CD33 expressing tumor cells. Calicheamicin (see Sect. 2.2.5.) binds to the minor groove of DNA, causing double strand DNA breaks and resulting in inhibition of DNA synthesis. Gemtuzumab ozogamicin was used for the treatment of elderly patients suffering from $CD33^+$ acute myeloid leukemia (AML) in their first relapse, who were not eligible for other chemotherapies. In this population, a combined response rate of 30% with a median relapse free survival of 7 months in responding patients was observed (Sievers and Linenberger 2001). The agent was withdrawn from the market in 2010.

Adverse Effects Myelosuppression is the most severe toxicity associated with gemtuzumab ozogamicin. Virtually all patients reach platelet nadirs of fewer than 25,000 cells/mm^3, with the time to platelet recovery ranging 35–75 days. Over 90% of patients have severe neutropenia (below 1000 cells/mm^3), with a median time to neutrophil recovery around 40 days. 50% of patients experience anemia (hemoglobin below 8 g/dL). Tumor lysis syndrome, including secondary renal failure, is a possible consequence of treatment. Hepatotoxicity, including severe venoocclusive disease, may arise. Patients should be monitored for rapid weight gain, right upper quadrant pain, hepatomegaly, ascites, and elevations

[1] Gemtuzumab ozogamicin was the first antibody-drug conjugate to reach the market in 2000.

in bilirubin or liver enzymes to identify and treat venoocclusive disease if it develops.

Brentuximab vedotin (SGN-35, cAC10-vcMMAE) <Adcetris> consists of the chimeric monoclonal antibody brentuximab, which targets CD30, linked to 3–5 units of the anti-mitotic (microtubule disrupting) agent monomethyl auristatin E (MMAE) via a protease-cleavable linker. Approved by the U.S. FDA in 2011, the agent is used for Hodgkin lymphoma and anaplastic large cell lymphoma. The recommended dose is 1.8 mg/kg administered as an intravenous infusion over 30 min every 3 weeks, continued over a maximum of 16 cycles, or until disease progression or unacceptable toxicity occurs.

Adverse Effects Adverse effects include peripheral neuropathy, neutropenia, fatigue, upper respiratory tract infection, nausea, and diarrhea. The drug is associated with progressive multifocal leukoencephalopathy due to JC virus reactivation.

Drug Interactions Monomethyl auristatin E (MMAE) is a substrate and an inhibitor of CYP3A4/5. Co-administration with ketoconazole, a potent CYP3A4 inhibitor, increases the exposure to MMAE by approximately 35 %. Co-administration with rifampin, a potent CYP3A4 inducer, reduces the exposure to MMAE by approximately 45 %. MMAE does not inhibit other CYP enzymes at clinical concentrations, nor is it expected to alter the exposure to drugs that are metabolized by CYP3A4 enzymes.

HuC242-DM4 is an immunotoxin of the humanized monoclonal antibody C242 (MoAb HuC242) conjugated with the derivative DM4 of the cytotoxic agent maytansine (see Sect. 3.1.6.). MoAb HuC242 recognizes the cell surface superantigen CA242[2], which is expressed on a variety of tumor cells. Upon binding and cellular uptake, the immunoconjugate releases the maytansinoid agent DM4, which binds to Tubulin, thereby affecting the dynamics of microtubule assembly and disassembly. As a result, this agent prevents cell division and reduces cell growth in cancer cells that express CA242.

MLN2704 is an immunoconjugate that consists of the humanized monoclonal antibody MLN591, which is directed to Prostate Specific Membrane Antigen (PSMA), linked to the maytansinoid DM1. The monoclonal antibody moiety binds to tumor cells expressing PSMA and is internalized. The DM1 maytansinoid moiety binds to Tubulin, inhibits Tubulin polymerization and microtubule assembly, resulting in a disruption of microtubule activity and cell division.

Ado-trastuzumab emtansine (trastuzumab emtansine, T-DM1) <Kadcyla>, consists of the monoclonal antibody trastuzumab <Herceptin> linked to the cytotoxic agent mertansine (DM1). The monoclonal antibody moiety binds to tumor cells expressing ERBB2 (HER2/NEU) and is internalized. Trastuzumab suppresses the growth of cancer cells, mertansine enters cells and destroys them by binding to Tubulin.Ado- trastuzumab emtansine (T-DM1) is indicated for the treatment of ERBB2-positive metastatic breast cancer in patients who have been treated previously with trastuzumab and a taxane (paclitaxel or docetaxel), and who have already been treated for metastatic breast cancer or developed tumor recurrence within 6 months of adjuvant therapy.

Adverse Effects The most common adverse effects of trastuzumab emtansine are fatigue, nausea, musculoskeletal pain, thrombocytopenia, headache, and constipation. Severe adverse events include hepatotoxicity (nodular regenerative hyperplasia, hepatic encephalopathy, rarely liver failure), heart damage (left ventricular dysfunction), interstitial lung disease (acute interstitial pneumonitis), and peripheral neuropathy.

The erb-38 immunotoxin is a 63 kD recombinant, bivalent fusion protein consisting of disulfide-stabilized Fv fragments of the anti-ERBB2 monoclonal antibody e23 and a truncated version of Pseudomonas Exotoxin A[3]. Erb-38 immunotoxin binds specifically to cells that over-express ERBB2, the antigenic target of the monoclonal antibody. The toxin moiety induces Caspase mediated apoptosis via a mechanism that involves mitochondrial damage. It also catalyzes the transfer of ADP ribose from nicotinamide adenine dinucleotide (NAD) to EF-2 (Elongation Factor-2), thereby inactivating EF-2 and inhibiting protein synthesis.

Adverse Effects The agent is hepatotoxic.

Mesothelin is a cell surface glycoprotein that may be over-expressed by ovarian cancers, mesotheliomata, lung adenocarcinomata, and some squamous cell carcinomata. The interactions of Mesothelin with CA-125 may promote the spread of ovarian cancer. SS1(dsFv)-PE38 immunotoxin is a recombinant conjugate consisting of the single chain anti-Mesothelin monoclonal antibody SS1(dsFv) linked to the Pseudomonas exotoxin A fragment PE38. The monoclonal antibody moiety of the agent binds to cells that express Mesothelin. After internalization, the exotoxin moiety inactivates translation via binding to EF-2 (Elongation Factor-2), thereby disrupting tumor cell protein synthesis. While SS1(dsFv)-PE38 immunotoxin has had modest success in

[2] CA242 is a sialilated carbohydrate associated with adenocarcinomata.

[3] A deletion of domain Ia, comprising amino acids 1–252, and part of domain Ib of Pseudomonas Exotoxin A produces the 38 kD protein PE38 that has low cytotoxicity because it cannot bind to Pseudomonas Exotoxin A specific cellular receptors.

clinical trials as first-line therapy it may be more promising as a second-line treatment after taxol.

BL22 immunotoxin (CAT-3888) is a recombinant protein consisting of the Fv portion of the anti-CD22 antibody RFB4 fused to the PE38 fragment of Pseudomonas exotoxin A. BL22 immunotoxin binds to CD22, an antigen expressed on B-cell malignancies, thereby delivering its toxin directly to the tumor cells. The exotoxin portion of the immunoconjugate is then released and lyses the cells.

- HA22 (CAT-8015) is an immunotoxin comprising a modified Pseudomonas exotoxin A and an engineered anti-CD22 antibody fragment. It was generated in an effort to increase the affinity of BL22, utilizing hot spot mutagenesis to alter specific regions of the anti-CD22 antibody. The Fv antibody fragment portion of the agent contains 3 modified amino acids to enhance the binding affinity for the target molecule. The drug is under study for the treatment of B-cell malignancies.

Several LMB immunotoxins (named after the Laboratory for Molecular Biology at the Center for Cancer Research, NIH, led by Ira Pastan) are under study for use in cancer therapy. LMB-2 immunotoxin is a fusion protein consisting of the Fv portion of a monoclonal antibody attached to a 38 kDa fragment of the Pseudomonas Exotoxin A (with amino acids 365–380 deleted). The antibody moiety targets the Interleukin-2 Receptor (IL-2R, CD25), which is expressed on activated untransformed T- and B-lymphocytes and macrophages and on the cells of various hematologic malignancies. The binding facilitates the entry of the exotoxin, which induces Caspase mediated apoptosis. It also blocks translational elongation via binding to EF-2. The agent has had some success in hairy cell leukemia.

Advanced adenocarcinomata of the colon, rectum, pancreas, esophagus, or stomach may over-express the antigen Lewis-Y.

- LMB-1 immunotoxin (B3-LysPE38) is a chimeric protein consisting of the Fv portion of a monoclonal antibody attached to a fragment of Pseudomonas Exotoxin A (lacking its cell binding region). LMB-1 immunotoxin targets B3, a Lewis Y related carbohydrate epitope. The antibody attaches to tumor cells and is internalized, then the released exotoxin stops protein synthesis by inactivating EF-2 (Elongation Factor 2).
- LMB-7 (B3(Fv)PE38) immunotoxin is a single chain chimeric protein consisting of a monoclonal antibody fragment attached to a portion of the Pseudomonas Exotoxin A.
- LMB-9 immunotoxin (B3(dsFv)PE38) is a recombinant disulfide-stabilized anti-Lewis Y IgG immunotoxin containing a 38 kD toxic element derived from the Pseudomonas aeruginosa Exotoxin A and a monoclonal antibody fragment.

The targeting moiety of an immunotoxin does not need to be an antibody or antibody fragment. TGFa-PE38 immunotoxin is a recombinant, chimeric toxin composed of TGF-α (Transforming Growth Factor α), fused to a fragment of Pseudomonas exotoxin (PE38) that lacks its cell binding domain. The TGF-α moiety of the agent attaches to tumor cells expressing EGFR. The exotoxin induces Caspase mediated apoptosis of tumor cells. It also inactivates EF-2 and inhibits protein synthesis.

Immunotoxins target cytotoxic drugs to transformed cells in order to achieve therapeutic concentrations in the cancer while reducing systemic adverse effects.
The targeting moieties are mostly antibodies (but may also be cytokine fragments), the targets are typically cell surface receptors.
If a suitable antigen is targeted, the conjugate is internalized via receptor mediated endocytosis and the free cytotoxic drug is released from the lysosomes into the cell.

11.2 Engineered Antibodies

The possibility to direct the immune system to fight cancer cells in virtually any location within the body with minimal adverse effects has attracted increasing research efforts. The high specificity and high binding affinity of antibodies have made them attractive as potential anti-cancer agents. For a long time, however, they were difficult to isolate in large quantities. The fusion of antibody producing cells with myeloma cells into hybridomas, accomplished by Cesar Milstein and Georges Koehler in the mid-1970s, remedied that. Yet, biotechnology had to advance to accomplish humanizing such antibodies before they became successful in therapy. In 1997, the U.S. FDA approved Rituxan, a monoclonal antibody to CD20 (developed by IDEC Pharmaceuticals) to treat non-Hodgkin lymphoma (McLaughlin et al. 1998). The process also led to the development of Herceptin, spearheaded by Dennis Slamon and Axel Ullrich, an antibody that targets the receptor ERBB2, which is over-expressed on the surface of about 30% of breast cancers. In further technical advances, molecular biology has allowed structural modifications of antibodies to alter their functions. Engineered antibodies take advantage of the targeting characteristics and combine them with various functionalities (Table 11.2).

Antibody-cytokine conjugates The hu14.18-IL2 immunocytokine (EMD 273063) recognizes the disialoganglioside GD2. It is under evaluation for the treatment of GD2-positive neuroblastoma and melanoma because of its ability to enhance tumor cell killing by antibody dependent cell mediated cytotoxicity (ADCC) and by anti-tumor cytotoxic T cells. hu14.18-IL2 binds to tumor cells via its antibody component. It increases cell-cell adhesion and activating immune

Table 11.2 Engineered antibodies

Cytokine conjugate		Cytokine	Antibody specificity	Characteristics
	hu14.18-IL2	IL-2	GD2	recombinant fusion protein
	Tucotuzumab celmoleukin	IL-2	EpCAM	recombinant fusion protein
Bispecific		*Antibody specificity*	*Antibody specificity*	
	Catumaxomab	CD3	EpCAM	Triomab
	Ertumaxomab	CD3	ERBB2	Triomab
	Bi20	CD3	CD20	Triomab
	Blinatumomab	CD3	CD19	BiTE
	MT110	CD3	EpCAM	BiTE
	2B1	CD16	ERBB2	
	MDX447	CD64	EGFR	(Fab)2
	rM28A	CD28	MAPG	Tandem single chain Fv fragments
Immunoliposome		*Drug*	*Antibody specificity*	
		Doxorubicin	ERBB2	

synapse formation with natural killer cells (NK cells) by engaging the IL-2 Receptors of the targeted immune system cells.

Tucotuzumab celmoleukin (huKS-IL2 immunocytokine) (EMD 273066) is a recombinant fusion protein comprised of a human monoclonal antibody directed to Epithelial Cell Adhesion Molecule (EpCAM, KS, CD326), linked to an active Interleukin-2 (IL-2) molecule. The humanized monoclonal antibody moiety of tucotuzumab celmoleukin recognizes and binds to a cell surface epithelial protein that is expressed on a wide variety of cancer cells, thereby concentrating the TH_1 cytokine IL-2 in EpCAM expressing tumor tissue. Subsequently, the localized IL-2 moiety of this fusion protein may stimulate a cytotoxic T-lymphocyte anti-tumor immune response. The agent can also enhance tumor cell killing by antibody dependent cell mediated cytotoxicity. The drug is under evaluation for the treatment of ovarian cancers and small cell lung cancer.

Bispecific antibodies A bispecific monoclonal antibody is composed of fragments of 2 distinct monoclonal antibodies and consequently binds to 2 different types of antigen. The potential of using bispecific antibodies to retarget effector cells toward tumor cells was developed in the 1980s (Karpovsky et al. 1984). Many bispecific antibodies direct one paratope to a tumor associated antigen and the other to a T-lymphocyte activating receptor. In the case of trifunctional antibodies, the Fc region additionally binds to a cell that expresses Fc receptors on the surface, such as a macrophage, a natural killer cell, or a dendritic cell. The recruitment and activation of immune system cells to the tumor is intended to generate an effective anti-cancer immune response.

- T-cell retargeting directs cytotoxic T-lymphocytes to tumors. Because the target cells do not express Fcγ receptors, antibodies that bind to CD3 may have the potential to redirect and activate circulating T-lymphocytes against tumors.
- A series of bispecific antibodies is directed to tumor associated antigens and FcγRI (CD64), which is prominently expressed on monocytes and macrophages and up-regulated upon activation on neutrophils.
- Antibodies with a hybrid rat/mouse Fc portion can efficiently interact with activating human Fc receptors (FcγRI and FcγRIII), but not inhibitory Fc receptors (FcγRIIB) (Lindhofer et al. 1995).

Several clinical trials were initiated in the early 1990s.

Catumaxomab (anti-EpCAM and anti-CD3) <Removab> was the first bispecific antibody to be approved for clinical use (2009 in the European Union). It is a trifunctional drug ("TriomAb") comprised of a rat-mouse hybrid monoclonal antibody, which binds simultaneously to EpCAM on tumor cells and CD3 on T-lymphocytes (Fig. 11.1). In addition, its Fc region (composed of the 2 immunoglobulin isotypes, mouse IgG2a and rat IgG2b) selectively binds to FcγI and FcγIII Receptors on innate immune cells, such as macrophages, dendritic cells, and natural killer cells. Catumaxomab became the first drug to be approved for the intraperitoneal treatment of malignant ascites in patients with EpCAM-positive carcinomata that are resistant to standard treatments. The peritoneum is of mesothelial origin and therefore lacks EpCAM expression. Overall survival may be positively affected in patients with ovarian or gastric cancers.

Pharmacokinetics The usual treatment of malignant ascites is to puncture the peritoneum and drain the accumulated fluid. Consecutively, catumaxomab is given as an intraperitoneal infusion. The procedure is repeated 4 times within 11 days. Alternative application routes may be intrapleural (for malignant pleural effusion) or intravenous (for non-small cell lung cancer).

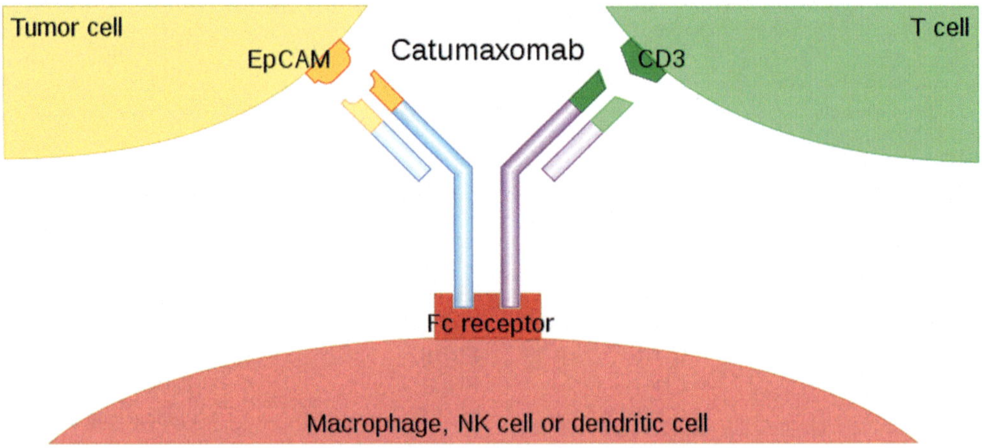

Fig. 11.1 Catumaxomab mechanism of action. Many types of cancer cells carry EpCAM (Epithelial Cell Adhesion Molecule) on their surface. By binding to such a cell via one arm, to a T lymphocyte via the other arm and to an antigen-presenting cell like a macrophage, a natural killer cell or a dendritic cell via the heavy chains, an immunological reaction against the cancer cell is triggered. Removing cancer cells from the abdominal cavity reduces the tumor burden which is seen as the cause for ascites in cancer patients. [http://en.wikipedia.org/wiki/Catumaxomab]

Adverse Effects Catumaxomab may cause fever, nausea, vomiting and abdominal pain due to cytokine release.

Ertumaxomab (anti-HER2 with anti-CD3) <Rexomun> is a trifunctional monoclonal antibody. It is comprised of a murine monoclonal antibody with 2 antigen recognition sites, for CD3 (a component of the T-cell antigen receptor) and for ERBB2 (a tumor associated antigen that promotes cell proliferation). The drug selectively cross-links tumor cells and immunologic effector cells. This mechanism results in the recruitment of cytotoxic T-lymphocytes to form a T-cell/tumor cell aggregate. Ertumaxomab is in clinical trials for peritoneal carcinomatosis and for metastatic breast cancer.

Drug Interactions Catumaxomab and ertumaxomab may be administered together intraperitoneally to patients with malignant ascites.

Bi20 (fBTA05) <Lymphomun> is a trifunctional monoclonal antibody that targets CD3 and CD20. CD20 is expressed during B-cell development and on B-cell malignancies. Bi20 is in clinical trials for chronic lymphocytic leukemia (CLL).

Bispecific T-cell engagers (BiTEs) are a type of tandem single chain Fv moieties aimed at activating T-lymphocytes. They are composed of an anti-CD3 single chain Fv fragment fused to an anti-tumor associated antigen single chain Fv fragment via the 5 residue peptide linker GGGGS. Bispecific T-cell engagers are active at a low concentration and do not require any kind of pre- or co-stimulation of effector T-lymphocytes. They are capable of inducing efficient tumor cell lysis at effector to target ratios of 1:10.

The first BiTE developed was blinatumomab (MT103), which is a murine anti-CD3 x anti-CD19. Doses of 5 μg/m^2/day can lead to an elimination of target cells in the blood of relapsed non-Hodgkin lymphoma patients. Blinatumomab is in clinical trials as a treatment of lymphoma and leukemia. Due to its small size (60 kD), the drug is rapidly cleared from the circulation and requires continuous infusion.

Pharmacokinetics Blinatumomab is characterized by a short blood half life of several hours, and so continuous intravenous infusion by portable mini-pumps is required.

MT110 is a bispecific T-cell engager comprised of anti-EpCAM and anti-CD3 tandem single chain Fv fragments. It is in clinical trials for lung, colorectal, and gastrointestinal cancer patients.

The bispecific antibody 2B1 is a monoclonal antibody specific for both, CD16 (Immunoglobulin G Receptor) and ERBB2. It may enhance cellular immune responses against ERBB2 expressing cells, resulting in increased tumor cell lysis.

The bispecific antibody MDX447 targets both, CD64 (the high affinity Immunoglobulin G Receptor) and EGFR (Epidermal Growth Factor Receptor). It may enhance cellular immune responses against EGFR-positive cells, resulting in increased tumor cell lysis.

Tandem single chain Fv fragments (TaFv) are 2 single chain Fv fragments linked by an interposed peptide linker that is deemed to confer good flexibility to each fragment. rM28A is a recombinant, bispecific, single chain antibody directed to both, the T-lymphocyte surface associated co-stimulatory molecule CD28 and Melanoma Associated Proteoglycan (MAPG, NG2). When activated, CD28 facilitates interactions between T-lymphocytes and other immune effector cells resulting in cytotoxic T-lymphocyte responses. MAPG is a surface antigen expressed on primary cutaneous, ocular, and metastatic melanomata. By targeting both CD28 and MAPG, the engineered antibody enhances cytotoxic T-lymphocyte recognition of melanoma cells, which may result in immune effector mediated tumor cell death. rM28A spontaneously forms stable dimers and is capable of inducing T-cell activation and effective tumor cell killing without a signal through the T-Cell Antigen Receptor (TCR) complex in a process called targeted supra-agonistic stimulation.

Pharmacokinetics This agent may have a long half-life in the blood secondary to the formation of dimers.

The Dock and Lock method creates bispecific antibodies. It relies on the spontaneous association of a dimer between the 45-amino acid peptide DDD2, derived from the regulatory subunit of cAMP-Dependent Protein Kinase (PKA) with the 21-amino acid peptide AD2, derived from the anchoring domains of A Kinase Anchor Proteins (AKAPs). Upon association, 2 disulfide bonds are created, resulting in a covalent complex that is stable for more than a week in situ.

TF2 is a molecule of 157 kD, comprising 2 Fab fragments (devoid of Fc fragments) derived from the humanized anti-CEA antibody hMN-14 and from the humanized antibody h679 that strongly binds the hapten histamine-succinyl-glycine (HSG). This bispecific Tri-Fab molecule (trimeric Fab fragments) contains the peptide IMP-288, which has 2 HSG epitopes. The divalent peptide is labeled with ^{177}Lutetium for radio-immunotherapy. ^{177}Lu has a half-life of 6.7 days. The emitted β radiation with a maximum energy of 498 keV is effective in destroying small tumors and metastases while sparing normal tissue.

Immunoliposomes Immunoliposomes combine the specificity of whole monoclonal antibodies or Fab fragments with the favorable pharmacokinetics and drug delivery of liposomes (Fig. 11.2). A pioneering approach exploited the conjugation of uncoated or PEGylated (polyethylene glycol-coated) liposomes to Fab fragments of trastuzumab to create immunoliposomes targeting ERBB2 (HER2/NEU) over-expressing cancers. Anti-ERBB2 liposomal doxorubicin selectively bound to ERBB2-positive cells, favoring the internalization of doxorubicin into the target cells compared with a less productive accumulation of liposome-encapsulated doxorubicin in the interstitium (Kirpotin et al. 1997; Drummond et al. 1999).

Molecular biology engineering of antibodies takes advantage of their targeting characteristics and combines them with various functionalities.
Antibody-cytokine conjugates target immunostimulatory cytokines to transformed cells in order to induce anti-tumor immunity.
Bispecific antibodies retarget immune effector cells toward tumor cells.
Bispecific antibody designs include triomabs, BiTEs, (Fab)$_2$s, and tandem single chain Fv fragments.
Immunoliposomes combine the specificity of antibodies with the favorable pharmacokinetics and drug delivery of liposomes.

11.3 Antigen Based Immunotherapy

Because anti-tumor immunity is predominantly cellular immunity, research has been directed toward turning T-lymphocytes against tumors. Steven A. Rosenberg focused his efforts to generate anti-cancer vaccines on tumor associated antigens. In a similar approach, Martin Kast studied the development of peptide based vaccines. Because the skin harbors relatively strong antigens, skin cancers (in particular melanoma) are frequently targeted in antigen-based immunotherapies.

Therapeutic peptide cancer vaccines (Table 11.3) aim at inducing strong CD8 and CD4 T-lymphocyte responses. They require the involvement of host antigen presenting cells to efficiently present the peptide antigens for activation of the required immune cell subsets. Cytotoxic T-lymphocytes represent the predominant effector cells for a tumor specific, immune mediated destruction of cancer cells. Cytotoxic T-lymphocytes recognize, engage and destroy target cells through the trimolecular interaction of the T-Cell Antigen Receptor (TCR) on the lymphocytes with peptides that are presented by the target cell in the context of the class I Major Histocompatibility Complex (MHC, Human Leukocyte Antigen, HLA)[4]. The recognition of an HLA/peptide complex by cytotoxic T-lymphocytes enables them to attack cancer cells expressing antigens that incorporate the presented peptide. The underlying concept of antigen based cancer vaccination is the introduction of tumor associated antigens in increased concentrations to the immune system, in order to deploy cytotoxic T-lymphocytes to destroy cancer cells. The use of one or a few peptide antigens in the therapeutic cancer vaccine is based on the assumption that the initial immune activation will evolve into a broad anti-tumor response. This however has not been the case in many cancer vaccine trials, presumably in part because tumor induced mechanisms suppress or block anti-tumor responses. Immune suppression through regulatory T cells, myeloid derived suppressor cells, or M_2 macrophages may contribute to immune escape.

The protein MAGE-3 is present in the cytosol of melanoma cells and lung adenocacrcinoma cells[5]. Its peptide epi-

[4] The class I Major Histocompatibility Complex is expressed on vitually all somatic cells. Expression of the class II Major Histocompatibility Complex is limited to antigen presenting cells.

[5] Melanoma Associated Antigens (MAGE) belong to a sub-group of the cancer testis antigen family that includes at least 55 closely related

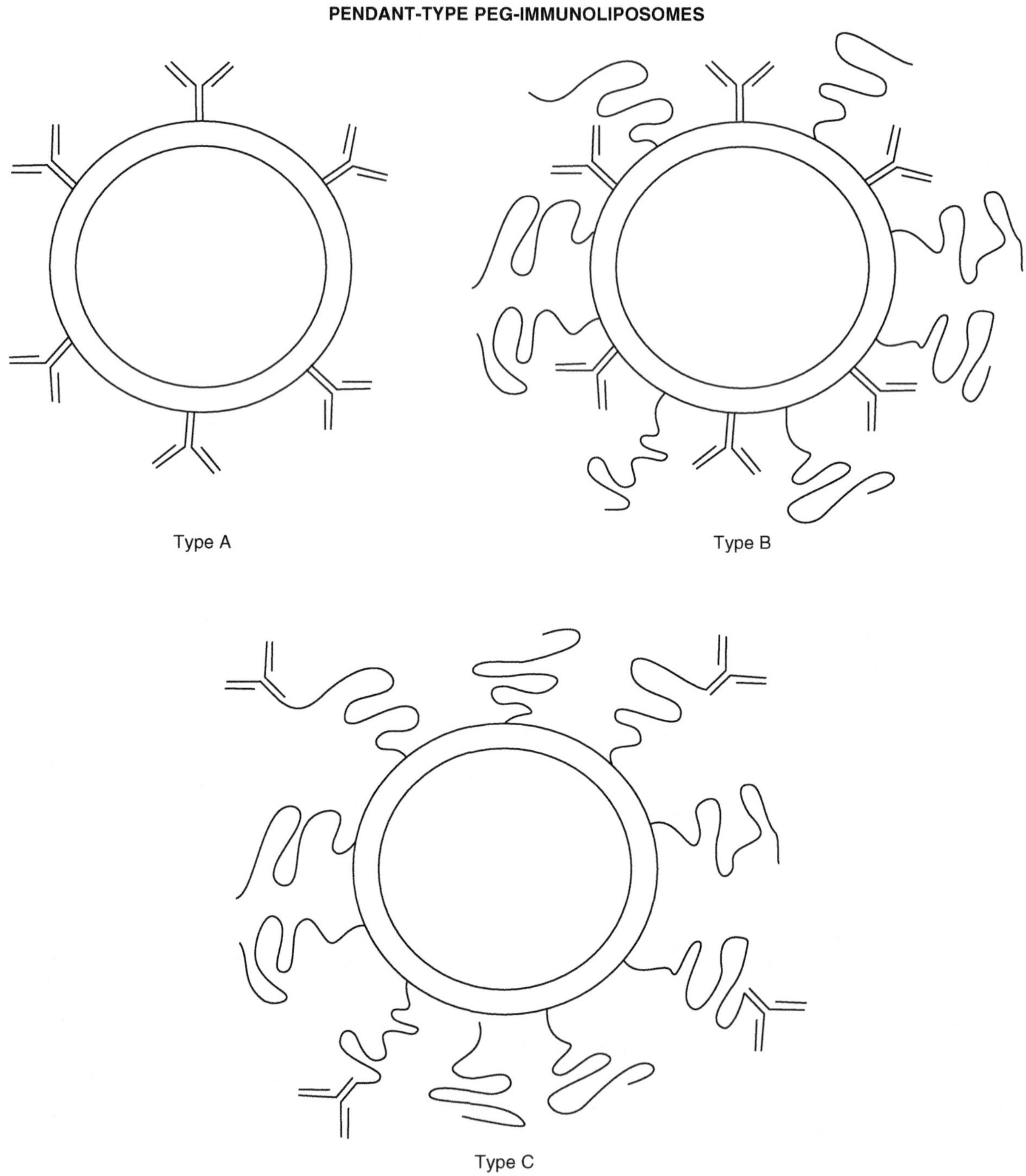

Fig. 11.2 Schematic illustration of antibody immobilization on liposomes. Type A: PEG-free immunoliposomes with the antibody covalently linked to the short anchor NGPE; Type B: PEG-immunoliposomes with the antibody covalently linked to NGPE; Type C: new type of PEG-immunoliposomes with antibody attached to the distal terminal of DSPE-PEG-COOH, so-called pendant-type PEG-immunoliposomes. (redrawn from Maruyama 2002)

topes are presented in class I MHC molecules on the cell surface. MAGE-3 may be expressed as the fusion protein D1/3-MAGE-3. D1/3-MAGE-3-His (GSK 2132231A) is a recombinant chimeric protein vaccine, which is produced by fusing MAGE-3 with a lipidated Protein D derived from Hemophilus Influenzae at its *N*-terminus and a sequence of several histidine residues at its *C*-terminus. This vaccine is recognized by specific cytotoxic T-lymphocytes. The fusion

proteins. MAGE proteins are characterized by a conserved signature domain (MAGE homology domain) that consists of a stretch of 200 amino acids (often located close to the *C*-terminus).

Table 11.3 Antigen based immunotherapy

Peptide vaccines		
Antigen	Tumor	Formulation
MAGE-3	Melanoma	Recombinant chimeric protein
MAGE-10.A2	Melanoma	Peptide
MAGE-A3	Melanoma	Coupled HPV-16 peptide
NY-ESO-1	Melanoma and others	Peptide
NY-ESO-1	Melanoma and others	Fowlpox virus
NY-ESO-1	Melanoma	Autologous dendritic cells
GP100	Melanoma	Plasmid DNA
GP100	Melanoma	Fused peptides
Tyrosinase	Melanoma	Vaccinia virus
Melan A VLP	Melanoma	Virus-like particles
MART-1	Melanoma	Peptide
tetanus toxin	Melanoma	Peptide adjuvant for tumor peptides
PSA	Prostate cancer	Fowlpox virus
PSA	Prostate cancer	Vaccinia virus
PSA	Prostate cancer	TRICOM (B7.1, ICAM-1, LFA-3)
G250	Renal cacrinoma	Peptide
MUC1	Breast cancer	Peptide
MUC1	Breast cancer	Vaccinia virus
MUC1 (BLP25)	Breast cancer	Liposome
ERBB2	Breast cancer	Peptide
ERBB2	Breast cancer	Recombinant peptide
CEA	Gastrointestinal, breast, lung cancers	Canarypox virus
CEA	Gastrointestinal, breast, lung cancers	Peptide
CEA	Gastrointestinal, breast, lung cancers	Dendritic cells
CEA, MUC1	Gastrointestinal, breast cancers	TRICOM (B7.1, ICAM-1, LFA-3)
AFP	Hepatocellular cacrcinoma	Plasmid DNA
WT1	Leukemia	Peptide
BCR-ABL	CLL	Peptide
Telomerase		Peptide
mutant P53		Pulsed dendritic cells

protein may boost anti-tumoral immune responses when used in the vaccine formulation.

HLA-A2 melanoma patients respond frequently with immune stimulation to the peptide MAGE-A$10_{254-262}$ (GLYDGMEHL). MAGE-10.A2 is a synthetic nonapeptide derived from this melanoma associated antigen. Vaccination with MAGE-10.A2 may stimulate a host cytotoxic T-cell response against tumor cells that express the antigen, resulting in tumor cell lysis.

There is a high prevalence of Melanoma Associated Antigen A3 (MAGE-A3) and human papillomavirus 16 (HPV-16) on squamous cell carcinoma of the head and neck. The MAGE-A3/HPV 16 peptide vaccine is a multi-epitope "Trojan antigen construct" vaccine consisting of MAGE-A3 and HPV-16 peptide epitopes linked by the Furin sensitive linker RVKR (arginine-valine-lysine-arginine). The Trojan antigen construct enters the cytoplasm of antigen presenting cells and is processed by the endoplasmic reticulum and the trans-Golgi network, where the Endopeptidase Furin releases the epitopes from the RVKR linker. This cleavage, together with various Exopeptidases, generates MHC class I binding peptides. Expressed on the cell surfaces of antigen presenting cells, these MHC class I binding peptides stimulate a cytotoxic T-lymphocyte response against tumor cells that display the same peptide epitopes on their cell surfaces.

The cancer testis antigen[6] NY-ESO-1 may be present on melanoma cells and on cancers of the prostate, bladder, brain, breast, esophagus, gastrointestinal tract, liver, kidney, lungs, and ovaries. The NY-ESO-1 peptide vaccine is a cancer vaccine consisting of an immunogenic peptide derived from NY-ESO-1. The peptide NY-ESO-1_{86-94} (RLLEFYLAM) is immunostimulatory. Vaccination with NY-ESO-1 peptide vaccine may stimulate the host immune system to mount a combined humoral and cytotoxic T-lymphocyte

[6] Cancer testis antigens are physiologically expressed in germ line cells and patho-physiologically in cancer cells. Over 140 such genes have been identified. The encoded proteins stimulate strong immune responses.

response to cells expressing the NY-ESO-1 antigen, which results in tumor cell lysis.

The Fowlpox-NY-ESO-1 vaccine is a cancer vaccine consisting of a recombinant fowlpox virus vector that encodes an immunogenic peptide derived from the cancer testis antigen NY-ESO-1. This antigen is expressed in normal testis and in various tumors. Vaccination with an NY-ESO-1 peptide vaccine may stimulate the host immune system to mount a humoral and cytotoxic T-lymphocyte response against tumor cells expressing the NY-ESO-1 antigen.

Dendritic cells act as gatekeepers of the immune system. Clinical trials at the Roswell Park Cancer Institute investigate an autologous NY-ESO-1 dendritic cell vaccine. The vaccine incorporates anti-DEC205-NY-ESO-1. The treated cells are then reinfused to the patient as a vaccine designed to recruit killer cells that destroy the cancer cells.

Glycoprotein 100 (GP100, Melanocyte Protein PMEL) is a transmembrane glycoprotein that is enriched in melanosomes and is involved in melanosome maturation. In melanoma, it may represent a tumor associated antigen.

MDX-1379 (BMS-734019) is made up of 2 peptides that are epitopes of the melanoma protein GP100. These peptides bind to HLA-A2, which is then recognized by T-lymphocytes. MDX-1379 has undergone clinical trials in conjunction with ipilimumab.

Gp100:209-217(210M) is a synthetic peptide cancer vaccine consisting of amino acid residues 209 through 217 of GP100, with a methionine substitution at position 210 to improve immunogenicity. Vaccination with gp100:209-217(210M) peptide may stimulate the host immune system to mount a cytotoxic T lymphocyte response against tumor cells that express GP100. Many clinical trials have studied the vaccine in conjunction with Interleukin-2. The gp100 cancer vaccine can also include other peptides derived from GP100, such as gp100:280-288(288V).

A *gp100* plasmid DNA vaccine consists of a plasmid DNA that encodes the melanoma associated antigen GP100. Upon administration, expressed GP100 antigen may stimulate cytotoxic T-lymphocytes to mount a HLA-A2.1 restricted immune response against tumor cells that express this antigen.

Tyrosinase is a melanocyte specific differentiation enzyme that catalyzes the synthesis of the melanin precursor L-3,4-dihydroxyphenylalanine (L-DOPA). Vaccinia-tyrosinase vaccine consists of a recombinant modified vaccinia virus Ankara that encodes the melanoma associated antigen Tyrosinase. Vaccination stimulates the host immune system to mount a cytotoxic T-lymphocyte response to cells expressing Tyrosinase.

MART-1 is a melanocytic differentiation antigen that is upregulated in most melanomata. MART-1 activates the immune system to exert a response, potentially resulting in tumor cell lysis of expressing cells. Vaccination with MART-1 antigen may stimulate a host cytotoxic T-lymphocyte response. Melan-A VLP vaccine consists of MART-1 (Melan A) and non-infectious virus-like particles (VLP). The virus-like particles stimulate the immune system and promote the cytolytic T-lymphocyte response.

MART-1:27-35 peptide vaccine is a natural or synthetic peptide cancer vaccine consisting of amino acid residues 27–35 of MART-1. Vaccination with MART-1:27-35 peptide may induce cytotoxic host immune responses against melanoma cells that express this peptide.

Pharmacokinetics The short half-life of the peptide may be overcome by terminal modifications. The vaccine injections are mixed with an oil-based substance <Montanide ISA-51>, which is intended to increase the immune response to the peptide antigen.

Tetanus peptide melanoma vaccine consists of peptides derived from melanoma associated antigens and a modified T-lymphocyte epitope derived from tetanus toxoid. Vaccination with this agent may stimulate a host cytotoxic and helper T-lymphocyte response against tumor cells that express melanoma associated antigens, resulting in decreased tumor growth.

Recombinant fowlpox-prostate specific antigen vaccine is a cancer vaccine consisting of a recombinant fowlpox virus that encodes PSA (Prostate Specific Antigen). Administration of this agent may stimulate a cytotoxic T-lymphocyte response against PSA expressing tumor cells.

Recombinant vaccinia prostate-specific antigen vaccine is a vaccine consisting of recombinant vaccinia virus that encodes PSA. Vaccination stimulates the host immune system to mount a cytotoxic T-lymphocyte response against tumor cells expressing PSA.

Vaccinia-PSA-TRICOM vaccine is a formulation consisting of a mixture of recombinant vaccinia virus that encodes PSA and recombinant vaccinia virus that encodes the 3 immuno-co-stimulatory transgenes B7.1, ICAM-1, and LFA-3 (TRICOM). This vaccine may enhance antigen presentation over preparations that lack co-stimulation, resulting in the augmentation of a cytotoxic T-lymphocyte immune response against tumor cells expressing PSA. The vaccinia and fowlpox vaccines may be combined and incorporate TRICOM (DiPaola et al. 2006) in <Prostvac-VF> on a prime and boost schedule.

The antigen G250 is a cell surface tumor associated antigen present on the majority of renal cell carcinomata. It contains an HLA-A2.1 restricted epitope that is recognized by cytotoxic T-lymphocytes. G250 peptide vaccine is a cancer vaccine consisting of a synthetic peptide. Vaccination with G250 peptide vaccine may stimulate the host immune system to mount a cytotoxic response against tumor cells that are positive for the antigen, resulting in decreased tumor growth.

The mammary-type Mucin (Mucin-1, MUC-1) is a high molecular weight transmembrane glycoprotein. A mid-region located on the extracellular domain is termed the tandem repeat domain, because it consists of a 20-amino acid sequence that is repeated multiple times. The tandem repeat domain of Mucin-1 is rich in proline, serine and threonine and contains several *O*-glycosylation sites at the serine and threonine residues. Mucin-1 is over-expressed and may be under-glycosyated on many tumor cells, particularly those of colon, breast, ovaries, prostate, lungs, and pancreas, as well as multiple myeloma. Thus, its expression pattern in tumor cells is different from untransformed cells. Mucin-1 in tumors promotes growth and survival, it is associated with disease progression and a poor prognosis.

MUC-1 peptide vaccine is a cancer vaccine that is comprised of a synthetic peptide derived from the antigen Mucin-1. Upon administration, MUC-1 peptide vaccine may stimulate the host immune system to mount a cytotoxic T-lymphocyte response against tumor cells that are positive for Mucin-1, resulting in decreased tumor growth.

Recombinant vaccinia-MUC-1 vaccine is a vaccine containing a recombinant vaccinia virus that carries the gene for human *mucin-1*. Upon administration, recombinant vaccinia-MUC-1 vaccine may elicit a Mucin-1 specific cytotoxic T-lymphocyte response against tumor cells that bear the antigen.

BLP25 liposomal vaccine (L-BLP25) is a liposome encapsulated peptide vaccine containing a synthetic peptide derived from the exposed core peptide of the tumor associated antigen Mucin-1. The BLP25 lipopeptide vaccine consists of

- a 25-amino acid Mucin-1 sequence (STAPPAHGVTSAPDTRPAPGSTAPP) that provides Mucin-1 specificity; it is slightly larger than one tandem repeat of the Mucin-1 protein and contains a palmitoyl lysine residue at the carboxyl terminus to enhance the incorporation of the lipopeptide into the liposome particle
- immunoadjuvant monophosphoryl lipid A, which is the Toll-Like Receptor-4 (TLR4) agonist that activates dendritic cells and macrophages
- 3 lipids (cholesterol, dimyristoyl phosphatidylglycerol, dipalmitoyl phosphatidylcholine) that serve as adjuvants.

The liposomal delivery system facilitates the uptake by antigen presenting cells for presentation through MHC molecules to specific T-lymphocytes that can identify and target cancer cells that express Mucin-1. Upon vaccination, MUC-1 peptide vaccine may stimulate the host immune system to mount a cytotoxic T-lymphocyte response against Mucin-1 expressing tumor cells. It thereby results in inhibiting tumor growth.

The 4 *erb* genes *erbB1* (*egfr*), *erbB2* (*her-2/neu*), *erbB3* (*her-3*), and *erbB4* (*her-4*) encode the family of EGF Receptor tyrosine kinases. They are composed of a cysteine-rich extracellular domain, a single transmembrane domain, and an intracellular catalytic domain. Although no ligand for ERBB2 has been identified, it may act by serving as the preferred hetero-dimerization partner of the other ERBB receptors. ERBB2 transduces signals through Phospholipase C, phosphatidylinositol 1,4,5-trisphosphate, diacylglycerol, and the cellular influx of calcium ions from the exterior. Thus, ERBB2 stimulates cell cycle progression as well as the expression of the anti-apoptotic regulators BCL-X_L and BCL-2. ERBB2 may constitute a tumor associated antigen that is over-expressed on a variety of carcinomata. The recognition and lysis of cancer cells by cytolytic T-lymphocytes often correlates with their expression levels of ERBB2. The immune system commonly recognizes 2 epitope peptides, of which GP2 (amino acids 654-662, IISAVVGIL) is shared by various epithelial tumors, including breast, ovarian, pancreas, and non-small cell lung cancers.

HER-2/NEU peptide vaccine is a cancer vaccine comprised of peptides that are derived from the extracellular domain of the tumor associated antigen ERBB2 (HER-2/NEU). HER-2/NEU peptide vaccine may induce specific antibodies with anti-tumor activity and elicit a specific $CD8^+$ T-lymphocyte response against ERBB2 expressing tumor cell types.

Recombinant dHER2 vaccine is a cancer vaccine consisting of a truncated recombinant ERBB2 peptide (dHER2). Upon administration, recombinant dHER2 vaccine may stimulate the host immune system to mount a cytotoxic T-lymphocyte response against tumor cells that over-express the ERBB2 protein, resulting in tumor cell lysis. dHER2 includes the extracellular domain and a part of the intracellular domain of the protein.

The precursor nature of the cells of origin for malignancy is evidenced by the frequent expression of fetal proteins in cancer. They include the glycoprotein Carcinoembryonic Antigen (CEA), which may be elevated in gastrointestinal, breast, lung, pancreas, and ovarian cancer, and in cases of bronchogenic and mammary carcinomata. The *cea* gene family encodes cell surface glycoproteins, belonging to the Immunoglobulin super-family of molecules, which are involved in cell adhesion.

A reduplication-defective avipox vaccine (ALVAC-CEA) contains the gene for Carcinoembryonic Antigen in a canarypox vector with the ability to infect human cells but inability to reduplicate. The vaccine has the ability to induce cytolytic T-lymphocyte responses in patients with advanced cancer. The vaccine is well tolerated and no substantial toxicity is attributed to the treatment.

Carcinoembryonic Antigen peptide 1-6D (CEA:571-579 (576D), mCEA Peptide) is a 9 residue HLA-restricted fragment of CEA. It comprises the amino acids 571-579, which have the sequence YLSGANLNL. The peptide vaccine may elicit a cytotoxic T-lymphocyte immune response against tumors expressing CEA.

Autologous vaccination with activated dendritic cells or peripheral blood mononuclear cells, which have been exposed to CEA peptide-1 in vitro may stimulate the host immune system to mount a cytotoxic T-lymphocyte response against tumor cells expressing CEA. A cancer vaccine consists of dendritic cells harvested from a patient with cancer and pulsed or transduced with a peptide fragment of CEA. When the altered dendritic cells are returned to the patient, they may stimulate the host immune system to mount a cytotoxic T-lymphocyte immune response against tumor cells expressing CEA.

Falimarev is a cancer vaccine comprised of

- a recombinant fowlpox viral vector that encodes CEA (Carcinoembryonic Antigen)
- MUC-1, a transmembrane glycoprotein secreted by glandular epithelial tissues
- TRICOM, comprised of the 3 co-stimulatory molecule transgenes B7-1, ICAM-1, and LFA-3.

This agent may enhance CEA and MUC-1 presentation to antigen presenting cells and activate a cytotoxic T-lymphocyte response against $CEA^{+}MUC\text{-}1^{+}$ tumor cells.

The AFP gene hepatocellular carcinoma vaccine is a cancer vaccine composed of naked plasmid DNA for the tumor associated antigen *afp* (*α-fetoprotein*). The protein α-Fetoprotein (AFP) acts as a specific immunologic target for hepatocellular carcinoma. This vaccine exerts an anti-tumor effect by inducing cytotoxic T-lymphocytes to attack AFP expressing tumor cells.

WT1, a tumor associated antigen, is over-expressed in most types of leukemia and in a variety of solid cancers. WT1 126-134 peptide vaccine is a synthetic peptide vaccine consisting of the amino acids 126-134 of the Wilms Tumor-1 (WT1) protein. Vaccination with WT1 126-134 peptide vaccine may induce a specific cytotoxic T-lymphocyte response against WT1 expressing cells, resulting in cell lysis and inhibition of cancer cell proliferation.

Fusion genes in chronic myelogenous leukemia (CML) typically result from the fusion of either *bcr* exon b2 or *bcr* exon b3 to *abl* exon a2, resulting in a b3a2 or a b2a2 fusion[7]. 4 peptides derived from amino acid sequences that cross the b3a2 breakpoint bind MHC class I molecules. HLA A3, A11, and B8 bind b3a2 derived peptide sequences.

A peptide vaccine consists of the BCR-ABL b2a2 fusion oncoprotein, frequently expressed in chronic myelogenous leukemia. Vaccination with the BCR-ABL b2a2 derived peptide vaccine (CML-VAX B2) or the BCR-ABL b3a2 derived peptide vaccine (CML-VAX B3) may stimulate the host immune system to mount a cytotoxic T-lymphocyte response against tumor cells that express the BCR-ABL fusion protein.

[7] The resulting fusion protein is a chimera of the Breakpoint Cluster Region (BCR) with the Abelson kinase (ABL) (see Sect. 4.1.2.).

Telomerase expression and activity (see Sect. 6.1.) is directly linked to tumor development. Its catalytic subunit is expressed in the majority of cancer cells, but in untransformed cells is largely limited to stem cells and germ line cells. Telomerase:540-548 peptide vaccine is a recombinant peptide consisting of the amino acid residues 540-548 of hTERT (human Telomerase Reverse Transcriptase). Vaccination with telomerase:540-548 peptide may stimulate cytotoxic T-lymphocytes to recognize and kill telomerase expressing cells.

Many tumor cells over-express mutant P53 proteins, which are responsible for the loss of apoptosis regulation and abnormal cell proliferation. Mutant P53 peptide pulsed dendritic cell vaccine is a cancer vaccine that consists of autologous dendritic cells, which have been pulsed with a mutant P53 peptide. Vaccination with mutant P53 peptide pulsed dendritic cells may stimulate the host immune system to mount a cytotoxic T-lymphocyte response against tumor cells that contain a somatic mutation in P53, thus resulting in tumor cell lysis.

Tumor associated antigens may turn T-lymphocytes against tumors.
Vaccines that incorporate tumor associated antigens (or their epitope peptides) may induce specific antibodies and elicit a specific $CD8^{+}$ cytotoxic T-lymphocyte response.

11.4 Cytokine Based Immunotherapy

Attack on cancer by focussing the immune response on the tumor has appeal because the immune system can equally well fight the primary tumor as metastases and the toxicity of this approach compared to chemotherapy or radiation is low. It is important, however, to trigger an efficient immune reaction since most tumors have low immunogenicity and some cancers even employ immunosuppressive mechanisms. Cytokines act as mediators and enhancers of immune responses. The cytokine profile (Th1 or Th2)[8] accompanying an immunotherapeutic regimen is an important determinant for successful outcome (Table 11.4). Both arms of

[8] There are 2 main sub-sets of T-lymphocytes, distinguished by the presence of the cell surface molecule CD4 (helper T-cells) or CD8 (effector T-cells). T-lymphocytes expressing CD4 support the immune response in part through cytokine secretion. This sub-set is further divided into Th1 and Th2 cells, the former stimulate a cellular immune response while the latter stimulate a humoral immune response.

Table 11.4 Basic types of immune responses

	Humoral response	Cellular response
Protection	Bacterial infections	Viral infections
Onset	Rapid (24–48 h)	Slower (about 72 h)
Induction	TH2 cytokines	TH1 cytokines
Effectors	B-lymphocytes, antibodies	T-lymphocytes, NK cells

the immune system can contribute to an efficient anti-tumor reaction. The transduction of irradiated tumor cells with cytokines is intended to not only activate the immune system but also direct the response to a predominantly cellular or humoral type. Suitably chosen cytokine treatment regimens may break the host tolerance to cancer cells (Table 11.5). Vaccination with cancer cells transfected with GM-CSF may have been particularly successful because this cytokine induces both cellular (Th1) and humoral (Th2) responses. The effect of GM-CSF is, however, compromised by its limited potency to induce cellular immunity. This may reflect the inability of GM-CSF to regulate the inducer cytokines IL-10 or IL-12. Its targeting of downstream effectors allows more distally acting cytokines to still direct the immune system toward cellular activation.

Glenn Dranoff demonstrated the high effectiveness of irradiated tumor cells transduced with the cytokine GM-CSF (Granulocyte Macrophage-Colony-Stimulating Factor) in stimulating anti-tumor immunity (Dranoff et al. 1993). GM-CSF binds to specific cell surface receptors on various immuno-hematopoietic cell types, enhancing their proliferation and differentiation and stimulating macrophage and dendritic cell functions in antigen presentation and anti-tumor immunity.

Table 11.5 Cytokine based immunotherapy

Granulocyte Macrophage-Colony-Stimulating Factor (GM-CSF)
Recombinant oncolytic adenovirus GM-CSF vaccine
Recombinant fowlpox GM-CSF vaccine
Allogeneic irradiated cancer cells transfected *gm-csf*
Autologous antigen presenting cells exposed to GM-CSF fused to PAP <Sipuleucel-T>
Interleukin-2 (IL-2)
Recombinant aldesleukin <Proleukin>
Recombinant fusion protein of IL-2 and diphtheria toxin denileukin diftitox <Ontak>
Interleukin-12 (IL-12)
Replication defective recombinant canarypox virus (ALVAC) encoding IL-12
Plasmid DNA encoding IL-12 embedded in polymer (EGEN-001)
Interferon (IFN)
IFN-α2
PEG-interferon α <Sylatron>
Recombinant adenovirus-hIFN-β
IFN-γ

- Oncolytic adenovirus encoding GM-CSF is a recombinant oncolytic adenovirus that carries the gene for the immune-hematopoietic cytokine GM-CSF. Upon administration, the oncolytic adenovirus selectively infects and reduplicates in tumor cells, which may result in tumor cells lysis. Synergistically, the expressed GM-CSF may promote a cytotoxic T-lymphocyte response against tumor cells that harbor the oncolytic adenovirus, resulting in immune mediated tumor cell death. This agent promotes antigen presentation, up-regulates antibody-dependent cellular cytotoxicity (ADCC), and increases Interleukin-2 mediated lymphokine-activated killer cell function. GM-CSF plasmid DNA is used as a vaccine adjuvant for melanoma, hepatocellular carcinoma, and pancreatic cancer.
- Recombinant fowlpox GM-CSF vaccine adjuvant is a cancer vaccine adjuvant consisting of a recombinant fowlpox virus that encodes GM-CSF. Administration of recombinant the fowlpox GM-CSF vaccine adjuvant may induce an immune response against tumor cells. The fowlpox virus vector is reduplication incompetent in mammalian cells.
- An allogeneic vaccine consisting of irradiated breast cancer cells (in some protocols 2 types of breast tumor cells developed from distinct patients) transfected with the *gm-csf* gene (GM-CSF BREAST VAC) is in use. Upon vaccination, the genetically modified cells secrete GM-CSF, thereby potentiating a tumor-specific T-lymphocyte response against breast cancer cell associated antigens. The vaccine is given in 12 injections into multiple sites.
- Sipuleucel-T (APC8015) <Provenge> is a cell-based vaccine composed of autologous antigen presenting peripheral blood mononuclear cells (enriched for a dendritic cell fraction) that have been exposed to a recombinant protein consisting of GM-CSF fused to Prostatic-Acid Phosphatase (PAP), a protein expressed by prostate cancer cells. Upon administration, the vaccine may stimulate an anti-tumor T-lymphocyte response against cancer cells expressing PAP.

Interleukin-2 (IL-2) was originally named T-Cell Growth Factor (TCGF) because it supports the proliferation of T-lymphocytes. This cytokine is involved in intercellular communication related to hematopoietic cell differentiation and proliferation, inflammation, and hormone release. Interleukin-2 binds to and activates specific receptors, triggering the expression of genes that may induce T-lymphocyte mediated tumor regression in some cancer types.

- As a therapeutic, the recombinant analog of endogenous Interleukin-2, aldesleukin <Proleukin>, is used to activate lymphocyte mediated anti-tumor reactions. The drug has been applied with some success in the treatment of renal cell carcinoma and melanoma. Its efficacy, however, has for the most part been limited to low response rates.
- Against melanoma, Interleukin-2 <Proleukin> offers the possibility of a complete and long lasting remission, although only in a small percentage of patients.
- Denileukin diftitox <Ontak> is a recombinant fusion protein that combines the active sections of both IL-2 and diphtheria toxin. Unconjugated diphtheria toxin is too toxic to administer. However, after conjugation its cytotoxic effects are directed toward cells that express the high-affinity form of the IL-2 Receptor (CD25), as is the case in persistent or recurrent cutaneous T-cell lymphoma, in which malignant cells express abundant CD25. Once denileukin diftitox interacts with the IL-2 Receptors, the toxin inhibits protein synthesis in the cancer cells and causes their death.

Adverse Effects Denileukin diftitox produces acute hypersensitivity reactions, influenza-like symptoms (sometimes with prominent diarrhea), and vascular leak syndrome. It differs from the vascular leak syndrome produced by high-dose IL-2 in that it occurs in fewer patients, is delayed in onset, is usually self-limited, and does not consistently recur on re-treatment. Patients with Albumin levels below 3 g/dL are at increased risk for vascular leak syndrome and the use of denileukin diftitox in these patients is not recommended.

The most common dose limiting toxicities of IL-2 are hypotension, fluid retention, and renal dysfunction. IL-2 decreases peripheral vascular resistance, producing vasodilation, tachycardia, and hypotension. A characteristic vascular leak syndrome (capillary leak syndrome) produces fluid retention, which can cause respiratory compromise. These toxicities require administration of vasopressors in most patients, judicious use of fluid support and diuretics, and supplemental oxygen. Patients with underlying cardiovascular or renal compromise are more susceptible to these adverse effects, and should be selected with caution for therapy. Most patients treated with high dose IL-2 experience thrombocytopenia, anemia, eosinophilia, reversible cholestasis, and skin erythema with burning and pruritus. In some patients neuropsychiatric changes, hypothyroidism, and bacterial infections are possible. In general, the toxicities from IL-2 therapy reverse quickly after discontinuation and can be managed by careful prospective monitoring and pharmacological supportive care. Patients need to be premedicated with an anti-histamine or acetaminophen prior to each infusion. They should be monitored for symptoms of capillary leak syndrome (hypotension, hypoalbuminemia, edema, weight gain).

Interleukin 12 (IL-12) is produced by dendritic cells, macrophages and B-lymphoblastoid cells in response to antigenic stimulation. The cytokine is involved in the differentiation of naïve T-cells into Th1 cells. It accomplishes this by stimulating the production of Interferon-γ (IFN-γ) and Tumor Necrosis Factor-α (TNF-α) from T-cells and natural killer (NK) cells, and by reducing the IL-4 mediated suppression of IFN-γ. IL-12 induces an enhancement of the cytotoxic activity of natural killer cells and $CD8^+$ cytotoxic T lymphocytes.

- Canarypox-hIL-12 melanoma vaccine consists of a reduplication defective recombinant canarypox virus (ALVAC) that encodes the gene for Interleukin-12. Vaccination with this agent may stimulate the host immune system to mount a response against tumor cells, thereby inhibiting tumor growth or metastasis. Canarypox-hIL-12 melanoma vaccine is intended to induce anti-tumor effects through the IL-12 mediated activation of natural killer cells, cytotoxic T-lymphocyte responses, and the release of Interferon-γ.
- EGEN-001 is a non-viral vector consisting of a plasmid DNA that encodes the *interleukin-12* gene, embedded in a biocompatible and biodegradable delivery polymer. EGEN-001 is designed to increase the local concentration of IL-12 in the tumor micro-environment, which may potentiate anti-tumoral functions of the host immune system, resulting in immune-mediated tumor regression.

Interferons (IFNs) constitute a large protein family, encoded by more than 300 genes. Interferons (Isaacs and Lindenmann 1957) are capable of inducing cell cycle arrest. Defects in their signal transduction pathways are associated with cellular immortalization, an important early event in the development of cancer. The immunologic anti-tumor activity of Interferons may be mediated by

- augmented lytic activity of immune effector cells. Both T-cell and natural killer cell expansion and lytic activity can be promoted by Interferons; Interferon-γ exerts its effects through the generation of tumor specific $CD4^+$ Th1 T-lymphocytes, supporting the generation of cytolytic T-cells and activation of cytocidal activity in macrophages,
- the migration of the T-cells to tumors, stimulated by Interferon-γ
- an enhanced immunogenicity of tumor cells; Interferon-γ up-regulates the expression of HLA-I and promotes tumor cell recognition and elimination by $CD8^+$ T-lymphocytes. Interferon-γ can also up-regulate the tumor associated antigens Carcinoembryonic Antigen (CEA) and TAG72.

Type I Interferons act through a cell surface receptor composed of 2 ubiquitously expressed transmembrane proteins, IFNAR1 and IFNAR2 (Interferon-α/β Receptors 1 and 2). IFN-γ is a single glycosylated protein of 140 amino acids that is designated as a type II Interferon. Like type I Interferons, it binds to 2 cytokine receptor proteins. IFNGR1 (Interferon-γ Receptor 1) has a JAK1 binding domain and a STAT1 docking site. IFNGR2 contains a JAK2 binding domain.

The initial U.S. FDA approval for the treatment of a chronic B-cell (hairy cell) leukemia with IFN-α2 was driven by publicity that resulted from its effectiveness in American Cancer Society trials. In hairy cell leukemia and chronic myelogenous leukemia (CML), IFN-α2 decreases marrow infiltration with malignant cells and normalizes peripheral hematologic cell counts. Over 90% of patients with chronic myelogenous leukemia with complete cytogenetic response remain in remission at 10 years. However, the survival advantage for IFN-α2 has now been exceeded by the effectiveness of the targeted inhibitor of the chimeric kinase BCR-ABL. There is therapeutic effectiveness of IFN-α2 in causing partial disease regression in myeloma, lymphomata, renal cell carcinoma, bladder carcinoma, melanoma, and Kaposi sarcoma (Borden et al. 2007). The combination of Interferon-α with bortezomib causes apoptosis in melanoma cells. Because this drug combination activates complementary death pathways it even kills cells with high levels of BCL-2 and MCL-1. Cure of metastatic malignancies can result when micro-metastases are eliminated in patients at high risk for recurrence after surgical removal of a primary tumor. This surgical adjuvant approach is the basis for administering IFN-α2 in patients at high risk for recurrence of melanoma. Intralesional administration of IFN-α into basal cell carcinomata may induce regression. Renal cell carcinoma is treated with immunomodulating agents, such as Interferon α2b <Intron A> and Interferon α2a <Roferon-A>,

PEG-interferon α <Sylatron> is a PEGylated Interferon. The polyethylene glycol (PEG) protects the molecule from proteolytic breakdown and increases the biological half-life of the Interferon protein. PEGylated Interferon α2b is used in the treatment of myeloproliferative neoplasms, of melanoma with nodal involvement after surgical resection, and of patients with neurofibromatosis to shrink the neurofibromata.

Recombinant adenovirus-hIFN-β is a recombinant, reduplication defective adenovirus, which encodes the gene for the cytokine Interferon-β (IFN-β). Once inserted into and reduplicating in host tumor cells, recombinant adenovirus-hIFN-β expresses Interferon-β, which may stimulate an anti-proliferative natural killer cell response against tumor cells and induce Caspase mediated tumor cell apoptosis.

Critical roles in the immune surveillance against and protection from cancer are played by Interferon-γ (Kaplan et al. 1998; Dighe et al. 1994; Shankaran et al. 2001). Interferon-γ induces increased susceptibility to apoptosis by FAS activators and cytotoxic chemotherapies in various cell types, including melanoma and colorectal carcinoma (Ugurel et al. 1999; Schwartzberg et al. 2002).

Adverse Effects Interferon toxicities are dose related and can be challenging at the high dose used for melanoma. With the initial dose, malaise, fever and chills, which last for a few hours, dominate, but tachyphylaxis occurs with subsequent injections. Fatigue and anorexia are often dose limiting with chronic administration. At higher doses, weight loss occurs and may be substantial (>10%). Reversible elevation of hepatic Transaminases can occur, as can hematologic effects, most markedly granulocytopenia (Borden et al. 2007).

Cytokines act as mediators and enhancers of immune responses.
The cytokine profile accompanying an immunotherapeutic regimen is important for outcome.
Cellular and humoral immunity can contribute to an efficient anti-tumor reaction.

11.5 Immune Response Modifiers

Biological response modifiers (BRMs) are compounds that are used to treat cancer by altering or augmenting naturally occurring processes within the body. Immunotherapy makes use of immune response modifiers (IRMs) for enhancing the activity of the immune system to increase the body's natural defense mechanisms against cancer (Table 11.6).

Table 11.6 Immune response modifiers

Name	Agent	Target cell	Function
Ipilimumab	Anti-CTLA-4	T-lymphocyte	Co-activation
Imiquimod	TLR-7 ligand		Stimulation of cytokine production
IMP321	High affinity ligand for MHC class II on dendritic cells	Dendritic cell	Maturation, antigen cross-presentation, migration to lymph nodes
Talactoferrin		Dendritic cell	Cell recruiter and activator
Talabostat mesylate	Dipeptidyl Peptidase inhibitor		Stimulation of cytokine and chemokine production
Virulizin		Macrophage	Activation

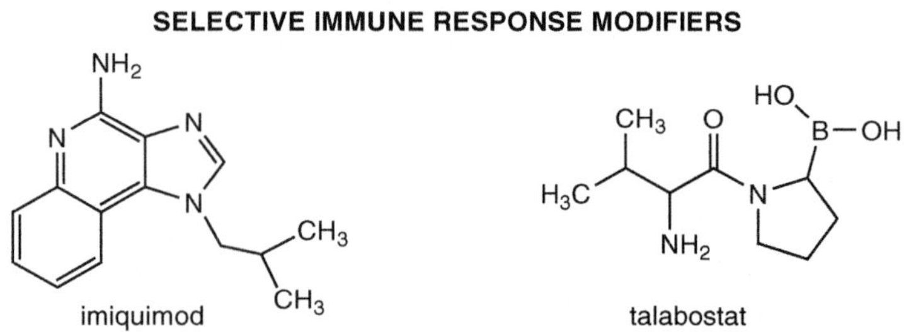

Fig. 11.3 Structures of immune response modifiers

Cytotoxic T lymphocytes can recognize and destroy cancer cells. This requires their activation through the T-Cell Antigen Receptor plus suitable co-stimulatory molecules. By contrast, the co-engagement of the inhibitory receptor CTLA-4 (Cytotoxic T-Lymphocyte Associated Antigen-4, CD152) on T-lymphocytes transmits a suppressive signal that limits activation and proliferation of T-lymphocytes. CTLA-4 was discovered in 1987. In 1996, James Allison showed that antibodies to CTLA-4 erased tumors in mice. In 2011, anti-CTLA-4 became the first treatment to prolong life in a randomized trial for advanced melanoma.

Ipilimumab (MDX-010) <Yervoy> is a monoclonal antibody directed to CTLA-4. By binding to its target, ipilimumab blocks the suppressive signal and enhances T-lymphocyte activation. It also induces the death of regulatory T-lymphocytes. The drug is under investigation for the treatment of late-stage melanoma (approved by the U.S. FDA in 2011, by Health Canada and the European Union in 2012), non-small cell lung carcinoma (NSCLC), small cell lung cancer (SCLC) and metastatic hormone-refractory prostate cancer.

Adverse Effects The T-lymphocyte activation and proliferation supported by ipilimumab treatment may cause severe immunological adverse events (typically based on autoimmune inflammation). Most of the common adverse effects are associated with the gastro-intestinal tract, comprising stomach pain, bloating, constipation, or diarrhea. The pituitary gland may suffer inflammation. Others include fever, difficulty breathing, or urinating problems. A risk evaluation and mitigation strategy has been developed for the use of ipilimumab. It consists of a communication plan to inform potential prescribers and supportive healthcare providers about serious adverse reactions.

PD-1 was discovered in the early 1990s. Monoclonal antibodies that antagonize the interaction of the negative regulatory receptor PD-1 (Programmed Death-1) with its ligands PD-L1 or PD-L2 may act in an immunostimulatory fashion. The anti-PD-1 antibodies nivolumab and lambrolizumab target PD-1 on T-lymphocytes. The antibody MPDL3280A binds to PD-L1 on tumor cells. By 2008, responses occurred in the first clinical trial of an anti-PD1 antibody. Some tumors keep responding even after discontinuation of the antibody, implying an active anti-tumor immune response.

Adverse Effects Blocking PD-1 prevents its interactions with PD1-L2 on antigen presenting cells in the lungs and may increase the risk for pneumonitis.

Imiquimod (1-(2-methylpropyl)-1*H*-imidazo[4,5-c]quinolin-4-amine) <Aldara, Zyclara, Beselna> is a synthetic agent with immune response modifying activity (Fig. 11.3). It activates immune cells through Toll-Like Receptor-7 (TLR7), a receptor that is commonly involved in pathogen recognition. As an immune response modifier, imiquimod stimulates the production of cytokines, especially Interferon, and enhances anti-tumor activity, particularly against cutaneous cancers. Also, a pro-apoptotic activity of imiquimod may be related to counter-acting the BCL-2 over-expression in susceptible tumor cells. The agent is indicated for actinic keratoses on the face or scalp and for superficial basal cell carcinoma when surgery is impractical. It received U.S. FDA approval in 1997.

Adverse Effects An anaphylactic event requires immediate medical attention. Adverse reactions include erythema, skin erosion, scabbing, edema, burning or soreness. The itching sensation caused by the drug can exacerbate the dermatitis. Headache, flu-like symptoms, myalgia, hypo- or hyper-pigmentation, and hyperkeratosis may occur.

Conditioning of the macrophage/dendritic cell network may be accomplished through the activation of Toll-Like Receptors as immunopotentiators or through the provision of ligands that enhance the antigen presenting activity of dendritic cells. Such ligands include CD40L and LAG-3 (Lymphocyte-Activation Gene 3, CD223). The clinical development of CD40L has been curtailed due to thrombosis induction (its receptor, CD40, is also expressed on platelets and endothelial cells). Thus, LAG-3 is presently the only protein available for this therapeutic approach.

The soluble LAG-3Ig fusion protein IMP321 <ImmuFact> is a recombinant T-lymp hocyte immunostimulatory factor derived from the soluble form of the protein LAG-3. Upon administration by repeated subcutaneous injections, alone or in combination with tumor antigens, IMP321 binds with high affinity to MHC class II molecules on dendritic cells and a fraction of macrophages. This interaction may result in dendritic cell maturation, dendritic cell migration to the lymph nodes, enhanced dendritic cell cross-presentation of antigens to T-lymphocytes, and anti-tumor cytotoxic T-lymphocyte responses. The drug effect is associated with the induction of various cytokines.

In the treatment of cancer, activated dendritic cells may identify tumor cells as targets and present this information to effector cells, with the consequence of triggering an anti-tumor immune response. The recombinant Lactoferrin, Talactoferrin α, is a targeted dendritic cell recruiter and activator. Orally administered, Talactoferrin is not absorbed. It binds to cells in the gut wall, leads to the release of cytokines and chemokines, and induces the recruitment of immature dendritic cells to the gut associated lymphoid tissue (GALT). Talactoferrin promotes the maturation of dendritic cells that have captured tumor antigens. Following their maturation, these dendritic cells activate natural killer cells of the innate immune pathway and $CD8^+$ lymphocytes of the adaptive immune pathway. Because the Talactoferrin effect is initiated distal to the tumor site it may be protected from immune evasion mechanisms used by the tumor cells, and may enhance the anti-tumor immune response initiated by dendritic cell-based immunotherapies. Talactoferrin α is indicated in combination with sunitinib for the first-line treatment of renal cell carcinoma.

Dipeptidyl Peptidases are involved in the activation of polypeptide hormones and chemokines. Talabostat mesylate ([(2R)-1-[(2S)-2-Amino-3-methylbutanoyl]pyrrolidin-2-yl] boronic acid mesylate) (PT-100) is the salt of an orally active small molecule with anti-neoplastic and hematopoiesis stimulating activities. By cleaving *N*-terminal X-proline or X-alanine residues, talabostat inhibits Dipeptidyl Peptidases, such as FAP (Fibroblast Activation Protein), resulting in the stimulation of cytokine and chemokine production with consecutive anti-tumor T-cell immunity. This agent may also stimulate the production of Colony Stimulating Factors, such as G-CSF (Ganulocyte Colony Stimulating Factor), resulting in the stimulation of hematopoiesis. It is under investigation for the treatment of lung, pancreas, and brain cancer.

Virulizin is a natural biological response modifier that constitutes a mixture of proteins and peptides extracted from bovine reticuloendothelial tissue. Virizulin activates macrophages and may enhance the cell mediated immune response to tumors. It is being developed for the treatment of pancreatic cancer, lung adenocarcinoma, advanced malignant melanoma, and Kaposi sarcoma in HIV patients. The agent may be given as first or second-line treatment in combination with chemotherapy drugs.

Biological response modifiers (BRMs) alter or augment naturally occurring processes within the body.
Immune response modifiers (IRMs) enhance the activity of the immune system to increase natural defense mechanisms against cancer.

11.6 Autologous Therapies

Sipuleucel-T <Provenge> is a cell based vaccine composed of autologous antigen presenting peripheral blood mononuclear cells (enriched for a dendritic cell fraction) after having been exposed to a recombinant protein consisting of Granulocyte-Macrophage Colony-Stimulating Factor (GM-CSF) fused to PAP (Prostatic-Acid Phosphatase), a protein expressed by prostate cancer cells. The therapeutic intent is to generate PAP-specific T-lymphocytes cells capable of recognizing and killing prostate cancer cells that express the antigen. After radical prostatectomy, the major remaining source of PAP in the body is the cancerous prostate tissue. The vaccine immunogen is formulated as PA2024, a fusion protein that combines recombinant PAP with recombinant GM-CSF. The triggered immune response is enhanced by the cytokine. In 2010, sipuleucel-T was the first targeted immunotherapeutic to be approved by the U.S. FDA for the treatment of patients with asymptomatic or minimally symptomatic metastatic castration-resistant prostate cancer. In these patients, sipuleucel-T prolongs the median survival by 4 months. At 3 years, the proportion of survivors may increase by 50%.

The PAP-GM-CSF fusion protein is incubated with autologous peripheral blood mononuclear cells obtained by leukapheresis. GM-CSF activates antigen presenting cells within these cell pools, which then induce the proliferation of PAP specific T-lymphocytes with the capacity to recognize and kill PAP expressing prostate cancer cells. 3 days after leukapheresis and after around 40 hours of incubation, the cells are washed to remove the fusion protein, and reinfused into the patient.

Adverse Effects Around 70% of patients experience acute infusion reactions, with most events being mild or moderate. The most common events, which occur in over 20% of patients, are chills, pyrexia, and fatigue. These effects generally arise within 1 day of an infusion and most are resolved within 2 days. Severe (grade 3) acute infusion reactions arise in fewer than 5% of patients and include asthenia, dyspnea, hypoxia, bronchospasm, dizziness, headache, hypertension, muscle ache, nausea, and vomiting. Fewer than 1% of patients are unable to receive all 3 infusions because of infusion related adverse effects.

Carcinoembryonic Antigen peptide 1-6D (CEA:571-579 (576D), mCEA Peptide) is a 9 residue HLA-restricted fragment of Carcinoembryonic Antigen. It comprises the amino acids 571-579, which have the sequence YLSGANLNL. A cancer vaccine consists of dendritic cells harvested from a patient with cancer and pulsed or transduced with the peptide fragment in vitro. Vaccination with these activated autologous dendritic cells or peripheral blood mononuclear cells may stimulate the host immune system to mount a cytotoxic T-lymphocyte response against tumor cells expressing Carcinoembryonic Antigen.

Table 11.7 Anti idiotype antibodies

Antibody	Antigen	Function	Cancer
105AD7	CD55	Decay accelerating factor for complement	Colon, breast, gastric, ovarian cancer
11D10	HMFG	Lipid delivery carrier	Breast cancer
Monoclonal antibody GD2 anti-idiotype vaccine	GD2	Component of the cell plasma membrane that modulates cell signal transduction events	Tumors of neuroectodermal origin (melanoma, neuroblastoma, sarcoma, small cell lung cancer)

The Center for Immunotherapy at Roswell Park Cancer Institute (RPCI) has initiated clinical trials of a NY-ESO-1 dendritic cell vaccine. Dendritic cells act as gatekeepers of the immune system. The vaccine incorporates a particular form of NY-ESO-1, anti-DEC205-NY-ESO-1. The treated cells are then reinfused to the patient as a vaccine designed to recruit killer cells that destroy the cancer cells.

Autologous dendritic vaccines have been primed with various tumor associated antigens, including epitope peptides of α-Fetoprotein (AFP) or mutant P53, and are under investigation.

Autologous therapies are matched to the patient.
Dendritic cells are effective antigen presenting cells in autologous therapies.
The implementation of autologous therapies is resource-intensive.

11.7 Other Regimens

Allogeneic idiotype vaccines Allogeneic dendritic cell-myeloma idiotype vaccine is a cell based vaccine composed of allogeneic dendritic cells pulsed ex vivo with an autologous myeloma idiotype. Upon administration, this vaccine may stimulate the host immune system to mount a specific cytotoxic T-lymphocyte response against myeloma cells, resulting in cell lysis.

Autologous immunoglobulin idiotype-KLH conjugate vaccine is a cancer vaccine composed of tumor specific idiotype determinants derived from patient tumor cells, which are conjugated to the immunostimulant carrier protein Keyhole Limpet Hemocyanin (KLH). When injected into the individual from whom the tumor cells were isolated, this vaccine may stimulate an anti-cancer cytotoxic T-lymphocytic immune response.

Anti-idiotype antibodies Idiotopes and allotypes are the 2 types of Immunoglobulin epitopes identified by monoclonal antibodies. Allotopes are mostly localized within the heavy and light chain constant regions of the Immunoglobulin and are inherited through the germline. Idiotopes are localized only in the hypervariable regions of the Immunoglobulin variable domains and are somatically generated. Whereas allotopes can be recognized as foreign because they are not shared by different individuals, idiotopes can be recognized as foreign because the extremely low abundance of them normally present in any individual is insufficient to elicit self-tolerance (Bendandi 2001). In 1982, Ron Levy and co-workers reported on the treatment of human B-cell lymphoma by means of a custom made, patient-, tumor- and idiotype-specific monoclonal antibody (Miller et al. 1982).

Monoclonal antibody 105AD7 anti-idiotype vaccine (Table 11.7) is a cancer vaccine consisting of a humanized monoclonal antibody that mimics the tumor associated antigen CD55 (791Tgp72). Vaccination with this agent may stimulate a host cytotoxic T-lymphocyte response against tumor cells that express CD55, resulting in tumor cell lysis.

Monoclonal antibody 11D10 anti-idiotype vaccine is a vaccine consisting of a monoclonal antibody directed to an idiotype that mimics a Human Milk Fat Globule (HMFG) membrane epitope. Vaccination with monoclonal antibody 11D10 anti-idiotype vaccine induces anti-anti-idiotype antibodies (Ab3), which may react with breast cancer cells that express the HMFG membrane epitope.

Monoclonal antibody GD2 anti-idiotype vaccine belongs to a class of vaccines that consist of anti-idiotype monoclonal antibodies against the tumor associated antigen disialoganglioside GD2. Vaccination with a monoclonal antibody GD2 anti-idiotype vaccine produces an Immunoglobulin response to GD2 with subsequent destruction of GD2 expressing tumor cells via antibody-dependent cellular cytotoxicity (ADCC). GD2 is over-expressed in melanoma, neuroblastoma, soft tissue sarcoma, and small cell carcinoma of the lung.

Mimotopes Non-peptidic epitopes may not stimulate an effective immune response when administered as vaccines. Synthetic peptides that mimic those epitopes (mimotopes) may substitute in active immunization strategies.

GD2 is a promising target for anti-tumor immunotherapy. However, the antigen itself cannot be used as an effective immunogen due to its glycolipid nature. Carbohydrates are mostly T-lymphocyte independent antigens. As they elicit no T-lymphocyte help, relatively low antibody titers and no memory responses are induced. In order to antigenically enhance GD2, the carbohydrate antigen has been translated into mimicking peptides. Decapeptide mimics, circularized by disulfide bonds between terminal cysteines, of an epitope on the GD2 antigen may serve as mimotopes.

References

Bendandi M (2001) Role of anti-idiotype vaccines in the modern treatment of human follicular lymphoma. Expert Rev Anticancer Ther 1:65–72

Borden EC, Sen GC, Uze G, Silverman RH, Ransohoff RM, Foster GR, Stark GR (2007) Interferons at age 50: past, current and future impact on biomedicine. Nat Rev Drug Discov 6:975–990

Busch W (1868) Aus der Sitzung der Medicinischen Section vom 13. November 1867. Berliner Klinische Wochenschrift 5:137

Coley WB (1893) The treatment of malignant tumors by repeated inoculations of Erysipelas, with a report of ten original cases. Am J Med Sci 105:487–511

Coley W (1896) Further observations upon the treatment of malignant tumours with the toxins of erysipelas and Bacillus prodigiosus with a report of 160 cases. Bull Johns Hopkins Hosp 7:57

Connell H (1935) The study treatment of cancer by proteolytic enzymes, a preliminary report. Can Med Assoc J 33:364–370

Dighe AS, Richards E, Old LJ, Schreiber RD (1994) Enhanced in vivo growth and resistance to rejection of tumor cells expressing dominant negative IFN g receptors. Immunity 1:447–456

DiPaola RS, Plante M, Kaufman H, Petrylak DP, Israeli R, Lattime E, Manson K, Schuetz T (2006) A phase I trial of Pox PSA vaccines (PROSTVAC®-VF) with B7–1, ICAM-1, and LFA-3 co-stimulatory molecules (TRICOM™) in patients with prostate cancer. J Transl Med 4:1

Doronina SO, Toki BE, Torgov MY, Mendelsohn BA, Cerveny CG, Chace DF, DeBlanc RL, Gearing RP, Bovee TD, Siegall CB, Francisco JA, Wahl AF, Meyer DL, Senter PD (2003) Development of potent monoclonal antibody auristatin conjugates for cancer therapy. Nat Biotechnol 21:778–784

Dranoff G, Jaffee E, Lazenby A, Golumbek P, Levitsky H, Brose K, Jackson V, Hamada H, Pardoll D, Mulligan RC (1993) Vaccination with irradiated tumor cells engineered to secrete murine granulocyte-macrophage colony-stimulating factor stimulates potent, specific, and long-lasting anti-tumor immunity. Proc Natl Acad Sci U S A 90:3539–3543

Drummond DC, Meyer O, Hong K, Kirpotin DB (1999) Papahadjopoulos. Optimizing liposomes for delivery of chemotherapeutic agents to solid tumors. Pharmacol Rev 51:692–743

Ehrlich P (1909) Ueber den jetzigen Stand der Karzinomforschung. Nederlands Tijdschrift voor Geneeskunde 53:273–290

Fehleisen VI (1882) Ueber die Zuechtung der Erysipelkokken auf kunstlichem Nahrboden und ihre Uebertragbarkeit auf den Menschen. Deutsche Medizinische Wochenschrift 8:553–554

Isaacs A, Lindenmann J (1957) Virus interference. I. The interferon. Proc R Soc Lond B Biol Sci 147:258–267

Jaracz S, Chen J, Kuznetsova LV, Ojima I (2005) Recent advances in tumor-targeting anticancer drug conjugates. Bioorg Med Chem 13:5043–5054

Kaplan DH, Shankaran V, Dighe AS, Stockert E, Aguet M, Old LJ, Schreiber RD (1998) Demonstration of an interferon γ-dependent tumor surveillance system in immunocompetent mice. Proc Natl Acad Sci U S A 95:7556–7561

Karpovsky B, Titus JA, Stephany DA, Segal DM (1984) Production of target-specific effector cells using hetero-cross-linked aggregates containing anti-target cell and anti-Fc gamma receptor antibodies. J Exp Med 160:1686–1701

Kirpotin D, Park JW, Hong K, Zalipsky S, Li WL, Carter P, Benz CC, Papahadjopoulos D (1997) Sterically stabilized anti-HER2 immunoliposomes: design and targeting to human breast cancer cells in vitro. Biochemistry 36:66–75

Lindhofer H, Mocikat R, Steipe B, Thierfelder S (1995) Preferential species-restricted heavy/light chain pairing in rat/mouse quadromas. Implications for a single-step purification of bispecific antibodies. J Immunol 155:219–225

Maruyama K (2002) PEG-Immunoliposome. Biosci Rep 22:251–266

McLaughlin P, Grillo-Lopez AJ, Link BK, Levy R, Czuczman MS, Williams ME, Heyman MR, Bence-Bruckler I, White CA, Cabanillas F, Jain V, Ho AD, Lister J, Wey K, Shen D, Dallaire BK (1998) Rituximab chimeric anti-CD20 monoclonal antibody therapy for relapsed indolent lymphoma: half of patients respond to a four-dose treatment program. J Clin Oncol 16:2825–2833

Miller RA, Maloney DG, Warnke R, Levy R (1982) Treatment of B-cell lymphoma with monoclonal anti-idiotype antibody. N Engl J Med 4:517–522

Morales A, Eidinger D, Bruce AW (2002) Intracavitary Bacillus Calmette-Guerin in the treatment of superficial bladder tumors. 1976. J Urol 167:891–893

Shintani Y, Sawada Y, Inagaki T, Kohjimoto Y, Uekado Y, Shinka T (2007) Intravesical instillation therapy with bacillus Calmette-Guerin for superficial bladder cancer: study of the mechanism of bacillus Calmette-Guerin immunotherapy. Int J Urol 14:140–146

Schrama D, Reisfeld RA, Becker JC (2006) Antibody targeted drugs as cancer therapeutics. Nat Rev Drug Discov 5:147–159

Schwartzberg LS, Petak I, Stewart C, Turner PK, Ashley J, Tillman DM, Douglas L, Tan M, Billups C, Mihalik R, Weir A, Tauer K, Shope S, Houghton JA (2002) Modulation of the Fas signaling pathway by IFN-g in therapy of colon cancer: phase I trial and correlative studies of IFN-g, 5-fluorouracil, and leukovorin. Clin Cancer Res 8:2488–2498

Shankaran V, Ikeda H, Bruce AT, White JM, Swanson PE, Old LJ, Schreiber RD (2001) IFNg and lymphocytes prevent primary tumour development and shape tumour immunogenicity. Nature 410:1107–1111

Sievers EL, Linenberger M (2001) Mylotarg: antibody-targeted chemotherapy comes of age. Curr Opin Oncol 13:522–527

Ugurel S, Seiter S, Rappl G, Stark A, Tilgen W, Reinhold U (1999) Heterogenous susceptibility to CD95-induced apoptosis in melanoma cells correlates with Bcl-2 and Bcl-x expression and is sensitive to modulation by interferon-g. Int J Cancer 82:727–736

Wei MQ, Mengesha A, Good D, Anné J (2008) Bacterial targeted tumour therapy-dawn of a new era. Cancer Lett 259:16–27

12 Anti-Angiogenesis

An adequate supply of oxygen and nutrients is critical for tissue homeostasis. These are delivered and metabolic end products are eliminated through the vascular system. Once a tumor grows to about 1–2 mm in diameter, the generation of new blood vessels becomes a prerequisite for further growth as the transport needs cannot be satisfied by diffusion beyond this size. Therefore, angiogenesis, the sprouting of new blood vessels from existing ones, is an essential process in the progression of cancer. It is initiated by a degradation of the extracellular matrix, followed by cell migration, proliferation and capillary tube formation of endothelial cells, and is completed by maturation. The secreted molecules and cell surface receptors that regulate this process constitute potential drug targets (Fig. 12.1).

Angiogenesis inhibitors induce only stabilization of disease—not eradication of cancer cells, but the induction of tumor dormancy is considered to be a clinically useful outcome that may increase overall survival. Because angiogenesis is also an essential component of metastasis, several agents that curb metastasis have suppressive effects on angiogenesis as well. The toxicity of angiogenesis inhibitors is generally modest.

A treatment concept for angiostatic therapy follows the paradigm of continuously (metronomically) dosed chemotherapeutics combined with pro-apoptotic biomodulators. Metronomic chemotherapy involves the administration of drugs at a reduced dose compared with traditional treatment regimens but at regular, more frequent intervals without extended rest periods (Kerbel and Kamen 2004). In contrast to the traditional maximum tolerated dose treatment, metronomic chemotherapy not only is cytotoxic against tumor cells but also exerts an anti-angiogenic effect toward the tumor associated endothelial cells. The anti-endothelial activity is due in part to the high intrinsic sensitivity of proliferating endothelial cells to chemotherapeutic drugs and in part to the induction of the endogenous angiogenesis inhibitor Thrombospondin-1 (TSP-1) (Bocci et al. 2003).

Angiogenesis is an essential process in cancer progression. The molecules that regulate this process constitute potential drug targets.
Angiogenesis inhibitors induce only stabilization of disease—not eradication of cancer cells.
Unlike the treatment cycles of traditional maximum-tolerated-dose chemotherapy, the dose schedule of anti-angiogenesis therapy is often metronomic.

12.1 VEGF Antagonists

12.1.1 VEGF Receptor Blockers

Secreted molecules that regulate the formation of new blood vessels include growth factors, adipocytokines, chemotactic cytokines, and guidance molecules. They act through cognate receptors on the target cell surface. Among these, the VEGF/VEGFR system is active early on in endothelial cell differentiation and angiogenesis. The cytokine Vascular Endothelial Growth Factor (VEGF, VPF) acts as a mitogen selectively on endothelial cells and promotes neo-vascularization. It is not mitogenic to fibroblasts or epithelial cells. The VEGF family includes the gene products VEGF-A, -B, -C, and -D, as well as Placenta Growth Factor (PLGF). VEGFs are homodimeric glycoproteins that bear 3 loops produced by 3 intramolecular disulfide bonds.

Angiogenic vessels express elevated levels of the tyrosine kinase receptors VEGFR-1(FLT-1), VEGFR-2 (KDR, FLK-1), and VEGFR-3 (FLT-4). VEGFR-2 is a high affinity receptor for VEGF-A and mediates most of its endothelial growth and survival signals. VEGFR-2 has a typical tyrosine kinase receptor structure. It utilizes a canonical signaling system for DNA synthesis in vascular endothelial cells. The Integrin $\alpha v\beta_3$ physically associates with VEGFR-2 and, after ligation, increases VEGF signaling. VEGFR-3 expression is restricted to the lymphatic endothelium in the adult and may have a role in lymphatic tumor spread. VEGFR inhibitors may suppress angiogenesis (Table 12.1, Fig. 12.2).

G. F. Weber, *Molecular Therapies of Cancer*, DOI 10.1007/978-3-319-13278-5_12,

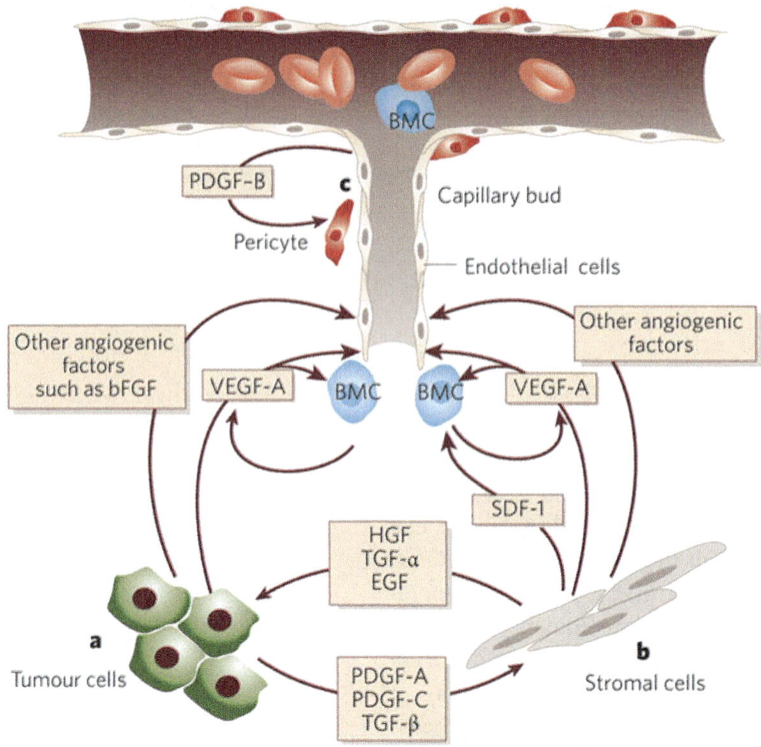

Fig. 12.1 Angiogenesis. **a** Tumor cells produce VEGF-A and other angiogenic factors such as bFGF, Angiopoietins, Interleukin-8, PlGF and VEGF-C. These stimulate resident endothelial cells to proliferate and migrate. **b** An additional source of angiogenic factors is the stroma. This is a heterogeneous compartment, comprising fibroblastic, inflammatory, and immune cells. Recent studies indicate that tumor associated fibroblasts produce chemokines such as SDF-1, which may recruit bone-marrow derived angiogenic cells (BMC). VEGF-A or PlGF may also recruit BMC. Tumor cells may release stromal cell-recruitment factors, such as PDGF-A, PDGF-C or Transforming Growth Factor (TGF)-β. A well-established function of tumor-associated fibroblasts is the production of growth/survival factor for tumor cells such as EGFR ligands, hepatocyte growth factor and Heregulin. **c** Endothelial cells produce PDGF-B, which promotes the recruitment of pericytes in the microvasculature after activation of PDGFR-β. *HGF* Hepatocyte Growth Factor. (Ferrara and Kerbel 2005 with permission)

Adverse Effects Hypertension and proteinuria are class effects of VEGF and VEGFR inhibitors. Some of the VEGFR kinase inhibitors cause severe skin reactions or visceral perforations.

Drug Resistance Infiltration of tumors by VEGFR-1 expressing macrophages is pro-angiogenic. Macrophage depletion makes tumors more sensitive to anti-VEGFR-2 mono-therapy, reflecting that the development of resistance to anti-VEGFR drugs is partly due to pro-angiogenic macrophages. Resistance to VEGFR inhibitors also develops by induction of angiogenic rescue, an event driven by genetic programs that are induced in response to severe intratumoral hypoxia.

Semaxanib (SU5416) is a small molecule tyrosine kinase inhibitor that targets VEGF Receptor 2 on endothelial cells, inhibiting VEGF mediated FLK1 signaling and the proliferation of endothelial cells. The drug also acts as a FLT3 (KDR, CD135) inhibitor. The maximum tolerated dose is 145 mg/m^2 given twice weekly. This agent was withdrawn from clinical development due to a lack of clinical benefit over standard cytotoxic treatment.

Adverse Effects Dose limiting toxicities consist of headache, nausea and vomiting, which have a high incidence but are reversible within 24–48 h of onset without sequelae.

Sunitinib malate (*N*-[2-(diethylamino)ethyl]-5-[(Z)-(5-fluoro-1,2-dihydro-2-oxo-3*H*-indol-3-ylidine)methyl]-2,4-dimethyl-1*H*-pyrrole-3-carboxamide) (SU11248) <Sutent> is the orally bioavailable salt of an indolinone based tyrosine kinase inhibitor. Sunitinib blocks the tyrosine kinase activities of VEGFR2, PDGFRβ, and c-KIT, thereby inhibiting angiogenesis and cell proliferation. This agent also blocks the phosphorylation of FLT3, a receptor tyrosine kinase expressed by some leukemic cells. Sunitinib was approved by the U.S. FDA for the treatment of renal cell carcinoma (RCC) and imatinib resistant gastrointestinal stromal tumor (GIST) in 2006. Thus, sunitinib was the first cancer drug simultaneously approved for two distinct indications. It has since become the standard of care for both of these cancers.

Table 12.1 Specificities of VEGFR inhibitors

Drug	VEGFR1	VEGFR2	VEGFR3	FLT3	c-KIT	PDGFRα	PDGFRβ	EGFR	HER2	RET	FGFR	ITK	B-RAF	TIE-2	MET	CHK-1/2	c-FMS
Semaxanib		S		S													
AEE788		S		S				S	S								
Sunitinib		S		S	S		S										
Motesanib	S	S	S		S		S			S							
Axitinib	S	S	S		S	S	S										
Pazopanib	S	S	S		S	S	S				S	S					
CHIR-265		S					S				S		S				
Vandetanib		S						S		S							
Cediranib	S	S	S														
Cabozantinib	S	S	S	S	S					S				S	S		
Lenvatinib		S	S			S	S				S						
Sorafenib		S		S	S		S			S			S				
regorafenib	S	S			S		S			S			S	S			
Vatalanib	S	S			S		S										S
XL844		S	S	S		S	S									S	

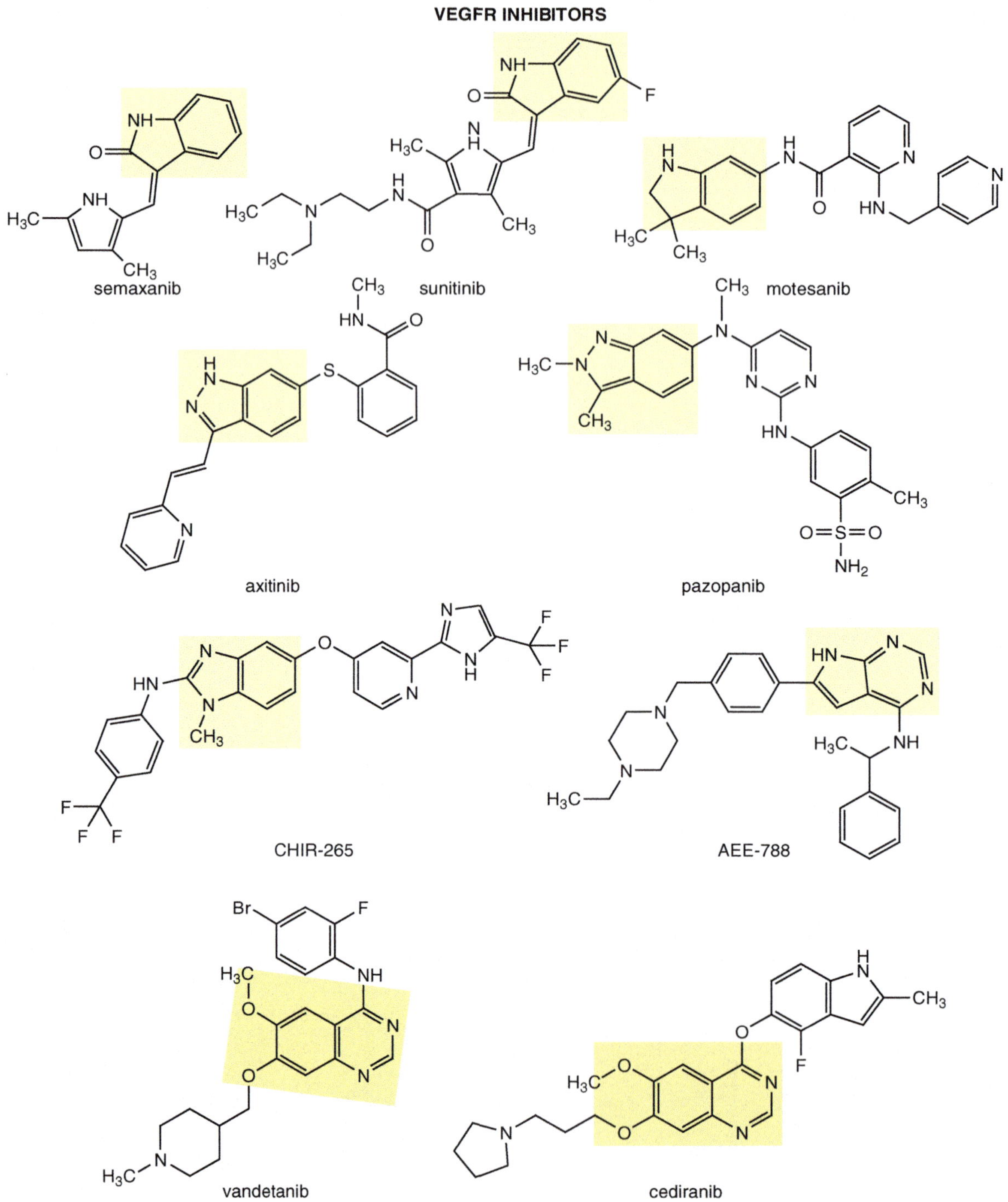

Fig. 12.2 Structures of VEGFR inhibitors. Because the agents act as small molecule receptor kinase inhibitors, many names and on -nib. The core structures shared among subgroups of agents are highlighted in *light* or *bright yellow*. The 1-residue difference between sorafenib and regorafenib is shown in *pink*

Motesanib diphosphate (*N*-(3,3-Dimethyl-2,3-dihydro-1*H*-indol-6-yl)-2-[(pyridin-4-ylmethyl)amino]pyridine-3-carboxamide) (AMG 706) is an orally administered, ATP-competitive small molecule antagonist of VEGF Receptors -1, -2, and -3. It also has activity as a RET, PDGFR, and KIT inhibitor. The drug is under investigation for thyroid cancer, breast cancer, and gastrointestinal stromal tumors.

Axitinib (AG-013736) <Inlyta> is a small molecule inhibitor of VEGFR-1, -2, and -3. It also inhibits c-KIT and

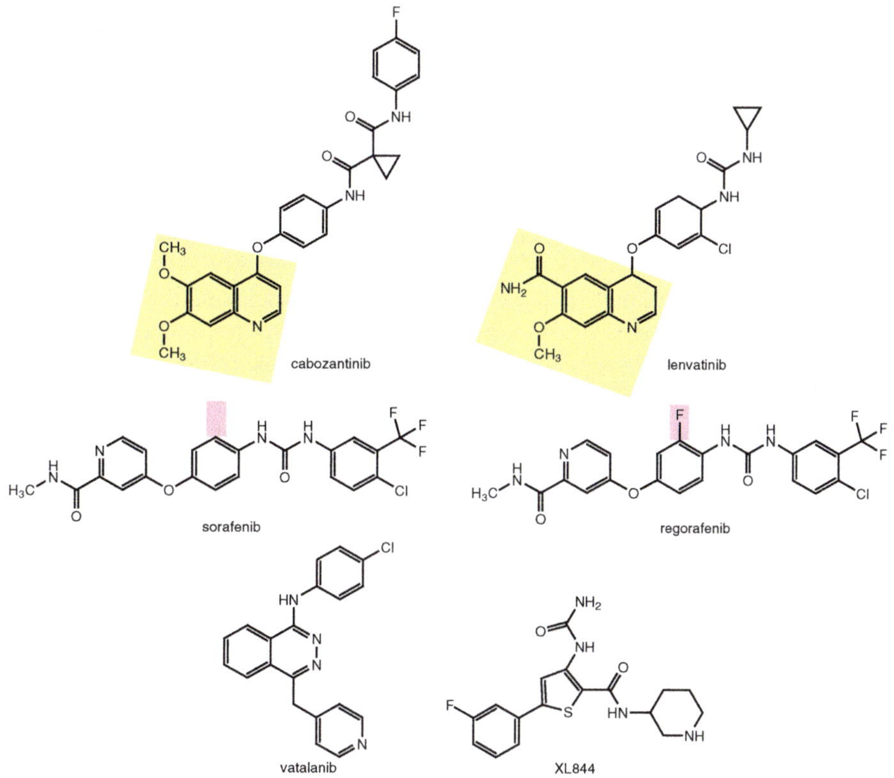

Fig. 12.2 (continued)

PDGFR. The agent is active when given orally. It typically exerts tumor cytostatic activity, which results in a limited efficacy in the mono-therapy setting. Axitinib is given orally, twice daily in 5 mg doses. The drug is indicated for the treatment of advanced renal cell carcinoma after failure of one prior systemic therapy. Axitinib in combination with gemcitabine is under study for advanced pancreatic cancer.

Adverse Effects The most common adverse events comprise diarrhea (55 %), hypertension (40 %), fatigue (40 %), decreased appetite (35 %), nausea (30 %), dysphonia (30 %), hand-foot syndrome (25 %), weight loss (25 %), vomiting (25 %), asthenia (20 %), and constipation (20 %).

Hypertension (including hypertensive crisis) may arise. Arterial and venous thrombotic events or hemorrhagia can be fatal (if any bleeding requires medical intervention, axitinib needs to be temporarily interrupted). Gastrointestinal perforation and fistula, including death, are rare but call for caution in patients at risk. Hypothyroidism may necessitate thyroid hormone replacement. Reversible posterior leukoencephalopathy syndrome is rare, but requires the permanent discontinuation of the drug.

Drug Interactions Concomitant use of strong CYP3A4/5 inhibitors may require axitinib dose reduction. Grapefruit or grapefruit juice may also increase the blood concentration of axitinib and should be avoided. Conversely, strong CYP3A4/5 inducers may require a dose increase.

Pazopanib hydrochloride (5-[[4-[(2,3-dimethyl-2*H*-indazol-6-yl)methylamino]-2-pyrimidinyl]amino]-2-methylbenzenesulfonamide monohydrochloride) <Votrient> is a salt of a small molecule inhibitor of multiple protein tyrosine kinases. Pazopanib selectively inhibits VEGFR-1, -2 and -3, c-Kit, PDGFR-α/β, FGFR, and ITK, which may result in the suppression of angiogenesis in tumors, in which these receptors are up-regulated. The drug is approved by the U.S. FDA for renal cell carcinoma and soft tissue sarcoma. It may also be active in ovarian cancer and non-small cell lung carcinoma. It is taken at 800 mg per day without food.

Pharmacokinetics Pazopanib is absorbed orally with median time to peak concentrations of 2–4 h after the dose and a mean half-life of 30 h after administration. Binding to plasma proteins is greater than 99 % over a wide concentration range. The agent is metabolized by CYP3A4, with minor contributions from CYP1A2 and CYP2C8. It is a substrate for ABCB1 (P-Glycoprotein, MDR) and ABCG2 (BCRP). Elimination is primarily via the feces (renal elimination accounts for less than 5 %).

Adverse Effects Common adverse reactions comprise hypertension, diarrhea, nausea and vomiting, abdominal pain, anorexia, fatigue, asthenia, and headache. Potentially serious adverse reactions to pazopanib include hepatotoxicity, hemorrhagic events, arterial thrombotic events, gastrointestinal perforation and fistula, torsades de pointes[1], and hypertensive crisis.

[1] Torsades de pointes are a form of ventricular tachycardia that displays distinct electrocardiographic characteristics.

Drug Interactions The concomitant use of strong CYP3A4 inhibitors (ketoconazole, ritonavir, clarithromycin) may increase pazopanib concentrations and should be avoided, or the pazopanib dose should be reduced to 400 mg. The concomitant use of strong CYP3A4 inducers (rifampin) may accelerate pazopanib disposition, resulting in ineffectively low concentrations.

CHIR-265 (RAF265) is an orally active small molecule that binds to and inhibits VEGFR-2, thereby disrupting tumor angiogenesis. It also has inhibiting properties against the kinases B-RAF and PDGFR-β (see Sect. 4.1.3). This agent is in clinical trials for the treatment of locally advanced or metastatic melanoma.

AEE788 ((R)-6-(4-((4-ethylpiperazin-1-yl)methyl) phenyl)-*N*-(1-phenylethyl)-7*H*-pyrrolo[2,3-d]pyrimidin-4-amine) is an orally bioavailable, reversible multiple receptor tyrosine kinase inhibitor that targets VEGFR2, ERBB1 (EGFR), ERBB2 (HER2), and FLT. The drug action causes receptor inhibition, and results in the suppression of cellular proliferation, induction of tumor cell apoptosis, and tumor associated endothelial cell apoptosis.

Vandetanib (N-(4-bromo-2-fluorophenyl)-6-methoxy-7-[(1-methylpiperidin-4-yl)methoxy]quinazolin-4-amine) (AZD6474, ZD6474) <Caprelsa, Zactima> is an orally bioavailable 4-anilinoquinazoline that inhibits the tyrosine kinase activity of VEGFR2, thereby blocking VEGF stimulated endothelial cell proliferation and migration and reducing tumor vessel permeability. This agent also blocks the tyrosine kinase activity of ERBB1 (EGFR), a receptor that mediates tumor cell proliferation and migration, as well as the tyrosine kinase RET, which may be associated with early transformation. Vandetanib is taken orally once per day.

- The agent is indicated for the treatment of symptomatic or progressive medullary thyroid cancer in patients with unresectable locally advanced or metastatic disease.
- Its use in patients with indolent, asymptomatic or slowly progressing disease should be carefully considered because of the treatment related risks of vandetanib.

Vandetanib has efficacy in combination with cytotoxic chemotherapy. In conjunction with docetaxel it increases the progression-free survival of non-small cell lung cancer patients.

Pharmacokinetics Vandetanib is administered at a dose of 300 mg. The peak blood concentration occurs after 6 h, and the half-life is 19 days. The drug accumulates approximately 8-fold on multiple dosing, with achievement of a steady state by approximately 3 months. The agent binds to Albumin and α1-Acid-Glycoprotein. *N*-desmethyl-vandetanib is primarily produced by CYP3A4 and vandetanib-*N*-oxide by FMO1 and FMO3. The *N*-desmethyl metabolite, representing 5–15 % of vandetanib exposure, has similar kinase inhibitory activity to the parent compound.

Adverse Effects The most common adverse drug reactions include hypertension, headache, nausea, fatigue, upper respiratory tract infections, decreased appetite, diarrhea, and abdominal pain. Mild to moderate skin reactions may manifest as rash, acne, dry skin, dermatitis, or pruritus. Severe skin reactions (including Stevens-Johnson syndrome), some leading to death, have occurred with vandetanib. Their treatment includes systemic corticosteroids and permanent discontinuation of the causative agent.

Vandetanib can prolong the QT interval. Torsades de pointes and sudden death are possible. The agent should not be used in patients with hypocalcemia, hypokalemia, hypomagnesemia, long QT syndrome, bradyarrhythmias or uncompensated heart failure.

Drug Interactions Vandetanib should not be used concomitantly with drugs that may prolong the QT interval, strong CYP3A4 inducers (dexamethasone, phenobarbital, phenytoin, carbamazepine, rifampin, rifabutin, rifapentine) or St. John's Wort.

Cediranib maleate (AZD-2171) <Recentin> is a relatively selective inhibitor of VEGFR-1, -2, and -3. It is under investigation for the treatment of ovarian cancer, gastrointestinal cancers, kidney cancer, cervical cancer, brain tumors, soft tissue sarcoma, and gall bladder and bile duct cancer.

Adverse Effects Adverse effects may include hypertension, diarrhea, nausea and vomiting, muscle pain and weakness, heart problems reflected in chest pain, increased risk of bleeding, fatigue, sore mouth hoarse voice.

Cabozantinib (S)-malate (XL184) <Cometriq> is an orally bioavailable, small molecule receptor tyrosine kinase inhibitor that strongly binds to and inhibits VEGFR2, which may result in the suppression of angiogenesis. This agent also inhibits TIE-2 (activated by Angiopoietins), FLT3, KIT, RET, and MET. Cabozantinib was approved by the U.S. FDA in 2012 for the treatment of medullary thyroid cancer. It is in clinical trials for melanoma, prostate, ovarian, brain, breast, non-small cell lung, hepatocellular, and kidney cancers. The drug has a long half-life of 60–120 h.

Adverse Effects Common adverse reactions include diarrhea, stomatitis, palmar-plantar erythrodysesthesia syndrome (PPES), weight loss, decreased appetite, nausea, fatigue, oral pain, hair color changes, dysgeusia (distortion of the sense of taste), hypertension, abdominal pain, and constipation.

Permanent discontinuation of cabozantinib is required in cases of development of visceral perforation or fistula formation, severe hemorrhage, serious arterial thromboembolic events (such as myocardial or cerebral infarction), nephrotic syndrome, malignant hypertension or hypertensive crisis, persistent uncontrolled hypertension despite optimized medical management, osteonecrosis of the jaw, reversible posterior leukoencephalopathy syndrome.

Drug Interactions Patients taking cabozantinib should not ingest grapefruit, grapefruit juice, or nutritional supplements that inhibit Cytochrome P450 enzymes, as this may increase the concentration of the drug in the blood. The concomitant administration of strong CYP3A4 inhibitors (ketoconazole, itraconazole, voriconazole, clarithromycin, telithromycin, atazanavir, nefazodone, saquinavir, ritonavir, indinavir, nelfinavir) is to be avoided.

Lenvatinib mesylate (E7080) is a synthetic, orally available inhibitor of the receptor tyrosine kinases VEGFR-2 and VEGFR-3. It blocks VEGFR activation by VEGF, resulting in inhibition of the VEGF Receptor signal transduction pathway. This leads to decreased vascular endothelial cell migration and proliferation, and vascular endothelial cell apoptosis. Lenvatinib also inhibits FGFR1, PDGFRα and PDGFRβ, respectively. The drug is in clinical trials for thyroid cancer and advanced liver cancer. It received orphan drug status in Japan in 2012.

Pharmacokinetics Lenvatinib is a 4-*O*-aryl quinoline derivative. As such, it undergoes conjugation with GSH, accompanied by the release of the *O*-aryl moiety. As a result of intra-molecular rearrangement, hydrolysis of the GSH conjugate yields *N*-cysteinyl-glycine and *N*-cysteine conjugates, rather than *S*-conjugates. Because the *N*-substituted derivatives possess free sulfhydryl groups, dimerization through disulfide bonds and a nucleophilic substitution reaction can result in the formation of disulfanyl dimers and an *N, S*-cysteinyl diquinoline derivative.

Adverse Effects The most frequent adverse events include hypertension (75 %), weight loss (55 %), diarrhea (55 %), and fatigue (55 %). Toxicities were managed with dose reduction in a fraction of patients.

Sorafenib tosylate (4-[4-[[4-chloro-3-(trifluoromethyl) phenyl]carbamoylamino] phenoxy]-*N*-methyl-pyridine-2-carboxamide) <Nexavar> is a synthetic compound that inhibits the VEGFR2/PDGFRβ signaling cascade, thereby blocking tumor angiogenesis. Sorafenib also inhibits wild-type and mutant forms of RAF, c-KIT (CD117), FLT3 (FMS-Related Tyrosine Kinase 3), RET, and PDGFRβ (Platelet-Derived Growth Factor Receptor β) (see Sect. 4.1.3). The drug was approved by the U.S. FDA in 2005, and received E.U. marketing authorization in 2006 to treat unresectable hepatocellular carcinoma and advanced renal cell carcinoma. The administration of sorafenib prolongs progression-free survival in patients with advanced clear cell renal carcinoma, in whom previous therapy has failed. Further, the agent is in testing for the treatment of soft tissue sarcoma.

Adverse Effects Common adverse effects include fatigue, weight loss, diarrhea, arthralgia or myalgia, alopecia, mucositis or stomatitis, hand-foot skin reactions, and skin rash or desquamation (in rare serious cases, Stevens-Johnson syndrome and toxic epidermal necrolysis).

Regorafenib (BAY 73–4506) <Stivarga> is an orally bioavailable multi-kinase inhibitor that targets VEGFR2 and the Angiopoietin Receptor TIE2, with additional activities against PDGFRβ, c-KIT, and RET. It increases the overall survival of patients with metastatic colorectal cancer and is under study for gastrointestinal stromal tumors.

Adverse Effects The most common adverse effects include weakness or fatigue, loss of appetite, palmar-plantar erythrodysesthesia (hand-foot syndrome), hypertension, diarrhea, mouth sores (mucositis), weight loss, infection, high blood pressure, and changes in voice volume or quality (dysphonia). There is a low risk for severe and fatal liver toxicity. Visceral perforations may occur.

Vatalanib (*N*-(4-chlorophenyl)-4-(pyridin-4-ylmethyl) phthalazin-1-amine) (PTK787, ZK 222584) is an orally bioavailable anilinophthalazine that binds to and inhibits the protein kinase domain of VEGFR-2 and to a lesser extent VEGFR-1 and -3. This agent also binds to and inhibits related receptor tyrosine kinases, including PDGFR, c-KIT, and c-FMS. It is under study for the treatment of imatinib resistant gastrointestinal stromal tumors and other solid cancers.

Pharmacokinetics The terminal elimination half-life for vatalanib in blood is 4–5 h. The drug is cleared mainly through oxidative metabolism. The metabolites, (4-chlorophenyl)-[4-(1-oxy-pyridin-4-yl-methyl)-phthalazin-1-yl]-amine and 4-[(4-chlorophenyl)amino]-α-(1-oxido-4-pyridyl)phthalazine-1-methanol, contribute mainly to the total systemic exposure. The parent drug and its metabolites are excreted rapidly and mainly via the biliary-fecal route. The area under the concentration-time curve for vatalanib pharmacokinetics declines over the first 2 weeks of treatment, likely due to auto-induction of CYP3A clearance.

Adverse Effects Adverse events attributable to vatalanib are generally similar to those of other VEGF pathway inhibitors. Most common are high blood pressure, gastrointestinal upset (diarrhea, nausea, and vomiting), fatigue, and dizziness. Thrombotic and embolic events of all grades may arise. Reversible posterior encephalopathy syndrome occurs in 1 % of the patients.

XL844 (EXEL-9844) inhibits VEGFR2 and VEGFR3, which are important mediators of tumor angiogenesis and lymphangiogenesis respectively. The compound also inhibits CHK1 and CHK2 (see Sect. 4.1.6), as well as FLT3 and

PDGFR. It is in clinical trials for advanced solid tumors or lymphomata, as a single agent or in combination with gemcitabine.

12.1.2 VEGF Inhibitors

VEGF dependent angiogenesis may be suppressed by agents that directly neutralize VEGF, that inhibit its signal transduction, or that block its induction (Fig. 12.3).

In 1989, Napoleone Ferrara at Genentech cloned the angiogenic growth factor Vascular Endothelial Growth Factor (VEGF). In 1993, his team used an antibody directed to VEGF to suppress angiogenesis in preclinical models. Consecutively, the antibody was humanized. Clinical trials began in 1997. The U.S. FDA approved bevacizumab as the first anti-angiogenic drug in 2004.

Bevacizumab <Avastin> is a recombinant humanized monoclonal IgG_1 antibody that binds to and inhibits the biologic activity of VEGF. It is used in the treatment of metastatic colorectal cancer in combination with intravenous 5-fluorouracil based chemotherapy. It is also indicated for first- or second-line treatment of patients with metastatic carcinoma of the colon or rectum, and in combination with carboplatin and paclitaxel for the first-line treatment of patients with unresectable, locally advanced, recurrent, or metastatic non-squamous, non-small cell lung cancer (U.S. FDA approval 2006). Bevacizumab improves the progression-free survival of patients with metastatic renal carcinoma when combined with Interferon-α for first-line therapy. In 2008, bevacizumab received U.S. FDA approval for the treatment of breast cancer based on measurements of tumor growth, not patient survival (almost simultaneously, the European EMA approved it for the same treatment.). The decision represented a deviation from previous standards. It was revoked in 2010 because the risks associated with the drug outweighed the benefits.

Bevacizumab is usually given at 10 mg/kg by infusion once every 2 weeks. The inhibition of VEGF may cause the following changes in the tumor vasculature:

- regression of existing micro-vessels, which arrests tumor growth
- normalization of the surviving mature vasculature, which makes it more conducive to effective anti-cancer chemotherapy,
- inhibition of neovascularization.

Adverse Effects The most common adverse events are proteinuria (risk increases with dose), weakness, abdominal pain, headache, diarrhea or constipation, nausea, vomiting, loss of appetite, mouth sores, upper respiratory infection, difficulty breathing, and skin irritation. Bevacizumab can result in the development of potentially serious gastrointestinal perforation, which requires permanent discontinuation. This event may occur throughout the course of treatment and can result in fatality. The antibody can lead to slow or incomplete wound healing (wound dehiscence). The appropriate waiting time between bevacizumab interruption and surgical intervention is undetermined. Some patients receiving the antibody with

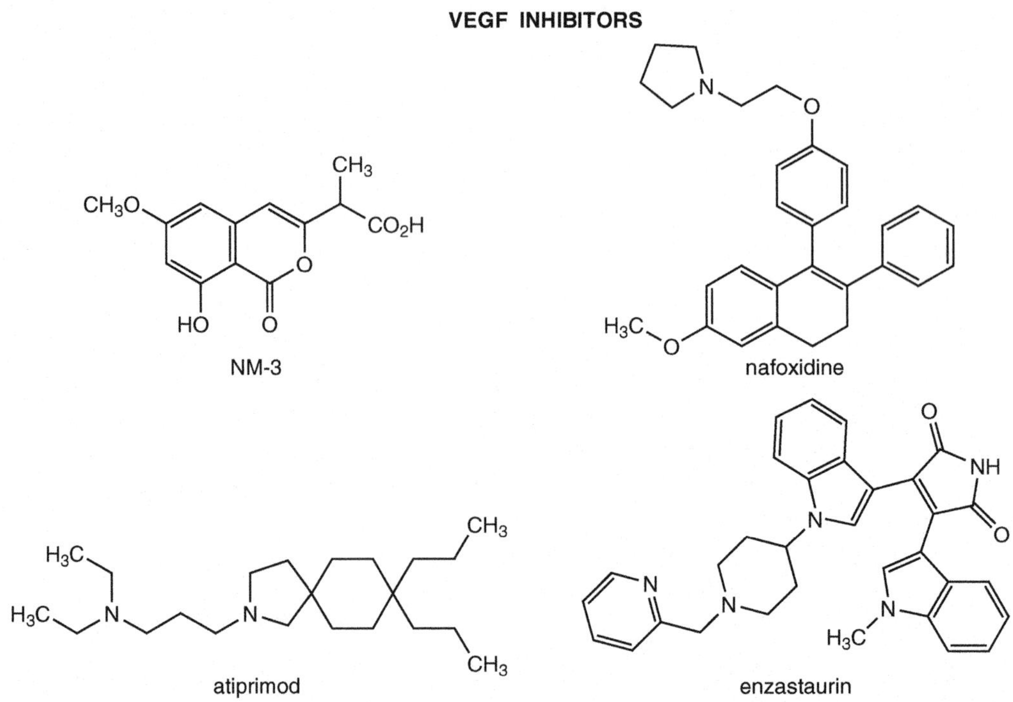

Fig. 12.3 Structures of VEGF inhibitors

chemotherapy for lung cancer experience hemoptysis or epistaxis. Additional serious adverse effects may include hypertensive crisis (risk increases with dose), reversible posterior leukoencephalopathy syndrome, neutropenia and infection, nephrotic syndrome, and congestive heart failure.

Venous thrombembolism is one of the leading causes of treatment induced morbidity in cancer patients. The use of bevacizumab increases this risk at 2.5 mg/kg/week. It is highest in the treatment of colon cancer, lower in non-small cell lung cancer and breast cancer, and lowest in renal cancer (Nalluri et al. 2008).

Drug Interactions Bevacizumab is associated with an increased risk of fatal adverse events in patients receiving taxanes or platinum agents, but not in conjunction with other agents. The most common causes are hemorrhage, neutropenia, and gastrointestinal tract perforation (Ranpura et al. 2011).

The isocoumarin NM-3 (2-(8-hydroxy-6-methoxy-1-oxo-1H-2-benzopyran-3-yl) propionic acid) was originally isolated from culture filtrate of Streptoverticillium eurocidicum. It is an anti-angiogenic derivative of cytogenin. The drug inhibits VEGF, thereby suppressing endothelial cell proliferation, migration, sprouting, and tube formation. This agent also induces apoptosis by a mechanism that involves reactive oxygen species. NM-3 is orally bioavailable and well tolerated.

VEGF and Fibroblast Growth Factor-2 (FGF-2, basic Fibroblast Growth Factor, bFGF) stimulate the proliferation of endothelial cells. Estrogen induces the transcription of their genes. Partial estrogen antagonists, such as tamoxifen, clomiphene, and nafoxidine, may suppress angiogenesis in a dose dependent manner by inhibiting the VEGF and FGF-2 stimulated endothelial cell growth.

Nafoxidine (1-[2-[4-(3,4-dihydro-6-methoxy-2-phenyl-1-naphthalenyl)phenoxy]ethyl]-pyrrolidine) (U-11,000A) is a non-steroidal partial estrogen antagonist that is structurally related to tamoxifen. It also inhibits angiogenesis in some tissues by blocking the expression and the effects of VEGF.

Adverse Effects Adverse effects include dryness of skin, photosensitivity reactions, and (less commonly) partial hair loss. In a paradoxical reaction, nafoxidine may enhance angiogenesis in uterine tissue[2].

Atiprimod (SK&F106615) is an orally bioavailable small molecule belonging to the azaspirane class of cationic amphiphilic agents. It antagonizes both the FGF-2 and VEGF induced proliferation and migration of endothelial cells, resulting in a disruption of tube formation. The atiprimod mode of action entails the inhibition of STAT-3 phosphorylation, blocking the signaling pathways of FGF-2 and VEGF, and down-regulating the anti-apoptotic proteins BCL-2, BCL-X_L, and MCL-1. These effects inhibit cell proliferation, induce cell cycle arrest, and lead to apoptosis. Atiprimod also lowers the blood levels of IL-6, VEGF, TNF-α, and IL-1. It is under evaluation for the treatment of multiple myeloma, metastatic carcinoid cancer, and hepatocellular carcinoma.

Enzastaurin hydrochloride (3-(1-methylindol-3-yl)-4-[1-[1-(pyridin-2-ylmethyl)piperidin-4-yl]indol-3-yl]pyrrole-2,5-dione) (LY317615) is the salt of a synthetic macrocyclic bisindolemaleimide. Binding to the ATP binding site of PKCβ (Protein Kinase C β), the agent inhibits this enzyme, which is involved in the induction of VEGF stimulated neo-angiogenesis. Enzastaurin also is a potent inhibitor of PKCα, PKCγ, and PKCε. The drug suppresses the phosphorylation of GSK3β, Ribosomal Protein S6S240/244, and AKT while having no direct effect on VEGFR phosphorylation. This agent may decrease tumor blood supply and consecutively tumor burden. Enzastaurin has orphan drug status in Europe for the treatment of diffuse large B-cell lymphoma.

Adverse Effects Adverse events associated with enzastaurin are fatigue, diarrhea, swelling, nausea.

Angiogenic vessels express elevated levels of the tyrosine kinase receptors VEGFR-1 through VEGFR-3.
VEGF dependent angiogenesis may be suppressed by agents that directly neutralize VEGF, that block its receptors, that inhibit its signal transduction, or that suppress its induction.
Various small molecule kinase inhibitors block VEGFR signaling.
Bevacizumab is a neutralizing antibody to VEGF.
Hypertension and proteinuria are class effects of VEGF and VEGFR inhibitors.Some VEGFR kinase inhibitors can cause severe skin reactions or visceral perforations.

12.2 FGF-2 Antagonists

The Fibroblast Growth Factor family consists of around 20 members. Because these proteins can bind to and have their biologic activities modulated by heparin or heparan sulfate proteoglycans, they are also termed Heparin Binding Growth Factors (HBGFs). The *fgf-2* (*basic fgf*) gene may generate 4 proteins of 18, 22, 23, and 24 kD through the use of alternate CTG start codons upstream from the ATG site. Mechanical stress triggers its release from the endothelium. FGF-2 engages the FGF Receptors -1, -2, -3, and -4. It induces angiogenesis through several pathways. Both low and high molecular weight forms activate endothelial cell proliferation and they may induce the expression of Integrin $\alpha v\beta_3$, chemotaxis, and matrix invasion by endothelial cells.

[2] Nafoxidine induces MMP-2, which aids in remodeling the basement membrane during angiogenesis, but also TIMP-1, which has anti-angiogenic activity in the late stages of tube formation.

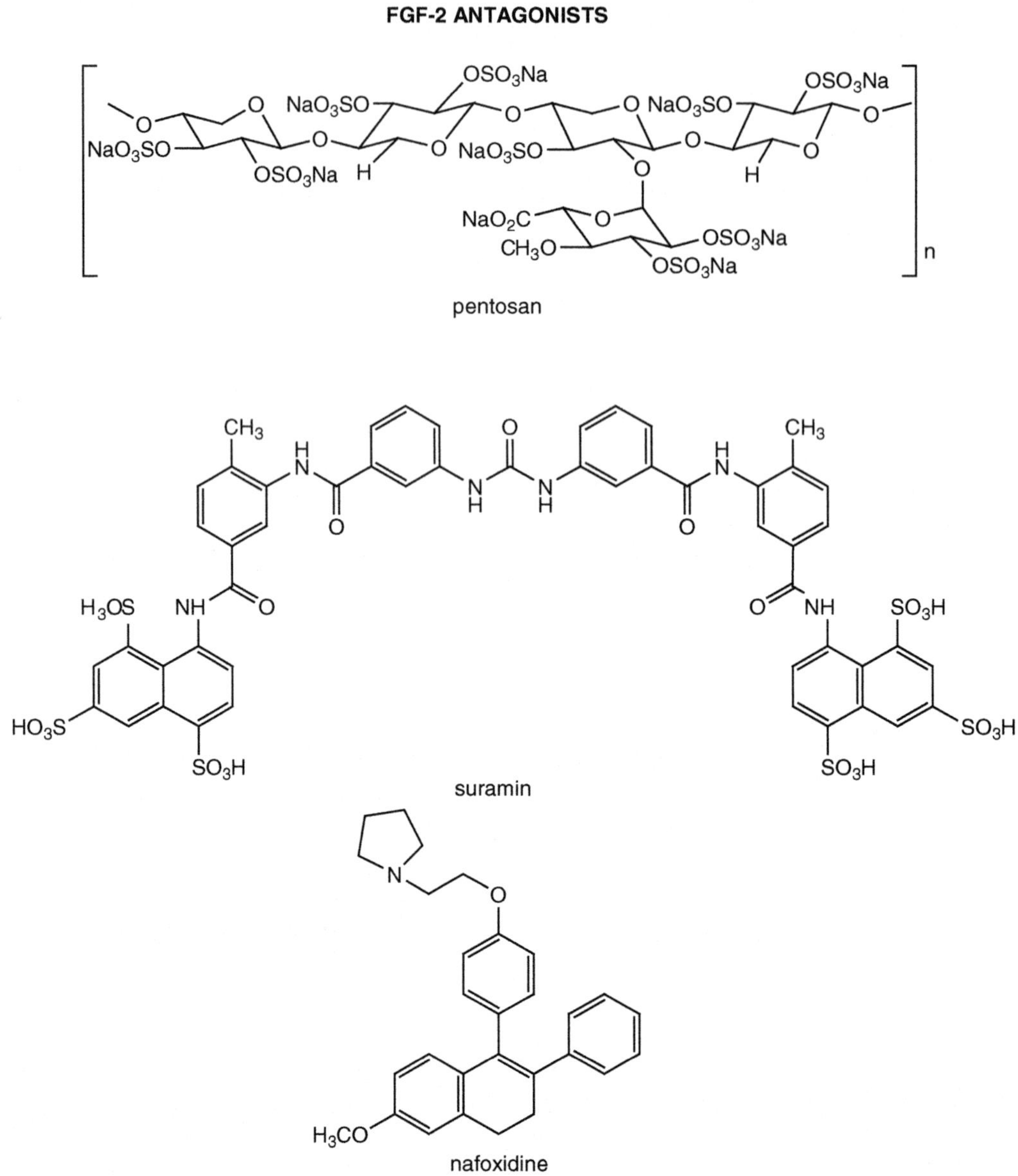

Fig. 12.4 Structures of FGF-2 antagonists

FGF-2 (basic Fibroblast Growth Factor, bFGF) is often over-expressed in gliomata, where it correlates with the degree of malignancy and vascularity. Kaposi sarcoma releases FGF-2 in response to various cytokines.

Oligosaccharides The capacity of various endogenous pro-angiogenic factors to interact with heparin or heparan sulfate raises the possibility that molecules which interfere with this interaction may act as angiogenesis inhibitors. This is the case for certain sugars.

Tecogalan sodium (D-gluco-D-galactan sulfate) (DS-4152, SP-PG) is a sulfated polysaccharide isolated from Arthrobacter species. The agent binds to FGF-2, thereby preventing the angiogenic growth factor from engaging its receptors. The disruption of this ligand-receptor interaction results in the inhibition of FGF-2 stimulated endothelial cell growth, proliferation, and migration.

Pentosan polysulfate is a polymer of xylose hydrogen sulfate that contains two sulfate groups per carbohydrate monomer (Fig. 12.4). It has affinity for heparin binding growth factors, including FGFs (pentosan polysulfate may be more effective in inhibiting FGF-4 than FGF-2 due to different structural requirements in their heparin interactions) and the heparin binding site of FGFR-1. Microvascular endothelium is more sensitive to inhibition by pentosan polysulfate than large vessel endothelium. The maximally tolerated dose, given by continuous intravenous infusion, is 3 mg/kg per day.

Adverse Effects Dose limiting toxic effects are characterized by reversible anti-coagulation and thrombocytopenia.

Malto-oligosaccharides and sulfated chitin derivatives exert their inhibitory activity by acting as heparin-like, poly-anionic compounds. They inhibit endothelial cell proliferation, chemotaxis, and morphogenesis. Thus they suppress neovascularization, resulting in the obstruction of tumor angiogenesis and growth.

Oligodeoxynucleotides Phosphorothioate oligodeoxynucleotides have the capacity to interact with heparin binding growth factors, including FGF-2, FGF-1, FGF-4, and VEGF. As poly-anions, they inhibit the binding of FGF-2 to heparin sulfate proteoglycans and to their cognate tyrosine kinase receptors, thus preventing mitogenic activity. The antagonist activity of phosphorothioate oligodeoxynucleotides depends only in part on their size and sequence and is independent of P-chirality. However, RNA ligands with defined consensus sequences and secondary structures interact specifically with FGF-2 at nanomolar affinity and in a manner that competes with heparin binding.

Others Suramin is a polysulfonated naphthylurea that suppresses endothelial cell proliferation and migration. The agent inhibits VEGF induced and FGF-2 induced angiogenesis. The agent also blocks the binding of various growth factors to their receptors, including IGF-1 (Insulin-Like Growth Factor 1), EGF (Epidermal Growth Factor), PDGF (Platelet-Derived Growth Factor), and TGF-β (Tumor Growth Factor β). This is due, at least in part, to the capacity of suramin to ligate the heparin binding regions of certain growth factors via one or more of its sulfate groups. Consistently, it is ineffective against angiogenesis elicited by non-heparin binding growth factors. Microvascular endothelium is more sensitive to inhibition by suramin derivatives than large vessel endothelium.

Adverse Effects A limitation on the clinical use of suramin is the high dose required to achieve anti-tumor activity. The half-life in the blood is 30–50 days. The drug dramatically increases tissue glycosaminoglycans, leading to mucopolysaccharidosis-like pathologic conditions. It elevates the concentration of circulating heparin and dermatan sulfates, thus inducing coagulopathy.

The proliferation of endothelial cells, induced by FGF-2 and VEGF, is under estrogenic regulation. Partial estrogen antagonists, such as tamoxifen, clomiphene, and nafoxidine, may suppress angiogenesis in a dose dependent manner by inhibiting the VEGF and FGF-2 stimulated endothelial cell growth. As this inhibition is not affected by the presence of estradiol, the anti-angiogenic action of the anti-estrogens does not occur via the Estrogen Receptor, but by a direct inhibition of growth factor stimulated endothelial cell growth.

Nafoxidine (U 11100A) inhibits angiogenesis in some tissues by blocking the effects of FGF-2 and VEGF. The drug also acts as a partial estrogen antagonist that binds to the cytoplasmic and nuclear forms of the Estrogen Receptor. Nafoxidine is under study for the treatment of breast cancer.

The Interferons-α and -β exert anti-angiogenic properties through inhibiting

- endothelial cell migration
- the secretion of such angiogenic factors as FGF-2 from tumor cells
- the transcription and translation of *fgf-1* by cancer cells
- MMP-2 (72 kD Gelatinase) production by suppression of its gene expression.

This compromises the formation of new blood vessels. Interferon can induce the regression of angiosarcomata and angioblastomata (Kaban et al. 2002; Marler et al. 2002). These tumors express high levels of FGF-2 as their major angiogenic mediator.

As various endogenous pro-angiogenic factors interact with heparin or heparan sulfate, molecules that interfere with this interaction may act as angiogenesis inhibitors.
Partial estrogen antagonists may suppress angiogenesis by inhibiting the VEGF and FGF-2 stimulated endothelial cell growth.

12.3 Thalidomide Related Drugs

Thalidomide (Fig. 12.5) was developed by the German pharmaceutical company Grünenthal in 1954. It was marketed in 1957 as a tranquilizer and painkiller, as well as a treatment for insomnia. Because the drug is an anti-emetic that has an inhibitory effect on morning sickness, it was commonly taken by pregnant women. In the late 1950s and early 1960s, more than 10,000 children worldwide were born with deformities, such as phocomelia, as a consequence of thalidomide use by pregnant women. The Australian obstetrician McBride reported in 1961 that nearly 20 % of women taking thalidomide during pregnancy had babies with multiple severe abnormalities (McBride 1961). The impact in the United States was minimized when Frances Oldham Kelsey, a reviewer for the U.S. FDA, refused approval for an application from Richardson Merrell to market thalidomide <Kevadon>. Despite pressure from the manufacturer (the drug had already been approved in Canada and over 20 European and African countries), she requested more testing due to safety concerns, thus protecting pregnant women in the U.S. from the adverse drug effects. In 1994, Robert D'Amato at Harvard Medical School reviewed organs with blood vessel

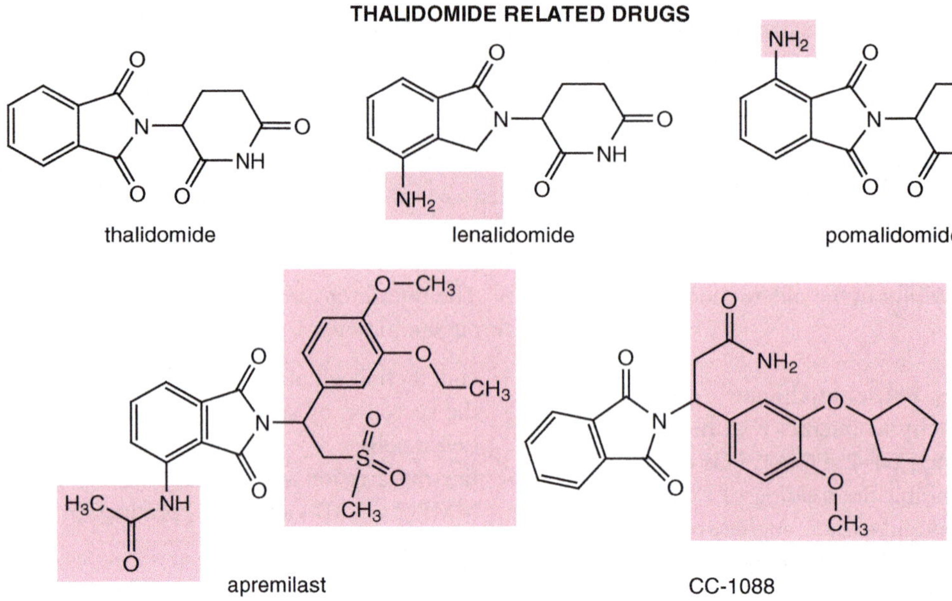

Fig. 12.5 Structures of thalidomide derivatives. The core motif is shared among all agents in this class. The difference in structure compared to thalidomide is shown in *pink*

development and drugs affecting these organs to identify potential angiogenesis inhibitors. Blood vessels grow in the uterus during the menstrual cycle and in the placenta during pregnancy. In the search for compounds that had been reported to stop menstruation and cause fetal malformations, two drugs stood out, retinoic acid and thalidomide. The discovery that thalidomide was a potent inhibitor of angiogenesis (D'Amato et al. 1994) not only provided an explanation for the drug's ability to cause birth defects, but also suggested a therapeutic use for thalidomide in inhibiting abnormal angiogenesis in diseases such as cancer. In 1995, New York cardiologist Ira Wolmer was diagnosed with multiple myeloma. After several treatment failures, his wife called Judah Folkman, who suggested trying thalidomide. Her husband's oncologist, Bart Barlogie, initially dismissed the idea, but Folkman convinced him of the potential. In 1997, Barlogie received permission to test thalidomide under tight safety protocols. Wolmer's cancer did not respond, and he died in the following year. A test in another patient, however, led to near-complete remission, causing Barlogie to expand to a larger trial, for which he reported a response to thalidomide in 1/3 of all patients in 1999.

Thalidomide (2-(2,6-dioxo-3-piperidyl)isoindole-1,3-dione) <Thalidomid>[3] inhibits angiogenesis by modulating the required cytokines VEGF, FGF-2 (basic Fibroblast Growth Factor), and IL-6. It may be anti-inflammatory by reducing the levels of TNFα (Tumor Necrosis Factor-α) produced by monocytes, as well as suppressing the pro-inflammatory cytokines IL-1, IL-6, and IL-12. Some of the effects are the result of intercalation of thalidomide into the guanine-rich DNA promoter sites of *fibroblastic growth factor-2* and the Integrin subunits α_V and β_3. The agent is effective for the treatment of multiple myeloma. The drug received approval for this use in Australia and New Zealand in 2003. In 2006, thalidomide received U.S. FDA approval in combination with dexamethasone for the treatment of newly diagnosed multiple myeloma. It may be given to keep the myeloma in remission after treatment, or to treat a recurrence of myeloma after first-line treatment. The use of thalidomide in multiple myeloma patients is accompanied by an increase in the number of circulating natural killer cells, and an increase in the blood levels of Interleukin-2 and Interferon-γ. Thalidomide therapy starts at 200 mg once daily, and is then increased to the maximum tolerated dose, which is usually 800 mg/day. Low doses are typically taken after a meal in the evening because drowsiness is a common effect, high doses are divided into four applications throughout the day. The agent is lipophilic and crosses the blood-brain barrier.

[3] Beside anti-angiogenesis, thalidomide and derivative compounds have multiple mechanisms of action.

- These drugs exert a toxic effect on multiple myeloma. They bind to Cereblon (CRBN), which activates a Ubiquitin E3 Ligase complex and causes the degradation of the transcription factors Ikaros (IKZF1) and Aiolos (IKZF3).
- Thalidomide and its structural and functional analogs are called IMiDs (immune modulating derivatives) because they also exert NK activating and T-lymphocyte co-stimulatory functions. Of note, in combination therapy with dexamethasone, the immunostimulatory activity is severely suppressed.
- Thalidomide is a sedative, hypnotic, and a potent teratogen.

Pharmacokinetics Despite poor aqueous solubility, the drug is orally bioavailable. Due to its slow absorption from the gastrointestinal tract, the mean time to peak blood concentrations is 3–5.5 h. In circulation, about 50 % of the drug is bound to plasma proteins. Thalidomide itself is not hepatically metabolized to any large extent, but undergoes non-enzymatic hydrolysis to multiple products in the blood. The drug does not induce or inhibit its own metabolism. The mean half-life of elimination ranges approximately 5–7 h.

Adverse Effects Adverse effects are constipation, orthostatic hypotension, and fatigue. High doses can lead to pulmonary edema, atelectasia, aspiration pneumonia, and refractory hypotension. Thalidomide also is associated with an increased risk of deep vein thrombosis and pulmonary embolism (1–5 % of patients receiving single-agent thalidomide), especially when combined with dexamethasone (10–15 % of patients) or other cytotoxic agents (25 % of patients). Prophylaxis with heparin, warfarin, or salicylate may be indicated. Peripheral neuropathy may occur with long term use and may necessitate the discontinuation of the medication. The agent has a well documented history of causing birth defects (phocomelia) when taken during pregnancy; it is therefore Pregnancy Category X. In the United States, the drug may be obtained only through practitioners and pharmacies registered in the System for Thalidomide Education and Prescribing Safety (STEPS) program.

Drug Interactions Thalidomide is often a component of combination chemotherapy. Doses greater than 200 mg/day are generally not indicated when thalidomide is combined with corticosteroids or chemotherapy.

Lenalidomide (3-(4-amino-1-oxo 1,3-dihydro-2H-isoindol-2-yl) piperidine-2,6-dione) <Revlimid> is a thalidomide analog that reduces the blood levels of the cytokines VEGF and FGF-2, inhibits TNF-α production, stimulates T-lymphocytes, and inhibits angiogenesis. This agent may also have a direct effect on malignant cells by promoting G_1 cell cycle arrest and apoptosis. Lenalidomide is used in combination with dexamethasone. In 2005, the U.S. FDA gave approval for lenalidomide as the first commercially useful derivative of thalidomide. The approved oral adult dose is 25 mg daily on days 1–21, along with 40 mg oral dexamethasone on days 1–4, 9–12, and 17–20 of each 28-day cycle. From cycle 5 on, dexamethasone is reduced to 40 mg/day on days 1–4.

- Lenalidomide in combination with dexamethasone is indicated for the treatment of patients with multiple myeloma who have failed prior therapy.
- Lenalidomide is indicated for the treatment of patients with transfusion dependent anemia due to myelodysplastic syndromes associated with a deletion of chromosome 5q.

The drug is only available in a restricted distribution setting to avoid its use during pregnancy (in the U.S.: RevAssist Program).

Pharmacokinetics Following single and multiple doses of lenalidomide, the maximum blood concentrations occur 0.5–6 h post-dose. Binding to plasma proteins is approximately 30 %. The mean half-life is 3–5 h. Lenalidomide is not a substrate for the multi-drug resistance proteins ABCC1 (MRP1), ABCC2 (MRP2, cMOAT), or ABCC3 (MRP3, cMOAT2) or for the organic ion uptake transporters OAT1, OAT3, OATP1B1, or OCT1. The agent is neither metabolized by nor inhibits or induces Cytochrome P450 enzymes. As lenalidomide undergoes limited metabolism, unchanged drug is the predominant circulating component in the blood. Metabolites are hydroxy-lenalidomide and N-acetyl-lenalidomide, each of which constitutes less than 5 % of the parent levels in circulation. Lenalidomide is extensively eliminated unchanged by the kidneys. Therefore, the risk of adverse events is higher in patients with renal dysfunction.

Adverse Effects Lenalidomide does not cause substantial somnolescence, constipation, or peripheral neuropathy. However, myelosuppression does occur and may reach grade three thrombocytopenia and neutropenia. In this case, dose interruption or reduction may be required. Venous thrombembolism is an adverse event in 5–20 % of patients, which can lead to pulmonary embolism. It has a higher incidence in patients undergoing combination therapy over mono-therapy. Allergic reactions and hepatotoxicity are possible.

Drug Interactions When digoxin is co-administered with multiple doses of lenalidomide, the digoxin disposition is reduced. Therefore, the digoxin blood levels should be monitored to avoid toxic levels. Concomitant therapies that may increase the risk of thrombosis, such as erythropoietic agents or estrogen containing therapies, should be used with caution in multiple myeloma patients receiving lenalidomide/dexamethasone.

Pomalidomide (3-amino-thalidomide) (CC-4047) <Pomalyst, Imnovid> is a thalidomide derivative. In addition to its anti-angiogenic properties, pomalidomide may also directly suppress the growth of myeloma cells. The drug is more potent in inhibiting TNFα than other thalidomide related drugs, and can therefore be given at a lower dose. The European EMA has granted pomalidomide an orphan designation for primary myelofibrosis, multiple myeloma, systemic sclerosis, post-polycythemia and post-essential thrombocythemia myelofibrosis. The drug has been approved by the U.S. FDA.

Selective cytokine inhibitory drugs (SelCIDs) inhibit Phosphodiesterase-4 (PDE4), an enzyme involved in TNF-α production. Apremilast (CC-10004) and CC-1088 are analogs of thalidomide that belongs to the functional class of SelCIDs. They inhibit the production of the pro-angiogenic cytokines

VEGF and IL-6 (Interleukin-6). Apremilast is in development for treating chronic inflammatory conditions. Its effects on cancer angiogenesis are under study. Apremilast reduces PDE4 activity leading to an increase in cyclic adenosine monophosphate (cAMP) concentrations in immune and non-immune cell types, partially inhibiting the production of many pro-inflammatory cytokines such as TNF-α, IFN-γ IL-2, IL-12 and IL-23 and elevating the production of the anti-inflammatory cytokine IL-10. The inhibition potency of apremilast in TNF-α production is similar to lenalidomide.

Thalidomide inhibits angiogenesis by modulating the required cytokines VEGF, FGF-2, and IL-6. It may be anti-inflammatory by reducing the levels of TNFa, IL-1, IL-6, and IL-12.

12.4 Integrin blockers

The Integrin $\alpha v\beta_3$ is absent from quiescent endothelial cells in established vessels, but its expression is induced on endothelial cells undergoing active angiogenesis. Integrin $\alpha_5\beta_1$ is expressed on endothelial cells and plays a crucial role in adhesion and migration. These same Integrins are present on metastasizing cells (see Sect. 5.1). Therefore, anti-metastasis drugs that target them also have anti-angiogenic properties.

Peptide inhibitors Cilengitide (EMD121974) is a small molecule blocker of Integrins on the surface of endothelial cells. It suppresses endothelial cell-cell interactions, endothelial cell-matrix interactions, and angiogenesis. The drug is under study for the treatment of prostate cancer, melanoma, myeloid leukemia, and brain tumors. The European EMA has granted cilengitide orphan drug status.

ATN-161 (ac-PHSCN-NH2) is a small peptide antagonist of Integrin $\alpha_5\beta_1$ that selectively binds to and blocks this receptor. It thereby prevents the engagement of Integrin $\alpha_5\beta_1$ by its cognate ligand. This receptor blockade may result in the inhibition of endothelial cell-cell interactions, endothelial cell-matrix interactions, angiogenesis, and thus tumor progression.

Antibodies Volociximab (Eos200–4, M200) is a chimeric neutralizing antibody that recognizes the Integrin $\alpha_5\beta_1$ and prevents the binding of Fibronectin. Volociximab inhibits endothelial cell-cell interactions, endothelial cell-matrix interactions, and angiogenesis. This induces apoptosis in proliferating endothelial cells. The antibody is under investigation for the treatment of metastatic kidney cancer.

Adverse Effects There is no dose limiting toxicity up to 10 mg/kg.

Integrin $\alpha v\beta_3$ is expressed on endothelial cells and plays a crucial role in endothelial cell adhesion and migration. A monoclonal antibody that inhibits this Integrin receptor is etaracizumab (MEDI-522) <Abegrin, Vitaxin>. It blocks the binding of ligands, such as Vitronectin or Osteopontin, resulting in the inhibition of metastasis and angiogenesis. Etaracizumab has been under study for the treatment of leiomyosarcoma and metastatic melanoma. It is also being investigated for the treatment of prostate cancer, ovarian cancer, and Kaposi sarcoma.

Others E7820 is an aromatic sulfonamide derivative. It acts as a modulator of the expression of *integrin* α_2 subunits in endothelial cells. This results in anti-angiogenic activity. E7820 is orally bioavailable.

The Integrin $\alpha v\beta_3$ is absent from quiescent endothelial cells, but is induced on endothelial cells undergoing angiogenesis. Integrin $\alpha_5\beta_1$ is expressed on endothelial cells and plays a crucial role in adhesion and migration. As these Integrins are expressed on metastasizing cells, anti-metastasis drugs that target them are also anti-angiogenic.

12.5 Endostatin and Angiostatin

Endostatin (O'Reilly et al. 1997), which is the COOH-terminal 20 kD fragment of Collagen XVIII, can inhibit angiogenesis and tumor growth by specifically targeting endothelial cells. It was discovered by Michael O'Reilly, who as a postdoctoral fellow had taken on a challenging project in the Judah Folkman laboratory (shunned by many of his predecessors) to identify angiogenesis inhibitors that are secreted by tumors. It was known that such molecules often were secreted in the urine and bound to heparin. Tumor-bearing mice were fed sugar water, which they liked and which increased their urine production. The excretions were then purified over heparin columns for analysis.

In 1998, the science reporter of The New York Times, Gina Kolata, attended a function with scientific dignitaries. She turned to Nobel Laureate James Watson and asked "what's new in cancer?". In response, Watson (known for his predisposition for unguarded comments) predicted that Judah Folkman "will cure cancer within two years". NCI director Richard Klausner declared Endostatin a "top priority" for the National Cancer Institute. This prophesy prompted a front-page New York Times story touting the discovery of Endostatin in the Folkman laboratory. The ensuing intense publicity created unrealistic expectations about the potential drug molecule, which was still early in development. Cancer patients called hospitals and asked to be put on this agent, which had not yet entered clinical trials. Problems with follow-up experiments and drug solubility soon caused a

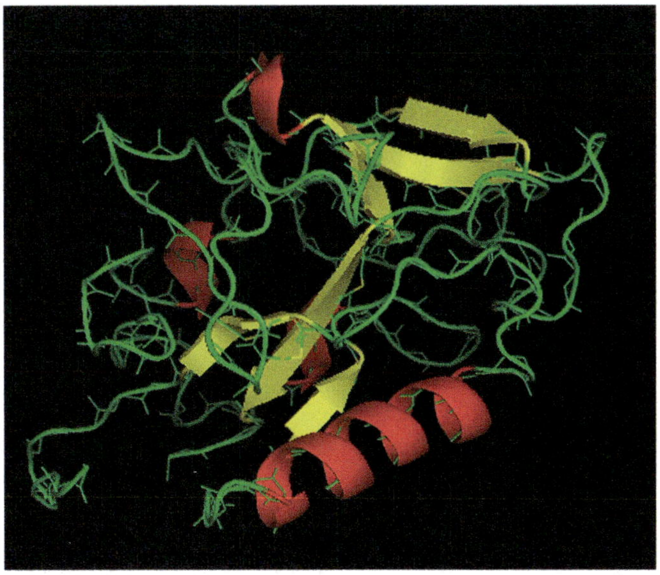

Fig. 12.6 The structure of Endostatin. The 3-dimensional structure of Endostatin was modeled using the program loopp and visualized with PyMOL

backlash against Endostatin. In 2004, the manufacturer, EntreMed, gave up on the lead and returned the rights to Children's Hospital in Boston.

In 2005, the government of China approved a modified version of Endostatin, Endostar, for patients with non-small cell lung cancer, once clinical trials revealed that it delayed disease progression when added to chemotherapy. Endostar had been developed by Luo Yongzhang, the only college graduate in a family of seven children from an impoverished Chinese village. Luo had promised a college friend who died of pancreatic cancer in his early 20s to devote himself to seeking a cure. Having received training at prestigious American Universities, he used his protein folding expertise to improve Endostatin. In 1999, he set up a joint venture with Yantai R.C. Pharmaceutical Co. On Christmas Eve that year, shortly after he succeeded in folding the protein properly, a power outage cut off electricity to the laboratory, where the drug specimens were kept in a freezer. Luo Yongzhang suffered frostbites when he connected extension cords from a nearby apartment to the laboratory freezer.

Endostatin is a proteolytic fragment of the C-terminal end of type XVIII Collagen. A recombinant version of Endostatin represents the candidate therapeutic agent (Fig. 12.6). The molecule induces microvascular endothelial cell apoptosis, and inhibits endothelial proliferation and migration. This leads to the suppression of angiogenesis, which may result in a reduction in tumor burden. This agent also may decrease hepatic metastasis by inhibiting VCAM (Vascular Cell Adhesion Molecule) dependent cell attachment to the hepatic microvasculature.

Angiostatin (O'Reilly et al. 1994) is a 38 kD internal fragment of Plasminogen. It is produced by auto-proteolytic cleavage of Plasminogen, involving extracellular disulfide bond reduction by free sulfhydryl donors or Phosphoglycerate Kinase. Urokinase Plasmiogen Activator (uPA) or Cathepsin D may generate Angiostatin. It is processed by the Matrix Metalloproteinases MMP-3, MMP-7, and possibly by MMP-2, -9, and -12. A shared mechanism of action for anti-angiogenic factors that are derived from extracellular matrix proteins and plasma proteins is their formation of complexes with adhesion proteins in the plasma to create an active anti-angiogenic substance. Angiostatin binds Fibrin and Vitronectin. The Integrins $\alpha v\beta_3$, $\alpha_9\beta_1$, and to a lesser extent $\alpha_4\beta_1$, on endothelial cells specifically bind to Angiostatin, with Integrin $\alpha v\beta_3$ being a predominant receptor. Angiostatin, but not Plasminogen, binds to ATP Synthase on the cell surface and thus down-regulates endothelial cell proliferation. A successful drug formulation of Angiostatin has not yet been developed.

12.6 Others

TNP-470 (AGM-1470) is a synthetic analog of fumagillin, an antibiotic isolated from the fungus Aspergillus fumigatus fresenius (Fig. 12.7). TNP-470 binds to and irreversibly inactivates Methionine Aminopeptidase-2 (MetAP2), resulting in the abrogation of amino-terminal processing of methionine, which may lead to endothelial cell cycle arrest late in the G_1 phase and consecutive inhibition of tumor angiogenesis. This agent may also induce the P53 pathway, thereby stimulating the production of the Cyclin-Dependent Kinase Inhibitor P21 and inhibiting blood vessel formation. TNP-470 is administered at a dose of 60 mg/m^2 as a 60-min intravenous infusion three times a week.

Adverse Effects The dose limiting complication is neurotoxicity.

Combretastatin A4 phosphate is a water soluble prodrug derived from the African bush willow (Combretum caffrum). It is directly cytotoxic to proliferating endothelial cells and tumor cells. After administration, the agent is dephosphorylated to its active metabolite, combretastatin A4, which binds to Tubulin and inhibits microtubule depolymerization, resulting in morphological changes in proliferating endothelial cells. As a result, the permeability of the tumor vasculature is increased, leading to reduced tumor blood flow and ischemic necrosis of the tumor tissue.

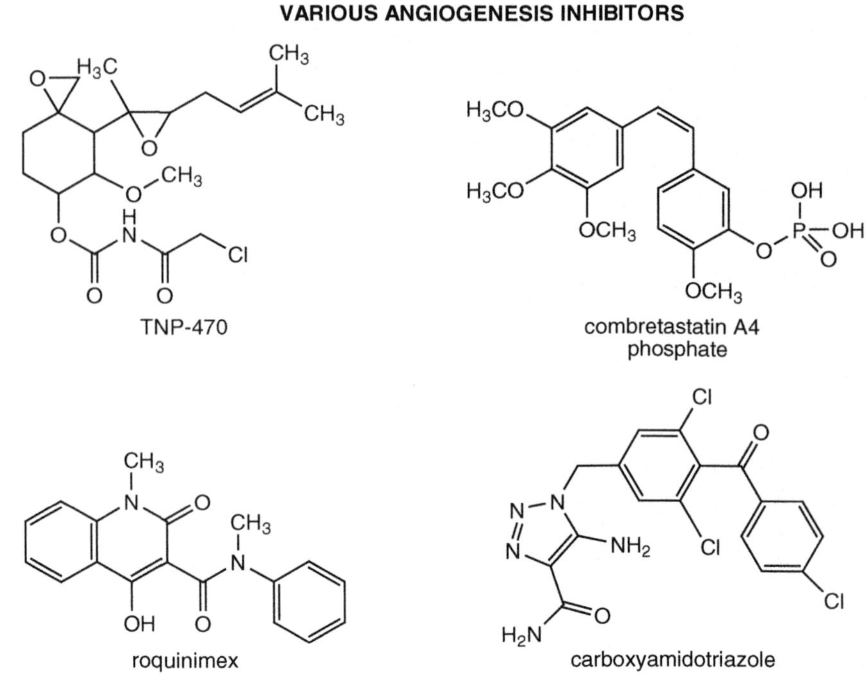

Fig. 12.7 Structures of various angiogenesis inhibitors

Roquinimex (4-hydroxy-*N*,1-dimethyl-2-oxo-*N*-phenyl-1,2-dihydroquinoline-3-carboxamide) (FCF 89, LS 2616) <Linomide> is a quinoline-3-carboxamide with anti-angiogenic properties. It inhibits endothelial cell proliferation, migration, and basement membrane invasion by reducing the secretion of the angiogenic factor TNF-α from tumor associated macrophages. This agent is also an immune modulator that may alter cytokine profiles and enhance the activity of T-lymphocytes, natural killer cells, and macrophages. Roquinimex is used in the treatment of chronic myelogenous leukemia (CML) with autologous bone marrow transplant. The agent is orally active.

Carboxyamidotriazole (CAI) may inhibit calcium mediated signal transduction. It is an inhibitor of receptor gated calcium channels, and results in the inhibition of Phospholipase C and Phospholipase A_2 phosphorylation. It blocks angiogenesis by inhibiting the FGF-2 dependent stimulation of endothelial cell proliferation.

A dysregulation of transcription factors is often associated with cancer. A key transcription factor involved in tumor angiogenesis, ID1 (Inhibitor of DNA Binding 1) is up-regulated in the endothelium of nearly all solid tumors, and is a downstream target of several pro-angiogenic factors, such as VEGF-A and FGF-2. Hence, inhibiting ID1 activity could have the advantage of short-circuiting multiple pathways involved in tumor angiogenesis. ID1 can be targeted by using a peptide-conjugated antisense oligonucleotide (PCAO).

Treatment of Myeloma

In myeloma, transformed plasma cells produce large quantities of M Protein (Myeloma Protein, which can be any of the Ig subclasses), leading to a stimulation of osteoclasts. The first pathogenetic step is the occurrence of monoclonal gammopathy of undetermined significance (MGUS). A more advanced stage is asymptomatic (smoldering) myeloma. Fully manifest myeloma is characterized by skeletal destruction, hypercalcemia, renal failure, and anemia (CRAB symptoms = hyper*c*alcemia, *r*enal insufficiency, *a*nemia, *b*one lesions), as well as infections and hyperviscosity[4].

In the early 1960s, the introduction of melphalan in combination with prednisone led to increased survival. In 1996, autologous stem cell transplantation was applied in the management of younger patients. One of the major treatment considerations was the assessment of the patient's ability to receive high dose chemotherapy followed by hematopoietic stem cell transplantation (Jagannath 2008; Schwartz 2008). Since the late 1990s, angiogenesis inhibitors

[4] The hyperviscosity constitutes a high risk for deep vein thrombosis and venous thromboembolism. Prophylactic anti-coagulation is frequently recommended by guidelines for patients with multiple myeloma.

and proteasome inhibitors have found increasing use. Thalidomide along with bortezomib changed the landscape of multiple myeloma treatment, such that toxic stem cell transplants may no longer be the standard treatment for this malignancy. Additionally, improved supportive care, including

- access to growth factors to treat anemia and thrombocytopenia
- decreased incidence of fractures and resultant complications due to the use of bisphosphonates
- improved management of patients with renal failure

has contributed to increased survival rates. Currently, initiation of treatment is determined largely by the stage of the disease.

Inhibition of cell proliferation Chemotherapy for multiple myeloma may be administered as frontline therapy, as induction therapy for transplant eligible patients, or as salvage therapy.

- Frontline therapy with curative intent is initiated in patients who are not transplant candidates.
- The aim of induction therapy has been to achieve a response in preparation for a hematopoietic stem cell transplant in eligible patients. As myeloma is a disease that arises predominantly in older adults, co-morbidities or compromised organ function may limit the options for stem cell transplants.
- Salvage therapy in patients who develop treatment resistance or relapse. Most individuals who have responded to initial therapy relapse within 10 years.

Historically, melphalan plus prednisone (MP) has been the standard treatment option for frontline therapy. Melphalan displays effectiveness in 50 % of cases at 0.2 mg/kg/day orally. These drugs have recently been combined with thalidomide (MPT) or bortezomib (MPB) to achieve higher response rates. However, the addition of thalidomide increases the incidence of thrombembolism.

The C-VAMP regimen is named after cyclophosphamide, vincristine, doxorubicin <Adriamycin>, and methylprednisolone. Cyclophosphamide is given as either an infusion or an injection. Methylprednisolone can be given as an infusion or as tablets. Following cyclophosphamide, vincristine and doxorubicin are administered together through a small portable pump over 4 days. The cycle is completed with additional cyclophosphamide on days 8 and 15, followed by a week of rest (to complete 3 weeks). Usually, 4–6 cycles are given over a period of 3–5 months.

A form of chemotherapy treatment for myeloma is VAD. The combination of vincristine, doxorubicin <Adriamycin>, and dexamethasone is used in some cases for frontline therapy or for induction therapy. VAD can be combined with cyclophosphamide in salvage therapy. On day 1, vincristine and doxorubicin are given together through a portable pump continuously for 4 days. Dexamethasone is then administered as tablets on days 1–4, 9–12, and 17–20. A rest period ensues for the next 8 days to complete a 4 week cycle. Usually, 4–6 cycles are given over a period of 4–6 months. Alternatively, liposomal doxorubicin plus vincristine and dexamethasone (DVD) is an option.

An aggressive regimen for salvage therapy comprises deaxamethasone, thalidomide, cisplatin, doxorubicin, cyclophosphamide, and etoposide (DT-PACE).

Elotuzumab (HuLuc63) is a humanized monoclonal antibody directed to CS1 (CD2 subset 1, CRACC, SLAMF7), which may trigger antibody-dependent cellular cytotoxicity (ADCC). CS1 is a cell surface glycoprotein that belongs to the CD2 subset of Immunoglobulin super-family receptors. It is abundantly expressed on multiple myeloma cells, but minimally on healthy cells.

Interference with myeloma-stroma interactions IL-6 (Interleukin-6) is an important mediator for the stromal cell interaction of myeloma cells. In many patients, the blood Interleukin-6 levels are elevated and the plasma cells express high levels of BCL-2. Both IL-6 and BCL-2 are inhibitors of apoptosis. Their over-expression may contribute to resistance to therapy. The adhesion of myeloma cells to stromal cells induces IL-6 secretion by the stromal cells, which in turn mediates the activation of signal transduction pathways for cell growth and transformation in the myeloma cells, such as the STAT, PKB and RAS pathways. Among these, the oncogene product RAS is a potential therapeutic target because *ras* mutations represent the most common gene mutation in multiple myeloma (Liu et al. 1996). Hence, Farnesyl Transferase inhibitors are in clinical studies for this disease.

Bisphosphonates protect from bone fractures by inhibiting the dissolution of hydroxyapatite crystals and down-regulating osteoclast function. Pamidronate (90 mg) is infused over 2–4 h once a month. Zolendronate is equivalent to pamidronate in bone protection. More potent, nitrogen containing bisphosphonates also reduce the production of IL-6 and have anti-tumor activity.

Adverse effects Adverse effects include fatigue, gastrointestinal effects, anemia, and skeletal pain. Avascular osteonecrosis of the jaw is a possible complication of bisphosphonate use.

Denosumab is a monoclonal antibody designed to inhibit RANKL (RANK Ligand), a protein that activates bone removal, thus counteracting bone loss. In multiple myeloma patients, denusomab <Xgeva> may be more effective than bisphosphonates in reducing bone fractures, limiting the need for bone radiation treatment, and preventing the worsening of pain in cancer patients with bone disease. However, denosumab is not indicated for the prevention of skeletal related events in patients with multiple myeloma.

The proteasome inhibitor bortezomib was introduced in 2003 as a representative of a new class of drugs. By blocking the transcription factor NF-κB, bortezomib inhibits the interaction between myeloma and bone marrow cells. Angiogenesis is also inhibited as a result. Further, myeloma cells are much more sensitive to proteasome inhibition than healthy peripheral blood cells. A current treatment of multiple myeloma is based on thalidomide and dexamethasone in conjunction with bortezomib. Bortezomib may also be combined with dexamethasone or dexamethasone plus doxorubicin for induction therapy.

Carfilzomib <Kyprolis> is a proteasome inhibitor for use in relapsed and refractory myeloma patients. It was approved by the U.S. FDA in 2012 for myeloma patients who have already been treated with at least bortezomib and either lenalidomide or thalidomide and who have also progressed on or within 60 days of completing their last therapy.

Anti-angiogenesis Increased bone marrow vascularity imparts a poor prognosis in myeloma. The use of the angiogenesis inhibitor thalidomide results in improved response rates and progression-free survival (Singhal et al. 1999). Thalidomide was originally used in conjunction with prednisone, later with dexamethasone. It may now be combined with bortezomib as frontline therapy or induction therapy.

Lenalidomide is an oral analog of thalidomide that has anti-myeloma activity but lacks the neurotoxic adverse effects associated with the prototype drug. Lenalidomide is approved in the U.S. and Europe for use in combination with dexamethasone in patients with at least 1 prior therapy. In these patients, this combination leads to a survival benefit over dexamethasone alone.

Pomalidomide <Pomalyst, Imnovid> in combination with low-dose dexamethasone may improve progression-free and overall survival for some patients with multiple myeloma that has progressed despite other treatments (typically bortezomib or lenalidomide).

Adverse effects Thalidomide derivatives cause birth defects (phocomelia) when taken during pregnancy. In the United States, the drugs may be obtained only through practitioners and pharmacies registered in the System for Thalidomide Education and Prescribing Safety (STEPS) program (renamed Thalidomid REMS program).

Supportive treatment Volume depletion, infection, and the use of non-steroidal anti-inflammatory agents (NSAIDs) for pain increase the risk of renal failure. A minimum intake of 2 l of fluid per day should be recommended.

Infection is a common complication of multiple myeloma. Up to 20 % of patients may develop varicalla-zoster virus infections. Varicella prophylaxis is recommended particularly with single-agent bortezomib. When corticosteroids are used, prophylactic broad-spectrum antibiotic therapy may be considered. Intravenous Immunoglobulin therapy should be considered in the setting of recurrent life-threatening infections.

Anemia often worsens during progressive disease, but may improve when the disease is controlled. Deficiencies in iron, folate, or vitamin B12 should receive treatment.

References

Bocci G, Francia G, Man S, Lawler J, Kerbel RS (2003) Thrombospondin 1, a mediator of the antiangiogenic effects of low-dose metronomic chemotherapy. Proc Natl Acad Sci U S A 100:12917–12922

D'Amato RJ, Loughnan MS, Flynn E, Folkman J (1994) Thalidomide is an inhibitor of angiogenesis. Proc Natl Acad Sci U S A 91:4082–4085

Ferrara N, Kerbel RS (2005) Angiogenesis as a therapeutic target. Nature 435:967–974

Jagannath S (2008) Pathophysiological underpinnings of multiple myeloma progression. J Manage Care Pharm 14:S7–S11

Kaban LB, Troulis MJ, Ebb D, August M, Hornicek FJ, Dodson TB (2002) Antiangiogenic therapy with interferon a for giant cell lesions of the jaws. J Oral Maxillofac Surg 60:1103–1111

Kerbel RS, Kamen BA (2004) The anti-angiogenic basis of metronomic chemotherapy. Nat Rev Cancer 4:423–436

Liu P, Leong T, Quam L, Billadeau D, Kay NE, Greipp P, Kyle RA, Oken MM, Van Ness B (1996) Activating mutations of N- and K-ras in multiple myeloma show different clinical associations: analysis of the Eastern Cooperative Oncology Group Phase III Trial. Blood 88:2699–2706

Marler JJ, Rubin JB, Trede NS, Connors S, Grier H, Upton J, Mulliken JB, Folkman J (2002) Successful antiangiogenic therapy of giant cell angioblastoma with interferon a 2b: report of 2 cases. Pediatrics 109:E37

McBride WG (1961) Thalidomide and congenital abnormalities. Lancet 2:1358

Nalluri SR, Chu D, Keresztes R, Zhu X, Wu S (2008) Risk of venous thromboembolism with the angiogenesis inhibitor bevacizumab in cancer patients: a meta-analysis. J Am Med Assoc 300:2277–2285

O'Reilly MS, Holmgren L, Shing Y, Chen C, Rosenthal RA, Moses M, Lane WS, Cao Y, Sage EH, Folkman J (1994) Angiostatin: a novel angiogenesis inhibitor that mediates the suppression of metastases by a Lewis lung carcinoma. Cell 79:315–328

O'Reilly MS, Boehm T, Shing Y, Fukai N, Vasios G, Lane WS, Flynn E, Birkhead JR, Olsen BR, Folkman J (1997) Endostatin: an endogenous inhibitor of angiogenesis and tumor growth. Cell 88:277–285

Ranpura V, Hapani S, Shenhong Wu S (2011) Treatment-related mortality with bevacizumab in cancer patients. J Am Med Assoc 305:487–494

Schwartz RN (2008) Current and emerging treatments for multiple myeloma. J Manage Care Pharm 14:S12–S18

Singhal S, Mehta J, Desikan R, Ayers D, Roberson P, Eddlemon P, Munshi N, Anaissie E, Wilson C, Dhodapkar M, Zeddis J, Barlogie B (1999) Antitumor activity of thalidomide in refractory multiple myeloma. New Engl J Med 341:1565–1571

Part V

Anti-Cancer Drug Pharmacokinetics

13 Drug Delivery and Drug Transport

Drug delivery is a key problem in the treatment of cancer. Most of the differences between tumor and host are quantitative, not qualitative. Therefore, untransformed cells have some sensitivity to many anti-cancer drugs. In particular, the conventional chemotherapy agents have high toxicity toward all proliferating cells, so it is essential that drug delivery maximize the drug concentration in the cancerous tissue while keeping it low in the rest of the body. Critical factors in this regard are route of administration and drug transport, both of which can be affected by a diversity of factors. Many anticancer agents that cannot be given orally are typically injected intravenously. Thrombosis and thrombophlebitis may result from direct contact of the drug with the intima of the injected vein. It is important to avoid high concentration and prolonged contact with these drugs, especially in cases of elevated pressure in the antebrachial vein, as is the case in mediastinal tumor compression from severe vena cava syndrome.

Delivery systems offer the potential to enhance the therapeutic index of anti-cancer agents by increasing the drug concentration in the tumor cells and decreasing the exposure in host tissues. One strategy to reduce the systemic toxicity of anti-cancer agents is the administration directly into the tumor via transcatheter arterial infusion. It depends on the capability of percutaneous selective catheter placement. Intra-arterial infusion has been effective in patients with carcinomata of the liver, bladder, prostate, uterus, ovary, and lung, in bone and soft tissue sarcomata, melanomata, and tumors of the brain. To prevent the administered drugs from leaching into the circulation via the venous drainage, the arterial infusion can be combined with embolization of the capillaries. Embolization may also have the benefit of clogging the blood supply of the tumor, thus leading to necrosis. The arterial infusion concept is compromised once a tumor has formed metastases.

Some delivery systems exploit the enhanced permeability and retention effect of tumor associated blood vessels. It is a consequence of the dysregulated nature of tumor angiogenesis, which characteristically involves structural and physiological defects that lead to hyper-permeability. Macromolecular agents with restricted volumes of distribution and the capacity for prolonged circulation (such as liposomes) preferentially extravasate from these abnormal vessels and accumulate in tumor tissue.

The blood-brain barrier, constituted by brain capillary endothelial walls, poses unique challenges for drug transport and delivery in the treatment of primary or metastatic brain cancers. Many highly water-soluble therapeutics (such as peptides and antisense oligonucleotides) do not readily enter the brain from the blood owing to poor transport through the blood-brain barrier. Strategies available for drug delivery to the brain include

- neurosurgical methods including intraventricular drug infusion or hyperosmotic opening of the blood-brain barrier
- pharmacological approaches, such as peptide lipidization or liposome encapsulation
- physiological ways, including the biochemical opening of the blood-brain barrier or the administration of chimeric peptides. Chimeric peptides are formed by the covalent coupling of a pharmaceutical peptide to a brain transport vector that undergoes absorptive mediated or receptor mediated transcytosis through the blood-brain barrier. The chimeric peptides are formed generally with chemical based linkers. However, avidin/biotin linkers allow for high yield coupling of drug to vector, and for the release of biologically active peptide following cleavage of the chimeric peptide linker.
- One of the currently most efficient brain transport vectors is a monoclonal antibody to the Transferrin Receptor, which achieves a brain volume of distribution approximately 15-fold greater than the plasma space by 5 h after a single intravenous injection (Partridge 1992).

G. F. Weber, *Molecular Therapies of Cancer,* DOI 10.1007/978-3-319-13278-5_13,

Conventional chemotherapy agents have high toxicity toward all proliferating cells, so drug delivery needs to maximize the drug concentration in the cancer while keeping it low in the rest of the body.
Critical factors in drug delivery are route of administration and drug transport.
Drug delivery systems enhance the therapeutic index of anti-cancer agents by increasing the drug concentration in the tumor cells and decreasing the exposure in host tissues.

13.1 Targeting with Drug Conjugates

Receptors that are present at high abundance on the tumor cell surface may be used for targeting anti-cancer agents predominantly to the cancer (Table 13.1).

DAB389 Epidermal Growth Factor is a recombinant fusion protein composed of Diphtheria Toxin with the receptor binding domain replaced by human Epidermal Growth Factor (ERBB1). When administered, EGF binds to its cognate receptor, which is up-regulated in many carcinomata. After binding to EGFR, the drug is internalized by the cell, where the Diphtheria Toxin moiety exerts its cytotoxic effect, inhibiting protein synthesis through ADP-ribosylation of EF-2 (Elongation Factor 2).

Improved targeted delivery of anti-cancer agents to a given neoplasm can be achieved by linking the drug to polymers that are recognized by receptors expressed in that particular tumor. PK2 is a doxorubicin formulation, that links the drug via a lysosomally degradable tetrapeptide sequence to hydrophilic *N*-(2-hydroxypropyl)methacrylamide (HPMA) copolymers bearing a galactosamine residue. Because the galactosamine is recognized by the hepatic Asialoglycoprotein Receptor, PK2 selectively accumulates in the liver. When used for the treatment of primary or metastatic liver cancer, the HPMA conjugate may lead to partial clinical responses, and it may be associated with improved cardiac safety.

Polyethylene glycol (PEG) is a polymer that facilitates the preferential accumulation of a drug in the tumor vasculature. The simple structure, flexible polymer size, and low toxicity of polyethylene glycol have made it a preferred material for drug conjugation and in excipient formulations. A number of anti-tumor agents have been bound to this polymer, including taxol, doxorubicin, camptothecin, and cisplatin.

Pegaspargase is a complex of polyethylene glycol conjugated with L-Asparaginase. L-asparagine is a non-essential amino acid that can be synthesized by most mammalian cells, except for those of certain lymphoid malignancies, which lack or have very low levels of the Synthetase enzyme required for L-asparagine formation. L-Asparaginase depletes existing supplies and inhibits protein synthesis. This results in tumor cell blockage of proliferation. PEGylation decreases the antigenicity of the enzyme.

PEGylated doxorubicin hydrochloride liposome is a formulation of doxorubicin <Doxil-Caelyx>, in which a drug containing liposome is surrounded by a layer of polyethylene glycol. This formulation preferentially accumulates in the tumor vasculature, resulting in a sustained targeted release of free doxorubicin into the tumor micro-environment. Peglyation increases the half-life of the liposome by inhibiting its phagocytosis in the reticuloendothelial system. Compared to other doxorubicin formulations, this form releases lower concentrations of free doxorubicin, thus increasing the safety profile.

An extracellularly tumor-activated prodrug (ETAP) incorporates both a tumor specific recognition site and a tumor selective enzymatic activation sequence. Drug delivery to tumors can be improved by coupling of suitable agents to ETAPs.

The bicyclic CDCRGDCFC (RGD-4C) peptide selectively binds to Integrins $\alpha_V\beta_3$ and $\alpha_V\beta_5$, which are highly over-expressed in invading tumor endothelial cells. Another tumor-specific sequence is the tripeptide APK (D-alanine-phenylalanine-lysine) that is recognized by the tumor associated protease Plasmin, an important factor of tumor invasion and metastasis. An aminocaproyl residue is incorporated as a spacer between the two peptide sequences, whereas a self-eliminating 4-aminobenzyl alcohol spacer is inserted between the Plasmin substrate and doxorubicin. This prodrug is designed to have Plasmin dependent cytotoxicity for endothelial cells and some tumor cells, but improvements in water solubility and bioavailability are needed for further development (de Groot et al. 2002).

Table 13.1 Drug conjugate targeting

Target	Vehicle	Drug
EGFR	EGF	Diphtheria toxin
Hepatic Asialo-Glycoprotein Receptor	N-(2-hydroxypropyl) methacrylamide	Doxorubicin
Tumor vasculature	Polyethylene glycol	L-Asparaginase
Tumor vasculature	Polyethylene glycol	Doxorubicin
Integrins $\alpha_v\beta_3$ and $\alpha_v\beta_5$	Bicyclic peptide CDCRGDCFC (RGD-4C)	Doxorubicin
Integrin α_v and NRP-1	Peptide iRGD (CRGDK/RGPD/EC)	Various
Tumor peptidases	N-glutaryl-[4-hydroxyprolyl]-Ala-Ser-cyclohexaglycyl-Glu-Ser-Leu	Doxorubicin
Tumor peptidases	N-succinyl-Ala-L-Leu-L-Ala-L-Leu	Doxorubicin
Tumor cells	Docosahexaenoic acid	Paclitaxel

The efficacy of anti-cancer agents is typically limited by their poor penetration into tumor tissue. In solid tumors, many drugs penetrate only 3–5 cell diameters from the blood vessels. The peptide iRGD (CRGDK/RGPD/EC), when chemically conjugated to a drug, can carry that drug deep into extravascular tissue. Because of its RGD motif, the peptide homes in on Integrin α_V, which is predominantly expressed on the endothelium of tumor vessels. iRGD is then proteolytically cleaved, with the truncated peptide gaining affinity for Neuropilin-1 (NRP-1). The NRP-1 binding triggers tissue penetration. The peptide may also enhance drug delivery when it is co-administered without being conjugated to the drug. This is independent of whether the drug is a small molecule, an antibody, or a nano-particle (Sugahara et al. 2010).

L-377,202 is a prodrug obtained by covalently linking the anthracycline antibiotic doxorubicin to *N*-glutaryl-[4-hydroxyprolyl]-Ala-Ser-cyclohexaglycyl-Glu-Ser-Leu. It belongs to a group of prodrugs that are unable to enter normal cells but are proteolytically activated by Peptidases that are rather selectively secreted by cancer cells (extracellularly tumor-activated prodrugs). In the presence of prostate cancer cells that secrete the serine protease PSA (Prostate-Specific Antigen), the peptide moiety of L-377,202 is hydrolyzed to release doxorubicin or Leu-doxorubicin, the latter being freely diffusible and activated to doxorubicin inside the target cells. L-377,202 is considerably more toxic to PSA-positive tumor cells than to PSA-negative healthy or tumor cells (Denmeade et al. 1998). Selective targeting of the treatment to prostate tumors occurs because the hydrolyzing PSA enzyme is localized to the prostate gland. Doxorubicin and leucine-doxorubicin intercalate into DNA and interact with Topoisomerase 2, thereby inhibiting DNA reduplication and repair, and RNA and protein synthesis. These agents also produce toxic free radical intermediates and interact with cell membrane lipids causing lipid peroxidation.

The extracellularly tumor-activated prodrug *N*-succinyl-Ala-L-Leu-L-Ala-L-Leu-DOX (CPI-0004Na) is a tetrapeptidic derivative of doxorubicin. CPI-0004Na does not undergo hydrolysis in blood nor does it enter the cells, but it is activated by tumor peptidases to yield *N*-(L-Leu-DOX), which eventually diffuses inside the cells. CPI-0004Na is significantly less toxic than doxorubicin due to its lower accumulation in the heart and other normal tissues (Trouet et al. 2001).

DHA-paclitaxel is a prodrug comprised of the naturally occurring Ω-3 fatty acid docosahexaenoic acid (DHA) covalently conjugated to the anti-microtubule agent paclitaxel. Because tumor cells take up docosahexaenoic acid, DHA-paclitaxel is delivered directly to tumor tissue. The conjugate exhibits improved pharmacokinetic and toxicity profiles when compared to conventional paclitaxel (Fig. 13.1).

Molecules that are produced in high abundance by cancer cells, such as receptors, may be used for targeting anti-tumor agents predominantly to the cancer.
Polyethylene glycol (PEG) preferentially accumulates in the tumor vaculature.
Extracellularly tumor-activated prodrugs (ETAPs) incorporate both a tumor specific recognition site and a tumor selective enzymatic activation sequence.
Tumor cells take up docosahexaenoic acid.

13.2 Radio-Targeting

Brachytherapy (brachys (Greek) = short distance) (sealed source radio-therapy, internal radio-therapy, endocurietherapy) is a form of radio-therapy where a radiation source is placed inside or in proximity to the area requiring treatment.

Salts Strontium chloride (^{89}Sr) is the salt of a radioactive strontium isotope. It is taken up and incorporated preferentially in metastatic lesions within bone, where it emits cytotoxic β radiation, resulting in a reduction of tumor growth and tumor related bone pain.

Samarium (^{135}Sm) lexidronam pentasodium is a salt of samarium, a therapeutic agent consisting of a medium energy β- and γ-emitting radioisotope and the teraphosphonate chelator ethylenediaminetetramethylene phosphonic acid (EDTMP). The chelator moiety of this drug associates with hydroxyapatite crystals concentrated in areas of bone turnover, thereby delivering cytotoxic radiation preferentially to osteoblastic bone metastases.

Because the vast majority of iodine in the body accumulates in the thyroid, radioiodine is used for the treatment of thyroid cancer.

The radiochemical iodine-131-meta-iodobenzylguanidine (^{131}I-MIBG) localizes to catecholamine secretion and is used to treat pheochromocytomata, paragangliomata, and carcinoid tumors. 90 % of neuroblastomata accumulate meta-iodobenzylguanidine and may be treatable with this drug. Before intravenous infusion, the MIBG carrier is attached to radioiodine. The drug is taken up by the cancer cells and exerts a cytotoxic effect. Blocking of the thyroid is important before this treatment regimen.

Radiopalladium (^{103}Pd) is a radioisotope of the metal palladium used in brachytherapy implants, called seeds. With a half-life of 17 days, radiopalladium allows continuous, site specific low energy irradiation to the tumor cell population while sparing healthy adjacent tissues from radiotoxicity.

Ruthenium (^{106}Ru) is a radioactive isotope of the rare element ruthenium, a member of the light platinum group. A

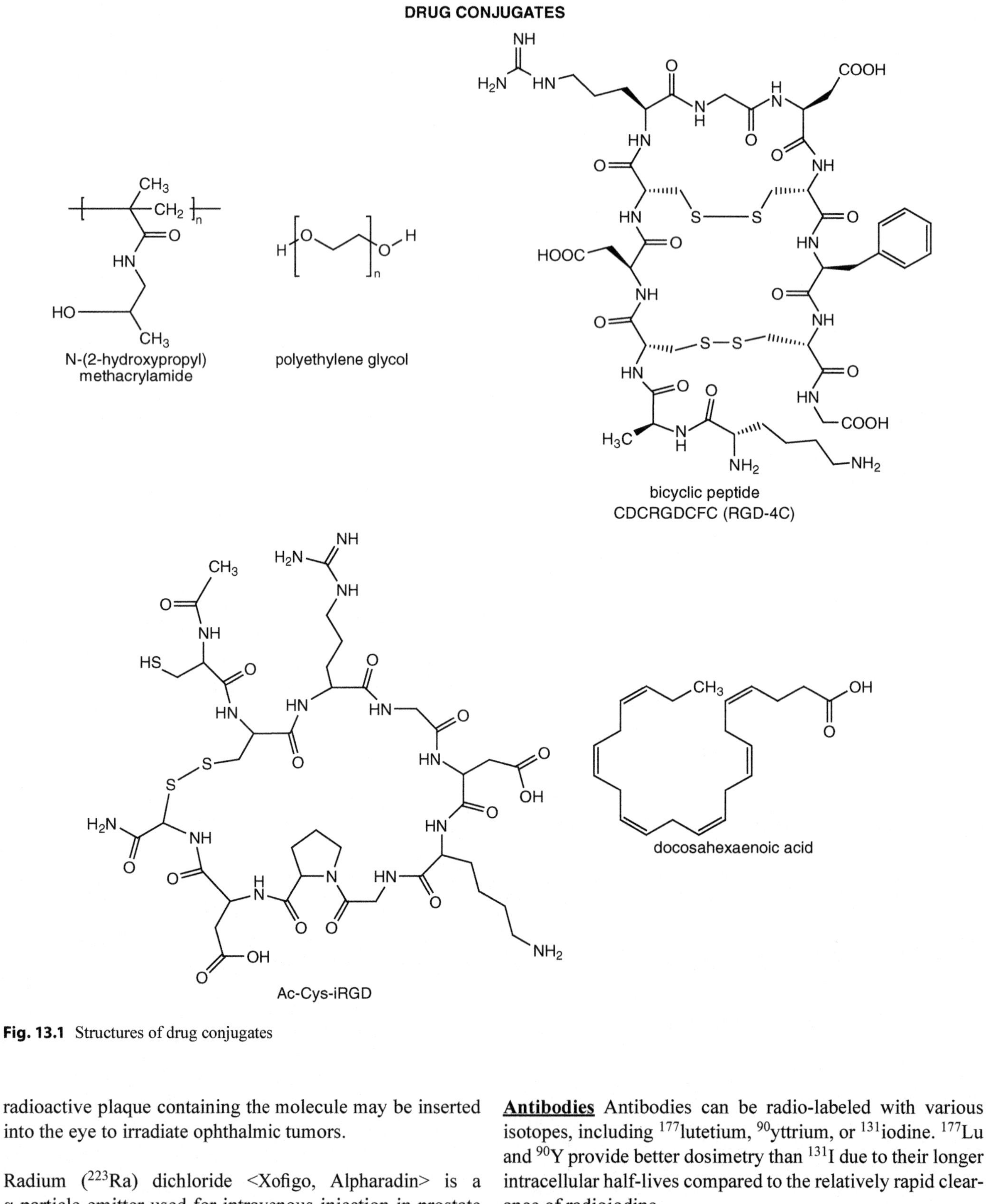

Fig. 13.1 Structures of drug conjugates

radioactive plaque containing the molecule may be inserted into the eye to irradiate ophthalmic tumors.

Radium (^{223}Ra) dichloride <Xofigo, Alpharadin> is a α-particle emitter used for intravenous injection in prostate cancer. The radiologic half-life is 11.5 days.

Adverse Effects The most common adverse effects include diarrhea, vomiting and swelling of the leg, ankle or foot. Blood cell counts may be reduced.

Antibodies Antibodies can be radio-labeled with various isotopes, including ^{177}lutetium, ^{90}yttrium, or ^{131}iodine. ^{177}Lu and ^{90}Y provide better dosimetry than ^{131}I due to their longer intracellular half-lives compared to the relatively rapid clearance of radioiodine.

Adverse Effects Radioisotopes used in the treatment of malignant effusions can cause severe serositis and may lead to slowly constricting and incapacitating fibrosis, particularly of the pleura.

^{131}I tositumomab <Bexxar> is a monoclonal antibody directed to CD20 (which is expressed on the surface of B-lymphocytes), radio-labeled with an isotope of iodine (^{131}I). ^{131}I emits both β andγ radiation and decays with a radiologic half-life of 8 days. The agent delivers radiation selectively to neoplastic CD20^{+} B-lymphocytes, thereby decreasing the systemic radio-toxicity. Tositumomab is used in the treatment of patients with CD20^{+} follicular non-Hodgkin lymphoma, whose disease is untreatable with rituximab and has relapsed following chemotherapy. The CD20 antigen is not shed from the cell surface and does not internalize upon antibody binding. The antibody is given intravenously at a dose that depends on distribution and clearance, which are determined by a test injection before the initiation of treatment (the dosimetric stage).

Adverse Effects At the beginning of the dosimetric stage, paracetamol and anti-histamine drips are administered to counteract possible anaphylactic reactions. Patients should be screened for human anti-mouse hypersensitivity antibodies (HAMA) to avoid the risk of serious immune reactions. Common adverse effects include mild flu-like symptoms, including fever, nausea, and asthenia. Blood counts are suppressed in 70% of patients, typically reaching their lowest point 6 weeks after treatment. The anemia can lead to fatigue, the low platelets can predispose to bleeding, and the reduced white cell pool can pose a risk for infections. Fluid intake is important (12 ounces every hour during the day for the first 2 days after administration). The treatment is combined with an oral iodine supplement, before initiation of treatment and continuing for 2 weeks, to block the ^{131}I effect on the thyroid gland.

Drug Interactions Patients should avoid aspirin, ibuprofen, ketoprofen, and naproxen, as these drugs may mask a fever or increase the risk of hemorrhaging. Additionally, anti-coagulants and agents that interfere with platelet function may increase the risk of bleeding. Tositumomab may decrease the response to and increase the risk of adverse reactions to live-virus vaccines.

Ibritumomab tiuxetan <Zevalin> is a monoclonal antibody radio-immunoconjugate treatment for some forms of B-cell non-Hodgkin lymphoma. The drug combines a mouse monoclonal $IgG_{1\kappa}$ directed to CD20 with the chelator tiuxetan, to which a radioactive isotope (either ^{90}yttrium or ^{111}indium) is bound. Tiuxetan is a modified version of diethylene triamine pentaacetic acid (DTPA), the carbon backbone of which contains an isothiocyanatobenzyl and a methyl group. The chelate, which tightly binds ^{90}Y, is covalently linked to ibritumomab. The β emission from ^{90}Y induces cellular damage by the formation of free radicals in the target and neighboring cells. Ibritumomab tiuxetan is indicated for the treatment of relapsed or refractory, low grade or follicular B-cell non-Hodgkin lymphoma, and for the treatment of previously untreated follicular non-Hodgkin lymphoma in patients who achieve a partial or complete response to first-line chemotherapy. Several hours before each dose of ibritumomab injection, rituximab is given as an integral part of the treatment.

Adverse Effects The most common adverse reactions to ibritumomab tiuxetan are decreases in blood counts (neutropenia, thrombocytopenia), fatigue, abdominal pain, nausea, diarrhea, inflammation of the nose and upper throat, infection, and fever. Among the most serious adverse reactions is prolonged and severe reduction in the number of blood counts. Deaths can occur within 24 h of rituximab infusion, an essential component of the ibritumomab tiuxetan therapeutic regimen. Such fatalities are associated with hypoxia, pulmonary infiltrates, acute respiratory distress syndrome, myocardial infarction, ventricular fibrillation, or cardiogenic shock. Secondary leukemia and myelodysplastic syndrome may arise.

A radio-immunoconjugate consists of the anti-CD22 monoclonal antibody epratuzumab chelated to the radioisotope yttrium-90 (^{90}Y). Yttrium Y 90 epratuzumab binds to tumor cells expressing CD22, it delivers a cytotoxic dose of β radiation. CD22 is a B cell-restricted antigen present on the surfaces of mature B cells; epratuzumab is a humanized version of the murine monoclonal antibody LL2.

^{90}Y-conjugated daclizumab is a synthetic radio-immunoconjugate that binds with high affinity to CD25 (a subunit of the IL-2 Receptor complex) and inhibits the binding of Interleukin-2, thereby blocking the activation of lymphocytes. Yttrium Y 90 daclizumab delivers radiation specifically to lymphocytes that express the IL-2 Receptor.

^{177}Lu monoclonal antibody J591 is a radio-immunoconjugate consisting of a humanized monoclonal antibody, directed to the extracellular domain of PSMA (Prostate-Specific Membrane Antigen), linked to a β-emitting radioisotope (lutetium-177). This conjugate binds to and selectively delivers β particle radiation to tumor cells that express the extracellular domain of PSMA, thus limiting the exposure of normal tissues to ionizing radiation.

Chelates and microspheres DOTA-TATE (DOTA-octreotate) is an amide of the acid DOTA (1,4,7,10-tetraazacyclododecane-1,4,7,10-tetraacetic acid) and (Tyr^{3})-octreotate, a derivative of octreotide. DOTA acts as a chelator for a radionuclide such as lutetium-177, (Tyr^{3})-octreotate binds to Somatostatin Receptors on the cell surfaces of various neuroendocrine tumors.

^{177}Lu DOTA-TATE is under study for the treatment of carcinoid and endocrine pancreatic tumor. Patients are treated with an intravenous infusion of 7.5 GBq of lutetium-177 octreotate. A course of therapy consists of four infusions at 3-monthly intervals.

Table 13.2 Nano-particles

Drug	Active agent	Formulation	Purpose	Cancer
Liposome-encapsulated carboquone	Cisplatin	Single lipid bilayer	Improved tumor bioavailability and toxicity profile	Non-small cell lung cancer
OSI-7904L	Benzoquinazoline folate analog OSI-7904	Liposome encapsulation	Improved efficacy and increased half-life	Various solid tumors
Liposomal cytarabine	Cytarabine	Liposome encapsulation	Intrathecal formulation	Lymphomatous meningitis
Vincristine sulfate liposomes	Vincristine	Rigid lipid bilayer of sphingomyelin	Prolonged maintenance of drug levels	Philadelphia chromosome negative acute lymphoblastic leukemia
Liposomal daunorubicin	Daunorubicin	Liposome encapsulation	Limited cardiotoxicity	AIDS-related Kaposi sarcoma, acute myeloblastic leukemia, multiple myeloma, non-Hodgkin lymphoma, breast cancer
Doxorubicin hydrochloride liposome	Doxorubicin	Multi-lamellar lipid particles with polyethylene glycol coating	Increasing the duration of therapeutic drug effects	Ovarian cancer, AIDS-related Kaposi sarcoma, multiple myeloma
Liposomal doxorubicin citrate	Doxorubicin	Liposome encapsulation	Possible use with trastuzumab due to limited cardiotoxicity	Breast cancer
Paclitaxel-loaded polymeric micelle	Paclitaxel	Poly(ethylene glycol)-poly(D,L-lactide) copolymer micelle	Increased water solubility	Breast cancer
Paclitaxel-polyglumex	Paclitaxel	Polyglutamate polymer	Increased water solubility	Ovarian cancer, glioblastoma
Doxorubicin-magnetic targeted carrier complex	Doxorubicin	Beads of activated carbon and iron		
Nab-paclitaxel	Paclitaxel	Albumin	Increased water solubility, prolonged circulation	Breast cancer
	Doxorubicin	Copolymer N-(2-hydroxypropyl) methacrylamide	Increased water solubility	

^{90}Y glass microspheres comprise an injectable formulation, consisting of glass microspheres that contain the radioisotope yttrium-90. When injected into the tumor vascular bed, these microspheres occlude tumor blood vessels and deliver a cytotoxic dose of β radiation to the tumor site, thereby reducing the neoplastic burden.

Radio-embolization involves the injection of radioactive microspheres into the tumor arteries with the goal to trap them in the tumor capillaries for localized delivery of the radiation. For the treatment of hepatic metastases, the microspheres are injected through a surgically implanted hepatic arterial port or through a transfemoral hepatic artery catheter. Radio-embolization may be combined with radiosensitizing systemic or locally administered chemotherapy.

Brachytherapy places a radiation source inside or in proximity to the area requiring treatment.
Radio-targeting may be accomplished through salts, antibodies, chelates or microspheres.

13.3 Nano-Particles

Nano-particles are under investigation as drug carriers because the technology promises prospects for treatment targeting. Candidate particles typically have a diameter of 50–100 nm (compared to diameters of 7–20 μm for most cells) and are readily taken up. The promise of nano-particles lies in their potential to concentrate the drugs they carry and reduce systemic exposure by releasing them at a designated site (targeting is accomplished by coupling specific moieties, such as antibodies, to the particle surface). The particles themselves are mostly designed to be inert with no drug action of their own. Limitations include the large particle size, charge, and surface structure. Nano-particle efficacy is often compromised due to recognition and clearance by the reticuloendothelial system prior to reaching the target. Formulations under study for cancer therapy include liposomes, carbon nano-tubes, metallic nano-structures, and magnetic nano-particles (Table 13.2).

- Liposomes are among the earliest nano-particles used in medical applications. They have applications for the delivery of small molecules, proteins or peptides, and DNA. The hydrophobic membranes of liposomes can fuse into cellular membranes and deliver their cargo molecules.
- Polymers can form micelles that may serve as drug carriers. Such polymers may facilitate the water solubility of otherwise poorly soluble drugs.
- Carbon nano-tubes have hydrophobic walls that can penetrate cell membranes and can be subjected to functionalization. Carbon nano-tubes have utility as multi-functional transporters and near-infrared agents for the selective destruction of cancer cells.
- Gold nano-particles are preferred metallic nano-structures because they are chemically inert and can be functionalized via Au(I)-thiolate linkages. Depending on their shape, gold nano-structures have strong scattering (spheres, shells) or absorption (rods, cages) cross-sections when irradiated with light. Absorbed photons are converted into phonons (lattice vibrations) that produce a localized temperature increase. This photothermal response can be exploited in cancer treatment as a means of hyperthermic therapy.
- Magnetic nano-particles, most commonly colloidal iron oxide, are used as contrast agents for magnetic resonance imaging (MRI). The particles can be functionalized with monoclonal antibodies. Their therapeutic utility needs to be further elucidated.

Unique challenges posed by this form of treatment include the off-target distribution of nano-particles in the reticuloendothelial system when administered systemically.

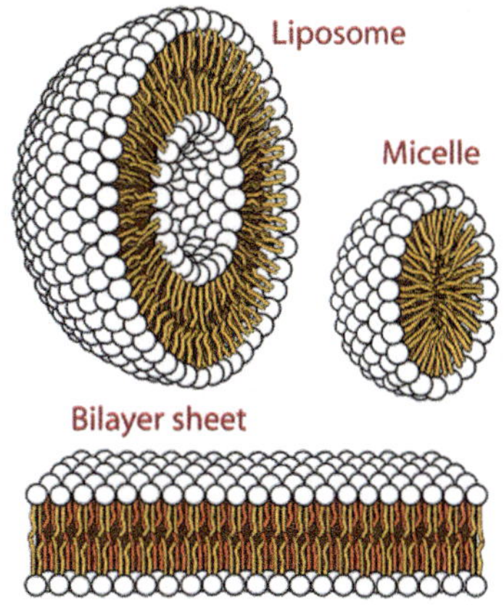

Fig. 13.2 Liposomes and micelles. Cross section view of the structures that can be formed by phospholipids in aqueous solutions (micelles are usually formed by single chain lipids since it is difficult to fit 2 chains into this shape). [http://upload.wikimedia.org/wikipedia/commons/c/c6/Phospholipids_aqueous_solution_structures.svg]

Liposomes and micelles Liposomes (synthetic fat globules) are multi-lamellar lipid particles, typically formed of lipid bilayers (Fig. 13.2). Liposomal treatment uses chemotherapy agents that have been packaged inside a fatty coating, which helps the drugs to penetrate cancer cells more selectively and decreases possible adverse systemic effects. After extravasation into the tumor tissue, these formulations remain within the tumor stroma as drug depots for sustained intra-tumoral drug release. Liposomes eventually become subject to enzymatic degradation or phagocytic attack, leading to the release of their cargo drugs.

A micelle is an aggregate of surfactant molecules dispersed in a liquid colloid. A typical micelle in aqueous solution forms an aggregate with the hydrophilic head regions in contact with surrounding solvent, sequestering the hydrophobic single tail regions in the micelle center. Drugs are entrapped, not covalently bonded, to the polymeric drug carrier micelle.

Liposomes or micelles with hydrophilic poly(ethylene glycol) (PEG) segments as the outer shell have high potential as a long circulating drug carrier system. The duration of such block co-polymer micelles in the blood compartment is greatly modulated by the PEG shell that sterically stabilizes the particles. Such entities are sometimes termed stealth liposomes or stealth micelles because they tend to avoid opsonin adsorption with subsequent uptake by the reticuloendothelial system (the mononuclear phagocytic system) in the liver and spleen. This translates into greatly increased blood circulation times. The longevity of the compounds in the blood stream enables the passive accumulation of entrapped chemotherapeutic reagents within tumor deposits by virtue of the relative increase in vascular permeability of the tumor vasculature over healthy vasculature (enhanced permeation and retention effect).

The cell membrane constitutes a barrier to the transportation of the anti-neoplastic agent cisplatin across and inside the tumor cell. A synthetic formulation, in which cisplatin is encapsulated in lipids, is cisplatin liposomal (liposome-encapsulated carboquone) <CQ-liposome, Lipoplatin>. It consists of small aggregates of cisplatin covered by a single lipid bilayer (110 nm diameter for Lipoplatin). Cationic liposomes (cationic lipoplexes) have favorable interactions with negatively charged cell membranes and DNA. The technology allows the liposome to empty its toxic payload (cisplatin) inside the cytoplasm to kill the tumor cell. Once inside the tumor mass, lipoplatin nano-particles can fuse with the cell membranes because of the presence of dipalmitoylphosphatidylglycerol (DPPG) in their lipid bilayer. Lipoplatin may also be taken up by endocytosis into tumor cells. The encasement in liposomes thus improves the tumor bioavailability and reduces the toxicity profile of the drug, while it does not directly affect its pharmacodynamic properties. Cisplatin liposomal has higher efficacy over cisplatin in combination with paclitaxel as a chemotherapy regimen in lung adenocarcinomata.

Pharmacokinetics Lipoplatin evades clearance by macrophages, circulates for long periods after intravenous administration (half-life around 120 h), and extravasates through the compromised endothelium of the vasculature in tumors created during the process of neo-angiogenesis.

- Stealth liposome-encapsulated cisplatin (SPI-77) is a long-circulating PEGylated liposome formulation.

Adverse Effects Nephrotoxicity is reduced compared to cisplatin.

OSI-7904L (GS7904L) is a liposome encapsulated formulation of the benzoquinazoline folate analog OSI-7904 ((S)-2-(5-(((3-methyl-1-oxo-1,2-dihydrobenzo[f]quinazolin-9-yl)methyl)amino)-1-oxoisoindolin-2-yl)pentanedioic acid). As a Thymidylate Synthase inhibitor, OSI-7904 noncompetitively binds to Thymidylate Synthase, resulting in the inhibition of thymine nucleotide synthesis and DNA reduplication. Liposome encapsulation improves the efficacy and increases the half-life of OSI-7904.

Adverse Effects Dose limiting toxicity occurs around 15 mg/m^2 and includes stomatitis, diarrhea, fatigue, tachyarrhythmia, rash, hand-foot syndrome, and potentially fatal neutropenic sepsis. Other toxicities, such as nausea and vomiting, are mild or moderate.

Liposomal cytarabine (liposomal Ara-C) <DepoCyt> is an intrathecal formulation of the anti-metabolite cytarabine. As a S-phase specific anti-metabolite, cytarabine is phosphorylated by Deoxycytidine Kinase to a triphosphate form, which then competes with thymidine for incorporation into the DNA. Cytarabine triphosphate incorporated into DNA may inhibit DNA Polymerase and so DNA synthesis, resulting in cell death. Liposomal cytarabine has a prolonged half-life and can be administered less frequently than the non-encapsulated drug. It is approved to treat lymphomatous meningitis, and is administered as intrathecal infusion (possibly via lumbar puncture) or intraventricular infusion (possibly with an Ommaya reservoir, which is a dome-shaped device with an attached catheter that is placed subcutaneously on the scalp).

Adverse Effects The most common adverse reactions include meningitis (steroids are given before and for 5 days after the injection to prevent or lessen this reaction), confusion or somnolescence (central neurotoxicity), headache, fatigue, nausea and vomiting, and fever.

Vincristine sulfate liposome injection <Marqibo> utilizes vincristine encapsulated in a rigid lipid bilayer of sphingomyelin for injection. Vincristine is a cell cycle specific agent, the activity of which depends on the duration of drug exposure. The active agent leaks out of the liposome slowly and efficacious drug levels are maintained for prolonged periods of time. In 2012, the U.S. FDA granted accelerated approval for vincristine sulfate liposome injection for the treatment of adult patients with Philadelphia chromosome negative acute lymphoblastic leukemia in second or greater relapse or whose disease has progressed following 2 or more anti-leukemia therapies. The drug is administered at a dose of 2.25 mg/m^2 intravenously over 1 h every 7 days.

Adverse Effects The most common adverse reactions, with an incidence over 30 %, include constipation or diarrhea, decreased appetite, nausea, pyrexia, fatigue, and insomnia. Patients should be monitored for peripheral motor and sensory, central and autonomic neuropathy, which may require dose reduction or discontinuation. Patients with preexisting severe neuropathy should be treated with vincristine sulfate liposome injection only after careful risk-to-benefit assessment. Neutropenia (especially febrile neutropenia), thrombocytopenia, or anemia may require dose reduction or interruption and supportive care measures.

Vincristine sulfate liposome injection is contraindicated in patients with demyelinating conditions, including Charcot-Marie-Tooth syndrome, and patients with hypersensitivity to the drug formulation. Vincristine sulfate liposome injection is contraindicated for intrathecal administration.

Anthracyclines are potent anti-cancer drugs which are constrained by substantial systemic toxicities. Drug delivery applications for these agents may enhance the efficacy against tumor cells while limiting the exposure of myocardium and bone marrow.

Daunorubicin citrate liposome injection (daunorubicin liposomal) <DaunoXome> is an encapsulated form of daunorubicin. The liposome provides extended circulation due to its size of 45 nm and its rigid bilayer. It utilizes the liposomal carrier system that provides a favorable pharmacokinetic profile at the site of lesions resulting in a 10-fold increase in concentration compared to that of non-encapsulated daunorubicin. Administration is intravenous. Daunorubicin citrate liposome injection is under investigation for the treatment of AIDS-related Kaposi sarcoma (first-line therapy), acute myeloblastic leukemia, multiple myeloma, non-Hodgkin lymphoma, and breast cancer.

Doxorubicin hydrochloride liposome <Doxil, Caelyx> is a PEGylated liposome encapsulated form of the doxorubicin hydrochloride salt. The liposomal delivery of the drug improves its penetration into tumors and decreases its clearance, thereby increasing the duration of the therapeutic effects. An intermittent 3-weekly schedule is common, and the maximum tolerated dose is 60–90 mg/m^2. Doxorubicin hydrochloride liposome is used primarily for the treatment of ovarian cancer, which has progressed or recurred after platinum based chemotherapy, for the treatment of AIDS-related Kaposi sarcoma, and for the treatment of multiple myeloma.

Pharmacokinetics Doxorubicin hydrochloride liposome is a small (around 100 nm) and rigid liposome, onto which a polymeric coat of polyethylene glycol is grafted. This PEGylated liposome displays inhibited interactions with plasma proteins and mononuclear phagocytes, and it consequently has greatly prolonged circulation times. This results in a terminal half-life of 55 h.

Adverse Effects The polyethylene glycol coating results in the preferential concentration of doxorubicin hydrochloride liposome in the skin, which is desired for the treatment of Kaposi sarcoma. However, it also causes the adverse effect of palmar plantar erythrodysesthesia (hand-foot syndrome). Following administration, small amounts of the drug can leak from capillaries in the palms of the hands and soles of the feet, leading to redness, tenderness, and peeling of the skin that can be uncomfortable. At 50 mg/m^2 dosing every 4 weeks, the incidence of hand-foot syndrome is about 50%. Liposome encapsulated doxorubicin is less cardiotoxic than unencapsulated doxorubicin.

Doxorubicin can only be used in sequential combination (not in concurrent combination) with trastuzumab <Herceptin>. Although their concurrent combination achieves a superior anti-tumor response, it results in a high risk of congestive heart failure. By limiting the cardiotoxicity of doxorubicin through liposomal encapsulation, it can be used safely in combination chemotherapy with other cardiotoxic drugs, such as trastuzumab.

Liposomal doxorubicin citrate (TLC D-99) <Myocet> is a liposome encapsulated form of the doxorubicin citrate salt. The liposomal delivery of the drug improves its penetration into tumors and slows the drug clearance, thereby increasing the duration of therapeutic drug effects. Liposomal doxorubicin citrate is approved in Europe and Canada for the treatment of metastatic breast cancer in combination with cyclophosphamide.

Pharmacokinetics Liposomal doxorubicin citrate has a different pharmacokinetic profile from doxorubicin, resulting in an improved therapeutic index (less cardiotoxicity with equal anti-cancer activity). The clearance is about 5-fold lower and the volume of distribution is about 10-fold lower than in patients receiving unencapsulated doxorubicin. The half-life (16–50 h) is much longer than that of conventional doxorubicin. Liposomes are lipid bilayers with a hydrophobic external surface, which compromises their ability to pass through healthy capillaries, thus decreasing the volume of distribution. Tumor capillaries are leaky, allowing the liposome to enter the malignant tissue, which is the basis for a relative selectivity and favorable pharmacokinetic properties.

Adverse Effects In patients on liposomal doxorubicin citrate, the frequency of congestive heart failure is reduced from 8 to 2% compared to carrier-free doxorubicin. The most substantial adverse effects are myelosuppression (especially thrombocytopenia), nausea and vomiting. Unlike doxorubicin hydrochloride liposome <Doxil>, liposomal doxorubicin citrate does not have a polyethylene glycol coating, and therefore presents a lower risk for hand-foot syndrome.

Polymers Because of its biocompatible and biodegradable nature, poly(lactide) (PLA) is a polymer with high potential for the design of a hydrophobic core for block co-polymer micelles with a programmed decaying property. Intravenously administered micelles from poly(ethyleneglycol)-PLA and poly(ethyleneglycol)-poly(lactide-co-glycolide) (PLGA) block co-polymers display improved circulation compared with simple poly(lactide) nano-particles.

Paclitaxel-loaded polymeric micelle <Genexol-PM> is a biodegradable poly(ethylene glycol)-poly(D, L-lactide) co-polymer (acetal-PEG-PDLLA) micelle nano-particle entrapped formulation of paclitaxel. The co-polymer residue increases the water solubility of paclitaxel and allows the delivery of higher doses than those achievable with paclitaxel alone.

Paclitaxel poliglumex is paclitaxel linked to a biodegradable, water soluble poly-L-glutamate polymer. The polyglutamate residue increases the water solubility of paclitaxel and allows delivery of higher doses than those achievable with paclitaxel alone.

Magnetic nano-particles Doxorubicin-magnetic targeted carrier complex (DOX-MTC) consists of doxorubicin bound to microscopic beads of activated carbon and iron (magnetic targeted carriers). With the placement of a magnet on the body surface overlaying a tumor site, this carrier complex delivers doxorubicin directly to the tumor, thereby prolonging the duration of the therapeutic effects while decreasing the systemic toxicity.

Various Nano-particles have emerged as a useful vehicle for poorly soluble agents such as paclitaxel. Nab-paclitaxel <Abraxane> is an Albumin-bound, nano-particle-sized form of the drug that allows a reduced use of solubilizer vehicles, such as Cremophor. This formulation permits the administration of larger doses of this agent, which would be toxic in an unbound or Cremophor ELP containing formulation. Nab-paclitaxel was approved by the U.S. FDA in 2005 for the treatment of breast cancer after failure of combination chemotherapy for metastatic disease or after relapse within 6 months of adjuvant chemotherapy. The agent is administered intravenously at 260 mg/m^2 over 30 min, every 21 days.

PK-1 is a conjugate of the water soluble, acrylamide based co-polymer *N*-(2-hydroxypropyl)methacrylamide and doxorubicin. Polymer associated anthracyclines have not achieved the same degree of prolonged circulation as sterically stabilized liposomal doxorubicin. However, their circulation surpasses that of free doxorubicin. Due to the enhanced permeability and retention effect of the tumor vasculature, prolonged circulation results in improved cancer accumulation.

Nano-particles have the potential to concentrate the drugs they carry and reduce systemic exposure by releasing them at a designated site.
Particles for therapeutic use typically have a diameter of 50–100 nm.
The particles are mostly designed to be inert with no drug action of their own.
Limitations include the large particle size, charge, surface structure, and clearance by the reticuloendothelial system.

13.4 Solubilizers

Cremophor ELP (Liebmann et al. 1993) is a non-ionic solubilizer that constitutes an excipient[1] for drug formulations to overcome poor water solubility. Cremophor (Fig. 13.3) is made by reacting castor oil with ethylene oxide in a molar ratio of 1:35, followed by a purification step. Cyclosporin, teniposide, paclitaxel and docetaxel are poorly soluble in aqueous solutions, and hence are formulated with vehicles, such as a 1:1 blend of cremophor EL (polyethoxylated castor oil) and ethanol, which is then diluted 5–20-fold in isotonic saline or 5 % dextrose solution for administration.

Pharmacokinetics Paclitaxel displays a non-linear pharmacokinetic behavior when formulated in cremophor-ethanol. The clearance is reduced compared to plain paclitaxel. Despite much higher blood levels of paclitaxel being reached when given in the cremophor EL-ethanol formulation, the tissue levels are similar among various drug preparations.

Adverse Effects Cremophor is associated with risks of hypersensitivity reactions, which can be severe and may be fatal. Premedication with corticosteroids (dexamethasone) and anti-histamines (both H_1 and H_2 receptor antagonists) increases drug safety by reducing the intensity and the incidence of serious hypersensitivity reactions in response to paclitaxel administration in cremophor[2]. Myelosuppression, nephrotoxicity, and neurotoxicity are associated with the solubilizer. Cremophor EL also has an influence on the function of endothelial and vesicular muscles and causes vasodilation, labored breathing, lethargy, and hypotension.

Polysorbate 80 (polyoxyethylene (20) sorbitan monooleate, (x)-sorbitan mono-9-octadecenoate poly(oxy-1,2-ethanediyl)) <Tween 80> is a non-ionic surfactant and emulsifier derived from polyethoxylated sorbitan and oleic acid. It serves as a solubilizer for drugs and an excipient to stabilize aqueous formulations of medications for parenteral administration. The compound is also a common food additive. Polysorbate 80 may be mixed with the surfactant pluronic L64, in the ratios of 3:1:6 (v/v/v) for enhanced solubilization.

Adverse Effects Although generally well tolerated, polysorbate 80 is allergenic, requires extensive premedication, and is responsible for most of the acute toxicities observed with taxane therapy (rather than the taxanes themselves). It can cause hypersensitivity particularly in patients with Crohn disease.

Cyclodextrins are cyclic oligosaccharides, which increase the solubility, dissolution rate, and bioavailability of poorly soluble drugs. They also increase the stability of labile drugs and improve the performance of intravenous formulations. Paclitaxel is more stable in cyclodextrin solution than in buffer solution of comparable pH (with maximum stability at the pH 3–5 range). An inclusion complex with hydroxy propyl-β-cyclodextrin enhances the solubility. Although paclitaxel can be complexed with α-cyclodextrins, the large cavities of β- and γ-cyclodextrins are more suitable to solubilize this drug. Paclitaxel forms predominantly second order complexes with the cyclodextrins, and the complexes with hydroxy propyl-β-cyclodextrin are more stable than those of hydroxy propyl-γ-cyclodextrin or γ-cyclodextrin. There is a further increase in solubility with the addition of ethanol.

Adverse Effects The passenger drug tends to precipitate out of the cyclodextrin complex on dilution with aqueous media. To overcome this, increased concentrations of cyclodextrin are required, which may cause hemolysis.

An emulsion type of delivery system can be formulated using triacetin as the internal phase in an oil-in-water emulsion. Triacetin is a very effective solubilizing vehicle. For drugs that do not precipitate, the emulsion is diluted before administration approximately 9-fold with 5 % dextrose in an intravenous piggyback system. Self-emulsifying formulations consist of a mixture of oil, surfactants and co-surfactants. Triacetin is a co-solvent, having affinity for both lipophilic and hydrophilic phases. It can serve a dual purpose of co-solvency as well as an emulsification aid.

Solubilizers may facilitate the administration of poorly water soluble drugs.
Hypersensitivity is a risk associated with many solubilizers.

[1] An excipient is an inactive substance added to the active ingredient of a formulation. It has the purpose of bulking it up, which facilitates dispensation and may favorably affect pharmacokinetics, including drug absorption or solubility.

[2] Note, however, that certain H_2 receptor antagonists (such as cimetidine and ranitidine) are inhibitors of Cytochrome P450s and have the potential to interfere with cancer drug metabolism.

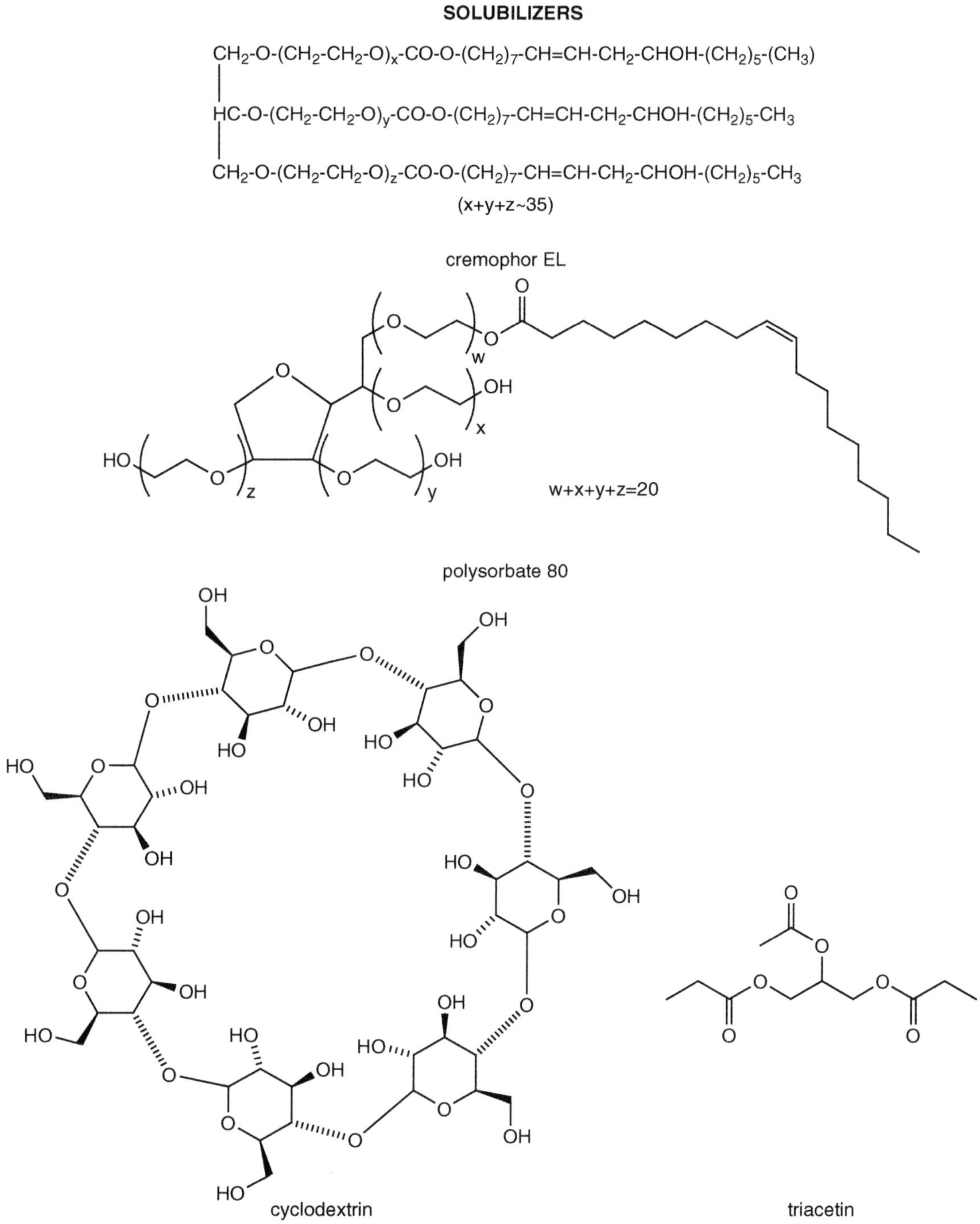

Fig. 13.3 Structures of solubilizers

13.5 Various

Hyperthermic therapy In 1898, Westermark used localized hyperthermia to produce tumor regression in patients (Westermark 1898). In hyperthermia (thermotherapy), tissue is exposed to high temperatures to damage proteins and structures within cancer cells, leading to a shrinkage of tumors. It is based on the notion that tumor cells are compromised in dissipating heat, due to their disorganized and compact vascular structure. Also, an acidic intra-tumor environment increases the response to hyperthermic treatment. By contrast, healthy tissues can more easily maintain a physiologic temperature. Various types of energy may be used in hyperthermic treatment, including focused ultrasound, infrared sauna, microwave heating, radiofrequency ablation, induction heating, magnetic hyperthermia, infusion of warmed liquids, or direct application of heat. For this technique to be effective, the temperatures must be high enough and sustained long enough to damage or kill the cancer cells. However, if the temperatures are too high or are kept elevated for too long, then serious adverse effects can result. To ensure that the desired temperature is reached, but not exceeded, the temperature of the tumor and surrounding tissue is monitored throughout hyperthermia treatment.

By itself, hyperthermia is generally ineffective, with only small numbers of patients receiving lasting benefit. The regimen is typically used with other forms of cancer therapy, such as chemotherapy (thermochemo-therapy) or radiation therapy (thermoradio-therapy). The elevated temperature increases the blood flow to the warmed area, thus increasing perfusion and enhancing the delivery of medications. Hyperthermia also increases oxygen delivery to the area, which may increase the sensitivity to radiation, as well as preventing cells from repairing the damage induced during a radiation session.

Hyperthermia may be applied locally, regionally, or to the whole body.

- In local hyperthermia (thermal ablation), heat is applied to a small area that contains the tumor. For tumors located in or just below the skin, energy is focused on the growth by external applicators to raise its temperature. Intraluminal or endocavitary methods may be used to treat tumors within or near body cavities, such as the esophagus or the rectum. Image guided interstitial techniques, requiring anesthesia, may treat tumors deep within the body.
- Regional hyperthermia targets large areas of tissue, such as a body cavity, organ, or limb. Deep tissue approaches may be used to treat cancers within the body, such as cervical or bladder cancer. Regional perfusion techniques remove blood from the patient, heat it, and perfuse it back into the limb or organ. Continuous hyperthermic peritoneal perfusion is a technique used to treat peritoneal carcinomatosis. During surgery, heated anti-cancer drugs flow from a warming device through the peritoneal cavity.
- Whole body hyperthermia is used to treat metastatic cancer that has disseminated throughout the body. This can be accomplished by the use of thermal chambers or hot water blankets.

Adverse Effects Due to regional differences in tissue characteristics, higher temperatures may occur in various spots, causing discomfort. External application of heat may cause blisters, which generally heal quickly, and burns, which heal slowly. Perfusion and moderate or high levels of hyperthermia can cause swelling, blood clots, and bleeding. Whole body hyperthermia usually results in diarrhea, nausea, vomiting, fatigue, and other symptoms of sunstroke. Rarely, it may also cause serious adverse effects, including cardiac and vascular disorders.

Gold nano-particles, magnetic nano-particles and carbon nano-tubes can efficiently generate heat upon electromagnetic stimulation after direct injection into tumors or preferential accumulation in tumors following systemic administration.

Magnetic iron oxide particles have been used for hyperthermia treatments since 1957 (Gilchrist et al. 1957). The application of a radio-frequency magnetic field around 150 kHz induces rapid oscillations and heating of the local environment.

Lyso-thermosensitive liposome doxorubicin is a formulation that contains the anthracycline antibiotic doxorubicin encapsulated in temperature sensitive liposomes. Upon intravenous administration, circulating thermo-sensitive liposomes are activated locally by heating the tumor to a temperature of 40 °C using an external heat source. The increased temperature causes composition changes in the liposome, thereby creating openings that trigger the release of the encapsulated doxorubicin. Compared to non-thermosensitive liposomes, lyso-thermosensitive liposomes deliver higher concentrations of the cytotoxic agent at the tumor site while diminishing drug concentrations at non-heat activated sites.

Thermodifferential chemotherapy consists of the systemic administration of anti-tumor drugs and local hyperthermia combined with general hypothermia. The general hypothermia applied not only enhances the local drug effect, it also reduces systemic toxicity. Cisplatin <Carboquone> displays good anti-tumor effects in this regimen, suggesting that its tumoricidal activity is enhanced under the acidic metabolic condition produced by hyperthermia (Kamura et al. 1979).

Other Methotrexate-e therapeutic implant is an injectable Collagen matrix gel containing the anti-metabolite methotrexate and the sympathicomimetic agent epinephrine. After intra-tumoral injection, the potent vasoconstrictor epinephrine enhances the penetration of methotrexate into the tumor tissue and reduces the dispersion to the surrounding tissues, thereby increasing the local concentration of methotrexate and improving its anti-tumor activity.

The majority of primary liver cancer is hepatocellular carcinoma. Several non-surgical treatment options, including transcatheter arterial embolization, have been developed and are widely used for unresectable hepatocellular carcinoma. However, these modalities are not indicated for patients with multifocal disease, invasion or thrombosis of major blood vessels, and poor liver function. Transcatheter arterial chemoembolization (TACE) is usually performed in the treatment of large tumors. It consists of an intra-arterial infusion of anti-neoplastic agents mixed with iodized oil (e.g. poppyseed oil <Lipiodol>). The greatest benefit is seen in patients with preserved liver function, absence of vascular invasion, and small tumors.

- Continuous local arterial infusion of 5-fluorouracil and cisplatin via an infuser pump and implanted reservoir prolongs the survival of patients with advanced hepatocellular carcinoma.
- Intra-arterial ^{131}I-lipiodol administration has efficacy in patients with unresectable tumors and those with portal vein thrombus. This treatment is also used as adjuvant therapy in resected patients (Lau et al. 1999).
- Radioembolization is a minimally invasive transcatheter therapy through which radioactive microspheres are infused into the hepatic arteries that supply tumor. These microspheres traverse the hepatic vascular plexus and selectively implant within the tumor arterioles. Embedded within the arterioles, the ^{90}Y or ^{188}Rh impregnated microspheres emit high energy and low penetrating radiation doses selectively to the tumor (Ibrahim et al. 2008).

References

de Groot FM, Broxterman HJ, Adams HP, van Vliet A, Tesser GI, Elderkamp YW, Schraa AJ, Kok RJ, Molema G, Pinedo HM, Scheeren HW (2002) Design, synthesis and biological evaluation of a dual tumor-specific motive containing integrin-targeted plasmin-cleavable doxorubicin prodrug. Mol Cancer Ther 1:901–911

Denmeade SR, Nagy A, Gao J, Lilja H, Schally AV, Isaacs JT (1998) Enzymatic activation of a doxorubicin-peptide prodrug by prostate-specific antigen. Cancer Res 58:2537–2540

Gilchrist RK, Medal R, Shorey WD, Hanselman RC, Parrot JC, Taylor CB (1957) Selective inductive heating of lymph. Ann Surg 146:596–606

Ibrahim SM, Lewandowski RJ, Sato KT, Gates VL, Kulik L, Mulcahy MF, Ryu RK, Omary RA, Salem R (2008) Radioembolization for the treatment of unresectable hepatocellular carcinoma: a clinical review. World J Gastroenterol 14:1664–1669

Kamura T, Aoki K, Nishikawa K, Baba T (1979) Antitumor effect of thermodifferential chemotherapy with carboquone on Ehrlich carcinoma. Gan 70:783–790

Lau W, Leung T, Ho S, Chan M, Machin D, Lau J, Chan A, Yeo W, Mok T, Yu S, Leung N, Johnson P (1999) Adjuvant intra-arterial iodine-131-labelled lipiodol for resectable hepatocellular carcinoma: a prospective randomised trial. Lancet 353:797–801

Liebmann J, Cook JA, Mitchell J (1993) Cremophor EL, solvent for paclitaxel, and toxicity. Lancet 342:1428

Partridge WM (1992) Recent developments in peptide drug delivery to the brain. Basic Clin Pharmacol Toxicol 71:3–10

Sugahara KN, Teesalu T, Karmali PP, Kotamraju VR, Agemy L, Greenwald DR, Ruoslahti E (2010) Coadministration of a tumor-penetrating peptide enhances the efficacy of cancer drugs. Science 328:1031–1035

Trouet A, Passioukov A, Van derpoorten K, Fernandez AM, Abarca-Quinones J, Baurain R, Lobl TJ, Oliyai C, Shochat D, Dubois V (2001) Extracellularly tumor-activated prodrugs for the selective chemotherapy of cancer: application to doxorubicin and preliminary in vitro and in vivo studies. Cancer Res 61:2843–2846

Westermark F (1898) Über die Behandlung des ulcerierenden Cervixcarcimons mittels konstanter Wärme. Zentralblatt für Gynäkologie 22:1335

Drug Metabolism

14

Interindividual differences in therapeutic efficacy and safety of anti-cancer agents may compromise treatment. In particular, variability in chemotherapy associated toxicity is a host related phenomenon that is largely a consequence of pharmacogenetic differences in absorption, distribution, metabolism, and elimination (ADME). The metabolic fate of a drug may depend on its route of administration.

Most drugs/xenobiotics undergo chemical modifications in the body before elimination. Biotransformation renders lipophilic drugs more hydrophilic to facilitate their elimination

- Phase I drug metabolizing enzymes introduce polar functional moieties (amino-, carboxyl-, sulfhydryl-, hydroxyl-) and typically decrease the chemical reactivity
- Phase II drug metabolizing enzymes catalyze the addition of small endogenous molecules (glucuronidation, sulfation, Glutathione conjugation, acetylation) to facilitate excretion.

The activities of many anti-cancer drugs can be modulated by drug metabolism. This may lead to the activation of prodrugs or inactivation of active drugs. Some alkylating agents, such as cyclophosphamide, ifosphamide, procarbazine, and dacarbazine are prodrugs that are converted to active cytotoxic agents as a consequence of oxidative metabolism catalyzed by Cytochrome P450s. Other alkylating agents, including melphalan, chlorambucil, and chloroethylnitrosoureas, can be transformed to inactive metabolites by the Glutathione S-Transferases.

Interindividual differences in therapeutic efficacy and safety of anti-cancer agents may compromise treatment.
Biotransformation occurs in phase I and phase II metabolism.
It renders lipophilic drugs more hydrophilic to facilitate their elimination.
The metabolic fate of a drug may depend on its route of administration.

14.1 CYP450

The Cytochrome P450 (CYP) super-family of enzymes that contain a heme-carbon monoxide complex with a maximal absorbance near 450 nm. They catalyze the oxidation of organic substrates, including metabolic intermediates (such as lipids and steroidal hormones), as well as xenobiotic substances (such as drugs and toxic chemicals). Cytochrome P450s are the major enzymes involved in drug metabolism. The range of functions necessitates many distinct *cyp* gene products (18 gene families encoding 57 enzymes) (Fig. 14.1). These enzymes are most abundant in the liver.

Genetic variations in the *cyp* genes may cause the absence of enzyme, diminished enzyme expression, enzyme with altered substrate specificity, or increased enzyme expression. Based on the composition of the alleles, the affected individuals can be categorized into poor metabolizers, intermediate metabolizers, extensive metabolizers, and ultrarapid metabolizers[1]. Although *cyp* genetics is a critical determinant of Cytochrome P450 activity, the expression of these enzymes is also highly responsive to environmental cues. The activities can be significantly affected by nutritional status, the presence of inflammatory conditions, concomitant medications or habits (caffeine, nicotine) that may induce or inhibit activity, and liver disease or hepatic metastases.

Various attempts have been made to modulate Cytochrome P450 activity in anti-cancer therapy to favor efficacy or lower toxicity of certain anti-cancer drugs. These approaches are still experimental.

CYP3A4 is generally the most abundant Cytochrome P450 in the liver and is often important in drug metabolism.

[1] CYP enzymes can roughly be divided into two classes: CYP1A1, CYP1A2, CYP2E1, and CYP3A4 are well conserved, do not have important functional polymorphisms, and are active in the metabolism of pre-carcinogens and drugs. CYP2B6, CYP2C9, CYP2C19, and CYP2D6 are highly polymorphic and active in the metabolism of drugs, but not of pre-carcinogens.

G. F. Weber, *Molecular Therapies of Cancer*, DOI 10.1007/978-3-319-13278-5_14,

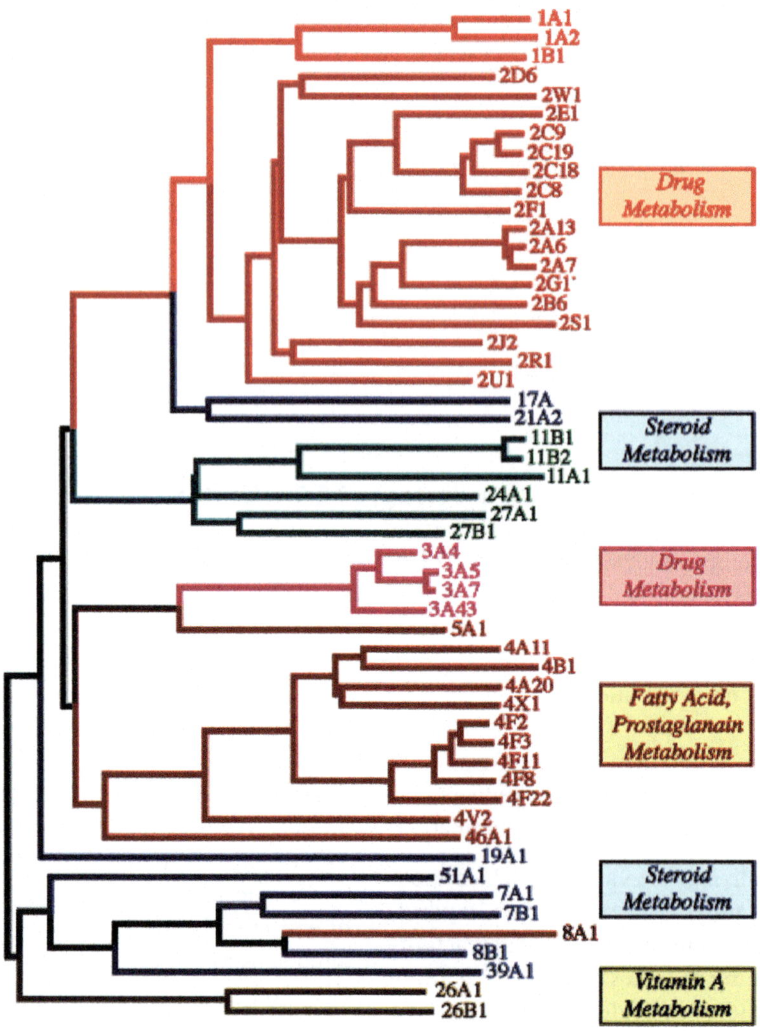

Fig. 14.1 Gene family of Cytochrome P450s. A phylogenetic tree of human Cytochrome P450 genes and their associated biological functions. (http://www.aist.go.jp/aist_e/aist_today/2002_04/hot_line/hot_line_23.html) There are instances where we have been unable to trace or contact the copyright holder. If notified the publisher will be pleased to rectify any errors or omissions at the earliest opportunity

Many anti-cancer drugs are metabolized predominantly by CYP3A4. Substances that are inducers of CYP3A4 activity (rifampicin) increase the metabolism of these drugs and decrease their blood concentrations. Substances that are potent inhibitors of CYP3A4 activity (ketoconazole, itraconazole) decrease the metabolic conversion and increase the blood concentrations.

Beside the impact of hepatic Cytochrome P450 on anti-cancer pharmacokinetics, Cytochrome P450 activity in the tumor cells can result in altered drug metabolism. The capacity of tumors to metabolize drugs is a potential mechanism of resistance to therapy via increased inactivation of anti-cancer drugs. CYP3A4 is involved in the oxidation of common chemotherapeutic agents, such as etoposide, ifosfamide, cyclophosphamide and doxorubicin. Consistently, the response to these drugs tends to be worse in tumors with high CYP3A expression. Therefore, the main drug metabolizing P450 enzymes expressed in cancer cells could influence the success of drug therapy. Other extrahepatic P450s that may be over-expressed in tumor tissue include CYP1B1, CYP2J2, CYP2W1, and CYP4Z1.

Drug interactions with grapefruit juice were discovered by serendipity in 1989 (Bailey 1989). During investigations whether alcohol could interact with felodipine <Plendil>, a solution of alcohol with grapefruit juice (intended to mask the taste of the alcohol for the study) revealed that the blood levels of felodipine were increased several-fold due to the intake of the grapefruit juice. The elevated blood levels caused higher drug effects and adverse effects of felodipine.

Grapefruits provide many nutrients (including vitamin C, potassium, and lycopene) but furanocoumarins (such as bergamottin, bergapten, bergaptol, and 6′,7′-dihydroxybergamottin)

in grapefruit juice and grapefruit pulp interfere with hepatic and intestinal Cytochrome P450 3A4 (CYP3A4), which metabolizes various drugs in the digestive system and limits their absorption into the body through a first-pass effect[2]. The result can be excessively altered levels of these agents in the blood and an increased risk of adverse events. Seville oranges (a type of bitter orange often used to make marmalade and compotes) and pomelos may have a similar effect.

One glass of grapefruit juice can suffice to elicit the maximum food-drug interaction effect, which may persist for longer than 24 h. Therefore, an effect may occur even if the intake of grapefruit juice and the susceptible medication is not simultaneous. The interaction can be avoided by separating the administration of grapefruit juice with susceptible drugs by 24 or more hours. Anti-cancer drugs affected include cyclophosphamide, etoposide, ifosfamide, tamoxifen, vinblastine, and vincristine.

The Cytochrome P450 (CYP) super-family of enzymes catalyzes the oxidation of organic substrates.
Cytochrome P450s are the major enzymes involved in drug metabolism.
Cytochrome P450 enzymes are most abundant in the liver, but may also play a role in the tumor.
Many anti-cancer drugs are metabolized predominantly by CYP3A4.

14.2 Flavin Monooxygenases

Flavin Monooxygenases (FMOs, Dimethylaniline Monooxygenases, Dimethylaniline *N*-Oxidases) are microsomal enzymes that catalyze the oxygenation of nucleophilic, hetero-atom containing xenobiotics (Fig. 14.2). This step serves to increase water solubility and generally decrease toxic potential. 3 of the 5 expressed *fmo* genes (*fmo1*, *fmo2*, and *fmo3*) exhibit genetic polymorphisms. These enzymes contribute to the metabolism of various anti-cancer agents, such as tamoxifen.

Sulindac is a non-steroidal anti-inflammatory drug with a chemopreventive effect in patients with familial adenomatous polyposis (FAP). The drug is inactivated by the hepatic microsomal enzyme Flavin Monooxygenase 3 (FMO3). Numerous polymorphisms exist in FMO3, which alter its enzymatic activity and subsequent substrate metabolism. Patients with the polymorphisms E158K and E308G have a greater reduction in both the size and number of polyps than others, suggesting that combined polymorphic changes in the E158K and E308G alleles may protect against polyposis in patients with FAP treated with sulindac (Hisamuddin 2005).

[2] Bioactive compounds in grapefruit juice may also interfere with ABCB1 (P-Glycoprotein, MDR-1) and organic anion transporting polypeptides (OATPs), thus either increasing or decreasing the bioavailability of a number of drugs.

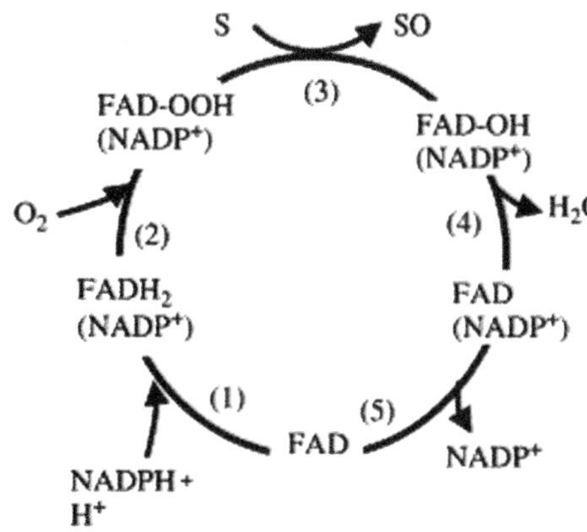

Fig. 14.2 Catalytic cycle of Flavin-Containing Monooxygenases. *1* FAD reduced by NADPH (fast). *2* $FADH_2$ reacts with O_2 (fast). Flavin-hydroperoxide is stable: likely the form in which FMO exists in the cell. *3* FAD-OOH reacts with any suitable nucleophile gaining access to active site, no substrate binding required. *4* One atom of O_2 is incorporated into substrate and the other into H_2O-FMO is a Monooxygenase. *5* FAD-OH is converted to FAD via release of H_2O (slowest step in the cycle determines V_{max}). The final step in the cycle is the release of $NADP^+$ (slow). (Krueger 2005)

Flavin Monooxygenases are microsomal enzymes that catalyze the oxygenation of nucleophilic, hetero-atom containing xenobiotics.

14.3 GST

The Glutathione S-Transferase super-family consists of cytosolic or membrane bound dimeric enzymes of 45–55 kD that are assigned to 6 classes including α, μ, π, θ, ζ and ω. Glutathione S-Transferases (GSTs) catalyze the conjugation of reduced Glutathione, via a sulfhydryl group, to electrophilic centers on various substrates (Fig. 14.3). This enhances their solubility and detoxifies endogenous or exogenous compounds, such as lipid peroxides and xenobiotics. Glutathione S-Transferases contribute to the Phase II metabolism of xenobiotics by conjugating typically electrophilic and slightly lipophilic compounds with reduced Glutathione (GSH) to facilitate dissolution in the aqueous cellular and extracellular media. The expression levels of these enzymes are a crucial determinant for the sensitivity of cells to a broad spectrum of toxic chemicals. Glutathione S-Transferases may also function as transport proteins. Like other gene products of the intermediary metabolism, the induction of Glutathione S-Transferase expression is very sensitive to environmental cues.

The arene oxides are very reactive. They may be generated in the Monooxygenase catalyzed metabolism of aromatic compounds. If these molecules escape enzymatic conversion, toxicity may result from their reactions with RNA, DNA, and proteins to generate covalent adducts. Glutathione S-Transferases detoxify reactive oxide derivatives, including

Fig. 14.3 Glutathione Transferase catalysis. Glutathione conjugation to a generic xenobiotic (X) via GST results in the formation of a glutathione-S conjugate. (Townsend 2003 with permission)

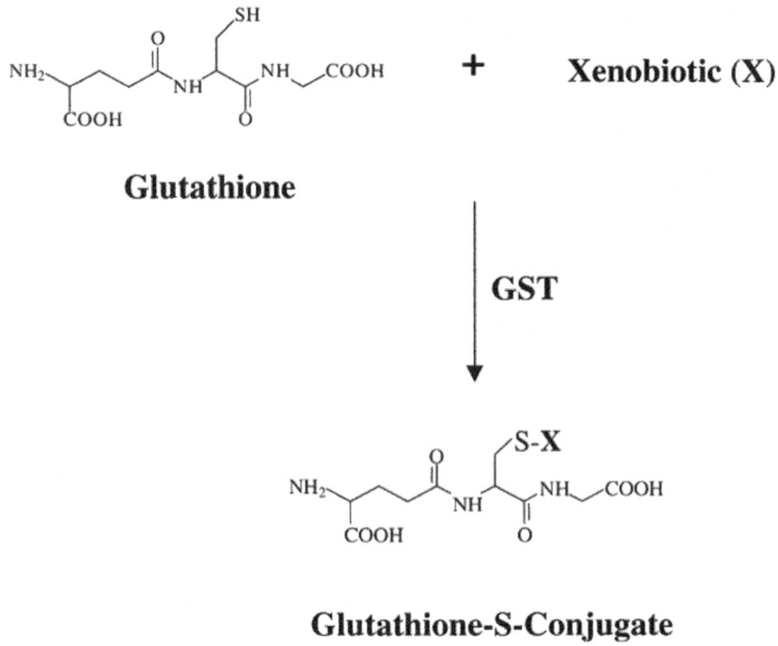

arene oxides. While this protects untransformed cells from genetic damage, the increased expression of Glutathione-S-Transferases in cancer cells is often associated with resistance to chemotherapeutic agents that form reactive oxides.

The over-abundance of certain Glutathione S-Transferases in some cancers may be exploited therapeutically. Glutathione S-Transferase P1-1 is an enzyme that is over-expressed in many malignancies. TLK286 is a modified Glutathione analog that is selectively activated by Glutathione S-Transferase P1-1 into an alkylating metabolite, which forms covalent linkages with nucleophilic centers in the DNA. Thereby the agent induces a cellular stress response and cytotoxicity, and is decreases tumor proliferation.

Glutathione S-Transferases conjugate reduced Glutathione, via a sulfhydryl group, to electrophilic centers on various substrates. This enhances their solubility and detoxifies endogenous or exogenous compounds.
Like other gene products of the intermediary metabolism, the induction of Glutathione S-Transferase expression is very sensitive to environmental cues.
Glutathione S-Transferases may contribute to drug resistance, but they may also represent therapeutic targets.

14.4 Others

Variable levels of the enzyme Thiopurine Methyltransferase (TPMT) in the population prompted the development of one of the earliest pharmacogenetic tests. Around 10 % of the population are heterozygous and produce a reduced quantity of functional enzyme. TPMT metabolizes 6-mercaptopurine and azathioprine, both of which are used in the treatment of childhood leukemia.

In patients with a deficiency in Thiopurine Methyltransferase, metabolism must proceed by alternative pathways, one of which leads to a metabolite that is toxic to the bone marrow, putting the affected individuals at risk of potentially fatal bone marrow suppression during the treatment. In 85–90 % of affected persons, this deficiency results from one specific variant allele[3]. 1 in 300 people have two variant alleles. These patients need only 5–10 % of the standard drug dose. For them, the underlying genotype predicts clinical outcome. The U.S. FDA recommends that patients who develop bone marrow suppression while receiving 6-mercaptopurine or azathioprine be tested for Thiopurine Methyltransferase deficiency.

N-Acetyl Transferases (NATs) are enzymes that catalyze the transfer of acetyl groups from acetyl-CoA to aromatic amines, heterocyclic amines, or hydrazine compounds. They have wide substrate specificity, and can also catalyze acetyl transfer between arylamines without CoA. The reaction pathway is catalyzed by the cytoplasmic *N*-Acetyl Transferase Type I (NAT1) and *N*-Acetyl Transferase Type II (NAT2). Genetic variation in *nat* genes modulates the acetylator status of individuals (slow, intermediate, or rapid acetylator phenotype) and therefore may impact upon their predisposition to anti-cancer drug efficacy or toxicity. The *nat* genes are located on chromosome 8p22, a region that is commonly deleted in cancers.

[3] Overall, the bearers of the variant allele are at greater risk of adverse effects, although as individuals their genotype is not necessarily predictive of their clinical outcome, which makes the interpretation of a clinical test difficult.

References

Bailey DG, Spence JD, Edgar B, Bayliff CD, Arnold JM (1989) Ethanol enhances the hemodynamic effects of felodipine. Clin Invest Med 12:357–362

Hisamuddin IM, Wehbi MA, Schmotzer B, Easley KA, Hylind LM, Giardiello FM, Yang VW (2005) Genetic polymorphisms of flavin monooxygenase 3 in sulindac-induced regression of colorectal adenomas in familial adenomatous polyposis. Cancer Epidemiol Biomarkers Prev 14:2366–2369

Krueger SK, Williams DE (2005) Mammalian flavin-containing monooxygenases: structure/function, genetic polymorphisms and role in drug metabolism. Pharmacol Ther 106:357–387

Townsend DM, Tew KD (2003) The role of glutathione-S-transferase in anti-cancer drug resistance. Oncogene 22:7369–7375

Prodrug Activation 15

15.1 Photodynamic Therapy

The first detailed scientific observation that photosensitive synthetic dyes, in combination with a light source and oxygen, could have potential therapeutic effects was made at the turn of the twentieth century in the laboratory of von Tappeiner. In 1903, von Tappeiner and Jesionek performed a trial with the photosensitizer eosin in patients with facial basal cell carcinoma and achieved substantial remission. The German physician Friedrich Meyer-Betz performed studies of photodynamic therapy with porphyrins in 1913 by testing the effects of hematoporphyrin use on his own skin. John Toth, product manager for Cooper Lasersonics, in 1981 wrote a white paper on early clinical argon dye lasers for their use in photodynamic therapy. Later research was done at the Mayo Clinic and Roswell Park Cancer Center, but did not become wide spread until Thomas Dougherty initiated clinical trials and formed the International Photodynamic Association, in 1986. Photodynamic therapy, which matured as a feasible medical technology in the 1980s at several institutions, is a ternary treatment for cancer involving three key components,

- a photosensitizer
- light
- tissue oxygen.

Photodynamic therapy applies light to induce chemical reactions that activate prodrugs in select tissues. In the absence of light, the photosensitizer is inactive. Photodynamic therapy requires a light source of a sufficiently long wavelength, which determines how far the external light can travel into the body. Compounds based on porphyrins, phthalocyanine dyes, or chlorophyll are the most promising photosensitizers. When light is directed at them, the photosynthesizer molecules become activated to produce singlet oxygen that destroys cancer cells within their proximity. In addition to directly killing tumor cells, two contributing mechanisms include damage to the tumor vasculature that prevents the tumor from receiving necessary nutrients, and activation of the immune system to attack the tumor cells. Drawbacks in photodynamic therapy include

- unfavorable biodistribution and lack of selective accumulation of photosensitizers in the target tissue
- the light needed to activate most photosensitizers cannot pass through more than about 1 cm of tissue, thus cannot treat deep seated tumors.

A key aspect in photodynamic therapy is the wavelength of the light used. If photoactivation of sensitizers located deep in a tissue is required, wavelengths above 600 nm are usually necessary. However, the extinction coefficient of many photosensitizers (e.g. porphyrins) is low in this range. The energy required to excite O_2 poses an upper limit in the infrared region for a photosensitizer to absorb light and induce singlet oxygen. This upper wavelength limit is 850–900 nm, depending on the energetic level of the photosensitizer triplet state. The therapeutic window is therefore 600–800 nm for treatment.

Photochemical internalization may improve the therapeutic effect of macromolecular sensitizers that accumulate in endocytic vesicles. Upon exposure to light, the contents of vesicles containing such photosensitizers are released into the cytosol in a functionally active form. The most efficient photosensitizers for use in photochemical internalization have an amphiphilic structure with a hydrophilic domain that inhibits penetration through cellular membranes. Upon exposure to light, singlet oxygen is formed and mediates the release of the contents of the endocytic vesicles.

Extracorporeal photopheresis is a type of photodynamic therapy, in which blood cells are collected by apheresis, treated outside the body with a photosensitizing agent, exposed to light, and then returned to the patient.

Porphyrins Tetrapyrroles are naturally occurring pigments. The presence in the center of tetrapyrroles of a coordinated metal ion and its electronic properties are of importance for the photocytotoxic potential. Porphyrins (Fig. 15.1) consist of 4 pyrrole subunits linked together by methine bridges. Porphyrins and porphyrin related dyes in photodynamic therapy have substituents in the peripheral positions of the pyrrole rings, on the 4 methine carbons, or on the coordinated metals. These derivatives influence water/lipid solubility, amphiphi-

G. F. Weber, *Molecular Therapies of Cancer*, DOI 10.1007/978-3-319-13278-5_15,

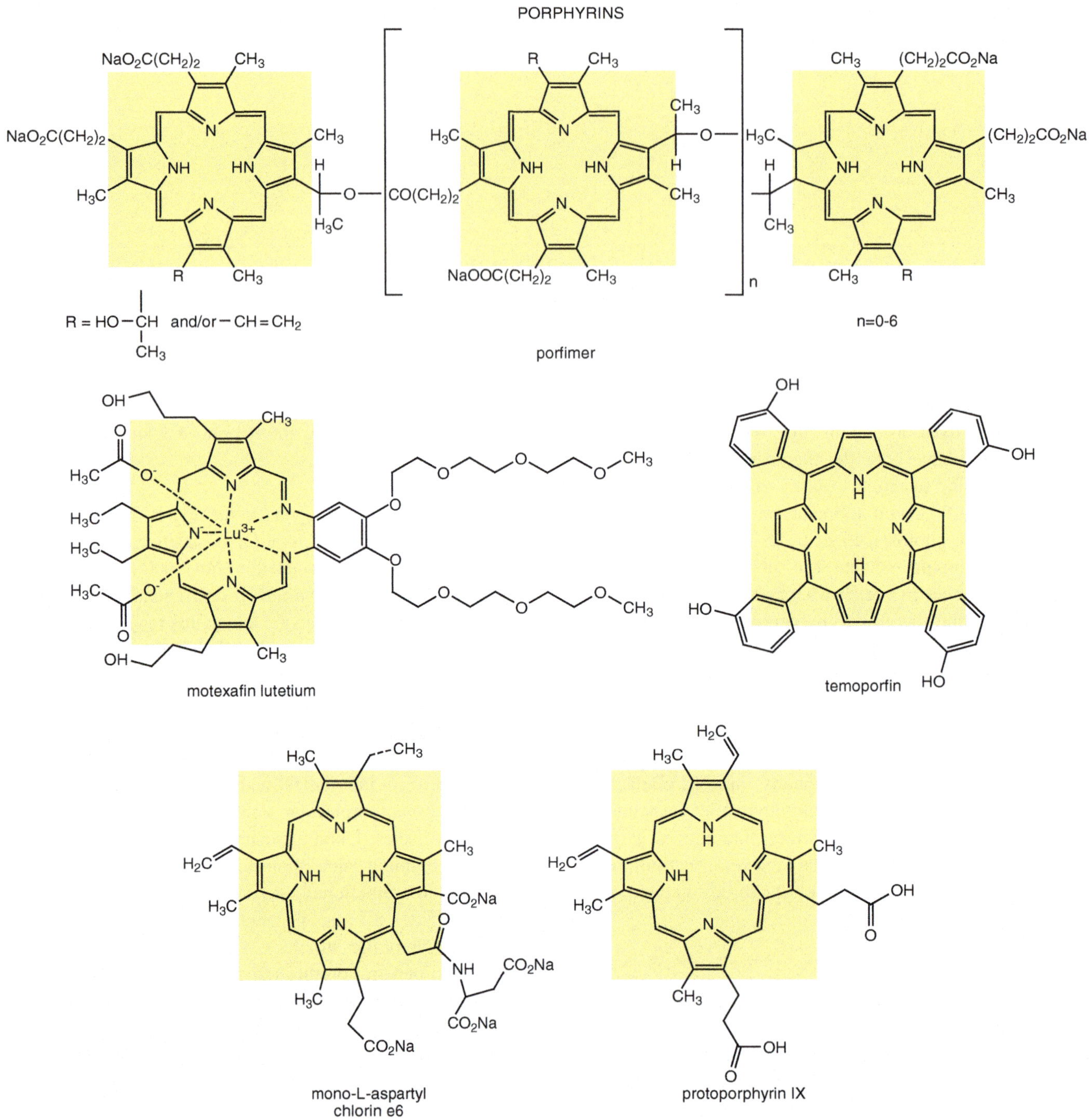

Fig. 15.1 Structures of porphyrin photosensitizers. The porphin core structure shared among all compounds in this class is highlighted in *yellow*. The presence of a coordinated metal ion in the tetrapyrrole center and its electronic properties are of importance for the photocytotoxic potential. Solubility, amphiphilicity, pKa, and stability of the compounds are conveyed by substituents in the peripheral positions of the pyrrole rings or on the methine bridges (or, in the case of motexafin, on the conjugated metal)

licity, pKa, and stability of the compounds. The physicochemical properties also determine the pharmacokinetic properties.

The first generation photosensitizer porfimer sodium <Photofrin> is a purified hematoporphyrin derivative. Porfimer sodium for injection is a mixture of oligomers formed by ether and ester linkages of up to eight porphyrin units. Porfimer sodium is given intravenously. It travels through the bloodstream to be absorbed by all cells in the body, including untransformed and cancer cells. Over days, the healthy cells exclude most of the drug. However, much of it remains in the cancer cells and in the cells of the skin. Light activation is required for cytotoxicity. This is typically accomplished by directing laser light via a fiber optic. To treat esophageal cancer or Barrett esophagus (a pre-cancerous lesion), the fiber optic is passed down the throat through an endoscope. For non-small cell lung cancer treatment, the fiber optic is passed through a bronchoscope. The light is applied for 5–40 min, depending on the size of the tumor. Any dead tissue remaining in the treated area is then removed during endoscopy or bronchoscopy 4–5 days later. The procedure is repeated as neccessitated. Patients treated with porfimer sodium should avoid direct sunlight and bright indoor light for at least 6 weeks, due to sensitivity of the skin and the eyes.

Adverse Effects The major adverse effects from porfimer sodium are photosensitivity reactions and swelling in the treated area, which may cause pain or trouble swallowing or breathing. Indications against the use of porfimer sodium are acute intermittent porphyria, allergy to porphyrins, a broncho-esophageal fistula, or a tumor eroding into a major blood vessel.

Motexafin lutetium <Antrin> is a pentadentate aromatic metallotexaphyrin that is photoactivated by 732 nm light. It preferentially accumulates in tumor cells due to their increased rates of metabolism and absorbs light, forming an extended high energy conformational state that produces high quantum yields of singlet oxygen. This results in local cytotoxic effects. The drug is used in the photodynamic therapy of prostate cancer.

Temoporfin (3,3′,3″,3‴-(2,3-dihydroporphyrin-5,10,15,20-tetrayl)tetraphenol, m-THPC) <Foscan> is a photosensitizer that is activated by 652 nm light. It is used in palliative photodynamic therapy for squamous cell carcinoma of the head and neck. It was approved in the European Union in 2001, but has not received approval in the United States. Following injection, the drug is given 90 h for distribution before activation by light exposure.

Adverse Effects Photosensitivity pertains for several weeks after treatment. Light exposure can cause retinal damage or symptoms akin to sunburn. Allergy to porphyrins is a contraindication.

Mono-L-aspartyl chlorin e6 (NPe6) is a second generation photosensitizer, which differs from benzoporphyrins and metallopurpurins in being hydrophilic and available in aqueous preparation. The drug has absorption peaks at 400 and 654 nm. Mono-L-aspartyl chlorin e6 is under study for recurrent adenocarcinoma of the breast, basal cell carcinoma, and squamous cell carcinoma.

Adverse Effects Mono-L-aspartyl chlorin e6 causes temporary generalized skin photosensitivity.

A main regulatory step in the heme synthesis pathway (Fig. 15.2) is linked to 5-Aminolevulinic Acid Synthase activity, which induces the formation of 5-aminolevulinate

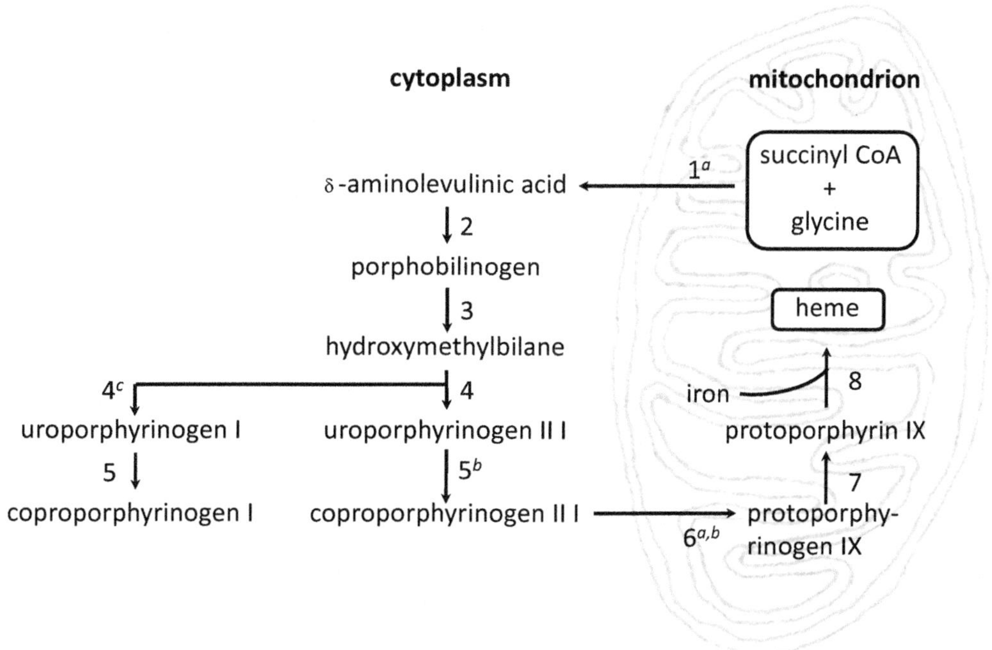

Fig. 15.2 Heme biosynthesis pathway. Numbers designate individual enzyme-catalyzed steps of heme biosynthesis. Enzyme name, *step 1*, ALA Synthase; *step 2*, ALA Dehydratase; step *3*, PBG Deaminase (Uroporphyrinogen Synthase); *step 4*, Uroporphyrinogen-III Cosynthase; *step 5*, Uroporphyrinogen Decarboxylase; *step 6*, Coproporphyrinogen Oxidase; *step 7*, Protoporphyrinogen Oxidase; *step 8*, Ferrochelatase. **a** ALA (5-aminolevulinate) is synthesized within mitochondria in *step 1* and then traverses to cytoplasm, where *step 2* occurs. Coproporphyrinogen III is synthesized in cytoplasm in *step 5* and then traverses into mitochondria, where *step 6* occurs. **b** Intermediate precursors not shown for *step 5* (7-, 6-, and 5-carboxyl porphyrinogens) or *step 6* (3-carboxyl porphyrinogen). **c** Alternative pathway at step *4* (hydroxymethylbilane to uroporphyrinogen I) is not enzymatically catalyzed. (Redrawn from http://www.herc.org/news/mcsarticles/daniell-full.html)

(5-ALA) from glycine and succinyl-CoA. Heme can inhibit the enzyme directly as well as its transcription, translation and protein transport into the mitochondria. The treatment of cells with 5-aminolevulinic acid or methyl aminolevulinic acid overrides this negative feedback and induces a high activity through the heme pathway. This results in the accumulation of porphyrins, which are not photochemically active, and protoporphyrin IX (PPIX), which sensitizes cells to photoinactivation. Esterification of the carboxyl group in 5-aminolevulinic acid may increase the rate of cellular uptake and tissue penetration. 5-Aminolevulinic acid may be applied topically or systemically, its esters are applied topically. The ensuing short photosensitivity period after application is favorable. Sufficient amounts of the endogenous photosensitizers accumulate in the neoplastic lesions within 1–3 h. The effect terminates when Ferrochelatase incorporates Fe^{2+} into protoporphyrin IX and converts it into the photochemically inactive porphyrin heme.

- Hexyl 5-aminolevulinic acid is the hexyl ester of 5-aminolevulinic acid with photodynamic properties. As a precursor of photoactive porphyrins, hexyl 5-aminolevulinate induces the endogenous production of the photosensitizer protoporphyrin IX, which accumulates selectively in tumor tissue. When exposed to specific wavelengths of light, protoporphyrin IX is activated and, depending on the applied wavelength and intensity, either fluoresces thereby allowing tumor imaging, or induces tumor cell apoptosis.

Chlorofylls Chlorophyll (chlorophyl) is a green chlorin[1] pigment produced by cyanobacteria, algae, and plants. In photosynthesis, it absorbs light most strongly in the blue portion of the electromagnetic spectrum, followed by the red portion. Chlorophyll is structurally similar to, and produced through the same metabolic pathway as porphyrins. At the center of the chlorin ring is a magnesium ion.

2-(1-hexyloxyethyl)-2-devinyl pyropheophorbide (HPPH) <Photochlor> is a lipophilic, chlorin based, second generation photosensitizer (Fig. 15.3). Upon intravenous administration, HPPH preferentially accumulates in the cytoplasm of cancer cells. A photodynamic reaction between HPPH and oxygen occurs when laser light is applied. As a result, reactants from the photodynamic activation trigger serial cytotoxic events, thereby killing the tumor cells. HPPH is used in adjuvant photodynamic therapy for esophageal cancer to prevent the recurrence of a tumor after surgical removal. It is under investigation for non-small cell lung cancer.

[1] A chlorin is a large heterocyclic aromatic ring, consisting at the core of 3 pyrroles and 1 pyrroline coupled through 4=CH- linkages.

Pharmacokinetics Compared to the first generation photosensitizer porfimer sodium, HPPH shows improved pharmacokinetic properties. It stays in the tumor for a prolonged time and clears faster from the rest of the system.

Adverse Effects HPPH causes only mild skin photosensitivity that declines over a few days.

Palladium-bacteriopheophorbide (WST09) <Tookad> is a palladium substituted bacteriochlorophyll derivative. Consecutive to administration, the inactive drug is activated locally when the tumor bed is exposed to photo-irradiation at 763 nm. The activated form induces local cytotoxic processes, resulting in tissue damage, disruption of the tumor vasculature, and tumor necrosis. Palladium-bacteriopheophorbide is used in the treatment of recurrent prostate cancer.

Talaporfin sodium (LS11, Pe6, mono-L-aspartyl chlorin e6) <Laserphyrin, Aptocine> is a natural, chlorophyll based, water soluble photosensitizer. The agent consists of chlorin e6, derived from chlorophyll, and L-aspartic acid, which has photosensitizing activity. The prodrug absorbs red light at 664 nm. After intratumoral activation by light emitting diodes, talaporfin sodium forms an extended high energy conformational state that generates singlet oxygen, resulting in free radical mediated cell death. Constant illumination can activate each molecule of talaporfin many times, resulting in a continuous supply of singlet oxygen molecules. The agent was approved in Japan in 2004, and is in clinical trials in the United States. It is used for bile duct carcinoma, esophageal cancer (local failure after chemotherapy), and malignant glioma.

The second generation photosensitizer tin ethyl etiopurpurin (rostaporfin, SnET2, Sn(IV) etiopurpurin) <Photrex, Purlytin> is a synthetic purpurin that preferentially accumulates in tumor cells due to an increased rate of metabolism. Upon exposure to a light source, this agent forms an extended high energy conformational state that produces high quantum yields of singlet oxygen with local cytotoxic effects. However, the photo-bleaching quantum yield of the agent is increased dramatically when it is bound to Albumin, thus limiting the production of singlet oxygen. Tin ethyl etiopurpurin is under study for the treatment of AIDS associated Kaposi sarcoma.

Phthalocyanines The photosensitizer aluminum (III) phthalocyanine tetrasulfonate (AlPcS4) <Photosense> has suitable photochemical properties to serve as a drug. However, its efficacy is compromised by its hydrophilicity that prevents it from reaching the critical intracellular targets. The efficacy may be improved in a photoimmunoconjugate,

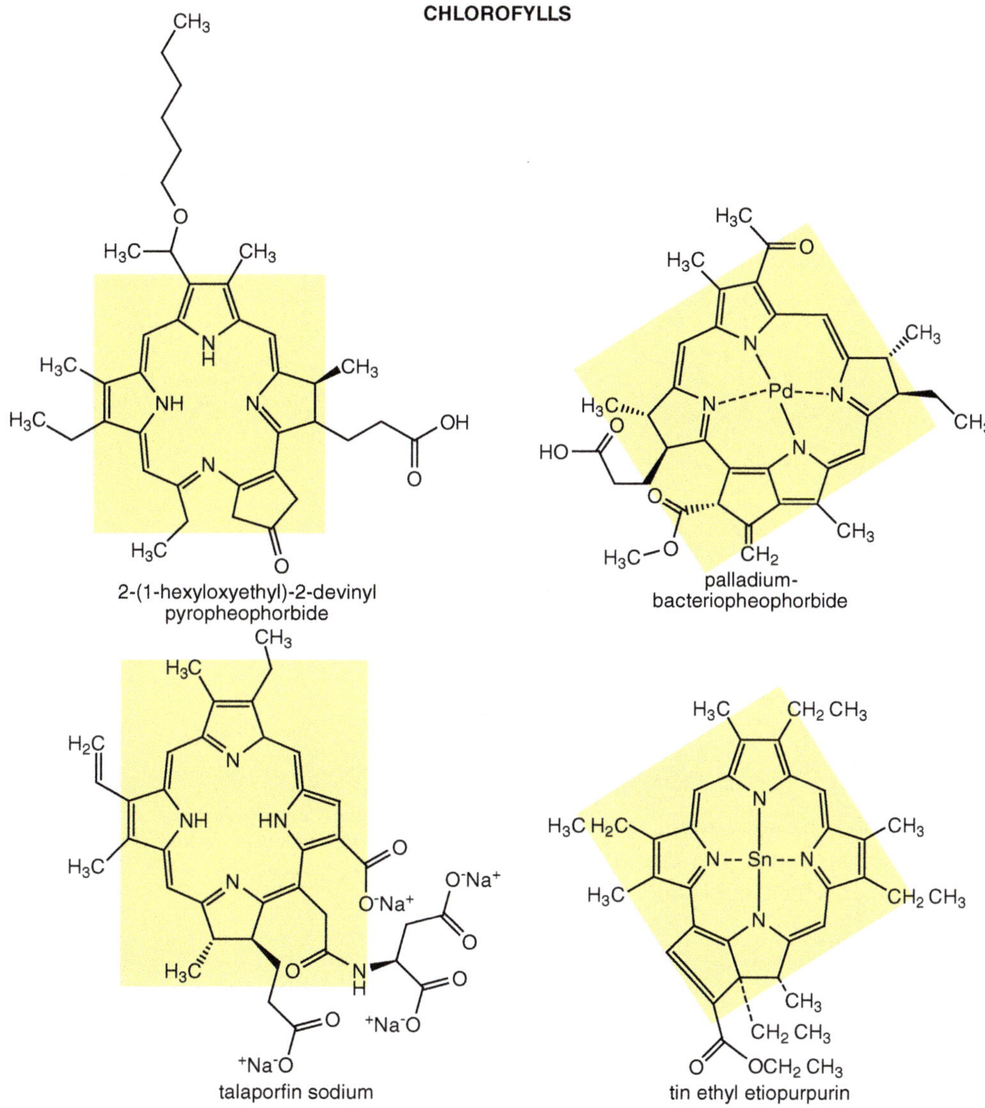

Fig. 15.3 Structures of chlorofylls. The core chlorin structure shared among all compounds in this class is highlighted in *yellow*. A metal, typically magnesium, is conjugated in the center of the core. Palladium-bacteriopheophorbide is an exception. The variable side chains convey distinctive properties to the individual members of this class of drugs

bound to an antibody that recognizes a tumor associated antigen. Aluminum phthalocyanine tetrasulfonate (Fig. 15.4) is under study for head and neck cancer.

Silicon phthalocyanine 4 (Pc-4) is a synthetic photosensitizer agent with peak absorption at 675 nm that contains a large macrocyclic ring chelated with silicon. It localizes primarily in mitochondrial cytosolic membranes. After photoexcitation, it forms reactive oxygen species that induce apoptosis.

<u>**Various**</u> Methoxsalen (xanthotoxin, 9-methoxy-7H-furo[3,2-g]chromen-7-one) <Oxsoralen, Deltasoralen, Meladinine> is a naturally occurring texaphyrin isolated from the seeds of the plant Ammi majus (Fig. 15.5). It belongs to the class of furanocoumarins (psoralens), consisting of coumarin annulated with furan. Upon photoactivation, methoxsalen binds covalently to and cross-links DNA. As the drug modifies the way skin cells receive UVA radiation it is used to treat cutaneous lymphoma.

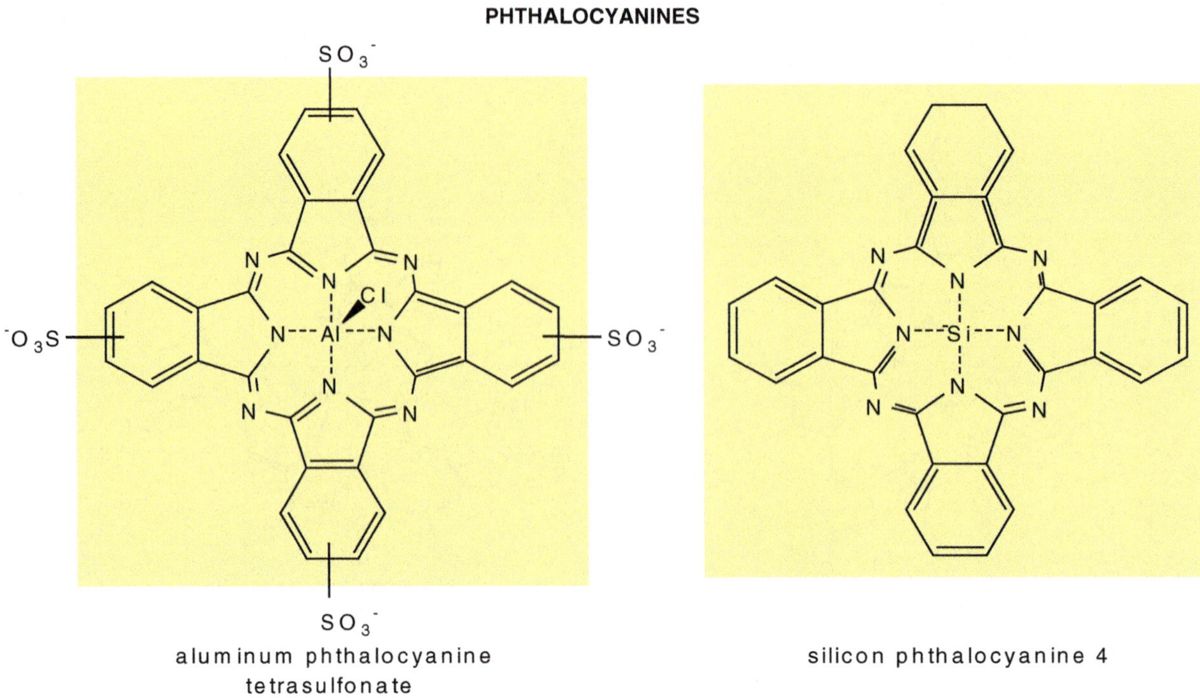

Fig. 15.4 Structures of phthalocyanines. The core structure shared by the compounds in this class is highlighted in *yellow*

Adverse Effects Methoxsalen causes nausea, headaches, dizziness, and in rare cases insomnia. The drug is classified as an IARC[2] Group 1 carcinogen, but is only cancerous when combined with Ultra Violet-A radiation. Patients with high blood pressure or a history of liver problems are at risk for inflammation and irreversible damage to liver and skin. While on treatment, the eyes must be protected from UVA radiation.

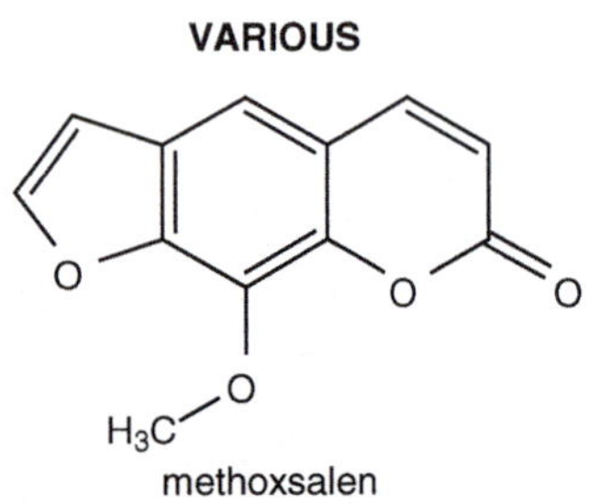

Fig. 15.5 Structures of various photodynamic therapy drugs

Other photosensitizers are at experimental stages of evaluation. The perylenequinone class of molecules includes phleichrome, the calphostins, hypocrellin A, and cercosporin. These compounds contain an extended oxidized aromatic subunit. Upon light activation, they produce singlet oxygen.

Photodynamic therapy induces chemical reactions that activate prodrugs in select tissues. It requires a photosensitizer, light, and tissue oxygen.

15.2 Radio-Sensitization

The use of radiation to fight cancer was under study early on. Soon after the discovery of X-rays (Roentgen 1895), Emil Grubbe in Chicago attempted to use X-rays to treat cancer (1896). The discovery the radioactive elements polonium and radium by Marie Curie in 1898 began to grow the field of radiation therapy in the early 1900s. Work by Maude Menton, Simon Flexner, and J.V. Jobling at the Rockefeller Institute lead to the publication of the monograph "Influence of Radium Bromide on a Carcinomatous Tumor of the White Rat" in 1910. By the 1950s, researchers at the Sloan-Kettering Institute in New York City became alarmed over thyroid cancers that were diagnosed in adolescents who had received radiation treatment of their thymus glands in childhood. Later reports began to document that thyroid cancers could develop about 20 years following childhood radiation therapy. The adverse effects of radiation treatment have led to strategies that aim at limiting the radiation effects to the tumor tissue. The radiation dose to the patient can be reduced if the tumor has previously received a radio-sensitizer.

<u>**Inducers of Reactive Oxygen**</u> Radiation damages cancer cells predominantly through the induction of reactive oxygen species. Short lived free radicals are obligate intermediates

[2] International Agency for Research on Cancer.

in the pathways to radiation induced cell death. Oxygen, a prototypical radio-sensitizer, is a biradical (containing two unpaired electrons). Severely hypoxic cells typically require 2-3-fold higher radiation doses to get killed compared to well oxygenated cells. Therefore, compounds that increase oxygen derivatives or decrease the antioxidant defenses may act as radio-sensitizers (Fig. 15.6). Cells at intermediate oxygen tensions are especially critical in defining the effects of hypoxic cell radio-sensitizers. Hypoxic cell sensitizers increase the radiation susceptibility of cells deficient in molecular oxygen. Their relative specificity is based on the premise that hypoxic cells are present mostly in tumors and rarely in healthy tissues. As tumors commonly include a substantial fraction of cells with low intracellular oxygen concentrations, improved oxygenation can often result in an increase in radio-sensitivity.

Carbogen is an inhalant consisting of a hyperoxic gas (95–98 % oxygen and 2–5 % carbon dioxide) with radio-sen-

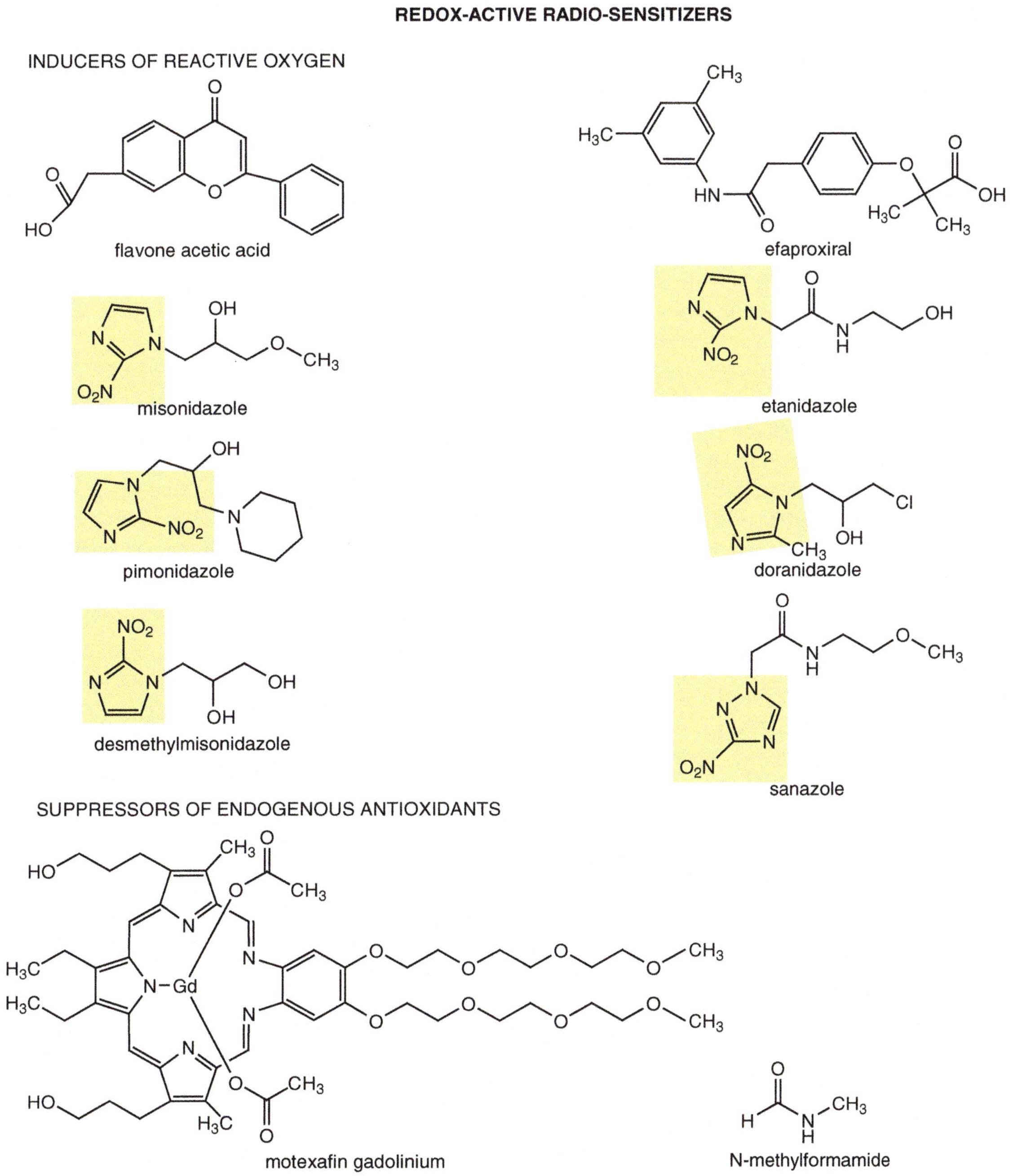

Fig. 15.6 Structures of redox modulators. (*Top panel*) Inducers of reactive oxygen. The common motif for the sub-class of nitrobenzenes and nitroimidazoles is highlighted in *yellow*. (*Bottom panel*) Suppressors of endogenous antioxidants

sitizing properties. Inhaled carbogen reduces diffusion-limited tumor hypoxia, thus increasing tumor radio-sensitivity. The enhanced availability of molecular oxygen facilitates cytotoxicity through radiation induced oxygen free radical production.

Nicotinamide in combination with carbogen and fractionated irradiation eliminates acute hypoxia (due to an intermittent closure of blood vessels upon exposure to carbogen), thus maintaining radio-sensitivity (nicotinamide was originally evaluated in radio-biology as an inhibitor of DNA repair via its interaction with Poly(ADP Ribose) Polymerase, but has found more value as a vasoactive agent). A common regimen is ARCON, consisting of accelerated radio-therapy (to inhibit repopulation of the cancer cells) with carbogen and nicotinamide.

Flavone acetic acid is a synthetic flavonoid with vascular targeting properties. It exhibits anti-proliferative effects on endothelial cells as a result of a superoxide dependent mechanism, which induces changes in permeability of the tumor vasculature. This agent may stimulate tumor necrosis and promote shunting of the blood flow to viable regions of the tumor, increasing their oxygenation and rendering them more susceptible to the anti-tumor effects of ionizing radiation.

Efaproxiral (RSR13) is a synthetic small molecule that increases the oxygen levels in hypoxic tumor tissues by binding non-covalently and allosterically to the Hemoglobin tetramer and decreasing the binding affinity between Hemoglobin and oxygen. The resulting increase in tissue oxygenation reduces tumor radio-resistance. The regimen is under study for metastatic brain cancer.

Electron-affinic radio-sensitizers have reactivity towards radiation-produced free radicals. Early prototypes were nitrobenzenes and nitroimidazoles (oxygen-mimetic radio-sensitizers) (drug names end on -nidazole). These nitroaromatic compounds bind preferentially to hypoxic cells via complex reductive chemistry involving an intermediate, oxygen-sensitive radical. Numerous nitroaromatic structures have been evaluated as alternatives to the prototypical misonidazole and its nitroimidazole analogs. Attempts to improve the therapeutic index by increasing hydrophilicity (to reduce the risk for peripheral neuropathy due to lower penetration into neural tissue and accelerated elimination) were only partially successful.

- The nitroimidazole misonidazole ((*RS*)-1-methoxy-3-(2-nitroimidazol-1-yl)propan-2-ol) (Ro 07-0582) induces the formation of free radicals and depletes radio-protective thiols, thereby sensitizing hypoxic cells to the cytotoxic effects of ionizing radiation. The single strand breaks in DNA induced by this agent result in the inhibition of DNA synthesis. Misonidazole has activity on cell survival, which determines local control and regrowth delay. Less than 25 % of the administered drug is eliminated in the urine. There is no general sensitization of healthy tissues, but mild hypoxia in the skin. Efficacy is reduced (but not eliminated) in multi-fractionated treatments because of re-oxygenation between treatments. The toxicity largely parallels the radio-sensitization efficacy, because the same property (electron affinity or reduction potential) dominates the structure-activity relationship.
- Etanidazole (SR2508) is a 2-nitroimidazole with radio-sensitizing properties. This agent also depletes Glutathione and inhibits Glutathione Transferase, thereby enhancing the cytotoxicity of ionizing radiation. Etanidazole may be useful as an imaging agent for identifying hypoxic, potentially drug resistant regions of primary tumors or metastases.
- Pimonidazole (Ro 03-8799) has enhanced radio-sensitizing efficacy compared to misonidazole without correspondingly enhanced cytotoxicity. Pimonidazole tends to reach higher nuclear concentrations than misonidazole.
- The 2-nitroimidazole radio-sensitizer doranidazole (PR-350) is highly water soluble.
- Desmethylmisonidazole (3-(2-nitro-1*H*-imidazol-1-yl)-1,2-propanediol) (Ro05-9963) is administered orally or intravenously. About half of the administered drug is eliminated in the urine.
- Sanazole (*N*-2′-methoxy ethyl)-2-(3″-nitro-1″-triazolyl) acetamide) (AK-2123) facilitates tumor cell killing in part by producing nitric oxide. It is under study for the treatment of squamous cell carcinoma of the uterine cervix. The drug has been linked to a chelating agent complexed with ^{177}Lu.

Various DNA targeted radio-sensitizing drugs include nitroimidazole/intercalator conjugates, nitroacridines, and nitroquinoline intercalators, minor groove binders, and polyamine conjugates. Diffusion limited hypoxic cells are distant from capillaries, so free diffusion unimpeded by binding to cells nearest capillaries is required for maximum efficacy, but has not yet been attained.

Suppressors of endogenous antioxidants Endogenous antioxidants scavenge and detoxify reactive oxygen intermediates. Thus they protect cells (in particular the genetic information stored in DNA) from lethal damage. In radiation therapy, the endogenous antioxidants within tumor cells compromise efficacy. The reduction of their levels before radiation exposure may improve the killing of the cancer cells.

Motexafin gadolinium is a synthetic metallotexaphyrin with radio-sensitizing and chemo-sensitizing properties. The agent accumulates preferentially in tumor cells due to their

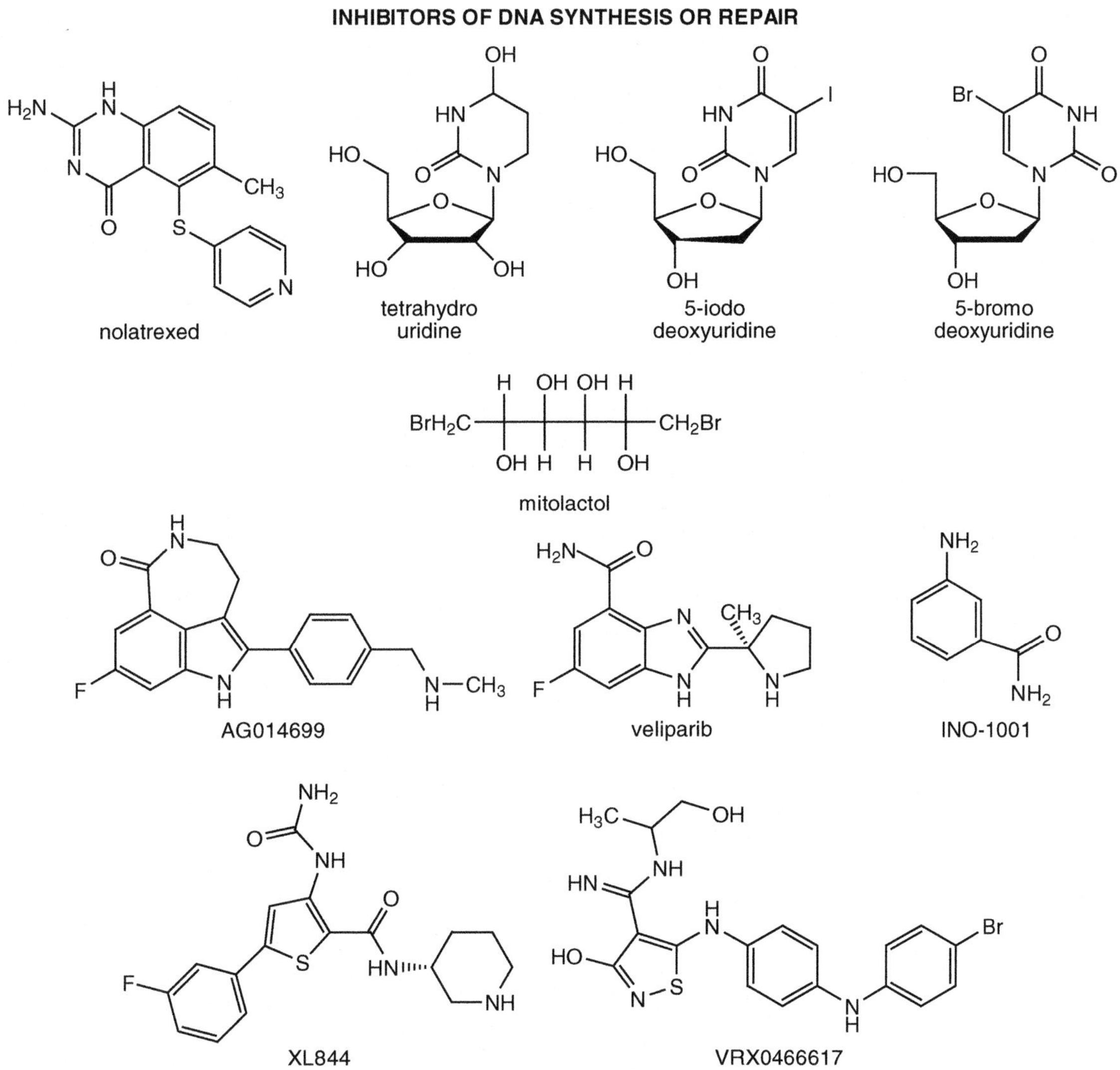

Fig. 15.7 Structures of inhibitors of DNA synthesis or repair

increased rates of metabolism, generating reactive oxygen species intracellularly and lowering the tumor cell apoptotic threshold to ionizing radiation and chemotherapy.

N-methylformamide is a water soluble organic solvent. As an adjuvant anti-neoplastic agent, *N*-methylformamide depletes cellular Glutathione, a key molecule involved in the protection form reactive oxygen intermediates, thereby enhancing the ionizing radiation induced DNA cross-linking of tumor cells.

Inhibitors of DNA synthesis or repair The use of halogenated pyrimidines in radio-therapy is based on the premise that tumor cells divide faster, and therefore incorporate more drug than the surrounding untransformed tissues. Some conventional anti-cancer drugs have radio-sensitizing properties.

- Nolatrexed dihydrochloride (2-amino-6-methyl-5-(4-pyridylthio)-1*H*-quinazolin-4-one) <Thymitaq> (Fig. 15.7) is a quinazoline folate analog that arrests cells in the S-phase of the cell cycle. This agent exhibits radio-sensitizing activity when cancer cells are exposed to it before irradiation, but is inactive if given after.
- Tetrahydro-uridine is a synthetic pyrimidine nucleoside analog that increases the efficacy of the radio-sensitizer cytochlor (5-chloro-2′-deoxycytidine) by inhibiting the enzyme Deoxycytidine Monophosphate Deaminase (dCMP Deaminase) and preventing the premature deamination of the cytochlor metabolite 5-chloro-2′-deoxycytidine monophosphate (CldCMP) to 5-chloro-2′-deoxyuridine monophosphate (CldUMP). This effect increases the tumor concentrations of CldUMP, which is then further anabolized

and incorporated into DNA as 5-chloro-2′-deoxyuridine (CldU).

- The antifolates 5-Iododeoxyuridine (IUDR) <Idoxuridine> and 5-Bromodeoxyuridine (BrUDR) are radio-sensitizers.

Mitolactol (dibromodulcitol) <Dibromdicil, Elobromol, Mitolac> is a synthetic derivative of hexitol that alkylates DNA via actual or derived epoxide groups, resulting in the inhibition of DNA and RNA synthesis. The drug has chemotherapeutic properties by itself and it may act as a radio-sensitizer.

DNA damaging strategies are among the most common treatments for cancer. The enzyme Poly(ADP-Ribose)Polymerase (PARP) can facilitate the repair of DNA damage caused by insult from chemotherapeutic agents or radiation. Increased PARP activity is associated with the survival of some cancer cells after chemotherapy. PARP inhibitors may potentiate the effects of radiotherapy and chemotherapy.

- The first PARP-1 small molecule inhibitor to enter clinical trials was AG-014699. The success of the treatment rationale adopted by current clinical trials of AG-014699 depends on the overall biological role of and necessity for PARP in cancer cells that are trying to repair the DNA damage induced by radiation or chemotherapy.
- Veliparib (2-[(*R*)-2-methylpyrrolidin-2-yl]-1*H*-benzimidazole-4-carboxamide) (ABT-888, NSC 737664) inhibits PARP-1 and PARP-2. It sensitizes cancer cells to ionizing irradiation, especially under hypoxic conditions. The sensitization is independent of the PTEN status or P53 status of the tumor. The drug also has chemosensitizing activity. Being devoid of anti-proliferative effects as a single agent at therapeutic concentrations, veliparib inhibits PARPs, thereby suppressing DNA repair and potentiating the cytotoxicity of DNA damaging agents. PARP nuclear enzymes are activated by DNA single or double strand breaks, resulting in the poly(ADP-ribosyl)ation of other nuclear DNA binding proteins involved in DNA repair.
- INO-1001 is an isoindolinone derivative and potent inhibitor of the nuclear enzyme PARP with chemo-sensitization and radio-sensitization properties. PARP inhibition may result in the suppression of tumor cell DNA repair mechanisms, and thus an amelioration of tumor cell resistance to chemotherapy and radiation therapy. PARP enzymes are activated by DNA breaks and thus are implicated in the repair of DNA. PARP inhibitors preferentially kill breast cancer cells with defects in the *brca* genes, which are normally involved in DNA repair.

Other PARP-1 inhibitors in early phase clinical trials include BSI-201, KU-59436, GPI-21016.

Inhibitors of the checkpoint kinases CHK-1 and CHK-2 suppress cell cycle arrest, which is required for DNA repair. They may thus act as radio-sensitizers.

- XL844 is a synthetic small molecule inhibitor of the checkpoint kinases CHK-1 and CHK-2. The agent inhibits cell cycle arrest and DNA repair, which ultimately leads to tumor cell apoptosis. XL844 increases cancer cell radio-sensitivity in a dose- and schedule-dependent manner through the promotion of mitotic catastrophe (an event in which a cell is destroyed during mitosis). Mechanistically, XL844 abrogates the radiation induced CHK-2 phosphorylation, induces the pan-nuclear Histone γ-H2A.X, and prolongs the presence of radiation induced γ-H2A.X foci, which may compromise the repair process.
- The selective CHK-2 inhibitor VRX0466617 is in pre-clinical development. VRX0466617 blocks the activation of CHK-2 and downstream degradation of MDM4 in response to ionizing radiation, and may thus act as a radio-sensitizer.

HDAC inhibitors (see Sect. 3.2.4.) are candidate radio-sensitizers because they decrease the cellular ability to repair DNA double strand breaks both by homologous repair and non-homologous end joining.

Others Boron neutron capture therapy (BNCT) was conceptualized in 1936 (Locher 1936). The first clinical trials took place at Brookhaven National Laboratory in the 1950s and early 1960s using boric acid and some of its derivatives as delivery agents. Neutron capture is based on the injection with a tumor localizing drug that contains a non-radioactive isotope with a high propensity for capturing neutrons. This is followed by irradiation of the patient with epithermal neutrons, which interact with the capture agent, resulting in a cytotoxic nuclear caption reaction.

Boron neutron capture therapy[3] is a selective, localized radio-targeting of tumor cells that aims at sparing adjacent normal tissues. Neutron capture by ^{10}boron nuclei results in fission of the generated ^{11}boron nuclei into ^{4}helium and ^{7}lithium ions. Both ^{10}B and ^{4}He nuclei have a very short range of effect, covering about one cellular diameter, and cause damage to the cancer cells, while largely sparing the surrounding healthy tissue.

- Boronophenylalanine-fructose complex (Fig. 15.8) is a boronated phenylalanine ((*L*)-4-dihydroxy-borylphenylalanine) complexed with fructose to increase its solubility. When exposed to neutron irradiation, boronophenylala-

[3] Boron is a non-metal in group 13, which has the stable isotopes ^{11}B and ^{10}B; the very large effective nuclear cross-section of the ^{10}B nucleus makes it amenable to the neutron capture process.

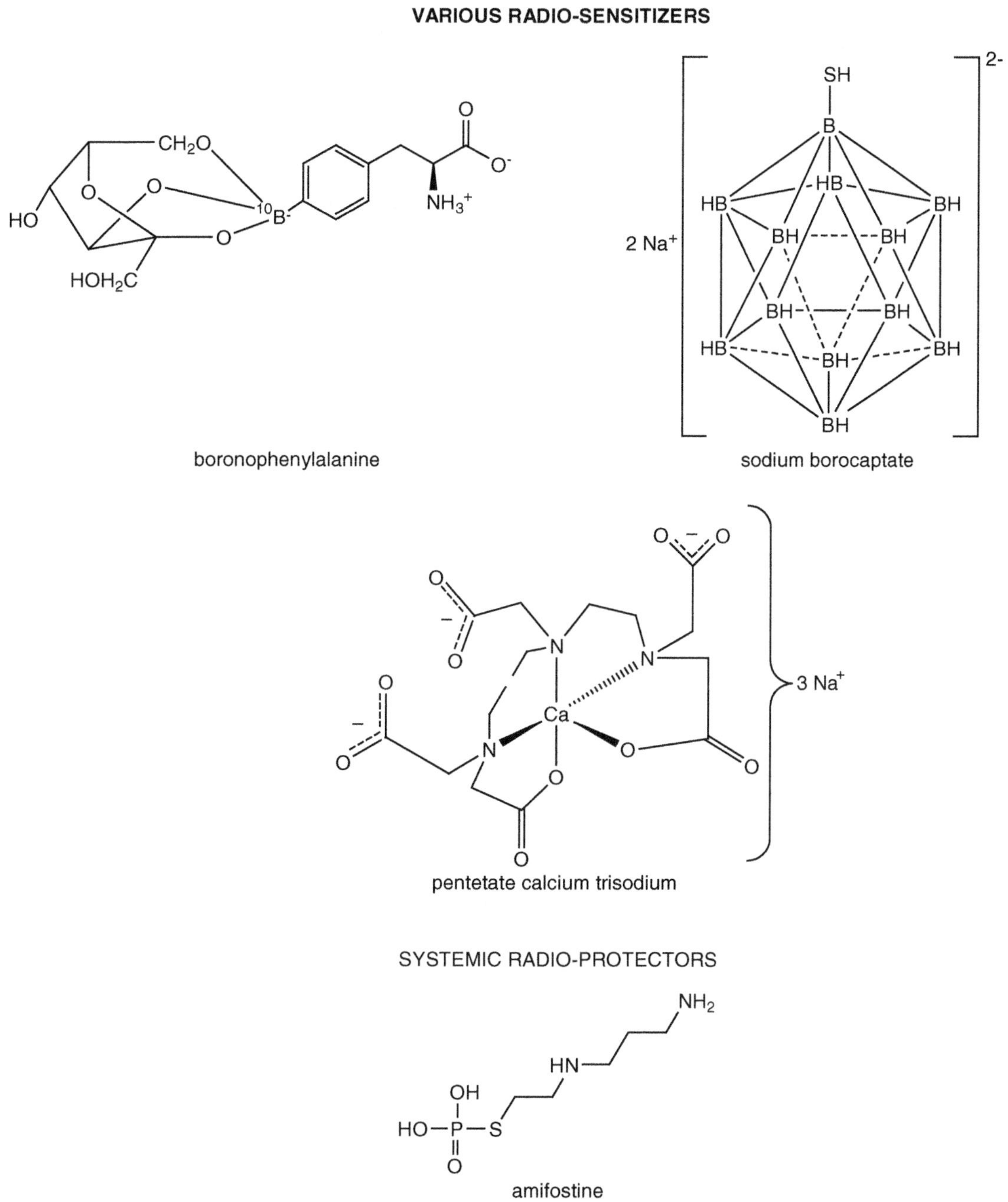

Fig. 15.8 Structures of various radiosensitizers and systemic radioprotectors

nine absorbs neutrons and decays, releasing short-range α radiation and recoil lithium in tumor cells. This results in α radiation induced tumor cell death.

- Sodium borocaptate (sodium mercaptoundecahydrocloso-dodecaborate) is a boron carrying compound. After parenteral administration, sodium borocaptate accumulates preferentially in tumor cells. When exposed, it absorbs the neutron irradiation and decays, releasing short range α radiation and recoil lithium in tumor cells, and resulting in cell death.

Pentetate calcium trisodium (trisodium calcium diethylenetriaminepenta-acetate) <Ca-DTPA> is a synthetic chelating agent related to ethylenediaminetetraacetic acid (EDTA). It chelates with the metallic radio-isotopic moieties of unbound, extracellular radio-immunotherapeutic agents. This mechanism results in higher specific tumor cell binding by these agents, and so improved tumor cell radio-cytotoxicity, while sparing healthy cells and tissues.

Various conventional chemotherapeutics, including taxanes, *N, N*-dimethylamino-benzoylphenylurea, and actinomycin D have possible radio-sensitizing properties.

One approach involves constructing prodrugs that comprise a bioreducible trigger (often a nitroaromatic moiety), which fragments to release active drug when reduced by cellular enzymes (donating an electron to form a radical anion). This release may be selective to hypoxia because the intermediate prodrug radical is oxygen reactive; oxygen inhibits drug release via a fast, free radical based reaction. Profiling drug release to oxygen tensions involves matching the rates of the reactions involved.

Systemic radio-protectors Chemical radio-protectors have the reverse effect of radio-sensitizers. The aim is to decrease the radio-sensitivity of healthy tissues. Clinical gain can be achieved either by a reduction in morbidity if the protection is conferred to untransformed cells, or by enhanced tumor cell kill if the drug allows the delivery of higher radiation doses. The thiol prodrug amifostine (WR-2721) is a radio-protector.

The radiation dose to the patient can be reduced if the tumor has been exposed to a radio-sensitizer.
Radiation damages cancer cells predominantly through the induction of reactive oxygen species.
Severely hypoxic cells typically require 2-3-fold higher radiation doses to get killed compared to well oxygenated cells.
Radio-sensitizers typically induce reactive oxygen, suppress endogenous antioxidants, or inhibit DNA synthesis or repair.

References

Locher GL (1936) Biological effects and therapeutic possibilities of neutrons. Am J Roentgenol Radium Ther 36:1–13

Drug Resistance 16

Drug resistance is a major obstacle in cancer treatment. It constitutes the insensitivity or reduced sensitivity to specific agents and can be intrinsic or acquired. Drug resistance is clinically reflected in progressive disease while on treatment (with or without an initial response), or in relapse within 6 months of completing a treatment. The ability of cancer cells to become simultaneously resistant to several, often diverse drugs (multi-drug resistance) remains a substantial impediment to successful chemotherapy. Gene expression signatures can frequently predict the sensitivity of cancer cells to chemotherapeutic drugs (Fig. 16.1).

Tumors consist of a heterogeneous population of cell types. The DNA repair mechanisms that maintain the integrity of non-transformed cells are often damaged in transformed cells. Because of the elevated genetic instability, mutations commonly occur (the mutator phenotype). Large tumors have undergone many cell divisions and harbor multiple cell mutations, resulting in genetically varied cell populations. These cytogenetic changes are highly associated with the ability of tumors to develop drug resistance (Buick 1994). The probability of developing resistant cell populations increases as tumor size increases.

Because of the genetic instability of cancer cells, even successful targeted therapies are likely to lose potency over time. The elevated mutation rate in cancer cells as compared to untransformed cells allows the generation and outgrowth of drug resistant cells in response to chemotherapy treatment. Resistant populations proliferate and eventually become the dominant cell types. Tumor cells that are exposed to chemotherapeutic agents will be selected for their ability to survive and grow in the presence of the cytotoxic drugs. This mechanism underlies the common phenomenon of an initial response to chemotherapy, followed by progressive tumor regrowth despite continuation of the same treatment regimen. Such events make it more likely for combination chemotherapy than mono-therapy to succeed in eradicating most cancer cells.

The RECIST criteria (Response Evaluation Criteria in Solid Tumors), established by the World Health Organization, unify response definitions in chemotherapy.

- Complete response means complete disappearance of all cancer without evidence of new disease for at least 1 month after treatment. The terms cure and complete response are not synonymous. Although an individual must have a complete response to be cured, many individuals who achieve a complete response will eventually relapse.
- A partial response is defined as a 30% or greater decrease in the tumor size or other objective disease markers, and no evidence of any new disease for at least 1 month. Overall objective response rates for a given treatment are calculated by adding the complete response and partial response rates.
- Progressive disease is defined as a 20% increase in the tumor size or the development of new lesions while receiving treatment.
- A patient whose tumor size neither grows nor shrinks by the above criteria is termed to have stable disease.
- Some patients may experience subjective improvement in the symptoms caused by their cancer without a defined response. Although clinically important, this does not indicate an objective response. The term clinical benefit response describes these subjective responses; it refers to patients who have clinical benefit as measured by decreases in pain or analgesic consumption, or improved quality of life or performance status.

The clinical readouts of full remission and overall survival are the gold standards of outcome measurements for anti-cancer drug treatment. Increasing emphasis is being placed on other survival end points that consider quality of life. These end points include disease free survival and progression-free survival, which measure the time the patient lives free of disease or its progression, respectively.

G. F. Weber, *Molecular Therapies of Cancer,* DOI 10.1007/978-3-319-13278-5_16,

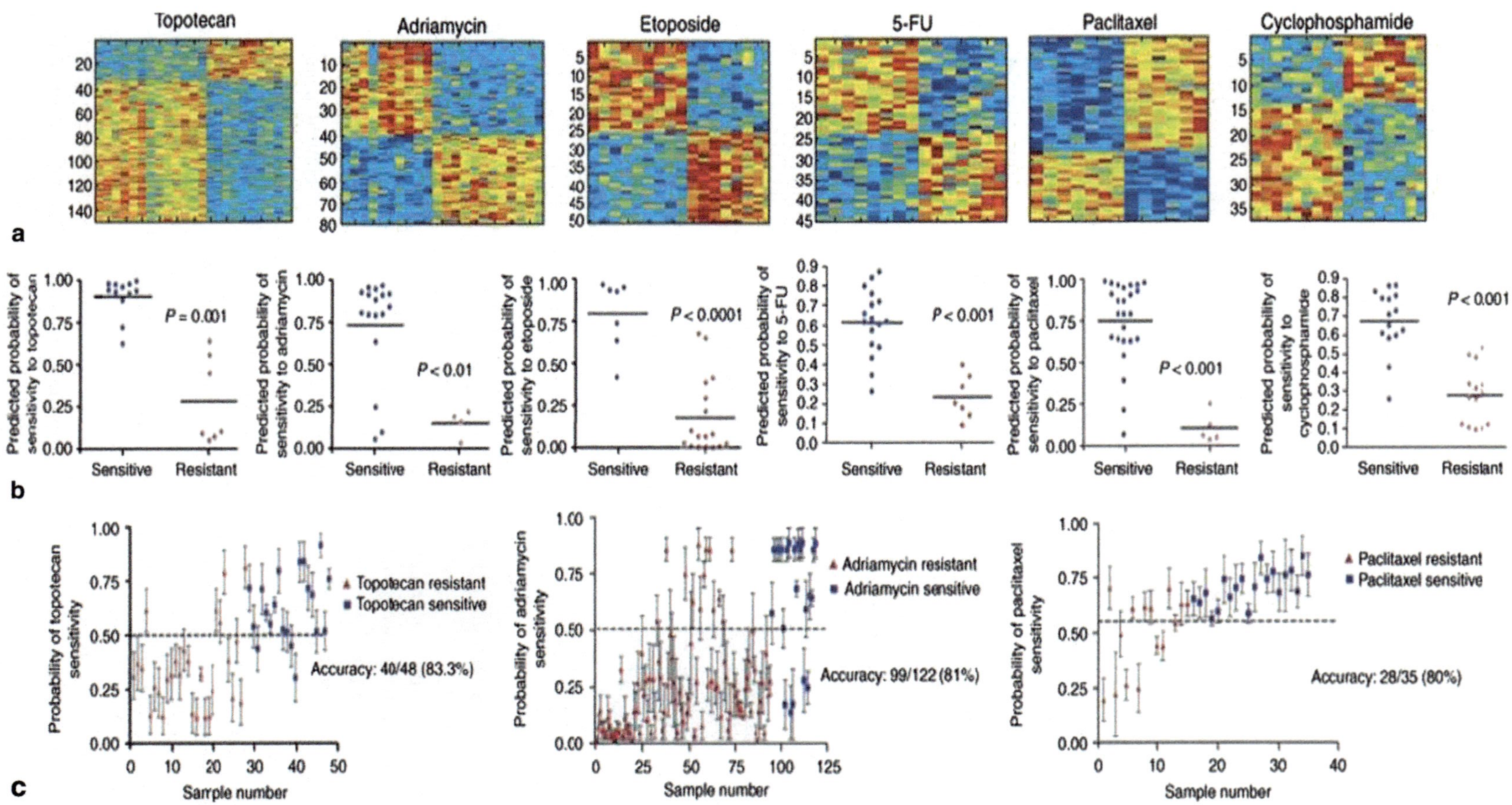

Fig. 16.1 Genomic signatures to guide the use of chemotherapeutics. Development of a panel of gene expression signatures that predict sensitivity to chemotherapeutic drugs. **a** Gene expression patterns selected for predicting response to the indicated drugs. **b** Independent validation of the chemotherapy response predictors. **c** Prediction of single-agent therapy response in clinical samples. *Left*, topotecan. *Middle*, the adriamycin predictor. *Right*, paclitaxel as salvage chemotherapy in advanced ovarian cancer. (Potti 2006 with permission)

16.1 Increased Efflux

The active outward transport of daunorubicin from drug resistant tumor cells was initially described in 1973 (Danø 1973). It constitutes a form of drug resistance that is mediated by high expression or activity of efflux transporters in the cell membrane. Membrane transporters play important roles in the absorption, distribution, and elimination of numerous compounds (Table 16.1). The efflux transporters typically have broad substrate specificity. Most contain two nucleotide binding domains, which capture the required chemical energy, and at least two transmembrane domains, the characteristics of which define the substrate specificity. They contribute to multi-drug resistance and belong to the ABC (ATP binding cassette) super-family. ATP hydrolysis provides the energy for substrate translocation. Efflux transporters prevent toxins from entering vital organs at the blood-brain barrier, the blood-testis barrier, the placenta, and the ovaries. In the intestines, efflux transporters mediate the ejection of resorbed molecules back into the lumen, thus limiting their bioavailability.

Table 16.1 Drug transporters

Efflux transporters
ABCA1 (ABC-Binding Cassette Protein A1, CERP): cholesterol efflux pump
ABCB1 (MDR1, P-Glycoprotein, PGY1): 2 transmembrane domains with 6 membrane spanning domains each
ABCCs (MRPs, MDR Associated Proteins)
– ABCC1 (MRP1) 3 transmembrane domains, transport of organic anions
– ABCC2 (MRP2, cMOAT) 3 transmembrane domains, transport of anionic conjugates
– ABCC3 (MRP3) 3 transmembrane domains, preference for the transport of glucuronide conjugates
– ABCC4 (MRP4) 2 transmembrane domains, transport of cAMP and cGMP
– ABCC5 (MRP5) 2 transmembrane domains, transports nucleotide analogs and glutathione conjugates
– ABCC6 (MRP6) 3 transmembrane domains, transports glutathione conjugates
– ABCC7 (MRP7, CFTR) transports 17β-estradiol glucuronide
– ABCC11 (MRP8)
– ABCC12 (MRP9)
ABCDs: peroxisomal transporters
– ABCD1
– ABCD2
– ABCD3
– ABCD4
ABCGs: efflux of cellular lipids, including cholesterol and phospholipids
– ABCG1, macrophages
– ABCG2 (MXR, Mitoxantrone Resistance Protein, Breast Cancer Resistance Protein, BCRP): a half-transporter that needs to dimerize to form a functional transporter
– ABCG5 (Sterolin-1) intestines and liver
– ABCG8 (Sterolin-2) intestines and liver
Uptake transporters (Solute Carrier Family, SLC)
Organic cation transporters: 2 families, OCT and OCTN, contain 12 transmembrane domains -only 11 in OCTN1, contain a nucleotide-binding motif
– SLC22A1 (OCT1)
– SLC22A2 (OCT2)
– SLC22A3 (OCT3)
– SLC22A4 (OCTN1)
– SLC22A5 (OCTN2)
Organic anion transporters: 2 families, OAT and OATP, contain 8-12 transmembrane domains
– SLC22A6 (OAT1)
– SLCC22A7 (OAT2)
– SLC22A8 (OAT3)
– SLC22A11 (OAT4)
– SLC21A3 (OATP1, OATP-A)
– SLC21A6 (OATP2, OATP-C, LST1)
– SLC21A8 (OATP8)
– SLC21A9 (OATP-B)
– SLC21A11 (OATP-D)
– SLC21A12 (OATP-E)
– SLC21A14 (OATP-F)

Table 16.1 (continued)

Nucleoside transporters: uptake of purine and pyrimidine nucleosides, equilibrative and concentrative transporters
– SLC29A1 (ENT1, Equilibrative Nucleoside Transporter 1)
– SLC29A2 (ENT2)
– SLC28A1 (CNT1, Concentrative Nucleoside Transporter 1)
– SLC28A2 (CNT2)
– SLC28A3 (CNT3)
Glucose transporters
– SLC2A1 (GLUT1)
– SLC2A2 (GLUT2)
– SLC2A3 (GLUT3)
Peptide transporters (hydrogen ion/peptide co-transporters): contain 12 transmembrane domains
– SLC15A1 (PEPT1)
– SLC15A2 (PEPT2)
Neurotransmitter transporters
– SLC6A1 (γ-amino butyric acid transporter)
– SLC6A2 (norepinephrine transporter)
– SLC6A3 (dopamine transporter)
– SLC6A4 (serotonin transporter)
– SLC6A5 (glycine transporter)
– SLC6A6 (taurine transporter)
– SLC6A7 (L-proline transporter)
– SLC6A8 (creatine transporter)
Cationic amino acid transporters: principal transporter of the cationic amino acids, arginine, lysine, and ornithine
– SLC7A1 (ATRC1, HCAT1)
– SLC7A2 (ATRC2, HCAT2)
– SLC7A3

16.1.1 ABC Transporters

ABC proteins (ATP binding cassette proteins) transport numerous endogenous substrates. They have important roles in protecting against blood-borne toxins and regulating the permeability into vital organs via the blood-brain barrier, the blood-tested barrier and the maternal-placental barrier. The blood-brain barrier is a principal limitation in the drug treatment of brain tumors. It is formed by the endothelial cells of capillaries, with ABCB1 located on the luminal surface, preventing the penetration of cytotoxins across the endothelium.

Classical multi-drug resistance (often resistance to natural-product hydrophobic drugs) may result from high level expressions of ATP-dependent efflux pumps with broad drug specificity. Even single amino acid substitutions in these transporters can affect their substrate specificity. Cancer chemotherapy may be affected by such substitutions that occur because of the mutator phenotype of cancer cells.

ABCB1 ABCB1 (P-Glycoprotein, PGP, P-170, MDR1, CD243) prevents the intracellular accumulation of many cytotoxic agents by exporting a wide variety of substrates across extra- and intracellular membranes. The protein is localized in the apical membranes of hepatocytes, where it transports toxins into the bile. In the gastrointestinal tract, ABCB1 is localized in the apical membranes of mucosal cells, where it extrudes toxins, forming a first line of defense and reducing the oral bioavailability of certain anti-cancer drugs. Additionally, ABCB1 actively secretes intravenously administered drugs into the gastrointestinal tract (Sparreboom 1997), and may thus limit the bioavailability of agents even if they are not administered orally. Substrates for ABCB1 include many of the most active natural products used in cancer therapy, including the anthracyclines, vinca alkaloids, mitoxantrone, and (to a lesser degree) the epipodophyllotoxin etoposide.

ABCB1 is highly expressed in colon, kidney, adrenocortical, and hepatocellular cancers. Cytotoxic agents derived from natural products can produce multi-drug resistance via up-regulation of ABCB1. A selection of cancer cells with natural product anti-cancer drugs, such as paclitaxel, doxorubicin, or vinblastine, frequently results in multi-drug resistance that is due to ABCB1 expression. The expression of this gene is often amplified in cells with resistance to multiple anti-cancer drugs (Fig. 16.2).

The role of ABCB1 in drug resistance is characterized as

- ABCB1 expression is highest in tumors that are dependent on its expression for survival
- ABCB1 expression impairs the response to chemotherapy
- ABCB1 expression levels increase as tumors become drug resistant (Gottesman 2002).

Inhibitors of ABC transporters, specifically of ABCB1, may enhance or sustain chemotherapy efficacy.

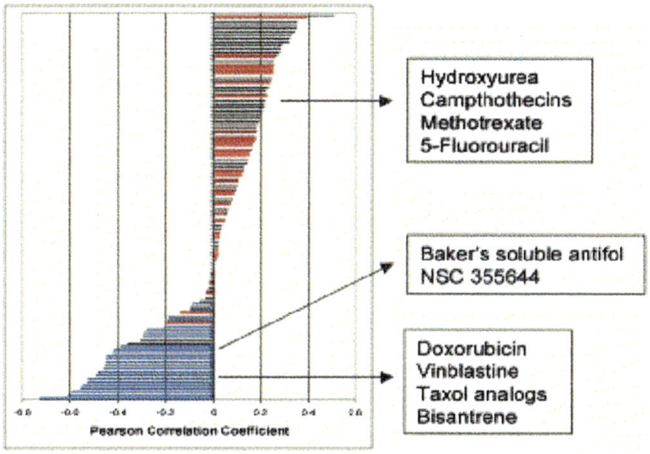

Fig. 16.2 The relationship between drug sensitivity and ABCB1 expression. Correlation between drug-induced growth inhibition and ABCB1 expression. *Blue bars* = known ABCB1 substrates; *red bars* = compounds shown not to be substrates of ABCB1; *black bars* = compounds for which data are not available. The drug names listed at the *top* and *bottom* are commonly used, representative agents from the classes shown by *red* and *blue bars* (NCI Developmental Therapeutics Program). ((Szakacs 2004) with permission)

Adverse Effects Concerns about the adverse effects of ABCB1 antagonists include the potential for bone marrow and neurological toxicity. Myelosuppression can occur in patients treated with ABCB1 inhibitors. Cerebellar ataxia can arise in patients treated with PSC-833, tamoxifen, or dexniguldipine administered alone, but other central nervous system toxicity is rare. Some of the pharmacokinetic complications associated with ABCB1 inhibitors may be due to the off-target effect of inhibiting other proteins involved in drug metabolism and disposition, such as Cytochrome P450.

Cyclosporin A <Sandimmune, Neoral> is a first generation inhibitor of ABCB1, ABCG2, and ABCC1. It may increase the exposure to anti-cancer drugs that are substrates for these transporters by 2–3-fold. Because cyclosporin A acts as a strong and non-specific immunosuppressant its use as an ABCB1 inhibitor is limited.

Valspodar (PSC833) <Amdray> is an analog of cyclosporin A but devoid of the immunosuppressive and nephrotoxic properties (Fig. 16.3). It inhibits ABCB1, the multi-drug resistance efflux pump, thereby restoring the retention and activity of some drugs in some drug-resistant tumor cells. Valspodar may substantially increase the concentration of paclitaxel in the brain. This agent also induces Caspase dependent apoptosis.

Pharmacokinetics Valspodar is a substrate for CYP2D6, CYP2C9, CYP2C19, CYP1A2, NAT2, and DPD.

Adverse Effects Adverse effects are transient and reversible. They include dizziness, numbness, tingling of the extremities, and nausea. Some patients may experience cerebellar dysfunction (difficulty walking, impairment of coordination) that is rapidly reversible. Liver functions may be affected.

Quinidine is a first generation ABCB1 inhibitor. It also inhibits Cytochrome P450 2D6 and acts as a class I antiarrhythmic. Thus, its application as a chemopotentiator that blocks drug export is compromised. Various derivatives hold more promise.

Among alkaloids, the aporphinoids constitute a broad subgroup of benzylisoquinoline compounds. Thalicarpine (thaliblastine) (NSC 68075) is a plant derived aporphine benzylisoquinoline vinca alkaloid that binds to and inhibits the multi-drug resistance efflux pump ABCB1. Thalicarpine can overcome multi-drug resistance in certain cancer cells because it has the capacity to increase cellular drug retention. The agent also induces single strand breaks in DNA and arrests cancer cells at the G_1 and G_2/M phase of the cell cycle.

Adverse Effects Common adverse effects include nausea and lethargy; less frequently vomiting, tachycardia, hypotension, pain distant from the infusion site, urticaria, chills, diarrhea, and mydriasis (dilation of the pupil) may arise.

Zosuquidar trihydrochloride (LY335979, RS 33295-198) is a difluorocyclopropyl quinoline that binds with high affinity to ABCB1 and inhibits ABCB1 mediated multi-drug resistance. The drug is only moderately active as an inhibitor of ABCB1 at the blood-brain barrier. It does not have anti-cancer activity by itself, but may enhance the retention of doxorubicin. Zosuquidar trihydrochloride is under study for enhancing the drug treatment of acute myeloid leukemia.

Tariquidar (XR9576) is a naturally occurring, orally bioavailable bisbenzylisoquinoline plant alkaloid with potential chemosensitization activity. An anthranilamide derivative, tariquidar binds non-competitively to the transporters ABCB1 and ABCG2, thereby inhibiting the transmembrane export of anti-cancer drugs. The inhibition of drug export may result in increased intracellular concentrations of various anti-cancer agents, thereby augmenting its cytotoxicity. As tariquidar inhibits the ATPase activity of ABCB1, the drug effect may be based on the inhibition of substrate binding or of ATP hydrolysis. The inhibition persists for 48 hours after a single dose.

Elacridar (*N*-(4-(2-(1,2,3,4-tetrahydro-6,7-dimethoxy-2-isoquinolinyl)ethyl)phenyl)-9,10-dihydro-5-methoxy-9-oxo-4-acridine carboxamide) (GF120918) is a third generation inhibitor of ABCB1 and ABCG2. If administered with anti-cancer drugs that are substrates for these efflux transporters the drug exposure increases approximately 2.5-

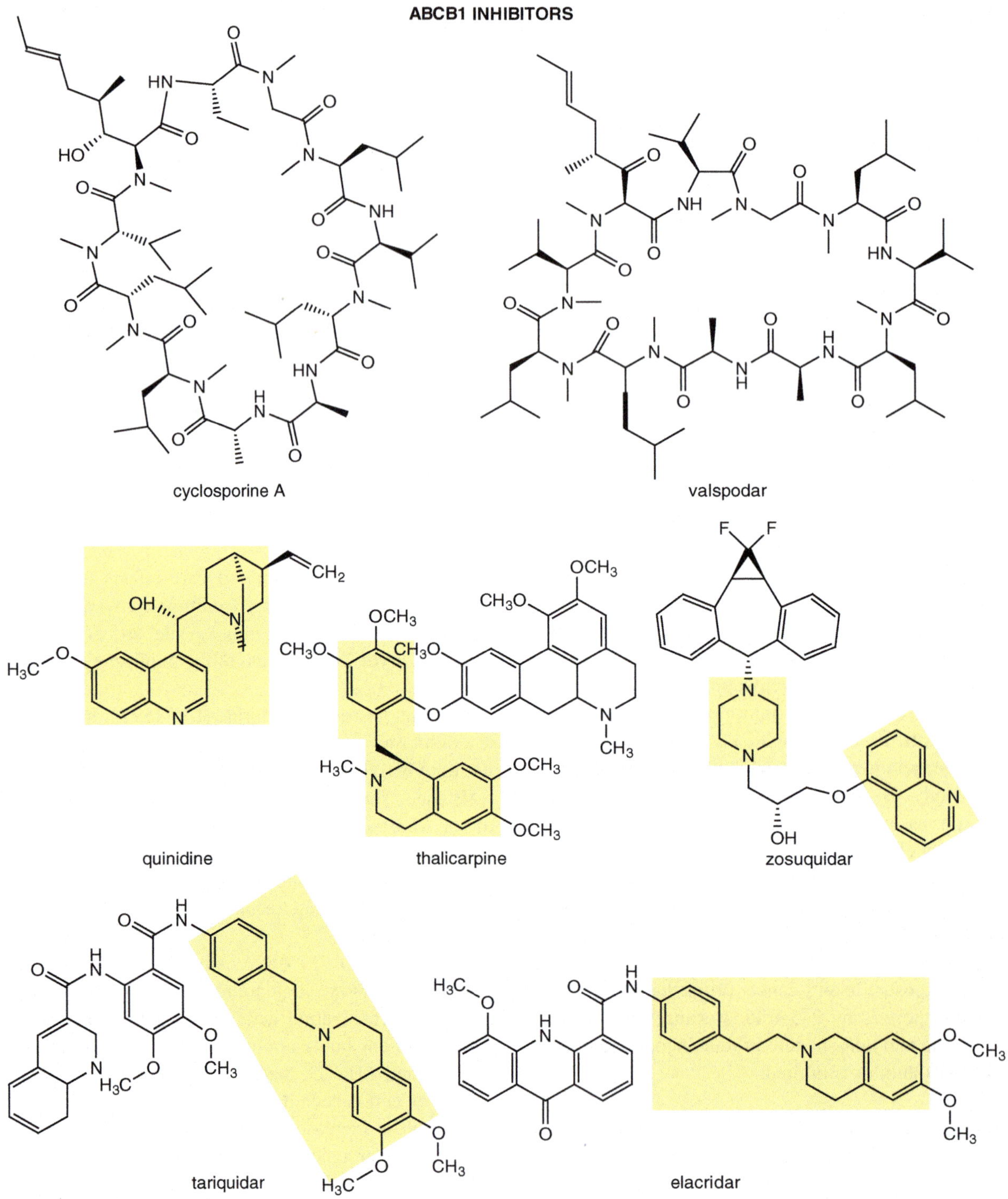

Fig. 16.3 Structures of ABCB1 inhibitors. A conserved benzylisoquinoline-derived motif of 2 connected 6-rings (containing various heteroatoms), a bridge and a 6-ring in a subset of drugs in this class is highlighted in *yellow*

fold. In anti-cancer therapy, the brain may present as a sanctuary site for cytotoxic drugs due to their inability to cross the blood-brain barrier. Elacridar may substantially increase the oral absorption (by inhibiting intestinal ABCB1) and the concentration of co-administered paclitaxel, topotecan, or the kinase inhibitors imatinib, dasatinib, gefitinib, sorafenib, sunitinib in the brain (by inhibiting ABCB1 at the blood-brain barrier). The agent is orally bioavailable.

Verapamil (dexverapamil) <Isoptin, Calan, Verelan, Covera-HS> is a first generation competitive inhibitor of ABCB1. It also is an L-type calcium channel blocker of

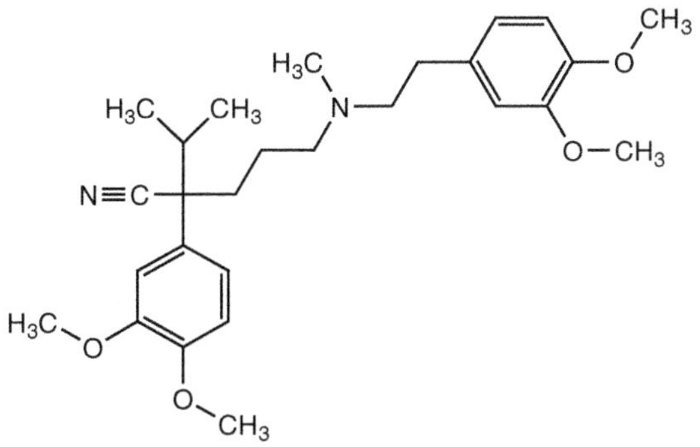

dexverapamil

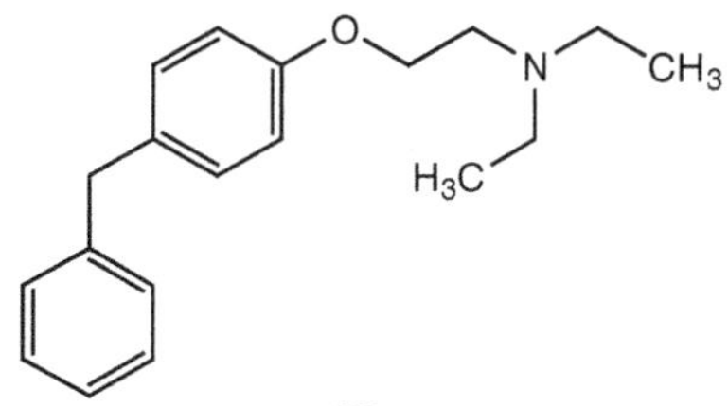

tesmilifene

Fig. 16.3 (continued)

the phenylalkylamine class. In clinical trials, verapamil has resulted in improved response rates and prolonged disease free and overall survivals.

Adverse Effects Common adverse reactions to orally administered verapamil comprise constipation, dizziness, nausea, headache, dyspnea, bradycardia, atrioventricular block, hypotension and edema. Verapamil has a negative inotropic effect, which in most patients is compensated by its afterload reduction (decreased systemic vascular resistance) properties without a net impairment of ventricular performance. In rare cases it can cause congestive heart failure or pulmonary edema.

Tesmilifene (*N, N*-Diethyl-2-[4-(phenylmethyl)phenoxy] ethanamine) is a small molecule chemopotentiator that targets ABCB1$^+$ multi-drug resistant cancer cells. In combination with various standard chemotherapy regimens, it may prevent ABCB1 mediated drug resistance. The agent can enhance the anti-tumor effects of anthracyclines and docetaxel. It also acts as an intracellular histamine antagonist. Tesmilifene is a substrate of CYP3A. It is under investigation for enhancing the chemotherapy of metastatic breast cancer.

ABCB1 inhibitory activity is exerted by the anti-depressants sertraline, desmethylsertraline, and paroxetine.

ABCG2 ABCG2 (MXR, Mitoxantrone-Resistance protein, BCRP, Breast Cancer Resistance Protein, ABC-P, ABC Transporter in Placenta) is abundant in the intestinal epithelium, liver canaliculi, the placental trophoblasts, mammary ducts and lobules, and endothelial cells of veins and capillaries. Its distribution conveys to it a substantial role in the pharmacokinetics of substrate drugs. Some anti-cancer drugs, such as mitoxantrone, doxorubicin, daunorubicin, and topotecan, are subject to encountering resistance based on up-regulation of ABCG2 in the target cells or in the path of drug distribution.

The diketopiperazine fungal toxin fumitremorgin C (FTC, tryptoquivaline), originally derived from Aspergillus fumigatus, is a potent and specific inhibitor of ABCG2 (Fig. 16.4).

Adverse Effects The neurotoxic effects of fumitremorgin C (induction of tremors and convulsions) preclude its use in patients. Being cell-permeable, it suppresses sphingolipid biosynthesis by inhibition of Sphingosine *N*-Acyl Transferase (Ceramide Synthase) preferentially in neuronal cells. The agent may have carcinogenic properties.

Ko143 is an ABCG2 inhibitor with more than 200-fold selectivity over the transporters ABCB1 and ABCC1. It increases intracellular drug accumulation and reverses ABCG2 mediated multi-drug resistance. When administered orally to inhibit intestinal ABCG2, Ko143 markedly increases the oral availability of topotecan.

The ABCG2 inhibitor lapatinib ditosylate (GW572016) <Tykerb, Tyverb> is a small molecule member of the 4-anilinoquinazoline class. Lapatinib also acts as a reversible kinase inhibitor for ERBB1, ERBB2, ERK-1, ERK-2, and PKB (see Sect. 4.1.1.). It also suppresses the Cyclin D protein levels in tumor cells. The drug is taken orally once a day.

The compound elacridar (*N*-[4-[2-(3,4-Dihydro-6,7-dimethoxy-2(1*H*)-isoquinolinyl)ethyl]phenyl]-9,10-dihydro-5-methoxy-9-oxo-4-acridinecarboxamide hydrochloride) (GF120918, GG918, GW0918) was developed as an ABCB1 inhibitor, but it also inhibits ABCG2. Clinically important substrate drugs of ABCG2 are often also ABCB1 substrates. Hence, a dual specificity inhibitor may be advantageous in some applications.

Others Estramustine is a nitrogen mustard derivative of estradiol. The transporter ABCA2 is over-expressed in estramustine resistant cells. It is located intracellularly in endosomal/lysosomal vesicles and may participate in steroid transport.

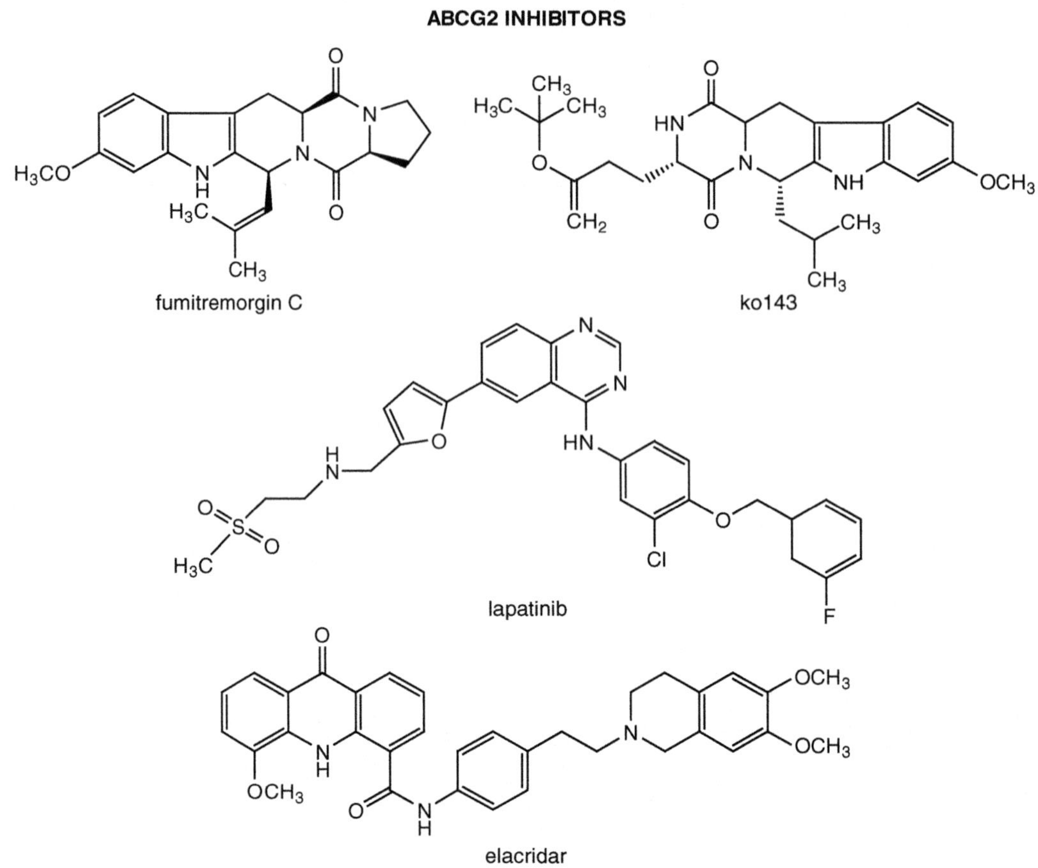

Fig. 16.4 Structures of ABCG2 inhibitors

ABCB4 (MDR2) functions as a Phosphatidylcholine Translocase, which reduces the toxicity of bile salts. Paclitaxel and vinblastine are substrates for ABCB4. ABCB11 (Bile Salt Export Protein, BSEP, SPGP) also confers low-level resistance to paclitaxel.

Many ABCC family members transport drugs and therefore have the potential to confer drug resistance (Borst 2000). ABCC1 (MRP1) is highly expressed in leukemias, esophageal carcinoma, and non-small-cell lung cancer. It transports Glutathione and other conjugates of these drugs. In some cases, such as for vincristine, ABCC1 co-transports unconjugated Glutathione.

ABCC2 (MRP2, cMOAT) localizes to the canalicular membranes of hepatocytes and the apical surfaces of epithelial cells. It has a primary role in the excretion of bilirubin-glucuronide and other organic anions into the bile. MRP2 is also capable of mediating drug efflux.

ABCC3 (MRP3) is present in the kidneys and intestines. ABCC3 is localized to the basolateral surface of hepatocytes, where it transports organic anions from the liver back into the bloodstream. It pumps out methotrexate, etoposide, doxorubicin, cisplatin, vincristine, and mitoxantrone.

The efflux transporter ABCC4 (MRP4) is expressed in prostate, testes, ovaries, intestines, liver, and adrenal glands. Its substrates include methotrexate and thiopurines.

ABCC5 (MRP5) is ubiquitously expressed. It contributes to the efflux of 6-mercaptopurine and 6-thioguanine.

16.2 Decreased Uptake

Drugs can reach their target cells by passive diffusion or by facilitated uptake (Fig. 16.5). Water soluble agents that use transporters and carriers to enter cells, or agents that enter by means of endocytosis may fail to accumulate when the molecules that facilitate their uptake are under-expressed. This is the case for cisplatin, the anti-folate methotrexate, doxorubicin, gemcitabine, paclitaxel, and nucleotide analogs (such as 5-fluorouracil and 8-azaguanine).

The members of the solute carrier (SLC) super-family of uptake transporters comprise approximately 360 biomolecules classified into 45 gene families. SLC molecules encode passive transporters, ion-coupled transporters, and exchangers.

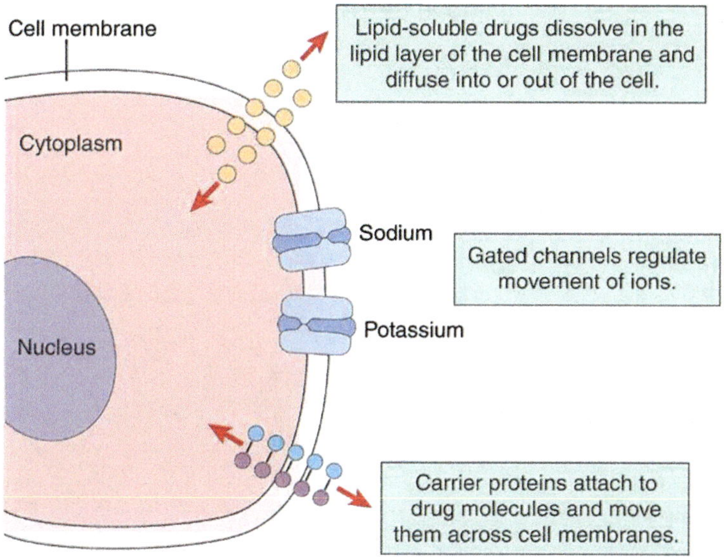

Fig. 16.5 Drug transport pathways. Drug molecules cross cell membranes to move into and out of cells by directly penetrating the lipid layer, diffusion through open or gated channels, or attaching to carrier proteins. (Instructor's Resource CD-ROM to Carlson J. Foundations of Clinical Drug Therapy 2005) There are instances where we have been unable to trace or contact the copyright holder. If notified the publisher will be pleased to rectify any errors or omissions at the earliest opportunity

- Decreased expression or polymorphisms in the gene encoding of SLC19A1 (Reduced Folate Carrier, hRFC1) affect the patient response to the anti-folate methotrexate.
- SLC22A1 (OCT1), SLC22A2 (OCT2), and SLC22A3 (OCT3) mediate the uptake of some platinum anti-cancer drugs.
- SLC22A4 confers sensitivity to doxorubicin in cancer cells.
- SLC29A1, SLC29A2 and SLC28A1 contribute to gemcitabine transport. SLC29A1 is a predictive marker for overall survival in patients with pancreatic cancer who have received gemcitabine. Cancers with reduced expression or mutants of SLC29A1, SLC29A2, or SLC28A1 may be resistant to this drug.
- SLCO1B3 (OATP1B3) mediates the uptake of paclitaxel, although paclitaxel pharmacokinetics is not linked to the polymorphisms T344G or G699A.

16.3 Anti-Apoptosis

In the transformation of normal cells to cancer cells, anti-apoptotic mechanisms play a central role. Drug resistance can also result from defective apoptotic pathways.

- Intrinsic drug resistance, based on anti-apoptosis, may occur as a result of the malignant transformation.
- Acquired drug resistance may be due to changes in apoptotic pathways during exposure to chemotherapy, such as the alteration of ceramide levels or changes in cell cycle checkpoints that prevent the initiation of apoptosis.

The BCL-2 family of proteins, which has more than 25 members comprising both pro-apoptotic (BAX, BAK) and pro-survival (BCL-2, BCL-X_L, MCL-1 and BCL-W) molecules, provides pivotal contributors to regulating programmed cell death. Often, drug resistance is caused by alterations in the components of the anti-apoptotic machinery. This may entail an elevated expression of pro-survival members in the BCL-2 family of proteins.

The BH3 domains of pro-apoptotic BCL-2 family members can neutralize anti-apoptotic BCL-2 family proteins, so that there is a level of mitochondrial priming that determines the threshold for depolarization of the mitochondria and consecutively chemosensitivity to cytotoxic anti-cancer agents (Ni Chonghaile 2011). Over-expression of the anti-apoptotic protein BCL-2 may render cancer cells resistant to various cytotoxic agents. Susceptible drugs are those that initiate signals, which impinge on a final common pathway for cell death that is blocked by BCL-2. Anti-apoptosis may be overcome by inhibitors of pro-survival BCL2 family members, including mimetics for the functionally critical BH3 domain. BCL-2 family inhibitors are discussed in Sect. 3.3.2.

Survivin, a member of the IAP (Inhibitor of Apoptosis) protein family, is often highly expressed in cancer while it is absent from most untransformed adult tissues (see Sect. 3.3.4.). The VEGF mediated induction of Survivin plays a pivotal role in preserving the microtubule network of tumor associated vascular endothelial cells and may act to shield tumor endothelial cells from the apoptotic effects of chemotherapy. Survivin is a major factor of drug and radia-

PRO-APOPTOTIC DRUGS

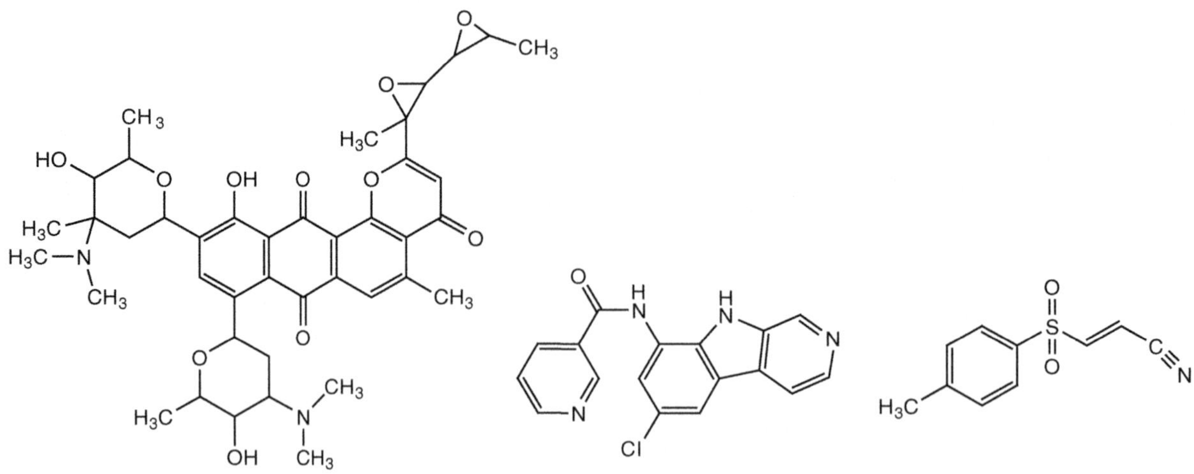

hedamycin PS1145 BAY-117082

Fig. 16.6 Structures of pro-apoptotic drugs

tion resistance, and hence constitutes a therapeutic target for cancer treatment, aimed at inducing apoptosis.

The transcriptional induction of *survivin* expression may be involved in drug resistance. Activated Estrogen Receptor α (ERα) interacts with P53 at its DNA binding site in the *survivin* promoter and de-represses the P53 mediated inhibition of *survivin* expression. Taxol induces Survivin and thus limits its own effectiveness to induce breast cancer cell death. Further, the down-regulation of Survivin expression in doxorubicin resistant cells may reverse drug resistance.

Hedamycin is an aromatic polyketide produced by Streptomyces griseoruber (Fig. 16.6). A member of the anthracyclines, hedamycin acts via reversible DNA intercalation and irreversible alkylation of a guanine residue at specific 5′-PyG-3′ motifs, with 5′-CGT sites favored over 5′-TGT sites. Transcriptional down-regulation of *survivin* expression by the GC-rich, DNA selective anti-cancer agent hedamycin is partially involved in its drug mediated apoptotic cell killing.

The stress-inducible transcription factor NF-κB exerts crucial functions in support of the cellular resistance to oxidants. Activation of NF-κB can contribute to the development and progression of certain cancers, and it can contribute to drug resistance. This may be overcome, in part, by compounds that suppress the NF-κB pathway. Pharmacological approaches to targeting NF-κB include the repression of NF-κB transactivating potential, the stabilization of I-κB by proteasome inhibitors, and the inhibition of upstream I-κB Kinases (IKKs).

I-κB Kinase (IKK) is a complex composed of the subunits IKKα, IKKβ, and IKKγ that phosphorylates two serines in the regulatory domain of I-κB proteins. Phosphorylation tags I-κB for poly-ubiquitination and degradation in the proteasome. The degradation of I-κB proteins then frees NF-κB to enter the nucleus, where it activates transcription. The unique properties of I-κB Kinase β (IKKβ) among the serine/threonine kinases have allowed the development of specific IKKβ inhibitors. In chronic myelocytic leukemia (CML) cells, NF-κB is a downstream component of the BCR-ABL initiated signaling pathway, the activity of which is associated with cellular resistance to imatinib.

- Treatment with the IKKβ inhibitor *N*-(6-chloro-9*H*-pyrido[3,4-b]indol-8-yl)-3-pyridinecarboxamide (PS1145) inhibits both basal and induced NF-κB activities. It may overcome imatinib resistance and induce apoptosis. The inhibition of NF-κB by PS1145 may also enhance docetaxel sensitivity in prostate cancer.
- (*E*)-3-(4-methylphenylsulfonyl)-2-propenenitrile (BAY-117082) selectively and irreversibly inhibits NF-κB activation by blocking the TNF-α induced phosphorylation of I-κBα without affecting the constitutive I-κBα auto-phosphorylation. Consecutively, the compound inhibits the TNF-α induced surface expression of the adhesion molecules ICAM-1, VCAM-1, and E-Selectin. BAY-117082 also stimulates the stress activated protein kinases, P38 and JNK-1. It induces apoptosis in leukemia cells through a mode that depends on reactive oxygen species but is independent of Caspases. However, in sarcoma cells, it may cause programmed cell death through mechanisms that are independent of NF-κB or reactive oxygen species, but depend on Caspases. The agent may be useful in combination with conventional chemotherapeutics, such as doxorubicin, to which resistance develops via NF-κB activation in some cancers.

P53 is an important regulator of the cell cycle. It mediates cell cycle arrest (often in the G_1 phase of the cell cycle) or apoptosis in response to DNA damage (genotoxic stress).

Drugs that convey DNA damage induce P53 mediated cell death. Loss of P53 function, which occurs in about 50 % of cancers, can be associated with resistance to those drugs. In breast cancer, a reduced expression of P53 modifies the response to paclitaxel and 5-fluorouracil. Reactivation of mutant *p53* may be an effective way of inducing tumor cell death.

MDM2 is a negative regulator of P53. It also may mediate anti-apoptosis via P53 independent pathways. In breast cancer, MDM2 may convey resistance to lapatinib treatment.

TRPM-2 is an anti-apoptotic Clusterin that is overexpressed by prostate cancer cells and is associated with chemoresistance. OGX-011 is a mixed-backbone antisense oligodeoxynucleotide with chemosensitizing properties. The agent inhibits *trpm-2* (*testosterone-repressed prostate message-2*). The administration of OGX-011 abrogates the anti-apoptotic effect of TRPM-2, thereby sensitizing cells to chemotherapy and resulting in tumor cell death.

16.4 Mutations in the Drug Target

Whereas most cellular polymers, including RNA, proteins and polysaccharides, are regularly turned over and re-synthesized based on the genetic blueprint, DNA cannot be turned over and requires repair when damaged. Because the genome is vulnerable to an array of damaging influences, various DNA repair pathways exist. Repair genes act as a second line of defense, and their lack of function can allow tumor cells to undergo genetic changes more rapidly than untransformed cells. This tendency is referred to as the mutator phenotype. Under the selective pressure of anti-cancer chemotherapy, the occurrence of mutations in the drug target may allow cancer cells to become drug resistant.

Gain of function of the Epidermal Growth Factor Receptor (EGFR) underlies transformation in various epithelial cancers. Reversible EGFR tyrosine kinase inhibitors are active in a subset of patients. However, most develop resistance and progress within the course of about 1 year. In nearly half of all cases, acquired resistance to kinase inhibitors is caused by the secondary EGFR mutation T790M. This amino acid change prevents erlotinib or gefitinib from binding to their drug target.

Erlotinib has limited efficacy in glioblastoma, where a distinct EGFR mutation, the variant III (vIII) in-frame deletion of exons 2–7, commonly arises.

Chronic myelogenous leukemia (CML) may be caused by the chromosome translocation t(9;22)(q34;q11) that generates the chimeric kinase BCR-ABL. The first line of treatment is constituted by small molecule kinase inhibitors (including imatinib) that are specific for this oncoprotein. Cases of leukemia that acquire drug resistance are often characterized by point mutations in BCR-ABL, which change the conformation of the kinase such that the treating drug becomes ineffective. Alternatively, amplification of the *bcr-abl* gene can induce resistance to non-toxic drug concentrations. In these cases, BCR-ABL is reactivated and cell proliferation remains dependent on BCR-ABL signaling. More than 70 point mutations fall into four major groups based on their location in the ATP binding loop (40 % of all mutations), the gatekeeper residue threonine 315 (25 % of all mutations), the catalytic domain (25 % of all mutations), or the activation loop (5 % of all mutations).

BCR-ABL contains the ATP binding P-loop and the activation loop, which stabilize the basal conformation. Mutations in these loops destabilize the structure, such that the kinase domain cannot assume the inactive conformation required for kinase inhibitor binding. Mutations in the P-loop region are the most common form of CML drug resistance, with T315I being completely resistant to multiple BCR-ABL directed therapies. The T315I substitution eliminates a critical oxygen molecule needed for hydrogen bonding between inhibitor and kinase. It also creates steric hindrance to the binding of most small molecule inhibitors.

- About 10 % of patients acquire drug resistance after an average of 18 months of imatinib treatment. Mutations in the kinase domain of BCR-ABL are the most prevalent underlying mechanism. Specifically, T315I leads to imatinib resistance.
- In acute phase/blast crisis of chronic myelogenous leukemia, 30–60 % of patients are refractory to nilotinib. Resistance to nilotinib is associated with a limited spectrum of BCR-ABL kinase mutations that mostly affect the P-loop and T315I.
- In acute phase/blast crisis of chronic myelogenous leukemia, 20–40 % of patients are refractory to dasatinib. Drug resistance to dasatinib occurs in patients with the BCR-ABL mutation T315I.

The development of an inhibitor for BCR-ABL^{T315I} has been challenging, because most ATP competitive inhibitors directly interact with threonine 315 via hydrogen bonding and with the specificity-imparting hydrophobic pocket, for which this residue serves as a gatekeeper.

Several BCR-ABL mutations in the active site, such as Y235F/H or E255K/V, also confer imatinib mesylate resistance. Small molecule inhibitors of Aurora Kinase, including MK-0457 (VX-680), XL228, and AT9713, can effectively inhibit such mutant enzymes.

Mutational frequencies increase as chronic myelogenous leukemia progresses from the chronic phase to the blast phase. The dasatinib resistant mutation V299L may develop

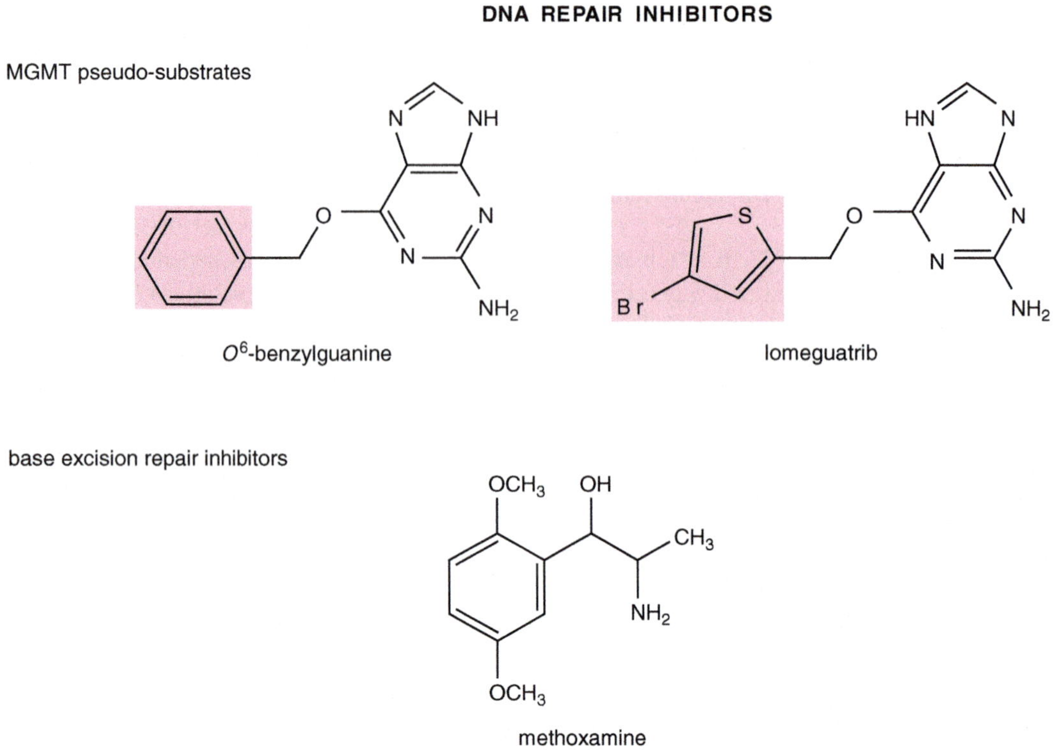

Fig. 16.7 Structures of DNA repair inhibitors. Two sub-classes comprise MGMT pseudo-substrates (*top* panel) and base excision repair inhibitors (*bottom* panel). The different structural elements between the MGMT pseudo-substrates are highlighted in *pink*

under treatment. This mutation regains sensitivity for imatinib but is also sensitive to the Aurora Kinase inhibitor tozasertib. The mutated leucine enhances the affinity of tozasertib for $BCR\text{-}ABL^{V299L}$.

16.5 Altered Repair of Drug Induced Damage

Because cancer cells typically proliferate more rapidly than their untransformed counterparts most anti-cancer drugs target cell cycle progression. Many chemotherapeutic agents kill proliferating cells by causing extensive DNA damage that ultimately leads to cell cycle arrest and cell death, either directly or following DNA reduplication during the S phase of the cell cycle. However, the efficacy of these drugs can be reduced by the ability of cells to repair DNA. DNA adducts, such as those created by alkylating agents, may be excised and repaired before they are confronted by the reduplication machinery. The network of interacting pathways to monitor the integrity of the DNA and coordinate responses to genetic damage includes sensor complexes that detect DNA breaks. MRE11-RAD50-NBS1 (MRN) recognizes DNA double strand breaks, while the RPA-ATRIP complex binds to single strand breaks. Kinases such as ATM and ATR are then recruited by MRN or RPA-ATRIP and activate other proteins, including the checkpoint kinases CHK1 and CHK2. This initiates a cascade that results in cell cycle arrest and DNA repair. Activated pathways include

- the direct damage reversal pathway (MGMT, ABH2, ABH3)
- the mismatch repair pathway
- the nucleotide excision repair pathway
- the base excision repair pathway (PARP)
- the homologous recombination pathway
- the non-homologous end joining pathway.

However, if the damage is irreparable the cell will enter senescence, apoptosis, or necrosis. Inducing these effects in cancer cells is the goal of cancer therapy.

DNA repair Defects in DNA damage checkpoint pathways (induced by inhibitors of DNA repair) result in increased sensitivity to a range of anti-cancer treatments. Therefore, inhibitors of specific DNA repair pathways may prove efficacious when used in combination with DNA damaging chemotherapeutic drugs. Under study are inhibitors of MGMT, PARP, base excision repair, and checkpoint kinases (Fig. 16.7).

The presence of O^6-Alkyl Guanine DNA Alkyl Transferase (AGT, O^6-Methyl Guanine Methyl Transferase, MGMT) protects cells from killing by methylating and chloroethylating agents, which are widely used in cancer chemotherapy.

Resistance to alkylating agents via direct DNA repair by MGMT (direct damage reversal) constitutes a barrier to the successful treatment with these classes of drugs. The resistance to O^6-alkylating agents can be overcome by depletion of MGMT activity. Pseudo-substrates for MGMT are in clinical trials as chemotherapy enhancers.

- The repair of DNA damage by MGMT is one of the most important mechanisms of resistance to alkylnitrosoureas (including BCNU and procarbazine) and alkyltriazenes (including temozolomide and DTIC), which are used to treat brain tumors, lymphomata, and malignant melanoma. The inactivation of MGMT by the inhibitor O^6-benzylguanine sensitizes cells to killing by these agents. O^6-benzylguanine binds the enzyme, transferring the benzyl moiety to the active site cysteine and resulting in the inhibition of MGMT mediated DNA repair. Co-administration of this agent potentiates the effects of chemotherapeutic agents that damage DNA.
- Lomeguatrib (O^6-(4-bromothenyl)guanine, PaTrin-2) is a more potent MGMT inhibitor than O^6-benzylguanine. It enhances the anti-cancer activity of temozolomide.

Adverse Effects When used in combination with cytotoxic chemotherapy, myelosuppression is substantially enhanced by O^6-benzylguanine and lomeguatrib, necessitating reductions in the doses of alkylating agents from those used in standard chemotherapy. On account of this lack of selectivity by the chemoenhancers for malignant tissue versus healthy bone marrow, no improvement in the therapeutic index has been demonstrated.

Poly(ADP-ribosyl)ation contributes to efficient DNA repair, leading to the survival of proliferating cells exposed to moderate genotoxic stresses. The enzyme PARP1 (Poly(ADP-Ribose) Polymerase 1) is required for the efficient base excision repair of apurinic sites, the intermediate DNA lesions induced by chemotherapeutic drugs like temozolomide. Specific inhibitors of PARP can prevent the repair of apurinic sites or the rejoining of DNA strand breaks. The combination of temozolomide with inhibitors of PARP1 (see Sect. 15.2.) is under investigation. Platinum chemotherapy is being tested with PARP inhibition in clinical trials.

Methoxyamine hydrochloride (TRC-102) is an inhibitor of base excision repair. It rapidly and covalently binds to apurinic/apyrimidinic sites generated during base excision repair. Methoxyamine-bound DNA causes Topoisomerase 2 dependent irreversible strand breaks and apoptosis, which are relatively selective for cancer cells as those cells typically over-express Topoisomerase 2. By contrast, in non-transformed cells with low Topoisomerase 2 expression, methoxyamine-bound DNA is excised and replaced by the long patch DNA repair system. The drug may potentiate the activity of other DNA repair inhibitors, including PARP inhibitors. It is under study for combination with temozolomide or pemetrexed.

CHK inhibitors are discussed in Sect. 4.1.6.

Defective mismatch repair Whereas most DNA repair pathways mediate resistance to drug induced DNA damage, mismatch repair is actually required for the toxicity of several anti-cancer drugs. A loss of mismatch repair (MMR) can result in drug resistance,

- directly by impairing the ability of the cell to detect DNA damage and activate apoptosis
- indirectly by increasing the mutation rate throughout the genome.

This may be caused by a futile repair cycle, in which mismatch repair removes the newly inserted intact base instead of the damaged base, triggering subsequent rounds of futile repair which can be deleterious to the cell. Mismatch repair deficient cells may be resistant to the methylating agents procarbazine and temozolomide, the alkylating agent busulfan, the platinum containing drugs cisplatin and carboplatin, the anti-metabolite 6-thioguanine, and the Topoisomerase 2 inhibitors etoposide and doxorubicin.

Methylating agents form a variety of DNA adducts, among which O^6-methyl-guanine is the most cytotoxic. The mismatch repair system recognizes the mis-pair that occurs after the erroneous incorporation of a thymine opposite the O^6-methyl-guanine during the next cycle of DNA reduplication. However, in the repair process a thymine is again incorporated opposite the persisting O^6-methyl-guanine. This causes the site to be once again recognized by the mismatch repair system, triggering a new round of attempted repair. This futile cycling may increase the risk for a double strand break, which leads to apoptosis during the next ensuing S phase.

Large numbers of O^6-methyl-guanine adducts are generated in the DNA by temozolomide, a mono-functional methylating imidazotetrazinone, and by procarbazine, a methylhydrazine derivative. The enzyme MGMT (O^6-Alkyl Guanine DNA Alkyl Transferase) can transfer the alkyl group from the O^6 position of the guanine residue to its own active site cysteine. In cells expressing this enzyme, this is the major route of repair. However, the cytotoxicity induced by many anti-cancer drugs depends on the activation of the mismatch repair system. Therefore, drug resistance may arise if the mismatch repair system is defective or MGMT is expressed at high levels.

16.6 Other Mechanisms

Prodrug activation and drug inactivation The underexpression of drug metabolizing enzymes can reduce drug efficacy in situations where an administered inactive prodrug has to undergo catalytic conversion to an active form.

- Arabinoside requires activation by Deoxycytidine Kinase. A loss or mutation of this enzyme renders this drug less effective.

An over-expression of drug metabolizing enzymes leads to resistance to those anti-cancer drugs that are their substrates.

- The increased production of Glutathione or ubiquitin contributes to inactivation of some drugs by forming conjugates that are excreted.
- Resistance to cisplatin in ovarian carcinoma cells is associated with increased expression of Dihydrodiol Dehydrogenase.

The orphan nuclear receptor SXR (Steroid and Xenobiotic Receptor) coordinately regulates drug metabolism and efflux (Synold 2001) by inducing the transcription of *cyp3A4* and *abcb1*. The SXR pathway is involved in colon cancer resistance to irinotecan. It is activated in response to SN-38, the active metabolite of irinotecan, translocates into the nucleus and associates with RXR. There, SXR induces the expression of genes for drug disposition.

Drug redistribution Vaults are large ribonucleoprotein particles that may confer drug resistance by redistributing drugs away from their intracellular targets. Major Vault Protein (MVP, Lung Resistance Protein, LRP) is expressed at high levels in the cytoplasm and on the nuclear membranes of drug resistant tumor cells. Specifically, it is associated with a poor response to chemotherapy in acute myeloid leukemia and ovarian carcinoma. The expression of MVP correlates with intrinsic resistance to vincristine and platinum compounds. It causes a redistribution of doxorubicin from the nucleus to the cytoplasm without changes in total drug intracellular concentrations.

The transcription factor STAT3 plays important roles in cancer progression. It may also contribute to the acquired drug resistance of gastric cancer to cisplatin. The vacuolar ATPase, a proton pump which interferes with the uptake of anti-cancer agents, is up-regulated by STAT3. The interruption of STAT3 signaling could reverse resistance to chemotherapy agents in gastric cancer.

- Auranofin <Ridaura> is an orally available, lipophilic, organogold compound. It interacts with a selenocysteine residue within the redox-active domain of mitochondrial Thioredoxin Reductase, thereby blocking its activity. Auranofin also inhibits the JAK1/STAT3 signal transduction pathway.
- Atiprimod is an orally bioavailable small molecule belonging to the azaspirane class of cationic amphiphilic agents. Atiprimod inhibits the phosphorylation of STAT3, thus inducing cell cycle arrest and apoptosis.
- Tipifarnib (R115777) <Zarnestra> is a non-peptidomimetic quinolinone that binds to and inhibits Farnesyl Protein Transferase. Tipifarnib may also target a survival pathway, reflected in reduced levels of phosphorylated PKB and STAT3 in bone marrow from patients, in whom these tumor survival pathways are constitutively active. The reduced phosphorylation correlates with disease stabilization.

Cancer cell heterogeneity The heterogeneity of cancers may underlie the eventual failure of cancer drug therapy in many patients. Relative drug resistance to conventional anti-cancer drugs (which generally target proliferating cells) may be caused by a low growth fraction of cancer cells. Cancer stem cells (CSCs, cancer initiating cells) are in this contingent. Because conventional anti-cancer drugs suppress cell division, cells that are not in the growth fraction are not effectively killed by these agents. Cancer stem cells acquire many multi-drug resistance mechanisms that are not present in the growth fraction. This may include the expression of efflux transporters, such as ABCA3 and ABCG2 in neuroblastoma cancer stem cells.

Drug resistance constitutes the insensitivity or reduced sensitivity to specific agents.
Drug resistance can be intrinsic or acquired.
Mutations in dug targets may lead to insensitivity.
Drugs that may overcome resistance include blockers of efflux transporters, inducers of apoptosis, and inhibitors of DNA repair pathways.
Such agents are referred to as chemoenhancers and are given together with chemotherapy.

References

Borst P, Evers R, Kool M, Wijnholds J (2000) A family of drug transporters: the multidrug resistance-associated proteins. J Natl Cancer Inst 92:1295–1302
Buick RN (1994) Cellular basis of chemotherapy. In: Von Hoff DD, Dorr RT (eds) Cancer chemotherapy handbook. Elsevier, New York, pp 3–14
Danø K (1973) Active outward transport of daunomycin in resistant Ehrlich ascites tumor cells. Biochim Biophys Acta 323:466–483
Gottesman MM, Fojo T, Bates SE (2002) Multidrug resistance in cancer: role of ATP-dependent transporters. Nat Rev Cancer 2:48–58

Ni Chonghaile T, Sarosiek KA, Vo TT, Ryan JA, Tammareddi A, Moore Vdel G, Deng J, Anderson KC, Richardson P, Tai YT, Mitsiades CS, Matulonis UA, Drapkin R, Stone R, Deangelo DJ, McConkey DJ, Sallan SE, Silverman L, Hirsch MS, Carrasco DR, Letai A (2011) Pretreatment mitochondrial priming correlates with clinical response to cytotoxic chemotherapy. Science 334:1129–1133

Potti A, Dressman HK, Bild A, Riedel RF, Chan G, Sayer R, Cragun J, Cottrill H, Kelley MJ, Petersen R, Harpole D, Marks J, Berchuck A, Ginsburg GS, Febbo P, Lancaster J, Nevins JR (2006) Genomic signatures to guide the use of chemotherapeutics. Nat Med 12:1294–1300

Sparreboom A, van Asperen J, Mayer U, Schinkel AH, Smit JW, Meijer DK, Borst P, Nooijen WJ, Beijnen JH, van Tellingen O (1997) Limited oral bioavailability and active epithelial excretion of paclitaxel (Taxol) caused by P-glycoprotein in the intestine. Proc Natl Acad Sci U S A 94:2031–2035

Synold TW, Dussault I, Forman BM (2001) The orphan nuclear receptor SXR coordinately regulates drug metabolism and efflux. Nat Med 7:584–590

Szakacs G, Annereau JP, Lababidi S, Shankavaram U, Arciello A, Bussey KJ, Reinhold W, Guo Y, Kruh GD, Reimers M, Weinstein JN, Gottesman MM (2004) Predicting drug sensitivity and resistance: profiling ABC transporter genes in cancer cells. Cancer Cell 6:129–137

Part VI
Supportive Therapy

In a broad sense, all chemotherapy is considered adjuvant. In cases where the complete resection of a tumor is the only prospect for a cure, drug therapy can play a supportive role.

- If a growth cannot be completely removed, but the tumor burden can be reduced by surgery, then adjuvant chemotherapy is suitable to clear the remaining malignant cells.
- Neo-adjuvant chemotherapy is chemotherapy administered before surgery to reduce the tumor burden and facilitate the prospects for complete resection.

In a restricted sense, adjuvant therapy synergizes with the actual chemotherapy to either enhance its anti-cancer effects or protect from its adverse effects[1]. As is evidenced by their origins, the conventional cancer chemotherapies are essentially poisons. Patients receiving these agents experience severe adverse effects (toxicity), which limit the doses that can be administered, and hence limit the beneficial anti-cancer effects (efficacy). The therapeutic window is narrow. Prominent toxicities are profound myelosuppression, nausea, and vomiting. Supportive drug therapy may ameliorate those adverse effects.

---

[1] To avoid confusion, the term "supportive therapy" is used here for agents given in conjunction with or preventive of chemotherapy.

17 Protection from Adverse Effects

The often severe adverse effects of chemotherapy are problematic in 2 ways. Tolerated dose limits cause treatment of cancers at sub-efficacious doses, resulting in morbidity and mortality from the malignancies. Drug toxicity itself is associated with morbidity and mortality.

The Cancer Therapy Evaluation Program (CTEP) provides a set of criteria, used to grade toxicities and adverse events. It has been refined in the Common Toxicity Criteria for Adverse Events (CTCAE). Adverse effects of cancer chemotherapeutics are often categorized using a numerical scale of 0–5. The grade number gets higher as the severity of the adverse event/toxicity increases.

0 = no adverse event/toxicity
1 = mild
2 = moderate
3 = severe
4 = life threatening
5 = fatal

The primary treatment for drug induced adverse effects is the discontinuation of the offending agent and provision of supportive care.

Tolerated dose limits cause treatment of cancers to occur at sub-efficacious doses (morbidity and mortality from the malignancies).
Drug toxicity is associated with morbidity and mortality.

17.1 Anti-Emetics

Emesis is regulated by 2 processing centers in the hind brain, the vomiting center and the chemoreceptor trigger zone, which communicate with each other. The vomiting center receives information about irritation of the gastrointestinal tract via serotonin (5-hydroxytryptamin, 5-HT). The chemoreceptor trigger zone receives information from the inner ear via histamine and acetylcholine and information about blood chemicals via dopamine and Substance P (Fig. 17.1). Most conventional anti-cancer agents cause very severe nausea (chemotherapy induced nausea and vomiting, CINV) that, while not directly causing patient deaths, is unbearable at higher drug doses. The development of drugs to prevent nausea (the prototype of which was ondansetron) has been of important practical use (Table 17.1).

Nausea and vomiting associated with chemotherapy may occur acute (within 24 h of therapy), delayed (later than 24 h, can persist for 6–7 days), or anticipatory (conditioned by prior exposure to chemotherapy and resulting from poor emetic control during previous therapy cycles). Anti-emesis drugs are antagonists of neurotransmitter receptors, including 5-HT_3 Serotonin Receptors (drug names end on -setron), D2 Dopamine Receptors (metoclopramide, phenothiazides, butyrophenones), Glucocorticosteroid Receptors (corticosteroids), Cannabinoid Receptors (cannabinoids), GABA Receptors (lorazepam), and NK1 Receptors (aprepitant). The acute phase emesis responds to 5-HT_3 antagonists. NK1 receptor antagonists elicit anti-emetic effect in the acute and delayed phases of emesis.

- Competitive serotonin 5-HT_3 Receptor antagonists comprise the carbazole derivative -setron drugs ondansetron <Zofran>, granisetron <Kytri>, dolasetron <Anzemet>, palonosetron <Aloxi>, and the indole tropisetron <Navoban>. They are available as tablets, solutions, and for injection. Treatment with -setrons results in the suppression of chemotherapy- and radio-therapy-induced nausea and vomiting and of vomiting triggered by gastrointestinal irritants. They act on 5-HT_3 Receptors peripherally in the gastrointestinal tract as well as centrally on vagal afferents in the area postrema of the central nervous system (the chemoreceptor trigger zone for vomiting). Typical adverse effects include diarrhea or constipation, headache, and dizziness.
- Metoclopramide (4-amino-5-chloro-*N*-(2-(diethylamino) ethyl)-2-methoxybenzamide) blocks 5-HT_3 receptors as

G. F. Weber, *Molecular Therapies of Cancer*, DOI 10.1007/978-3-319-13278-5_17,

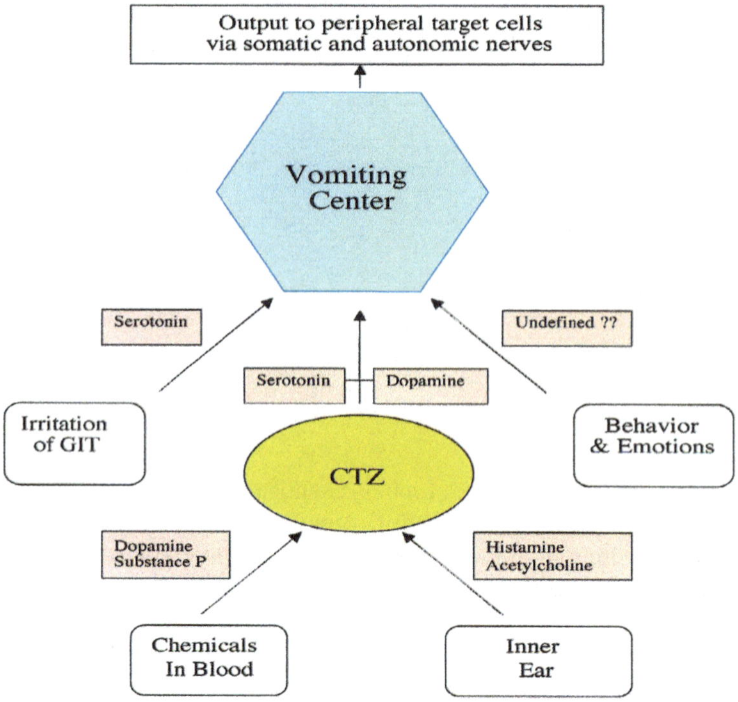

Fig. 17.1 Vomiting pathways in the central nervous system. The chemoreceptor trigger zone and the vomiting center receive input from various peripheral signals, including the gastrointestinal tract, the inner ear, the blood (chemical), and from emotional cues. They communicate via the use of neurotransmitters. These neurotransmitters and their receptors are drug targets for anti-emesis. *GIT* gastrointestinal tract, *CTZ* chemoreceptor trigger zone

Table 17.1 Antiemetic treatment guidelines. CINV, chemotherapy-induced nausea and vomiting; 5-HT3, serotonin type 3; NK-1, neurokinin-1. (adapted from Grunberg 2007)

Current treatment guidelines for prophylaxis against CINV		
Emesis risk	Acute phase (day 1)	Delayed phase (days 2–5)
High	5-HT_3 antagonist corticosteroid and NK-1 antagonist[a]	Corticosteroid and NK-1 antagonist[a]
Moderate	5-HT_3 antagonist and corticosteroid (and NK-1 antagonist)[a]	Monotherapy with 5-HT_3 antagonist or corticosteroid or metoclopramide (or corticosteroid and NK-1 antagonist)[a]
Low	Corticosteroid	None
Minimal	None	None

[a] The more recent guidelines by Multinational Association of Supportive Care in Cancer and National Comprehensive Cancer Network recommend using an NK-1 antagonist in combination with a 5-HT_3 antagonist or corticosteroid for all patients receiving highly emetogenic chemotherapy and for selected patients receiving moderately emetogenic chemotherapy

well as the Dopaminergic Receptors in the trigger zone on the floor of 4th ventricle, thus exerting anti-emetic and gastroprokinetic effects. Further, metoclopramide acts as an antagonist of muscarinic receptors and as an agonist of 5-HT_4 receptors. Common adverse drug reactions include akathisia, focal dystonia, fatigue and drowsiness. Rare but serious adverse events are agranulocytosis, supraventricular tachycardia, hyperaldosteronism, neuroleptic malignant syndrome, and tardive dyskinesia.

- Phenothiazine (dibenzothiazine, thiodiphenylamine) is a 3-ring structure compound, in which 2 benzene rings are joined by a sulfur and nitrogen atom at non-adjacent positions. Phenothiazines act as D2 Dopamine Receptor antagonists, which comprise the largest class of neuroleptic anti-psychotic drugs. Often, these agents also have anti-emetic properties. The group of -azine drugs includes prochlorperazine <Compazine> and triflupromazine <Vesprin>. They can be administered orally, by injection, or as suppositories (for cases where retention after oral administration is uncertain). The primary adverse effects are drowsiness and substantial weight gain. These drugs may also cause severe adverse effects such as akathisia (restlessness), tardive dyskinesia, extrapyramidal symptoms, and the rare but potentially fatal neuroleptic malignant syndrome.

- Butyrophenones are a class of drugs that block Dopamine Receptors and are used to treat various psychiatric disorders (such as schizophrenia), as well as acting as moderately effective anti-emetics. The butyrophenone derivative haloperidol <Haldol, Aloperidin, Duraperidol> exerts competitive blockade of postsynaptic D2 Receptors in the mesolimbic dopaminergic system. Adverse effects include dry mouth, lethargy, muscle stiffness or cramping, tremors, and weight gain. Other adverse effects may cause extrapyramidal symptoms (akinesia, akathisia). The risk of tardive dyskinesia is below 5 %.
- Corticosteroids are commonly used to control and prevent nausea and vomiting caused by chemotherapy. Dexamethasone exerts central anti-emetic effects through the action of Glucocorticosteroid Receptors in the nucleus of the solitary tract in the medulla. Methylprednisolone may also suppress the release of 5-hydroxytryptamine (5-HT). Dexamethasone and methylprednisolone are effective as mono-therapy or in combination with other anti-emetic agents.
- The CB1 cannabinoid receptors are expressed predominantly in central and peripheral neurons and receptor stimulation is implicated in the reduction of chemotherapy induced nausea. Levonantradol is a synthetic cannabinoid analog of Δ^9-tetrahydrocannabinol (Δ^9-THC). The agent may bind and activate the cannabinoid receptors CB1 or CB2 and exert anti-emetic effects. Nabilone is a synthetic cannabinoid and dibenzopyrane derivative that acts as a selective and strong agonist for the cannabinoid receptors CB1 and CB2, both of which are coupled to $G_{i/o}$ proteins.
- Lorazepam <Ativan> binds to central benzodiazepine receptors, which interact allosterically with GABA receptors. Lorazepam has the intrinsic benzodiazepine effects of anti-emesis, anxiolysis, anterograde amnesia, sedation/hypnosis, anti-convulsion, and muscle relaxation. Long-term effects of benzodiazepines include tolerance, dependence, a benzodiazepine withdrawal syndrome, and cognitive impairments.
- Aprepitant <Emend> is an antagonist of the G-Protein Coupled Receptor NK1 (Substance P, Neurokinin 1) Receptor. This receptor is located at the brain stem nuclei of the dorsal vagal complex and is a crucial regulator of vomiting. Aprepitant is used in combination with corticosteroids or -setron drugs.

Most conventional anti-cancer agents cause severe nausea and vomiting.
Chemotherapy induced nausea and vomiting may occur acute, delayed, or anticipatory.
Anti-emesis drugs are antagonists of neurotransmitter receptors, including 5-HT3 Serotonin Receptors, D2 Dopamine Receptors, Glucocorticosteroid Receptors, Cannabinoid Receptors, GABA Receptors, and NK1 Receptors.

17.2 Protection from Anemia

Factors that may cause anemia in cancer patients include the damage to hematopoiesis by chemotherapy or radiation therapy, chronic gastrointestinal blood loss, nutrient deficiency (particularly of iron or folate), bone marrow invasion by the tumor, hemolysis, or renal dysfunction. The bone marrow is critically sensitive to many anti-neoplastic agents. Conventional anti-cancer drugs kill rapidly dividing bone marrow progenitor cells, resulting in acute reversible neutropenia, thrombocytopenia, and anemia within 4–20 days. The repopulation of the marrow progenitor niche precedes the recovery of blood cell counts by several days.

Red blood cell count Anemia can lead to hypoxia, which is problematic in cancer chemotherapy. Low oxygen may promote tumor progression by inducing angiogenesis. The up-regulation of survival factors in hypoxic cancer cells may interfere with the ability of chemotherapeutics to kill them. For most effective anti-cancer treatment, the hematocrit and hemoglobin levels should be in the upper 1/3 of the normal range. Measures to normalize the blood cell count should be considered for patients not meeting this criterion. The mainstay for the acute management of chemotherapy induced anemia is red blood cell transfusions. For the long-term management, drugs are available.

Erythropoiesis stimulating agents treat chemotherapy induced anemia in patients with non-myeloid malignancies. They often improve the quality of life by increasing hemoglobin and hematocrit and decreasing transfusion requirements. Epoetin α was the first agent to be approved for this indication in 1993, followed by the approval of Darbepoetin α in 2002, while Epoetin β is available outside of the United States.

These drugs are commonly used in conjunction with iron supplementation, depending on baseline Ferritin, B12, folate, iron, and total iron binding capacity levels. Intravenous iron sucrose, ferric gluconate, or iron dextran are suitable. Intravenous iron supplementation improves the hematologic response to therapy with erythropoiesis stimulating agents, and it reduces treatment failures in patients with chemotherapy related anemia and normal iron status. Iron supplements are given intravenously rather than orally because of superior efficacy. The additional toxicity is low, however iron dextran has been associated with a higher rate of adverse events.

Adverse Effects Adverse effects related to erythropoietic products are generally mild and include pain at the injection site, rash, influenza-like symptoms, and hypertension (very rarely resulting in hypertensive encephalopathy). However, a serious adverse effect of the erythropoiesis stimulating agents is venous thrombembolism and possibly resulting mortality (Bennett et al. 2008). Pure red cell aplasia is possible. According to the U.S. FDA, patients may only receive Erythropoiesis stimulating agents when their Hemoglobin level is below 10 g/dl. These agents are not indicated for patients when the anticipated outcome of their cancer treatment is cure. Blood transfusion are preferred in cancer patients with a reasonably long life expectancy. This is due to a higher rate of death in patients with breast cancer and head and neck cancer, who received an Erythropoiesis stimulating agent as compared to patients who did not (Henke et al. 2003; Leyland-Jones 2003).

Erythropoietin (EPO) is a glycoprotein cytokine that acts on precursor cells to stimulate erythropoiesis. The molecule exerts additional actions including vasoconstriction-dependent hypertension, angiogenesis, and the induction of neuronal protection during hypoxic conditions. It is primarily produced in response to hypoxia by cells of the peritubular capillary endothelium of the kidneys. Circulating Erythropoietin binds to its cognate receptors on the surface of committed erythroid progenitors in the bone marrow, resulting in their reduplication and maturation into functional erythrocytes.

- Recombinant Erythropoietin has a variety of glycosylation patterns giving rise to the forms α, β, δ, and ω. The substitutions affect the half-lives. Epoetin α <Procrit, Epogen> is a recombinant therapeutic agent that is almost identical to the endogenous cytokine Erythropoietin. It is typically started at 40,000 units once each week.
- Epoetin β <NeoRecormon> is a synthetic recombinant form of Erythropoietin that is marketed in Europe.
- Methoxy polyethylene glycol Epoetin β <Mircera> is a PEGylated form of recombinant human Erythropoietin with long-acting Erythropoietin Receptor activating properties.
- Darbepoetin α <Aranesp, Cresp> is a recombinant analog of the endogenous cytokine Erythropoietin. Similar to Erythropoietin, darbepoietin α binds to and activates Epoetin Receptors, thereby inducing the differentiation and maturation of erythrocyte progenitors and supporting endothelial cell proliferation. It also stimulates B-lymphocyte proliferation and Immunoglobulin production. Darbepoetin α is given at a dose of 200 μg every other week or 500 μg every 3 weeks. The agent was approved by the European EMA for cancer applications in 2001. Due to possessing 2 *N*-linked oligosaccharide chains in addition to the endogenous cytokine (substitutions at N57, T59, V114, N115, and T117), darbepoetin α exhibits a 3-fold longer half-life compared to Erythropoietin (which has a half-life of 5 h).

Nandrolone decanoate is a salt form of an anabolic steroid analog of testosterone. It has androgenic, anabolic, and Erythropoietin stimulating effects. Responsive tissues include the prostate, seminal vesicles, scrotum, penis, larynx, hair follicles, muscle, and bone. Upon entering its target cells, nandrolone binds to and activates specific Androgen Receptors. The resulting activated hormone receptor complex translocates into the nucleus and binds to androgen response elements in the promoter regions of targeted genes, where it supports a gene expression pattern necessary for maintaining male sex characteristics. Mimicking the negative feedback mechanism of testosterone, nandrolone decanoate also suppresses the secretion of Luteinizing Hormone (LH). Furthermore, this agent also stimulates Erythropoietin expression by enhancing the production of erythropoiesis stimulating factors.

Platelet count The normal value for blood platelets ranges from 150,000 to 400,000 per μl (mm^3). Thrombocytopenia is diagnosed at a value below 20,000/μl. It can result in bleeding from the nose, gums, urinary tract, or gastrointestinal tract. The usual time for a low platelet count to occur is 10–21 days after the initiation of chemotherapy. In order to reduce the risk of bleeding during anti-cancer drug treatment it is important to avoid drugs that can affect platelet function, such as salicylic acid <Aspirin>, ibuprofen <Advil>, naprosyn <Aleve>.

Platelet transfusions are the mainstay of management. They are mostly reserved for patients with a platelet count below 10,000 cells/μl, unless they are actively bleeding, must undergo a surgical procedure, or have documented infections or fever, in which case the threshold is higher.

In patients who have a low trend to thrombocytopenia, the recombinant Interleukin-11 (IL-11) preparation oprelvekin <Neumega> may prevent a further decline in the platelet counts. It may serve as secondary prophylaxis in patients with non-myeloid malignancies, who have experienced significant thrombocytopenia with a prior cycle of chemotherapy. Oprelvekin is not glycosylated and lacks the amino-terminal proline. Adults without severe renal impairment are given 50 μg/kg subcutaneously once daily.

Adverse Effects Interleukin-11 is associated with substantial adverse effects, mostly related to fluid retention (edema, dilutional anemia, dyspnea, pleural effusions). Cardiac toxicity, especially tachycardia and atrial fibrillation, can arise. The most frequent serious adverse events are neutropenic fever, syncope, and pneumonia. The drug can cause allergic or hypersensitivity reactions, including anaphylaxis, and should be permanently discontinued in affected patients. Oprelvekin is not indicated following myeloablative chemotherapy, due to low efficacy and increased toxicity.

Thrombopoietin (TPO, THPO, Megakaryocyte Growth and Development Factor, MGDF) is a glycoprotein hormone produced mainly by the liver and the kidneys. It stimulates the production and differentiation of the megakaryocyte

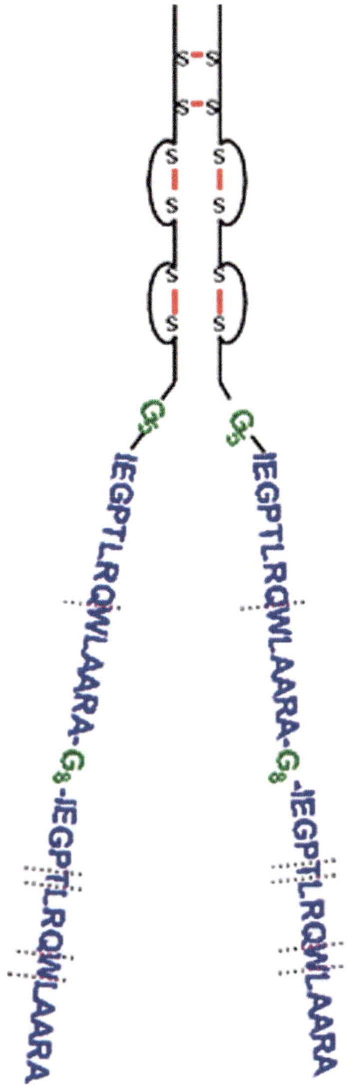

Fig. 17.2 Structure of romiplostim. Fc region is shown in black, TMP regions in *blue*, linkers in *green*, and disulfide bridges in *red*. Proteolytic points are noted by hashed lines. (Hall et al. 2010)

precursors to thrombocytes. Mimetics that stimulate the Thrombopoietin Receptor (cMPL) are treatment options for thrombocytopenia.

- Romiplostim (AMG531) <Nplate>is a peptibody molecule that contains 2 identical single-chain human IgG_1 Fc subunits, covalently linked at their carboxyl-terminus to a peptide containing 2 Thrombopoietin Receptor binding domains (Fig. 17.2). While the bacterial recombinant romiplostim molecule has no amino acid sequence homology to endogenous Thrombopoietin, it activates signaling pathways that lead to increased platelet production. Serious adverse reactions are bone marrow Reticulin deposition and worsening thrombocytopenia after romiplostim discontinuation. Common adverse effects entail pain in the extremities or shoulders (25 %), arthralgia (25 %), myalgia (15 %), dizziness (15 %), insomnia (15 %), abdominal pain (10 %), dyspepsia (5 %), and paresthesia (5 %). As a protein drug, romiplostim may be immunogenic. The drug is Pregnancy Category C.
- Eltrombopag olamine (SB-497115-GR) <Promacta, Revolade> is a small molecule Thrombopoietin Receptor agonist for oral administration. The agent interacts with the transmembrane domain of the Thrombopoietin Receptor leading to increased platelet production. Eltrombopag may cause hepatotoxicity.

Conventional anti-cancer drugs kill rapidly dividing bone marrow progenitor cells, resulting in acute reversible neutropenia, thrombocytopenia, and anemia.
The repopulation of the marrow progenitor niche precedes the recovery of blood cell counts by several days.
Blood transfusions or growth factors may aid the reversal of anemia.

17.3 Immune Recovery

Myelosuppression is the most common dose limiting adverse effect of cytotoxic agents. In the process of destroying cancer cells, conventional chemotherapy can also cause damage to other rapidly dividing cells, such as the cells of the bone marrow. White blood cells, especially neutrophil precursors, are most significantly affected because of their high proliferation rate and short life span of 8–24 h. Platelets (5–10 day life span) are affected to a much lower extent than neutrophils. Erythrocytes, with a 120 day life span, are compromised the least. Myelosuppression may be evidenced according to

- the total number of white blood cells below 3,000/μl
- the absolute neutrophil count below 1,500/μl.

Bone marrow suppression does not usually arise immediately after chemotherapy administration. Usual nadirs (lowest blood cell counts) occur at 10–14 days following chemotherapy administration. Because of their short life span white blood cells are affected particularly rapidly, reaching their nadir 10–14 days after the completion of a treatment cycle. This leads to an increased risk of infections. Recovery typically takes 3–4 weeks, but there is variation.

- The nitrosoureas, mitomycin C, gemtuzumab, and radiolabeled antibodies exhibit a delayed pattern of nadir (4–6 weeks) and recovery (6–8 weeks).
- Patients with leukemia or receiving a stem cell transplant may have a more rapid nadir of about 5–7 days.
- Patients who have received multiple prior courses of other myelotoxic chemotherapy regimens or extensive radiation therapy, especially to the pelvis, may have a decreased bone marrow reserve. They are more sensitive to the myelosuppressive effects of chemotherapy, and normal doses may produce profound marrow toxicity (DiPiro et al. 2008).

The risk of infection is directly proportional to the duration and severity of neutropenia. Usual signs and symptoms of infection, such as pus, abscesses, and infiltrates on chest radiography, are often absent as a result of the lack of white blood cells. Due to the risk of sepsis in neutropenia, the basic approach to the management of febrile neutropenic cancer patients is the prompt initiation of empiric antibiotics, which are chosen based on reliable coverage of the most likely organisms, antibiotic sensitivities at the institution, and the patient's symptoms.

Growth factors Colony stimulating factors (CSFs) are naturally occurring proteins, which are essential for the normal growth and maturation of various blood cell types. In cases where the recovery from chemotherapy induced myelosuppression is too slow, it may be necessary to delay the next cycle and administer colony stimulating factors to support hematopoiesis and prevent infections. By mimicking endogenous hormones, these factors reduce the incidence, magnitude, and duration of neutropenia. The therapeutic effects are accompanied by a modest decrease in febrile days, infections, days on antibiotics, and may result in a decreased incidence of mucositis.

Colony stimulating factors for treatment are produced by recombinant DNA technology in bacteria, yeast, or mammalian cells. The differences in posttranslational modifications among various source cells do not result in clinically discernible effects on neutrophil production. These growth factors may be used in either primary or secondary prophylaxis of neutropenia.

- Primary prophylaxis refers to the use of colony stimulating factors to prevent neutropenia with the first cycle of chemotherapy.
- Secondary prophylaxis refers to the use of growth factors to prevent recurrent neutropenia in patients who have experienced neutropenia with the prior cycle of chemotherapy. It is recommended that secondary prophylaxis be reserved for patients with chemosensitive cancers, where dose reduction may affect disease free or overall survival.
- The role of colony stimulating factors in the treatment of established neutropenia is not well defined. There may be only minimal clinical benefit from their use in treating neutropenia. Therefore, these agents should not be routinely employed in patients with established neutropenia, regardless of the presence of fever (DiPiro et al. 2008).

Adverse Effects The most common toxicity of the colony stimulating factors is bone pain (20–25 %), usually in the sternum or hips. Patients experiencing bone pain may take acetaminophen or a non-steroidal analgesic to ease the symptoms. Additional adverse effects include low grade fever, myalgia, arthralgia, lethargy, and mild headache. At higher doses, pleural and pericardial effusions, capillary leak syndrome, and thrombus formation can occur. Liver function may be compromised. A first-dose reaction, consisting of dyspnea, facial flushing, hypotension, hypoxia, and tachycardia, may arise especially after intravenous infusion of bacterial GM-CSF (Granulocyte-Macrophage Colony Stimulating Factor). Growth factors should not be used in patients receiving concomitant chemotherapy or radio-therapy, especially if the radiation involves the mediastinum. These patients are at risk to experience more significant thrombocytopenia when administered colony stimulating factors.

- The recombinant GM-CSFs sargramostim <Leukine> and molgramostim promote the proliferation of granulocytes (neutrophils and eosinophils) and monocytes/macrophages. The agents are administered subcutaneously or intravenously for 14 days at 250 μg/m^2.
- The recombinant G-CSFs (Granulocyte Colony Stimulating Factors) filgrastim <Neupogen, Grafeel, Neugraf, Neukine>, tbo-filgastim (non-glycosylated methionyl G-CSF) <Granix>, and lenograstim <Euprotin, Granocyte, Lenobio, Neutrogin> specifically stimulate the production of neutrophilic granulocytes. G-CSF is given at 5 μg/kg/day until the absolute neutrophil count reaches 10,000/μl (or as long as it is clinically safe). Subcutaneous injection is the most effective route. It is started 24–72 h after chemotherapy and stopped the day before the next cycle. The half-life of filgrastim is 3–4 h.
- A single dose of the polyethylene glycol conjugated, long-acting G-CSF pegfilgrastim <Neulasta, Neulastim> has a half-life of 15–80 h. The effects it provides are equivalent to 10–11 days of daily G-CSF, with a similar adverse event profile. Pegfilgrastim is administered at 6 mg as a single dose. It needs to be stopped within 14 days of the next chemotherapy dose.

Thymopentin is a synthetic pentapeptide (L-arginyl-L-lysyl-L-α-aspartyl-L-valyl-L-tyrosine) that covers the active site of the naturally occurring hormone Thymopoietin. Thymopentin enhances the production of thymic T-lymphocytes and may help restore immunocompetence in immunosuppressed subjects. This agent also augments the effects of ionizing radiation by arresting cancer cells in the G_2/M phase of the cell cycle.

Bone marrow transplantation The myelotoxicity of conventional chemotherapy is dose limiting. It is possible to apply very high doses of chemotherapy if the patient's bone marrow is first harvested, the chemotherapy administered, and the harvested marrow then returned to the patient a few days later. This approach of autologous bone marrow transplantation was devised to be beneficial to a wide group of patients. However, it has failed to convey this benefit for solid tumors, and therefore autologous transplantation is no longer widely used. The curative benefits of high doses of chemotherapy afforded by autologous bone marrow rescue are limited to patients with hematologic malignancies, who have failed treatment with conventional combination chemotherapy.

Colony stimulating growth factors may accelerate hematopoietic engraftment and treat graft failure following hematopoietic stem cell transplantation. They initially enhance demargination and mobilization of mature cells from the marrow and then provide constant stimulation of stem cell progenitors.

Hypersensitivity prophylaxis The immune system can respond to chemotherapy treatment with a hypersensitivity reaction (allergy, anaphylaxis) that results in local or systemic tissue injury. It may manifest in shortness of breath, wheezing, closing up of the throat, swelling of facial features, itching, or hives. Immediate discontinuation of the drug is a mandatory first response. Treatment comprises anti-histamines of the group of H_1 Receptor blockers (diphenhydramine <Benadryl>, hydroxyzine, cyproheptadine), corticosteroids (beclomethasone <Beclovent>, methylprednisolone <Solumedrol>), and bronchodilators (albuterol <Proventil>, or terbutaline <Brethine>).

Myelosuppression is the most common dose limiting adverse effect of cytotoxic agents.
The risk of infection is directly proportional to the duration and severity of the neutropenia.
Colony stimulating factors may aid the recovery from chemotherapy induced myelosuppression.
Bone marrow transplantation is a strategy to be considered in some cases.

17.4 Cardiovascular Protection

Cardiotoxicity can be caused by chemotherapy treatment. Cardiac events induced by anti-cancer agents may include cardiomyopathy and congestive heart failure, myocardial infarction, arrhythmias (supra-ventricular tachyarrhythmias, atrial and ventricular ectopy, ventricular tachycardias), myocarditis or pericarditis. They can develop in an acute, subacute, or chronic manner.

- Anthracyclines (including doxorubicin) can generate congestive heart failure and left ventricular dysfunction in a dose and schedule dependent manner. The risk is increased after mediastinal X-ray therapy or when anthracycline chemotherapy is administered concurrently or before adjuvant treatment with trastuzumab.
- The anthraquinone mitoxantrone induces acute myocarditis and arrhythmia during infusion.
- Anti-metabolite agents, such as capecitabine or cytarabine, can induce ischemia, pericarditis, congestive heart failure, and cardiogenic shock. Dose dependent cardiotoxicity can be induced by fluoropyrimidines (5-fluorouracil) and become manifest in myocardial ischemia.
- Microtubule disturbing drugs (paclitaxel, vinca alkaloids) can cause sinus bradycardia, atrioventricular block, ventricular tachycardia, hypotension, congestive heart failure, or ischemia.
- Heart failure that occurs after high dose cyclophosphamide or ifosfamide treatment is manifested by neuro-humoral activation without concomitant cardiomyocyte necrosis. Mild functional mitral regurgitation may also develop.

- Various anti-cancer drugs prolong the QT interval, including eribulin, small molecule kinase inhibitors (nilotinib, dasatinib, tozasertib, sorafenib, vemurafenib, AT7519, vandetanib, cizotinib, BMS-641988), and abarelix[1].

Damage to the circulation may manifest in thrombosis and embolism, hypo- or hypertension.

Cardiomyopathy and heart failure Cardiotoxicity is the occurrence of heart muscle damage under chemotherapy. The heart becomes weaker and less efficient in pumping the circulating blood. One treatment strategy for preventing left ventricular dysfunction associated with cancer therapy is the co-administration of standard heart failure medications. This approach focusses on neuro-hormonal antagonism (including β-blockers, Angiotensin Converting Enzyme inhibitors, Angiotensin II Receptor blockers, aldosterone antagonists). Cardiac transplantation is an option in patients with cancer treatment induced end-stage heart disease.

Doxorubicin has adverse cardiac effects, which can lead to dilated cardiomyopathy and congestive heart failure. The risk is increased at a total cumulative dose above 450 mg/m^2. It may be ameliorated if the drug is administered in a liposomal formulation. Also, treatment or prevention of cardiotoxicity may be possible with combination therapy, consisting of cardiac glycosides (digoxin), β-blockers, diuretics, and afterload reduction (Angiotensin Converting Enzyme inhibitors).

- Cardiac glycosides increase the force of heart contractions, which can be beneficial in congestive heart failure and for irregular heart beats. In the treatment of doxorubicin induced cardiomyopathy and congestive heart failure, the efficacy of digoxin is temporary.
- β-Blockers (such as metoprolol, bucindolol, labetalol, and practolol) have some success in children with systolic dysfunction. Carvedilol is a unique β-blocker in that it produces a non-selective β-Receptor and α_1 Receptor blockade, as well as exerts an anti-oxidant effect. Carvedilol reduces the risk of progression and death for cardiac causes in adult patients with congestive heart failure.
- Diuretics reduce the burden on the heart action by lowering the total volume of the blood. They comprise Carbonic Anhydrase inhibitors, thiazides, loop diuretics, aldosterone antagonists, and potassium sparing diuretics.
- ACE (Angiotensin-Converting Enzyme) inhibitors, such as enalapril <Vasotec, Enaladex> and captopril <Capoten>, may be indicated in patients with elevated afterload and asymptomatic left ventricular dysfunction. However, the enalapril induced improvement in left ventricular structure and function is transient and prone to inexorable deterioration, likely because the short term improvement is related to lowered diastolic blood pressure rather than to inhibited myocardium remodeling (Minotti et al. 2004).
- The Topoisomerase 2-inactive bisdioxopiperazine[2] ICRF-161 is a protective agent against doxorubicin induced cardiomyopathy. In patients under doxorubicin treatment, dexrazoxane hydrochloride ((*S*)-4,4′-(1-methyl-1,2-ethanediyl)bis-2,6piperazinedione) (ICRF-187) <Zinecard, Totect> limits the mean decrease from baseline in left ventricular ejection function (LVEF) and lowers the incidence of congestive heart failure. As a derivative of EDTA, dexrazoxane readily penetrates cell membranes. It chelates iron and reduces the iron catalyzed production of reactive oxygen species. The appropriate dose of dexrazoxane is dependent on the dose of doxorubicin used in chemotherapy. Equilibrium is reached within 2–4 h after injection. The drug is not bound to plasma proteins. Urinary excretion plays an important role in the elimination of dexrazoxane, accounting for about 40 % of the administered dose. Drug clearance is reduced in patients with renal dysfunction. As hyper-bilirubinemia requires a doxorubicin dose reduction, the dexrazoxane dosage is to be proportionately reduced in patients with hepatic impairment (maintaining a 10:1 ratio). Dexrazoxane may add to the myelosuppression caused by chemotherapeutic agents (likely due to the inhibition of Topoisomerase 2). The use of dexrazoxane concurrently with FAC (fluorouracil, doxorubicin <Adriamycin PFS>, cyclophosphamide) therapy interferes with the anti-tumor efficacy of the regimen, and is not recommended.

Pericarditis Pericarditis in cancer patients can be caused by the malignancy (often lymphomata or lung cancers; malignant pericardial effusions occur in up to 20 % of cancer patients), by radiation therapy of the chest, or by drugs. Pericarditis causes chest tightness, sharp or burning chest pain that may radiate, sweating, dizziness, and fatigue. Pericardial effusions are often a pre-terminal event.

[1] The QT interval describes the time between the start of the Q wave and the end of the T wave in the electrical cycle of the heart beat. It represents the electrical depolarization and repolarization of the ventricles. In long QT syndrome, delayed repolarization of the heart following a beat increases the risk of ventricular tachyarrhythmias. Such episodes may lead to fainting and sudden death.

[2] Bisdioxopiperazines, such as ICRF-159 and ICRF-193, are under study as inhibitors of DNA Topoisomerase 2 (see Sect. 2.3.2.). However, not all compounds in the class of bisdioxopiperazienes have this activity.

- Non-steroidal anti-inflammatory drugs (NSAIDs) are given to decrease the inflammation in the lining of the heart, and to provide comfort. Specifically salicylate <Aspirin> may also act as blood thinner. Ibuprofen is a drug of choice as it acts as an anti-inflammatory and as an analgesic (however, ibuprofen is contraindicated for heart attacks with pericarditis because it may interfere with cardiac healing). If NSAID agents are incompatible with the chemotherapy administered, acetaminophen <Tylenol> up to 3000 mg per day may help.
- Antibiotics are indicated if a bacterial origin of the pericarditis is likely.
- ACE inhibitors (enalapril maleate <Vasotec, Enaladex>, fosinopril sodium <Monopril>, captopril <Capoten>, lisinopril <Zestril>) work by dilating the arteries. They lower the blood pressure and improve the blood flow to the kidneys, thus lessening the symptoms.
- β-blockers (metoprolol <Lopressor>, propranolol <Inderal>, atenolol <Tenormin>) can be used to slow down the heart rate and improve the blood flow through the body, thus lessening the symptoms of pericarditis. This is of particular benefit if there is arrhythmia or high blood pressure.
- Calcium channel blockers (verapamil <Calan>, diltiazem <Dilacor XR>) may be given to treat chest pain, high blood pressure, or irregular heart beats.

Thrombosis Cancer patients are 6 times more likely to develop venous thromboembolism than the healthy population, with specific cancers (ovarian, brain, and pancreatic cancers) and advanced stages (metastatic disease) being more prone to this condition than others. A tumor may compress or invade adjacent vessels, resulting in blood stasis. Hypercoagulability may be triggered by phlebitis (secondary to vascular wall damage) or circulatory stasis (reduced or altered blood flow). Tumors that produce Thrombin or elevate the levels of Factor VIII or Fibrinogen are at high risk for thromboembolism. Further, age, surgery, central line placement, immobilization, dehydration, and comorbid conditions may also predispose to thrombotic complications in patients with cancer. Anti-cancer drugs may be a factor:

- Life-threatening hemorrhage and arterial thromboembolism can arise in patients being treated with broad-spectrum angiogenesis inhibitors, such as bevacizumab or thalidomide derivatives.
- The alkylating agent cisplatin can trigger platelets to aggregate, enhance thromboxane formation, and activate arachidonate pathways.
- The risk of hemorrhage and thromboembolisms increases with the use of drugs that modify the expression pattern of adhesion molecules, such as Integrins and Cadherins, on endothelial cells. Doxycycline targets the adherens junction in vascular endothelial cells by inducing the expression and suppressing the phosphorylation of vascular endothelial Cadherins.

A thrombus can occur in any vein of the body, but usually forms in the lower limbs. Thrombi of the larger veins above the knee often break off to form pulmonary embolism (more than 95 % of emboli originate as thrombi in the deep veins of the lower limbs). Thromboembolism may also become manifest as Trousseau syndrome (chronic disseminated intravascular coagulopathy associated with microangiopathy, verrucous endocarditis, and arterial emboli in patients with cancer), Budd-Chiari syndrome (hepatic vein obstruction), or portal vein thrombosis. It is a leading cause for mortality in cancer patients, making it appropriate to initiate anticoagulant therapy for prevention. Classes of drugs used in the prevention and treatment of thromboembolism comprise anti-coagulants, anti-platelet agents, and thrombolytic drugs (Pruemer 2006).

- Vitamin K antagonists (the 4-hydroxycoumarin warfarin <Coumadin, Jantoven, Marevan, Lawarin, Waran, Warfant>, the aromatic trans-fixed β-diketone fluindione) can be given orally and do not require dose adjustment in renal impairment. Warfarin is a standard treatment for long-term prophylaxis, however, the narrow therapeutic range poses dosing challenges.
- Platelet inhibitors (aspirin, clopidogrel bisulfide <Plavix>) are usually administered for the relatively specific prophylaxis against arterial thrombosis, myocardial infarction, and stroke.
- Unfractionated heparin is a glycosaminoglycan consisting of a heterogeneous mix of polysaccharide chains that vary in molecular weight[3]. The initial prophylactic dose is 5,000 units every 8–12 h.
- Low molecular weight heparins (LMWH, drug names end on -parin), including nandroparin, enoxaparin (1.5 mg/kg/day), dalteparin (initially at 200 U/kg/day, maintenance 150 U/kg/day), and tinzaparin, preferentially inhibit Factor Xa. They do not require extensive monitoring because of greater bioavailability, longer half-life, lower protein binding, and primarily non-saturable renal elimination of low molecular weight heparins compared to unfractionated heparin. This results in more consistent anti-coagulation and makes standardized 1–2 daily subcutaneous administrations possible.

[3] Any penta-saccharide containing a heparin chain can inhibit the action of Factor Xa by binding to Antithrombin and causing a conformational change. In contrast, to inactivate Thrombin, heparin must form a ternary complex with Antithrombin and Thrombin, which requires at least 18 saccharide units. Whereas most of the chains of unfractionated heparin are at least 18 saccharide units long, in low molecular weight heparins fewer than half of those are of sufficient length.

- Factor Xa antagonists, including fondaparinux <Arixtra> and apixaban <Eliquis>, compare to heparin in effectiveness.

The use of low molecular weight heparin is recommended (by the American Society for Clinical Oncology, ASCO, in 2007) for the initial treatment of venous thromboembolism for 5–10 days, followed by anti-coagulant protection for at least 6 months. After 6 months, indefinite anti-coagulation should be considered in high risk patients. Inferior vena cava filters are reserved for patients with contraindications for anti-coagulation and for patients who had pulmonary embolism despite adequate long-term low molecular weight heparin.

Adverse Effects The primary adverse effect of anti-coagulant therapy is the risk of bleeding. Heparin induced thrombocytopenia is characterized by a drop in platelet count below 150,000/μL or by a more than 50 % reduction from the baseline platelet count. It occurs in 1–5 % of patients receiving heparin for at least 1 week.

Drug Resistance Neither low dose warfarin nor aspirin can prevent thromboembolic events in patients treated with thalidomide plus steroids or plus chemotherapy.

Leucostasis is associated with acute and chronic myeloid leukemias. It causes hyper-viscosity of the blood with capillary plugging, circulatory stagnation, and subsequent blood vessel rupture. Disseminated intravascular coagulation can also arise, resulting in a widespread formation of thrombi in the micro-circulation, which may cause ischemic damage and necrosis. The incidence is up to 10 % of cancer patients. In severe cases, it may result in uncontrollable hemorrhage due to the consumption of clotting factors.

Plasmin is produced by the liver in the inactive pro-form Plasminogen. Tissue Plasminogen Activator (tPA) and Urokinase convert Plasminogen to the active Plasmin, thus allowing fibrinolysis to occur. Many cancer patients before surgery or chemotherapy display excess fibrinolysis, which warrants correction with appropriate administration of 6-aminocaproic acid (ε-aminocaproic acid, 6-aminohexanoic acid) <Amicar>(Knock 1967).

Hypertension High blood pressure is the most common comorbid condition in cancer patients. Some tumors cause inessential hypertension via an ectopic secretion of hormones that are involved in the control of blood pressure. Surgery or radiation therapy that involves the head or neck can lead to baroreflex failure and to associated difficult-to-treat labile hypertension and hypertensive crisis. As symptoms occur late, hypertension is widely undertreated. The main complications include vision impairment, stroke, myocardial infarction, blood vessel damage, and kidney failure. Anti-hypertensive agents regulate the blood volume (diuretics), the blood vessel tone (ACE inhibitors, ACE Receptor blockers, β-blockers, calcium channel blockers), or the heart action (channel blockers, β-blockers, nitrates, glycosides).

An adverse effect of treatment with anti-angiogenic agents (bevacizumab), alkylating agents (cisplatin), or kinase inhibitors (sorafenib, sunitinib, pazopanib) is the exacerbation of hypertension, with potentially acute or long-term health effects. Hypertension may be caused by anti-angiogenesis agents that inhibit Vascular Endothelial Growth Factor (VEGF) through decreased Nitric Oxide Synthase activity and consequently reduced nitric oxide (NO) production. As nitric oxide is a natural vasodilator, its blocked production in the walls of arterioles and other resistance vessels promotes vasoconstriction, increases the peripheral vascular resistance, and raises the blood pressure. Also, the decreased endothelial Nitric Oxide Synthase activity may stimulate Plasminogen Activator Inhibitor-1 (PAI-1) expression, which results in an increased risk of hypertension. Furthermore, endothelial dysfunction can be associated with increased vascular and renal Endothelin production.

17-Spironolactone is a synthetic corticosteroid with anti-hypertensive, potassium sparing diuretic, and anti-androgen activities. Spironolactone competitively inhibits the activity of aldosterone in the distal renal tubules, the myocardium, and the vasculature. This agent may inhibit the pathophysiological effects of aldosterone, produced in excess by various types of malignant and benign tumors, thus aiding in maintaining a low blood pressure.

Cardiotoxicity can be caused by chemotherapy treatment. It may manifest in cardiomyopathy, myocardial infarction, arrhythmias, or carditis.
Damage to the circulation may manifest in thromboembolism, hypo- or hypertension.

17.5 Anti-Oxidants

Free radicals are chemically very reactive molecules as they have unpaired electrons in their outer shells. Because of the nature of oxygen as a biradical and the human dependence on this molecule, the most common forms of free radicals originate from oxygen. Oxidative metabolism, exposure to various environmental factors, or anti-cancer drugs can lead to reactive oxygen intermediates and oxygen derived free radicals, which cause damage to biomolecules, including DNA. Such damage may become irreversible and lead to cell death or cell transformation.

Anti-oxidants neutralize the electrical charges of free radicals, prevent them from taking up electrons from other molecules, and thus protect from damage to the cells. The use of anti-oxidants in cancer chemotherapy needs to be weighed carefully as free radical damage to the transformed cells is often part of the therapeutic action, while free radical damage to the untransformed host cells leads to potentially serious adverse effects.

Anthracyclines induce cardiotoxicity via free radical injury to cardiac myocytes. Dexrazoxane hydrochloride (ICRF-187) <Zinecard, Totect> is the hydrochloride salt of a bisdioxopiperazine, which possesses cardioprotective activities. After hydrolysis by Dihydropyrimidine Aminohydrolase to an active form that is similar to ethylenediaminetetraacetate (EDTA), dexrazoxane chelates iron, thereby preventing the metal-catalyzed formation of reactive oxygen radicals induced by anthracycline antibiotics.

Adverse Effects Dexrazoxane may potentiate hematologic toxicity induced by chemotherapy or radiation.

Dimesna and mesna detoxify through their thiol groups. Both are very hydrophilic. They do not leave the vascular compartment and are excreted by the kidneys, where they exert their anti-oxidant protective actions.

- Dimesna <Tavocept> is a synthetic derivative of dithioethane sulfonate. Its anti-oxidant properties can be uroprotective when used with ifosfamide. In the kidney, dimesna undergoes reduction to the free thiol compound, mesna, which reacts chemically with the urotoxic ifosfamide metabolites acrolein and 4-hydroxy-ifosfamide, resulting in their detoxification. This agent also inhibits cyclophosphamide induced hemorrhagic cystitis, and it may alleviate cisplatin nephrotoxicity.
- Mesna (sodium-2-mercaptoethane sulfonate) <Uromexitan, Mesnex> protects bladder and kidneys from the toxic effects of oxazaphosphorines (cyclophosphamide, ifosfamide, or trofosfamide).

The water soluble organic triphosphate thiol prodrug, amifostine (WR-2721) <Ethyol> can act as an anti-oxidant. It decreases the cumulative nephrotoxicity by cisplatin. Amifostine is dephosphorylated by Alkaline Phosphatase in various tissues to the pharmacologically active free thiol, which readily scavenges reactive oxygen species.

N-acetyl-*L*-cysteine (NAC) <Assist, Parvolex, Acetadote> is a thiol and a precursor building block for the intracellular tripeptide Glutathione (glutamyl-cysteinyl-glycine). *N*-acetyl-*L*-cysteine is broadly effective as an anti-oxidant, and is therefore widely used as a nutrition supplement. The agent may ameliorate the adverse effects of ifosfamide, but likely not of doxorubicin.

- RK-0202 is an oral polymer matrix based rinse formulation that contains *N*-acetyl-*L*-cysteine, an anti-oxidant amino acid derivative with anti-inflammatory properties. RK-0202 may alleviate the symptoms of radiation induced oral mucositis.
- *N*-acetyl-*L*-cysteine <Fluimucil, Mucomyst, Mucosil> is inhaled for mucolytic therapy or ingested for nephroprotection.

Adverse Effects *N*-acetyl-*L*-cysteine may induce nausea and vomiting, diarrhea or constipation. Rarely, it can cause rashes, fever, headache, drowsiness, low blood pressure, or liver impairments. When inhaled, it may cause swelling in the mouth, runny nose, drowsiness, and chest tightness. *N*-acetyl-*L*-cysteine is metabolized to S-nitroso-*N*-acetylcysteine (SNOAC), which at very high doses leads to pulmonary artery hypertension. There is a concern that *N*-acetyl-*L*-cysteine might cause bronchospasm in people with asthma if inhaled or taken orally.

The over-production and resulting destructive effect of superoxide is a basic characteristic of carcinogenic DNA damage. The metalloenzyme Superoxide Dismutase (SOD) catalyzes the disproportionation of the cytotoxic superoxide radical to oxygen and hydrogen peroxide. It plays a crucial role in the protection of cells against the damage caused by the reactive oxygen species. There are 2 forms of Superoxide Dismutase, characterized by either manganese or zinc and copper in the catalytic center. The important role of this enzyme in organism protection has made it a model compound for the design of low molecular antioxidants on the basis of copper or manganese complexes mimicking the active site of the metalloenzyme, thus achieving Superoxide Dismutase like activity.

- The conjugate ethylenediaminetetraacetic acid bis-(5-aminosalicylic acid methyl ester) (EBAME) chelates copper^{2+} or manganese^{2+} ions in a 1:1 ratio, and achieves Superoxide dismutase activity.
- Kinetin (N^6-furfuryladenine) is a naturally occurring phytohormone in the family of Cytokinins. Kinetin can act both as an inhibitor of radical oxygen species formation and as a scavenger. Copper^{2+} chlorido complexes involving kinetin as a ligand can exhibit high Superoxide Dismutase mimic activity based on the possible synergic effect of the ligand and redox active copper centers.
- Copper complexes involving methoxy-benzyl derived N^6-benzyladenines have potential as anti-oxidant drug candidates.
- Manganese porphyrins, such as Mn^{3+} meso-tetrakis(*N*-*n*-butoxyethylpyridinium-2-yl)porphyrin, mimic the mitochondrial Superoxide Dismutase (MnSOD). Their lipophilicity can be optimized. However, when used at high single or cumulative doses they become toxic, in

part due to their micellar properties (caused by the presence of polar cationic nitrogens and hydrophobic alkyl chains). The replacement of a CH_2 group by an oxygen atom in each of the 4 alkyl chains disrupts the porphyrin micellar character. The modifying oxygens become heavily solvated, which leads to a significant drop in the lipophilicity of porphyrin. However, when the oxygen atoms are buried deeper within the long heptyl chains, their excessive solvation is precluded and the lipophilicity preserved. Porphyrin complexes can act as DNA intercalators, and can display phototoxicity or hepatotoxicity.

- A group of manganese complexes that can act as SOD mimics contain salen-type ligands. These ligands are obtained from the condensation reactions of a hydroxybenzaldehyde and 1,2-diamino ethane to produce a tetradentate proligand, which forms a complex containing the manganese.
- Polyaza-macrocyclic manganese^{2+} complexes contain 7-coordinate manganese with a trans arrangement of the Cl^- ligands. They may have SOD activity.

Silymarin is a mixture of flavonolignans (including silibinin, isosilibinin, silicristin, silidianin) extracted from the milk thistle plant Silybum marianum. Silymarin may act as an anti-oxidant, protecting hepatic cells from chemotherapy related free radical damage. This agent may also support the growth of new hepatic cells.

Free radicals are chemically very reactive due to unpaired electrons in their outer shells.
Reactive oxygen intermediates and oxygen derived free radicals cause damage to various biomolecules, including DNA.
The use of anti-oxidants in cancer chemotherapy needs to be weighed carefully as they may protect the host but compromise the drug action in cancer cells.

17.6 Anti-Cachexia Drugs

Cancer cachexia describes a syndrome of progressive weight loss, anorexia, and persistent erosion of host body cell mass, which affects especially the skeletal muscle, in response to malignant growth. The fundamental physiological derangement leading to cancer associated weight loss is a decline in food intake relative to energy expenditure. Alternatively, abnormalities in the host metabolism lead to continued mobilization and ineffective repletion of tissue, despite adequate nutritional support.

Cachexia can be mediated by the release of factors from the tumor. Also, cytokines can be produced as a defense against malignancy and act as signaling molecules in cachexia. Such molecules include Tumor Necrosis Factor-α (TNF-α, Cachectin), Interleukin-1β (IL-1β), Interleukin-6 (IL-6), Ciliary Neurotropic Factor (CNTF), and Proteolysis Inducing Factor (PIF).

- Nutritional support is often effective in maintaining the body weight of cachectic cancer patients, but ineffective in maintaining lean body mass. Oral omega-3 (n-3) fatty acid supplements may benefit by improving appetite and maintaining body weight. Specifically, a supplement of eicosapentaenoic acid down-regulates the production of pro-inflammatory cytokines, such as IL-6, IL-1 and Tumor Necrosis Factor-α, as well as Proteolysis Inducing Factor, and may help cancer patients to retain muscle mass.
- Insulin therapy may preserve host composition by preferential feeding of the host over the tumor.
- Cachexia may be treated with corticosteroids, such as dexamethasone (3–8 mg/d), which increase appetite and may reverse weight loss, but do not reverse muscle loss. Substantial toxicities associated with long-term administration include myopathy, peptic ulcer disease, infection, adrenal suppression, and hyperglycemia. Many patients with advanced cancer anorexia and cachexia, however, do not survive long enough to suffer from these adverse effects.
- Cachexia may be treated by progesterones, such as megestrol or medroxyprogesterone, which increase appetite and may reverse weight loss. These drugs show efficacy in a matter of days, and they are effective anti-emetics. Progestational agents can cause adrenal suppression or increase the risk of thromboembolic phenomena.
- Hydrazine sulfate is the synthetic sulfate salt of a derivative of ammonia. Hydrazine inhibits the enzyme Phosphoenol Pyruvate Carboxykinase, thereby blocking gluconeogenesis. This agent decreases the excessive energy needs and cachexia of cancer patients. Hydrazine sulfate is also a weak inhibitor of MAO (Mono-Amine Oxidase). However, the drug itself may be carcinogenic.
- The anti-serotonergic drug cyproheptadine is a relatively strong appetite stimulant in patients with carcinoid syndrome, because it directly counteracts the large amounts of serotonin secreted in these patients.

Cancer cachexia entails progressive weight loss, anorexia, and persistent erosion of host body cell mass.
Cachexia can be mediated by the release of factors from the tumor, or by a cytokine defense against the malignancy.

17.7 Protection from Hepatotoxicity

Chemotherapy can exert damage to the liver. In addition, paraneoplastic phenomena (such as hepatitis through colony-stimulating factors secreted from tumors, cholestasis in association with renal cell carcinoma), immunosuppression, infectious diseases, metastases, and poly-pharmacy can contribute. Although many pharmaceuticals can cause liver injury, most hepatotoxic drug reactions are idiosyncratic, due to immunologic mechanisms or variations in the host

Table 17.2 Dose modification with hepatic disease. *ULN* upper limit of normal, *ALT* Alanine Amino Transferase, *AST* Aspartate Amino Transferase

Agent	Dose Modification	Bilirubin	Aminotransferases
Hydroxyurea, vincristine, vinblastine	Reduce dose by 50%	>1.5 mg/d	
	Reduce dose by 75%	>3.0 mg/dL	
Vinorelbine	Reduce dose by 50%	>2.0 mg/dL	
	Reduce dose by 75%	>3.0 mg/dL	
Gemcitabine	Reduce dose by 20%	>1.6 mg/dL	
irinotecan	Contraindicated	>2 mg/dL	>3 × ULN (without liver metastases) or >5 × ULN (with liver metastases)
Doxorubicin, daunorubicin	Reduce dose by 25%	20-51 μM	ALT or AST 2-3 × ULN
	Reduce dose by 50%	51-85 μM	ALT or AST >3 × ULN
	Contraindicated	>85 μM	
Etoposide	Reduce dose by 50%	25-51 μM	AST>180
5-fluorouracil	Contraindicated	>85 μM	
Procarbazine	Contraindicated	>85 μM	ALT or AST>180
Paclitaxel	Reduce dose by 25%	<1.5 mg/dl	AST 2 × ULN
	Reduce dose by 60%	1.6-30 mg/dl	
	Reduce dose by 75%	73 mg/dl	
Docetaxel	Contraindicated	>1.5 × ULN	>1.5 × ULN

metabolic response. These reactions are not stringently dose dependent.

Symptoms include fatigue, abdominal pain, excessive bleeding, and swollen feet and ankles. Bilirubin is a chemical released into the blood during the breakdown of red blood cells. It is used in the liver to make bile. If the liver is damaged its bilirubin utilization is compromised, which leads to a buildup in bilirubin blood levels and manifests in jaundice (ikterus).

There are no drugs to specifically treat the elevated bilirubin or liver enzyme levels, unless there is an infection, blockage, or tumor. The treatment is aimed at correcting the underlying cause and minimizing further damage to the liver. With severe liver damage, diuretics and pain relievers may be prescribed. Patients should avoid alcohol and acetaminophen <Tylenol>.

In patients with liver dysfunction, the dosing of some conventional chemotherapeutics needs to be adjusted (Table 17.2).

Chemotherapy can exert damage to the liver.
In patients with liver dysfunction, the dosing of some chemotherapeutics requires adjustment.

17.8 Protection from Urinary Toxicity

Nephrotoxicity of chemotherapy Rapid tumor lysis leading to acute uric acid nephropathy, hyper-kalemia, and hyper-phosphatemia may complicate the treatment of patients with chemotherapy-responsive tumors. Aggressive management with intravenous hydration, urinary alkalinization and administration of allopurinol can ameliorate these complications of therapy.

Compromised renal function in cancer patients is a common complication. Several anti-neoplastic agents are potentially nephrotoxic. Previous renal impairment and combinations of nephrotoxic drugs may increase the risk of renal failure during chemotherapy.

- Methotrexate induces renal damage most frequently with high-dose therapy; it can be avoided by forced alkaline diuresis and administration of folinic acid.
- Cisplatin nephrotoxicity is dose related and may be dose limiting.
- Renal dysfunction caused by semustine is related to cumulative doses in excess to 1.2 g/m^2; the onset may be delayed and renal failure can progress after drug discontinuation.
- Streptozotocin is nephrotoxic, it may cause proteinuria and renal tubular acidosis; progressive renal failure can be prevented by drug discontinuation.
- Mitomycin mediated renal failure is frequently associated with micro-angiopathic hemolytic anemia; renal failure is usually delayed, but may be rapidly progressive even after stopping the drug treatment.
- Cyclophosphamide and ifosfamide exert toxic effects to the bladder and the ureter; cystitis may arise in up to 10% of patients receiving intermittent or chronic low dose cyclophosphamide and in up to 40% of patients receiving cyclophosphamide in a high dose bone marrow transplant program.

Table 17.3 Dose modifications with renal disease. Cl_{cr} creatinine clearance (DiPiro et al. 2008)

Empiric Dose Modifications in Patients with Renal Disease	
Agent	Suggested Dose Modification
Methotrexate, cisplatin	In proportion to lowered creatinine clearance (normal = 60 mL/min per m^2)
	Clcr < 10 mL/min, contraindicated
Carboplatin	Dose (mg) = area under the curve × (Clcr + 25)
Cyclophosphamide	Clcr < 25 mL/min; reduce dose by 50 %
Bleomycin	Clcr < 25 mL/min; reduce dose by 50–75 %
Capecitabine	Clcr 30–50 mL/min; reduce dose by 25 %
	Clcr <30 mL/min, contraindicated
Cytarabine (high dose: > 1 g/m2)	For creatinine 1.5–1.9 mg/dL, reduce dose by 50 %
	For creatinine > 2.0 mg/dL, reduce dose by 95 %
Topotecan	Clcr 20–39 mL/min; reduce dose by 25 %
Cladribine, fludarabine	In proportion to lowered creatinine clearance

Protection is best achieved through frequent voiding and vigorous hydration to dilute the toxic metabolites in the urine. The treatment of hemorrhagic cystitis may require bladder irrigation with saline or formalin.

The uroprotectant drug mesna (sodium 2-mercaptoethane sulfonate) <Uromitexan, Mesnex> (discovered in 1978) can be administered as an adjuvant for chemotherapy with cyclophosphamide or ifosfamide. It reduces the incidence of hemorrhagic cystitis and hematuria by neutralizing the urotoxic drug metabolite acrolein via binding through its sulfhydryl moieties. It also increases the urinary excretion of cysteine.

Adverse Effects Adverse effects include taste change (reversible upon completion of the treatment), limb and joint pain, skin rash, headache, fatigue, diarrhea, and mood swings.

Dose adjustment in renal dysfunction In patients with kidney dysfunction, the dosing of some conventional chemotherapeutics needs to be adjusted (Table 17.3). Based on the glomerular filtration rate (GFR in mL/min) and desired drug area under the concentration-versus-time curve (AUC in mg/mL min), the appropriate dose adjustment (total dose in mg) can be calculated as

$$\text{total dose} = (\text{desired AUC}) \cdot (\text{GFR} + 25).$$

Chemotherapeutics may exert toxic effects to the kidneys or bladder.
Rapid tumor lysis can cause acute uric acid nephropathy, hyper-kalemia, and hyper-phosphatemia.
In patients with renal dysfunction, the dosing of some chemotherapeutics requires adjustment.

17.9 Protection of the Gastrointestinal Tract

The gastrointestinal mucosa is composed of epithelial cells with a high mitotic index and rapid turnover rate, making it highly sensitive to anti-proliferative agents. Mucosal damage can occur at any point along the gastrointestinal tract. During and after chemotherapy, mucositis may range from xerostomia (dry mouth) to ulcers or local infection. Patients at high risk are those receiving 5-fluorouracil, doxorubicin, or methotrexate. The effects may impact on oral comfort and ability to eat or drink, but can be minimized by adequate care. Basic mouth hygiene, initiated before chemotherapy starts, is of primary preventive importance (high-risk patients should have a dental evaluation prior to chemotherapy). Xerostomia can be easily treated with drinking fluids, sucking ice chips, eating fresh fruits, or chewing gum. Following chemotherapy, patients should rinse their mouths frequently with salt water, baking soda, or chlorhexidine (in patients undergoing radiation to the head and neck, chlorhexidine rinses are detrimental to the oral mucosa). Once mucositis or mouth sores have developed, treatment is mostly supportive for 7–14 days until the cells regenerate themselves.

Analgesics and anesthetics can be employed if they do not contain irritants (such as peroxides).

- Lidocaine (lignocaine) <Xylocaine> is a local anesthetic. It can be applied as a gel or spray, but it has a short duration of action. It should not be used prior to meals, as it can cause choking.
- Diphenhydramine liquid <Benadryl> is a first generation anti-histamine with anti-cholinergic, anti-tussive, anti-emetic, and sedative properties. As a topical anesthetic, it can treat mucositis.
- Dyclonine is a topical anesthetic commonly employed.

Protective drugs can prevent the progression of the damage.

- RK-0202 is an oral polymer matrix based rinse formulation that contains *N*-acetyl cysteine, an antioxidant amino acid derivative with anti-inflammatory properties. RK-0202 may alleviate the symptoms of radiation induced oral mucositis.
- Protective agents, such as sucralfate <Carafate> or bismuth subsalicylate (attapulgite) <Kaopectate, Pepto

Table 17.4 Management of Diarrhea

Focus on
Preventing excessive water and electrolyte losses
Dietary care
Relieving symptoms
Treating curable causes
Treating secondary disorders

Table 17.5 Anti-Diarrhea Drug Groups

Anti-motility (loperamide)
Adsorbents (polycarbophil)
Anti-secretory compounds (bismuth subsalicylate)
Antibiotics
Enzymes
Intestinal microflora (Lactobacillus)

Bismol>, can be applied to cover ulcers and decrease irritation.

Regenerative agents accelerate the mucosal healing.

- Velafermin (CG-53135) is a recombinant Fibroblast Growth Factor-20 (rhFGF-20) protein with pro-proliferative activity. Velafermin stimulates DNA synthesis and cell proliferation, specifically promoting epithelial and mesenchymal cell proliferation, and may prevent radiation induced or chemotherapy induced oral mucositis.
- The Keratinocyte Growth Factor palifermin <Kepivance> is administered to patients receiving high dose chemo-radio-therapy prior to hematopoietic stem cell transplantation. Palifermin is given intravenously at a dose of 60 μg/kg per day for 3 consecutive days immediately before the initiation of conditioning therapy and then again for 3 days after hematopoietic stem cell transplantation to reduce the risk for oral mucositis. The use of palifermin in non-hematologic cancers is not recommended.

Topical steroids are contraindicated as they may facilitate infections. In addition, patients should not take in spicy, hot, or coarse foods, or acidic juice.

A disruption of the gastrointestinal mucosal barrier may provide an avenue for systemic microbial invasion that requires antibiotic therapy.

Anti-cancer drugs can damage the digestive tract, leading to diarrhea. Specific drugs that are particularly associated with loose or liquid bowel movements include 5-fluorouracil, methotrexate, cytarabine, capecitabine, and irinotecan. However, it is often difficult to predict which patients will develop diarrhea. The management is symptomatic and needs to include electrolyte replacement (Table 17.4). Adequate fluid intake is critical in order to prevent dehydration. While oral fluid replacement is preferred, intravenous fluid support may be indicated in severe cases of dehydration. If required, diarrhea can be controlled with diphenoxylate/atropine <Lomotil> or loperamide hydrochloride <Imodium>, unless it is caused by an infection (Table 17.5).

Diarrhea caused by irinotecan is treated in a unique manner. If it occurs less than 24 h after the infusion, atropine is given to control the symptoms. For late onset diarrhea, the patient should take 4 mg loperamide after the first episode of loose stools, followed by 2 mg every 2 h until the diarrhea subsides. During night time, the patients take 4 mg every 4 h.

In some cases, constipation can be a consequence of anticancer treatment. It may be prompted by

- narcotic analgesics, which can cause a substantial decrease in bowel movements by inhibiting the nerves in the gastrointestinal tract; oral morphine <MS Contin>, oral oxycodone <Oxycontin>, fentanyl <Duragesic> topical patch, or hydrocodone <Dilaudid> are implicated
- vinca chemotherapy drugs, which frequently cause constipation beginning within 7 days of therapy; elderly patients are particularly susceptible
- calcium containing antacids <Tums> taken to counteract chemotherapy-induced gastric reflux.

Any patients started on these drugs should also take in adequate fluids and fruits to stimulate bowel function. In addition, a stimulant laxative along with a stool softener should be taken Table 17.6.

Heartburn (gastric reflux, acid indigestion, dyspepsia, gastro-esophageal reflux disease, GERD) may arise during chemotherapy. It can be aggravated by stress, smoking, certain foods (e.g. caffeine), or medications. Gastric reflux is caused by a flow of food from the stomach into the esophagus, which results in a burning discomfort that radiates from the stomach upwards. The primary modes of treatment are lifestyle

Table 17.6 3 General Classes of Laxatives

1	Agents that cause softening of feces in 1–3 days: osmotic laxatives (methylcellulose, polycarbophil, psyllium), Polyethylene glycol 3350, emollients (lactulose, sorbitol)
2	Agents that result in soft or semifluid stool in 6–12 h: bisacodyl, senna, magnesium sulfate (low dose)
3	Agents that cause watery evacuation in 1–6 h: magnesium citrate, magnesium hydroxide, magnesium sulfate (high dose), sodium phosphates, bisacodyl, polyethylene glycol preparations

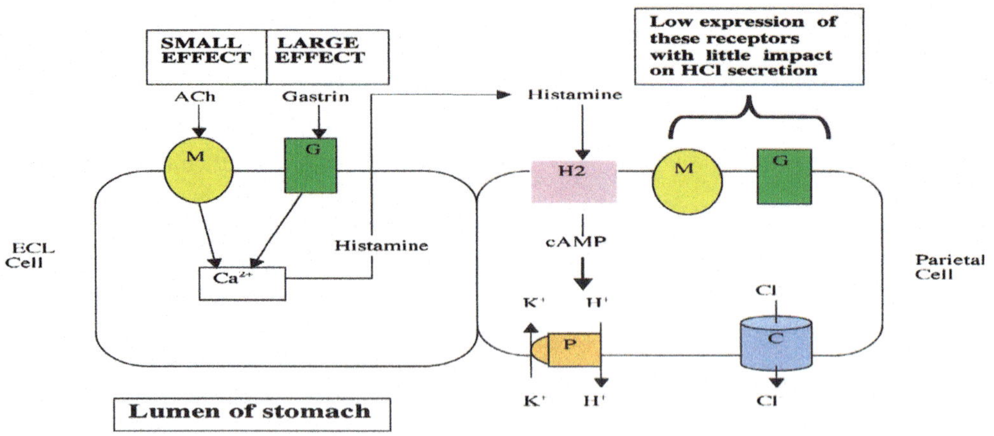

Fig. 17.3 The control of gastric acid secretion. The enterochromaffin-like cells communicate hormonal signals to the parietal cells, which respond to the secretion of HCl into the stomach lumen. *M* Muscarinic Receptor, *G* Gastrin Receptor, *H* Histamine H2 Receptor, *P* proton pump (active transport), *C* chloride channel (passive transport), *ECL* enterochromaffin-like cell

changes, which can include sleeping with elevated head, not eating 2–3 h before going to bed, limiting caffeine intake and smoking, and weight loss. If it is permissible with the chemotherapy regimen, antacids containing calcium carbonate, aluminum hydroxide, magnesium hydroxide, or magladrate may be tried. In severe cases, drugs that affect the endocrine regulation of gastric acid secretion (Fig. 17.3) may be appropriate.

- H_2 Receptor blockers in the family of -tidines (cimetidine <Tagamet>, famotidine <Pepcid>, nizatidine <Axid>, ranitidine <Zantac>) compete with histamine at the H_2 Receptors on the interstitial side of the parietal cells, which are located in the lining of the stomach and the small intestine. This inhibition decreases gastric acid secretion.
- Proton-pump inhibitors in the group of -prazoles (omeprazole <Prilosec>, lansopraxole <Prevacid>, esomeprazole <Nexium>, pantoprozole <Protonix>, rabeprazole <Aciphex>) suppress gastric acid secretion by inhibiting the enzyme pump process, which is the final step in the production of gastric acid. They are suitable for short term use to treat active ulcers or reflux disease.

Mucosal damage is treatable with anesthetics, protective agents, or regenerative drugs.
Various gastrointestinal symptoms can be managed with symptomatic therapy.

17.10 Treatment of Dermatologic Reactions to Chemotherapy

Chemotherapy can cause various skin reactions. Vesicant drugs (mustards, vinca alkaloids, Topoisomerase inhibitors, anthracyclines and their liposomal preparations) can cause local skin reactions when injected but precautions and antidotes can minimize these reactions.

Infusion reactions, such as pain, phlebitis, induration, and swelling, are common adverse events after intravenous drug administration. Because of the toxicity of most anti-cancer agents, the extravasation of drugs given intravenously may constitute an emergency as they can necrotize the surrounding tissue. Topical cooling with ice packs may help to limit the tissue damage.

- Dimethyl sulfoxide (DMSO) may be administered topically as an anti-oxidant protective.
- Dexrazoxane hydrochloride <Totect> is used as an intravenously delivered antidote following the extravasation of anthracyclines (it should not be used together with topical DMSO as this may worsen the tissue injury).

The hand-foot syndrome (palmar-plantar erythrodysesthesia) was first reported in association with chemotherapy in 1974 (Zuehlke 1974). The reaction comprises a painful redness, irritation, and fissuration of the hands and soles that may arise with capecitabine, 5-flurouracil, continuous-infusion doxorubicin, doxorubicin liposomal, or high dose Interleukin-2. The symptoms can occur days to months after exposure to the offending medication, depending on the dose and speed of administration. The likely cause is that during chemotherapy small amounts of drug leak out of the capillaries in the palms of the hands and the soles of the feet. Exposure to heat as well as friction on the palms and soles increases the blood flow and consecutively the amount of drug leakage. The areas affected display redness (erythema) and tenderness, can become dry and peel, with numbness or tingling sensation developing.

Prevention involves the reduction of heat exposure or friction to the hands and feet for about 1 week after intravenous chemotherapy treatment. Cooling may provide temporary relief from pain and tenderness. Treatment of this syndrome is mainly supportive and comprises

- moisturizing of the affected regions with creams and emollients such as <Aveeno>, <Lubriderm>, petroleum jelly <Vaseline>, 8-hydroxyquinoline sulfate in petrolatum/lanolin (udder cream) <Bag Balm>
- pain relievers such as acetaminophen <Tylenol> may ameliorate discomfort, for more severe cases corticosteroids have some efficacy
- vitamin B6 (pyridoxine) may be beneficial, as it is linked to vascular integrity by decreasing the formation of homocysteine.

Radiation recall is an inflammatory reaction that sometimes occurs when a patient receives chemotherapy following radiation therapy. The most common type of reaction is radiation recall dermatitis. The anti-cancer drugs most commonly associated with radiation recall include, doxorubicin <Adriamycin>, docetaxel <Taxotere>, paclitaxel <Taxol>, gemcitabine <Gemzar>, capecitabine <Xeloda>. The symptoms can occur within days or years after the completion of radiation therapy, affecting close to 10% of patients. The skin reaction appears at the site of radiation treatment and is caused by inflammation. Prolonging the interval between completion of the radiation therapy and initiation of the chemotherapy can mitigate the risk.

The treatment for a radiation recall reaction is primarily supportive care to manage the symptoms. Eliminating the drug source of the reaction is often the first step. Medications such as oral or topical corticosteroids and anti-inflammatory preparations may be used to decrease the inflammation.

Chemotherapy can cause adverse skin reactions. They include infusion reactions, hand-foot syndrome, and radiation recall.

17.11 Electrolyte Balance

A strong initial response to chemotherapy may cause massive tumor breakdown and the resultant systemic release of intracellular contents. This effect may constitute a basis for the severe metabolic disturbances, which constitute the tumor lysis syndrome. The metabolic derangement is characterized by the development of hyperkalemia, hypocalcemia, hyperuricemia, and hyperphosphatemia. The patient may present with lethargy, weakness, paralysis, nausea, vomiting, renal colic, and joint pain. The syndrome ultimately leads to the development of acute renal failure and may require the patient to undergo continuous hemodialysis. Associated complications can include arrythmias, seizures, tetany, and sudden death. The tumor lysis syndrome most commonly occurs upon treatment of high grade lymphomata or acute leukemias. Steroids are potent anti-leukemic agents that may provoke a rapid breakdown of tumor cells in previously untreated patients. Because early recognition and management can be lifesaving, prophylactic measures should be instituted when abnormal laboratory results arise. Electrolyte abnormalities should be treated appropriately. Preventive measures include hyper-hydration with aggressive intravenous fluid therapy, administration of allopurinol, Rasburicase (recombinant Urate Oxidase) <Uricozyme, Elitek, Fasturtec>, and alkalinization of the urine. Institution of these measures is particularly critical during the first 24–48 h. Loop diuretics may be administered.

Hyperuricemia may develop during cancer treatment with alkylating agents. The adverse effect of urate precipitation should be anticipated, particularly in lymphoma patients, and adequate control of hyperuricemia should be instituted. A basic precaution is abundant fluid intake before treatment.

Calcium strengthens bones and teeth, supports muscle function, and helps blood clot. Parathyroid hormone mobilizes calcium from the kidneys and bone, while calcitrol (a form of vitamin D) enhances the intestinal absorption of calcium. Healthy kidneys are capable of filtering large amounts of calcium, which are subsequently reabsorbed in the tubuli to the extent required for homeostasis.

Hypercalcemia is a common complication of cancer (most often in breast cancer, lung cancer, multiple myeloma, and lymphoma or leukemia), arising in 10–20% of adult patients but rarely in children. If hypercalcemia is not treated, it may lead to coma and death. To prevent hypercalcemia, patients should drink sufficient amounts of fluids, get enough salt in the diet, control nausea and vomiting, control fever, and avoid drugs that can induce elevated calcium levels.

The treatment of moderate hypercalcemia includes the replacement of fluids as the first and most important step, which helps to improve symptoms, such as confusion, nausea, and vomiting. Specific drugs may reduce the breakdown of bone and the release of calcium into the blood.

- Bisphosphonates suppress bone resorption.
- Calcitonin blocks bone resorption and increases urinary calcium excretion (by inhibiting the tubular reabsorption).
- Plicamycin (mithramycin) suppresses bone resorption. The drug was occasionally used for hypercalcemia, but has been discontinued due to a risk for severe thrombocytopenia.
- Gallium nitrate ($Ga(NO_3)_3$) <Ganite> inhibits bone resorption and changes the structures of bone crystals. It is in clinical trials for use in lymphomata to treat the hypercalcemia of malignancy.

- Glucocorticosteroids increase urinary calcium excretion and decrease intestinal calcium absorption.
- Phosphates can correct the hypophosphatemia associated with hypercalcemia, which aids in lowering the blood calcium.

Dialysis may be required for patients with kidney failure.

Various anti-estrogens may cause tumor flare in a fraction of breast cancer patients with bone metastases during the first weeks of treatment. Tumor flare is a syndrome of diffuse musculoskeletal pain and erythema with tumor lesions that initially increase in size, but later regress. It is often accompanied by hypercalcemia. The condition may force discontinuation of the anti-estrogenic treatment and require supportive measures.

Electrolyte imbalance may arise in tumor lysis syndrome or tumor flare syndrome.
Fluid replacement is a basic measure to control electrolyte imbalance.
Supportive treatment with specific drugs may aid in restoring homeostasis.

17.12 Reproductive Protection

The majority of young breast cancer patients receive chemotherapy, hormone therapy, or both. These patients are at high risk for transient or permanent amenorrhea, and a long term risk of premature ovarian failure. Alkylating agents, particularly the combination regimen of CMF (cyclophosphamide, methotrexate, 5-fluorouracil) or CEF (cyclophosphamide, epirubicin, 5-fluorouracil), are associated with the highest risk of ovarian failure, reaching 90% in women over the age of 40. As the adverse effect targets predominantly cells with a rapid turnover, hormonal methods to suppress gonadal function may reduce the gonadotoxicity of chemotherapy.

- The continuous exposure to Luteinizing Hormone Releasing Hormone (LHRH) analogs decreases the secretion of Follicle Stimulating Hormone (FSH) and suppresses gonadal function. A large fraction of pre-menopausal patients receiving the LHRH analog goserelin before and during chemotherapy are protected from premature menopause, with women under 40 years of age benefiting more than older patients.
- Triptorelin <Decapeptyl, Diphereline, Gonapeptyl, Trelstar> is an agonistic decapeptide analog of Gonadotropin Releasing Hormone (GnRH) (see Sect. 10.2.4.). By causing a constant stimulation of the pituitary, triptorelin decreases the secretion of the Gonadotropins (Luteinizing Hormone and Follicle Stimulating Hormone). It can temporarily suppress the ovaries during chemotherapy, which leads to a reduced incidence of early menopause.

Chemotherapy or radiotherapy can affect fertility potential by causing azoospermia. While spermatogenesis often returns in affected men, the time frame ranges from months to years. Approximately 15–30% of childhood cancer survivors are permanently sterile following therapy. Cyclophosphamide or procarbazine containing regimens result in azoospermia in the vast majority of patients. The treatment of testicular cancer with cisplatin and carboplatin regimens leads to temporary azoo- and oligozoospermia in most patients, with a recovery to normospermia in 80% of cases within 5 years. High dose chemotherapy used as preparation before bone marrow transplant is also associated with irreversible germinal epithelial failure in the majority of men. Anti-cancer drugs can affect spermatogenesis via

- inhibition of the normal overall rate and sequence of development (kinetic damage),
- direct action on a cell type resulting in its subsequent death and depletion from the system (cellular damage),
- interference with cell morphology resulting in a change in either testicular or epididymal phases (morphological damage),
- a change manifest during cleavage of an egg fertilized by an affected spermatozoon, resulting in the death of embryos during gestation (early genetic damage),
- damaging action resulting in genetic changes in the progeny (late genetic damage),
- an effect on the structural matrix of the testicular tissue including Leydig and Sertoli cells (matrix damage) (Fox and Fox 1967).

The cryopreservation of spermatozoa is the only reliable method for protecting fertility from the effects of chemotherapy.

Chemotherapy or radiotherapy can affect fertility potential by causing azoospermia.
As cells with a rapid turnover are predominantly affected, hormonal methods to suppress gonadal function may reduce the gonadotoxicity of chemotherapy.

17.13 Others

An increase in intracranial pressure affects many cancer patients as a consequence of their disease (primary brain tumors, cerebral metastases, infections, encephalopathies, vascular disorders) or of the associated therapy. Cerebral irritation may result from the effects of tumor cell breakdown or from cerebral necrosis secondary to the results of total body irradiation. Corticosteroids are given to reduce brain swelling.

The anti-estrogen tamoxifen <Novaldex> is primarily used in the treatment of breast cancer, ovarian cancer, pancreatic cancer, and malignant melanoma. Dose dependent ocular adverse effects are common over 180 mg/day, but rare up to 20 mg/day. They include corneal opacities, retinal or macular yellow or white refractile opacities, edema, degeneration, pigmentary changes, and hemorrhages.

- Acute manifestations usually occur within a few weeks after initiation of therapy, likely due to estrogenic activity that leads to venous thrombembolism. Symptoms include vision loss, retinal edema, retinal hemorrhage, and optic disc swelling.
- Typical tamoxifen retinopathy most commonly occurs after more than 1 year of therapy with a cumulative total of more than 100 gm of the drug. The retinopathy can include cystoid macular edema, punctuate macular retinal pigment epithelial changes, parafoveal hemorrhages, and peripheral retinal pigment epithelium changes. These lesions are not likely to regress when the drug is discontinued. Visual acuity loss is often progressive, dose dependent, and irreversible. Corneal deposits are seldom clinically significant and are usually reversible.

Substantial color vision loss may provide valid grounds for discontinuing the drug. If the medication is stopped for 3 months and color vision returns to normal, tamoxifen may be re-started. If there is no rebound or if the visual adverse effects continue to progress, a substitute for tamoxifen needs to be considered.

Potential ocular adverse effects of Interferon α2b <Intron A> include decreased vision, ocular pain, conjunctivitis, retinal changes, and optic neuritis. Diabetics and patients with hypertension may be more severely affected.

- A transient decrease in vision may occur within 15 min of the first exposure. Patients often are subjectively aware of this. Some patients experience intense ocular or orbital pain.
- Conjunctivitis arises in about 5 % of patients taking Interferon.
- If there are retinal changes, such as capillary non-perfusion or cotton wool spots due to vascular occlusions, they characteristically manifest between 2 weeks and 3 months after the initiation of drug therapy. They may spontaneously regress while the patient is still on the drug or may require the discontinuation of treatment.
- Eyelash growth from 2.0 to 6.5 cm in length can occur.
- Only a small percentage of patients encounter permanent changes, such as rare cases of optic neuritis.

Depression may accompany a large fraction of cancers. There is a correlation among increasing pain, impaired quality of life, and depressive symptoms. Treatment usually includes tricyclic anti-depressants, selective serotonin reuptake inhibitors (SSRIs), or a combination of both. Selective serotonin reuptake inhibitors have fewer adverse effects than tricyclic anti-depressants. In particular, the anti-cholinergic symptoms (dry mouth) and somnolence are reduced, but these drugs lack the analgesic efficacy.

Cancer related fatigue is a distressing persistent sense of tiredness or exhaustion, caused by the disease or its treatment. Psychostimulants, such as methylphenidate, can ameliorate fatigue.

References

Bennett CL, Silver SM, Djulbegovic B, Samaras AT, Blau CA, Gleason KJ, Barnato SE, Elverman KM, Courtney DM, McKoy JM, Edwards BJ, Tigue CC, Raisch DW, Yarnold PR, Dorr DA, Kuzel TM, Tallman MS, Trifilio SM, West DP, Lai SY, Henke M (2008) Venous thromboembolism and mortality associated with recombinant erythropoietin and darbepoetin administration for the treatment of cancer-associated anemia. J Am Med Assoc 299:914–924

DiPiro JT, Talbert RL, Yee GC, Matzke GR, Wells BG, Posey LM (2008) Pharmacotherapy: a Pathophysiologic Approach. 7. McGraw-Hill

Fox BW, Fox M (1967) Biochemical aspects of the actions of drugs on spermatogenesis. Pharmacol Rev 19:21–57

Grunberg SM (2007) Antiemetic activity of corticosteroids in patients receiving cancer chemotherapy: dosing, efficacy, and tolerability analysis. Ann Oncol 18:233–240

Hall MP, Gegg C, Walker K, Spahr C, Ortiz R, Patel V, Yu S, Zhang L, Lu H, DeSilva B, Lee JW (2010) Ligand-binding mass spectrometry to study biotransformation of fusion protein drugs and guide immunoassay development: strategic approach and application to peptibodies targeting the thrombopoietin receptor. AAPS Journal 12:576–585

Henke M, Laszig R, Rübe C, Schäfer U, Haase KD, Schilcher B, Mose S, Beer KT, Burger U, Dougherty C, Frommhold H (2003) Erythropoietin to treat head and neck cancer patients with anaemia undergoing radiotherapy: randomised, double-blind, placebo-controlled trial. The Lancet 362:1255–1260

Knock FE (1967) Anticancer agents. Springfield, Charles C. Thomas

Leyland-Jones B (2003) BEST Investigators and Study Group. Breast cancer trial with erythropoietin terminated unexpectedly. Lancet Oncol 4:459–460

Minotti G, Menna P, Salvatorelli E, Cairo G, Gianni L (2004) Anthracyclines: Molecular Advances and Pharmacologic Developments in Antitumor Activity and Cardiotoxicity. Pharmacol Rev 56:185–229

Pruemer J (2006) Treatment of cancer-associated thrombosis: Distinguishing among antithrombotic agents. Sem Oncol 33(suppl 4):S26-S39

Zuehlke, R (1974) Erythematous eruption of the palms and soles associated with mitotane therapy. Dermatologica 148:90–92

18 Pain Management

Pain can be associated with both localized tumors and metastatic cancer. It becomes more pervasive as the disease progresses. Tumor invasion of the bone, which commonly occurs in breast cancer, prostate cancer, and multiple myeloma, accounts for pain in approximately half of these patients. Most other causes of tumor related pain comprise nerve compression or infiltration (neuropathic pain), or tumor involvement in the gastrointestinal tract or soft tissue (somatic pain).

The actions of chemotherapeutic drugs may be the cause of pain.

- Platinum drugs, vinca alkaloids, taxanes, proteasome inhibitors, thalidomide, or epothilones can affect some vulnerable nerves, causing peripheral neuropathy, which can last from months to years after the completion of chemotherapy. The neuropathy is often felt as a burning in the hands and feet. In addition, the impaired sensation can compromise simple motor skills. The management of this form of pain requires drugs specific for neuropathy.
- The withdrawal of steroid medication can lead to joint pain and diffuse muscle pain, accompanied by fatigue. The symptoms typically resolve with the re-commencement of steroid therapy. The chronic administration of steroids can result in aseptic necrosis of the humoral or femoral head with pain and reduced motion. Aromatase inhibitors can cause diffuse muscle and joint pain and stiffness. It may increase the likelihood of osteoporosis and consequent fractures.

Pain may require alleviation with drug treatment or some other intervention for relief. While 90–95 % of patients receive adequate pain control using the WHO guidelines, there are still 5–10 % who do not.

18.1 Non-Steroidal Drugs

Adjuvant Strategies for pain management comprise non-steroidal anti-inflammatory drugs (NSAIDs) and acetaminophen. Mild pain (pain score of 1–4) should be treated at step 1 with analgesics in this class.

The prototypic non-steroidal anti-inflammatory drug, acetyl-salicylic acid, was introduced into medicine by Bayer AG in 1899. This class of therapeutics has since expanded. The non-steroidal anti-inflammatory drugs (NSAIDs) comprise salicylates (including acetyl-salicylate <Aspirin>), propionic acid derivatives (including ibuprofen <Advil>, naproxen <Aleve>), acetic acid derivatives (including indomethacin <Indocin>), enolic acid derivatives (including piroxicam <Feldene, Roxam, Dolonex>, tenoxicam <Mobiflex>), and fenamic acid derivatives (including meclofenamate <Meclomen>, tolfenamate <Clotam Rapid, Tufnil>). They have analgesic, anti-pyretic, and anti-coagulative effects. Their mode of action is to inhibit COX-1 and COX-2 enzymes, thus blocking prostaglandin formation. Prostaglandins act as mediators of inflammation and are partially responsible for bone pain from metastasis.

Selective COX-2 inhibitors (including celcecoxib <Celebrex>, parecoxib <Dynastat>) were initially developed to avoid the adverse effects on the stomach lining and risk for ulcers associated with the combined COX-1 and COX-2 inhibitors. However, the lack of COX-1 inhibition has conferred to these drugs a higher risk for blood clotting, which has led to the withdrawal of two representatives from this class.

Acetanilide <Antifebrin> is the original representative of the class of aniline analgesic drugs, introduced into medical practice by Cahn and Hepp in 1886. However, its propensity to induce methemoglobinemia has limited its clinical utility. In 1893, Joseph von Mehring identified phenacetin as a viable alternative. Although phenacetin was a popular analgesic and antipyretic, it causes nephropathy and hematologic toxicity and has carcinogenic potential. Acetaminophen is

G. F. Weber, *Molecular Therapies of Cancer,* DOI 10.1007/978-3-319-13278-5_18,

the active metabolite of phenacetin, and research around 1947–1949 found it to be an efficacious analgesic. Acetaminophen was first marketed in the United States in 1953.

Acetaminophen (paracetamol, para-acetylaminophenol) <Tylenol, Panadol, Anacin-3, Tempra, Datril, Ofirmev, Acamol, Efferalgan, Doliprane, Crocin> is an analgesic and anti-pyretic that inhibits COX enzymes in the central nervous system. Though acetaminophen is used to treat inflammatory pain, it is not classified as a non-steroidal anti-inflammatory drug, because it exhibits only weak anti-inflammatory activity. The drug may be administered orally, rectally, intravenously, or intramuscularly. The common adult dose is 500–1000 mg/day.

Adverse Effects Acetaminophen toxicity due to acute over-dosing can manifest as hepatotoxicity or as hemolytic anemia. Patients with Gilbert syndrome have enhanced susceptibility to acetaminophen toxicity.

Drug Interactions The drug is eliminated primarily by glucuronidation, which prevents its Cytochrome P450 catalyzed bioactivation to a hepatotoxic reactive intermediate. Reduced glucuronidation (which may be caused by anti-cancer drugs, such as imatinib mesylate) leads to enhanced bioactivation and may result in excessive drug levels.

18.2 Opioid Drugs

Opioid Receptors are a group of G-Protein Coupled Receptors with opioids[1] as their cognate ligands. These receptors are distributed widely in the brain, the spinal cord, and the digestive tract. Opioids, resembling morphine in their pharmacological effects, bind to the μ-Opioid Receptors within the central nervous system. Their analgesic effects are due to decreased perception of pain, decreased reaction to pain as well as increased pain tolerance.

Opioid regimens are agents of first choice in cancer pain management, progressing from weak opioids to those of greater strength. Three steps are recommended in establishing a therapeutic opioid regimen,

- initiating therapy: The initial treatment and titration with opioids in opioid-naive patients should include immediate-release preparations. The prolonged absorption of a sustained-release product may result in prolonged adverse effects in a patient who is receiving opioids for the first time. This concern is particularly relevant in the elderly
- consolidating therapy: As pain levels are reduced with the use of either shorter-acting products alone or both shorter- and longer-acting products, analgesic therapies should be consolidated. The therapeutic opioid regimen should be based on longer acting products, administered at regular dosing intervals. Dosing with sustained-release products assists in patient compliance
- maintaining therapy: Patients who do not achieve adequate analgesia throughout the dosing interval are more likely to benefit from an increase in dose rather than a decrease in the dosing interval. For patients who achieve excellent analgesia that is not sustained for the full dosing period, a decrease in the dosing interval may help to maintain an adequate level of the opioid (Cleary 2000).

The route of opioid administration may be oral, sublingual, subcutaneous or intravenous injection, or by enema. The parenteral administration of opioids may be necessary in patients who cannot swallow, who have intractable adverse effects (the steady blood concentrations resulting from intravenous administration may reduce the adverse effects), or in whom rectal delivery is not desirable. Fewer than 5 % of cancer patients have a need for the direct delivery of opioids to the central nervous system. Patients with unmanageable adverse effects may benefit from the epidural or intrathecal administration, which require only a fraction of the intravenous dose. Sustained-release products are available to treat cancer pain.

Adverse Effects Prophylaxis against and treatment of the adverse opioid effects foster quality of life and continued compliance with the medications. Patient responses can be highly variable.

- While not all patients will develop nausea and vomiting (particularly after the initial ingestion or injection), anti-emetic agents should be available to them. Metoclopramide can minimize opioid induced nausea and vomiting, haloperidol is an anti-emetic agent that also treats agitation.
- Opioids act on the myenteric plexus in the intestinal tract, reducing gut motility, and causing constipation. The gastrointestinal effects are mediated primarily by μ-Opioid Receptors in the bowel. By inhibiting gastric emptying and reducing propulsive peristalsis of the intestine, opioids decreases the rate of transit. Reduction in gut secretion and increased intestinal fluid absorption also contribute to the constipating effect. Opioids also may act on the gut indirectly through tonic gut spasms consecutive to the inhibition of nitric oxide generation. Preventing constipation, which occurs in almost all patients who use opioids (in rare cases leads to ruptured bowel), reduces hospitalizations. Bowel management should consist of the combination of both stimulants and stool softeners. The use of bulking agents while on opioids is contraindicated as it may increase the risk of constipation in cancer patients

[1] Endogenous opioids are dynorphins, enkephalins, endorphins, endomorphins, nociceptin.

(many cancer patients do not maintain adequate food and liquid intake to allow these agents to work, especially as the performance status decreases).
- In a small percentage of patients, fatigue and sedation may be intractable.
- Confusion is an adverse effect of opioids. Near the end of life, the addition of haloperidol to the regimen may correct confusion and delirium without affecting the pain outcome. An effective pharmacological measure in controlling adverse drug symptoms is rotating or switching opioids.

Opioids are potential drugs of abuse as they produce a feeling of euphoria. Continued intake may lead to tolerance, dependence can develop with ongoing administration, leading to a withdrawal syndrome upon abrupt discontinuation. The U.S. FDA defines opioid tolerance as occurring when a patient uses 60 mg or more of morphine per day.

Drug Interactions Central nervous system depressants, such as anesthetics, sedatives, hypnotics, barbiturates, phenothiazines, chloral hydrate, dimenhydrinate, or glutethimide may enhance the depressant effects of opioids. Anti-depressants in the class of Monoamine Oxidase Inhibitors (MAO inhibitors, such as phenelzine <Nardil>, tranylcypromine <Parnate>, isocarboxazid <Marplan>, or selegiline <Emsam>) may cause coma, slow or shallow breathing, low blood pressure, excitability, seizures, or shock if codeine is given within 2 weeks of the last dose. First generation anti-histamines (brompheniramine, promethazine, diphenhydramine, chlorpheniramine), β-blockers, or alcohol may also enhance the depressant effect of opioids. For combined therapy, the dose of one or both agents should be reduced.

18.2.1 Weak Opioids

For moderate pain (pain score of 5–6), weak opioids are indicated, with codeine, oxycodone, or hydrocodone usually administered as combination formulations. Propoxyphene, butophanol <Stadol>, nalbuphine <Nubian>, and pentazocine <Talwin> also belong to this class of drugs.

Codeine <Codrix> binds to opiate receptors in the central nervous system, which changes the perception of pain as well as the emotional response to it.

Adverse Effects Adverse effects include drowsiness, dizziness or lightheadedness, mood changes, and dry mouth. Less common are mental clouding, low blood pressure (which can cause dizziness when sitting or standing up), decreased heart rate, flushing, itching, sweating, difficulty urinating, trouble breathing, and abdominal pain.

Drug Interactions Buprenorphine <Subutex, Suboxone>, butorphanol <Stadol>, nalbuphine <Nubain>, or pentazocine <Talwin, Talacen>may decrease the effects of codeine or abrogate its action. If taken with codeine, tricyclic antidepressants (such as amitriptyline, desipramine, doxepin, imipramine, nortriptyline) can raise the risk of bowel blockage and trouble passing urine.

Freund and Speyer at the University of Frankfurt, Germany first synthesized the opioid analgesic oxycodone from thebaine (paramorphine) in 1916, a few years after the German pharmaceutical company Bayer had stopped the mass production of heroin due to hazardous use and dependence. Oxycodone was developed with the intent to improve on the existing opioids, morphine, diacetylmorphine (heroin), and codeine. The first clinical use of the drug was documented in 1917. It was first introduced to the U.S. market in 1939.

Oxycodone <OxyContin, Oxy-IR, Oxynorm, Percodan, Roxicodone> is a semi-synthetic opioid that acts on κ-Opioid Receptors as a narcotic analgesic for the relief of moderate pain. The drug can be administered orally or parenterally. A controlled release oral tablet form is indicated for cancer and intended to be taken every 12 h. Suppositories, available in Australia, contain 30 mg of oxycodone pectinate.

Pharmacokinetics Oxycodone and its metabolites are mainly excreted in the urine and sweat. Therefore, the drug accumulates in patients with renal impairment.

Adverse Effects The most commonly occurring adverse effects include memory loss, anxiety, headache, dizziness, dry mouth, pruritus, and diaphoresis (excessive sweating). The risk of severe withdrawal symptoms is high if a patient discontinues oxycodone abruptly. Therefore, in cases where the drug has been taken regularly over an extended period of time, use should be discontinued gradually.

Hydrocodone is a semi-synthetic opioid, derived from codeine, with narcotic and analgesic properties. As a narcotic, hydrocodone relieves pain by binding to Opioid Receptors in the central nervous system. It acts primarily on μ-Opioid Receptors, with about 6-fold lower affinity to δ-Opioid Receptors. It is approximately 1.5-fold less potent than oxycodone.

- A common formulation is hydrocodone/acetaminophen <Vicodin, Vicodin ES, Vicodin HP, Anexsia, Lortab, Lorcet, Lorcet Plus, Norco, Zydone>.

Pharmacokinetics Hydrocodone is orally available. Its analgesic action begins 20–30 min after intake and lasts 4–8 h. In the blood, 20–50 % of the drug is bound to protein and has a half-life of 4 h. Hydrocodone is biotransformed in the liver by Cytochrome P450 2D6, which converts it into the more potent hydromorphone. Ultrarapid CYP2D6 metabolizers may have an increased response to the drug. A major metabolite, norhydrocodone, is predominantly formed by a CYP3A4 catalyzed oxidation. Approximately 40 % of the agent is metabolized independently of Cytochrome P450.

Adverse Effects Common adverse effects of hydrocodone are dry throat, difficulty urinating, drowsiness, anxiety, mood swings, and rash. Serious adverse effects include slowed or irregular breathing and chest tightness.

Drug Interactions Patients consuming alcohol, other opioids, anti-histamines, anti-psychotics, anti-anxiety agents, or other central nervous system depressants together with hydrocodone may exhibit an additive effect.

Dextropropoxyphene <Darvon, Dolene> is suited to treat moderate pain. It also has anti-tussive and local anesthetic effects.

- Dextropropoxyphene is sometimes combined with paracetamol or acetylsalicylic acid <Darvocet-N, Di-Gesic, Co-Proxamol, Capadex, Lentogesic, Di-Antalvic>.

Adverse Effects The drug has been taken off the market in Europe and the U.S. due to concerns over fatal overdoses and arrhythmias. It may lead to stomach pain, skin rash, mood changes, drowsiness, and headache. A serious adverse effect is difficulty breathing.

18.2.2 Strong Opioids

Severe pain (pain score of 7 or higher) should be treated with full doses of strong opioids such as morphine, hydromorphone, or fentanyl. Levorphanol <Levo-Dromoran>, meperidine <Demerol>, methadone <Dolophine>, oxymorphone <Numorphan> also are strong opioids.

Morphine (named after Morpheus, the Greek god of dreams) was isolated in 1804 by Friedrich Sertürner and first distributed by him in 1817. It became more widely used after the invention of the hypodermic needle in 1857.

Morphine <MS Contin, MSIR, Avinza, Kadian, Oramorph, Roxanol, Kapanol> is a potent opiate analgesic drug that represents the prototypic narcotic agent. It is used to relieve acute and chronic severe pain. Morphine interacts predominantly with μ-Opioid Receptors that are discretely distributed in the brain, with high densities in the posterior amygdala, hypothalamus, thalamus, nucleus caudatus, putamen, and select cortical areas. Immediate release morphine is beneficial in reducing the symptom of acute shortness of breath due to cancer. In the setting of breathlessness at rest or on minimal exertion from advanced cancer, low-dose sustained release morphine safely reduces the symptoms, with its benefits being maintained over time. The duration of analgesia is about 3–4 h when administered via intravenous, subcutaneous, or intramuscular routes and 3–6 h when given orally.

Adverse Effects Morphine has a high potential for addiction. Although physiological dependence may take several months to develop, psychological dependence develops rapidly. Tolerance to respiratory depression and euphoria evolves faster than tolerance to analgesia, and many chronic pain patients are maintained on a stable dose for years.

Hydromorphone (dihydromorphinone) hydrochloride <Palladone, Dilaudid> is a semi-synthetic hydrogenated ketone of morphine. It represents a centrally acting analgesic opioid that is used to relieve moderate to severe chronic pain. Hydromorphone, a μ-Opioid Receptor agonist, produces its major effects on the central nervous system and gastrointestinal tract. These include analgesia, drowsiness and mental clouding, changes in mood (euphoria or dysphoria), increased parasympathetic activity, cough suppression, and decreased gastrointestinal motility.

Hydromorphone is commonly administered intravenously because its bioavailability orally, rectally, and intranasally is very low. Sublingual administration is usually preferable to swallowing for absorption. Hydromorphone is superior to morphine and diamorphine in solubility, speed of onset, efficacy, and lower dependence liability. It is a common alternative for patients who tend to have hallucinations from fentanyl.

Pharmacokinetics Hydromorphone is extensively glucuronidated in the liver, with greater than 95 % of the dose metabolized to hydromorphone-3-glucuronide along with minor metabolism of 6-hydroxy reduction. Hydromorphone does not produce the toxic metabolites of other methadone class opioids, such as norpethidine.

Adverse Effects The major hazards of hydromorphone include dose related respiratory depression and sometimes circulatory depression. Common adverse effects include light-headedness, dizziness, nausea and vomiting, itching, and sweating.

Most patients who suffer from cancer pain are given relief treatment with long-acting, strong analgesics, such as morphine. Despite this medication, a large fraction of these patients also experiences episodes of transient pain attacks (breakthrough pain), either spontaneously or induced by activity. During a sudden attack of cancer related pain, fentanyl preparations that are absorbed through the mucous membranes of the mouth, gums, and tongue may provide fast relief.

- <Abstral, Fentora> are fast-dissolving tablet formulations of fentanyl citrate that are placed under the tongue. The effect is thereby faster and more predictable than oral tablets or injections of fentanyl pain medications. The European EMEA recommended approval in 2008 and the U.S. FDA approved the drug in 2011.

- <Actiq> is an oral swab formulation of fentanyl citrate that dissolves slowly in the mouth for absorption across the buccal mucosa.
- <Onsolis> is a fentanyl buccal soluble film indicated for the management of breakthrough pain in cancer patients of 18 years and older for underlying persistent cancer pain.
- <Durogesic, Duragesic> are 72 h continuous release fentanyl patches for transdermal delivery.

Adverse Effects Transmucosal opioid medications may only be given to opioid tolerant patients who are already taking opioid medications on a regular basis to control cancer pain. Non-tolerant patients have a high risk for fatal respiratory depression. The use together with CYP3A4 inhibitors may increase the exposure dose and cause fatal respiratory depression.

While opioids are the mainstay of cancer pain management, adjunct medications may permit a decrease in opioid dose with an associated decrease in adverse effects. Non-steroidal and opioid pain killers are combined in oxycodone/acetaminophen <Percocet, Depalgos>, hydrocodone/acetaminophen <Vicodin, Lortab>, codeine/acetaminophen (co-codamol) <Tylenol-Codeine, Tylex CD, Panadeine, Captin, Disprol, Dymadon, Fensum, Hedex, Mexalen, Nofedol, Paralen, Pediapirin, Perfalgan, Solpadeine>, dihydrocodeine/acetaminophen (co-dydramol) <Paramol, Paracod, Remedeine>, dextropropoxyphene/acetaminophen <Darvon with APAP, Di-Gesic, Capadex, Lentogesic, Di-Antalvic>, and dextropropoxyphene/acetylsalicylic acid <Darvon with ASA>. A combination of paracetamol, codeine, and the calmative doxylamine succinate <Syndol, Mersyndol> may be used.

18.3 Others

Peripheral neuropathy is caused by sensory nerve damage, a potential complication of treatment with platinum drugs, taxanes, or bortezomib. The disorder comprises numbness and tingling of the arms, hands, legs, and feet. Neuropathic pain may be associated with dysesthesias and allodynia (pain produced by normally non-painful stimuli). It may have continuous and paroxysmal components. A subset of afflicted patients progresses to a chronic, painful form of the condition, which is continuous and exacerbated by touch or temperature. Painful chronic chemotherapy-induced peripheral neuropathy (CCIPN) substantially reduces the quality of life for cancer patients.

- Anti-depressants, such as amitriptyline <Elavil> and desipramine (desmethylimipramine) <Treyzafagit, Norpramin, Pertofrane>, are useful adjuncts for all cancer pain, but they are particularly beneficial in treating neuropathic pain.
- Anti-convulsants such as carbamazepine have been used as second-line treatment for neuropathic pain, but they usually require 3–4 weeks to reach effectiveness (Cleary 2000).
- Neuropathic pain is not resistant to opioids, but high doses may be needed.
- The cannabinoid nabiximols <Sativex> is an oromucosal spray containing a fixed dose combination of δ-9-tetrahydrocannabinol and cannabidiol. The product is approved in Sweden and Canada as adjunctive treatment for the symptomatic relief of neuropathic pain in cancer.
- The anti-oxidants Glutathione and α-lipoic acid may ameliorate the symptoms of peripheral neuropathy.
- KRN5500, a compound in development to treat a painful form of chronic chemotherapy-induced peripheral neuropathy, is an intravenously administered, non-opioid analgesic with rapid onset of action and prolonged pain mitigation. KRN5500 is under development to treat painful chemotherapy-induced peripheral neuropathy, which is characterized by the persistence of chemotherapy-associated pain for at least 12 weeks after chemotherapy has stopped.

Bone metastases can weaken bones and lead to pathological fractures or spinal cord compression. They may be a source of intense pain, belonging to the class of dull, deep somatic pain that cannot be localized accurately by the patient. Bone pain in cancer patients requires treatment.

- For mild to moderate pain (grade 1–3), non-opioid pain killers (including acetaminophen and non-steroidal anti-inflammatory drugs) are the first choice.
- Patients with moderate to severe pain (grade 4–6) who have not responded to prior treatment should receive an opioid, possibly with acetaminophen or a non-steroidal anti-inflammatory drug.
- Bisphosphonates may prevent or treat skeletal problems from bone metastases. They decrease pain while also reducing bone damage and risk for fracture. They are usually given by intravenous infusion.
- The neutralizing antibody denusomab <Prolia> acts as a RANKL inhibitor. Thereby, denosumab inhibits the maturation of osteoclasts and protects from bone loss. It is injected subcutaneously.
- Corticosteroids may be useful in the management of bone pain, but their prolonged use causes deleterious side effects.

Duloxetine hydrochloride <Cymbalta> is a serotonin and norepinephrine reuptake inhibitor (SNRI). It works by raising the levels of serotonin and norepinephrine in the brain.

Duloxetine is used to treat depression, anxiety, and chronic pain. The drug can help patients who develop a painful adverse effect from chemotherapy.

By reducing pressure on the liver capsule, the cause of hepatic pain, corticosteroids are particularly useful in managing painful liver metastases.

Nerve blocks, either with chemicals or other neuroablative methods, may be useful in the pain management of some patients.

References

Cleary JF (2000) Cancer pain management. Cancer Cont 7 120–131

19 Preventive Treatment

19.1 Vaccines

Hepatitis B is a major risk factor for hepatic cancer, as chronic infection with hepatitis B causes 80 % of primary liver cancers. The virus is transmitted through contact with body fluids from infected individuals. It is therefore an occupational hazard for health care workers.

A vaccine against hepatitis B has been available since 1982 and was called the "first cancer vaccine" by the U.S. FDA. Hepatitis B vaccine is a non-infectious mixture containing recombinant hepatitis B surface antigen (HBsAg) in a liquid vehicle. Immunization with the vaccine induces the formation of specific anti-viral antibodies and active immunity against hepatitis B infection. The vaccine can be given in three or four separate doses, as part of existing routine immunization schedules. It is 95 % effective in preventing infection and its chronic consequences. In areas where mother-to-infant spread of the hepatitis B virus is common, the first dose should be given within 24 h after birth. The complete vaccine series induces protective antibody levels in more than 95 % of infants, children and young adults. The protection lasts at least 20 years.

Human papilloma virus (HPV) is spread mainly through sexual contact. While infection usually causes no symptoms and is cleared within 2 years, rare cases can develop into genital warts and cancer in both men and women. There are more than 100 types of human papilloma virus, of which about 15 are known to cause cervical cancer. Vaccines protect against the strains HPV-16 and HPV-18, which cause 70 % of cervical cancers, 80 % of anal cancers, 60 % of vaginal cancers, 40 % of vulvar cancers, most human papilloma virus induced oral cancers, and some rare genital cancers.

- Human papillomavirus 16/18 L1 virus-like particle/AS04 vaccine (GSK-580299) <Cervarix>was approved by the U.S. FDA in 2009. It constitutes a recombinant, bivalent human papillomavirus vaccine, containing virus-like particles for HPV types 16 and 18 linked to the adjuvant ASO4[1] (Table 19.1). Upon administration, this vaccine generates humoral and cellular immunity against human papilloma virus strains 16 and 18, and has a 70 % likelihood of immunizing against cancers caused by other strains of the virus. In addition, this agent may stimulate an anti-tumoral cellular immune response against cervical cancer associated with human papilloma virus infection. Adverse effects are mostly mild, including pain and swelling at the injection site, fatigue and headache.
- Recombinant human papillomavirus quadrivalent (Types 6, 11, 16, and 18) vaccine <Gardasil> was approved by the U.S. FDA in 2006. Gardasil protects against HPV-16 and -18, and also defends against HPV-6 and -11 that cause 90 % of condylomata acuminata (genital warts). The vaccine is given as three injections over 6 months, the second dose comes 2 months after the first dose, and the third dose comes 6 months after the first dose. Adverse effects include pain, swelling, itching, bruising, and redness at the injection site, headache, fever, nausea, dizziness, vomiting, and rarely fainting.

19.2 Chemoprevention

19.2.1 Nutrition

Dietary intake of soy products tends to be high in Asia. Among Chinese breast cancer patients, a high soy diet lowers the risk of recurrence and breast cancer death. Eating more than 15 gm of soy protein per day is associated with a 30 % lower risk of recurrence compared to intake of less than 5 gm of soy protein per day (Shu et al. 2009). While the benefit of late-onset soy consumption is unknown, it is unlikely that dietary soy would be associated with adverse effects.

[1] Adjuvant System 04 (ASO4) is a combination of aluminum hydroxide (enhances the antibody response) and monophosphoryl lipid A (a TLR4 agonist derived from bacterial cell walls).

G. F. Weber, *Molecular Therapies of Cancer*, DOI 10.1007/978-3-319-13278-5_19,

Table 19.1 Vaccine adjuvants

Adjuvant	Description	Effect
Individual		
Aluminum hydroxide	Salt	Higher and more prolonged antibody responses
Aluminum phosphate	Salt	Higher and more prolonged antibody responses
Potassium aluminum sulfate	Salt	Higher and more prolonged antibody responses
Monophosphoryl lipid A	Detoxified form of LPS, derived from the bacterial cell wall	TLR4 agonist, stimulates TH1 response
3′-cytidine 5′-guanosine dinucleotide	Common in bacterial or viral DNA	TLR9 Agonists
QS21	Saponins (glycosides), derived from tree bark	Induce IL-2 and gamma IFN secretion and TH1 response
Cholera toxin	Protein	
Combinations		
ASO4	Alum + MPL	
ASO3	Squalene + D,L-α-tocopherol + polysorbate 80	
ASO2	MPL + QS21 + oil/water emulsion	
AS01E	MPL + QS21 + liposomes	
MF59	Oil based emulsion (including squalene)	Uptake by dendritic cells, stimulate cytokine production, induce TH2 response
Freund's complete adjuvant	Emulsion	Immunostimulant

Omega-3 fatty acids may reduce the risk of developing colon, breast, or prostate cancers. Cold water fish, such as salmon or halibut, are sources of omega-3 fatty acids. Moderate doses of fish oil can help reduce the growth rate of colon cancer cells, but high doses can increase the risk of bleeding.

Most malignancies are driven by genetic alterations that directly affect the function of critical cell cycle regulators. Phytochemicals, which can either modulate signaling pathways leading to cell cycle regulation or directly alter cell cycle regulatory molecules, may support cancer therapy and prevention. The polyphenol curcumin (diferuloylmethane) is derived from the turmeric plant (curcuma longa). In chemoprevention or chemotherapy, cell cycle regulation can be modulated by curcumin to exert anti-proliferative or apoptotic effects with low inherent toxicity.

19.2.2 Nutrition Supplements

The susceptibility to various cancers has been associated with nutritional habits. This has triggered efforts to supplement nutrition with protective agents. Increased environmental health awareness in the 1970s caused the recognition that while the intake of some foods can increase the risk for specific malignancies, others can act in a chemopreventive fashion (Sporn et al. 1976). In the U.S., the Dietary Supplement Health and Education Act was signed into law in 1994[2]. The legislation classified dietary supplements as a sub-category of food and allowed manufacturers to market products without submitting proof of safety or efficacy to the FDA (Denham 2011). The growing public health conscience in the late years of the twenteeth century, combined with insights into the potential carcinogenic properties of reactive oxygen intermediates prompted multiple studies into cancer preventive capacities of anti-oxidants. Numerous nutrition supplements are marketed with claims to cancer prevention. The levels of underlying scientific support vary widely.

Vitamin E, a fat soluble antioxidant nutrient, is an essential compound in cell membranes. It is absorbed together with lipids, packed into chylomicrons, in the proximal part of the intestine and enters the circulation via the lymphatic system, which transports it to the liver. The distinct forms of vitamin E comprise four tocopherols (α, β, γ, and δ) and four tocotrienols (α, β, γ, and δ). There are several stereoisomers of α-tocopherol, the most widely distributed being RRR-α-tocopherol (d-α-tocopherol). It had been hypothesized that vitamin E can reduce cancer risk, but high-dose dietary supplementation with vitamin E significantly increases the risk of cancer.

Background fortification of the food supply with folic acid began as a policy in the United States in 1998 to reduce the risk of neural tube defects. It has improved the folate

[2] In the United States, the Proxmire Amendment is a law passed in 1976 that curbed the ability of the FDA to regulate vitamin dosage. In 1989, an outbreak of eosinophilia-myalgia syndrome occurred among L-tryptophan users (caused by impurities in the supplement). It led to the death of 38 individuals and produced adverse reactions in 1500 people. When the U.S. FDA was perceived as heavy-handed in response to the incident, industry lobbyists applied pressure on lawmakers to protect their products from regulation.

status in the population. Folate, vitamin B6, and vitamin B12 are important for the 1-carbon metabolism. This metabolic process is essential for DNA synthesis and methylation, which are critical for upholding DNA integrity and regulating gene expression. Deficiencies in B vitamins may increase the probability of DNA damage and subsequent gene mutations, as well as cause aberrant methylation patterns. Therefore, these nutrients have potentially important roles in inhibiting cancer development. However, empirical results have been conflicting, ranging from an inverse association between intake or blood level of folate, vitamin B6, and vitamin B12 and the risk of cancer (Giovannucci 2002; Harnack et al. 2002; Johansson et al. 2010) via no significant effect of combined folic acid, vitamin B6, and vitamin B12 treatment on overall risk of invasive cancer (Zhang et al. 2008) to a possible increased risk by folic acid supplementation for neoplasia (Cole et al. 2007).

Vitamin C is a water soluble enzyme cofactor present in plants and some animals. There are two chemical forms of vitamin C, the reduced form (ascorbate) and the oxidized form (dehydroascorbate). Ascorbate is a potent anti-oxidant that efficiently quenches reactive oxygen intermediates, but at high concentrations or in the presence of transition metals it can acquire pro-oxidant properties. Unlike most mammals, humans do not have the ability to synthesize this nutrient endogenously and therefore must obtain vitamin C through the diet. The use of vitamin C in clinical practice began in the 1970s when Ewan Cameron, Linus Pauling, and Allan Campbell used high doses of vitamin C as a supplement for cancer patients.

Arsenic trioxide inhibits Glutathione Peroxidase, possibly through the generation of arsenic-GSH conjugates, and consecutively increases the cellular hydrogen peroxide levels. Consistently, vitamin C, which can increase the cellular hydrogen peroxide content, enhances the arsenic trioxide induced apoptosis of lymphoma cells, but not of healthy bone marrow cells.

19.2.3 Others

Close to ¾ of breast cancers need estrogen to grow. Anti-estrogen therapies such as tamoxifen and raloxifene, have been approved by the U.S. FDA as preventive therapies for women at high breast cancer risk.

The Aromatase inhibitor exemestane <Aromasin>blocks the production of estrogen and reduces the risk of breast cancer in high risk post-menopausal women by more than 50 % (Goss et al. 2011).

References

Cole BF, Baron JA, Sandler RS, Haile RW, Ahnen DJ, Bresalier RS, McKeown-Eyssen G, Summers RW, Rothstein RI, Burke CA, Snover DC, Church TR, Allen JI, Robertson DJ, Beck GJ, Bond JH, Byers T, Mandel JS, Mott LA, Pearson LH, Barry EL, Rees JR, Marcon N, Saibil F (2007) Folic acid for the prevention of colorectal adenomas: a randomized clinical trial. J Am Med Assoc 297:2351–2359

Denham BE (2011) Dietary supplements–regulatory issues and implications for public health. J Am Med Assoc 306:428–429

Giovannucci E (2002) Epidemiologic studies of folate and colorectal neoplasia: a review. J Nutr 132(suppl):2350S–2355S

Goss PE, Ingle JN, Alés-Martínez JE, Cheung AM, Chlebowski RT, Wactawski-Wende J, McTiernan A, Robbins J, Johnson KC, Martin LW, Winquist E, Sarto GE, Garber JE, Fabian CJ, Pujol P, Maunsell E, Farmer P, Gelmon KA, Tu D, Richardson H, the NCIC CTG MAP.3 S (2011) Exemestane for breast-cancer prevention in postmenopausal women. N Engl J Med 364:2381–2391

Harnack L, Jacobs DR, Nicodemus K, Lazovitch D, Anderson K, Folsom AR (2002) Relationship of folate vitamin B-6, vitamin B-12, and methionine intake to incidence of colorectal cancers. Nutr Cancer 43:152–158

Johansson M, Relton C, Ueland PM, Vollset SE, Midttun Ø, Nygård O, Slimani N, Boffetta P, Jenab M, Clavel-Chapelon F, Boutron-Ruault MC, Fagherazzi G, Kaaks R, Rohrmann S, Boeing H, Weikert C, Bueno-de-Mesquita HB, Ros MM, van Gils CH, Peeters PH, Agudo A (2010) Serum B vitamin levels and risk of lung cancer. J Am Med Assoc 303:2377–2385

Shu XO, Zheng Y, Cai H, Gu K, Chen Z, Zheng W, Lu W (2009) Soy food intake and breast cancer survival. J Am Med Assoc 302:2437–2443

Sporn MB, Dunlop NM, Newton DL, Smith JM (1976) Prevention of chemical carcinogenesis by vitamin A and its synthetic analogs (retinoids). Fed Proc 35:1332–1338

Zhang SM, Cook NR, Albert CM, Gaziano JM, Buring JE, Manson JE (2008) Effect of combined folic acid, vitamin B6, and vitamin B12 on cancer risk in women: a randomized trial. J Am Med Assoc 300:2012–2021

Index

G. F. Weber, *Molecular Therapies of Cancer*, DOI 10.1007/978-3-319-13278-5,

B

C

F

I

J

K

N

O

PEG

Q

R

S